English-Chinese Collegiate Textbooks in Traditional Chinese Medicine for Institutions of Traditional Chinese Medicine of Higher Learning
Edited by Beijing University of Traditional Chinese Medicine

普通高等中医药院校英汉对照中医本科系列教材
北京中医药大学　主编

Traditional Chinese Internal Medicine

中医内科学

Academy Press [XueYuan]
學苑出版社

图书在版编目(CIP)数据

中医内科学 / 田德禄，邹建华主编. -北京：学苑出版社，2000.1(2007.4 重印)
(普通高等中医药院校英汉对照中医本科系列教材)
ISBN 978-7-5077-1268-1

Ⅰ. 中… Ⅱ. ①田… ②邹… Ⅲ. 中医内科学-医学院校-教材-英、汉 Ⅳ. R242

中国版本图书馆 CIP 数据核字(2000)第 13611 号

责任编辑：陈 辉 东 青
封面设计：李 戎 张致民
出版发行：学苑出版社
社 址：北京市丰台区南方庄 2 号院 1 号楼
邮政编码：100079
网 址：www.book001.com
电子信箱：xueyuan@public.bta.net.cn
销售电话：010-67675512、67602949、67678944
经 销：新华书店
印 刷 厂：北京市广内印刷厂
开本尺寸：787×1092 1/16
印 张：64
字 数：1436 千字
版 次：2000 年 1 月北京第 1 版
印 次：2007 年 4 月北京第 2 次印刷
印 数：3001—6000 册
定 价：128.00 元($)

English-Chinese Collegiate Textbooks in Traditional Chinese Medicine for Institutions of Traditional Chinese Medicine of Higher Learning
Edited by Beijing University of Traditional Chinese Medicine

普通高等中医药院校
英汉对照中医本科系列教材
北京中医药大学　主编

General Chief Editor: Long Zhixian
Associate Chief Editors: Zheng Shouzeng
He Min
He Xingdong
Suo Runtang
Liu Jinsheng
Gao Baozhong
Chen Jing
Chief Reviewers of Chinese: Wang Yuchuan
Yan Zhenghua

总 主 编: 龙致贤
副总主编: 郑守曾　何　珉
贺兴东　索润堂
刘金生　高宝忠
陈　静
中文主审: 王玉川　颜正华

TRADITIONAL CHINESE INTERNAL MEDICINE
中医内科学

Chief Editor of Chinese: Tian Delu
Chief Editor of English: Zou Jianhua
Associate Chinese Editors: Wu Weiping Yang Jinxiang Sun Suolun

Translators: (In the order of the number of Chinese strokes in the surnames)
Wang Youjing Wang Yuqin
Liu Linxiang Liu Junling
Li Yajun Yang Yong
Yang Yikun Zhuo Qin
Zou Jianhua Hu Yanmin
Xiang Manjun Duan Shumin

中文主编: 田德禄
英文主编: 邹建华
中文副主编: 武维屏 杨晋翔 孙塑伦
英文译者: (以下按姓氏笔画为序)
王友京 王玉芹 刘林祥
刘俊岭 李亚俊 杨 勇
杨怡坤 卓 勤 邹建华
胡艳敏 项曼君 段树民

Specially Invited International Editors

Chief Reviewer: Nengyu Fang
Associate Reviewer: Concetta Maria Pirrone
Advisor: George Francis Mclean

特邀外籍审校人员

英文主审校: 方能御
协　　　校: 康西特·玛丽亚·皮罗尼
顾　　　问: 乔治·弗郎西斯·麦克林

Preface

Beijing University of Traditional Chinese Medicine under the auspices of the Department of Science and Education for the State Administration of Traditional Chinese Medicine has compiled the English-Chinese textbook series in Traditional Chinese Medicine (TCM) for undergraduate of college. These textbooks include Basic Theories of Traditional Chinese Medicine, Diagnostics of Traditional Chinese Medicine, Chinese Materia Medica, Formulas of Traditional Chinese Medicine, Traditional Chinese Internal Medicine, Acupuncture & Moxibustion and an English-Chinese Dictionary of Traditional Chinese Medicine. This project is very scholastic and now is coming into publication for the first time domestically and abroad.

Traditional Chinese Medicine possesses a unique theoretical system, rich clinical experience and excellent clinical effects. It has made great contributions to the health of mankind. Either now or future, based on its own potential, TCM will play an increasingly important role in promoting the development of a world medicine, and more attention of people in the world. More and more international friends are interested in TCM and they are studying and practicing TCM throughout the world. In order to overcome the language barrier and to understand TCM correctly they are eager for a set of TCM textbooks. They want these textbooks to be suitable for use in colleges of higher learning and with accurate in English translation.

Beijing University of Traditional Chinese Medicine is a key university among the TCM teaching institutions of higher learning in China. The university began to enroll foreign students in 1957. Since then about one thousand foreign students coming from more than 70 countries and regions in the world graduated form it. At present, there are nearly 300 foreign students from 41 countries and regions studying at the university. The university has accumulated rich experience in teaching foreign students and understands their special needs in the study of TCM. These years of practice in teaching has greatly helped the compilation of the TCM textbooks.

The authorities of the university highly evaluate the task of compiling and translating the TCM textbook series and organized a special working group of experienced professors and other professionals to compile the series. Based on the fifth edition of relevant all-China TCM textbooks of higher learning, the TCM textbooks absorb the latest achievements of scientific research in TCM lay more stress on logicality, scientificality and practicality, make every effort to contain more information and to build a rational framework of the content in an understandable and readable manner. This TCM textbook series in suitable for both foreign and Chinese students and all those who are interested in TCM, both at home and abroad.

In order to ensure academic standards and accurate English translation of this textbook series, we invited well-known TCM experts Prof. Wang Yuchuan and Prof. Yan Zhenghua to examine and review the Chinese language, experts Fang Nengyu, Concetta Maria Pirrone and George Francis Mclean to review the English translation.

Internal medicine of Traditional Chinese Medicine (TCM), a bridge course between basic theory of TCM and clinical departments, plays a role of connecting the precedence to the following. Only by further studying and clinically practicing internal medicine, can basic theory be deeply understood and grasped. Only on the basis of internal medicine, can characteristics and skills of clinical departments be better known. This is the importance of internal medicine.

During the long-term development of TCM, importance has been always attached to internal medicine. Through long-term accumulation and reorganization, the knowledge of internal medicine, including etiology, pathology, taxonomy and therapeutic, has developed widely and deeply, formed a complete theoretical system, and can effectively direct clinical practice.

Internal medicine of TCM is a discipline to systematically deal with internal diseases by using principle of diagnosis and treatment based on an overall analysis of the illness and the patient's condition under the guidance of TCM theory. Its extremely wide contents mainly consist of two major types of diseases, seasonal diseases caused by exogenous factors and miscellaneous diseases due to internal injury. With different etiology, pathology, clinical characteristics, diagnostic and therapeutic methods, the tow major types of diseases are linked to and transformed into each other. Therefore, internal medicine must be systematically studied and comprehensively grasped.

Finally, any correction to errors and suggestions concerning its contents and format will be appreciated. We will take them into careful consideration in the next edition and we believe that with such help, these TCM textbooks will be much improved in the next edition.

During the compilation of the TCM textbook series, we have been greatly helped by the relevant official departments and experts and we would like to express our profound thanks to them.

The compiler and translator

前言

北京中医药大学受国家中医药管理局科技教育司的委托，编译高等中医药院校英汉对照中医本科系列教材，包括《中医基础理论》、《中医诊断学》、《中药学》、《方剂学》、《中医内科学》、《针灸学》及《英汉中医药学词典》7种。这是中医高等教材汉译英方面空前盛大的工程，是一项大型科研活动。

中国医药学以其独特的理论体系、丰富的医疗实践、卓越的临床疗效，为人类的健康事业作出了巨大贡献。当今和未来，中医药学将发挥出更大的潜力，推动世界医学向前发展，引起世界人民更多更大的重视与关注。近年来，外国朋友中学习、研究、应用中医中药的人越来越多，但由于语言文字的差异，给学习带来一定的困难，他们迫切需要一套专业层次高、翻译准确的英汉对照教材，以便更好学习中医中药。

北京中医药大学是唯一的中国重点中医药大学，自1957年接受外国留学生以来，已为世界70多个国家和地区培养了近千名留学生。目前在校外国留学生近3百人，分别来自41个国家和地区，多年来，北京中医药大学积累了丰富的培养外国留学生的教学经验，了解他们学习的规律和特点，这为编写这套教材打下了良好的基础。

北京中医药大学领导十分重视这套教材，专门组织了教学经验丰富的专家、教授和专业骨干从事编写工作。全套教材在全国高等中医院校五版教材的基础上，扬长避短，吸收了中医药的最新科研成果，强调逻辑性、科学性、实用性，努力做到内容充实，重点突出，通俗易懂。

本套教材适用于留学生、国内学生及国内外研究中医药的学者。

为保证这套教材的学术与翻译水平，中文内容特请全国著名中医学专家王玉川教授、颜正华教授审定，英文译文特邀美籍专家 Fang Nengyu(方能御)，Concetta Maria Pirrone，George Francis Mclean 审校。

中医内科学是中医基础理论与临床各学科的桥梁课程，具有承上启下的作用。基础理论知识只有通过内科学的进一步讲授和临床实习，才能达到深入理解和掌握；临床各学科则必须以内科学作基础，才能更好地熟悉本学科的特点和技能。这就是内科学重要性之所在。

在源远流长的祖国医学发展进程中，内科学一直受到人们的重视，经过长期的积累和整理，使内科学知识，包括病因学、病理学、分类学、治疗学等项内容，在广度和深度上都得到了发展，形成了较为完整的理论体系，能够有效地指导临床实践。

中医内科学是在祖国医学理论指导下，运用辨证论治的法则，系统地阐述和处理内科病证的一门学科。其内容极为广泛，主要包括外感时病和内伤杂病两大类疾病，二者各有其病因病理、临床特点、诊治方法，但二者又是相互联系、相互转化的，因此必须系统学习，全面掌握。

由于时间紧迫，水平有限，不妥之处在所难免，真诚地欢迎国内外同道提出批评意见，以便再版时进行修改补充，使这套教材更加完善。

编译工作过程中，得到有关部门和专家的大力支持与协助，在此深表谢意。

编译者

CONTENTS

General Discussion

Systematic Considerations

目　录

总　论

各　论

General Discussion

Chapter 1 The Development of Traditional Chinese Internal Medicine

The Traditional Chinese Internal Medicine, known as "Da Fang Mai" in ancient times, an important part of the Chinese medical treasure house, has been constantly accumulated and gradually formed in long-term medical practices.

Due to its special position in the Chinese medicine, Traditional Chinese Internal Medicine, like the Chinese medicine, can be traced back to the primitive society. For example, names and symptoms of internal diseases, such as "wind", "symptom", "epidemic" and "abdominal pain", can be seen in the medical book "Shan Hai Jing". However, the formation of a medical theory needs a certain level of productive forces. Only in feudal society, could the theory of Traditional Chinese Internal Medicine be gradually formed. In slave society, slaves produced richer and richer wealth, creating conditions for the development of science and culture. The appearance of classes and further expansion of division of social labor made all walks of life increasingly specialized, enabling Traditional Chinese Internal Medicine to gradually become an independent discipline in medical practices. According to "Zhou Rituals Tian Guan", then court medical practitioners were divided into physicians, dietitians, surgeons and veterinarians. Physicians were practitioners specializing in Traditional Chinese Internal Medicine. Bian Que has been considered as a pioneer in the division of disciplines. Because of wide spread existence of internal diseases and deep development of medical practices, the theoretical knowledge and clinical experience of Traditional Chinese Internal Medicine were rapidly developed. "The Yellow Emperor's Internal Classic" has been regarded as the summary of medical knowledge before the Warring States Period.

The theories of yin-yang and five elements were naive materialism in Yin and Zhou Dynasties and were widely used to expound and explain all natural phenomena in the Spring and Autumn Period and the Warring States Period. They were also adopted in TCM to study and recognize physiological and pathological phenomena of the human body, thus promoting the development of medicine and laying a solid and reliable theoretical foundation for TCM. Therefore, from the Warring States Period to Qin and Han Dynasties was the foundation-laying period for TCM theoretical system.

"The Yellow Emperor's Internal Classic", consisting of "Plain Questions" and "Miraculous Pivot", has 18 volumes, each with 81 articles. Its basic theory can be summarized as follows. (1) A whole conception is stressed: The human body is an organic whole; Health and diseases have certain relations to natural environment. (2) The theories of yin-yang and five elements are applied to physiology, pathology, diagnosis and treatment to find out rough laws on diseases and their treatment. (3) Importance is attached to viscera, channels and collaterals to expound the physiological functions, pathological changes and their relations of five zang-organs and six fu-organs, twelve main channels and eight extra channels. (4) Under the guidance of the above-mentioned theories, descriptions are made on six exopathic factors, seven emotions, diet, internal injury caused by overstrain, and other causes of diseases, as well as on the pathological changes of viscera, six kinds of natural factors, channels and collaterals. (5) Descriptions are made on four diagnostic methods of inspection, auscultation and olfaction, interrogation, pulse feeling and palpation, and their concrete contents. and (6) therapeutic principles are determined on preventively treating diseases, taking measures in line with different time, local condition and individual, treating superficiality and origin, applying routine treatment, treating a disease contrary to the routine, prescribing a recipe, imposing dietetic restraint, and conducting psychotherapy and acupuncture. In a relatively systematic theoretical system thus formed, an embryonic form of theory, therapy, recipe and drug became the theoretical source of TCM internal medicine.

In addition, "The Yellow Emperor's Internal Classic" briefly describes more than 200 internal diseases in etiology, pathology, transformation, prognosis and other respects. Some diseases are discussed in special articles, such as "On Fever", "On Cough", "On Flaccidity", "On Malaria" and "On Arthralgia", thus laying the foundation for the development of Traditional Chinese Internal Medicine.

Zhang Zhongjing inherited the basic theories of "Internal Classic" and other classic medical books. He used the six channels to discuss exogenous febrile diseases, used viscera to discuss miscellaneous diseases, put forward a relatively systematic principle of diagnosis and treatment, including theory, therapy, recipe and drug, and closely combined the basic theory with clinical practice, making the Traditional Chinese Internal Medicine develop scientifically.

Using the six channels to discuss exogenous febrile diseases, "Treatise on Febrile Diseases" discusses the characteristics and treatments of various diseases, expounds their transformation, combined syndromes and complications, and describes diagnosis and treatment of deteriorated cases caused by no or erroneous treatment. In accordance with the theory of the six channels, febrile diseases can be differentiated into exterior or interior, cold or heat, deficiency or excess syndromes, which are then summarized with Yin-Yang, thus laying a foundation for later analysis and differentiation of pathological conditions in accordance with the eight principal syndromes.

"Synopsis of Prescriptions of the Golden Chamber" uses viscera to discuss miscellaneous diseases and expounds the diagnosis and treatment of pulmonary abscess, consumptive lung disease, phlegm retention, jaundice, dysentery, edema and other diseases in special articles.

Zhang Zhongjing pioneered diagnosis and treatment based on overall analysis of the illness and the patient's condition. In clinical practice, he determined therapy according to syndrome, gave recipe according to therapy, prescribed drugs according to recipe, and paid attention to influence of dosage form on curative effect. In "Treatise on Febrile and miscellaneous diseases", there are 375 recipes, of which quite a few famous recipes have been used so far with very high curative effects. Therefore, the medical book occupies an important position in the development of Traditional Chinese Internal Medicine.

In Sui and Tang Dynasties, thanks to the development of TCM theory and practice, medical education also reached a relatively perfect level. Court medical schools stipulated that students should first learn basic courses, such as "Plain Questions", "Shen Nong's Herbal Classic" and "The Pulse Classic", and then study clinical disciplines including internal medicine, thus organically relating theory to practice. It can thus be seen what position Traditional Chinese Internal Medicine occupied and what scale it had at that time. In Sui and Tang Dynasties, many internal diseases were described in detail. For example, certain experiences were accumulated in treating exogenous febrile disease, apoplexy, epidemic disease, epidemic febrile disease, tinea pedis and endemic goiter; and relatively high levels were also reached in the prevention and treatment of cestodiasis, leprosy, shashitsu and rabies. "The Medical Secrets of an Official" describes the urine of diabetics as sweet, observes the curative effect for jaundice, and raises: "A white cloth is soaked in urine every night, and its changed color can be used as an indicator." Sun Simiao further summarized the pathogenic process of diabetes and its treatment with drug and food, and stipulated some contraindications on diet and daily life. "General Treatise on the Causes and Symptoms of Diseases", the earliest existing treatise in China on etiology, pathology and syndrome, records 784 symptoms of internal diseases in 27 volumes, and deeply studies and summarizes etiology, pathology and symptoms for each disease. For example, contrary to the past, it separately discusses diarrhea and dysentery, phlegm syndrome and fluid retention syndrome; and deeply recognizes the etiology of proglottid of tapeworm, the classification of malaria and clinical symptoms of leprosy.

Song Dynasty attached more importance to the selection and training of medical talents, and stipulated the proportion of practitioners in various disciplines. According to "Yuan Feng Bei Dui", in the time of Song Shen Zong, "there were 300 students of nine disciplines in the Bureau of Imperial Physicians" with 120 students majoring in internal medicine known as Da Fang Mai and 80 others in specialty of wind diseases. It can thus be seen what importance was attached to internal medicine at that time. Song, Jin, Yuan and Ming Dynasties set up Da Fang Mai discipline, a specialty for treating various internal diseases in adults, promoting the development of TCM internal medicine. It is particularly worth noting that in Jin and Yuan Dynasties, four famous physicians summarized medical theory and treatment with characteristics according to the social situation at that time, conditions of the human body and pathogenic features. For example, Liu Wansu deeply studied the theory of five elements' evolutions and six kinds of natural factors in "Internal Classic". According to experience in clinical practice and in reference to the spirit of nineteen items of pathogenesis in "Internal Classic", he regarded "pathogenic fire" as an important cause of diseases, strove to advocate the mechanism of pathogenic fire causing diseases, and created "the theory of pathogenic fire". He was very good at using cold and cool drugs to treat diseases, so he has been known as "the cold and cool medical school". Influenced by and bringing into play Liu Wansu's theory, Zhang Zihe held that diseases were radically caused by pathogenic factors. As soon as external or internal pathogenic factors invaded the human body, they should be expelled and should not be allowed to stay in the human body to cause diseases. He widely applied the methods of diaphoresis, emesis and purgation to clinical practice with his unique view. Because he mainly used expelling pathogenic factors to treat diseases, he has been known as "purgationist school". Li Gao lived in Jin and Yuan Dynasties, when civil war and social disturbance made people lose means of livelihood and suffer hunger, cold and feebleness, thus making the position of spleen and stomach in the human body more important. Therefore, he pointed out: "Internal injury of the spleen and stomach can cause diseases." He mainly used drugs of invigorating qi and elevating Yang to treat diseases. Because he was good at warming and invigorating the spleen and stomach, he has been known as "the school of invigorating the earth". Zhu Danxi studied academic ideas and works of ancestral physicians, synthesized various theories and independently created "ministerial fire theory" and "the theory of yang sufficiency and yin deficiency". Because he strongly stood for using the method of nourishing Yin and reducing pathogenic fire to treat diseases, he has been known as "nourishing Yin school". The four physicians formed four major schools with the largest influence on the later ages.

Apart from their academic value, the four major schools were bold in and good at studying and summarizing diseases clinically and theoretically and put forward their views. They proved that TCM was inherited in the process of its development and developed in the process of its inheritance, providing the greatest inspiration to later generations.

Since four famous physicians in Jin and Yuan Dynasties launched the prevailing practice of academic contention, physicians in later generations have aired their views one after another, making TCM theory and practice increasingly deep, mature, systematic and complete. For example, in the past dynasties, debate made the recognition of apoplexy more explicit. The deliberation of reinforcing the spleen, nourishing the kidney and replenishing both the spleen and the kidney enabled people to more clearly recognize the physiology and pathology of the spleen and the kidney, their importance in the human body, and their relations. From "damp-heat theory" of Dongyuan and Danxi and "fire decline theory" of Zhao Yangkui and Sun yikui to "the theory of water accumulation, qi stagnation and blood stasis" of Yu Chang, the pathogenesis of tympanites was analyzed more thoroughly, thus better guiding clinical practice and enhancing curative effect.

The achievements in Jin and Yuan Dynasties were not just confined to the four famous physicians. Meanwhile, "General Collection for Holly Relief" has 18 volumes specializing in winds, reflecting that the monographic study of "wind syndrome" reached a certain level at that time. "Ji Feng Pu Ji Recipe" written by Zhang Rui divides edema into many types, distinguishes different types of edema and applies different treatments according to characteristics of its original location. In addition, there were some treatises on internal diseases. For example, "General Program for Treatments of Beriberi", written by Dong Ji in Song Dynasty, expounds the causes, conditions and treatments of beriberi, and prescribes 64 recipes. It is an existing relatively comprehensive treatise on beriberi. In "A Miraculous Book of Ten Prescriptions", a treatise on treating tuberculosis, written by Ge Kejiu in Yuan Dynasty, 10 famous recipes with effects of arresting bleeding, relieving cough, removing phlegm and replenishing nutrients respectively summarize a set of experiences in classifying and treating tuberculosis.

Important progress was also made in etiology at that time. On the basis of classifying causes of diseases in "Treatise on Febrile Diseases" and in combination with the theory of "Internal Classic", "Prescriptions Assigned to the Three Categories of Pathogenic Factors of Diseases" written by Chen Wuze creates the theory of three categories of exopathic, endopathic and non-endo-exopathic etiologic factors. The theory with strong summarization has been used so far for clinical applications.

After Jin and Yuan Dynasties, an atmosphere of development and creation was formed in TCM academic circle. For example, new studies on the physiology and pathology of an internal organ of the human body, importance attached to its metabolic products, and new breakthroughs constantly made in the view on diagnosis and treatment of an internal disease enabled Traditional Chinese Internal Medicine to rapidly develop in width and depth.

Academic achievements made in Jin and Yuan Dynasties were inherited and developed in Ming Dynasty. For example, academically influenced by Li Gao who was good at warming and recuperating, "Summary of Internal Medicine" written by Xue Ji developed Traditional Chinese Internal Medicine, becoming the earliest book on internal medicine in China. "Orthodox Medical Problems" written by Yu Tuan developed the theory of Zhu Danxi. Wang Lun explicitly pointed out: "Diseases due to exopathy are treated with methods of Zhongjing, diseases due to internal injury with methods of Dongyuan, febrile diseases with methods of Hejian and miscellaneous diseases with methods of Danxi", summarizing the academic idea of Traditional Chinese Internal Medicine at that time. In addition, "Longevity and Life Preservation" written by Gong Tingxian describes basic theory, clinical practice, recipes and medical cases, with rich materials, elaborated discussion, practicable recipes and applicable reference to clinical practice of internal medicine. "Complete Works of Zhang Jingyue" corrects the prejudice in favor of using cold and cool drugs to treat diseases by Liu and Zhang in Jin and Yuan Dynasties. It advocates that qi and yang dominate the human life, points out that in the human body, "Yang is not usually redundant while the genuine Yin is often deficient", and holds that warming and recuperating methods should be used to treat diseases. The complete works have 28 volumes on the diagnosis and treatment of more than 70 miscellaneous diseases of internal medicine with quoted ancient theories and the author's own view for each disease. The author most incisively analyzed and summarized the pathology of many internal diseases and prescribed many recipes with his own view. He fully expounded the theory of warming and recuperating in combination with diseases.

The formation and development of the theory of epidemic febrile diseases In Ming and Qing Dynasties occupies a particularly outstanding position in the medical history, making the practice and theory of exopathic diseases of internal medicine enter a higher and more perfect realm. Wu Youke, who wrote "Treatise on Pestilence", an early treatise on infectious diseases in China, thought that different from other febrile diseases, epidemic was caused not by "six kinds of natural factors" but mainly by "epidemic pathogenic factors" and dysfunction of the body. He pointed out that "epidemic pathogenic factors" were infected by means of contact with the human body or through the mouth and nose, and that anyone, old and young, strong and weak, who contacted them, would fall ill. This recognition is a breakthrough in the development of TCM. "Treatise on Epidemic Febrile Diseases", written by Ye Tianshi, laid a theoretical, diagnostic and curative foundation for the development of theory of epidemic febrile diseases. His contributions are as follows. Firstly, he raised the theory: "When attacking the upper-jiao, the pathogenic warm first invades the lung and then the heart", summarizing the invasive route and infectious rule of epidemic febrile diseases and becoming a program of epidemic febrile diseases caused by exopathogen. Secondly, he divided the course of pathogenic changes of epidemic febrile diseases into four stages of wei, qi, ying and xue, forming a program of diagnosis and treatment based on overall analysis of the illness and the patient's condition. Thirdly, he summarized predecessors' experiences in diagnosing epidemic febrile diseases and creatively developed the methods of observing the tongue, inspecting teeth and distinguishing exanthema maculosum from miliaria alba. These contributions laid a theoretical and practical foundation for the theory of epidemic febrile diseases. On the basis of Ye's theory, Wu Jutong wrote "Treatise on Differentiation and Treatment of Epidemic Febrile Diseases". He used triple-jiao as a program and names of diseases as items to describe the diagnosis and treatment of nine kinds of epidemic febrile diseases, including wind-warm syndrome, warm-heat pathogen and infectious epidemic diseases. He also raised various treatments, such as removing heat from the lung channel, clearing up the ying system and nourishing yin, making the theory of epidemic febrile diseases more systematic and complete, and establishing a system of diagnosis and treatment for epidemic febrile diseases. In his book "Damp-heat Syndrome", Xue Shengbai fully studied damp-warm syndrome. In his book "Compendium on Epidemic Febrile Diseases", Wang Mengying divided epidemic febrile diseases into two main types, new affection and incubation pathogen, for diagnosis and treatment. They developed and supplemented the theory of epidemic febrile diseases, promoting its development.

In Ming and Qing Dynasties, some progress was made in studying miscellaneous diseases of internal medicine. In his book "Draft of Difficult Clinical Records", Yu Chang raised his view on close relations between occurrence of diseases and back ground of the time, deeply recognizing the nature of occurrence of diseases, improving the diagnosis and treatment of diseases and enhancing theoretical level. In addition, "Classified Treatment", written by Lin Peiqin, is very practicable. Xiong Hu wrote "On Apoplexy". You Zaijin wrote "The Essence of the Synopsis of the Golden Chamber" to describe apoplexy. "Shen Rou Wu Shu" written by Hu Shenrou and "Li Xu Yuan Jian" written by Qi Shi analyze consumptive disease. "Jie Nue Lun Shu", written by Lu Zhiyi, studies malaria. All the treatises on internal medicine are of a certain academic level. At that time, new breakthrough was made in recognition of blood troubles. For example, "Corrections on the Errors of Medical Works", written by Wang Qingren, describes blood stasis and creates recipes of promoting blood circulation to remove blood stasis. He particularly pioneered "Decoction of Invigorating Yang for Recuperation" for supplementing qi and activating blood circulation to treat qi deficiency and blood stasis. The book has so far had the highest practicable value. "A Treatise on Blood Troubles", written by Tang Rongchuan, further recognizes blood troubles and raises four major methods to treat them, exerting relatively great influence on later generations.

After the Opium War, China gradually became a semi-colonial and semi-feudal society. The Western medicine entering China inevitably influenced the development of TCM. It was under such circumstances that a sect of integrating Chinese and Western medicine was formed. It was impossible for the fatuous and incompetent reactionary ruling class of old China to correctly guide Chinese and Western medicine to learn from each other. On the contrary, it most erroneously attempted to strangle TCM.

After liberation, under the guidance of Chairman Mao's thought of "making the past serve the present and foreign things serve China", new progress has been constantly made in inheritance and development of TCM. The establishment of TCM colleges, schools and hospitals has enabled internal medicine and other disciplines to make progress day after day. The unified textbook of "TCM Internal Medicine" has been revised several times. A number of famous TCM physicians have written books. For example, "Lecture Notes of Qianzhai on Medicine" written by Qin Bowei, "Medical Records" and "Medical Notes" written by Pu Fuzhou and "Collection on Medicine" written by Ren Yingqiu have certain insight and elaboration. Inspired by the Party's spirit of "vitalizing TCM", there will surely be more and more and better and better books of this kind. "Hengyang conference" in 1983 and "Hefei conference" in 1985 have played tremendous promoting role in vitalizing TCM. Particularly, the decision of the secretariat of the central committee of the Communist Party of China on health work has explicitly pointed out: "Chinese and Western medicine should be put on the same important position. TCM is a unique feature and advantage of the Chinese medical and health cause, and it should not be abandoned and must be preserved and further developed. However, TCM should make active use of advanced science and technology and up-to-date means to promote its development." The decision has been responded nationwide. TCM schools and hospitals have sprung up like mushrooms. TCM rank has constantly grown. A large number of professional talents on internal medicine have been brought up. Higher and newer theory of internal medicine has been created to better guide clinical practice and promote the rapid development of the internal medicine.

Questions for Review

1. What contributions have "The Yellow Emperor's Internal Classic", "Treatise

on Febrile and Miscellaneous Diseases" and "General Treatise of the Causes and Symptoms of Diseases" made to the formation of TCM internal medicine?

2. What promoting roles have four famous physicians in Jin and Yuan Dynasties played in the development of TCM internal medicine?

3. What are the contents of the decision of the secretariat of the central committee of the Communist Party of China on health work declared at "Hefei conference" in 1985?

Chapter 2 The Basis of Traditional Chinese Internal Medicine

Section 1 Etiology

TCM etiological theory gradually developed in the struggle between medicine and witchcraft in ancient times. Yi He, a famous physician in Qin State in the Spring and Autumn Period, raised his etiological theory of six kinds of natural factors, and pointed out that excessive obscene could cause interior heat diseases. This is a relatively primitive theory on etiology. "Internal Classic" already clearly recognized relations of diseases to natural environment and raised disease-preventing knowledge, confirming relatively deep recognition of etiology at that time. "Treatise on Febrile and Miscellaneous Diseases" roughly divided complexetiology into three types. It points out: "There are no more than three types of causes for a thousand diseases. Firstly, pathogenic factors invade viscera through channels and collaterals, forming endopathic cause. Secondly, blood circulation in four limbs and nine orifices is obstructed, forming exopathic cause. Thirdly, injury is caused by sexual strain, sword, insects or animals." In Sui Dynasty, Chao's "General Treatise on the Causes and Symptoms of Diseases", known as the earliest treatise on etiology and pathology in China, scientifically and thoroughly describes etiology and pathology of diseases. It explicitly points out that some parasitoses are related to diet, for example, taeniasis is caused by eating half-cooked meat, that some infectious diseases are caused by harmful substances, and that some diseases are related to allergic constitution, for example, dermatitis rhus is caused by contact with lacquer. Later medical books, such as "Peaceful Holy Benevolent Prescriptions" and "General Collection for Holy Relief", first discuss causes of diseases, then pulse conditions, symptoms, prescriptions and drugs, indicating that people already attached importance to etiology.

In Song Dynasty, on the basis of Zhongjing's theory on etiology and in combination with the theory of"Internal Classic", Chen Yan deeply studied etiology and wrote"Prescriptions Assigned to the Three Categories of Pathogenic Factors of Diseases", the first treatise on etiology in China. Systematically expounding"the theory on three categories of etiological factors", it points out that endopathic factors are seven emotions, i. e., joy, anger, melancholy, anxiety, grief, fear and terror. "Persistent and violent emotions injure the viscera and manifest themselves in the limbs and body." Exopathic factors are six climatic conditions, i. e., wind, cold, summer-heat, dampness, dryness and fire. Exogenous febrile disease, summer-heat, epidemic and other diseases invade the viscera through channels and collaterals. Non-endo-exopathic factors are hunger or eating one's fill, damage to qi by cry, injury by insects or animals, poisoning, injury by sword, and injury from fall, press or drowning. This method of classification clearly and specifically conforms to clinical practices. In combination with the influence of social background on diseases, later physicians steadily developed concrete pathogenic factors, such as Wu Gao's "improper diet and excessive fatigue", Zhu Danxi's "melancholia" and "sexual strain", Wu Youke's "epidemic pathogenic factors", and Wang Mengying's "new affection" and "incubative pathogen". However, they did not go beyond the theory of three categories of etiological factors, which has been used so far.

(A) Six Climatic Conditions

Wind, cold, summer-heat, dampness, dryness and fire are main factors for exopathic diseases. Affected by six climatic conditions in excess as pathogenic factors, people will fall ill.

1. Wind is moving and changeable, and prevails most widely. In different season and weather, wind can be divided into wind-warm, wind-cold, wind-heat and wind-dryness. Wind often combines with other pathogenic factors to form wind-dampness or wind-fire. Therefore, our ancestors regarded "wind as the chief cause for various diseases".

Wind pathogen affecting the upper jiao causes mild disease called common cold, while wind pathogen affecting channels, collaterals and the viscera causes serious disease called "wind-stroke syndrome".

2. Cold is yin pathogen with spasm as its main nature. Cold attacking the exterior of the body causes exogenous febrile disease, while cold directly attacking the interior of the body causes "syncope due to pathogenic cold".

3. When the surface of the body is exposed to summer-heat and wind, the pathogen affects the upper jiao. When people walk or work for a long time in a scorching sun, summer-heat can cause heatstroke, also called yang summer-heat syndrome. On the contrary, yin summer-heat syndrome is caused by calmness in

summer. Summer-heat often combines damp pathogen, so ancient physicians often treated both summer-heat and damp-syndrome.

4. Dampness, a heavy and turbid pathogen, is sticky and difficult to be removed. Wet weather, wad, drench, moist residence and sweat in clothes can cause damp pathogen to invade the human body. Dampness, belonging to yin, combines wind pathogen to form wind-dampness, combines cold pathogen to form cold-dampness, and combines heat pathogen to form damp-heat.

5. Dryness, a main pathogen in autumn and residual pathogen of fire, can be divided into warm-dryness and cool-dryness. In early autumn, dryness and warm-heat invade the human body to cause warm-dryness syndrome. In late autumn, dryness and cold invade the human body to cause cool-dryness syndrome.

6. Fire is caused by excess of yang. Fire and heat are caused to different extent by exopathic warm-heat pathogen. Our ancestors said that the five pathogens of wind, cold, summer-heat, dampness and dryness could be transformed into fire pathogen.

In addition, pestilence is one of the exopathic factors. People, old and young, can be infected with epidemic diseases with similar symptoms. Poisonous epidemic pathogenic factors in the nature are more detrimental to the human body and different from six climatic conditions.

Immediate onset of the epidemic febrile disease after invasion by six climatic conditions is called "new affection". Not immediate onset of the epidemic febrile disease after invasion of six climatic conditions and symptoms appearing after a period is called "incubative pathogen". New affection and incubative pathogen are distinguished mainly by exterior from interior, mild from serious, and chronic from acute symptoms.

(B) Seven Emotions

Seven emotions are joy, anger, melancholy, anxiety, grief, fear and terror. Persistent and violent emotions as pathogenic factors can cause dysfunction of the viscera, yin, yang, qi and blood, leading to diseases. "Internal Classic" points out: "Anger causes qi to flow upward, joy causes qi to flow slowly, grief causes qi to eradicate, fear causes qi to flow downward, and anxiety causes qi to stagnate." "Joy impairs the heart, anger impairs the liver, anxiety impairs the spleen, melancholy impairs the lung, and fear impairs the kidney." The description indicates the general rule of seven emotions causing diseases. Pathogenic changes caused by seven emotions first manifest themselves in the changes of qi and then affect blood because of the relations of qi to blood.

Diseases caused by seven emotions are related to strong or weak stimulation, and constitution and sensitivity of the patient. In addition, the patient's emotions fluctuate abnormally, often causing acute exacerbation.

(C) Diet

Diet is the main source of nutrients for the human body. Unrestricted, unclear and prejudicial diet often causes disease due to dysfunction of the spleen and stomach. Impairment by overeating can cause gastrointestinal diseases. "Internal Classic" says: "Overeating can impair the intestine and stomach." Impairment by overeating can also cause dampness accumulation, phlegm formation, heat generation, parasitoses and other diseases.

(D) Five Endogenous Pathogenic Factors

Five endogenous pathogenic factors, i. e., endogenous wind, endogenous cold, endogenous dampness, endogenous dryness and endogenous fire (heat), are pathological products and pathogenic factors caused by dysfunction of the viscera.

1. Endogenous wind is mainly caused by hyperactivity of liver-yang, deficiency of yin and excess of phlegm-fire, often giving rise to dizziness, convulsion, syncope, numbness and opisthotonus.

2. Endogenous cold is mainly caused by deficiency of qi and yang. For example, insufficiency of heart-yang, deficiency of lung-qi, insufficiency of spleen-yang and insufficiency of kidney-yang can cause diseases called cold of insufficiency type, often giving rise to vague pain in the abdomen, diarrhea, cold limbs and weak pulse.

3. Endogenous dampness is caused by overeating fatty diet, raw fruit, and sweet and greasy food or by exogenous dampness entering the interior. Endogenous dampness can cause dysfunction of the spleen-qi in transport, often giving rise to oppressed feeling in the chest, epigastric distention and stuffiness, anorexia, nausea, vomiting, scanty urine, loose stool, and edema in the face and limbs.

4. Endogenous dryness is caused by depletion of body fluid and blood after febrile disease, or by overtaking warm and hot drugs, or by profuse sweating and excessive vomit and purgation. Dryness syndrome often causes dry skin, parched lips, dry eyes, dry-heat in nostrils, thirst, hunger, dry throat, dysphagia,

constipation, flaccidity syndrome, phthisical cough and convulsive seizure.

5. Endogenous fire can be divided into two types: fire of excess type and fire of deficiency type. Fire of excess type is mainly caused by hyperfunction of five zang-organs, often giving rise to aphthae, vexation, insomnia, conjunctival congestion, bitter taste in the mouth, dizziness, headache, abdominal pain, constipation, hematemesis, sore throat, hemoptysis, yellowish phlegm, dark urine, seminal emission and stranguria. Fire of deficiency type is mainly caused by deficiency of yin-blood, often giving rise to hectic fever, night sweat, flushed checks, tinnitus, vexation and insomnia.

(E) Retention of Phlegm and Fluid

Retention of phlegm and fluid is mainly caused by dysfunction of the lung, spleen and kidney and by dysbolism of water. Phlegm is sticky while fluid is thin. Phlegm exists everywhere with various symptoms while fluid easily stay in cavities and porous tissues.

(F) Blood Stasis

Blood stagnating in the body is called blood stasis. Blood stasis is mainly caused by stagnation of qi, deficiency of qi, blood-cold, blood-heat, deficiency of yin-blood, insufficiency of yang-qi and external injury, often giving rise to prickling pain, tumor, squamous and dry skin, purple lips and tongue and ecchymosis.

(G) Excessive Fatigue or Leisure

Excessive fatigue or leisure can cause diseases. Fatigue includes excessive labor, overtax and sexual strain. Leisure includes no work and no exercise for a long time, causing qi and blood not to flow smoothly and functions of spleen and stomach to weaken. "Internal Classic" says: "lying for a long time will impair qi."

(H) External Injury

External injury can be caused by bullet, sword, fall, beat, heavy load, burn, scald, cold, insect, animal, food poisoning or drug poisoning. These factors can cause not only surgical diseases but also dysfunction of the viscera, giving rise to internal diseases.

Pathogens of six climatic conditions belong to exopathic causes. Seven emotions, diet, five endogenous pathogenic factors, retention of phlegm and fluid and blood stasis belong to endopathic causes. Excessive fatigue and leisure and external injury belong to non-endo-exopathic causes.

Section 2 Pathology

"The Yellow Emperor's Internal Classic" laid a foundation for TCM theory, deeply expounded physiology and pathology of the human body, and created conditions for the development of pathology in later ages. "Treatise on Febrile and Miscellaneous Diseases" creatively developed pathology and raised the method of "analyzing and differentiating exogenous febrile diseases in accordance with the theory of the six channels, and analyzing and differentiating miscellaneous diseases according to pathological changes of the viscera and their interrelations". Physicians in later ages applied analysis and differentiation of exogenous febrile diseases in accordance with the theory of six channels to miscellaneous diseases. Analysis and differentiation of miscellaneous diseases according to pathological changes of the viscera and their interrelations increasingly deepened and developed. Particularly, four famous physicians in Jin and Yuan Dynasties deeply expounded the above-mentioned theory in various aspects. Thanks to persistent efforts by physicians of the past dynasties, analysis and differentiation of miscellaneous diseases according to pathological changes of the viscera and their interrelations has been gradually perfected. Moreover, products of pathological changes of the viscera, such as qi, blood, wind, fire, phlegm, dampness and blood stasis, have been deeply recognized, systematized and completed through constant rearrangement and replenishment. In Ming and Qing Dynasties, the doctrine of epidemic febrile diseases was developed. Specific contents of analyzing and differentiating epidemic febrile diseases by studying conditions of the four systems (wei, qi, ying and xue) and analyzing and differentiating syndromes according to the pathological changes of triple-jiao were raised and perfected, forming a complete pathological theory. People have recognized in practices that rich pathological theory of TCM can be applied to different types of diseases. For example, the six channels, the four systems and triple-jiao are mainly applied to exopathic diseases, while the viscera, qi, blood, wind, phlegm and dampness are mainly applied to diseases caused by internal injuries. However, the two can also influence and permeate each other. Physicians in later ages have gradually recognized that various methods of analyzing and differentiating diseases can be unified to the physiology and pathology of the viscera. of Course, this work is to be further studied and will surely promote the steady development of pathology.

A. Basic Concept of Pathogenesis and Syndromes of the Viscera

Pathogenesis of the viscera is the mechanism for pathological changes of visceral functions in the course of illness. Syndromes of the viscera are clinically symptomatic complexes reflected in the pathological changes of visceral functions.

In terms of pathophysiology of the viscera, the heart governs vessels and controls mental activities. Full blood supply will make complexion rosy and glowing. The tongue is the sprout and specific orifice of the heart. The heart and the small intestine are interior-exteriorly related to each other. Heat syndrome of the heart often causes red tongue tip. Heat syndrome of the small intestine often causes boil of the tongue, vexation and scanty dark urine. Pericardium is the external membrane to protect the heart. The invasion of pericardium by exopathogen causes diseases. The lung governs qi and controls respiration. It is related to the skin and hair, and has its orifice in the nose. The lung is a delicate zang-organ intolerable to cold or heat, so exopathic diseases often first invade it. The lung and the large intestine are interior-exteriorly related to each other. The large intestine depends on the purifying and descending function of the lung-qi to excrete smoothly. On the contrary, constipation can influence the purifying and descending function of the lung-qi. The spleen and stomach provide the material basis of the acquired constitution and the source of generation of qi and blood. They receive food, transform food into chyme and transport nutrients. The spleen governs blood and controls the limbs and muscles. The spleen lifts lucid yang, and the stomach transports food downward. Their dysfunction will surely affect the reception and digestion of food to cause gastrointestinal diseases. The liver is firm in nature, governs the normal flow of qi, stores blood, nourishes tendons and nails, and has its orifices in eyes. Its channels link up with the gallbladder, converge to the vertex and run round the external genital. The gallbladder attaches to the liver, and they are interior-exteriorly related to each other. Hyperactivity of the liver-yang causes excessive gallbladder-fire with symptoms such as flushed face, conjunctival congestion and headache. Deficiency of the liver-blood causes weak gallbladder-qi with symptoms such as dizziness, xenophthalmia, hypopsia and night blindness. The kidney is a zang-organ of water and fire. The gate of life attaches to the two kidneys with the kidney-yin and the kidney-yang in it. The kidney stores reproductive essence and food essence, and has the function of warming and moistening the five zang-organs. As the source of quintessence of the human body, the kidney is called the origin of congenital constitution. The consolidation of kidney-qi manifests itself in healthy brain, consolidated bones, thick hair and firm teeth. The kidney governs fertility, development and menstruation, and reflects sufficiency or deficiency of the kidney-qi. The kidney and the bladder are interior-exteriorly related to each other. The bladder serves as a reservoir responsible for storage of fluid. The functional activity of qi depends on if the kidney-qi is consolidated. Therefore, the diseased kidney can cause unconsolidated bones, unhealthy brain, thin hair, poor hearing ability, loose teeth, developmental retardation, suspension of menstruation, disturbance of childbirth and dysfunction of qi activity, with dyspnea, swelling, retention of urine and enuresis and other symptoms.

Zang-fu is a closely related whole in the human body, five zang-organs promote and restrict one another, and zang and fu are interior-exteriorly related to each other. Therefore, in the course of illness, pathological changes and syndromes of the viscera are extremely complicated. Particularly, changes of pathogenesis, deficiency, excess, cold and heat are all key points of diagnosis and treatment. If a physician can clearly recognize the basic concept of visceral pathogenesis, he will be able to differentiate syndromes of internal miscellaneous diseases. He will also be able to distinguish primary from secondary conditions of illness and its deficient from excessive nature, and recognize its pathological transformation. In so doing, he can consistently use theory, therapy, recipe and drug, and lay a solid foundation for clinical practice and deep research.

Key points for physiology, pathology, syndromes and symptoms of the heart and small intestine, lung and large intestine, spleen and stomach, liver and gallbladder, kidney and bladder and other zang-fu organs as well as diagnosis and treatment are described respectively as follows. Pericardium, the external membrane of the heart, and triple-jiao, basically including the visceral pathogenesis and syndromes, are not discussed in separate topics.

(A) The Heart (and the Small Intestine)

1. Physiology: The heart in the chest with pericardium as its external membrane is interior-exteriorly related to the small intestine. Its channels link up with the small intestine. The tongue is the orifice of the heart. The heart governing blood is the center of life activities of the human body. The heart controlling

mentality is the center of thinking activities.

2. Pathology: Because the physiological function of the heart is mainly to govern blood and control mentality, clinical symptoms always link up with disturbance of blood circulation and abnormality of thinking activities. Warm pathogen often affects pericardium. Heart diseases are mainly caused by internal injuries. Congenital deficiency, weak functional activities of the zang-organs, lack of proper care after an illness, excessive anxiety and damage to the heart and spleen can all cause deficiency of the heart-yin and insufficiency of the heart-yang. The main pathogenesis of deficiency of the heart-yin is depletion of the heart-blood, while the main pathogenesis of insufficiency of the heart-yang is deficiency of the heart-qi. Both can manifest themselves in irritability. Excessive anxiety, stagnation of qi, accumulation of fluid, transformation of phlegm into fire, mental disturbance due to phlegm-fire, obstruction of collaterals by blood stasis, or hindrance of the heart-yang by fluid retention can all cause heat syndrome and excess syndrome of the heart.

3. Symptoms mainly are palpitation, cardialgia, amnesia, insomnia, seminal emission, madness, coma, asthma, haematemesis, apostaxis, boil of the tongue, and hematuria.

4. Classification of Syndromes:

(1) Deficiency Syndrome

(a) Insufficiency of the Heart-yang

Treatment: Yang Xin Decoction, or Si Ni Decoction ang their like are used to warm and invigorate the heart yang, tonify heart qi.

Summary of Pathogenesis: caused by overtaxing nerves due to anxiety, excessive mental activity and weak heart-qi.

Main Pulse Conditions and Symptoms: Palpitation, asthma, cardialgia, whitish fur, and thready and feeble pulse are main symptoms for insufficiency of the heart-yang. Palpitation is characterized by accelerated and arrhythmic heartbeat, particularly in motion. Asthma manifests itself in fits of seizure and short breath, particularly in motion. Cardialgia suddenly breaks out with symptoms of cold limbs, fast and confused pulse. In serious conditions, hands, feet, lips and nose turn dark purple, or the patient has pale complexion, spontaneous perspiration and cold body.

(b) Deficiency of the Heart-yin

Schematic Diagram for Pathological Mechanism of the Heart

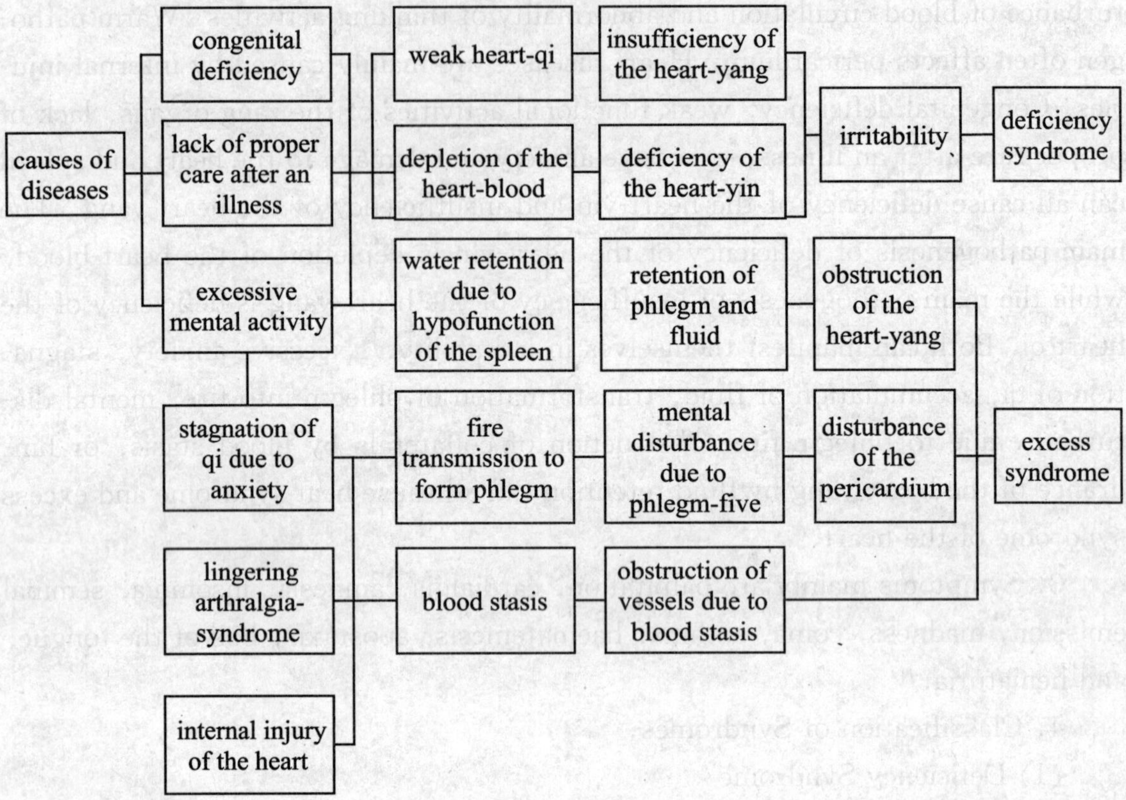

Summary of Pathogenesis: Excessive mental activity causes deficiency of blood, depletion of yin-essence, failure of yin to keep yang well, and floating heart-yang.

Main Pulse Conditions and Symptoms: Palpitation, cardialgia, insomnia, confused heartbeat, pink tongue, scanty fur or dry and red tongue tip are main symptoms for deficiency of the heart-yin. The characteristics of palpitation and cardialgia are vexation, vague pain and restlessness. Insomnia is often accompanied with dreaminess. Confused heartbeat manifests itself in scorching heat in the heart as if the patient is hungry. In addition, there are amnesia, nocturnal emission, night sweat, suspicion, anxiety and other symptoms.

Treatment: Tian Wang Bu Xin Pill or Zhu Sha An Shen Pill and their like are used to replenish yin, nourish the heart and tranquilize the mind.

(2) Excess Syndrome

(a) Mental Disturbance due to Phlegm-fire

Summary of Pathogenesis: stagnation of qi due to anxiety, accumulation of fluid to form phlegm, or dysfunction of the spleen in transport, long retention of damp phlegm to cause fire-transmission, mental disturbance due to phlegm-heat; in serious cases, disturbance of the pericardium and irritability.

Main Pulse Conditions and Symptoms: Palpitation, madness, insomnia, red parched tongue, yellow fur, slippery and rapid pulse are its main symptoms. Palpitation is often accompanied with dysphoria. Madness is characterized by dementia, or by impetuosity and anger, or by variable laugh and cry in serious cases. Insomnia is often accompanied with nightmare and agitation. In addition, there are other symptoms, such as flushed face, thirst for cold drinks, hematemesis, epistaxis, hot dark urine, hematuria and stranguria with pain.

Treatment: Huang Lian Wen Dan Decoction or Meng Shi Gun Tan Pill is used to clear away the heart-fire and remove phlegm.

(b) Obstruction of the Heart-yang due to Fluid Retention

Summary of Pathogenesis: Obstruction of the heart-yang is caused by long retention of water in the chest.

Main Pulse Conditions and Symptoms: Palpitation, dizziness, vomiting, white and greasy fur, and slippery or deep and tense pulse are its main symptoms. Palpitation is accompanied with oppressed feeling in the chest and disturbance of visceral function. Dizziness is often accompanied with nausea. Vomit is all phlegm. Sometimes there are symptoms of aversion to cold, hypochondriac mass and bowel sound.

Treatment: Xiao Ban Xia Jia Fu Ling Decoction or Ling Gui Zhu Gan Decoction and their like are used to warm yang and remove fluid retention.

(c) Stagnation of the Heart Blood

Summary of Pathogenesis: impairment of the heart due to fatigue, unconsolidated heart-qi, stagnation of qi, or long arthralgia syndrome in the heart, stagnation of blood, and disorder of collaterals.

Main Pulse Conditions and Symptoms: palpitation with restlessness, prickling pain in the chest, hypochondria, shoulders and back, dark red tongue with purple petechiae, scanty fur, or purple face, lips and nails, and uneven pulse.

Treatment: Shi Xiao Powder or Xue Fu Zhu Yu Decoction and their like are used to promote blood circulation and remove blood stasis.

(3) Accompanying Syndromes

(a) Deficiency of Qi and Blood in the Heart and Spleen: sallow complexion, anorexia, fatigue, dyspnea, lassitude, amnesia, severe palpitation, insomnia, irregular menstruation, thready, soft and powerless pulse, white fur and pale tongue. Gui Bi Decoction and its like are used to replenish the heart and spleen.

(b) Breakdown of the Normal Physiological Coordination between the Heart and the Kidney: insomnia due to vexation, nocturnal emission, tidal fever, night sweat, dry throat, dizziness, tinnitus, lassitude in loin and legs, polyuria, red tongue without fur, and feeble and rapid pulse. Huang Lian A Jiao Decoction or Jiao Tai Pill and its like are used to coordinate the heart and the kidney.

(c) Accumulation of Phlegm and Blood Stasis: insomnia due to vexation, dreaminess with susceptibility to fright, anorexia, nausea, dizziness, feeling of stuffiness and tightness in the chest and stomach, prickling pain in the chest, chest pain through to the back, dark purple tongue with ecchymosis, greasy fur and slippery pulse. Wen Dan Decoction, Dan Sheng Decoction and their like are used to resolve phlegm and remove blood stasis.

(d) Invasion of the Small Intestine by Heat: Refer to excessive heat in the small intestine for detailed information.

5. Key Points of Diagnosis and Treatment:

(1) Deficiency of the heart-qi and depletion of the heart-blood are main pathogenesis of insufficiency of the heart-yang and deficiency of the heart-yin.

(2) Deficiency of both yin and yang or deficiency of both qi and blood should be treated simultaneously. For example, Zhi Gan Cao Decoction is used to nourish both yin and yang, and Shi Quan Da Bu Decoction is used to replenish both qi and blood.

(3) Both insufficiency of the heart-yang and obstruction of the heart-yang due to fluid retention are also related to dysfunction of the spleen-yang. Therefore, they should be also treated with drugs to warm the spleen-yang, strengthen the spleen and nourish the heart.

(4) Both deficiency of the heart-yin and disturbance of the heart due to phlegm-fire are also related to deficiency and excess of the liver channel. The former is deficiency of the liver-qi due to deficiency of blood, and the latter is liver-fire due to phlegm-fire. Therefore, they should be treated as a whole.

(5) Both phlegm and blood stasis are caused by the heart-fire or by deficiency of both the heart and the spleen. Therefore, phlegm stagnation and blood stasis can take place at the same time. They should be treated with drugs of replenishing the heart and the spleen to resolve phlegm and remove blood stasis.

(6) Deficiency syndrome can be generally treated with drugs of tranquilizing the mind and relieving mental stress, such as date, arborvitae seed, poria with hostwood, and longan aril. Excess syndrome can be treated with drugs of tranquilizing the mind and inducing recuscitation, such as dragon's teeth, oyster shell, curcuma root, calamus and amber.

(7) The small intestine disease due to the heart-heat belongs to excess syndrome. It should be treated with drugs of clearing away the heart-fire to induce heat to move downward. The disease of small intestine channel is often related to the spleen, stomach and large intestine. It should be diagnosed in combination with them.

The diagnosis and treatment of heart diseases are shown in a simplified table as follows.

Simplified Table for Diagnosis and Treatment of Heart Diseases

symptoms	deficiency syndrome		excess syndrome		
	insufficiency of the heart-yang	deficiency of the heart-yin	phlegm-fire	fluid retention	blood stasis
pathogenesis	deficiency of the heart-qi	deficiency of the heart-blood	disturbance of the heart due to phlegm-fire, mental confusion due to phlegm	obstruction of the heart-yang due to fluid retention	obstruction of the vessel due to blood stasis
consciousness	susceptibility to calmness and aversion to motion, qi deficiency and cold body, pale complexion and edema of face	doubting mania, dim complexion	dementia, dysporia, divagation	aversion to cold, cold back, twitching of muscles, vomiting due to phlegm accumulation	restlessness due to pain, purple nails
palpitation	palpitation with hollow feeling	palpitation with restlessness of deficiency type	palpitation with fidgetiness, dysporia with smothery sensation in the chest	palpitation with oppressed feeling in the chest or with asthma	palpitation with fits of cardialgia

symptoms	deficiency syndrome		excess syndrome		
cardialgia	vague pain	vague pain or excessive pain	oppressed pain or burning pain	oppressed pain or epigatric pain	with palpitation prickling pain
sleep	lethargy	insomnia with dreaminess	insomnia with dysporia, dreaminess	difficulty in sleep due to dyspnea and palpitation	difficulty in sleep due to pain
perspiration	spontaneous perspiration	night sweat	spontaneous perspiration	spontaneous perspiration	perspiration due to severe pain
fur	pale tongue	pink tongue, or red tongue with scanty fur	red tongue with yellow and thick fur	white and greasy fur	dark purple tongue sometimes with ecchymosis
pulse condition	feeble, full and hollow pulse	thready and rapid pulse	slippery and rapid pulse	deep, tense or slightly slippery pulse	uneven pulse
treatment	replenishing the heart-qi and warming the heart-yang	nourishing the heart-yin	clearing away the heart-fire and resolving phlegm	removing fluid retention and resolving phlegm	promoting blood circulation to remove blood stasis and remove obstruction in the channels
recipes	Yang Xin Decoction, Si Ni Decoction	Tian Wang Bu Xin Pill, Zhu Zha An Shen Pill	Xiao Xian Xiong Decoction, Meng Shi Gun Tan Pill	Xiao Ban Xia Jia Fu Ling Decoction, Ling Gui Zhu Gan Decoction	Shi Xiao Powder, Xue Fu Zhu Yu Decoction

Small Intestine

1. Physiology: The small intestine is connected upward to pylorus leading to the stomach and downward to the large intestine with ileocecal junction at their convergence. Its channels are connected to the heart. The small intestine receives digested food from the stomach, transports nutrients to various parts, and sends wastes to the bladder and the large intestine.

2. Pathology: Diseases of the small intestine are mainly caused by improper diet to damage the spleen and stomach. The small intestine and the heart are

interior-exteriorly related to each other. Therefore, heat can be transferred from the heart to the small intestine. The pathological manifestations of the small intestine mainly are indiscrimination of nutrients and wastes and disturbance of transportation with symptoms of disturbance of urination and diarrhea. Diseases of small intestine are clinically divided into cold of insufficiency type, heat of excess type and pain due to disorder of qi.

3. Classification of Diseases:

(1) Cold of insufficiency type in the small intestine: vague pain in lower abdomen and preference for massage, bowel sound, diarrhea, frequent and difficult urination, pale tongue with thin and white fur, thready and slow pulse. Wu Zhu Yu Decoction and its like are used to warm and clear the small intestine.

(2) Heat of excess type in the small intestine: vexation, aphtha, sore throat, deafness, difficulty in micturition with dark urine or pain in the penis, abdominal distention slightly alleviated after passing flatus, red tongue, yellow fur, and slippery and rapid pulse. Dao Chi Powder or Liang Ge Powder and their like are used to eliminate excessive heat.

(3) Pain due to disorder of qi in the small intestine: acute pain in the lower abdomen affecting the waist, back and testicle, white fur, deep and taut or taut and slippery pulse. Tian Tai Wu Yao Powder and its like are used to promote the circulation of qi to resolve mass.

(B) The Liver (and the Gallbladder)

1. Physiology: The gallbladder attaches to the liver under hypochondria. The liver is in charge of the tendons and has its orifice in the eye. Its channels connect to eyes and converge to the vertex. Its function is to store blood, regulate blood supply and nourish the eye with good sight. The liver governs the bend and stretch of tendons and joints of the whole body. Firm in nature, the liver likes optimism and dislikes depression. The regulation of mental functions is closely related to the liver-qi.

2. Pathology: The pathological manifestations of the liver can be summarized as deficiency syndrome and excess syndrome with the latter frequently seen. Sad emotion causes the stagnation of the liver-qi, giving rise to fire-syndrome. Hyperactivity of the liver-yang brings about endogenous wind. Wind and fire invade vertex or channels and collaterals, causing blood not to circulate in the vessels but to go up with qi and fire. According to conditions of illness, syndromes of excessive

heat can be divided into stagnation of the liver-qi, flaming-up of the liver-fire and hyperactivity of the liver-yang. Deficiency of the kidney-yin, essence failing to produce blood, and malnutrition of the liver can cause deficiency syndrome of insufficiency of the liver-yin and upward floating of yang in deficiency condition. Invasion of the liver-channel by exogenous cold also belongs to excess syndrome of the liver.

Schematic Diagram for Pathogenesis of Liver Diseases

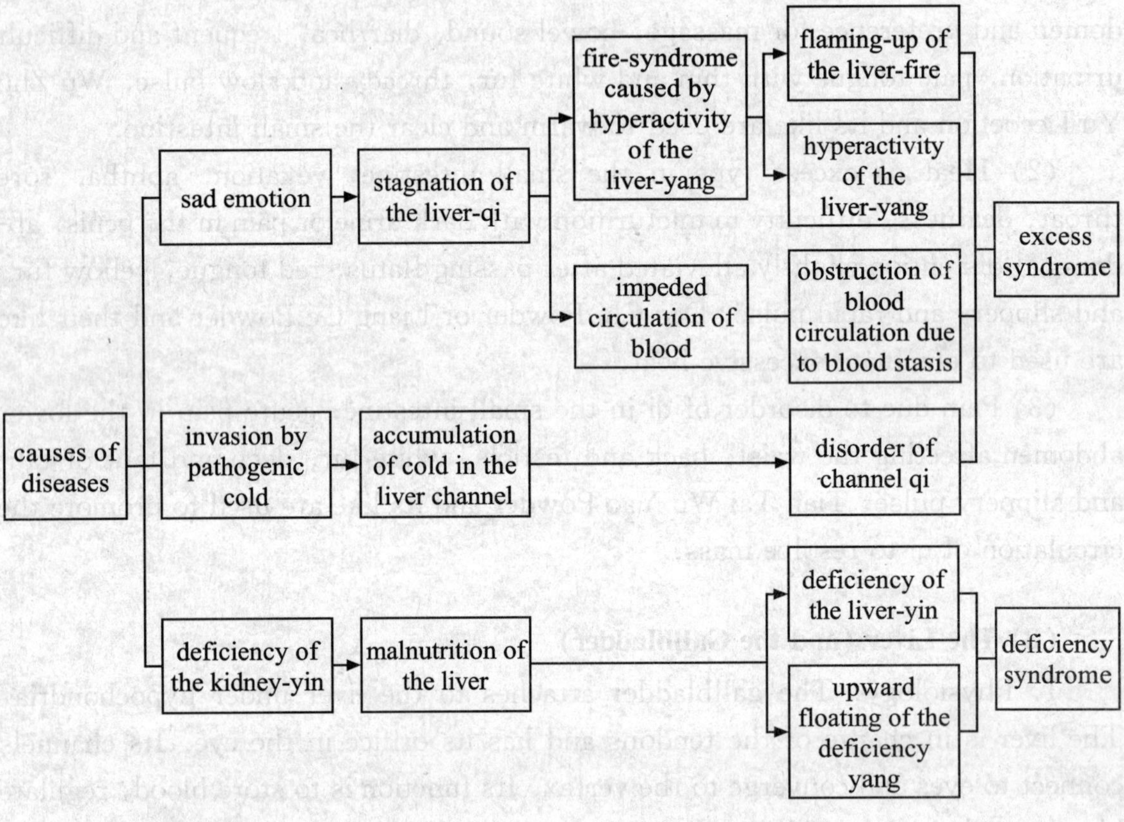

3. Scope of Symptoms: Clinically pathological changes of the liver and gallbladder mainly are apoplexy, dizziness, headache, spasm, epilepsy, syncope, abdominal mass, deafness, tinnitus, hernia, hematemesis, apostaxis, panic, insomnia, numbness and tremor.

4. Classification of Syndromes:

(1) Excess Syndrome

(a) Stagnation of the Liver-qi

Summary of Pathogenesis: impairment of the liver due to depression and anger, dysfunction of the liver, transverse invasion by the hyperactive liver-qi, obstruction and stagnation of the liver-qi, pain, abdominal mass, obstruction of blood circulation due to blood stasis, blockage of channels, and hypochondriac lump.

Main Pulse Conditions and Symptoms: hypochondriac pain, vomiting, abdominal pain, diarrhea, abdominal mass, thin fur and taut pulse are main symptoms. Hypochondriac pain is characterized by uncomfortable oppressed feeling in the chest, wandering pain and inability of turning round. Vomiting is characterized by adverse flow of qi, regurgitation of acid, and vomiting of yellow, green and bitter watery fluid. Abdominal pain and diarrhea are characterized by uncomfortable pain in the lower abdomen without alleviation after diarrhea. Abdominal mass is under the hypochondria and hypochondriac lump moves left or right, converges or diverges uncertainly, with distending pain or prickling pain. In addition, there are other symptoms of liability to anger and anorexia.

Treatment: Chai Hu Shu Gan Powder or Xue Yu Pill and their like are used to sooth the liver and regulate the circulation of qi, and to dissolve lump and resolve mass.

(b) Flaming-up of the Liver-fire

Summary of Pathogenesis: dysfunction of the liver and gallbladder, fire-syndrome caused by stagnation of qi, scurry of fire with qi, upward invasion of the vertex by the liver-fire.

Main Pulse Conditions and Symptoms: hypochondriac pain, vomiting, dizziness, headache, fury, deafness, tinnitus, conjunctival congestion, hematemesis, apostaxis, red smooth tongue, yellow or dry greasy fur, and taut and rapid pulse are main symptoms. Hypochondriac pain is characterized by burning pain and vexation. Vomiting is characterized by bitter or yellow watery fluid. Dizziness and headache are characterized by intolerable dizziness, pulse feeling of tendon and muscle, heat in the forehead with chopping pain or distending pain. Tinnitus and deafness are characterized by sudden fits with tidal sound in the ear without alleviation under massage. Conjunctival congestion is characterized by acute pain and swelling. Hematemesis and apostaxis are characterized by sudden fits with a large amount of blood gushed from the mouth. In addition, there are other symptoms of difficulty in micturition with hot dark urine, hot red face, and dry mouth with bitter taste.

Treatment: Long Dan Xie Gan Decoction and its like are used to clear away heat from the liver and gallbladder.

(c) Hyperactivity of the Liver-yang

Summary of Pathogenesis: fire-syndrome caused by hyperactivity of the liver-qi, sudden expansion of yang-qi, scurry of fire with qi, transverse invasion of channels and collaterals by the hyperactive liver-qi, blood ascending with qi to the vertex.

Main Pulse Conditions and Symptoms: syncope, spasm, numbness, dizziness, headache, taut pulse, crooked, quivered and reddened tongue, and thin and yellow fur are main symptoms. Syncope is characterized by sudden fall with unconsciousness, or convulsion or salivation. Spasm is characterized by neck stiffness, acute spasm in the limbs unable to bend and stretch, and opisthotonus. Numbness is characterized by a feeling as if ants crawl on hands, feet, face, lips and other parts. Dizziness and headache are characterized by floating walking and throbbing pain in the head. In addition, there are other symptoms of crooked mouth and eyes, dysphasia and hemiparalysis.

Treatment: Tian Ma Gou Teng Decoction and its like are used to calm the liver and stop wind.

(d) Stagnation of Cold in the Liver Channel

Summary of Pathogenesis: invasion of Jueyin liver channel by exopathic cold, dysfunction of the liver-qi, and obstruction of the channel-qi.

Main Pulse Conditions and Symptoms: distending pain in the lower abdomen, dropping distension of the testicle or shrink of the scrotum, moistened and smooth tongue, white fur, and deep and taut or slow pulse are main symptoms. Distending pain in the lower abdomen is characterized by acute dropping pain in the testicle, which is aggravated in cold exposure and alleviated in heat exposure. Shrink of the scrotum is characterized by stagnation of cold in Jueyin, causing spasm in channels of the lower abdomen. Therefore, shrink of scrotum is often accompanied with distending pain in the lower abdomen. In addition, the patient is weak and timid and curls up.

Treatment: Nuan Gan Decoction and its like are used to warm the liver channel.

(2) Deficiency Syndrome

Deficiency of the Liver-yin

Summary of Pathogenesis: As a firm zang-organ, the liver is nourished by the kidney-yin. Deficiency of the kidney-yin, failure of essence to produce blood, and failure of blood to nourish the liver can cause deficiency of the liver-yin and hyperactivity of the liver-yang.

Main Pulse Conditions and Symptoms: dizziness, headache, tinnitus, deafness, hypochondriac pain, numbness, tremor, nyctalopia, red dry tongue, scanty saliva, scanty fur, taut, thready and rapid pulse are main symptoms. Dizziness and headache are characterized by tottering and continuous distending pain. Tinnitus and deafness gradually occur with constant low sound, and they can be alleviated with massage. Numbness can be lessened with massage. Hypochondriac vague pain can be weakened with massage. Tremor is characterized by muscular contracture, conscious or unconscious shiver, or spasm of the limbs. Nyctalopia is characterized by dry eye, drastically reduced sight at night or night blindness. In addition, there are other symptoms of burning heat in the face, red checks in the afternoon, dry mouth and throat, insomnia and dreaminess.

Treatment: Yi Guan Decoction or Da Bu Yin Pill and their like are used to nourish the liver and replenish the kidney, and nourish yin and suppress the excessive yang.

(3) Accompanying Syndromes

(a) The Hyperactive Liver-qi Attacking the Stomach: stiff and oppressed feeling in the chest and stomach with wandering pain in hypochondria, indigestion, eructation and acid regurgitation, thin and yellow fur, and taut pulse. Si Ni Powder and Zuo Jin Pill and their like are used to quench fire in the liver and regulate the stomach.

(b) Incoordination between the Liver and the Spleen: anorexia, abdominal distension with bowel sound, loose stool, white and greasy fur, and taut and slow pulse. Xiao Yao Powder and its like are used to coordinate the liver and the spleen.

(c) Disturbance of the Liver and the Gallbladder: insomnia due to vexation, dreadful nightmare, susceptibility to fright, short breath, lassitude, blurred sight, bitter taste in the mouth, thin and white fur, and taut and thready pulse. Suan Zao Ren Decoction and its like are used to nourish the liver, remove heat from the gallbladder, and tranquilize the mind. Huang Lian Wen Dan Decoction is used to treat accumulation of phlegm and heat in the lung, greasy and yellow fur, and taut and slippery pulse.

(d) Yin Deficiency of the Liver and Kidney: sallow complexion, pink cheeks, dizziness, dry eyes, lassitude in loin and knees, sore throat, night sweat, dysphoria with feverish sensation in chest, palms and shoes, dyschesia, seminal emission, irregular menstruation or leukorrhea, red tongue without fur, and thready pulse. Qi Ju Di Huang Pill and its like are used to nourish yin and reduce pathogenic fire.

(e) Invasion of the Lung by the Liver-fire: prickling pain in the chest and hypochondria, fits of cough, hematemesis, impetuosity and susceptibility to anger, dysphoria with smothery sensation, bitter taste in the mouth, dizziness, conjunctival congestion, thin fur, red tongue, and taut and rapid pulse. Dai Ge Powder or Xie Bai Powder and their like are used to remove heat from the liver and the lung.

5. Key Points for Diagnosis and Treatment:

(1) As a firm zang-organ, the liver belongs to wood, governs wind and prefers ascension. Therefore, liver diseases mainly are syndromes of the liver-yang. Cold syndrome of the liver is merely seen in accumulation of pathogenic cold in the lower abdomen and Jueyin liver channel.

(2) In excess syndrome of the liver, stagnation of the liver-qi, flaming-up of the liver-fire, and hyperactivity of the liver-yang come from the same source. They are mainly caused by emotional depression, fire-syndrome due to hyperactive liver-qi, hypoactive yin-blood and hyperactive yang. The three are closely related to one another, and can not be separated categorically. Primary cause should be clinically distinguished from secondary ones in diagnosis and treatment of diseases.

(3) Hyperactivity of the liver-yang is a life-threatening syndrome with upward invasion of the vertex and transverse invasion of channels and collaterals. The former is appropriately treated with drugs to calm the endogenous wind and suppress the exuberant yang. The latter should be treated with drugs to regulate channels and tranquilize the endogenous wind. Accumulation of phlegm should be treated with drugs to remove phlegm.

(4) Lingering excess syndrome easily depletes the liver-yin to cause the syndrome of deficiency in origin and excess in superficiality, which is clinically often seen and should be noticed in diagnosis and treatment.

(5) Deficiency syndrome of the liver is mainly caused by deficiency of the kidney-yin, failure of the essence to produce blood, deficiency of the liver-yin and hyperactivity of the liver-yang. It should be carefully distinguished from excess syndrome. Its pathogenesis is very closely related to deficiency of the kidney-yin. Therefore, the treatment of both the liver and the kidney is clinically often used.

Diagnosis and treatment of liver diseases are shown in the following table.

Brief Table for Diagnosis and Treatment of Liver Diseases

syndromes	deficiency syndrome	excess syndrome			
pathogenesis	deficiency of the liver-yin	stagnation of the liver-qi	flaming-up of the liver-fire	hyperactivity of the liver-yang	invasion of the liver-channel by cold
	deficiency of the liver-yin, malnutrition of the liver	disorder of qi, abnormal flow of qi	fire-syndrome due to stagnation of qi, flaming-up of the liver-fire	ascension of blood with qi, transverse invasion of channels	accumulation of cold in Jueyin channels and collaterals
dizziness	dizziness with no desire to open eyes	occasional fit of dizziness	dizziness and distension with fits of burning heat in the head	dizziness, carebaria, floating walking	dizziness with falling trend
headache	lingering pain	slightly distending pain on both sides	hot forehead with cutting pain	convulsion and pain in the vertex	occasional fit of migraine
tinnitus	gradual fit of tinnitus as if a cicada is chirping in the ear, and tinnitus can be alleviated with massage	occasional fit of tinnitus	tidal tinnitus, which can not be alleviated with massage	roaring tinnitus	occasional tinnitus
expression	depression	depression or liability to anger	fury or arrogance	facial hemiparalysis, dysphasia, even coma	aversion to cold, and curling up
pain in the heart, hypochondria and abdomen	uncomfortable vague pain in the hypochondria	wandering and distending pain in the hypochondria	vexation and burning pain		abdominal pain affecting hypochondria with a comfortable feeling when the abdomen is warmed

syndromes	deficiency syndrome	excess syndrome			
eye symptoms	dry eyes and night blindness	blurred sight sometimes	conjunctival congestion with acute pain or swelling	strabismus	blurred sight sometimes
urination and defecation	dyschesia with dry feces	constipation or diarrhea	dry feces and hot dark urine	enuresis	dropping distension of the testicle or shrink of the scrotum, clear urine
fur	red tongue with scanty fur, or split tongue	thin and white or thin and yellow fur	red tongue, yellow fur and scanty saliva	crooked, quivered and reddened tongue with yellowish fur	moistened tongue with white fur
pulse conditions	taut, thready and rapid pulse	taut pulse	taut and rapid pulse	taut, slippery and powerful pulse	deep and taut pulse
treatment	replenishing yin and nourishing the liver	soothing the liver and regulating the circulation of qi	removing heat from the liver and gallbladder	calming the liver to stop the wind	warming the liver-channel
recipes	Qi Ju Di Huang Pill	Chai Hu Shu Gan Powder	Long Dan Xie Gan Decoction	Tian Ma Gou Teng Decoction	Nuan Gan Decoction

Gallbladder

1. Physiology: The gallbladder attaches to the liver and stores bile. Gallbladder channels connect to the liver. The clean bile is different from turbid fluid in other fu-organs. Therefore, Prescriptions Worth a Thousand Gold for Emergencies calls the gallbladder "clean fu-organ". The gallbladder is one of the six fu-organs, and also one of the extraordinary fu-organs. Upright in nature, the gallbladder controls the power of decision. Plain Questions says: "The gallbladder,

an upright organ, controls the power of decision."

2. Pathology: Gallbladder diseases mainly are syndromes of hyperactive yang and excessive fire. Pathogenic fire can turn fluid into phlegm, so gallbladder diseases are often accompanied with phlegm syndrome. Mental disturbance due to phlegm-fire should be treated with drugs to remove heat from the gallbladder, resolve phlegm, clear away the heart-fire and tranquilize the mind.

3. Classification of Syndromes:

(1) Deficiency Syndrome of the Gallbladder: dizziness, nausea, liability to fright, insomnia, blurred sight, thin and smooth fur, and taut and thready pulse. Suan Zao Ren Decoction and its like are used to nourish the heart, calm the mind, and regulate the gallbladder and the stomach.

(2) Excess Syndrome of the Gallbladder: dizziness, deafness, fullness sensation in the chest, hypochondriac pain, bitter taste in the mouth, vomiting of bitter watery fluid, vexation, liability to anger, insomnia, dreaminess, alternate attacks of chill and fever, sallow complexion, taut, rapid and forceful pulse, yellow fur and red tongue. Long Dan Xie Gan Decoction and its like are used to remove heat from the gallbladder. Yin Chen Hao Decoction is used to treat jaundice. Vexation, liability to anger, dysphoria, insomnia, dreaminess, sticky phlegm, anorexia, greasy and yellow fur, and taut and slippery pulse should be treated with Huang Lian Wen Dan Decoction and its like to remove phlegm-heat.

(C) Spleen (and Stomach)

1. Physiology: The spleen and the stomach are connected with a membrane in the abdomen, and interior-exteriorly related to each other. They are digestive organs, nourish the muscles and have their orifice in the mouth. The stomach receives food and transforms it into chyme. The spleen transports nutrients to the whole body and sends down wastes. The spleen also has important physiological functions of supplementing qi, governing the blood, and nourishing the muscles and limbs. Therefore, our ancestors called the spleen and the stomach "the basis of the acquired constitution".

2. Pathology: Functions of the spleen and the stomach mainly are to receive food and transport and transform nutrients. Their pathogenic factors mainly are hunger, fullness and fatigue, affecting digestion and absorption of food and resulting in their dysfunction in receiving food, transforming it into chyme, and transporting nutrients. Diseases of the spleen channel are nothing but deficiency,

excess, cold and heat. For example, insufficiency of the spleen-yang and deficiency of qi in middle jiao belong to deficiency syndrome, while invasion of the spleen by cold-dampness and retention of damp-heat belong to excess syndrome. Insufficiency of the spleen causes water retention in the body, so spleen diseases are often related to dampness, showing syndromes of deficiency in origin and excess in superficiality. Insufficiency of the spleen usually affects other organs, causing accompanying syndromes.

Schematic Diagram for Pathogenesis of the Spleen Channel

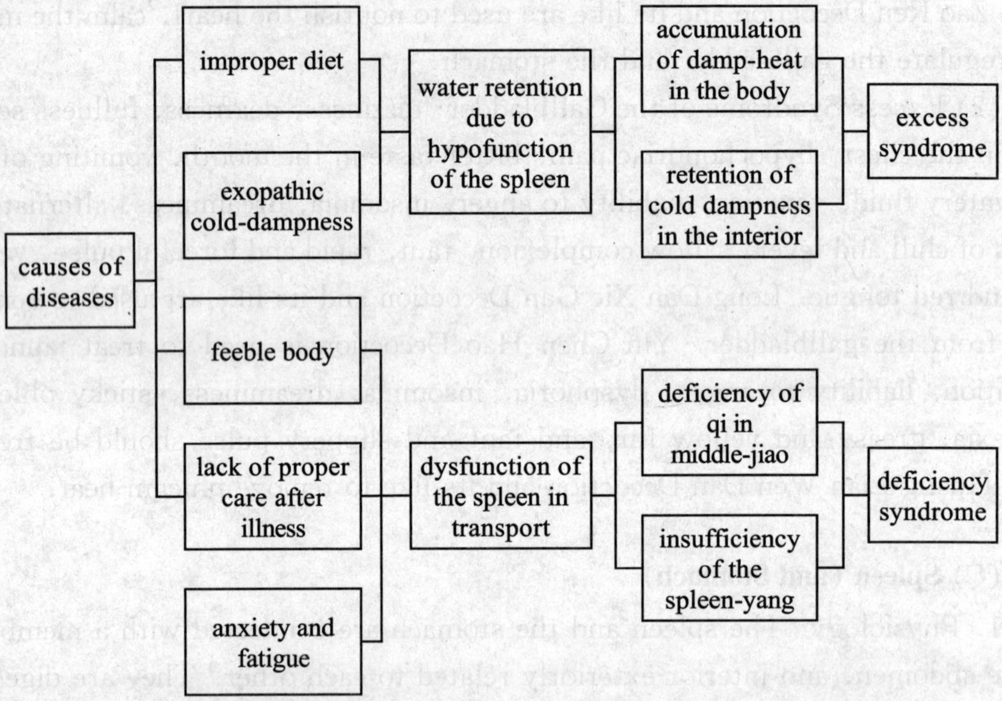

3. Scope of Diseases: Clinically common diseases of the spleen and the stomach are diarrhea, cholera, jaundice, stomachache, vomiting, hiccup, edema, tympanites, phlegm retention, hematemesis, hemafecia, metrorrhagia and metrostaxis.

4. Classification of Syndromes:

(1) Deficiency Syndrome

(a) Insufficiency of the Spleen-yang

Summary of Pathogenesis: lingering gastropathy, eating uncooked, cold, fatty and sweet food, overdosing cold and cool drugs, old age, feeble body, lack of proper care after illness, insufficiency of the spleen-yang, and dysfunction of the spleen to transport and transform nutrients.

Main Pulse Conditions and Symptoms: sallow and dim complexion, susceptibility to warmness and hot drink due to cold stomach, loose stool, clear urine, magersucht, aversion to cold, cold limbs, disinclination to talk due to deficiency of qi, pale tongue, white fur, and slow and feeble pulse.

Treatment: Li Zhong Decoction and its like are used to warm yang in middle jiao.

(b) Deficiency of Qi in Middle Jiao

Summary of Pathogenesis: deficiency of qi, depletion of the spleen-qi and the stomach-qi due to lingering disease, and failure to send up nutrients and send down wastes.

Main Pulse Conditions and Symptoms: low voice and short breath, acratia in the limbs, bowel sound and abdominal distension, frequent loose stool, pale tongue with thin and white fur, and slow and feeble pulse, or magersucht, qi stagnation in the waist and abdomen, and proctoptosis.

Treatment: Si Jun Zi Decoction and its like are used to strengthen the spleen and replenish qi. Sinking of qi in the middle qi should be treated with Bu Zhong Yi Qi Decoction to replenish qi and elevate the spleen-yang.

(2) Excess Syndrome

(a) Invasion of the Spleen by Cold-dampness

Summary of Pathogenesis: wading, drenching, sitting or lying on a wet ground, or excessive endogenous dampness, obstruction of yang in middle jiao, failure of the spleen to transport and transform nutrients.

Main Pulse Conditions and Symptoms: anorexia, fullness and tightness sensation in the stomach, sweet taste and sticky feeling in the mouth, carebaria and lassitude, loose stool or diarrhea, white and greasy fur, slow and feeble pulse.

Treatment: Wei Ling Decoction and its like are used to activate the spleen and eliminate dampness.

(b) Retention of Damp-heat in the Body

Summary of Pathogenesis: impairment of the spleen and the stomach due to affection of exopathogen or addiction of wine, dysfunction of the spleen in transport, heat caused by retention of dampness, dampness in combination with heat as a pathogenic factor, and failure of qi to ascend and descend.

Main Pulse Conditions and Symptoms: chest stuffiness and abdominal distension, anorexia, sticky and greasy feeling in the mouth, nausea and vomiting, carebaria and lassitude, difficulty in micturition with dark urine, yellow and greasy fur, and soft and rapid pulse, or thirst and bitter taste in the mouth.

Treatment: Xiao Xian Xiong Decoction or Lian Po Decoction and their like are used to clear away heat and induce diuresis.

(3) Accompanying Syndrome

(a) Incoordination between the Spleen and the Stomach: stuffiness and fullness sensation in the stomach with lingering vague pain, indigestion, eructation and hiccup, nausea and vomiting, loose stool or frequent defecation, thready pulse, and thin and white fur. Ban Xia Xie Xin Decoction and its like can be used to nourish qi in middle jiao and coordinate the spleen and the stomach.

(b) Yang Insufficiency of Both the Spleen and the Kidney: disinclination to talk due to deficiency of qi, aversion to cold, cold limbs, spontaneous perspiration, loose stool, diarrhea before dawn, lassitude in loin and knees, pale tongue, thin and white fur, and deep and thready pulse. Li Zhong Decoction and Si Shen Pill and their like are used to strengthen the spleen and warm the kidney.

(c) Invasion of the Lung by Dampness in the Spleen: cough with phlegm, chest tightness, short breath, anorexia, white and slightly greasy fur, and slippery pulse. Er Chen Decoction or Ping Wei Powder and their like are used to eliminate dampness and resolve phlegm.

(d) Deficiency of Qi and Blood in the Heart and Spleen: See accompanying syndrome of the heart.

5. Key Points for Diagnosis and Treatment:

(1) Deficiency syndrome of the spleen is the opposite of its excess syndrome. Failure to transport nutrients due to deficiency of the spleen, and water retention mainly belong to deficiency in origin and excess in superficiality, which should be clinically noticed. Mild case should be first treated with drugs to strengthen the spleen and eliminate dampness. Syndromes of excess in superficiality should be treated with drugs to purge and nourish simultaneously.

(2) Spleen diseases are very closely related to dampness. Regardless of deficiency, excess, cold or heat syndrome, accompanying syndrome of dampness can be seen. For example, invasion of the spleen by cold-dampness belongs to cold syndrome, retention of damp-heat in the body belongs to heat syndrome, retention of water in the body belongs to excess syndrome, and failure of the spleen to transport dampness belongs to deficiency syndrome. Therefore, spleen diseases should be treated with drugs to eliminate dampness, induce diuresis, dispel

retained water and resolve dampness according to illness conditions. With dampness eliminated, the function of the spleen will naturally return to normal.

(3) Pathology of the spleen and the stomach can be relatively observed. Our ancestors believed: "Yangming disease occurs in strong people while Taiyin disease occurs in weak people." Therefore, spleen diseases are mainly deficiency and cold syndromes, while stomach diseases are mainly excess and heat syndromes.

(4) Judging from the whole concept of the viscera, the pathological changes of the spleen are related not only to the stomach and intestine but also to other internal organs. For example, lingering spleen diseases often affect other internal organs, and likewise, diseases of other internal organs often affect the spleen as well. Therefore, treatment of spleen diseases can improve diseases of other internal organs, and treatment of diseases of other internal organs can contribute to recovery from spleen diseases.

The diagnosis and treatment of spleen diseases is shown in the following brief table.

Brief Table for Diagnosis and Treatment of Spleen Diseases

differentiation	deficiency syndrome		excess syndrome	
	insufficiency of the spleen-yang	deficiency of qi in middle jiao	invasion of the spleen by cold-dampness	retention of damp-heat in the body
pathogenesis	depletion of qi in middle jiao, insufficiency of the spleen-yang	weakness of the spleen and the stomach, deficiency or even sinking of qi in middle jiao	failure of the spleen to transport and transform nutrients due to invasion of the spleen by cold-dampness	failure to send up nutrients and send down wastes due to damp-heat
main symptoms	cold stomach and abdominal distension with vague pain, aversion to cold, cold limbs, thirst for hot drink, disinclination to talk due to deficiency of qi, clear urine, and loose stool	short breath, low voice, anorexia, lassitude, frequent loose stool, dropping distension in the waist and abdomen, even proctoptosis	fullness and tightness sensation in the stomach, anorexia, nausea, vomiting, carebaria, lassitude, sweet taste and sticky feeling in the mouth, loose stool or diarrhea	feeling of stuffiness and distension in the chest, nausea, vomiting, sticky and greasy feeling in the mouth, loose stool, difficulty in micturition with dark urine, heaviness sensation in the limbs, lassitude

differentiation	deficiency syndrome		excess syndrome	
fur	pale enlarged tongue with thin and white fur	pale tongue with white fur	white and greasy fur	yellow and greasy fur
pulse conditions	deep, thready and slow pulse	thready, slow and powerless pulse	soft and thready pulse	soft and rapid pulse
treatment	warming the middle-jiao and strengthening the spleen	nourishing qi, strengthening the spleen and elevating yang	activating the spleen to eliminate dampness	eliminating damp-heat
recipes	Li Zhong Decoction	Si Jun Zi Decoction, Bu Zhong Yi Qi Decoction	Wei Ling Decoction	Xiao Xian Xiong Decoction

Stomach

1. Physiology: The stomach under diaphragm connects upward to the esophagus and downward to the small intestine. Its channels lead to the spleen. Its upper opening is cardia, also known as the upper part of the gastric cavity, its lower opening is pylorus, also known as the lower part of the gastric cavity, and the area between the two is called the middle part of the gastric cavity. The three parts altogether is called the gastric cavity. The function of the stomach is to receive food and transform it into chyme, while the function of the spleen is to transport and transform nutrients. Therefore, the spleen and the stomach are interior-exteriorly related to each other, and jointly send up nutrients and send down wastes. Miraculous Pivot says: "The stomach is an organ to receive food."

2. Pathology: The stomach is a reservoir of foodstuff. Improper diet, overeating or going hungry, and inappropriately cold or hot food can influence the gastric function, causing pathological changes. The stomach, corresponding to dry earth, likes moisture and dislikes dryness. Therefore, indigestion and stagnated heat are generally treated with drugs to normalize the functions of the stomach and spleen and send down abnormally ascending qi. Gastric diseases easily have symptoms of adverse flow of qi, eructation and vomiting.

3. Classification of Syndromes:

(1) Cold Syndrome of the Stomach: distension and fullness in the stomach

with lingering pain, susceptibility to heat and massage, vomiting of watery fluid, hiccup, white and smooth fur, and slow pulse. Liang Fu Pill and its like are used to warm the stomach and disperse cold.

(2) Heat Syndrome of the Stomach: thirst for cold drink, hyperorexia, vomiting, halitosis, swelling pain, decay and bleeding in the gum, red tongue, yellow fur, scanty saliva, and slippery and rapid pulse. Qing Wei Powder and its like are used to clear away heat from the stomach.

(3) Deficiency Syndrome of the Stomach: fullness in the stomach, indigestion, eructation, loose stool, soft and feeble pulse, and scanty fur. Jian Zhong Decoction and its like are used to replenish qi and strengthen the spleen.

(4) Excess Syndrome of the Stomach: indigestion, distension and fullness in the stomach and abdomen, difficulty in defecation, halitosis with decaying smell, vomiting, thin and yellow fur, and slippery pulse. Xiang Su Decoction or Bao He Pill and their like are used to promote digestion and remove stagnated food, normalize functions of the stomach and the spleen, and send down abnormally ascending qi.

(D) Lung (and Large Intestine)

1. Physiology: The lung in the chest connects upward to the trachea and has the nose as its orifice, forming the pulmonary system. The lung is in charge of the skin. Its channels lead to the large intestine. The lung and the large intestine are interior-exteriorly related to each other. The lung governs qi, has defensive function, forms pectoral qi, controls respiration, and helps the heart function normally. Plain Questions says: "The lung, an auxiliary organ, helps the heart function normally."

2. Pathology: Because the lung governs qi, its pathological changes mainly are disorder of qi. Because the lung is a tender organ intolerable to cold and heat and a respiratory passage, exopathic disease and pulmonary tuberculosis often first invade the lung. Because the lung-qi flows through channels to other internal organs, diseases of other internal organs often affect the lung.

Syndromes of the lung can be divided into two main types: deficiency syndrome and excess syndrome. Deficiency syndrome can be subdivided into deficiency of yin and deficiency of qi. Deficiency of yin mainly results from consumption of fluid and malnutrition of the lung. Deficiency of qi is mainly caused by a lingering illness or affected by diseases of other internal organs. Excess syndrome is attributed to accumulation of phlegm and fluid, and invasion of the lung by pathogenic cold or pathogenic heat.

Schematic Diagram for Pathogenesis of Lung Diseases

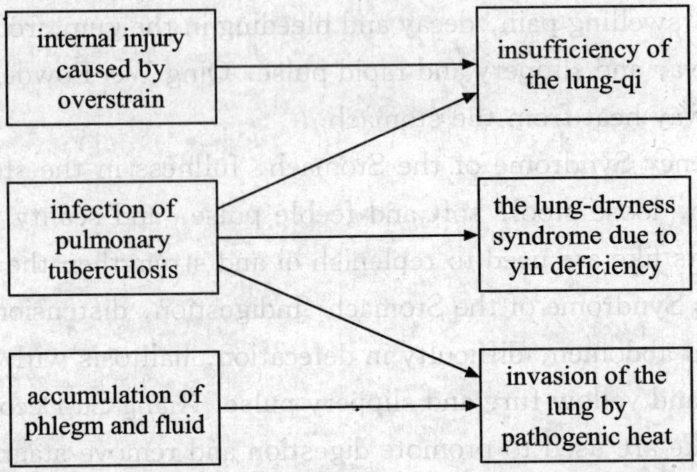

Scope of Symptoms: Diseases of the pulmonary system often have clinical symptoms of common cold, cough, asthma, pulmonary abscess, pulmonary tuberculosis, consumptive lung disease, hemoptysis, aphonia, epistaxis, and chest pain.

3. Classification of Syndromes:

(1) Deficiency Syndrome

(a) The Lung-dryness Syndrome due to Yin Deficiency

Summary of Pathogenesis: exopathic dryness, pulmonary tuberculosis, and impairment of the lung by lingering cough cause deficiency of the lung-yin and damage to the lung by fever of deficiency type.

Main Pulse Conditions and Symptoms: cough, dyspnea, adverse flow of qi, sticky phlegm with blood streak or blood clot, tidal fever, night sweat, red cheeks in the afternoon, insomnia, dry mouth and throat, red tongue. scanty fur, and thready and rapid pulse.

Treatment: Bai He Gu Jin Decoction and its like are used to nourish yin and moisten the lung.

(b) Insufficiency of the Lung-qi

Summary of Pathogenesis: internal injury caused by overstrain, failure of primordial qi to recover after illness, impairment of the lung due to lingering cough.

Main Pulse Conditions and Symptoms: cough, short breath, thin phlegm, disinclination to talk due to lassitude, low voice, pale complexion, aversion to wind, spontaneous perspiration, pale tongue, thin and white fur, and feeble pulse.

Treatment: Bu Fei Decoction and its like are used to replenish and restore the lung-qi.

(2) Excess Syndrome

(a) Stagnation of Phlegm in the Lung

Summary of Pathogenesis: Accumulation of fluid and phlegm causes disorder of qi.

Main Pulse Conditions and Symptoms: cough, asthma, rale in the throat, sticky and thick phlegm, so serious fullness and pain in the chest and hypochondria that the patient can not lie down, greasy and yellow fur, and slippery pulse.

Treatment: San Zi Yang Qin Decoction or Ting Li Da Zao Xie Fei Decoction is used to remove retained phlegm and send down abnormally ascending qi.

(b) Invasion of the Lung by Wind-cold Pathogen

Summary of Pathogenesis: obstruction of the lung-qi due to attack by exopathic wind-cold, or impairment of purifying and descending function of the lung due to interior obstruction by cold-fluid retention.

Main Pulse Conditions and Symptoms: The patient attacked by exopathic wind-cold suffers from fever, aversion to cold, pain in the head and body, no sweat, nasal obstruction, rhinorrhea, cough, thin phlegm, thin and white fur, and floating and tense pulse. The patient with interior obstruction by cold-fluid retention suffers from frequent acute cough, short breath, heaviness sensation in the limbs, abundant white sticky sputum, fever, aversion to cold, white and smooth fur, and floating and tense pulse.

Treatment: San Ao Decoction is used to disperse wind-cold, and Xiao Qing Long Decoction is used to warm and resolve cold-fluid retention.

(c) Invasion of the Lung by Pathogenic Heat

Summary of Pathogenesis: wind-heat syndrome, or heat syndrome caused by cold stagnation, or accumulation of phlegm and heat in the lung, obstruction of the lung by pathogenic heat, impairment of purifying and descending function of the lung.

Main Pulse Conditions and Symptoms: loud cough, asthma, short breath, yellow sticky phlegm, spitting pus and blood with stinking small, cough with chest pain affecting the back. dry nostrils, epistaxis, nares flaring, thick nasal discharge, hot exhalation, fever, extreme thirst for drinking, sore throat, dry feces, difficulty in micturition with dark urine, red dry tongue, dry and yellow fur, and rapid pulse.

Treatment: Sang Bai Pi Decoction or Qian Jin Wei Jing Decoction and their like are used to clear away heat from the lung.

(3) Accompanying Syndromes

(a) Deficiency of the Spleen Affecting the Lung: anorexia, loose stool, cough, abundant phlegm, lassitude, edema in the face and feet, white fur, soft and feeble pulse. Si Jun Zi Decoction and its like are used to strengthen the lung by means of reinforcing the spleen.

(b) Deficiency of Both the Lung and the Kidney: acute cough at night, lassitude in loin and legs, short breath in motion, hectic fever due to yin-deficiency, night sweat, seminal emission, red tongue with less fur, and thready and rapid pulse. Sheng Mai Powder and its like are used to nourish yin and moisten the lung.

4. Key Points for Diagnosis and Treatment:

(1) The lung governs qi. Pungent, bitter and warm drugs can be used to disperse and purge the lung-qi. Pungent and sour drugs can be used to arrest persistent cough and nourish qi. Drugs for the blood system are generally not used unless necessary.

(2) The lung is a tender organ. Light and clean recipes should be chosen instead of heavy and turbid ones. "Upper jiao is as light as a feather, so none other than light drugs should be used to treat it." Purifying and descending methods should be mainly used to treat diseases of the lung-qi. The lung is a tender organ intolerable to cold and heat, so it is most appropriate to use pungent, calm, sweet and moist drugs.

(3) The lung governing qi is a tender organ. Therefore, for the treatment of deficiency syndrome of the lung, it is inappropriate to use warm and dry drugs to reinforce the lung, and it is strictly forbidden to use greasy drugs to moisten the lung.

(4) Lung diseases can be indirectly treated through visceral relations. For example, deficiency syndrome can be treated by means of reinforcing the spleen and nourishing the kidney, while excess syndrome can be treated by means of removing fire from the liver.

(5) The lung and the large intestine are interior-exteriorly related to each other. Therefore, excess syndrome and heat syndrome of the lung channel can be treated with purging the large intestine of pathogenic fire, enabling the lung-heat

to excrete from the large intestine and qi to purify and descend. For patients with constipation caused by no fluid in the large intestine due to insufficiency of the lung-qi, methods of nourishing the lung-qi can be used to clear and moisten the large intestine.

(6) Diseases of the lung channel can be etiologically divided into exopathic affection and internal injury, and clinically classified into deficiency and excess syndromes, which are subdivided into cold, heat and phlegm syndromes. Physicians should grasp the gist to diagnose and treat flexibly. The diagnosis and treatment of lung diseases is shown in the following brief table.

Brief Table for Diagnosis and Treatment of Lung Diseases

classification of syndromes	excess syndrome			deficiency syndrome	
pathogenesis	stagnation of phlegm in the lung	invasion of the lung by wind-cold pathogen	invasion of the lung by pathogenic heat	the lung-dryness syndrome due to yin deficiency	insufficiency of the lung-qi
pathogenesis	obstruction of the lung-qi due to retention of fluid and phlegm	impairment of purifying and descending function of the lung-qi due to wind-cold pathogen and cold retention	heat syndrome caused by cold accumulation, or phlegm-fire, flaming-up of pathogenic wind-heat	pulmonary tuberculosis, impairment of the lung by pathogenic dryness, deficiency of yin-fluid	internal injury caused by overstrain, impairment of qi by lingering cough
cough	cough with low voice and abundant thick sputum	frequent acute cough with loud voice and abundant thin sputum	cough with loud voice and yellow sticky sputum	cough and dyspnea with sticky sputum and difficulty in spitting	powerless cough with thin phlegm
breath	difficulty in breathing, even so severe that the patient can not lie down	short breath	heavy breath, nares flaring and hot exhalation	dysphoria and slightly short breath	short breath and fright, severer in motion

classification of syndromes	excess syndrome			deficiency syndrome	
chest pain	chest pain and tightness, fullness in the hypochondria	chest tightness or pain	pain in the chest and back due to cough	vague pain in the chest and hypochondria	vague pain in the chest and hypochondria
hemoptysis	phlegm with red or dark red blood, hemoptysis with abundant fresh red blood	phlegm with blood filament or blood clot, sometimes with abundant red blood	occasional phlegm with reddish blood		
cold and heat	unremarkable cold and heat	heavy cold and light heat without sweat	fever, flushed face, dysphoria with smothery sensation and desire for drink, perspiration	tidal fever, night sweat	aversion to cold, cold limbs, spontaneous perspiration
throat	rale	dumbness	dryness, swelling and pain	dryness, itch and pain	
fur	greasy or yellow fur	thin, white and smooth fur	red tongue with yellow and dry fur	red tongue with scanty fur	pale tongue with white fur
pulse conditions	slippery pulse	floating and tense pulse	rapid pulse	thready and rapid pulse	feeble pulse
treatment	removing phlegm from the lung	dispersing wind-cold, resolving phlegm and relieving cough	removing heat from the lung	nourishing yin to moisten the lung	replenishing and restoring the lung-qi

classification of syndromes	excess syndrome			deficiency syndrome	
recipe	San Zi Yang Qin Decoction, or Ting Li Da Zao Xie Fei Decoction	San Ao Decoction, Xiao Qing Long Decoction	Sang Bai Pi Decoction, "Qian Jin" Wei Jing Decoction	Bai He Gu Jin Decoction	Bu Fei Decoction

Large Intestine

1. Physiology: The large intestine consists of the ileum and rectum. The ileum connects upward to the ileocecal junction and downward to rectum with the anus at its lower end. The large intestine channel connects the lung. The large intestine is in charge of transporting and excreting wastes. Plain Questions says: "The large intestine, a transport organ, excretes wastes."

2. Pathology: Because the large intestine is a "transport organ", its pathological changes are mainly reflected by defecation, constipation in particular. All heat syndromes can deplete fluid to cause constipation. Impairment of purifying and descending function of the lung, deficiency of the kidney-yin and lack of fluid in the intestine can also cause constipation. In addition, Because the large intestine belongs to the spleen-stomach system, weakness of the spleen and stomach and dysfunction of the spleen in transport can also directly affect the large intestine to cause its dysfunction in transport.

3. Classification of Syndromes:

(1) Cold Syndrome: abdominal pain, bowel sound, loose stool, clear urine, slow pulse, and white and smooth fur. Wei Ling Decoction and Liang Fu Pill and their like are used to disperse cold and stop pain.

(2) Heat Syndrome: dry mouth, parched lips, constipation, foul feces, burning heat and swelling pain in the anus, scanty dark urine, yellow and dry fur, and rapid pulse. Liang Ge Powder and its like are used to relax the bowels and purge heat. Diarrhea with reddish and whitish discharge or mucus and blood, tenesmus, fever, heaviness sensation in the limbs, slippery and rapid pulse, and yellow and greasy fur are symptoms of dysentery due to damp-heat pathogen. Shao Yao Decoction or Bai Tou Weng Decoction and their like are used to purge

heat and induce diuresis.

(3) Deficiency Syndrome: diarrhea due to lingering dysentery, prostoptosis, cold limbs, pale tongue with thin fur, and thready and rapid pulse. Zhen Ren Yang Zang Decoction and its like are used to nourish the intestine and induce astringency.

(4) Excess Syndrome: abdominal pain unable to be massaged, fever, vomiting, constipation, difficulty in defecation, yellow fur, and deep and forceful pulse, Cheng Qi Decoction and its like are used to clear away heat and resolve stagnation.

(E) Kidney and Bladder

1. Physiology: There are two kidneys in the human body, one on the left and the other on the right. The gate of life attaches to the kidney. With the kidney-yin and kidney-yang in it, the kidney is an internal organ of water and fire. Its channel connects to the bladder. The kidney and the bladder are interior-exteriorly related to each other. The kidney is in charge of the bone and has its orifice in the ear. The physiological function of the kidney is to store reproductive essence and food essence, control reproduction and development, regulate water metabolism, and govern the growth of the bone and marrow. The hearing function of the ear relies on the nourishment by the kidney-qi. The physiological function of the kidney is so important that our ancestors said: "The kidney is the origin of congenital constitution." This means that the kidney is actually the root of the life.

2. Pathology: Because the kidney is the origin of congenital constitution, it is appropriate to reinforce the kidney and inappropriate to purge it. Therefore, kidney diseases are mainly manifested in deficiency syndrome and caused by depletion of the kidney-qi due to fatigue, intemperance in sex, and loss of nutrients from lingering illness. There are two main types of their clinical manifestations: deficiency of yin and insufficiency of yang. Insufficiency of yang includes unconsolidated kidney-qi, failure of the kidney to receive qi, insufficiency of the kidney-yang, and edema due to the kidney insufficiency. Deficiency of yin includes deficiency of the kidney-yin and hyperactivity of fire due to yin deficiency. Because the kidney and the bladder are interior-exteriorly related to each other, deficiency of the kidney-qi directly affects the function of the bladder. Therefore, the deficiency syndrome of the bladder is also a pathological manifestation of deficiency of the kidney.

Schematic Diagram for Pathogenesis of Kidney Diseases

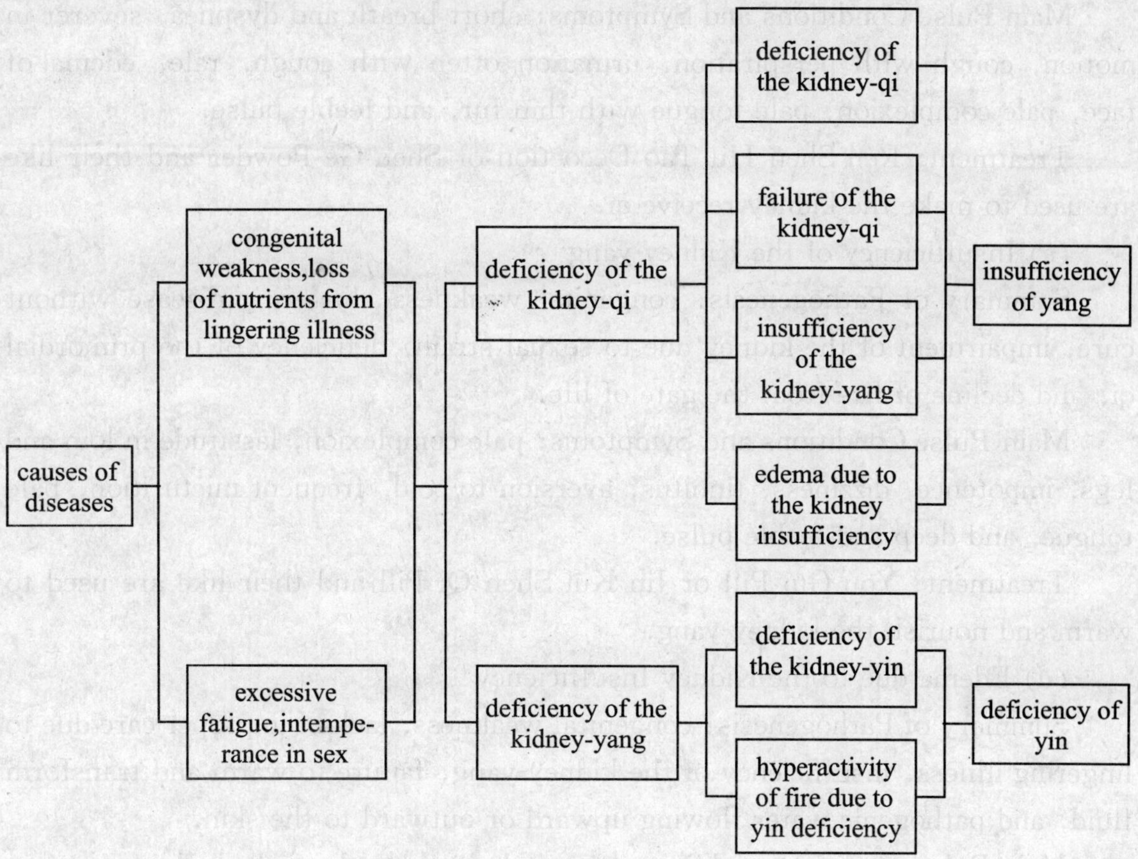

3. Classification of Syndromes:

(1) Insufficiency of Yang

(a) Unconsolidated Kidney-qi

Summary of Pathogenesis: insufficiency of the kidney-yang, internal injury due to overstrain, loss of nutrients from lingering illness, deficiency of the kidney-qi, and dysfunction of the kidney in storing essence and inducing astringency.

Main Pulse Conditions and Symptoms: pale complexion, lassitude in loin and spine, hypoacusis, frequent micturition with clear urine, even urinary incontinence, spermatorrhoea, premature ejaculation, dribbling urination, pale tongue with thin and white fur, and thready and feeble pulse.

Treatment: Da Bu Yuan Decoction and its like are used to reinforce and astringe the kidney-qi.

(b) Failure of the Kidney to Receive Qi

Summary of Pathogenesis: internal injury of the kidney-qi due to overstrain, deficiency of qi due to lingering illness, lack of primordial qi, and failure of the kidney to arrest discharge and receive qi.

Main Pulse Conditions and Symptoms: short breath and dyspnea, severer in motion, cough with perspiration, urination often with cough, rale, edema of face, pale complexion, pale tongue with thin fur, and feeble pulse.

Treatment: Ren Shen Hu Tao Decoction or Shen Ge Powder and their like are used to make the kidney receive qi.

(c) Insufficiency of the Kidney-yang

Summary of Pathogenesis: congenital weakness, lingering disease without cure, impairment of the kidney due to sexual strain, deficiency of the primordial qi, and decline of fire from the gate of life.

Main Pulse Conditions and Symptoms: pale complexion, lassitude in loin and legs, impotence, dizziness, tinnitus, aversion to cold, frequent micturition, pale tongue, and deep and feeble pulse.

Treatment: You Gui Pill or Jin Kui Shen Qi Pill and their like are used to warm and nourish the kidney-yang.

(d) Edema due to the Kidney Insufficiency

Summary of Pathogenesis: congenital weakness, lack of improper care due to lingering illness, insufficiency of the kidney-yang, failure to warm and transform fluid, and pathogenic water flowing upward or outward to the skin.

Main Pulse conditions and Symptoms: edema throughout the body due to water flowing outward to the skin, particularly in the lower limbs like mud when pressed. distension and fullness in the waist and abdomen, oliguria. excessive water turning into phlegm, cough, abundant thin sputum, dyspnea in motion. pale tongue, and deep and slow pulse.

Treatment: Zhen Wu Decoction or Ji Sheng Shen Qi Pill and their like are used to warm yang and promote diuresis.

(2) Deficiency of Yin

(a) Deficiency of the Kidney-yin

Summary of Pathogenesis: indulgence in drinking and sex, excessive anxiety, and depletion of the kidney-yin after long term illness.

Main Pulse Conditions and Symptoms: feebleness, dizziness, tinnitus, insomnia, amnesia, lassitude in loin and legs, seminal emission, dry mouth, red tongue with scanty fur, and thready pulse.

Treatment: Liu Wei Di Huang Decoction and its like are used to nourish the kidney-yin.

(b) Hyperactivity of Fire due to Yin Deficiency

Summary of Pathogenesis: hyperactivity of sexual desire, depletion of the kidney-yin after febrile disease, interior heat due to yin deficiency, and insufficiency of water leading to excess of fire.

Main Pulse Conditions and Symptoms: red cheeks and lips, tidal fever, night sweat, lassitude in loin and spine, insomnia due to vexation, nocturnal emission, dryness and pain in the mouth and throat, cough, yellow urine, constipation, red tongue with scanty fur, and thready and rapid pulse.

Treatment: Zhi Bai Di Huang Decoction and its like are used to nourish yin and reduce pathogenic fire.

(3) Accompanying Syndromes

(a) Decline of Earth due to Kidney Deficiency: loose stool, indigestion, diarrhea, abdominal distention, anorexia, lassitude, cold body, pale tongue with thin fur, and deep and slow pulse. Si Shen Pill and its like are used to supplement fire and invigorate earth.

(b) Invasion of the Heart by Kidney Water: palpitation, restlessness, edema, distention and fullness in the chest and abdomen, so serious cough with short breath that the patient can not lie down, purple fingers and lips, cold limbs, pale tongue with thin fur, and feeble and rapid pulse. Zhen Wu Decoction and its like are used to warm and resolve water.

4. Key Points for Diagnosis and Treatment:

(1) In general, the kidney has no exterior syndrome and excess syndrome. Heat in the kidney is caused by yin deficiency, and cold in the kidney results from yang insufficiency. This should be clinically grasped.

(2) The deficiency syndrome of the kidney is generally divided into yin deficiency and yang insufficiency. The general principle of its treatment is "to reinforce its deficiency and not to reduce its sufficiency". Yin deficiency syndrome should not be treated with pungent, dry, bitter and cold drugs but with sweet and moist drugs to invigorate water and nourish yin to match yang, reducing fire of deficiency type to make yang return to yin. Yang insufficiency syndrome should not be treated with cool, moist, pungent and dispersing drugs but with sweet and warm drugs to replenish qi and nourish yang to match yin, making yin disperse and subordinate to yang. Deficiency syndrome of yin and yang and of qi and blood should be treated with drugs of nourishing yin and yang.

(3) Deficiency of the kidney-yin often results in hyperactivity of the ministerial fire, which is caused by interior heat produced by deficiency. It should be

treated with drugs to nourish yin and purge ministerial fire. Insufficiency of the kidney-yang should be treated with drugs to warm the kidney, supplement fire, replenish essence and strengthen the body.

(4) The kidney and the bladder are interior-exteriorly related to each other. Pathological changes of the bladder belonging to cold of insufficiency type are mainly caused by insufficiency of the kidney-yang and disturbance in qi transformation. They should be mainly treated with drugs to warm the kidney and normalize the function of qi. Syndrome of difficulty in urination due to heat of excess type can be caused by heat transferred by another zang-organ, or by stagnation of damp-heat in the bladder itself. It should be mainly treated with drugs to remove heat, promote diuresis, and clear passage.

(5) The Kidney is very closely related to other visceral organs. Deficiency of the kidney-yin can cause failure of water to promote wood, hyperactivity of the liver-yang, or illness of the child organ involving the mother organ, impairment of the lung-yin, or failure of water to flow upward, and breakdown of the normal physiological coordination between the heart and the kidney. Insufficiency of the kidney-yang can result in failure of fire to promote earth and insufficiency of the spleen-yang. For the above-mentioned syndromes, treatment of the kidney and other visceral organs is of very important significance for recovery.

Diangosis and treatmaent kidney diseases is shown in the following brief table.

Brief Table for Diagnosis and Treatment of Kidney Diseases

syndrome	insufficiency of yang				deficiency of yin	
	unconsolidated kidney-qi	failure of the kidney to receive qi	insufficiency of the kidney-yang	edema due to the kidney insufficiency	deficiency of the kidney-yin	hyperactivity of fire due to yin deficiency
pathogenesis	depletion of the kidney-qi, failure to store essence and astringe	failure of the kidney to receive qi and form primordial qi	insufficiency of the kidney-yang, decline of the fire from the gate of life	decline of the fire from the gate of life, failure to warm and resolve, retention of water	internal injury caused by overstrain, long term illness, depletion of the kidney-yin	deficiency of the kidney-yin, flaming-up of fire of deficiency type

syndrome	insufficiency of yang				deficiency of yin	
physique	pale complexion	white complexion	pale complexion	edema in the limbs and body, particularly in lower limbs	feeble physique	red cheeks and lips
mind	lassitude, hypoacusis	cough, dyspnea, restlessness	cold physique, aversion to cold, tinnitus	disinclination to talk due to deficiency of qi	dizziness, tinnitus, amnesia, insomnia	insomnia due to fire of deficiency type, tidal fever, night sweat
loin and legs	lassitude in loin and spine	lassitude in loin and spine	lassitude in loin and legs	distention and fullness in the waist and abdomen	lasssitude in loin and legs	lassitude in loin and spine
cough, dyspnea		short breath, dyspnea, more exhalation and less inhalation, severer in motion, cough with perspiration	dyspnea, asthma, thin phlegm with foam	dyspnea, abundant white thin phlegm with foam		dry throat, cough
seminal emission	seminal emission, premature ejaculation		impotence		seminal emission	nocturnal emission
urination and defecation	dribbling after urination	urine often obstructed and discharged with cough	frequent micturition	oliguria	yellow urine	yellow urine, constipation
fur	pale	pale and thin	pale	pale	red tongue with scanty fur	red thin tongue with scanty fur

syndrome	insufficiency of yang				deficiency of yin	
pulse conditions	thready and feeble pulse	feeble pulse	deep and feeble pulse	slippery and slow pulse	thready pulse	thready and rapid pulse
treatment	reinforcing and astringing the kidney-qi	receiving qi to the kidney	warming and nourishing the kidney-yang	warming yang to promote diuresis	nourishing the kidney-yin	nourishing yin to reduce pathogenic fire
recipes	Da Bu Yuan Decoction	Ren Shen Hu Tao Decoction	You Gui Pill	Zhen Wu Decoction	Liu Wei Di Huang Pill	Zhi Bai Di Huang Pill

The Urinary Bladder

1. Physiology: The bladder is in the lower abdomen, and its channel leads to the stomach. Its main physiological function is to store fluid, promote the circulation of qi and induce diuresis. Plain Questions says: "The bladder serves as a reservoir to store fluid. Qi circulation makes urine excreted from the body." Fluid is the source of urine. Residual fluid entering the bladder and excreted from the body is called urine.

2. Pathology: Pathological changes of the bladder are mainly manifested in disturbance of qi circulation, retention of urine, difficulty in urination, frequent micturition and urinary incontinence. The kidney controls fluid. The kidney and bladder are interior-exteriorly related to each other. Deficiency of the kidney-qi will surely influence the functional activity of qi in the bladder. This is the main pathogenesis of deficiency syndrome of the bladder. Excess syndrome of the bladder is caused by heat transferred from other visceral organs or by accumulation of damp-heat in the bladder.

3. Classification of Syndromes:

(1) Cold of Deficiency Type: frequent micturition, dribbling urination, enuresis, pale tongue, moist fur, and deep and thready pulse. Sang Piao Xiao Powder and its like are used to reinforce and astringe the kidney-qi.

(2) Heat of Excess Type: scanty dark or turbid urine, difficulty in urination, heating pain in the penis during urination, even dribbling urination, or urine with mucus, blood and sand, red tongue, yellow fur, and rapid pulse. Ba Zheng Powder and its like are used to remove damp-heat.

B. Basic Concept on Pathogenesis and Syndromes of Qi and Blood

Qi and blood, the motive forces and sources of the life activities of the human body, is not only the reflection of visceral functions but also products of visceral activities. Pathological changes of the human body are all related to qi and blood. Therefore, only by recognizing and analyzing the pathogenesis and syndromes of qi and blood, can the pathological changes of the viscera be deeply studied. This is of important significance to the guidance of clinical practice.

(A) Qi

1. Physiology: Qi bestowed by parents is called primordial qi in the kidney. Qi acquired from essence of water and food is called visceral qi, which is distributed by the spleen and stomach to visceral organs. The primordial qi and visceral qi in combination become a motive force of the life activities of the human body. Miraculous Pivot says: "Congenitally bestowed genuine qi and food qi in combination fulfill the body."

Qi is divided into primordial qi, pectoral qi, ying-qi, defensive qi and visceral qi. Primordial qi is derived from congenital essence, originates from the kidney and is distributed by triple-jiao to the whole body to activate the visceral functions. Pectoral qi is formed in the chest by essence of water and food combined with fresh air in the nature. It controls respiration through the throat and activates the heart to circulate qi and blood. Ying-qi is also acquired from water and food, originates from the spleen and stomach and circulates in channels to nourish visceral organs, limbs and bones. Like ying-qi, defensive qi is also produced by water and food and originates from the spleen and stomach, but moves outside channels to nourish muscles and skin. Its main function is to protect the surface of the body from invasion by oxopathogen. Visceral qi is the specific manifestations of the visceral functions.

Pathology: The scope for activities of qi is wide, so the occurrence and development of a disease is very closely related to qi. Plain Questions says: "Diseases are all caused by qi."

Qi diseases are caused by exopathogen or by internal injury. In diseases due to exopathogen, invasion by wind-cold causes obstruction of the lung-qi and cough. Cold in combination with qi gives rise to hernia and abdominal mass. Flaring-up of wind-heat leads to impairment of purifying and descending function of the lung-qi with cough, yellow phlegm and nares flaring. Invasion of the pericardium by pathogenic heat results in disorder of the heart-qi with coma and infantile convulsion. Retention of dampness in the qi system causes obstruction of the lung-qi with dyspnea and salivation, and collapse of the spleen-qi with diarrhea. In diseases due to internal injury, overstrain leads to depletion of qi and deficiency of blood. Improper diet gives rise to failure of the stomach-qi to descend. Anger causes qi to ascend, joy causes qi to flow slowly, grief causes qi to disappear, fear causes qi to descend, fatigue causes qi to deplete, and anxiety causes qi to stagnate. Fatigue, improper diet and emotional stress also have some relations to qi diseases. To sum up, exopathogen and internal injury can cause qi diseases, and because of different etiology and pathogenesis, their pathological changes have different syndromes.

Qi diseases are very closely related to the viscera. Qi originates from the spleen and kidney. The lung controls qi to ascend, descend, exit and enter. The liver governs the normal flow of qi. The heart controls blood to circulate in vessels. Therefore, visceral diseases can directly or indirectly reflect pathological changes of qi, causing different symptoms of qi diseases. For example, obstruction of the lung-qi causes asthma and cough, deficiency of the lung-qi causes lassitude and short breath, disorder of the heart-qi causes coma and madness due to mental disturbance, and depletion of qi and blood causes severe palpitation due to deficiency of the heart-qi. Incoordination between the spleen and stomach causes nausea and vomiting due to adverse ascension of the stomach-qi. Failure of the spleen to transport and transform nutrients causes anorexia, diarrhea and dampness and phlegm due to insufficiency of the stomach-qi. Stagnation of the liver-qi causes disturbance of mental activity due to flaming-up of the liver-fire and hyperactivity of the liver-yang. Deficiency of the liver-qi causes deficiency of the gallbladder-qi, leading to dizziness, palpitation, timidity and numb limbs. Deficiency of the kidney-qi causes seminal emission due to failure to astringe. Failure of the kidney to receive qi causes dyspnea in motion. Failure of qi to discharge water causes retention of water, leading to phlegm and edema.

Although qi diseases can be divided into deficiency syndrome and excess syndrome, they are mainly caused by changes in ascension, descension, exit and entry of qi. These are basic forms of the movement of qi and fundamental manifestations of visceral functions, such as descension of the heart-fire, and ascension of the kidney-yin. The liver controls elevation and dispersion. The lung governs purification and descension. The spleen is in charge of sending up essence. The stomach is responsible for sending down digested food. The lung controls respiration. The kidney governs receiving qi. The spleen and stomach are the center of ascension and descension of qi. The liver and lung are passages for qi to ascend and descend. The Heart and kidney are the motive force of ascension and descension of qi. It is appropriate to descend qi in the heart, lung and stomach, and to ascend qi in the liver, spleen and kidney. Visceral coordination maintains ascension, descension, exit and entry of qi. Pathologically, visceral dysfunction influences ascension, descension, exit and entry of qi, hence diseases.

2. Qi Syndromes: Pathology of qi syndromes is directly related to the viscera. Therefore, qi syndromes are also included in visceral syndromes and can be divided into deficiency syndrome and excess syndrome.

(1) Deficiency Syndrome of Qi: Internal injury caused by overstrain, and malnutrition due to lingering illness cause depletion of primordial qi. Its main symptoms are disinclination to talk due to deficiency of qi, low voice, spontaneous perspiration, severe palpitation, dizziness, tinnitus, lassitude, anorexia, clear urine, frequent micturition, and feeble and weak or feeble and full pulse. Deficiency of qi is easily to collapse, and lingering illness causes insufficiency of yang. Therefore, proctoptosis and dysteroptosis also fall into the category of deficiency of qi.

(2) Excess Syndrome of Qi: It is mainly caused by phlegm-fire, indigestion, and stagnation of damp-heat, or by improper treatment of exopathic diseases. Its main symptoms are oppressed feeling in the chest, stuffy sensation in the stomach, abundant phlegm, asthma, difficulty in breath, abdominal distention, constipation, and taut and slippery or rapid and forceful pulse. Reverse ascension of qi cause nausea, vomiting, hiccup, eructation and dysphagia. Excessive qi is easily to turn into fire.

3. Treatment of Qi Diseases: Its fundamental principle is to reinforce qi for deficiency syndrome of qi, and to regulate the flow of qi, promote the circulation of qi, and send down abnormally ascending qi for excess syndrome of qi. Deficiency syndrome of qi should be treated with drugs to reinforce qi in the lung, kidney and spleen. Because the spleen and stomach are the source of primordial qi, deficiency of the spleen and stomach causes deficiency of primordial qi, leading to deficiency of other visceral organs. Li Dongyuan said: "Diseases are caused by unconsolidated primordial qi due to impairment of qi in the spleen and stomach."

The lung is a child organ of the spleen, so deficiency of the spleen-qi most easily leads to abnormal ascension, descension, exit and entry of the lung-qi, aggravating the condition of illness. The kidney is the origin of congenital constitution, stores reproductive essence and food essence, and controls receiving qi. Deficiency of the kidney-qi can give rise to a series of syndromes with disturbance of transformation of fluid. Therefore, qi diseases are mainly treated with drugs to reinforce qi in the lung, spleen and kidney according to different pathogenesis of qi deficiency. Si Jun Zi Decoction or Bu Zhong Yi Qi Decoction is often used to reinforce qi in the spleen and stomach. Bu Fei Decoction is often used to reinforce the lung-qi. Da Bu Yuan Decoction or Jin Kui Shen Qi Pill is often used to reinforce the kidney-qi. Deficiency syndrome complicated with excess symptom of phlegm-fire should be treated according to specific conditions.

Excess syndrome of qi, mainly caused by stagnation of qi, adverse flow of qi, and exopathogen, is closely related to the liver, lung and spleen. Therefore, it is mainly treated with drugs to remove fire from the liver, regulate the function of spleen, promote the dispersing function of the lung, lower the adverse flow of qi, expel cold and dissolve lumps. Excess syndrome of qi is often complicated, so it should be treated according to its relations with visceral organs. For example, obstructed lung-qi should be relieved, stagnated stomach-qi should be guided, adversely ascending liver-fire should be removed, stagnated liver-qi should be soothed, obstructed gallbladder-qi should be regulated, hyperactive fire of liver and gallbladder should be removed, and qi stagnation with pain should be recuperated. Excess syndrome of qi complicated with dampness, indigestion, phlegm and fire should be treated according to specific conditions

(B) Blood

1. Physiology: Blood originates from essence of water and food, and circulates in the vessels through functions of the spleen and stomach. Blood is very closely related to the kidney. "The kidney is a water zang-organ, stores essence and transforms it into blood." The main function of blood is to nourish the whole body. Sight of the eye, walk on foot, motion of the hand, sensation of the skin, and coordination of the visceral function rely on nourishment of blood.

The unceasing circulation of blood in vessels is not only directly related to the function of heart but also closely related to the function of qi. Blood belongs to yin, and its circulation relies on yang-qi. Movement of qi causes circulation of blood, stagnation of qi leads to blood stasis, and exhaustion of qi gives rise to loss of blood. Therefore, "blood circulates with qi, and qi is the commander of blood."

2. Pathology: Blood diseases are generally divided into bleeding, blood stasis and blood deficiency. Their etiology and pathology are different but related. For example, bleeding is not only the etiology of blood deficiency but also the pathogenesis of blood stasis. Their pathology is described as follows:

(1) Bleeding: Normally, blood circulates in vessels. If a vessel is injured, blood flowing out of it is called bleeding, such as hemoptysis, hematemesis, epistaxis, hemafecia, hematuria, and metrorrhagia and metrostaxis.

Bleeding is mainly caused by fire or by qi deficiency. The pathogenesis of bleeding can be summarized as impairment of vessels by wind, fire, dryness and heat; excessive drinking, overeating pungent, fatty and sweet food; disturbance of seven emotional factors, flaring-up of fire of five emotions; depletion of the kidney-yin and impairment of vessels by deficiency fire due to lingering blood disease and sexual indulgence; and injury due to fall, beat or overburden.

(2) Blood Stasis: Blood stasis can be formed by blood flowing out of vessels but staying in the body, or by blood in vessels obstructed by pathogenic factor, phlegm-fire or damp-heat. Its pathogenesis can be summarized as pathogenic poison entering ying or obstructing vessels; improper treatment of bleeding with residual blood staying in the body; lochiostasis after delivery; injury of vessels, and other qi diseases or blood diseases.

(3) Deficiency of Blood: It is mainly caused by excessive bleeding or deficient hematosis. Hematemesis, epistaxis, postpartum hemorrhage, traumatic bleeding, weak spleen and stomach unable to turn essence into blood, lingering illness, malnutrition due to parasitic infection in the intestine, and consumption of ying-blood can cause malnutrition of the viscera and blood vessels, leading to a series of pathological reactions of blood deficiency.

3. Syndromes of Blood Diseases:

(1) Bleeding: It is classified according to its location or organ. For example, blood spitted out with phlegm in cough is called bleeding of the pulmonary system. Blood vomited out with food is called gastric bleeding. Blood discharged with feces and urine is called hemafecia and hematuria. Blood flowing out of the nose is called epistaxis. Profuse menstruation or polymenia is called metrorrhagia and metrostaxis. Bleeding can also take place in gum, ear, eye and skin. Clinical

symptoms of bleeding are different, depending on its etiology, pathogenesis and location.

(2) Blood Stasis: It is mainly manifested in prickling pain at a fixed place where blood stasis is. The pain is often accompanied by feeling of stuffiness, tightness, distention and fullness, by dyspnea with smothery sensation, by black eyelids, parched lips, purple spots in the skin, or blood streak, even by squamous and dry skin, darkish tongue, ecchymosis, thready and uneven pulse.

(3) Blood Deficiency: pale complexion, pale and dim lips, tongue and nails; dizziness, severe palpitation, weak and short breath, lassitude, numb limbs, and thready pulse.

4. Treatment of Blood Diseases:

It is appropriate to enrich blood for blood deficiency, to stop bleeding for hemorrhage, and to promote blood circulation to remove blood stasis.

(1) Bleeding: Bleeding caused by extreme heat is mainly treated with drugs to purge heat and stop bleeding. Bleeding due to flaming-up of fire in the liver and gallbladder is treated with Long Dan Xie Gan Decoction and its like. Bleeding due to blood-heat is treated with Xi Jiao Di Huang Decoction and its like. Bleeding due to flaming-up of the stomach-fire is treated with Jin Kui Xie Xin Decoction and its like. Hemoptysis caused by hyperactivity of fire due to yin deficiency is treated with Sha Shen Mai Men Dong Decoction and its like. Hematochezia is treated with Huai Hua Powder and its like. Hematuria due to heat in the lower-jiao is treated with Xiao Ji Yin Zi and its like. Bleeding due to failure of the spleen to govern blood or due to failure of qi to astringe blood is treated with Gui Pi Decoction or Bu Zhong Yi Qi Decoction and their like to replenish qi and astringe blood.

(2) Blood Stasis: Accumulation of blood stasis is treated with Tao Ren Cheng Qi Decoction or Di Dang Decoction and their like to promote blood circulation to remove blood stasis. Obstruction of blood stasis is treated with Xue Fu Zhu Yu Decoction and its like to promote the circulation of qi and blood to remove blood stasis. Blood stasis due to stagnation of cold in channels is treated with Wen Jing Decoction and its like to warm channels and promote blood circulation. Blood stasis due to weakened body resistance is treated with Bu Yang Huan Wu Decoction and its like to strengthen body resistance and eliminate blood stasis.

(3) Blood Deficiency: Ren Shen Yang Rong Decoction or Shi Quan Da Bu Decoction is mainly used to replenish qi and enrich blood. Si Wu Decoction or Dang Gui Bu Xue Decoction and their like are used to treat blood deficiency in

women. Deficiency of both essence and blood should be treated with drugs to nourish the kidney and replenish essence.

C. Basic Concept on Pathogenesis and Syndromes of Wind, Fire, Dampness and Phlegm

Wind, fire, dampness and phlegm are not only among six climatic conditions in excess as pathogenic factors, but also products of pathological changes of the viscera, and clinical manifestations of visceral diseases. Therefore, they are directly or indirectly endopathic and exopathic factors.

(A) Wind

Wind can be divided into endopathic wind and exopathic wind. Exopathic wind is one of six external etiological factors. Endopathic wind, caused by yang-qi of the human body, is mainly manifested in a series of symptoms of disorder of qi and blood due to hyperactivity of fire-heat, hyperactivity of the liver-yang, or deficiency of yin-blood.

1. Characteristics of Wind Syndrome:

(1) Exopathic Wind: acute fit, fever, thirst, cough, aching pain in the body and limbs, swelling joints, wandering pain, rubella with itch, wry mouth and stiff tongue.

(2) Endopathic Wind: It is mainly caused by the liver-yang, liver-wind, deficiency of yin-blood, or by improper emotion, diet and life, with symptoms of dizziness, spasm, tremor, madness, coma, facial hemiparalysis, dysphasia, and hemiplegia.

2. Pathogenesis of Wind Syndrome:

(1) Exopathic Wind: Wind is the chief of six climatic conditions in excess as pathogenic factors. It can invade people all the year round. Wind entering mouth and nose often first invades the pulmonary system. Wind entering the skin often first invades channels and then attacks the viscera due to weakened body resistance and hyperactive pathogenic factors. Wind can invade people through mouth and nose as well as through the skin at the same time.

Wind pathogen invades people rarely by itself alone but often with other pathogens or with prevalent epidemic pathogens, such as cold pathogen in winter. In warm season, wind pathogen and warm pathogen invade people to cause epidemic febrile diseases. In damp season or at a damp residence, wind pathogen and damp pathogen attack people. Sometimes, wind, cold and dampness affect people at the same time to cause diseases. Wind is yang pathogen with its moving and changeable nature. It invades channels and joints with wandering pain. Wind-heat often invades the head and throat. Wind-dampness usually affects the lower limbs. Strong wind often suddenly attacks people and stagnates in channels to cause wry mouth, stiff tongue, contracture, crampy pain and other symptoms.

(2) Endopathic Wind

(a) Wind Syndrome Caused by Extreme Heat: Extreme heat surely consumes fluid and ying-blood, causing diseases of the heart and liver with symptoms of convulsion and coma.

(b) Up-stirring of the Liver: Emotional depression can cause stagnation of the liver-qi, flaming-up of the liver-fire, bleeding resulting from reversed flow of qi, invasion of channels and vertex by hyperactive liver-qi, and disturbance of mental activity, with symptoms of dizziness, convulsion or coma.

(c) Endopathic Wind due to Blood Deficiency: The liver, a blood-storing organ, is nourished by blood. Blood deficiency can cause hypoactivity of the liver-yin, hyperactivity of the liver-yang and endopathic wind, with symptoms of clonic convulsion, dizziness and infantile convulsion.

Endopathic wind syndrome is mainly related to the heart, liver and kidney, with its origin at the liver and kidney, and with its superficiality at the heart. Endopathic wind is also related to phlegm. Stagnation of the phlegm-fire more easily causes endopathic wind. Ascension of phlegm due to up-stirring of the liver easily causes coma. Pathogenesis of phlegm will be described later.

3. Diagnosis and Treatment of Wind Syndromes:

(1) Exopathic Wind Syndrome

(a) Wind-cold Syndrome: Invasion of the lung by exopathic wind-cold causes symptoms of severe pain in the vertex, aversion to cold, fever without sweat, stuffy nose, thin and white fur, and floating and tense pulse. Cong Chi Decoction or Jing Fang Bai Du Powder and their like are used to expel wind and disperse cold.

(b) Wind-heat Syndrome: Exopathic wind-heat often attacks the upper-jiao. Its symptoms are distension of the head, sore throat, fever without aversion to cold, slightly sweating with aversion to wind, conjunctival congestion with distending pain and photophobia, cough with yellow phlegm, red face with swelling pain, tonsillitis, and rhinorrhea with turbid discharge. Impairment of channels by wind-heat can cause hemoptysis, yellow urine, and full and rapid pulse. Sang Ju Decoction or Yin Qiao Powder and their like are used to expel wind and remove heat.

(c) Wind-dampness Syndrome: Its symptoms are headache, carebaria, wandering pain in joints, eczema, chickenpox, bowel sound, abdominal pain, and diarrhea. Syndrome in superficial channels is treated with Qiang Huo Sheng Shi Decoction and its like, and syndrome in the intestine and stomach is treated with Huo Xiang Zheng Qi Powder and its like, to dispel wind and remove dampness.

(2) Endopathic Wind Syndromes

Mild cases mainly have dizziness, dysphoria, and shivering of the limbs. Severe cases suddenly have coma, facial hemiparalysis, opisthotonus, and hemiplegia. Wind syndrome due to extreme heat is surely accompanied with symptoms of extreme heat. Stirring-up of endopathic wind of deficiency type is surely accompanied with symptoms of yin deficiency of the liver and kidney, and hyperactivity of the liver-yang. Wind syndrome due to blood deficiency is surely accompanied with symptoms of endopathic dryness due to blood deficiency.

Wind syndrome due to extreme heat is treated with Tian Ma Gou Teng Decoction and its like to calm the liver and stop the wind. An Gong Niu Huang Pill, Zhi Bao Pill and Zi Xue Pill can be added according to conditions. Hyperactive yang of deficiency type is treated with Da Ding Feng Zhu Decoction and its like to nourish yin and suppress hyperactive yang. Wind syndrome due to blood deficiency is treated with Jia Jian Fu Mai Decoction and its like to nourish yin and stop wind.

(B) Fire

Fire is extreme heat. It is one of six climatic conditions in excess as pathogenic factors, and can also be caused in the process of illness. It can be divided into deficiency fire and excess fire. Excess fire is often directly caused by heat, or by other pathogens. Deficiency fire, a product of pathological changes of the viscera, is mainly caused by depletion of yin-fluid and by deficiency of essence and blood.

1. Characteristics of Fire Syndromes: Fire is extreme heat, so fire syndromes are similar to but severer than heat syndromes.

Excess Fire: It is usually caused by exopathy, with acute disease and short course. Its main symptoms are high fever, flushed face and ears, thirst, vexation, preference for cold drinks, even mania, delirium, coma, scanty dark urine, constipation, parched lips, yellow, dry and prickly fur, and full and rapid pulse.

Deficiency Fire: It is mainly caused by internal injury, with chronic disease and long course. Its main symptoms are tidal fever, night sweat, red cheeks in the afternoon, insomnia due to vexation, dry mouth and throat, cough without phlegm or with phlegm and blood, tinnitus, amnesia, lumbago, seminal emission, red tongue with scanty saliva, no fur, and thready and rapid pulse.

2. Pathogenesis of Fire Syndromes: Physiologically, the visceral activities are nourished by essence of water and food to produce fire called "junior fire". The human body relies on the heat energy to transform food into chyme, generate vital essence and maintain the life. Pathologically, fire produced by depletion of essence and blood, visceral dysfunction, imbalance between yin and yang, and hyperactivity of the visceral yang is called "sthenic fire". Internal Classic says: "Sthenic fire consumes qi, while junior fire generates qi." This means that junior fire, a normal fire, supports the life, while sthenic fire, an abnormal fire, can damage the vital qi to cause diseases.

Fire syndrome is caused by internal injuries or by external pathogens. Fire syndrome can be directly caused by pathogenic fire or by other external pathogens. Fire syndrome due to pathogenic fire is caused by depletion of fluid and yin-blood and by impairment of the viscera. Fire syndrome due to other external pathogens is caused by gradually producing heat and heat generating fire. For example, pathogenic cold produces heat, and extreme heat generates fire. Dampness combines with heat or accumulates to produce heat, and extreme damp-heat generates phlegm-fire. Fire caused by external pathogens generally belongs to excess fire.

Fire syndrome can be caused by internal injuries, such as overstrain, depression and hyperactive sexual desires. These factors can influence normal function of the viscera, causing depletion of yin-fluid. Fire syndrome can also be caused by deficiency of essence and blood due to malnutrition after a long-term illness. Fire caused by internal injuries mainly belongs to deficiency fire.

3. Diagnosis and Treatment of Fire Syndromes:

Deficiency fire syndrome or excess fire syndrome should be first diagnosed carefully. It is appropriate to nourish for deficiency fire syndrome, to conduct fire back to its origin for floating fire syndrome, and to remove fire for excess fire syndrome.

(1) Excess Fire

(a) Flaming of the Heart-fire: Its main symptoms are flushed face and ears; dysphoria with feverish sensation in the chest, palms and soles; dry mouth and fissured lips; tongue erosion; even abnormal laugh, delirium, coma, hematemesis and epistaxis. Xie Xin Decoction and its like are used to remove fire from the heart.

(b) Excessive Fire in the Liver and Gallbladder: Its main symptoms are hypochondriac pain, deafness, insomnia, dreaminess, dizziness, conjunctival congestion, bitter taste in the mouth, myasthenia, stranguria with turbid urine, and hematuria. Long Dan Xie Gan Decoction and its like are used to remove fire from the liver and gallbladder.

(c) Hyperactive Lung-fire: Its main symptoms are difficulty in breath, nares flaring, cough with thick phlegm, extreme thirst for drinking, dried feces, epistaxis, and hemoptysis. Qian Jin Wei Jing Decoction or Sang Bai Pi Decoction and their like are used to remove fire from the lung.

(d) Excessive Stomach-fire: Its main symptoms are extreme thirst for drinking, gum erosion with pain and bleeding, vomiting, gastric discomfort with acid regurgitation, and polyorexia. Qing Wei Powder and its like are used to remove heat from the stomach.

(e) Large Intestinal Fire: Its main symptoms are constipation, spouting diarrhea, and burning heat in the anus. Da Cheng Qi Decoction and its like are used to remove accumulated heat.

(f) Small Intestinal Fire: Its main symptoms are dropping pain in the lower abdomen, and stranguria with turbid urine and blood. Dao Chi Powder and its like are used to remove heart-fire.

(g) Flaming of the Spleen fire: Its main symptoms are dry mouth and lips, extreme thirst, and polyorexia. Xie Huang Powder and its like are used to remove spleen-fire.

(h) Bladder-fire: Its main symptoms are retention of urine, dribbling urination, enuresis with turbid urine, hematuria, and abdominal pain. Ba Zheng Powder and its like are used to remove fire.

(i) Disturbance of Mental Activity due to Heart-fire: Its main symptoms are coma, delirium, and clonic convulsion. An Gong Niu Huang Pill or Zhi Bao Pill and their like are used to remove heart-fire and restore consciousness.

(2) Deficiency Fire

(a) Kidney-fire of Deficiency Type: Hyperactivity of the ministerial fire is caused by deficiency of the kidney-yin, with hectic fever and other symptoms due to yin deficiency. Zhi Bai Di Huang Pill and its like are used to nourish yin and remove fire. Qing Gu Powder and its like are used to treat hectic fever due to yin deficiency.

(b) Deficiency Fire of the Spleen and Stomach: Its main symptoms are gastric discomfort with acid regurgitation, dry mouth with no desire to drink, hunger with no desire to eat, and dry feces. Yi Wei Decoction and its like are used to nourish yin and remove the stomach-fire.

(C) Dampness

Dampness is divided into endopathic dampness and exopathic dampness. Exopathic dampness, one of six climatic conditions in excess as pathogenic factors, often first attacks the lower limbs, and stagnates in the body to cause damp-heat, cold-dampness, diarrhea or edema. Endopathic dampness is closely related to the pathological changes of the spleen.

1. Characteristics of Damp Syndrome:

Dampness, a yin pathogen, can be removed by warm and by yang. However, dampness can not be removed easily and rapidly, so damp syndrome often relapses repeatedly.

Exopathic Dampness: Exopathic damp syndrome is related to climate and environment. It can easily caused in wet season and at a place full of fog, dew and dampness. It can also easily caused in people with weak function of the spleen and stomach. Its main symptoms are heaviness sensation in the limbs; lassitude in the body; pain in fixed joints; even difficulty in stretch, bend and twist; white and slightly greasy fur; and soft and slow pulse.

Endopathic Dampness: Endopathic damp syndrome is related to the spleen and stomach. Its main symptoms are tasteless and greasy sensation in the mouth; anorexia; feeling of stuffiness and tightness in the chest and stomach; eructation; diarrhea; lassitude and heaviness sensation in the limbs; headache; white, thick and greasy fur; and soft and feeble pulse.

2. Pathogenesis of Damp Syndrome:

Exopathic dampness often in combination with cold, heat and wind invades the skin, muscle, joints, and the viscera. Dampness combines with yin to form cold and with yang to form heat, depending on visceral function, congenital bestowal and improper treatment. Dampness is easily to form cold in people who have deficiency of the kidney-yin or overeat cold and cool food. Dampness is easily to form heat in people who have stomach-heat or overeat warm and dry food.

Endopathic dampness is mainly caused by improper diet. Overeating uncooked, cold, fatty and sweet food can damage the spleen and stomach, cause dysfunction of transporting fluid, make dampness accumulated, and lead to diarrhea, edema or phlegm retention. Internal Classic says: "All kinds of edema are caused by the spleen." People with endopathic dampness are more easily affected by exopathic dampness. The interaction between the two can cause all kinds of damp syndromes.

3. Diagnosis and Treatment of Damp Syndromes:

(1) Exopathic Dampness

(a) Cold-dampness: Its symptoms are pain all over the body, severe pain in joints, difficulty in motion, no sweat, loose stool, edema in the limbs, white and greasy fur, and soft and slow pulse. Juan Bi Decoction and its like are used to remove stagnation and clear channels.

(b) Wind-dampness: See diagnosis and treatment of wind syndromes.

(c) Damp-heat: Its symptoms are fever, vexation, thirst, spontaneous perspiration, swelling pain in joints, fullness sensation in the chest, jaundice, dark urine, yellow and greasy fur, and soft and rapid pulse. Cang Zhu Bai Hu Decoction and its like are used to remove heat and dampness. Gui Zhi Bai Hu Decoction and its like are used to treat damp-heat syndrome with swelling pain in joints as its main symptom. Yin Chen Wu Ling Powder and its like are used to treat damp-heat syndrome with jaundice as its main symptom.

(d) Summer Dampness: Its main symptoms are vomiting, diarrhea, fever with sweat, tightness sensation in the chest, fullness feeling in the abdomen, anorexia, white and smooth fur, feeble and soft pulse. Huo Xiang Zheng Qi Powder and its like are used to remove dampness.

(2) Endopathic Dampness

(a) Water Retention due to Hypofunction of the Spleen: Its main symptoms are heaviness sensation in the limbs, lassitude, tightness and distension feeling in the stomach, loose stool, vomiting, feeble and soft pulse, and white and greasy fur. Wei Ling Decoction and its like are used to regulate the spleen and remove dampness.

(b) Damp-heat: Stagnation of damp-heat in the heart-channel will cause ulceration of the mouth and tongue. Retention of damp-heat in the lower-jiao will cause dysentery, stranguria with turbid urine, hematuria, urine retention, and leukorrhea. Invasion of the skin by damp-heat will cause skin diseases. Attack on joints by damp-heat will cause swelling pain. Damp-heat syndrome can be treated in reference to the treatment of fire syndromes and with drugs to remove dampness according to conditions. Skin diseases caused by damp-heat can be treated with Ku Shen Decoction or She Chuang Zi Powder and their like to remove toxin and dampness.

(D) Phlegm

Phlegm and fluid retention, products of pathological changes, are two different syndromes with water retained in the body. Ancient people said: "Water accumulates into fluid retention, and retained fluid coagulates into phlegm." The difference among the three is that phlegm is thick, retained fluid is thin, and water is thinner. The production of phlegm and fluid retention is very closely related to the spleen, lung and kidney.

1. Characteristics of Phlegm and Fluid Retention: In terms of affecting area, fluid retention mainly occurs in the chest, abdomen and limbs, and is closely related to the spleen and stomach. Phlegm syndrome affects the whole body, and is related to the visceral diseases. Zhang Jingyue said: "fluid retention only occurs in the intestine and stomach, while phlegm goes anywhere. Fluid retention syndrome is totally caused by the spleen and stomach. Phlegm syndrome is caused by visceral injuries." Symptoms of phlegm syndrome and fluid retention syndrome are described as follows:

(1) Main Symptoms of Phlegm Syndrome: feeling of stuffiness and tightness in the chest, distending pain in the hypochondria, cough with abundant phlegm, nausea, vomiting, diarrhea, palpitation, dizziness, madness, numb skin, pain or swelling in joints, subcutaneous nodule or abscess, diabrosis with pus flowing out, no cure for a long time, white smooth or thick fur, and slippery pulse.

(2) Main symptoms of fluid retention syndrome: Clinical symptoms mainly depend on area of fluid retention. Symptoms of phlegm retention in the intestine and stomach are epigastric fullness and rigidity, salivation, and bowel sound. Symptoms of fluid retention in the chest and hypochondria are hypochondriac pain in cough and spitting, and difficulty in twist. Symptoms of fluid retention in the

limbs are heaviness sensation and edema in the limbs. Symptoms of fluid retention in hypochondria and epigastrium are asthma, cough, salivation, and inability to lie down.

2. Pathogenesis of Phlegm and Fluid Retention: Physiologically, Through the function of the spleen, lung, kidney and triple-jiao, essence of water and food is transformed into blood or fluid to nourish the whole body, or into sweat, qi or urine to be excreted from the body. Pathologically, visceral dysfunction makes essence of water and food meet yin-cold to form fluid retention, and meet fire to form phlegm. Insufficiency of the spleen, failure of the middle-jiao yang, failure to transport and transform nutrients, and abnormal distribution of essence of water and food can form fluid retention or phlegm. Heat generated by deficiency of yin, and fire produced by stagnation of the liver-qi can make fluid form phlegm. Heat and dryness due to invasion of the lung by wind-cold and due to visceral dysfunction can make fluid in the lung form phlegm. Mental confusion due to phlegm can cause coma and epilepsy. Invasion of the lung by phlegm can cause cough with abundant phlegm. Stagnation of phlegm in the middle-jiao can cause bowel sound and diarrhea. Invasion of the muscle and bone by phlegm can cause scrofula and subcutaneous nodule. Fluid retention in the muscle can cause edema. Fluid retention in the hypochondria can lead to hypochondriac pain in cough and spitting, and to epigastric fullness and rigidity. Fluid retention in the epigastrium can cause cough, asthma, and inability to lie down. Fluid retention in the intestine can cause bowel sound.

3. Diagnosis and Treatment of Phlegm Syndrome and Fluid:
Retention Syndrome

(1) Phlegm Syndrome

(a) Cough due to Wind-phlegm: Common cold with cough and phlegm can be treated with Xing Su Powder and its like to ventilate the lung and resolve phlegm.

(b) Invasion of the Lung by Phlegm-dampness: Cough with abundant, white and thin phlegm can be treated with San Zi Yang Qin Decoction and its like to remove dampness and resolve phlegm.

(c) Accumulation of Phlegm-Heat in the Lung: Accumulated heat in the lung, and sticky and yellow phlegm can be treated with Qing Jin Hua Tan Decoction and its like to remove heat and resolve phlegm.

(d) Mental Confusion due to Phlegm: Sudden coma and accumulated phlegm and saliva can be treated with Xi Yan Powder and its like to resolve phlegm and restore consciousness.

(e) Subcutaneous nodule and scrofula under the neck can be treated with Xiao He Powder and its like to resolve phlegm and remove nodule.

(f) Interaction between Phlegm and Qi: Stagnation of qi, accumulation of phlegm, asthma, cough, short breath, and obstruction of the epigastrium can be treated with Su Zi Jiang Qi Decoction and its like to send down abnormally ascending qi and resolve phlegm.

(2) Fluid Retention Syndrome.

(a) Phlegm Retention: Its symptoms are no desire to drink water, bowel sound, vomiting clear water, feeling of distension and fullness in the chest and abdomen, white fur, and taut and slippery pulse. Ling Gui Zhu Gan Decoction and its like are used to warm and resolve phlegm retention.

(b) Fluid Retention in the Hypochondria: Its symptoms are hypochondriac pain due to cough and spit, difficulty in twist, fever with sweat, white or greasy fur, and taut pulse. Shi Zao Decoction and its like are used to eliminate water retention.

(c) Fluid Retention in the Limbs: Its symptoms are retching, fever, thirst, edema in the face and limbs, heaviness sensation and pain in the limbs, white or yellowish fur, and floating and scattered pulse. Xiao Qing Long Decoction and its like are used to induce diaphoresis and eliminate fluid retention.

(d) Fluid Retention in the Hypochondria and Epigastrium: Its symptoms are cough with dyspnea, short breath, inability to lie down, slight edema in the body, taut and thready pulse, and white fur. Ting Li Da Zao Xie Fei Decoction and its like are used to remove heat from the lung and eliminate fluid retention.

D. Basic Concept on Pathogenesis and Syndromes of the Six Channels

On the basis of inheriting Internal Classic, Classic on Medical Problems, and other ancient medical knowledge, Zhang Zhongjing created a system of diagnosis and treatment based on analyzing and differentiating febrile diseases in accordance with the theory of the six channels. He divided clinical manifestations of febrile diseases into six different types of Taiyang, Yangming, Shaoyang, Taiyin, Shaoyin and Jueyin. Clinical manifestations of febrile diseases are pathological reflections of visceral channels caused by exopathgens, mainly wind and cold. It is imperative to grasp and apply such a law. Because of difference in exopathogen, focus, constitution and age, and because of yin and yang of the viscera and channels, there are syndromes of cold, heat, deficiency and excess. It is necessary to flexibly apply the theory on its original basis in diagnosis.

There are two kinds of clinical significance in analyzing and differentiating febrile diseases in accordance with the theory of the six channels. One is summarization of different syndromes of the six channels at different stages of the development of exopathic wind-cold diseases, namely, syndromes of Taiyang, Yangming, Shaoyang, Taiyin, Shaoyin and Jueyin. The other is a general law governing the transformation of the focus of exopathic wind and cold, namely, from Taiyang syndrome to Yangming syndrome, to Shaoyang syndrome, to Taiyin syndrome, to Shaoyin syndrome, and to Jueyin syndrome. The theory shows the six stages of illness conditions from exterior to interior and from shallow to deep area.

The basic contents of analyzing and differentiating febrile diseases in according to the theory of the six channels are summarized as follows.

(A) Taiyang Syndrome

It is mainly an exterior syndrome and the initial stage of exopathic disease caused by invasion of the skin by wind and cold.

1. Outline: Taiyang syndrome has symptoms of floating pulse, severe pain in the vertex, and aversion to cold.

2. Pathology: Channel syndrome is caused by invasion of the skin by wind and cold, and by incoordination between ying and wei. Fu-organ syndrome is caused by affection of channel syndrome on the bladder. Water retention syndrome is caused by invasion of the qi system by pathogen. Blood retention syndrome is caused by invasion of the blood system by pathogen.

3. Diagnosis and Treatment:

(1) Channel syndromes are divided into wind-stroke syndrome and exogenous febrile disease.

Wind-stroke syndrome is also called exterior syndrome of deficiency. Its symptoms are aversion to wind, fever, perspiration, severe pain in the vertex, and floating and slow pulse. Gui Zhi Decoction is used as a main recipe to regulate ying and wei.

Exogenous febrile disease is also called exterior syndrome of excess. Its symptoms are aversion to cold, fever, no sweat, headache, pain throughout the body, stiffness of the nape and back, and floating and tense pulse. Ma Huang

Decoction, pungent in taste and warm in nature, is used as a main recipe to relieve exterior syndrome.

(2) Fu-organ syndromes are divided into water retention syndrome and blood retention syndrome.

Water retention syndrome has symptoms of aversion to wind, fever, difficulty in urination, extreme thirst for drinking, vomiting immediately after drinking, and floating pulse. Wu Ling Powder is used as a main recipe to relieve exterior syndrome and induce diuresis.

Blood retention syndrome has symptoms of aversion to wind, fever, stiffness and fullness feeling in the lower abdomen, enuresis, mental disorder, even madness, and deep and thready pulse. Tao He Cheng Qi Decoction is used as a main recipe to remove blood stasis.

(B) Yangming Syndrome

It is mainly an interior syndrome caused by exopathic wind- cold invading from exterior to interior and transforming into extreme heat.

1. Outline: Yangming syndrome is in the stomach.

2. Pathology: Exopathic cold invades from exterior to interior and transform into heat accumulated in the stomach and intestine. Channel syndrome has no dry feces in the intestine, while fu-organ syndrome has dry feces in the intestine.

3. Diagnosis and Treatment:

(1) Channel syndrome has symptoms of high fever, spontaneous perspiration, aversion to heat, extreme thirst for drinking, full and rapid pulse, and yellow and dry fur. Bai Hu Decoction is used as a main recipe to remove heat.

(2) Fu-organ syndrome has symptoms of fullness sensation and pain in the abdomen, constipation, tidal fever, delirium, and deep and forceful pulse. Zhu Cheng Qi Decoction is used as a main recipe to remove heat and clear the viscera.

(C) Shaoyang Syndrome

It is mainly a half-exterior and half-interior syndrome. Pathogen has left the exterior of Taiyang but has not entered the interior of Yangming.

1. Outline: Shaoyang syndrome has symptoms of bitter taste in the mouth, dry throat and dizziness.

2. Pathology: Pathogen goes from exterior to interior or from interior to exterior, or comes from the channel and stay between the exterior and interior,

causing disturbance of visceral function.

3. Diagnosis and Treatment: Shaoyang syndrome has symptoms of alternate attacks of chill and fever, fullness sensation in the chest and hypochondria, anorexia, vexation, vomiting, bitter taste in the mouth, dry throat, and dizziness. Xiao Chai Hu Decoction is used as a main recipe to treat Shaoyang syndrome. Combined syndrome of the Taiyang and Shaoyang channels also has symptoms of headache, pain throughout the body, and perspiration. Chai Hu Gui Zhi Decoction is used as a main recipe to relieve exterior syndrome. Combined syndrome of the Shaoyang and Yangming channels also has symptoms of distension, fullness, stuffiness and stiffness sensation in the stomach and abdomen, and constipation or diarrhea. Da Chai Hu Decoction is used as a main recipe to treat the syndrome.

(D) Taiyin Syndrome

It is mainly deficiency of the spleen-yang caused by impairment of the spleen and stomach due to disease of three yang channels or direct invasion by pathogen. Taiying syndrome is the early stage of invasion of yin by pathogen.

1. Outline: Its symptoms are fullness sensation in the abdomen, vomiting, anorexia, abdominal pain, and stiffness feeling in the chest.

2. Pathology: Cold pathogen goes from exterior to interior to damage the spleen and stomach, causing deficiency of the spleen-yang and failure to transport and transform nutrients.

3. Diagnosis and Treatment: Taiyin syndrome, with symptoms of fullness sensation and pain in the abdomen, diarrhea, anorexia and vomiting, should be treated with Li Zhong Decoction as a main recipe to warm the middle-jiao and strengthen the spleen. Taiyin syndrome accompanied with exterior syndrome should be treated with drugs to first relieve exterior syndrome and then warm the interior or to relieve exterior syndrome and warm the interior at the same time according to conditions.

(E) Shaoyin Syndrome

It is mainly deficiency of yin and yang in the heart and kidney caused by pathogen invading Shaoyin to damage the heart and kidney. It can also be caused by other channel syndrome. Shaoyin syndrome is the late stage of serious illness.

1. Outline: Shaoyin syndrome has symptoms of feeble and thready pulse, and desire to sleep.

2. Pathology: Pathogen goes deeply to damage the heart and kidney, causing depletion of yang-qi to produce cold of insufficiency type, or causing deficiency of yin-blood to form heat of deficiency type. Shaoyin syndrome is mainly cold of deficiency type and rarely heat of deficiency type.

3. Diagnosis and Treatment:

(1) Shaoyin syndrome with cold of deficiency type has symptoms of aversion to cold, curling up the body, cold limbs, listlessness, desire to sleep, feeble and thready pulse, diarrhea with undigested food in stool, and clear urine. Si Ni Decoction is used as a main recipe to recuperate depleted yang and rescue the patient from collapse.

(2) Shaoyin syndrome with heat of deficiency type has symptoms of vexation, insomnia, dry mouth and throat, red tongue, scanty fur, and thready and rapid pulse. Huang Lian A Jiao Decoction is used as a main recipe to nourish yin and remove heat.

(3) Shaoyin syndrome with edema has symptoms of palpitation, dizziness, myospasm, shivering all over the body, trend to fall down, even edema, difficulty in urination, heaviness sensation and pain in the limbs, diarrhea, and abdominal pain. Zhen Wu Decoction is used as a main recipe to warm yang and induce diuresis.

(4) Shaoyin syndrome accompanied with Taiyang syndrome or with Yangming syndrome should be both treated respectively with Ma Huang Fu Zi Xi Xin Decoction of restoring yang and relieving exterior syndrome or with Da Cheng Qi Decoction of timely purgation to preserve yin.

(F) Jueyin Syndrome

It is mainly simultaneous occurrence of cold and heat syndromes. Jueyin syndrome is the late stage of febrile disease. Pathogen goes inside to seriously damage functions of qi, blood, fluid and viscera, causing complicated condition of illness with alternate attacks of chill and fever and with yin-yang interlocking.

1. Outline: Jueyin syndrome has symptoms of diabetes, reflux of qi to the heart, pain and heat in the heart, hunger but with no desire to eat, vomiting ascaris after eating, and continual diarrhea.

2. Pathology: Pathogen damages qi, blood and fluid and causes visceral dysfunction, imbalance between yin and yang, and simultaneous occurrence of cold and heat syndromes.

3. Diagnosis and Treatment:

(1) Simultaneous occurrence of cold and heat syndromes, with symptoms of vexation, vomiting after eating, even vomiting ascaris, should be treated with Wu Mei Pill as a main recipe to eliminate cold and dampness.

(2) Cold syndrome of Jueyin, with symptoms of retching, salivation, headache, cold limbs, and thready and extremely weak pulse, should be treated with Dang Gui Si Ni Jia Wu Zhu Yu Sheng Jiang Decoction as a main recipe to nourish blood, promote blood circulation, warm channel and dispel cold.

(3) Heat syndrome of Jueyin, with symptoms of dysentery of heat type, thirst for drinking water, and rapid pulse, should be treated with Bai Tou Weng Decoction as a main recipe to remove heat, dampness and toxin.

E. Basic Concept on Pathogenesis and Syndromes of Wei, Qi, Ying and Xue

The pathogenesis of wei, qi, ying and xue is to study the mechanism of development of an epidemic febrile disease in four stages of wei, qi, ying and xue from mild to serious cases. In Treatise on Epidemic Febrile Diseases, Ye Tianshi pointed out: "In general, wei is followed by qi, and ying is followed by xue", summarizing a law governing the transformation of an epidemic febrile disease. Syndromes of wei, qi, ying and xue are four different stages of invasion by warm-pathogen, namely, syndrome at wei stage, syndrome of qi system, syndrome at ying stage, and syndrome of blood system. The general law for their changes from mild to serious cases is from wei stage to qi system, to ying stage, and to blood system; and from serious to mild cases is from ying and blood to wei and qi.

(A) Syndrome at Wei Stage

Syndrome at Wei stage is mainly seen at the first stage of an epidemic febrile disease with warm-pathogen entering the mouth, nose and skin to invade the lung.

1. Main symptoms are fever, slight aversion to wind and cold, headache, no or scanty sweat, cough, thirst, red tongue edge, thin and white fur, and floating and rapid pulse.

2. Pathology: Attack of warm-pathogen on the upper-jiao or skin causes impairment of purifying and descending function of the lung.

3. Diagnosis and Treatment:

(1) Wind-warm syndrome at wei stage with the above-mentioned main symptoms should be treated with Yin Qiao Powder, pungent in taste and cool in nature, as a main recipe to relieve exterior syndrome.

(2) Autumn-dryness syndrome at wei stage has symptoms of aversion to cold, fever, headache, no sweat, dry mouth, parched lips, dry nose, cough, thin, white and dry fur, and floating and thready pulse. Autumn-dryness is divided into cool-dryness and warm-dryness. Cool-dryness should be treated with Xin Su Powder as a main recipe to dispel cold, relieve exterior syndrome, promote the dispersing function of the lung, and moisten dryness. Warm-dryness should be treated with Sang Xin Decoction, pungent in taste and cool in nature, as a main recipe to relieve exterior syndrome, promote the dispersing function of the lung, and moisten dryness.

(3) Summer-warm or damp-warm syndrome at wei stage can be treated in reference to upper-jiao syndrome.

(B) Syndrome of Qi System

Syndrome of Qi system is mainly seen when warm-pathogen goes inside from wei to transform into heat, affecting the stomach, spleen, intestine, gallbladder and diaphragm. Extreme heat in Yangming is often seen.

1. Main symptoms are vigorous heat, aversion to heat, abundant sweat, thirst for cold drinks, yellow and dry fur, and full pulse.

2. Pathology: Pathogen enters qi system in Yangming to deplete fluid.

3. Diagnosis and Treatment:

(1) Accumulation of heat in the lung and stomach with the above-mentioned main symptoms should be treated with Bai Hu Decoction as a main recipe to remove heat and produce fluid. Depletion of fluid and qi due to abundant sweat can be treated with Ren Shen Bai Hu Decoction. Yellow and thick phlegm, chest pain and asthma can be treated with Ma Xin Shi Gan Decoction and drugs to remove phlegm-heat. Constipation or diarrhea with yellow, foul and watery discharge, and abdominal pain can be treated with Tiao Wei Cheng Qi Decoction. Impairment of yin can be treated with Zeng Ye Cheng Qi Decoction.

(2) Internal heat and dampness syndrome can be treated in reference to middle-jiao syndrome.

(C) Syndrome at ying stage

Syndrome at ying stage mainly comes from syndrome at wei stage or of qi system, or occurs by itself. It is the serious stage of an epidemic febrile disease.

1. Main symptoms are fever or high fever, thirst with no desire to drink, insomnia due to vexation, delirium, red tongue, and thready and rapid pulse.

2. Pathology: Warm pathogen goes inside to form extreme heat, damage ying-yin, disturb mental activity, or cause wind syndrome.

3. Diagnosis and Treatment:

(1) Consumption of ying-yin by heat, with the above-mentioned main symptoms, or with skin eruption, red tongue and no fur, should be treated with Qing Ying Decoction as a main recipe to clear up the ying system and remove heat.

(2) Invasion of the pericardium by heat with symptoms of high fever, coma, delirium, cold limbs and clonic convulsion should be treated with Qing Ying Decoction and An Gong Niu Huang Pill or Ju Fang Zhi Bao Pill to remove heat from the heart and restore consciousness.

(3) Occurrence of wind syndrome due to extreme heat has symptoms of high fever, dysphoria, clonic convulsion, spasm of limbs, stiffness of nape, opisphotonus, tremor of the tongue, red tongue, and taut and rapid pulse. Bai Hu Decoction plus antelope's horn and hooked uncaria and their like should be used to remove heat and expel wind.

(D) Syndrome of Blood System

Syndrome of blood system mainly comes from syndrome at ying stage, or at wei stage, or of qi system, or occasionally occurs by itself. It is the life-threatening stage of an epidemic febrile disease.

1. Main symptoms are hematemesis, epistaxis, hemafecia, hematuria, dense skin eruptions, fever or low fever, heat in palms and soles, dry mouth and tongue, parched lips, dysphoria, coma, delirium, red and glossy tongue, clonic convulsion of limbs, and infantile convulsion.

2. Pathology: Invasion of blood system by extreme heat causes accumulation of heat and stasis, depletion of yin-fluid, and stirring-up of endopathic wind of deficiency type.

3. Diagnosis and Treatment:

(1) Invasion of blood system by heat with the above-mentioned main symptoms

should be treated with Xi Jiao Di Huang Decoction as a main recipe to remove heat from the blood and toxic material from the body.

(2) Intense heat in both qi and blood systems has symptoms of vigorous heat, thirst, vexation, dysphoria, even madness, delirium, hematemesis, epistaxis, skin eruptions, red tongue, yellow and dry fur, and rapid pulse. Hua Ban Decoction is used to clear qi, remove heat from the blood, and eliminate skin eruptions. Invasion of the viscera and channels by toxic heat has symptoms of shiver with cold, high fever, extreme thirst for cold drinks, severe headache, dysphoria, delirium, coma, and bleeding. Qing Wen Bai Du Decoction is used as a main recipe to clear qi, and remove heat from the blood and toxic material from the body.

(3) Blood-heat in combination with wind has symptoms of vigorous heat, coma, dizziness, distending pain in the head, clonic convulsion of the limbs, stiffness of nape, opisthotonus, dry and red tongue, and taut and rapid pulse. Ling Yang Gou Teng Decoction is used as a main recipe to remove heat from the liver and calm wind.

(4) Impairment of yin by blood-heat should be treated with drugs to remove heat from the blood or to nourish yin and increase fluid according to the strength of pathogenic qi and different depletion of yin-fluid.

Section 3 Taxonomy

As practitioners have been deepening medical practice and accumulating medical knowledge, diseases studied by TCM internal medicine have been increasing. In order to facilitate study and clinical application, people have long attached importance to the classification of internal diseases. In Synopsis of Prescriptions of the Golden Chamber, diseases are roughly classified to facilitate diagnosis and treatment. General Treatise on the Causes and Symptoms of Diseases, the first existing treatise on syndromes and symptoms in China, has 1739 cases in "symptoms", showing detailed classification of syndromes and symptoms. Prescriptions Worth a Thousand Gold carries out preliminary summarization. Prescriptions of Peaceful Benevolent Dispensary, a book of set recipes in Song Dynasty, classifies diseases. Prescriptions Assigned to the Three Categories of Pathogenic Factors of Diseases, written by Chen Yan in Song Dynasty, imperfectly classifies diseases into three categories, namely, exopathic, endopathic and non-endo-exopathic categories. Classified Medical Records of Famous Physicians emphatically discusses common internal diseases.

Three Therapeutic Methods and Six Categories, written by Zhang Congzheng, etiologically classifies diseases into wind, cold, summer heat, dampness, dryness, fire, internal injury, external injury, internal mass and external mass, exerting considerable influence on Principle and Prohibition for Medical Profession. The book classifies the first six and miscellaneous diseases. Compendium of Medicine classifies visceral organs. It can be seen that the authors worked hard on taxonomy, and their books have great value. Diagnosis for Causes and Feeling Pulse for Treatment classifies diseases into exopathy and internal injury. Overall Supplement to Diagnosis and Treatment classifies internal diseases into 8 categories. Medicine Is Easy Indeed classifies diseases into exterior, interior, cold, heat, excess and deficiency syndromes.

There is no unified view on classification of diseases. In order to direct clinical practice, it is imperative to seek a relatively reasonable classification. After liberation, physicians believe that it is appropriate to classify internal diseases according to etiological causes and pathological changes. According to etiological causes, internal diseases can be classified into exopathy and internal injury. Exopathic diseases are caused by six external etiological factors. Internal injury diseases are pathological products caused by mental stimulation, improper diet, excessive fatigue, irregular life and visceral dysfunction. For example, they can be induced by phlegm and blood stasis produced by abnormal distribution of qi, blood and fluid. Of course, Exopathic diseases and internal injury diseases can be transformed into each other at some stage of illness. According to pathological changes, internal diseases can be classified into febrile diseases and miscellaneous diseases. Febrile diseases comprise all pathological changes in six channels, triple-jiao, wei, qi, ying and xue. Miscellaneous diseases mainly comprise visceral dysfunction.

Etiological classification facilitates clinical diagnosis. Pathological classification helps grasp the law governing the occurrence and development of diseases. Pathological changes are mainly caused by visceral dysfunction, so diseases can be further classified according to visceral organs.

Pathological classification is based on and a supplement to etiological classification. Therefore, the two classifications can be clinically combined into exopathic febrile diseases and internal injury miscellaneous diseases.

(A) Classification of Exopathic Febrile Diseases

According to affection by different exopathogens, exopathic febrile diseases can be classified into exogenous febrile diseases and epidemic febrile diseases. Epidemic febrile diseases can be further divided into warm-heat diseases and damp-heat diseases. Warm-heat diseases comprise wind-warm, spring-warm, winter-warm, autumn-dryness, virulent heat and virulent contagious diseases. Damp-heat diseases comprise damp-warm, summer-heat and summer-fever diseases. Epidemic febrile diseases can also be classified into those occurring immediately after invasion by exopathogens and those occurring after incubation. Epidemic febrile diseases occurring immediately after invasion by exopathogens comprise wind-warm, winter-warm, summer-fever and autumn dryness diseases. Epidemic febrile diseases occurring after incubation comprise spring-warm and summer-heat diseases.

(B) Classification of Internal Injury Miscellaneous Diseases

Its theoretical basis is viscera-state doctrine. The human body is an organic whole with the viscera as its center, with limbs, bones, five sense organs, and nine orifices outside, with qi, blood and fluid as material basis, and with channels as passages. Therefore, the pathological changes of internal injury miscellaneous diseases are caused by dysfunction of the viscera, by obstruction of channels, and by abnormal generation, circulation and distribution of qi, blood and fluid. According to pathological changes of the viscera, internal injury miscellaneous diseases should be classified into those of the lung system, heart system, liver system, kidney system, channel system, qi and blood system, and fluid system.

Common internal diseases are classified as follows:

1. Exopathic Diseases: common cold, cholera and malaria.

2. Internal Injury Diseases:

(1) Diseases of the Lung System: cough, dyspnea, asthma, pulmonary abscess, consumptive lung disease, lung distension, pulmonary tuberculosis.

(2) Diseases of the Spleen and Stomach: stomachache (and acid regurgitation), vomiting, hiccup, dysphagia, abdominal pain, diarrhea, dysentery, constipation and parasitosis.

(3) Diseases of the Liver System: dizziness, apoplexy, hypochondriac pain, jaundice, tympanites and convulsion.

(4) Diseases of the Heart System: palpitation, chest pain, insomnia, dreaminess, madness and epilepsy.

(5) Diseases of the Kidney System: edema, stranguria, retention of urine, seminal emission (and impotence), lumbago, tinnitus and deafness.

(6) Diseases of the Channels: arthralgia syndrome, flaccidity syndrome and headache.

(7) Diseases of the Qi, Blood and Fluid Systems: perspiration, diabetes, phlegm retention, abdominal mass, fever due to internal injury, consumptive disease, goiter, blood troubles, syncope and melancholia.

Section 4 Therapeutics

The therapeutics of TCM internal medicine is theoretically rigorous and methodologically diversified. Its contents comprise therapeutic principles and methods. Therapeutic principles can be summarized as treating the human body as an organic whole, searching for the primary cause of disease in treatment, and implementing treatment with a dynamic viewpoint. Therapeutic methods can be summarized as two main types of internal and external treatments, each with many specific methods.

Prescriptions for Fifty-two Kinds of Diseases, earlier than Internal Classic, records internal treatments such as decoction and medicated wine, and external treatments such as medicated bath, fumigation, steaming, hot medicated compress, stone needling, moxibustion and massage. Synopsis of Prescriptions of the Golden Chamber has dosage forms of Chinese drugs such as decoction, pill, powder, medicated wine, lotion, fumigant, ear drops, nasal insufflating power, nasal perfusate, ointment, rectal suppository and pessary. Treatise on febrile Diseases deeply studies drug-taking methods. Rhymed Discourses on External Therapy comprehensively summarizes external treatments. All the improved treatments are aimed at enhancing curative effect, facilitating medication and reducing toxic side effects.

Chinese drugs and recipes are main means for internal treatments. Collected are 365 drugs in Shen Nong's Herbal Classic and 1892 drugs in Compendium of Materia Medica. Through efforts made by physicians of later dynasties, new Chinese drugs have been discovered and clinically applied. Especially since the founding of the People's Republic of China, medicine has entered an entirely new stage, and 5 000 Chinese drugs have been used. In addition, progress in methods of processing Chinese drugs has strengthened their potency and reduced their toxicity. Lei's Treatise on Preparation of Drugs in the 5th century records 17 drug-preparing methods, such as steaming, cooking, parching, baking, stir-frying with liquids, stir-baking, calcining, infusing and refining powder with water. Afterwards, drug-preparing methods have been increasing. Particularly after liberation, new dosage forms have been made, such as tablet, granule or powder taken after being infused in boiling water, and injection, more easily facilitating clinical application.

The composition of recipes has been produced and developed under the guidance of TCM theory. The recipe-composing principle in Internal Classic stipulates 4 kinds of drugs, namely, monarch, minister, adjuvant and conductant drugs. On the basis of Internal Classic and in accordance with illness conditions and drug properties, Cheng Wuji raised 7 kinds of recipes, namely, heavy prescription, minor prescription, slow-acting prescription, quick-acting prescription, prescription with odd-numbered ingredients, prescription with even-numbered ingredients, and compound prescription. Concise Exposition on Exogenous Febrile Diseases classifies recipes into 10 types according to their effects, namely, dispersing, obstruction-removing, nourishing, purgative, light diaphoretic, heavy, lubricating, astringent, drying and moistening prescriptions. Collection of Prescriptions with Notes classifies recipes into 21 kinds. They are nourishing, diaphoretic, vomiting-causing, purgative, diaphoretic and purgative, regulating, qi flow regulating, blood circulation regulating, wind expelling, cold dispelling, summer heat eliminating, diuresis inducng, moistening, fire removing, phlegm relieving, digestion promoting, astringing, parasites destroying, eyesight improving, large carbuncle, and gynecologic and obstetric prescriptions, with good first-aid recipes. This classification of recipes facilitates clinical applications and is also related to classification of Chinese drugs, so it is welcomed among physicians. On the basis of this classification, through summarization and in combination with illness nature, Medicine Comprehended classifies recipes into 8 treatments, namely, diaphoretic, emetic, purgative, warming, heat clearing, nourishing, resolving and regulating therapies. Therefore, this concise classification has been used among later physicians.

The production and development of recipes are based on enhancement of clinically curative effects. "Prescriptions for Fifth-two Kinds of Diseases" collects more than 280 recipes. "Peaceful Holy Benevolent Prescriptions" in Song Dynasty collects 16834 recipes. "General Collection for Holly Relief" collects over 20000 recipes. "Prescriptions for Universal Relief" is the existing largest medical formulary in China with 61730 recipes in it. It can thus be seen how rich TCM recipes are. In order to facilitate clinical application, it is indispensable to screen recipes. According to clinical needs, "Revised Prescriptions of Peaceful Benevolent Dispensary" selects 297 recipes. In order to facilitate application, recitation and memory, "Collection of Prescriptions with Notes", "Recipes in Verse", "Popular Recipes in Verse" and other medical books make new selection of recipes, thus also having considerable reference value.

A. Therapeutic Principles

Therapeutic principles, stipulated in the spirit of a whole concept and diagnosis and treatment based on overall analysis of symptoms and illness conditions according to TCM basic theory, has instructive significance for working out a therapy, prescribing a recipe and taking a drug during the process of treatment. Its contents can be summarized as treating the human body as an organic whole, searching for the primary cause of disease in treatment, implementing treatment with a dynamic viewpoint, combining treatment with nursing care, and using 8 therapies.

(A) Treating the Human Body as an Organic Whole

The viscera, channels, body and orifices constitute an organic whole, and are closely related to the nature. Therefore, disease at any part will often influence the whole body, it is inadequate to purely treat the part, and more attention should be paid to nursing the whole body to achieve the objective of treating local pathological changes. In addition, treatment should be comprehensively considered in combination with climate, locality, constitution and other factors. Only by taking an appropriate therapeutic method according to different time, locality and person, can better curative effect be achieved.

(B) Searching for the Primary Cause of Disease in Treatment

Primary and secondary causes of disease are relative. Vital qi is primary cause, while pathogen is secondary cause. Old illness and primary disease are primary causes, while new illness and secondary disease are secondary causes.

Through analyzing and differentiating symptoms, the physician can recognize the nature of disease, distinguish primary from secondary causes, and determine corresponding therapy. To use the principle of searching for the primary cause of disease in treatment, it is necessary to grasp "routine treatment and treatment contrary to the routine", "treatment of symptoms and treatment of causes", "strengthening the body resistance and eliminating pathogenic factor" and "giving priority to prevention".

1. Routine Treatment and Treatment Contrary to the Routine:

(1) Routine treatment, a therapeutic principle of treatment with recipes opposite to the nature of disease, is applicable to diseases with its nature identical to its symptoms.

(2) Treatment contrary to the routine is a therapeutic principle of treatment with recipes identical to the nature of disease. For example, drugs hot in nature are used to treat cold syndrome with pseudo-heat symptoms. Drugs cold in nature are used to treat heat syndrome with pseudo-cold symptoms. Tonic drugs are used to treat deficiency syndrome with pseudo-excess symptoms. Purgative drugs are used to treat excess syndrome with pseudo-deficiency symptoms.

2. Treatment of Symptoms and Treatment of Causes: The general principle is to treat acute symptoms with quick-acting drugs, treat causes with slow-acting drugs, and treat the symptoms and causes simultaneously.

(1) To Treat Acute Symptoms with Quick-acting Drugs: Acute symptoms, if not resolved promptly, will threaten life or influence treatment. Therefore, it is necessary to alleviate symptoms as soon as possible.

(2) To Treat Causes with Slow-acting Drugs: After acute symptoms are alleviated or when no obvious life-threatening symptoms exist, the fundamental cause of disease, or a primary disease, can be treated. Therefore, this principle is of important significance for chronic diseases or for the restoration stage of an acute disease.

(3) To Treat Symptoms and Causes Simultaneously: When symptoms and causes are equally important, it is necessary to treat them simultaneously without neglecting any one of them. For example, drugs are used to supplement qi and expel exogenous factors, or to expel both exopathic and endopathic factors.

There are both principle and flexibility in treating symptoms and causes. However, the ultimate goal is to grasp the main contradiction of a disease in searching for the primary cause in its treatment.

3. Strengthening the Body Resistance and Eliminating Pathogenic Factors: The occurrence and development of a disease are the manifestation of struggle between the body resistance and pathogenic factors. Therefore, the treatment of a disease is to strengthen the body resistance and eliminate pathogenic factors, thus gradually improving the condition and eventually curing the disease.

(1) Strengthening the Body Resistance: This principle is applicable to deficiency syndrome with weak resistance as the main contradiction and with hypoactive pathogenic factors.

(2) Eliminating Pathogenic Factors: This principle is applicable to excess syndrome with hyperactive pathogenic factors as the main contradiction and with normal body resistance.

First strengthening the body resistance and then eliminating pathogenic factors is applicable to syndromes with weakened body resistance unable to withstand while attacking hyperactive pathogenic factors. First eliminating pathogenic factors and then strengthening body resistance is applicable to syndromes with body resistance still able to withstand while attacking hyperactive pathogenic factors, or with strengthening body resistance able to help pathogenic factors instead. Strengthening the body resistance and eliminating pathogenic factors at the same time is applicable to syndromes with strengthening body resistance unable to help pathogenic factors and eliminating pathogenic factors unable to impair body resistance.

4. Giving Priority to Prevention: Measures should be taken to prevent occurrence and development of diseases.

(1) Preventing Occurrence of Diseases: Occurrence of diseases depends on body resistance and pathogenic factors, so strong body resistance keeps pathogenic factors away. Maintaining and strengthening body resistance mainly relies on nursing health to calm mind and normalize visceral function, on doing physical exercise to build up constitution and invigorate qi and blood, and on leading a regular life to conserve strength and store up energy to deal with harmful stimulation and injury. In addition, it is also important to prevent diseases with drugs, implement artificial immunity, pay attention to hygiene and prevent pollution to environment, water source and food.

(2) Preventing Development of Diseases: Disease should be diagnosed and treated as early as possible to prevent it from developing and changing.

(C) Implementing Treatment with A Dynamic Viewpoint

A disease can be improved or deteriorated, so it should be observed and handled with a dynamic viewpoint. During clinical practice, it is necessary to grasp common therapies and main recipes, and change recipes according to changes of illness conditions, so as not to treat a disease with a therapy and a recipe through to the end.

Exopathy and internal injury diseases have certain stages. Only by familiarizing the characteristics of every stage and knowing the law governing the change of an illness, can the physician treat the disease in accordance with the change of symptoms.

(D) Combining Treatment with Nursing Care

The curative effect is very closely related to nursing care, so it is vital important to strengthen nursing care in the mind, diet, daily life, and medication during treatment. Necessary nursing measures should be taken according to characteristics of a disease to enhance curative effect.

B. Using 8 Therapies

8 therapies are referred to as clinically common used 8 therapeutic methods, namely, diaphoretic, emetic, purgative, regulating, warming, heat-removing, nourishing, and resolving therapies.

(A) Diaphoretic Therapy

It is a therapeutic method of dispersion and purgation of muscular striae to expel pathogens out of the body.

Diaphoretic therapy is applicable to the early stage of common exopathy, edema and skin diseases, and to the stage of promoting skin eruption.

(B) Emetic Therapy

It is a therapeutic method of vomiting pathogens or toxic substances from the mouth.

Emetic therapy is applicable to phlegm accumulation, indigestion, nausea and food poisoning.

(C) Purgative Therapy

It is a therapeutic method of purging stagnation and relaxing the bowels.

Purgative therapy is applicable to pathogens in the stomach and intestine, constipation, heat accumulation in the body, water retention, blood retention, phlegm stagnation, and parasitosis.

(D) Regulating Therapy

It is a therapeutic method of eliminating pathogenic factors and strengthening body resistance without impairment of the body resistance by eliminating pathogenic factors.

Regulating therapy is very widely applicable to Shaoyang syndrome, combined syndrome of Taiyang and Shaoyang combined syndrome of Shaoyang and Yangming, incoordination between the liver and stomach, irregular menstruation due to stagnation of the liver-qi, and abdominal pain and diarrhea due to affection of functions of the spleen and stomach by hyperactivity of the liver.

(E) Warming Therapy

It is a therapeutic method of eliminating cold pathogen and replenishing yang-qi. It is mainly used to recuperate depleted yang to rescue the patient from collapse, and warm the middle-jiao to dispel cold.

Warming therapy is applicable to stagnation of cold pathogen, and cold syndrome transformed from heat syndrome.

(F) Heat-removing Therapy

It is a therapeutic method to treat common heat syndrome with effects of reducing fever, removing fire, reserving fluid, eliminating vexation and quenching thirst.

Heat-removing therapy is applicable to all heat syndromes with excessive internal heat in qi system or ying-blood due to internal injury or exopathy.

(G) Nourishing Therapy

It is a therapeutic method to treat deficiency of yin, yang, qi, blood, or a visceral organ.

Nourishing therapy is applicable to feeble patients with deficiency of qi, blood, yin and yang, and those with body resistance too weakened to eliminate pathogenic factors.

(H) Resolving Therapy

It is divided into dispersion and destruction with their effect similar to and different from that of purgative therapy.

Resolving therapy is applicable to food stagnation or chronic abdominal mass inappropriate to be purged and appropriate to be dispersed. It is also applicable to stagnation of qi, blood, phlegm and food.

C. TCM Therapeutic Methods

(A) Internal Treatment

Its dosage forms are decoction, powder, pill, ointment, pellet, wine, tablet, granule, oral liquid, and injection.

(B) External Treatment

Its methods are sticking, plastering, topical application, compress, hot medicated compress, fumigation, infusing, washing, rubbing, steaming, powder-applying, sneezing, blowing, inhaling, chiropractic, plugging, lying, pillow, full-filling, inducing, wearing, scrapping, cupping, massage and moxibustion.

Correctly using and actively spreading internal and external treatments will surely enhance curative effect.

Questions for Review

1. Try to describe the contents of "Theory on Three Categories of Etiological Factors" raised by Chen Yan, and its influence on later etiological theories.
2. How to recognize that phlegm and blood stasis are not only pathological products of visceral dysfunction but also etiological factors?
3. Briefly describe main syndromes of five zang-organs.
4. Briefly describe commonly used recipes for five zang syndromes.
5. How to grasp the pathology of five zang syndromes?
6. How to recognize deficiency and excess of qi syndrome? What relations exist between disorder of qi and the viscera?

7. What are pathological changes of bleeding, blood stasis and blood deficiency?
8. What are pathological changes of wind, fire, phlegm and dampness?
9. What is the clinical significance of analyzing and differentiating febrile diseases in accordance with the theory of six channels? What are the contents of six channel syndromes?
10. How to clinically use the pathology of wei, qi, ying, blood and triple-jiao?
11. How to grasp and use internal and external treatments? Can external treatment be used for miscellaneous diseases due to internal injury? Try to explain with examples.

Chapter 3 Methods of Clinical Practice and Writing of Medical Record in Traditional Chinese Internal Medicine

Section 1 Method of Clinical Practice in Traditional Chinese Internal Medicine

Internal medicine is the basis of all clinical disciplines. In the process of teaching internal medicine, apart from teaching theoretical knowledge and clinical application of diagnosis and treatment of internal diseases, teaching method of clinical practice is a very important link.

Method of clinical practice is how to use TCM theoretical knowledge to diagnose and treat diseases. TCM clinical practice is generally summarized as examination, diagnosis and treatment. The whole process comprises the physician's thinking activity and the writing of medical record as stipulated. This is the actual reflection of a physician's theoretical knowledge and clinical skill.

The requirements for clinical practice are to diagnose and treat rapidly and correctly, to closely relate theory, method, recipe and drug, and to bring curative effect to patients. Therefore, to train, grasp and familiarize method of clinical practice is indispensable for every student.

A. Examination

Its contents mainly are four diagnostic methods, namely, inspection, auscultation and olfaction, interrogation, and pulse-feeling and palpation. Through four diagnostic methods, the physician obtain all the information needed for diagnosis, including the patient's general condition, such as name, sex, age, place of birth, occupation, work unit, and marriage. The physician should also know the patient's disposition, recreation, belief, and residential condition, and deeply understand pathogenic condition, the most painful symptoms, diagnosis, treatment, curative effect and all the diseases the patient is suffering from. TCM diagnosis is very closely related to chief complaint, including the most painful symptoms, ailing pain to be most urgently relieved, and the time of its occurrence and continuation. Meanwhile, the physician should also know anamnesis, conditions of illness and death of family members, personal history, history of menstruation, leukorrhea, pregnancy and delivery, and history of drug allergy. Medical check-up should be carried out through inspection, auscultation and olfaction, and pulse feeling and palpation to discover positive signs. With scientific progress, the methods and contents of TCM inspection, auscultation and olfaction, and pulse feeling and palpation have been gradually enriched and developed. For example, pathological changes of gastric mucosa observed with gastrofiberscope have been included in the contents of inspection. Results of X-ray, B-ultrasonic and assay have been also recognized and used by TCM, enriching the contents of TCM four diagnostic methods and enhancing the level of TCM diagnosis and treatment.

Illness history should be collected comprehensively, systematically, explicitly and concisely. By comprehensively, we mean that the physician should patiently and carefully understand the whole process of occurrence and development of illness, including its causes, initial symptoms, diagnosis, treatment, curative effect, the most outstanding symptoms, and anamnesis. By systematically, we mean that pondering while interrogating, the physician should systematize illness conditions to diagnose if the patient is suffering from a disease due to exopathy or internal injury. A disease due to internal injury should be diagnosed as mainly in the heart system, or in systems of the heart and liver, or in systems of the heart, liver and spleen. If necessary, the physician should ask the patient to give illness history and introduce illness conditions in detail. At the same time, the physician should guard against subjective judgement or induce the patient to describe illness conditions. By emphatically, we mean that the physician should emphatically write the patient's symptoms in its medical record.

Medical check-up should be performed regularly, gently and skillfully. It is necessary to practise repeatedly. With inspection, auscultation and olfaction, and pulse feeling and palpation in TCM as main methods, and with inspection, touch, knock and listening in Western medicine as auxiliary methods, Western medicine should serve TCM diagnosis.

B. Diagnosis

Using TCM theory, the physician should analyze, summarize, infer and judge all the information obtained with four diagnostic methods to determine the focus, nature, pathogenesis, syndrome and symptoms of a disease.

Internal diseases are divided into two main types of diseases due to exopathy and internal injury. During its development for a long time, TCM has formed the richest diagnostic methods. Diseases due to exopathy are generally diagnosed in accordance with the theory of the six channels, the condition of wei, qi, ying and blood, and the pathogenic changes of triple-jiao. Diseases due to internal injury are often diagnosed according to pathogenic changes of the viscera, the state of qi and blood, and the condition of wind, fire, phlegm and dampness. However, both types of diseases are interrelated, with visceral physiology and pathology as their basis, and with 8 principal syndromes as their general program.

There are many methods to clinically analyze illness condition. Comprehensively analyzing method is often used to diagnose an internal disease. According to the information obtained with the four diagnostic methods on main symptoms, accompanying symptoms, tongue picture, pulse condition and other medical check-up, the physician should use TCM basic theoretical knowledge to analyze pathological changes, to infer the focus, nature and pathogenesis of a disease, and finally to make diagnosis.

Diagnosis should be made reasonably, evidentially, concisely and accurately. In writing TCM medical records, sentences can be traditionally made with four or six Chinese characters. or analysis can be made point by point, to finally get conclusion.

Resulting from differentiation of symptoms, diagnosis of a disease or syndrome is very closely related to chief complaint, and diagnosis of symptoms and signs involves nature and pathogenesis of illness. For example, a disease is diagnosed as stomachache, and symptoms are diagnosed as incoordination of the spleen and stomach, and heat in the upper and cold in the lower.

C. Treatment

According to diagnosis, the physician should determine therapeutic pattern, principle and method, main or basic recipe, composition and dosage of drug, drug-decocting and drug-taking method, recuperative medical care and dietetic restraint.

Therapeutic pattern is the general design of treatment, such as pure Chinese drug, or Chinese drug accompanied with acupuncture, massage or dietetic therapy; pure purgation or nourishment, or first purgation and then nourishment, or first nourishment and then purgation, or purgation and nourishment at the same time. Therapeutic principle includes routine treatment or treatment contrary to the routine, treating superficiality or origin, slow or quick acting treatment, visceral purgation or nourishment, and treatment according to three categories of etiological factors. Therapeutic method includes internal or external treatment, and commonly used twelve kinds of prescriptions. It is particularly imperative for beginners to choose a most appropriate ancient recipe or self-prescribed recipe as the main recipe under the guidance of therapeutic method. Otherwise, they would piece together a recipe at random without methodology to influence curative effect. The physician should use the main recipe plus or minus ingredients to make it more applicable to the patient's specific condition. A physician with more clinical experience will be more flexible in increasing or decreasing ingredients to make the recipe more effective. Dosage should be adjusted according to ancient and modern experience. Drug-decocting and drug-taking method, recuperative medical care and dietetic restraint are also vitally important to curative effect. Therefore, this component of treatment should bot be missed or neglected.

In treatment, it is imperative to flexibly determine therapy according to disease, select recipe according to therapy, and give drugs according to recipe, making theory, therapy, recipe and drugs consistent.

Method of clinical practice is a clinical skill that clinical physicians should grasp. Only by repeated practice, can skill come from practice to enhance curative effect.

Section 2 General Requirements for Traditional Chinese Internal Medicine Record

Written in TCM medical record closely combining TCM theory with clinical practice are changes of illness condition, therapeutic pattern and curative effect, medical check-ups, and ideas of physicians. Medical record is an important basis for correct diagnosis and treatment and for inferring prognosis, a valuable material for medical, teaching and scientific research work, and an important reference material for proficiency assessment and for administrative and judicial organizations.

To strengthen the management of TCM medical records and enhance the requirements for writing them is an important link in the management of a hospital, an important measure to raise the level of TCM clinical diagnosis and treatment, and a content for students to practise basic skill in teaching hospitals.

The general requirements for writing TCM medical records are summarized as follows:

1. A complete TCM medical record should include three major contents, namely, social condition, examination with the four diagnostic methods, and diagnosis and treatment. Diagnosis by physicians of western medicine should be also included as required by health administration department at present.

2. A TCM medical record should be written in TCM terms, under the guidance of TCM theory to carry out diagnosis and treatment, making theory, therapy, recipe and drugs consistent.

3. A medical record should be seriously written item by item without missing. It should be comprehensively, systematically, concisely, accurately and neatly written with a pen and in neat and coherent writing.

4. A medical record written by a resident should be checked, approved, revised with a pencil and signed by an attending doctor. Too much revised medical record should be re-written by the resident. A medical record written by an intern or a training physician should be revised with a pencil and signed by a resident or an attending doctor. Too much revised medical record should be re-written.

5. An in-patient medical record should be written within 24 hours, and an out-patient medical record should be written immediately.

Section 3 Written Form and Contents of In-patient Internal Medical Record

A. Form and Contents

Name: Sex:
Age: Place of Birth:
Nationality: Marriage:
Address: Pathogenic Season:
Admission Date: History-taking Date:
Informant: Reliability:
Diagnostic Interrogation:
Chief Complaint: the most painful symptoms suffered by the patient and

their locations, nature and time, namely, main reason for going to a doctor.

History of Present Illness: The physician should record the whole process of occurrence, development and change of an illness with the main symptoms as its center. Symptoms should be described in TCM terms. TCM and Western medical diagnosis and treatment should be written.

Present symptoms should be thoroughly and accurately recorded as the main basis for diagnosis and treatment.

Anamnesis: general health condition, time of illnesses suffered by the patient in the past and condition of their treatment.

Personal History: place of birth, environmental condition of residence, condition of life and work, dietary habit, and specific hobby.

History of Menstruation, Leukorrhea, Pregnancy and Delivery (for female patients): time of menarche, menstrual cycle, amount, color and nature, marriage age, and condition of pregnancy and delivery.

Family History: health and illness conditions of relatives and friends closely related to the patient, and causes of death of relatives and their ages.

The Whole Body: spirit, color, shape and state.

Localities: head, face, hair, five sense organs, throat, neck, chest, abdomen, spine, waist, back, the limbs, nails, skin, and specific conditions of the fourteen channels.

Excreta: phlegm, vomiting substances, sweat, urine, feces, nasal discharge, tear, and secretion from the body surface.

Inspection of the Tongue: changes of shape, texture, fur, frenulum and dorsum of the tongue,

Diagnostic Auscultation and Olfaction:

Voice: pronunciation, phonetics, breath, cough, hiccup, vomiting, sighing, moan, and bowel sound.

Smell: air from the mouth, sweat, phlegm, saliva, vomiting substances, urine and feces.

Pressing the Skin: head, face, neck, chest, hypochondria, abdomen, body, four limbs and pressure pain points.

Pulse Feeling and Palpation: Pulse conditions of cun, guan and chi on left and right hands should be recorded thoroughly and respectively. Pulse conditions of three portions and nine pulse-taking points should be depicted if necessary. Diagnostic method of three portions should be applied to critical patients to record conditions of Renying pulse and Fuyang pulse and pay attention to the manifestation of the stomach-qi, spirit and root in pulse condition.

Summary of Four Diagnostic Methods:

Analysis of Syndrome: focus, property of syndrome, and change of pathogenesis.

TCM Diagnosis: differentiation of disease and syndrome, including main disease and syndrome as well as accompanying disease and syndrome. The type of syndrome should be written in the brackets immediately after the name of disease.

Therapeutic Principle and Method: including therapeutic steps.

Recipe: main recipe:

Medicinal Ingredients: ××× (decoction of a wrapped drug), ×× (decocted first), ×× (decocted later), ×× (melted by heat and taken after being infused in boiling water in several times), ×××, ×××, ×××, ×××, ××× (minutes).

Nursing care: including medication, food restraint, dietetic therapy, and daily life.

Physiochemical Examination: for positive signs.

Diagnosis by Western Medical Physician: main disease and accompanying disease (stage, type and nature).

Diagnostic Basis:

Arrangement of Treatment: mainly supportive, expectant and emergency treatment.

Signature of physician

At (time) on (date)

B. Concrete Requirements for In-patient Medical Record

1. Social condition should be clearly written item by item. Pathogenic season should be recorded according to the theory of correspondence between man and universe, so as to summarize the relations between occurrence of illness and seasons.

2. Four Diagnostic Methods:

(1) Main Symptoms: the most painful symptoms suffered by the patient, and their locations, nature and time, demonstrating the main reason for the patient to see a doctor.

(2) History of Present Illness: The physician should record the whole process of occurrence, development and change of main and accompanying

symptoms, which should be described in TCM terms. TCM and Western medical diagnosis and treatment should be included.

(3) Anamnesis: Attention should be paid to TCM characteristics in recording personal history, history of menstruation, leukorrhea, pregnancy and delivery, and family history. For example, relations between congenital deficiency and family history should be recorded in detail.

(4) Diagnostic Inspection: Stress should be put on inspection of the tongue. Changes of shape, texture and fur of the tongue should be recorded in detail. Spirit and color of the face and five sense organs should be emphatically observed. Importance should be attached to inspection of localities and excreta.

(5) Diagnostic Auscultation and Olfaction: Sound and smell should be comprehensively recorded.

(6) Pulse Feeling and Palpation: Stress should be put on pulse feeling. Pulse conditions at cun kou should be recorded in detail. Pulse conditions at three portions and nine pulse-taking points should be depicted if necessary. Diagnostic method of three portions should be applied to critical patients to record conditions of Renying pulse and Fuyang pulse and pay attention to the manifestation of the stomach-qi, spirit and root. Pulse conditions at cun kou can be recorded at cun, guan and chi on left and right hands respectively.

3. Diagnosis and Treatment:

(1) Summary of Four Diagnostic Methods: Symptoms on the admission date should be especially recorded in detail to accurately reflect the characteristics of illness, providing basis to TCM diagnosis and treatment.

(2) Analysis of Symptoms: Clinical information obtained with four diagnostic methods can be grouped with main symptoms, tongue picture and pulse condition as key points and according to organic relations between symptoms. The physician should use TCM theory to analyze the cause, focus, syndrome, pathogenesis and development of illness. The writing should be reasonable, evidential, concise and correct. By reasonable and evidential, we mean that the analysis should be carried out according to TCM basic theory and disease-differentiating method.

(3) TCM Diagnosis: Diseases are arranged in order of importance. The physician should write names of diseases, main symptoms (if disease names unavailable) and syndrome types. Two or three paragraphes should be used in diagnosis. For example:

Jaundice (occupying one line)

Yin jaundice occupying another line and drawn back by one (Chinese character)

Stagnation of cold-dampness and blood stasis in the body (occupying another line)

(4) Therapeutic Principle and Method: The physician should clearly write superficiality and origin, order of priority, and the arrangement of therapeutic steps.

(5) Recipe and Drugs: The physician should write the name of a main recipe. The name is allowed unwritten for a self-prescribed recipe. 4 drugs should be written in one line, with decocting, taking and preparing method written on the upper right side of every drug, and dosage written on the lower right side of every drug. Drugs are arranged in the order of monarch, minister, adjuvant and conductant drugs as well as compatibility of drugs.

(6) Nursing Care: The physician should explicitly write contraindication of drug and food, nursing measures and dietetic therapy, especially nursing requirements on admission date and in hospital.

C. Example of In-patient Internal Medical Record

Name: Mr. Hu

Age: 45 Sex: male

Nationality: Man Place of Birth: Beijing

Occupation: worker Marital Status: married

Address: 2 Dongsongnian, Dongcheng District

Work Unit: The 4th factory of Beijing Passenger Car Refit Company

Admission Time: at 5:30 PM on February 22, 1982

Pathogenic Season: 3 days before Rain Water

Informant: the patient himself

Medical Record Writing Time: at 5:30 PM on February 22, 1982

Reliability: reliable

Diagnostic Interrogation:

Main Symptoms: fever, aversion to cold, cough for 2 days, and drawing pain in the right chest for half a day.

History of Present Illness: On February 20, due to careless wear, the patient had headache affecting the vertex and face, nasal obstruction, low voice, watery nasal discharge, slight cough, serious aversion to cold, and low fever without sweat. He thought that he was suffering from common cold and took analgesic with no effect. He still persisted in work without rest. In the next morning, his symptoms were aggravated, with headache affecting neck and back, and lassitude throughout the body. At 3 PM in the afternoon, he suddenly had shiver with cold, frequent cough with sticky and yellow phlegm, turbid nasal discharge, no appetite, constipation, and dark urine. He hurried to the hospital for emergency treatment. A physician took his body temperature of 39 Celsius degrees, diagnosed him as having "upper respiratory tract infection", and gave him "common cold preparation to be taken after being infused in boiling water, oral compound sinomin, and compound aminopyrine for intramuscular injection". The patient also took "APC" by himself with abundant sweat but without alleviating fever. His suffering increased with aversion to wind and cold, difficulty in breath, vexation, and thirst for cold drinks. Symptoms became severer at night. This morning, he felt drawing pain in right chest, did not dare to breathe deeply, and coughed out "dark red" phlegm. He paid a return visit to the hospital. Emergency examination discovered temperature: 39 Celsius degrees, WBC: 29800 per cubic millimeter, N79%, L3%, and signs of upper right lobar pneumonia. The emergency department admitted him to my ward.

Anamnesis: The patient was in good health with no history of pulmonary tuberculosis and other infectious diseases, chronic bronchitis, and drug and food allergy.

Personal History: He was born in Beijing, and has been to Guangdong, Northeast China, Suzhou, Hangzhou and other places. His residence is not wet. He likes pungent food, smokes for over 10 years with 10 cigarettes a day, and drinks a little wine. He is optimistic and talkative.

History of Marriage: He got married at the age of 29. His wife has repeated relapses of cough and hemoptysis for many years. She is in good health. They have a son and a daughter.

Family History: His mother, 70 years old, is in good health. His father died of encephalomalacia in 1980.

Diagnostic Inspection:

The Whole Body: consciousness, lassitude, painful expression, sallow complexion, thinness, flashing eyes, inclination to move in bed, and free carriage.

Localities: Thin lustrous gray hair. Slightly sunken sockets of eyeball, no yellow color in eyeballs, no blood streak in the white of eye, and equally sized and round pupils. Slight nares flaring. Ruddy helixes, and no otorrhea and sore. Dark red dry cracked lips. Yellow odontolite, odontoloxy, a lower left molar tooth missing, no dental caries, and no gingival bleeding. Pink pharynx, and no tonsillitis. Symmetric soft neck without deformity, goiter and scrofula. Flat thorax, pigeon chest, difficulty in breathing even so serious as to pound the chest with a fist. Relaxed abdomen with no tympanites and vessels seen. Straight spine with two sides symmetric. Four limbs without edema. No arthroncus of knee and clubbed finger. Lustrous nails and skin. No jaundice, no skin eruption, no subcutaneous nodule, no miliaria alba, no furuncle, no carbuncle, no nail-like boil, and no cellulitis.

Excreta: yellow and sticky phlegm without blood streak and clot, turbid and white nasal discharge, constipation for 3 days, dark urine, and perspiration all over the body.

Tongue Picture: red and normally sized tongue with yellow and slight greasy fur, dark red and normally sized lingual frenulum.

Diagnostic Auscultation and Olfaction:

Voice: high-pitch and forceful voice, low voice in speaking, difficulty in respiration and short breath, occasional cough with loud sound, no fading murmuring, no delirium, and no moan.

Smell: slight helitosis, sweat smell, and foul smell of urine.

Pulse Feeling and Palpation:

Pressing the Skin: moist and soft skin without sunken area, extreme heat in the forehead and skin, and no goiter and scrofula in the neck, armpit and groin.

Pressing the Chest and Abdomen: The patient felt pain when right chest and upper abdomen were slightly pressed. No stiff mass was found.

Pulse Feeling

	cun	guan	chi
left	taut, slippery, slightly rapid	taut, slippery, slightly rapid	taut, thready, slippery, slightly rapid
right	floating, lightly rapid	taut, slippery, slightly rapid	taut, slippery, slightly rapid

Summary of Four Diagnostic Methods:

The existing symptoms are as follows: Fever, aversion to cold, occasional shiver with cold. Lassitude in the body. Sweating after taking diaphoretic. Headache. Nasal obstruction and nasal discharge. Cough with yellow and sticky phlegm. Difficulty in respiration with slight dyspnea. Drawing pain in the right chest is aggravated during deep breath. Thirst for cold drinks. Constipation lasted 3 days. Scanty dark urine. Red tongue and yellow and slightly greasy fur. Floating and slightly rapid pulse at right cun; taut, slippery and slightly rapid pulse at left cun. Sober but painful emotion. Tired sallow complexion and thinness. Moistened lustrous skin. Slightly sunken sockets of eyeball, no blood streak in the white of eye, no yellow eyeballs. Slight nares flaring. Dark red dry cracked lips. Yellow odontolite. Pink pharynx with no tonsillitis. High-pitch low voice in speaking. Difficulty in short breath with occasional cough. Slight helitosis, sweat smell, foul smell of urine. High fever in the forehead and skin. No goiter and scrofula in the neck, armpit and groin. The patient felt pain when right chest and upper abdomen were slightly pressed. No stiff mass was found.

Analysis of Symptoms:

The patient is thin, likes pungent food, and has accumulated heat in his spleen and stomach. In early spring, it is still cold and windy. Careless in wear, he was attacked by exopathic wind and cold with symptoms of headache, aversion to cold, fever and lassitude. The lung has purifying and descending function with the nose as its orifice. Obstruction of the lung-qi and stagnation of phlegm-heat in the lung cause its dysfunction with cough and nasal obstruction. The lung and the large intestine are interior-exteriorly related to each other. Obstruction of the lung-qi and fu-qi, stagnation of heat in the lung and stomach and depletion of body fluid cause constipation and scanty dark urine. Red tongue, yellow and slightly greasy fur, and taut, slippery and slightly rapid pulse are signs of phlegm-heat; while floating pulse at right cun is a sign of exopathy.

Judging from pulse condition, the focus should be at the lung, stomach and large intestine with heat of excess type as the main cause. The disease involves both exterior and interior, with exopathogen unrelieved, heat stagnated in the lung and stomach, and fu-qi obstructed.

TCM Diagnosis: wind-warm syndrome
in both wei and qi systems
with exterior cold and interior heat

Therapeutic Principle and Method: dispelling wind to induce diaphoresis, and removing heat from the lung to dissolve phlegm, supplemented with removing obstruction in the channels to relieve pain.

Recipe and Drugs:

(1) Qing Jie Ye 60cc
55G, N, S 500cc/gttVst

(2) Qing Kai Ling 40cc
Ringer's solution 500cc/gttVst

(3) Jing Fang Bai Du Ji 2cc im st

(4) Decoction: Yin Qiao Powder and Ma Xing Shi Gan Decoction Jia Jian
ephedra 3g, gypsum 30g (decocted first), forsythia fruit 10g,
honeysuckle flower 10g, peppermint 5g (decocted later),
fresh reed rhizome 30g, apricot kernel 10g,
parched arctium fruit 10g, scutellaria root 10g, and
trichosanthes fruit 30g, luffa 10g. 2 portions were decocted.

(5) Acupuncture: Main points are selected at Urinary Bladder Channel of Foot-Taiyang and Large Intestine Channel of Hang-Yangming to dispel wind, induce diaphoresis and remove heat.

Point Selection: Quchi (Li11), Hegu (Li4), Fengmen (B12) and Dazhui (Du14). Needles are retained for 20 minutes.

Nursing Care: to keep warm, avoid wind and cold, prohibit eating uncooked and cold food, carefully guard against lingering high fever and sudden collapse of qi and yin, and closely observe changes of perspiration, pulse condition, complexion and breath.

Western Medical Examination:

T: 38 Celsius degrees, P: 82 times per minute, R: 20 times per minute, Bp: 130/90mmHg.

Normal development, moderate nutrition and sober consciousness. No xanthochromia, no ulcer, no rash and no furuncle in dermal mucosa. Normal sized lymph nodes. Normal sized skull. Darkish complexion. Flushed face with high fever. No pressure pain on mastoid process and nasal sinuses. Slight nares flaring and light nasal obstruction with small amount of white and sticky secretion, no abnormal secretion in external auditory canal. Normal oral mucosa. Tooth 3 and 4 missing. Light congestion of throat. Normal tonsil. Soft neck, without abnormal pulsation in the neck, with trachea in the middle and normal thyroid. Symmetric thorax, and basically even respiratory movement. Bubbling sound under the 4th right rib with strengthened voice conduction. Slight rough respiratory sound in the left lung without obvious rales. Apex beat 0.5cm inside midclavicular line and under the 5th left rib. Normal sized heart with heart rate 82 times per minute, no arrhythmia, no pathologic murmur in auscultation area. Soft abdomen with no pressure pain, no touch of the liver and spleen under ribs. Murphy's sign (−). Normal sized spine and four limbs, Existence of physiologic reflex, and no pathologic reflex.

Laboratory Examination: WBC: 29800/cubic millimeter, N:97%, L:3%.

Fluoroscopy of Chest: upper right lobar pneumonia.

Western Medical Diagnosis and Basis:

Diagnosis: upper right lobar pneumonia.

Basis:

(1) History of illness: acute disease for 2 days.

(2) Symptoms: fever, aversion to cold, pain in the chest, cough with phlegm, difficulty in respiration, and dyspnea.

(3) Body signs: vocal fremitus and strengthened voice conduction above the 4th right rib, resonance, percussion pain, and bubbling sound.

(4) Laboratory Examination: WBC: 29800/cubic millimeter, N: 97%, L: 3%.

(5) Fluoroscopy of Chest: upper right lobar pneumonia.

Western Medical Treatment:

Supporting Treatment:

10%G·S	500cc
5%G·N·S	1000cc
5%G·S	1000cc
Vitc	2g/V1time/day

Expectant Treatment: physical cooling and alcohol bath if necessary.

Other Examination:

(1) blood Rt, urine Rt, feces Rt.

(2) Phlegm cultivation + drug allergy.

(3) Fluoroscopy of Chest: eutopic chest roentgenogram.

Recorder: ×××

at 17:20 on February 22, 1982

Section 4 Written Form and Contents for the First Medical Record of Internal Outpatient

Name: Sex:

Age: Occupation:

Work Unit: Consulting Time:

Diagnostic Interrogation:

Chief Complaint:

History of Illness:

Inspection, Auscultation and Olfaction, Pulse Feeling and Palpation:

Analyzing and Differentiating Symptoms:

Diagnosis (syndrome type is written in brackets after names of disease and syndrome):

Therapy:

Recipe and Drugs (recipe name, ingredients and dosage):

Medical Order:

Somatoscopy and Physicochemical examination:

Diagnosis by modern medicine: (name(s) of disease(s), the principal one comes first)

Signature of doctor: ×××

O'clock Min Date

Questions for Review

1. What are the general requirements for writing out a case record of the TCM internal department?
2. How to master contents of the in-patient record of the TCM internal department?
3. Which part of the case record of the internal department do the characteristics of TCM reflect?
4. What are your understandings and comments on writing a case record of the internal department?
5. What are the form and content for writing an out—patient record for the first time?

Systematic Considerations

Common Cold

〔Simple Introduction〕

Common cold is referred to a disease resulted from attack of the body by pathogenic wind, manifested in clinic mainly by nasal stuffiness and nasal discharge, sneezing, headache, chills, fever, malaise in the whole body, etc.. In mild case, it is also termed as "shangfeng" (wind-impairment i. e. impaired by wind evil) or "maofeng" (affection by wind) or "maohan" (affection by cold); and in severe case, it is also termed as "severe shangfeng" (severe common cold). In a certain period of time, it spreads extensively and a lot of people have similar symptoms, which is named as influenza. This disease occurs all the year round, particularly in the winter and spring. Because of changes of the climate during four seasons in a year, variance of the pathogens and patients' constitutions, common cold may be mild or severe in severity and can be divided into two major categories, i. e. wind-cold and wind-heat. It may be complicated with dampness or summer-heat in some cases and also occurs in some patients with weak constitution.

For treatment of the upper respiratory tract infection and influenza termed in modern medicine, please consult contents of the present chapter.

〔Cause of Disease and Pathogenesis〕

Common cold often results mainly from affection of the body by pathogenic wind or pestilential evils, particularly from abrupt change of the climate, abnormal cold or warmth, and deficiency of the vital energy of the body.

1. Affection by pathogenic wind and pestilential toxicity

Wind evil is the first one of the six pathogenic factors, but in different seasons, it often invades the human body along with the seasonal pathogenic factors. For instance, in winter, the wind evil mostly belongs to wind-cold, during spring, it mostly to wind-heat; during summer, it is often mixed with summer-heat and dampness pathogens; during autumn, it is often accompanied by dryness pathogen; and during plum rain season, it is frequently combined with dampness pathogen. In any one of the four seasons, if the climate gets abnormal, common cold or flu may occur. For example, in spring, the weather should be warm but is still cold; in summer, it should be hot, but gets very cool; in autumn, it should be cool, but gets hot; and in winter, it should be cold but becomes rather warm, under the circumstances, pathogenic wind, or cold, or summer-heat or dampness may invade the human body to induce common cold or influenza. Those indicate that affection by external wind-evil is the main cause of common cold, but wind-evil injuries the human body to produce disease often in combination with seasonal or non-seasonal evils or with non-seasonal evils plus pestilential toxicity.

2. Weakness of the body resistance and dysfunction of the lung and wei-system

If one gets abnormal in daily life habit, including irregularity in keeping cold and warmth and excessive fatigue, the defensive function of the muscles and skin will be injured and the regulative functions of the lung and wei-system will fall into disorder and the human body will protect itself from attack of pathogenic factors. As a result, he or she is very liable to catch a cold due to weak constitution. Additionally, the nature of the pathogenic factors affected is closely related to the character of the patient's own constitution, for example, people with yang-deficiency constitution are likely to catch win-cold type common cold, those with yin-deficiency constitution likely to catch wind-heat or dry-heat type common cold, those with hyperactivity of dampness liable to be affected by external damp-evil, and those with hyperactivity of damp-heat liable to be affected by summer-heat, etc.

In a word, common cold is located in the lung and wei-system. The wind is roving in nature. When the exopathogens invade the human body, the lung and wei-system are the first organs to be affected, resulting in suppression of the defensive-yang and disharmony between ying and wei. The resultant struggle between the vital energy and the pathogenic factors induces aversion to cold, fever, headache, pantalgia etc.; and the resultant failure of the lung-qi in dispersing and descending leads to nasal stuffiness, nasal discharge, cough and sore throat, etc.

Because of variance of affection by sudden changes of the climate of the four seasons in a year and due to difference of patients' constitutions, clinical syndromes have wind-cold or wind-heat type, or one of the two types with coexistence of dampness, summer-heat, dryness, or deficiency. And during development of the disease, transformation or coexistence of cold and heat syndromes is often met.

〔Differentiation of Syndromes and Treatment〕

1. Main points for differentiating different syndromes

1) Wind-cold or wind-heat

Wind-cold type common cold is often seen in patients with general or yang-deficiency constitution and occurs mostly during winter, manifested as aversion to cold being severer, fever being mild, headache, pantalgia, nasal stuffiness and nasal clear discharge, throat itching, white fur, superficial and tense pulse, no thirst and no throat swelling or pain. Wind-heat type common cold is frequently seen in patients with ordinary, or yin-deficiency or yang-excess constitution and occurs mostly in spring, marked by fever being severer, aversion to cold being mild, nasal stuffiness, nasal yellowish discharge, thirst, sore throat, superficial and rapid pulse.

2) Differentiation of accompanied syndromes

Common cold complicated with dampness is often seen in plum rain season, marked by recessive fever, head distension being as wrapped by a piece of cloth, osteodynia, chest choking sensation, tastelessness or sweet taste.

Common cold complicated with summer-heat is frequently seen in the last month of summer (long summer), characterized as fever, sweating, irritability, thirsty, scanty dark urine, yellow greasy tongue coating, etc.

Common cold complicated with dryness is frequently met in autumn, manifested as fever, headache, dry nose and throat, cough without or with less sputum, thirst, red tongue, etc.

Common cold with concomitant indigestion is often met in patients with overeating, manifested as fever, gastric distension, poor appetite, nausea, diarrhea, greasy fur, etc.

3) Differentiation of mildness and seriousness, deficiency and excess

Common cold mostly belongs to exterior-excess syndrome, with the state of illness being milder and the duration being shorter. In patients with weak physique, common cold mostly belongs to the type of coexistence of deficiency and excess, the state of the disease is closely related to patients' physique and pathogenic factors, and the duration of disease is longer. Influenza mostly belongs to excess syndrome, the state of illness is more serious and the duration is difficult to be estimated. The comparison among them is shown as follows:

	Common cold	Common cold of deficiency type	Influenza
Age	mostly in youth and middle aged people	mostly in the middle aged and the aged people	in people with any age
Constitution	sthenia	weakness	weakness
Chronic disease	generally not existing	mostly existing	uncertain
Evoked factors	disorder of cold and warmth, excessive fatigue	slight careless-ness	in the period of seasonal pestilence, contact with influenza patients
Characters of syndromes	good constitution, excess of evils, excess of symptoms, excess of syndromes	coexistence of deficiency and excess, coexistence of cold and heat, variance in the state of illness	mostly being excess-syndrome, or coexistence of deficiency and excess, variance in the the state of illness
Infectivity	no	no	yes

4) Differentiation of common cold and exogenous febrile disease orepidemic febrile disease

Common cold is generally lighter in severity and locates in the topical lung-wei system. While febrile diseases and epidemic diseases are very serious in the state of illness, marked mainly by aversion to cold and fever. When they attack, the pathogenic factors of febrile diseases develop from the exterior to the interior of the body and the progress process of epidemic febrile diseases is from wei-fen to qi-fen, ying-fen and xue-fen respectively.

Diagrammatic Sketch of the Etiology and Pathogenesis of Common Cold

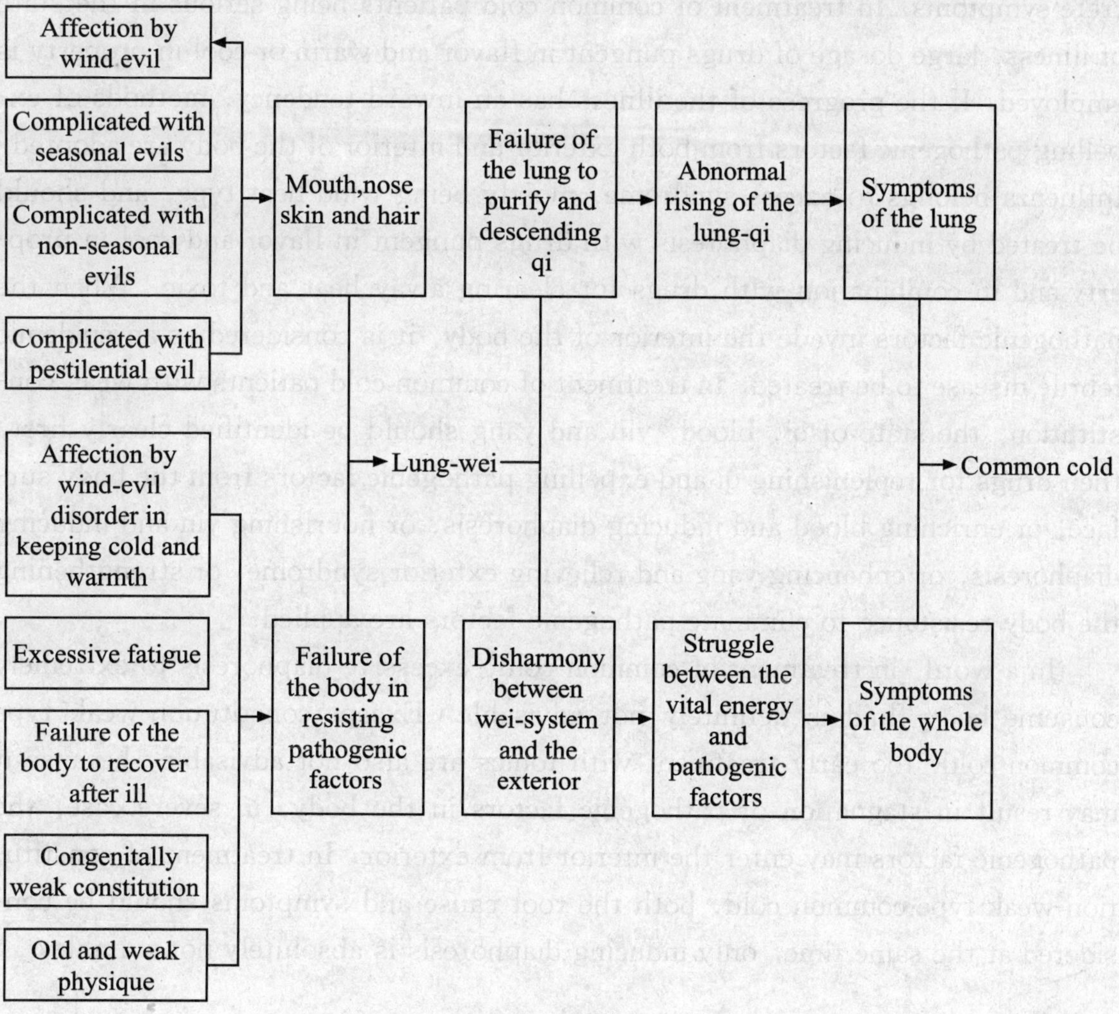

2. Typing and Treatment

Concerning common cold, the pathogenic factors are in the lung and wei-system. Generally speaking, common cold mostly belongs to excess-syndrome and should be treated with inducing diaphoresis to eliminate pathogenic factors. For treatment of wind-cold type common cold, inducing diaphoresis with drugs pungent in flavor and warm in property is used; for treatment of wind-heat type common cold, relieving the exterior syndrome with drugs pungent in flavor and cool in property is given; for common cold complicated with summer-heat and dampness, eliminating summer-heat and dampness from the body by diaphoresis is employed; for common cold with dryness syndrome transformed from dampness, some other Chinese medicinal herbs are added or subtracted according to the concrete symptoms. In treatment of common cold patients being serious in the state of illness, large dosage of drugs pungent in flavor and warm or cool in property is employed. If the progress of the illness has an inward tendency, methods of expelling pathogenic factors from both exterior and interior of the body are adopted. Influenza belongs to excess-syndrome, mostly being wind-heat type, and should be treated by inducing diaphoresis with drugs pungent in flavor and cool in property and in combination with drugs for clearing away heat and toxic. When the pathogenic factors invade the interior of the body, it is considered as an epidemic febrile disease to be treated. In treatment of common cold patients with weak constitution, the state of qi, blood, yin and yang should be identified clearly first, then drugs for replenishing qi and expelling pathogenic factors from the body surface, or enriching blood and inducing diaphoresis, or nourishing yin and inducing diaphoresis, or enhancing yang and relieving exterior syndrome, or strengthening the body resistance to eliminate pathogenic factors are applied.

In a word, in treatment of common cold, excessive diaphoresis to extremely consume body fluid is definitely not advisable. Except constitution-weak type common cold, too early treatment with tonics are also not advisable, because it may result in stagnation of pathogenic factors in the body, in severe case, the pathogenic factors may enter the interior from exterior. In treatment of constitution-weak type common cold, both the root cause and symptoms should be considered at the same time, only inducing diaphoresis is absolutely not suitable.

1) Wind-cold type common cold

Main symptoms: nasal stuffiness, muffled voice, sneezing, running nose, itching throat, whitish thin sputum, etc. in mild cases; aversion to cold being severer, mild fever, anhidrosis, headache, arthralgia etc. in serious cases.

Concomitant symptoms:

(1) common cold complicated with dampness: heavy head, fatigue, chest distress, nausea, poor appetite, diarrhea, tastelessness without thirst;

(2) that complicated with sputum: cough, profuse sputum, chest distress, poor appetite;

(3) that complicated with qi-stagnation: chest distress and discomfort, and pain in the hypochondria in severe case;

(4) that complicated with interior-fire: symptoms of both severe cold-

syndrome and interior-heat syndrome may be seen at the same time, such as cough, shortness of breath, yellowish sticky and thick sputum, irritability, deep dark urine, constipation.

Tongue picture and pulses: Thin white tongue with moisture, and superficial or superficial tense pulse may be seen in patients with common cold; for common cold complicated with dampness or sputum, white greasy coating, and slippery pulse can be seen; and if being complicated with qi-stagnation, taut pulse often appears; and for cold type common cold complicated with interior-fire syndrome, yellow tongue coating and superficial rapid pulse will appear.

Analysis: Wind and cold pathogens invade the upper-jiao of the body to result in stagnation of the lung-qi, manifested as nasal stuffiness, muffled voice, running nose, itching throat, and cough. Cold evil is a yin pathogen, so patients have no thirst or have thirst with desire of drinking hot water, and white clean and thin sputum. Cold pathogen invades the superficial part of the body, leading to closed interspace of muscle, suppression of defensive yang, thus, aversion to cold, fever and anhidrosis. The resultant stagnation of clear yang and impairment of collateral branch of the meridian induce headache and arthrodynia of extremities. Thin white tongue coating with moisture, and floating-tight pulse are signs of exterior cold syndrome.

Therapeutic principles: Relieving the exterior syndrome with pungunt and warm herbs, promoting the dispersing function of the lung and clearing away pathogenic cold.

Recipe and drugs: Supplemented Congchi Decoction or Modified Jingfang Baidu San are used. In the former recipe, Bulbus Allii Fistulosi is employed to activating yang to expel cold; Semen Sojae Paraeparatum used to remove pathogenic factors from the exterior; Folium Perillae (larger dose) and Semen Armeniacae Amarum are used to ventilate the lung and resolve phlegm; Herba Schizonepetae and Radix Ledebouriellae used to increase the dispersing power of the herbs pungent in flavor and warm in property. Supplemented Congchi Decoction is mostly used to treat mild type common cold. In the later recipe, Herba Schizonepetae, Radix Ledebouriellae and Rhizoma Zingiberis Recens are pungent in flavor and warm in property and used to expel cold; Herba Schizonepetae and Herba Menthae are used to dispel exterior syndrome and remove fever; Rhizoma Chuanxiong is used to promote blood circulation and dispel wind for treatment of headache; Radix Peucedani, Radix Platycodi, Fructus Aurantii, Poria and dried Radix

Glycyrrhizae are used to ventilate the lung, regulate qi, resolve sputum and stop cough; Zhizoma seu Radix Notopterygii and Radix Angelicae Pubescent function in expelling wind and clearing away cold, as well as eliminating dampness at the same time and are the important herbs for treatment of pain in the extremities. Radix Ginseng of this recipe is used to enhance body resistance to eliminate pathogenic factors and is thus not used for common cold patients with excess syndrome. this recipe is mostly used to treat severe common cold. For common cold complicated with dampness syndrome, Cortex Magnoliae Officinalis, Pericarpium Citri Reticulatae, Rhizoma Atractylodis and Rhizoma Pinelliae are added, or Modified Qianghuo Shengshi Decoction is employed to dispel wind and remove dampness; for that complicated with sputum syndrome, Erchen Decoction is supplemented to resolve sputum and dampness; for that complicated with qi-stagnation, Rhizoma Cyperi, Caulis Perillae, etc are supplemented to regulate qi and soothe the liver; for that with mixture of exterior -cold and interior-heat syndromes, Maxing Shigan Decoction is employed to relieve the exterior-cold and interior-heat syndromes, and if the exterior-cold is severer, Herba Schizonepetae and Radix Ledebouriellae are used to relieve the exterior-syndrome, and if the interior-heat is severer, Radix Scutellariae, Rhizoma Anemarrhenae and Frutus Gardeniae are employed to clear away heat; and that with both exterior- and interior-excess, Modified Fangfeng Tongsheng Powder is employed.

Recipe example:

Fermented Soybean 10g, Folium Perillae 10g, Herba Schizonepetae 10g, Radix Ledebouriellae 10g, Radix Platycodi 6g, Rhizoma Cynanchi Stauntonii 10g, Rhizoma Ligustici Chuanxiong 10g, Radix Glycyrrhizae 6g, Semen Armeniacae Amarum 10g, Fructus Aurantii 10g and Rhizoma Zingiberis Recens 10g.

2) Wind-heat type common cold

Main symptoms: Fever, slight aversion to cold, obstructed sweating, headache, nasal stuffiness, nasal discharge, dryness of mouth, thirst, reddish swelling and sore throat, cough, and yellowish sticky sputum.

Concomitant symptoms:

(1) In severe wind-heat type of common cold patients or affected by seasonal evils, high fever without declining of body temperature, aversion to cold or chill, headache, dryness of nose and throat, thirst and irritability are often seen;

(2) in wind-heat type common cold patients with concurrent dampness, head

heaviness, tiredness, chest distress, nausea and dark urine may be seen;

(3) in those with concurrent summer-dampness, higher fever, sweating without lowering of body temperature, heaviness of extremities, thirst, scanty or dark urine are frequently seen; and

(4) in those with concurrent autumn-dryness, dryness of mouth, lips, nose and throat, thirst, dry cough without sputum or with hard expectorated sputum can be seen.

Tongue pictures and pulses: Thin yellowish tongue coating and superficial rapid pulse are seen in wind-heat type common cold patients; if wind-heat type common cold is serious, reddish tongue with yellowish coating often appears; if this type common cold is complicated with dampness, yellowish greasy tongue coating is seen; if it is combined with summer-heat, yellowish greasy fur and soft rapid pulse will be seen; and if it is combined with dryness, red tongue with less moisture, slight rapid pulse will be seen.

Analysis: Wind and heat pathogens invade the superficial part of the body and heat accumulates in the skin and muscles, resulting in dysfunction of the wei-system, which is manifested as fever, slight aversion to wind-cold, sweating without declining of fever; up-disturbing of wind-heat leads to distending-pain in the head; wind-heat pathogens fumigate the throat to induce swelling pain, dryness and thirst, turbid nasal discharge; wind-heat invades the lung to bring about dysfunction of purifying and descending of lung-qi, and cough with sticky or yellowish sputum. White and sight yellowish fur and floating rapid pulse are signs of invasion of the lung by wind-heat.

Therapeutic principles: Relieving exterior syndrome by using herbs pungent in flavor and cool in property, dispelling pathogenic factors from the lung.

Recipes and drugs: Modified Yinqiao Powder, from which Flos Lonicerae and Fructus Forsythiae are pungent in flavor and cool in property and are used to dispel pathogenic factors from the exterior and remove heat and toxic materials; Herba Menthae, Herba Schizonepetae and Semen Sojae Praeparatum are employed to dispel wind, relieve exterior syndrome and drive pathogenic factors out; Radix Platycodi, Fructus Arctii and Radix Glycyrrhizae are used to ventilate the lung, resolve sputum and reduce pharyngeal swelling; Herba Lophatheri and Rhizoma Phragmitis are sweat in flavor and cool in property and function in promoting production of body fluid to quench thirst. For common headache, Folium Mori and Flos Chrysanthemi are supplemented to remove wind-heat from the head and improve vision; for cough with profuse sputum, Semen Armeniacae and Bulbus Fritillariae Cirrhosae as well as Pericarium Trichosanthis are supplemented to relieve cough and reduce sputum; for severe red swelling sore-throat, Radix Isatidis, Lasiosphaera seu Calvatia and Radix Scrophulariae are added to clear away heat, relieve exterior syndrome and the sore-throat; for severe wind-heat type common cold or epidemic common cold, on the basis of applying Yinqiao Powder, Radix Puerariae is supplemented to expel pathogenic factors from muscles and skin; Radix Scutellariae and Gypsum Fibrosum are supplemented to clear away heat; Rhizoma Anemarrhenae and Radix Trichosanthis supplemented to promote production of body fluid to quench thirst. For wind-heat common cold combined with dampness, on the basis of applying Yinqiao Powder, Herba Agastachis and Herba Eupatorii are added to remove dampness. In summer, for treatment of wind-heat type common cold with summer-heat and dampness, Modified Xinjia Xiangru Decoction is used, additionally and according to the characters of seasonal climate, fresh Folium Nelumbinis, Petiolus Nelumbinis, fresh Herba Agastachis and Herba Eupatorii, Exocarpium Citrulli, Liu Yi Powder etc. can be selected to eliminate summer-heat and dampness. In autumn, wind-heat type common cold with concurrent dryness, Yinqiao Powder is used in combination with Semen Armeniacae, pear peel, Pericarpium Trichosanthis, etc. or, Modified Sang Xing Decoction is used to dispel wind and remove dryness, clear away lung-heat and nourish lung-yin.

Example of recipe:

Herba Schizonepetae 10g, Herba Menthae 6g (decocted later), Semen Sojae Praeparatum 10g, Flos Lonicerae 10g, Fructus Forsythiae 10g, Radix Platycodi 6g, Radix Glycyrrhizae 6g, prepared Fructus Arctii 10g, fresh Rhizoma Phragmitis 30g, Bilbus Fritillariae Thunbergii 10g and Semen Armeniacae 10g.

3) Somatasthenia type common cold

(1) Qi-deficiency type common cold

Main symptoms: Aversion to cold, fever, headache, nasal stuffiness, cough with white sputum, lassitude and weakness, shortness of breath, indolence of speaking.

Concomitant symptoms: Obesity and hyperhidrosis, dim complexion, old or chronic asthma, chronic epigastralgia etc.

Tongue picture and pulse: Pale tongue with thin white fur, floating weak pulse.

Analysis: Qi-deficiency results in failure of the body to resist exopathogens; and wind-cold tightening the exterior induces obstruction of the lung-qi, as a result, the exterior syndrome occurs. Due to original qi-deficiency or weakness of body-resistance, shortness of breath, indolence of speaking, lassitude and weakness are thus seen. The aforementioned tongue picture and pulse suggest qi-deficiency and also indicate that pathogenic factors are located at the wei-fen or the exterior of the body.

Therapeutic principles: Replenishing qi and relieving exterior syndrome.

Recipe and drugs: Modified Shen Su Decoction. In this recipe, Radix Codonopsis Pilosulae is often used instead of Radix Ginseng, Poria and Radix Glycyrrhizae are used to replenish qi, and strengthen the body resistance to eliminate pathogenic factors; Folium Perillae and Radix Puerariae are used to dispel wind and relieve exterior syndrome; Radix Peucedani, Radix Platycodi, Fructus Aurantii, Rhizoma Pinelliae and Pericarpium Citri Reticulatae employed to ventilate the lung, regulate qi, resolve sputum and relieve cough. If deficiency of qi is severer, Radix Astragali seu Hedysari is supplemented or Bu Zhong Yiqi Decoction used in combination with Folium Perillae, etc for supplementing qi and expelling pathogenic factors from the body surface. For patients with qi-deficiency and spontaneous perspiration and susceptible to be affected by exogenous pathogenic factors, Yu Pingfeng Powder is selected to replenish qi, consolidate superficial resistance, suppress sweating and expel wind.

Example of recipe: Folium Perillae 10g, Radix Codonopsis Pilosulae 10g, Poria 10g, Radix Glycyrrhizae 6g, Radix Peucedani 10g, Radix Platycodi 6g, Fructus Aurantii 10g, Rhizoma Pinelliae 10g, Pericarpium Citri Reticulatae 10g, Semen Armeniacae 10g and Rhizoma Ligustici Chuanxiong 10g.

(2) Yang-deficiency type common cold

Main symptoms: Lighter fever, severer aversion to cold, headache, pantagia, pale complexion, cold limbs, feeble voice of speaking, etc.

Concomitant symptoms: Old and general asthenial or accompanied by chronic diarrhea before dawn, edema, deficiency of both spleen and kidney-yang due to consumption.

Tongue picture and pulse: Pale and bulgy tongue with white thin fur, deep and weak pulse.

Analysis: Insufficiency of yang-qi can not warm and nourish muscles and skin, thus, external cold symptoms, such as feeble voice of speaking, cold limbs, pale and bulgy tongue, deep and weak pulse appear. After affection by wind-cold pathogens, the exterior-cold syndrome is more serious, manifested by severer cold and lighter fever. Wind-cold pathogens tighten the exterior to result in suppression of yang-qi and dysfunction of the collateral branches of meridians, inducing headache and pantalgia.

Therapeutic principles: Strengthening yang and relieving exterior syndrome

Recipes and drugs: Modified Shenfu Zaizhao Pill. Aconiti Praeparata and Ramulus Cinnamomi from this recipe are used to strengthen yang. Qi belongs to yang, when yang is deficient, qi is also insufficient, so, Radix Genseng, Radix Astragali seu Hedysari and prepared Radix Glycyrrhizae are used; Rhizoma seu Radix Notopterygii, Radix Ledebouriellae and Herba Asari are used to relieve exterior syndrome and dispel cold. The present recipe functions in strengthening yang, replenishing qi and clearing away pathogenic cold from the exterior of the body, and induces diaphoresis without impairment of the body resistance and supplements yang and qi without remains of pathogens. If the patient has aversion to cold without sweating and lighter deficiency of yang, Modified Mahuang Fuzhi Xixin Decoction can also be applied.

Example of recipe: Sliced Aconiti Praeparata 6g, Ramulus Cinnamomi 10g, Radix Codonopsis Pilosulae 10g, dried Radix Astragali seu Hedysari 15g, Rhizoma seu Radix Notopterygii 10g, Radix Ledebouriellae 18g, Herba Asari 3g, Radix Platycodi 6g, Radix Glycyrrhizae 6g, Semen Armeniacae 10g and Radix Peucedani 10g.

(3) Blood-deficiency type common cold

Main symptoms: Headache, fever, slight aversion to cold, anhidrosis, dim complexion, pale lips and finger nails, palpitation and dizziness.

Concomitant Symptoms: Postpartum stage or hypermenorrhea, hematohidrosis, hemafesia, etc.

Tongue picture and pulse condition: Pale tongue with white coating, thready pulse or weak floating pulse.

Analysis: Due to deficiency of yin and blood, dizziness, palpitation, pale complexion, pale lips and finger nails are often seen. Because of deficiency of blood, Ying- and wei-systems are unable to protect the body against pathogenic factors, the human body is susceptible to affection by exopathogens, manifested as headache, fever, slight aversion to cold, anhidrosis, pale tongue, thready or weak floating pulse.

Therapeutic principles: Nourishing blood and relieving exterior syndrome.

Recipes and drugs: Modified Congbai Qiwei Powder; in the recipe, Bulbus Allii Fistulosi, Semen Sojia Praeparatum, Radix Puerariae and Rhizoma Zingiberis Recens are used to relieve exterior syndrome; and Radix Rehmanniae and Radix Ophiopogonis used to nourish yin and supplement blood. Inducing sweating while supplementing blood does not injure yin and blood. If being severer in aversion to cold, the above mentioned recipe or Siwu Decoction is used in combination with Folium Perillae and Herba Schizonepetae; if being severer in fever, the above mentioned recipe is used in combination with Flos Lonicerace and Fructus Forsythiae or Radix Scutellariae; or Chai Hu Si Wu Decoction is used; and for continuous bleeding, Colla Corii Asini, Nodus Nelumbinis Rhizomatis, Rhizoma Bletillae, Radix Notoginseng, etc are added.

Example of recipe: Radix Angelicae Sinensis 10g, Redix Rehmanniae 10g, Radix Paeoniae Alba 10g, Rhizoma Ligustici Chuanxiong 10g, Herba Schizonepetae 10g, Radix Ledebouriellae 10g, Radix Bupleuri 10g, Radix Glycyrrhizae 6g, Semen Armeniacae 10g and Radix Purerariae 10g.

(4) Yin-deficiency type common cold

Tongue picture and pulse condition: Red tongue with exfoliative fur or without fur, and a thready and rapid pulse.

Main symptoms: Headache, fever, slight aversion to wind-cold, anhidrosis or mild sweating, or night sweating, dizziness, irritability, thirst, dryness of throat, feverish sensation in the palms and soles, dry cough with less sputum, or with blood-tinged sputum.

Concomitant symptoms: Dysphoria with feverish sensation in chest, palms and soles, insomnia, constipation, etc. (often seen in patients with yin-deficiency constitution or with weak physique after falling ill)

Analysis: Yin-deficiency produces heat in the interior of the body, resulting in dizziness, irritability, feverish sensation in palms and soles; yin-deficiency and less body fluid lead to thirst, dryness of throat, dry cough with less sputum; yin-deficiency physique with additional affection by exopathogen and heat-transformation leads to headache, fever and slight aversion to cold, wind-heat syndrome is thus often seen. Red tongue with exfoliative fur or without fur, thready and rapid pulse are signs of internal heat due to yin-deficiency.

Therapeutic principles: Nourishing yin and relieving exterior syndrome.

Recipes and drugs: Modified Weirui Decoction. In this recipe, Rhizoma Polygouati Odorati is used to nourish yin and promote production of body fluid for increasing the source of sweating; Bulbus Allii Fistulosi, Semen Sojia Praeparatum, Radix Platycodi and Herba Menthae are employed to induce sweating and relieve exterior syndrome for dispelling exopathogens; Radix Cynanchi Atrati is used to clear away heat, normalize yin and expel pathogenic factors from the exterior; Fructus Ziziphi Jujubae and Radix Glycyrrhizae are sweet in taste and moist in property and are employed to regulate the middle-jiao and to help Rhizoma Polygouati Odorati to nourish yin. The aforementioned recipe induces sweating without impairment of yin and nourish yin without keeping pathogenic factors. For severer exterior syndrome, this recipe is used in combination with Herba Menthae and Herba Schizonepetae for dispelling wind pathogen from the exterior of the body. For dryness of throat, cough with difficult expectoration, Fructus Arctii and Pericarpium Trichosanthis are supplemented to relieve sore-throat and resolve sputum; and for severer irritability and thirst, Herba Lophatheri and Radix Trichosanthis supplemented to eliminate heat and stop irritability, promote production of body fluid to quench thirst.

Example of recipe: Rhizoma Polygouati Odorati 15g, Radix Cynanchi Atrati 10g, Radix Ophiopogonis 10g, Radix Adenophorae 15g, Radix Scrophulariae 12g, Radix Glycyrrhizae 6g, Semen Oroxyli 5g, fried Fructus Arctii 10g, Rhizoma Phragmitis 30g, Rhizoma Imperatae 30g, Radix Schizonepetae 10g.

Although the above-mentioned deficiency type common cold is subdivided into qi-, blood- yang- and yin-deficiency types, insufficiency of both qi and yin, insufficiency of qi and blood, and deficiency of both yin and yang are also seen in clinic. It is thus needed to differentiate different syndromes carefully and select related herbs.

〔Measures for Prevention and Nursing〕

1) Keep air in the room fresh and temperature suitable; 2) Keep a regular daily life, be careful about changes of temperature, and take regular exercise to enhance one's health; 3) Patients with serious common cold (aversion to cold and fever) should be confined to bed, and patients with influenza should be isolated; 4) Pay attention to changes of patients' body temperature, sweating, pulse condition, tongue picture, etc.; 5) Drink more warm boiled water and have light food; for patients with light fever, half-liquid diet is suitable and after decline of body

temperature, meat dish and half-liquid food or common food are preferable; and 6) Drugs for prevention and treatment of common cold:

(1) During winter and spring when wind and cold weather is prevalent, Rhizoma Dryopteris Crassirhizomae 10g, Folium Perillae 10g, Herba Schizonepetae 10g and Radix Glycyrrhizae 3g are decocted in water and taken one dose daily, continuously for 3 days.

(2) During summer, when summer-heat and dampness are prevalent, Herba Agastachis 10g, Herba Eupatorii 10g and Herba Menthae 5g (for fresh herbs, larger does are used) are decocted in water and serve as a drink to be taken.

(3) If seasonal pathogens are in vogue for a time, Rhizoma Dryopteris Crassirhizomae 15g, Radix Isatidis (or Folium Isatidis) 12g and dried Radix Glycyrrhizae 3g are decocted in water and taken one dose daily. For preventing infection, vinegar fumigating method can be used in rooms by heating mixed solution of vinegar 5～10ml plus water 10～20ml for 2 hours, once every other day.

〔Typical Case〕

Zhang ××, male, adult. His first visit was on February 25, 1995.

Clinical manifestations and diagnosis: Aversion to cold, fever, headache, osteodynia, frequent vomiting, thin greasy tongue coating and floating pulse, suggesting an exopathetic disease with accumulation of damp-heat in the interior and failure of the stomach-qi in descending. It was treated with dispelling pathogenic factors from the exterior, ventilating the lung and eliminating dampness.

Prescription: Soya-bean sprouts 12g, Caulis Perillae with leaves 4.5g, Herba Menthae 2.4g (decocted later), Folium Mori (collected in winter) 9g, fried Flos Chrysanthemi 4.5g, tender Radix Peucedani 4.5g, Bulbus Fritillariae Thunbergii 9g, Rhizoma Coptidis (prepared with fresh ginger) 1g, and Ganlu Xiaodu Pill (decocted by wrapping), 2 doses.

Second consultation: Both cold-aversion and fever abated, headache and vomiting were relieved, but, the patient still could not sleep well and had bitter taste in mouth, suggesting existence of damp-heat and disorder of stomach-qi. It was treated by regulating the stomach-qi to tranquilize the mind and eliminating dampness and heat.

Prescription: Poria cum Ligno Hospite 9g, prepared Radix Polygalae 3g, fried Semen Ziziphi Spinosae 9g, Fructus Tritici Levis 12g, fried Radix Stellariae 3g, prepared Rhizoma Pinelliae 4.5g, alcohol-fried Radix Scutellariae 4.5g,

Exocarpium Citri Reticulatae 4. 5g, fried Caulis Bambusae in Taeniam 4. 5g, fried husked kaoliang (decocted by wrapping up) 9g, fried Fructus Hordei Germinatus 12g, two doses.

Note: The present case is a common cold complicated with damp-heat and is treated mainly by relieving exterior syndrome and eliminating fever. Radix Scutellariae (imitating the usage of Xiao Caihu Decoction) and Rhizoma Pinelliae (imitating the usage of Erchen Decoction), Rhizoma Coptidis (fried with fresh ginger) and Rhizoma Pinelliae (imitating the usage of heart-fire-purging method) are used together for treatment of both the interior and exterior pathogens at the same time. In this way, exopathogens and dampness, heat and turbid sputum are removed and the therapeutic effect is achieved rapidly. Dispelling pathogenic wind or removing dampness can isolate the condition of heat and shorten the duration of fever.

In conclusion, common cold is a frequently-seen exopathic disease, manifested mainly as nasal stuffiness, nasal discharge, sneezing, cough, headache, aversion to cold, fever, general malaise, etc. In etiology, it results from attack of the lung and wei-system by six evils, seasonal pestilential evils and from weakening of defensive function and inability of the body in regulation and adaptation. According to differentiation of syndromes, properties of pathogenic factors, patients' physique, the exterior-excess syndrome can be divided into wind-cold, wind-heat, summer-heat-dampness and physique-deficiency type common cold, and are treated mainly by dispelling pathogenic factors from the exterior. For wind-cold type, herbs pungent in flavor and warm in property are used; for wind-heat type, herbs pungent in flavor and cool in property used; for summer-heat and damp type, it is treated by clearing away summer-heat and dampness; and for physique-weak type, it is treated by considering the symptoms and cause as a whole and avoiding excessively dispersing. Generally, for treatment of common cold, excessive dispersing should be prohibited, and in addition to physique-weak type, reinforcing and astringing are also excluded.

In short, in treatment of common cold, cold, heat, deficiency and excess should be identified first, followed by fully understanding the concomitant symptoms or complicated syndromes and corresponding treatment.

Questions for Review

1. Try to narrate the difference between common cold and febrile disease and

between common cold and epidemic febrile disease.

2. Try to narrate the differentiation of syndromes and therapeutic principles of wind-cold type and wind-heat type common cold.
3. Try to narrate the differentiation of syndromes and therapeutic principles of qi-deficiency type and yin-deficiency type common cold.

Cough

〔Simple Introduction〕

Cough is one of the important symptoms of pulmonary diseases. It is not only a dependant syndrome but also a symptom of many kinds of disease of the lung. Generally speaking, cough is accompanied by sound production and sputum or no sputum which are difficult to be separated each other in clinic. Cough without sputum is called as dry cough.

In the past dynasties of China, there were quite a few names in regard to nomenclature of cough, while Zhang Jingyue, a famous physician of Ming Dynasty, divided it into two major categories: exopathic cough and internal injury cough.

The exopathic cough and internal injury cough are different and should be strictly distinguished. When treated, it should be carefully analyzed by combining the history and cause of disease, clinical manifestations and necessary physiological and chemical examinations. Exopathic cough is often accompanied by exterior syndrome of the lung-wei, while internal injury cough mostly combined with dysfunction of the internal organs.

Cough discussed in the present chapter is referred to diseases manifesting mainly as cough, which can be consulted mutually with the contents of the concurrent cough of other diseases. Chronic cough can result in asthma, manifesting as deficiency-cold of lung or latent cold fluid-retention in lung, which can be used for reference with contents of asthma and sputum-rheum described in the following parts.

Differentiation of syndromes, diagnosis and treatment of cough in the present chapter may be used for consultation in treatment of cough, a main concurrent symptom induced by upper respiratory tract infection, acute and chronic bronchitis, pneumonia, bronchiectasis, pulmonary tuberculosis, pneumonectasis, pulmonary abscess, etc.

〔Pathogenic Factors and Pathogenesis〕

Cough results from diseases of the lung and from abnormal rising of lung-qi. Its focus is located in the lung but closely related to the liver, spleen and kidney. To sum up, the pathogenic factors of cough are exopathic and internal-injury causes and are introduced briefly as follows:

1. Exopathic cough: It is referred to cough because of invasion of the lung by six exogenous pathogenic factors. When any one of the six exogenous pathogenic factors invades the human body, cough will be initiated, but in clinic, it is most closely related to wind, cold, dryness and heat.

The lung is in charge of qi and is compared to a canopy of the five zang-organs. It connects with throat, opens into nose and is an organ for respiration. It is associated with the skin and hair and communicates with the outside world of the body directly. When attacked by exogenous pathogenic factors, no matter by way of mouth, nose or the skin, the lung-qi is accumulated and obstructed and is unable to function in purifying and descending, leading to abnormal production of sputum-rheum, impeding the free flow of air in the respiratory tract and inducing cough. Due to difference in patients' yin- or yang-constitution and changes of seasonal climate, the exogenous pathogenic factors are various in property. Wind evil is the first and the foremost of the six pathogenic factors, when invading the human body, the other exopathogens often indulge in wanton massacre along with wind evil. Thus, in clinic, cough contains wind-cold, wind-heat and dry-heat types.

2. Internal injury type cough: Internal injury type cough is referred to cough induced by functional disorders of the zang- or fu-organs. When the lung is in hypofunction or gets into trouble due to dysfunction of other zang- or fu-organs, cough occurs immediately. In clinic, a few kinds of its common pathogenesis are:

1) Hypofunction of lung In case of consumption of lung-yin, the lung loses nourishment, inducing adverse rising of qi to evoke cough with less sputum. In case of insufficiency of lung-qi, the lung is incapable of functioning in purifying and descending and dominating qi, resulting in cough and shortness of breath.

2) Dysfunction of spleen When the spleen falls into disorder in transformation and transportation, food is unable to be transformed into essence, or rather becomes sputum pathogen. The resultant damp-sputum accumulates in the lung, causing the lung to lost its functions in dispersing and descending and inducing obstruction of lung-qi. As a result, cough occurs. In addition, the spleen and

lung are mother - and son-organ relationship and belong to Earth and Gold respectively according to the theory of the five elements. The spleen provides the material basis of acquired constitution. When the Earth is weak in function, it can not give birth to the Gold, i.e. when the spleen gets into hypofunction, the lung-qi is insufficient and the lung is incapable of purifying and descending normally, resulting in cough.

3) Attack of the lung by hyperactive liver-fire The Liver Meridian distributes bilaterally in the hypochondrium and costal areas and enters the lung. When the liver-qi is depressed for a long time, it will transform into fire. The resultant fir evil impairs the lung and transforms the body fluid into sputum, hindering the descending ability of the lung to induce cough; and

4) Insufficiency of kidney The kidney has the function of promoting inspiration and is an organ of water and is the source of qi-transformation. If kidney-qi is weak, it will lost its function in accepting qi, inducing reverse rising of qi and inability of qi-transformation. As a result, the water in the body can not flow along the normal way, if accumulating in the lung, it will induce cough immediately. The lung and kidney are mother- and son-organs separately and the lung-yin and kidney-yin nourish the kidney and lung each other. Insufficiency of kidney-yin leads to hyperactivity of fire, consuming lung-yin. The deficient-fire burns the body fluid to turn it into sputum, obstructing the descending function of the lung-qi to produce cough.

In brief, cough can be divided into two major categories of exopathy and internal-injury. The focus of exopathic cough is located in the lung and this type of cough belongs to excess syndrome. It often results from affection of the lung by exogenous pathogenic factors and stagnation of lung-qi. If treated not in time or improperly, it will become a chronic disease to consume and impair lung-qi and lung-yin. As a result, exopathic cough may turn into internal-injury cough. The focus of the internal-injury type cough is also mainly located in the lung, but, has a close relation with the liver, spleen and kidney. This type of cough often belongs to coexistence of evil-excess and body resistance weakness and its pathogenic factors chiefly are sputum and fire. But the sputum contains cold and heat syndromes and the fire includes deficiency and excess types. The sputum can be transformed into fire (or heat) due to accumulation being for a longer period of time. The resultant fire burns the body fluid and turns it into sputum. If other viscera fall into disorder in functional activity to involve the lung, cough occurs often due to evil-excess-induced weakness of the body resistance. For instance, the liver-fire attacks the lung to consume body fluid and impairs the lung, the body fluid will becomes sputum. In case of invasion of the lung by sputum-dampness, it mostly results from dysfunction of the spleen in transportation. Under the circumstances, water and food in the body can not be transformed into essence to be transported to and to nourish the lung and accumulate to become sputum. The resultant sputum stores in the lung and obstructs flow of lung-qi, inducing adverse rising of qi and cough. If this situation develops continuously, deficiency of both spleen-qi and lung-qi will happens, leading to inability of the qi to transform body fluid and causing production of sputum. In severe case, it will results in hypofunction of all the kidney, lung and spleen, impeding normal circulation of qi and blood. In case of insufficiency of lung-yin, it will give rise to flaring-up of fire of deficiency type, consuming body fluid and turning it into sputum, inability of the lung to be moistened and adverse flow of qi to induce cough. In case of deficiency of lung-qi, the lung-qi is unable to function in descending and in transforming body fluid, arousing accumulation of body fluid to become sputum and inducing adverse rising of qi to evoke cough. Moreover, cough patients of internal injury type are liable to attack of exogenous pathogenic factors to get exopathic cough due to hypofunction of zang- or fu-organs and weakness of the ying- and wei-system, which combines together to become coexistence of deficiency- and excess-syndrome. In a word, in spit of variance in the cause of disease and etiology, the pathogenesis still lies in failure of the lung in dispersing and descending abilities and adverse rising of the lung-qi.

〔Differentiation of Syndromes and Treatment〕

1. Main points for differentiating syndromes

1) Differentiation of internal injury type or exopathic type cough

Generally, exopathic type cough has characters of onset being acute, duration of disease being shorter and cough accompanied by exterior syndrome and belongs to excess-syndrome; while internal injury type cough manifests as slow onset, longer duration of disease and cough accompanied by internal-injury syndrome of zang- or fu-organs and belongs to coexistence of deficiency- and excess-syndrome.

2) Differentiation of cold, heat, deficiency and excess

(1) Differentiation of existence or no existence, shape, property, color, texture, amount and taste of sputum.

(a) Dry cough with or without sputum implicates dryness and fire.

(b) Cough with sputum: In case of cough due to impairment of the lung by wind-dryness or wind-cold, the sputum is white in color and is accompanied by thin foam; in case of impairment of lung by wind-heat, the sputum is accompanied by sticky foam; in case of impairment of the lung by heat (deficiency-heat or excess-heat, internal injury or exopathy), the sputum is less in amount, yellow in color and sticky and thick in texture; in case of severe heat or insufficiency of body fluid (mostly due to internal injury), the sputum presents little lump-like shape; in case of obstruction of the lung by wind-dampness, the sputum is profuse and white and is accompanied by bubbles; in case of obstruction of the lung by cold sputum and excessive fluid, the sputum is clear and thin, and if becomes sticky and thick, it indicates a tendency of heat-transformation. Abundant, yellowish and thin expectoration suggests damp-heat or wind-heat; sticky and thick sputum suggests impairment of the lung by heat (deficiency-heat or excess-heat); and pus-like sputum suggests impairment of the lung by fire-heat (excess-heat).

(c) Sweetish sputum suggests spleen-heat; sour and hot sputum means attack of the lung by liver-qi and salt sputum signifies edema due to kidney-deficiency.

(2) Differentiation of cough sound

Cough in a lower, vague voice often implies wind-cold or coexistence of dampness; cough in a loud voice mostly suggests wind-heat; cough in a hoarse voice frequently implies dry-heat; paroxysmal gusts of cough mostly suggest hyperactivity of the liver and gallbladder-fire; cough in a low, muffled voice just like sending forth from a jar often suggests dry-heat and wind-heat; cough in a lower tone mostly belongs to wind-cold; cough in a weak, low voice and attacking now and then, or intermittently implies internal injury, including insufficiency of lung-yin or weakness of lung-qi.

(3) Differentiation of onset time of cough

When cough worsens in winter or due to attack by wind-cold and becomes better in summer, it implies cold- or yang-deficiency-syndrome; if cough worsens in summer and autumn, it often suggests summer-heat- and dampness- or dryness-syndrome; if cough occurs mostly in the morning, it indicates a stomach-fire or excess-heat of the stomach; if cough occurs mostly in the afternoon, it often suggests a yin-deficiency-syndrome; if cough occurs mostly in the dusk, it belongs to hyperactivity of fire due to yin-deficiency, usually being lung-fire; if cough happens mostly during daybreak, it usually implies a sputum-retention; if cough lasts shorter in duration, happens unceasingly day and night, it belongs to affection by exopathogens; and if cough is chronic and attacks continuously, it belongs to internal injury.

Schematic Diagram of Causes and Pathogenesis of Cough

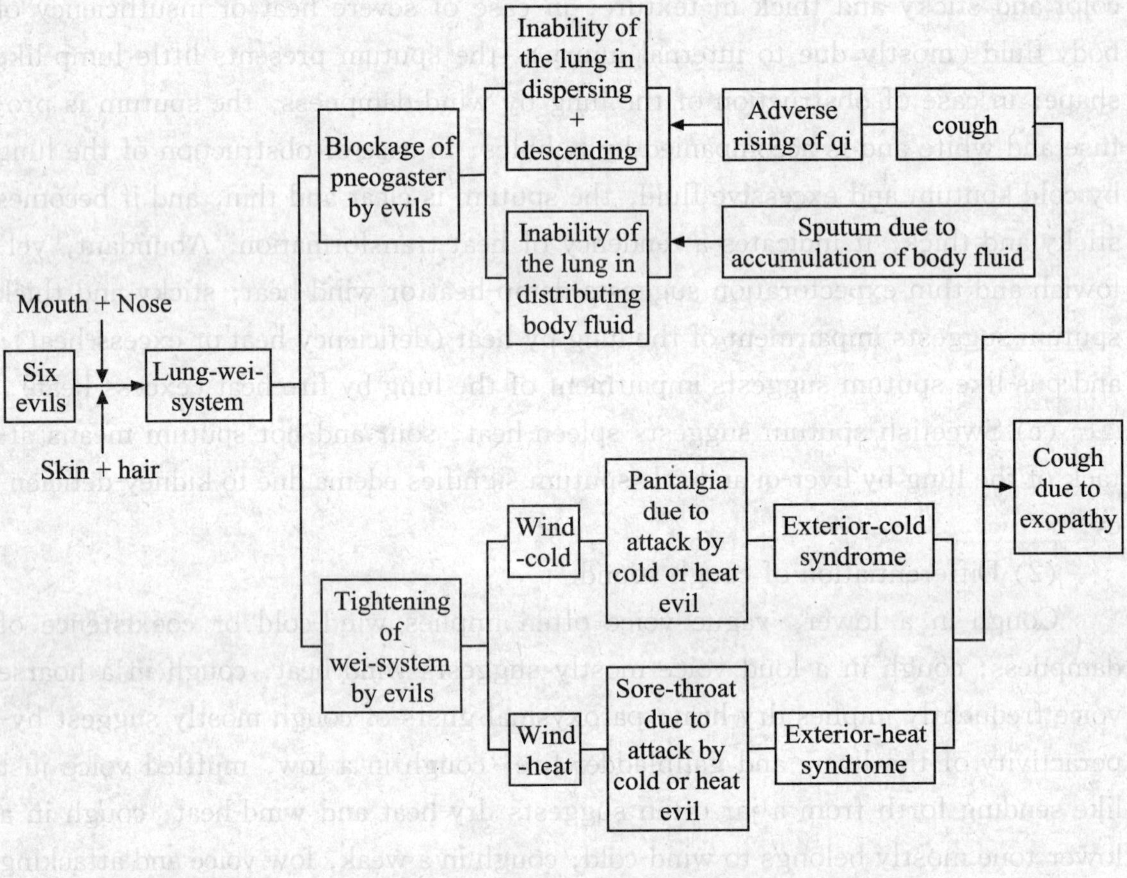

(4) Differentiation of main complicated syndromes of cough

Cough with itching throat often indicates attack of the lung by additional wind evil; cough with polyuria often suggests a concomitant unsolidation of kidney-qi; cough with excessive fatigue suggests existence of qi-deficiency; repeatedly coughing implies existence of dry-heat or liver-fire; cough with exterior syndrome is considered as affection by exopathogen; and, cough with hectic fever and flushing of zygomatic region implies existence of hyperactivity of fire due to yin-deficiency.

Schematic Diagram of Causes and Pathogenesis of Cough

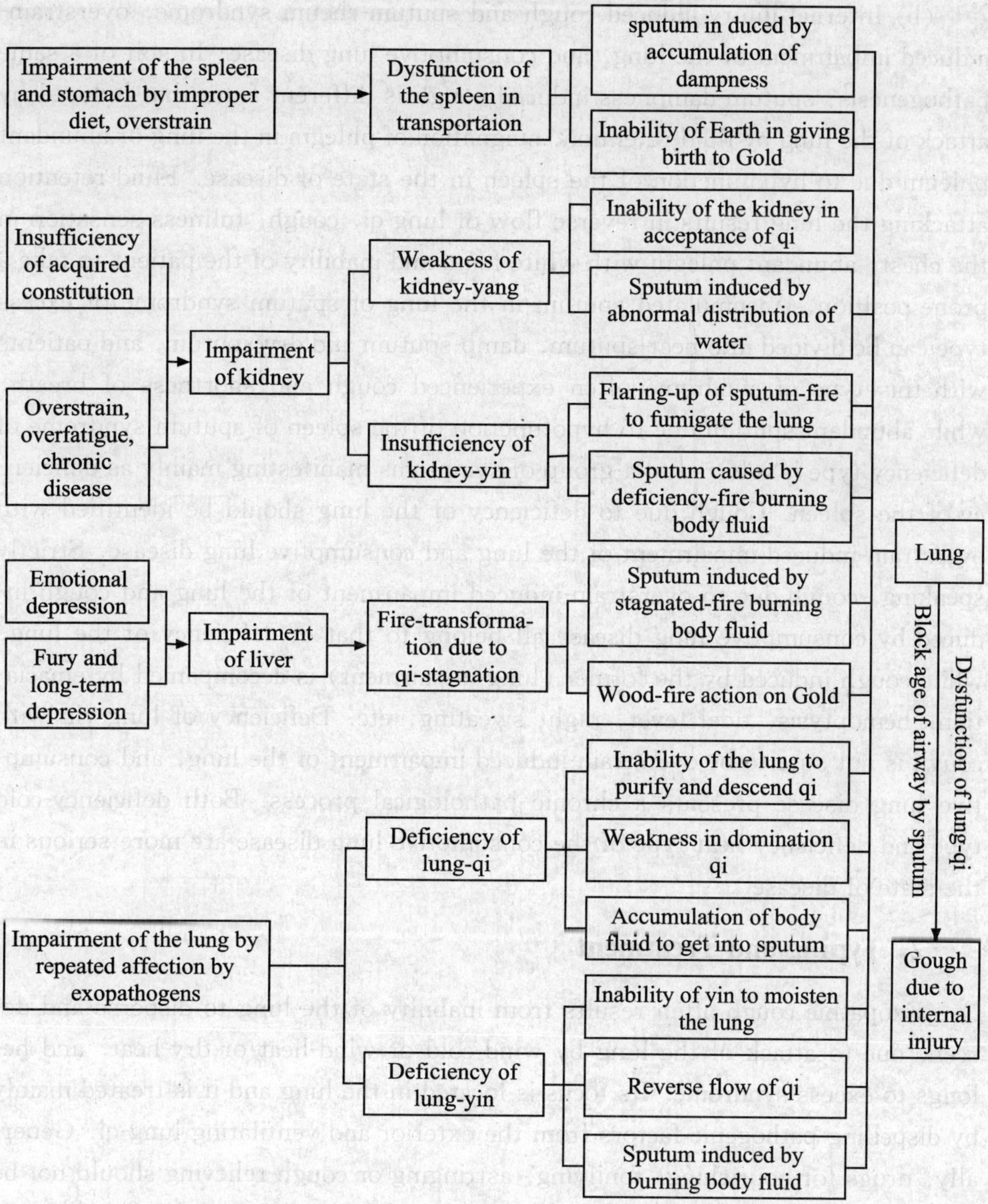

(5) Differentiation of cough and common cold, sputum-rheum, overstrain-in-

duced impairment of the lung, and consumptive lung disease.

(a) Exopathy-induced cough and common cold: Exopathy-induced cough always manifests itself mainly as cough, while common cold chiefly as exterior-syndrome of the lung wei-system.

(b) Internal injury-induced cough and sputum-rheum syndrome, overstrain-induced impairment of the lung, and consumptive lung disease: In spit of a same pathogenesis, sputum-dampness induced cough is different from that induced by attack of the lung by fluid-retention, stagnation of phlegm in the lung or abundant phlegm due to hypofunction of the spleen in the state of disease. Fluid-retention attacking the lung results in reverse flow of lung-qi, cough, fullness sensation in the chest, abundant phlegm with white foam and inability of the patient to take a prone position. Accumulated sputum in the lung of sputum syndrome of excess type can be divided into heat-sputum, damp-sputum and dry-sputum, and patients with this type of syndrome often experienced cough and shortness of breath; while abundant sputum due to hypofunction of the spleen of sputum syndrome of deficiency type is referred to a group of symptoms manifesting mainly as deficiency of the spleen. Cough due to deficiency of the lung should be identified with overstrain-induced impairment of the lung and consumptive lung disease. Strictly speaking, cough due to overstrain-induced impairment of the lung and cough induced by consumptive lung disease all belong to that of deficiency of the lung, while cough induced by the former (lung-impairment) is accompanied by emaciation, hemoptysis, tidal fever, night sweating, etc. Deficiency of lung-yin with cough is not sure to be overstrain-induced impairment of the lung, and consumptive lung disease presents a chronic pathological process. Both deficiency-cold type and deficiency-heat type of the consumptive lung disease are more serious in the state of disease.

2. Typing and Treatment

Exopathic cough often results from inability of the lung to disperse and descend due to attack of the lung by wind-cold or wind-heat or dry-heat, and belongs to excess-syndrome. Its focus is located in the lung and it is treated mainly by dispelling pathogenic factors from the exterior and ventilating lung-qi. Generally, drugs for nourishing, tonifying, astringing or cough-relieving should not be used too early for avoiding retaining pathogenic factors. Internal injury-induced cough results from inability of lung-qi in dispersing and descending due to involvement of the lung by disorders of the other zang - or fu-organs, and is considered as coexistence of deficiency and excess. In spit of the focus being situated in the lung, it still has close relation with the liver, spleen and kidney. Treatment of cough should be given mainly by regulating functional activities of zang - or fu-organs, such as strengthening spleen, eliminating liver-fire, nourishing lung, tonifying lung, etc. Cough due to attack of the lung by liver-fire or sputum-rheum often is a coexistence of deficiency- and excess-syndrome, and should be treated according to the greater or lesser urgency of the symptoms and cause of disease. Then, both symptoms and cause of disease are treated simultaneously or only symptoms treated first.

1) Exopathic cough

(1) Wind-cold type cough

Main symptoms: Newly-occurred cough, coughing sound being lower and vague, white and thin sputum.

Concurrent symptoms: Headache, nasal stuffiness, nasal clear discharge, painful sensation in the joints, aversion to cold and anhidrosis.

Tongue picture and pulse condition: White, thin tongue coating, floating pulse.

Analysis: When wind-cold attacks the lung, the lung-qi is not able to flow freely and loses its function in dispersing, thus, cough happens, accompanied by lower and vague voice, white thin sputum, nasal stuffiness and nasal clear discharge. The cold-evil induces contraction. When wind-cold invades the superficial part of the body, the interspace of muscles, sweat pores, etc. are stuffed and meridians obstructed, thus, aversion to cold, fever, anhidrosis, headache, pantalgia, etc. appear. Because pathogenic factors are situated in the exterior, thus, white and thin tongue coating and floating pulse present.

Therapeutic principles: Dispelling wind, removing cold, and ventilating lung-qi.

Recipes and drugs: San Ao Decoction and Modified Xing Su Powder. In the former recipe, Herba Ephedrae, Semen Armeniacae and Radix Glycyrrhizae are used to ventilate the lung to relieve cough; in the later recipe, Folium Perillae and Rhizoma Zingiberis Recens function in dispelling wind-cold; Radix Peucedani and Radix Platycodi function in ventilating the lung, resolving phlegm and regulating qi; Pericarpium Citri Reticulatae, Fructus Aurantii, Rhizoma Pinelliae and Poria are used to regulate qi, remove dampness and resolve sputum. In treatment of severer wind-cold syndrome, Herba Ephedrae is used in a larger dose to strengthen the power of ventilating lung and dispelling cold; for abundant sputum, both Pericarpium Citri Reticulatae and Rhizoma Pinelliae are employed in a larger dose; for lesser sputum, both Radix Platycodi and Radix Glycyrrhizae are used in a larger dose or Modified Jin Fu Cao Powder is used. In case of cough with sore and dry throat, thirst, thick sputum difficult to be expectorated, coughing with a louder voice, severer fever, white or yellowish greasy fur, and floating-rapid pulse, which suggest wind-cold attacking exterior and stagnated lung-heat in the interior (which is also called as cough of coexistence type of external cold and internal heat or cough of fire wrapped by cold), Supplemented Ma Xing Shi Gan Decoction or the aforementioned San Ao Decoction plus Modified Xing Su Powder is used after ruling out Cortex Mori Radicis, Fructus Arctii and Radix Scutellariae.

Recipe example:

Prepared Herba Ephedrae 3～6g, Semen Armeniacae 10g, Caulis Perillae 10g, dried Radix Glycyrrhizae 5g, Radix Platycodi 8g, Radix Peucedani 10g, Exocarpium Citri Reticulatae 10g, Rhizoma Pinelliae 5g and Fructus Aurantii 10g.

(2) Wind-heat type cough

Main symptoms: Cough with loud voice, sputum being thick in texture and yellowish in color.

Concurrent symptoms: Fever and aversion to wind (in most cases), headache, sweating, sore throat, thirst.

Tongue picture and pulse condition: Thin and yellow tongue coating, floating-rapid pulse.

Analysis: When attacked by wind-heat, the lung loses its normal function in dispersing and descending, inducing acute cough with louder voice. If heat evil bakes the body fluid to cause it to become sputum, the resultant sputum is sticky in texture and yellow in color. Because the evils are situated in the body surface, thus, cough with aversion to wind, fever or headache happens. Due to consumption of body fluid by lung-heat, thirst and sore throat occur. Because of wind-heat being in the lung and the exterior, thin yellow tongue coating and floating-rapid pulse present.

Therapeutic principles: Dispelling wind, clearing away heat, ventilating the lung and resolving sputum.

Recipes and drugs: Modified Sang Ju Xin. In this recipe, Folium Mori, Flos Chrysanthemi and Herba Menthae are pungent in flavor and cool in property and are used to expel wind-heat; Semen Armeniacae, Radix Platycodi and dried Radix Glycyrrhizae are used to ventilate the lung-qi; Rhizoma Phragmitis is used to clear away heat and promote production of body fluid. For aversion to cold, Herba Schizonepetae and Radix Ledebouriellae are added to relieve the exterior syndrome; for severer lung-heat, Radix Scutellariae and Gypsum Fibrosum are supplemented to remove heat; for severer cough, Fructus Arctii and Radix Peucedani are added for strengthening lung-ventilating effect; for epistaxis, Rhizoma Imperatae and Nodus Nelumbinis Rhizomatis are added to remove heat from blood; for sore throat, Fructus Arctii, Lasiophaera seu Calvatia and Radix Isatidis are used in combination for eliminating heat and relieving the sore throat; and for difficult expectoration, Semen Benincasae, and Fructus Trichosanthis are used together. In case of appearing wind-heat type cough with abundant sputum, chest distress, sweating, white, greasy tongue coating with yellowish color in its middle part, soft-rapid pulse, it is considered as impairment of the lung by wind-heat and damp evils and treated with Sang Ju Decoction from which Semen Coicis and Semen Armeniacae or lesser amount of Cortex Magnoliae Officinalis are used to ventilate the lung and remove dampness. Wind-heat type cough often happens in the summer. If cough is accompanied by chest distress, irritability, thirst, dark urine, red tongue with yellow fur, soft-rapid pulse, it denotes impairment of the lung by wind-heat combined with summer-heat and dampness and treatment is given by using wind-heat-eliminating and dampness-removing methods. Aromatics Herba Agastachis, Herba Eupatorii, Radix Peucedani and Liu Yi Powder for dispelling wind and clearing away summer-heat are thus chosen. If the dampness is preponderant in comparison with heat, Modified Huoxiang Zhengqi Powder is used for removing dampness and ventilating the lung; if the heat is severer, Lian Pu Decoction or Supplemented Huangqin Huashi Decoction is used to clear away heat and eliminate dampness.

Recipe example:

Herba Schizonepetae 10g, Herba Menthae 5g (decocted later), Radix Platycodi 10g, Fructus Forsythiae 10g, Fructus Arctii 10g, Radix Peucedani 10g, Bulbus Fritillariae Thunbergii 10g, dried Radix Glycyrrhizae 5g, Folium Mori 10g and Flos Chrysanthemi 10g.

(3) Dry-heat type cough

Main symptoms: Newly-occurred cough with a hoarse or splitting voice, dry cough without sputum or with less sticky sputum being difficult to be expectorated.

Concurrent symptoms: Dryness of the nose and throat, or cough with blood-tinged sputum, or cough-induced chest pain, or aversion to wind and fever.

Tongue picture and pulse condition: Redness of the tongue-tip, thin, yellow and dry tongue coating, slightly-rapid pulse.

Analysis: Dry-heat type cough is often seen in the dry seasons i.e. at the end of summer and the beginning of autumn. When dry-heat injuries the lung, the lung-fluid is consumed, resulting in failure of lung-qi to disperse. Thus, cough with hoarse voice, itching throat, dry cough without phlegm, dry nose, dry throat, and dry tongue with less moisture appear. Because dry-heat injuries the lung and consumes body-fluid, functional activities of the lung including dispersing and descending fall into disorder, resulting in cough and related chest pain. In case of impairment of the pulmonary blood vessels by dry-heat, bloody expectoration appears.

Therapeutic principles: Clearing away heat and moistening (by using drugs for slight dispersing and moistening).

Recipe and drugs: Supplemented Sang Xing Decoction. In this recipe, Folium Mori is used to clear away dryness from the lung; Semen Armeniacae functions in moistening the lung and relieving cough; Radix Glehniae, pear peel and Pericarpium Fructus Gardeniae are employed to promote production of body fluid, moisten dryness and eliminate heat, combined with Semen Sojae Praeparatum for dispelling wind and ventilating lung, and with Bulbus Fritillariae Thunbergii for clearing away lung-heat and resolving phlegm. In addition, Fructus Trichosanthis, or Radix Ophiopogonis, Fresh Reed Rhizoma, etc. for eliminating heat and moistening lung can also be added in the light of concrete situations. For severe cough and itching throat, Radix Peucedani, Periostracum Cicadae, Radix Platycodi and Radix Glycyrrhizae are used in combination for ventilating lung and removing pathogenic factors. For chronic dry cough, red tongue with less moisture, and emaciation, Modified Qingzhao Jiufei Decoction may be used. For severer fever, Gypsum Fibrosum and Rhizoma Anemarrhenae are supplemented. For hemoptysis, hemostats are used. In case of dry cough with less expectoration, dry throat and dry nose, accompanying with aversion to cold, fever, headache, anhidrosis, thin, white and dry tongue coating which belong to cold-dryness impairing lung (i.e. combination of wind-cold and wind-dryness), Qing Zao Jiufei Decoction is used by taking off Pericarpium Fructus Gardeniae, pear peel and Bulbus Fritillariae Thunbergii; or Xing Su Powder is used in combination with Herba Schizonetae, Radix Ledebouriellae, Radix Asteris and Flos Farfarae for removing cold, ventilating lung, eliminating dampness and resolving phlegm.

Recipe example:

Folium Mori 10g, Semen Armeniacae 10g, Radix Glehniae 12g, Radix Peucedani 10g, prepared Folium Eriobotryae 10g, Rhizoma Anemarrhenae 10g, Bulbus Fritillariae Thunbergii 10g, dried Radix Glycyrrhizae 5g and Radix Asteris 10g.

If the aforementioned symptoms of exopathic cough are not cured for a long time or cured temporarily but relapse, manifesting as itching throat, cough with difficult expectoration, or severer cough with flushed face and vomiting, and if the exterior syndrome is not evident, Modified Zhi Shou Powder may be used. In this recipe, Herba Schizonepetae pungent in flavor and neutral in nature is used to dispel wind-evil, Radix Stemonae, Rhizoma Cynanchi Stauntonii and Radix Asteris is bitter in taste and warm and moistening in nature function in lowering lung-qi; Radix Glycyrrhizae and Radix Platycodi function in regulating qi and resolving phlegm. The present recipe contains drugs both warm and cool in property is particularly suitable for treatment of exopathic cough patients still with evils left, marked by inability of the lung to disperse and descend with less phlegm, etc.

2) Internal-injury type cough

(1) Phlegm-dampness attacking lung

Tongue picture and pulse condition: White and sticky tongue coating, soft and smooth pulse.

Analysis: The dysfunction of spleen in transportation and transformation results in accumulation of phlegm and dampness. Upward attack of phlegm and dampness on the lung is the cause of cough with abundant sputum being white in color and stick in texture. Since chronic cough may harm the lung and phlegm-dampness retains inside, the failure of lung in dispersion and descent function leads to chest distress. Poor attetite, tiredness, weakness and frequent loose stool are the consequences of stagnant phlegm-dampness in spleen and deficiency of spleen qi. White and sticky tongue coating, soft and smooth pulse are the signs of phlegm-dampness.

Main symptoms: Chronic cough, abundant sputum being white in color and stick in texture and easy to be expectorated.

Concurrent symptoms: Chest distress, poor appetite, tiredness, weakness and frequent loose stool.

Therapeutic principles: Strengthening the spleen, removing dampness, resolving phlegm and relieving cough.

Recipe and drugs: Supplemented Erchen Decoction. Erchen Decoction is an original recipe for treatment of phlegm-dampness syndrome. In case of profuse phlegm and stuffy chest, Rhizoma Atractylodis, Cortex Magnoliae, Semen Armeniacae and Semen Coicis are supplemented to strengthen the spleen, remove dampness and resolve phlegm; for severer cough, Herba Ephedrae, Semen Armeniacae, Fructus Perillae and Radix Cynanchi Stauntonii are added to ventilate the lung and descend qi; in case of clear fatigue, pale tongue and weak pulse due to deficiency of spleen, Radix Codonopsis Pilosulae, Rhizoma Atractylodis Macrocephalae or Modified Liu Junzi Decoction; and for cough with striking reverse flow of qi, Erchen Decoction and Sanzi Yangqin Decoction are used together. Phlegm-dampness attacking lung is often subject to cold- or heat-transformation changes, so, if the spleen-yang is weak or the patient had too much cold food, it may turn into chronic cough due to cold transformation of latent fluid-retention or phlegm. In the event of over-intake of pungent and hot food or affection by heat-evil, etc., it will lead to heat-transformation to become a chronic cough of phlegm-heat accumulated in lung type. The cold-transformation type cough is marked by aversion to cold, cold limbs, loose stool, pale -bluish complexion, pale tongue, white greasy and slippery fur, taunt-slow pulse and should be treated with Ping Wei Powder plus Modified Erchen Decoction, combined with Herba Asari, Rhizoma Zingiberis, and Fructus Schisandrae, or with Supplemented Linggui Zhugan Decoction for warming and resolving phlegm-dampness, regulating qi and relieving cough. If cold phlegm is latent in the interior with coexistence of wind-cold attack, marked by aversion to cold, fever and headache, Xiao Qinglong Decoction is used to relieve exterior syndrome, warm the interior, warm and resolve phlegm-rheum. In the event of heat-transformation, the phlegm-heat accumulates in the lung, resulting in cough with yellow greasy sputum or with difficult expectoration stinking in smell, shortness of breath, bitter taste, thirst, yellow greasy tongue coating, slippery-rapid pulse, Qingjin Huatan Decoction is used to clear away heat, resolve phlegm and relieve cough. In this recipe, Cortex Mori Radicis, Radix Scutellariae, Fructus Gardeniae and Rhizoma Anemarrhenae function in removing lung-heat; Bulbus Fritillariae Cirrhosae, Fructus Trichosanthis and Radix Platycodi are used to eliminate lung-heat and relieve cough; and Radix Ophiopogonis, Exocarpium Citri Reticulatae, Poria and Radix Glycyrrhizae are used to nourish yin and resolve phlegm.

Recipe example:

Pericardium Citri Reticulatae 10g, Poria 10g, Rhizoma Pinelliae 10g, dried Radix Glycyrrhizae 4g, Semen Armeniacae 10g, Cortex Magnoliae 6g, Semen Coicis 15g, Caulis Perillae 10g and Fructus Perillae 10g, combined with Herba Asari 3g, Rhizoma Zingiberis 6g and Fructus Schisandrae 5g for cold-transformation; with Radix Scutellariae 10g, Fructus Trichosanthis 15g and Fructus Gardeniae 10g for heat-transformation.

(2) Accumulation of phlegm-heat in lung

Main symptoms: Cough, shortness of breath, yellow greasy phlegm.

Concurrent symptoms: Cough-induced distending and painful sensations in the chest and hypochondrium, bitter taste, dry mouth, thirst, stinking phlegm or bloody phlegm, or fever.

Tongue picture and pulse condition: Yellow greasy tongue coating, slippery rapid or taut rapid pulse.

Analysis: When phlegm-heat accumulates in the lung and obstructs lung-qi, impairment of purifying and descending functions of the lung happens, resulting in cough, shortness of breath, and yellow greasy phlegm. Due to accumulation and fumigation of phlegm-heat, the sputum is thus stinking. In case of impairment of the pulmonary vessels and disorder of qi, distending pain in the chest and hypochondrium or bloody expectoration happens. Accumulation of lung-heat in the interior is responsible for fever, bitter taste, dry mouth and thirst. Yellow greasy tongue coating and slippery rapid pulse are all signs of sputum-heat.

Therapeutic principles: Clearing away lung-heat, resolving sputum and lowering lung-qi.

Recipe and drugs: Modified Qingjin Huatan Decoction. This recipe functions in resolving sputum and removing lung-heat. Cortex Mori Radicis, Radix Scutellariae, Fructus Gardeniae and Rhizoma Anemarrhenae are used to clear away lung-heat; Bulbus Fritillariae Cirrhosae, Fructus Trichosanthis and Radix Platycodi are used to resolve sputum, remove lung-heat and relieve cough. Exocarpium Citri Reticulatae is used to resolve sputum and regulate qi; Poria is used to eliminate dampness; Radix Ophiopogonis and Radix Glycyrrhizae are used to nourish yin and moisten the lung. In the event of yellow, thick, stinking and pus-like sputum, Herba Houttuyniae, Rhizoma Fagopyri Cymosi, Fructus Forsythiae, Semen Benincasae and Semen Coicis are used to eliminate heat and resolve sputum. If cough due to reverse flow of qi, fullness feeling in the chest, and cough worsening while lying, etc. happen, Semen Lepidii seu Descurainiae and Natriisulfas are used to purge lung-heat and remove sputum; and if sputum-heat consumes body fluid to result in dry mouth, thirst and red tongue, Radix Glehnia, Radix Trichosanthis and Daige Powder are used to nourish yin, clear away heat and resolve sputum.

Recipe example:

Fructus Trichosanthis 20g, Radix Scutellariae 10g, Rhizoma Anemarrhenae 10g, Bulbus Fritillariae Cirrhosae 10g, Charred Fructus Gardeniae 10g, Rhizoma Pinelliae 10g, Arisaema cum Bile 6g, Radix Platycodi 6g, Semen Lepidii seu Descurainiae 10g and Cortex Mori Radicis 10g.

(3) Liver-fire attacking lung

Main symptoms: Paroxysmal cough due to reversed flow of qi, dry cough without sputum or with less sputum, cough induced pain involving the chest and hypochondrium.

Concurrent symptoms: Flushed face, dry throat, dry mouth; Generally, symptoms are more or less along with changes of emotional activity.

Tongue picture and pulse condition: Red margin of the tongue, yellow thin tongue coating with less moisture, taut rapid pulse.

Analysis: When the liver-qi stagnates to transform fire, the qi and fire rise adversely to attack the lung. Deficiency of Gold (lung) can not suppress Wood (liver) and the lung fails in purifying and descending, leading to cough because of liver-fire attacking lung. So, the patient often feels reverse flow of qi reaching the throat and experiences cough. Flaming-up of liver-fire is responsible for flushed face. The lung connects with the throat, so, when fire-heat consumes body fluid, the patient feel dry in the throat. In case of liver-fire burning Gold (lung), the body fluid is consumed and becomes sputum, the sputum is thick and sticky and difficult to be expectorated. The hypochondrium is the site where the Liver Meridian passes through, so, when liver-qi falls into disorder, the resultant cough often induces painful sensation involving the hypochondriac region. Yellow thin tongue coating with less moisture and taut rapid pulse are signs of hyperactivity of the liver, lung-heat and consumption of body fluid.

Therapeutic principles: Clearing away lung-heat, soothing the liver, lowering the adverse flow of qi and removing fire.

Recipes and drugs: Xie Bai Powder plus Modified Dai Ga Powder. The former recipe is used to clear away lung-heat and the latter one used to remove liver-fire and resolve sputum. Cortex Mori Radicis is used to eliminate the accumulated heat in the lung; Cortex Lycii Radicis used to clear away latent fire in the lung; polished round-grained rice and Radix Glycyrrhizae are used to nourish the stomach and normalize functions of the spleen and stomach to help the lung-qi. Dai Ga Powder functions in eliminating liver-fire and resolving long-term accumulated sputum. Pericarpium Citri Reticulatae and Pericarpium Citri Reticulatae Viride can be added to normalize activity of qi, Radix Scutellariae and Fructus Gardeniae are used to get rid of heat, Bulbus Fritillariae Thunbergii and Fructus Trichosanthis used to resolve sputum.

Recipe example:

Cortex Mori Radicis 10g, Cortex Lycii Radicis 10g, Radix Scutellariae 10g, Fructus Trichosanthis 15g, Dai Ga Powder (wrapped up in a piece of cloth and then decocted) 12g, Radix Stemonae 10g, Fructus Gardeniae 10g and dried Radix Glycyrrhizae 5g.

(4) Lung-deficiency type

Insufficiency of both lung-yin and -qi all can lead to cough. But in patients with qi-deficiency, asthma and cough are often seen at the same time. For detail, please consult the chapter of asthma. Here, only lung-yin-induced cough is introduced as follows.

Main symptoms: Chronic cough, dry cough with less sputum or with bloody sputum, afternoon tidal fever.

Concurrent symptoms: Flushed cheeks, feverish sensation in the palms and soles, insomnia, night sweating, lack of vitality, tiredness and restlessness.

Tongue picture and pulse condition: Red tongue with less coating, thready rapid pulse.

Analysis: In the event of deficiency of lung-yin, the lung is unable to be moistened to produce dry-heat, so, dry cough with less sputum, dry mouth and dry throat present. Impairment of the pulmonary vessels results in bloody sputum or hemoptysis. Hyperactivity of yin-deficiency is responsible for signs of deficiency-heat including afternoon tidal fever, flushed cheeks, feverish sensation in the palms and soles, restlessness, insomnia, night sweating, red tongue with less coating and thready rapid pulse.

Therapeutic principles: Nourishing yin, clearing away lung-heat, resolving sputum and relieving cough.

Recipe and drugs: Modified Shashen Maidong Decoction. Radxi Glehnia, Radix Ophiopogonis, Rhizoma Polygonati Odorati and Radix Trichosanthis of the recipe are used to nourish yin and promote production of body fluid, moisten the lung and relieve cough; Semen Dolichoris and Radix Glycyrrhizae are used to strengthen the spleen and reinforce the middle-jiao. If cough is severer, Semen Armeniacae and Bulbus Fritillariae Cirrhosae are supplemented to resolve sputum and relieve cough. For treatment of hemoptysis, Cacumen Biotae, Herba Agrimoniae, Nodus Nelumbinis Rhizomatis, Rhizoma Bletillae, Colla Corii Asini and Radix Notoginseng are supplemented to stop bleeding; in case of afternoon tidal fever and flushed cheek, Radix Stellariae, Cortex Cycii Radicis, Radix Scutellariae and Radix Cynanchi Atrati are used to clear away hectic fever; in cases of yellow sputum, Radix Scutellariae, Rhizoma Anemarrhenae and Concha Meretricis seu Cyclinae are used to get rid of heat and resolve sputum; in case of cough and asthma due to chronic deficiency of both qi and yin of the lung and kidney, Radix Rehmanniae Praeparata, Fructus Corni, Fructus Schisandrae, Radix Ginseng and Gecko are used to reinforce the kidney toimprove inspiration.

Recipe example:

Radxi Glehnia 12g, Radix Ophiopogonis 10g, Fructus Schisandrae 6～10g, Semen Armeniacae 10g, prepared Folium Eriobotryae 10g and Bulbus Fritillariae Cirrhosae 10g, Radix Asteris 10g and prepared Radix Glycyrrhizae 6g.

In addition, if the internal injury type cough lasts for quite some time, and the activity of pathogenic factors have subsided clearly and the lung-qi has been consumed, drugs for astringing the lung to stop cough as Fructus Schisandrae, Galla Chinensis, Fructus Chebulae, Pericarpium Papaveris, etc. are supplemented on the basis of differentiation of syndromes, which is also called as cough-stopping method. In recent years, through abundant studies on treatment and prevention of chronic bronchitis, it is demonstrated that during remission stage, continuous treatment in a longer period of time by adopting body resistance-enhancing therapy mainly for tonifying the spleen and kidney is rather effective for internal injury type cough, though it is refractory and attacks repeatedly in spit of long term treatment or sometimes, it is cured temporarily but relapses time and again. Thus this therapy is worthy of being taken seriously.

〔Measures for Prevention and Nursing〕

1) Understanding patient's conditions in detail and completely, identifying pathogenic factors and predisposing cause of a disease and then dealing with them separately.

2) Keeping a suitable temperature and humidity in the ward; ordering the patient to be careful about his or her daily life and diet, to avoid exogenous evils, and to have an appropriate regular physical exercise; and advising the patient to give up smoking. In the ward, smoking should be prohibited, the room is well ventilated and kept in fresh air frequently. Asking the patient to pay attention to personal hygiene, particularly to keep his or her oral hygiene.

3) Patients with wind-heat type exopathy should have light diet and easily-digestible food; those with spleen-deficiency should pay more attention to having easily-digestible food and have less greasy and hot food for avoiding impairing the spleen further; those with kidney-deficiency-cold syndrome may have much warm-tonic food such as beef, mutton, etc.; those with deficiency of both lung - and kidney-yin may have more fruits or drink boiled water-soaked yin-nourishing herbs as glehnia root, lilyturf root etc. liquid instead of tea; and those with hyperactivity of liver-fire should easy and console themselves frequently.

4) Urging the patient with abundant phlegm to try his or her best to get rid of phlegm, helping the patient with severe qi-deficiency to spit phlegm out by turning his or her body posture and tapping the back, if necessary, measures for aspirating sputum are adopted but excessive stimulation or impairment of the pharyngeal portion should be avoided. Antitussives with violent power are definitely not used for avoiding even more difficult expectoration of sputum in spit of cough-relief.

5) When being severer, cough can be treated by employing the following measures.

a) Acupuncture therapy; common acupoints used are Feishu (BL 13), Lieque (LU 7), Tiantu (RN 22), Neiguan (PC 6), Zusanli (ST 36), etc.

b) Cupping, performed on the back of the body.

c) Simple recipe: a peeled and pit-removed pear, some crystal sugar (just the right amount) and a little of fritillary bulb powder are steamed and taken for resolving sputum and stopping cough. This recipe can be used frequently.

〔Analysis of A Typical Case〕

Sun You, female. failure of the lung to disperse in water metabolism, manifested by cough with thick sputum, thready taunt pulse, and yellow thin tongue coating. Treatment was given by clearing away lung-heat and resolving sputum.

Drugs used were: Pericarpium Trichosanthis 6g, Radix Curcumae 4. 5g, Bulbus Fritillariae Thunbergii 6g, Fructus Aristolochiae 4. 5g, dried Radix Asteris 9g, Semen Sterculiae Scaphigerae 2 grains, Fructus Liquidambaris 6g, crude Ochra Haematitum 9g, Rhizoma Pinelliae Praeparata 4. 5g, Herba Menthae 0. 3g and frosted Folium Mori 6g.

Second treatment:

The patient's sputum-heat still existed and cough abated. She had a delayed menstruation and slight abdominal distension, which were due to rising of qi and fire. Examination showed yellow, greasy tongue root and taunt pulse (on the right side). It was treated by nourishing the liver, lowering fire, removing stagnation of qi and blood and restoring menstrual flow.

Dried Rhizoma Corydalis 6g, Pericarpium Citri Reticulatae Viride 4. 5g, Rhizoma Pinelliae Praeparata 6g, Radix Angelicae Sinensis 4. 5g, fresh Semen Persicae 9g, Herba Lycopi 6g, prepared Fructus Crataegi 6g, dried Radix Asteris 9g, Fructus Aristolochiae 4. 5g, fried Herba Schizonepetae 4. 5g, Semen Leonuri 9g and Pericarpium Trichosanthis 6g.

Third Treatment:

The patient still had no menstrual onset but her abdominal distension disappeared and she got better in appetite and had nasal turbid discharge. Examination showed taunt pulse on the right side and yellow thin fur on the middle of the tongue, which suggested stagnated heat in the lung. She was treated with nourishing yin and strengthening the spleen and clearing away lung-heat to treat the secondary aspect of the disease.

Fried Fructus Corni 4. 5g, Fructus Lycii 6g, Cortex Eucommiae 6g, Bulbus Fritillariae Thunbergii 3g, Fructus Aristolochiae 3g, dried Cortex Mori Radicis 6g, frosted Folium Mori 6g. fresh Caulis Bambusae in Taeniam 4. 5g, prepared Herba Schizonepetae 4. 5g, dried Radix Asteris 9g, prepared Fructus Ligustri Lucidi 12g, Radix Linderae 7. 5g and Herba Lycopi 6g.

Note: The present case has no exterior syndrome but suffers from cough and greasy thick sputum which suggests stagnated heat in the lung and belongs to internal injury type cough. It is treated by removing heat, resolving sputum, and ventilating the lung to lower qi first, and then by nourishing yin and strengthening the spleen. In this way, if the patient is weak in constitution and when the state of disease gets better gradually, i.e. in the stage of weakness of body's resistance and less pathogenic factors, reinforcing and reducing methods are used in combination. (selected from《Collections of Medical Prescriptions》)

Summary:

Cough is one of symptoms of the lung diseases but in etiology it can be divided into two major categories: exopathic type and internal injury type. The exopathic type cough results from attack of the lung by six pathogenic factors, while the internal injury type from inability of the lung in dispersing and descending functions, and reverse flow of lung-qi due to functional disorders of zang- or fu-organs.

When making differentiation of syndromes, exopathic or internal injury type cough should be identified clearly first. Generally, exopathic type cough happens newly and belongs to excessiveness of pathogens; the focus is at the lung and treatment should be aimed at eliminating pathogens and removing lung-heat. While internal in jury type cough mostly belongs to weakness of body resistance and excessiveness of pathogens; its focus is chiefly at the lung but is also associated with the liver, spleen and kidney, and treatment should be aimed at getting rid of pathogens, relieving cough, strengthening body resistance and reinforcing deficiency, i.e. dealing with the primary aspect first and then the secondary.

When treating cough, in addition to considering the topical lung, an integrated therapy for regulating functions of the liver, spleen and kidney should be emphasized. For treatment of exopathic cough, generally, astringing method may result in stagnation of pathogenic factors in the body and is thus definitely not advisable. According to the circumstances, if the functional disturbance of the lung-qi is relieved, cough will stop spontaneously. In treatment of internal injury type cough, excessively ventilating the lung will impair the vital energy of the body, so, measures for reasonable regulation and protection of the vital-qi are necessary.

In short, cough is a pathological sign of the lung disease and is also a physiological manifestation of the human body in driving pathogenic factors out, therefore, treatment can not simply follow the method for treating cough when meeting it. On the basis of different causes of the disease, corresponding measures are adopted. Generally speaking, mildness or seriousness of cough may reflect the state of the disease, but under certain circumstances, i.e. pathogenic factors can not be driven out due to weakness of body resistance, in spit of mildness of cough in appearance, in fact, the state of the disease is serious, this situation should be taken seriously.

Questions for review

1. How to identify exopathic type cough and internal injury type cough?
2. What are the differences and differentiation and treatment of wind-cold type and wind-heat type cough?
3. How many kinds of internal injury type cough? How to differentiate syndromes and treat them?
4. What are the differences and treatment of sputum-damp type cough and lung-deficiency type cough?

Bronchial Wheezing Syndrome

〔Simple Introduction〕

Bronchial Wheezing Syndrome is a paroxysmal gasp with phlegm-wheezing, characterized by wheezing sound in the throat, rapid breathing, dyspnea, and even being unable to lie flat in severe case. In the ancient documents of traditional Chinese medicine, both wheezing syndrome and panting syndrome belongs to dyspnea-tachypnea, in fact, they are different in property. When treated, they should be distinguished first by combining the cause of disease, pathology and clinical manifestations with necessary physical and laboratory examinations. In clinic, wheezing is sure to be accompanied by panting, thus, wheezing and panting are generally called as asthma, but panting is not always accompanied by wheezing.

In modern medicine, asthma various patterns, such as bronchial asthma, asthmatic bronchitis or other causes induced asthma, like cardiac asthma, hypereosinophilic syndrome, etc. When they are treated, contents of differentiation of syndromes and treatment methods described in this chapter can be used for reference, if symptoms are similar.

〔Cause of Disease and Pathogenesis〕

Wheezing syndrome belongs to a paroxysmal disease and results from obstruction of the airway and reverse flow of the lung-qi due to old sputum-retention latent in the lung, combined with additional factors as exopathy, improper diet, abnormal emotional activity, over-exertion, etc.

1. Attack by exogenous pathogenic factors

In case of affection by wind-cold or wind-heat, and if the pathogens are not dispelled from the exterior of the body in time, they will accumulate in the lung to obstruct flow of lung-qi, resulting in inability of qi to distribute body fluid and formation of phlegm. Besides, in patients with special constitution, when they inhale pollen, fume, etc. the lung-qi fails in performing dispersing and descending functions, causing body fluid to accumulate to form sputum. The resultant phlegm-rheum stagnates in the interior to induce wheezing;

2. Improper diet

Clinging to raw and cool food may lead to stagnation of cold fluid-retention in the interior. Addicting to sour, salty, sweet or greasy food can also generate accumulation of sputum and pathogenic heat. Improper intake of sea food often lead to dysfunction of the spleen in transportation and transformation, causing the food unable to be transformed into essence and generation of sputum in the interior. The resultant sputum goes up to the lung to block regular flow of lung-qi, resulting in wheezing; and

3. Weak constitution and Copos

In patients with acquired weak constitution, or somatasthenia after illness, such as infantile measles, paroxysmal cough, or repeated attack of common cold and chronic cough, etc. the lung-qi is consumed and fails in transformation of body fluid, generating sputum-rheum in the interior; or, yin-deficiency-induced hyperactivity of fire consumes body fluid and causes accumulation of liquid, and thick sticky sputum. If wheezing onset is due to weak constitution, deficiency of both liver and kidney are predominant; while if wheezing occurs because of copos, deficiency of both lung and spleen as well as accumulation of sputum in the interior are often seen. The internal wind very often stirs up in patients with a constitution of deficiency of both liver-yin and kidney-yin. If so, disorders of liver-qi and lung-qi in ascending and descending are seen.

Schematic Diagram of the Cause of Disease and Pathogenesis of Wheezing Syndrome

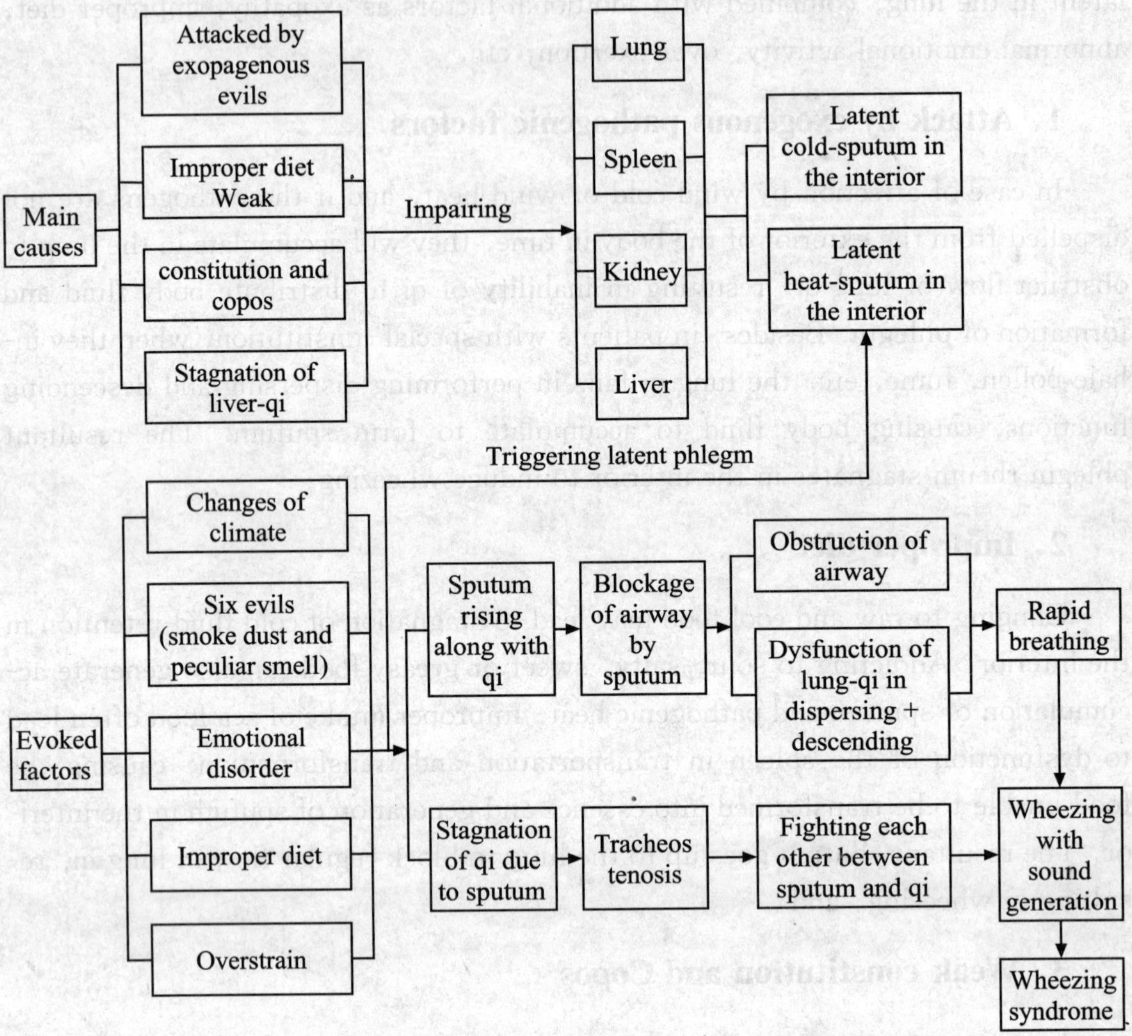

To sum up, sputum is a chief pathogenic factor responsible for onset of wheezing and results from accumulation of body fluid due to failure of the lung in dispersing and distributing body fluid, or inability of the spleen to transport essence, or inability of the kidney to transform water liquid. The resultant sputum is stored in the lung and becomes the latent and fundamental factor of wheezing. Thereafter, in case of sudden changes of the climate, improper diet, emotional disturbance, fatigue, smoke dust, peculiar smell factor, etc wheezing will be evoked. These factors, especially abrupt change of the climate, are often interrelated in evoking wheezing.

The pathogenesis of wheezing lies in that originally, the latent old sputum exists in the interior, when any one of the evoked factors invades the body, the old sputum goes up with qi, resulting in combination of qi and sputum, obstruction of the airway and tracheostenosis. In this way, dysfunction of lung-qi in dispersing and descending, and failure of the stagnated sputum to be removed or resolved, and dyspnea and tachypnea with a loud phlegmatic sound will occur. The basic link of onset of wheezing is stagnation of phlegm to obstruct the air-passage, characterized by excessiveness of pathogen. If wheezing occurs because of cold-evil attack or yang-deficiency constitution and subsequent cold-transformation of phlegm-evil, it is called as wheezing of cold type; and if it happens due to heat-evil attack or yang-exuberance constitution and subsequent heat-transformation of phlegm-evil, it is termed as wheezing of heat type. Besides, wheezing syndrome of cold wrapping fire type, i. e. stagnation of phlegm-heat in the interior and wind-cold tightening the exterior, is also not rare in clinic. If wind-evil stirs, both the internal and external wind can result in wind type wheezing. Similarly, if blood stasis stays in the interior of the body to cause the lung to be unable to function in dispersing and descending, wheezing of blood stasis type will happen. If wheezing attacks repeatedly, cold-sputum impairs spleen-yang and kidney-yang or sputum-heat consumes lung-yin and kidney-yin, the excess syndrome may transform into deficiency syndrome, presenting a series of symptoms of deficiency of lung-qi, spleen-qi and kidney-qi. In case of hypofunction of lung, the lung is unable to dominate qi and the lung-qi can not transform body fluid, resulting in stagnation of sputum in the interior and failure of the lung in dispersing and descending. Under the circumstances, the human body loses its consolidated defensive ability, and is thus liable to be invaded by exogenous pathogenic factors and to have wheeze subsequently. In case of hypofunction of the spleen, water and food can not be transformed into nutrient substances to distribute upwards to the lung and rather, they become dampness and sputum, the resultant sputum stores in the lung to hinder the up- and down-flow of lung-qi. In case of insufficiency of kidney-qi and kidney-essence, the kidney fails in governing acceptance of air and water metabolism, resulting in generation of sputum due to yang-deficiency or due to depletion of body fluid by exuberant fire because of yin-deficiency. The resultant sputum interferes in pulmonary function to induce disorders of lung-qi in governing respiration. The three zang-organs affect each other in functional activities, therefore, deficiency of both lung-qi and spleen-qi, deficiency of both lung-yin and kidney-yin, and deficiency of both spleen-yang and kidney-yang are frequently seen in clinic. During intermittent period of wheezing, the patient often feels week, has gasp of breath and light uninterrupted wheezing. Once the patient has a grand mal, wheezing attacks continuously, excess of pathogens and weakness of body resistance appear at the same time, marked by deficiency of both spleen and kidney and abundant sputum-rheum. In severe cases, the lung can not function normally in transporting blood and conducting gas exchange and in regulating circulation of the heart-blood, and the fire from the gate of life and the heart loses its balance. As a result, the heart-yang is impaired, causing asthma-prostration syndrome.

〔Differentiation of Syndromes and Treatment〕

1. Main points for differentiation

1) Differentiation of cold and heat

Wheezing type of asthma can transform chiefly into cold - and heat-syndrome. Thus, there a saying that "wheeze contains cold - and heat-types while panting is made up of deficiency - and excess-types". When differentiating cold - or heat-type, situations of sputum should be made clear first. Generally, wheezing with thick, yellow and sticky sputum being difficult to be expectorated is considered as heat type; while that with white sticky sputum or thin foamy sputum considered as cold type. Secondly, the predisposing causes of onset of this disease can be used as reference. Under ordinary circumstances, onset of wheezing due to invasion of summer-heat mostly belongs to heat type; that occurred due to attack of cold-evil mostly belongs to cold type; if wheezing is a cold-wrapping-fire syndrome, the accompanying symptoms should be also noted at the same time. For instance, wheezing accompanied by aversion to cold, fever, anhidrosis, headache (exterior-cold syndrome) is mostly considered as cold type wheezing or cold-wrapping-fire type wheezing; and if that accompanied by headache, sore throat, fever, slight aversion to wind, it is mostly considered as heat-type wheezing.

2) Differentiation of deficiency and excess

From pathology, newly-occurred wheezing mostly belongs to excess-syndrome, while chronic wheezing belongs to deficiency-syndrome. In the stage of attack, wheezing mostly belongs to excess-syndrome while during intermission, weakness of patient's body resistance is predominant. Speaking from symptoms, accumulation of qi due to stagnation of sputum, wheezing sound and phlegm-induced stridor in the throat, being comfortable when sputum being spitted out, thick greasy tongue coating and taunt slippery pulse are attributed to excess-syndrome. Stagnation of qi, chest stuffiness and fullness, distending pain at the hypochondrium, feeling comfortable if having a long expiration, shrill wheezing at a high tone, red tongue with thin coating and taunt pulse are also attributed to excess-syndrome. Spontaneous sweating, aversion to wind, being easily to catch common cold, attack of wheezing due to abrupt change of climate, or pale complexion, fatigue, poor appetite, epigastric fullness, shortness of breath while making excertion, soreness of waist and weakness of limbs are attributed to deficiency-syndrome.

3) Differentiation of wind, sputum, qi and blood

If wheezing syndrome results from attack of wind-evil, the predisposing factor is clear, the onset of disease is acute and it is often associated with the acquired constitution. In patients with liver-yin- and kidney-yin-deficient constitution, endogenous wind symptoms are often seen. In case of insufficiency of lung-qi, the defensive function of the body surface is weak, so, the exogenous wind-evil is readily to invade the human body.

Internally-stagnated phlegm-rheum induced wheezing may transform into cold type or heat type on the basis of the nature of phlegm, which has been mentioned above in 1.

If manifesting mainly as stagnation of qi, wheezing often results from exogenous wind-evil or internal wind-evil, characterized by choking and fullness sensations in the chest, wheezing in the throat without phlegm, distending pain at the hypochondrium, being comfortable after having an long expiration. It is readily to attack if the patient gets angry or depressed. If so, taunt pulse will be seen.

If manifesting chiefly as blood stasis, the wheezing mostly belongs to chronic and refractory type, dim complexion, cyan-purple lips and nails, deep red tongue or with ecchymoses, and pain sensation from the hypochondrium.

4) Differentiation of wheezing- and panting-syndrome

Both wheezing and panting syndromes manifest as hasty breathing but can be distinguished according to the aforementioned clinical characters of wheezing.

(1) Breath of wheezing syndrome is short, combined with rattles due to phlegm in the throat.

Panting patients manifest mainly as rapid breathing without production of louder sound, while wheezing patients mainly as louder sound in the throat because of obstruction of qi by phlegm.

(2) Wheezing syndrome has its perennial root and predisposing causes, while panting syndrome has no perennial root. Excess type of panting results from invasion of evils. When evils are removed, panting will be relieved immediately. Deficiency type of panting mostly results from chronic disease, characterized by hypofunction of zang-organs.

(3) Wheezing syndrome is of characters of paroxysm, repeated attack and obstinacy, while panting syndrome has no these.

(4) Wheezing syndrome is an independent disease, while panting syndrome may be a complication of multiple chronic diseases. Wheezing is certainly accompanied by panting while panting is not always accompanied by wheezing. If lasting for a long period time, wheezing will develop to become a sustaining asthma with wheezing sound due to phlegm, which is attributed to the category of panting syndrome.

2. Typing and treatment

When wheezing syndrome attacks, the excess type is frequently seen and treated according to differentiation of cold or heat property of the disease first and then mainly by adopting therapeutic principles of dispelling pathogenic factors, removing phlegm and regulating qi. Cold type wheezing should be treated by warming and resolving the cold-phlegm and ventilating the lung, while heat type wheezing is fit to be treated by clearing away lung-heat and removing phlegm. If induced by wind-evil, wheezing will be treated by eliminating wind; while if induced due to blockage of meridians by blood stasis, it is treated predominantly by promoting blood circulation. In patients with chronic wheezing accompanied with deficiency syndrome, treatment should be aimed chiefly at strengthening body resistance in spit of no acute attack and is conducted by tonifying the lung, invigorating the spleen or reinforcing the kidney after understanding the principal and secondary involvement of the three organs. At the same time, deficiency of yang or yin should be also understood. In treatment of yang-deficiency type wheezing, warming-reinforcing method is applied and in treatment of yin-deficiency type, nourishing method is adopted to relieve or control onset of this disease. In case of coexistence of cold, heat, deficiency and excess syndromes, treatment should be given by considering all these aspects.

Stage of attack

(1) Cold type wheezing

Main symptoms: Asthmatic breathing with wheezing sound in the throat, white, greasy phlegm or thin, foamy phlegm, stuffiness and fullness in the chest, dim and bluish complexion, absence or existence of thirst, preference of warm drink.

Concurrent symptoms: (Attack often due to cold weather or affection by cold), headache, fever, aversion to cold, anhidrosis or cold limbs.

Tongue picture and pulse condition: White greasy or white slippery tongue coating, floating and tense pulse.

Analysis: In addition to cold-phlegm hiding in the lung, some predisposing factors may contribute to the attack of wheezing. If so, qi stagnates in the lung due to accumulation of phlegm, and fighting between phlegm and qi leads to asthmatic breathing with wheezing sound in the throat. When lung-qi is obstructed to lose its function in dispersing, phlegm is unable to be expectorated, so, stuffiness and fullness feeling in the chest, white, greasy sputum or thin, foamy sputum present. Hyperactivity of yin in the interior causes yang-qi to be unable to spread to the body surface, thus, dim and bluish complexion, cold limbs and aversion to cold happen. In case of hyperactivity of yin-cold in the interior and no heat-transformation, the patient has no desire of thirst and likes warm drink. The abovementioned tongue picture and pulse condition both suggest cold sputum. The external cold-evil is liable to trigger noxious activity of the internal sputum-retention. Therefore, wheezing often occurs in cold weather or the patient is attacked by cold-evil, presenting a series of symptoms of exterior-cold syndrome, such as headache, fever, aversion to cold, anhidrosis, etc.

Therapeutic principles: Warming the lung, dispelling cold, removing sputum and regulating qi.

Recipes and drugs: Modified Shegan Mahuang Decoction. Rhizoma Belamcandae and Herba Ephedrae of this recipe are used to ventilate the lung, relieve panting and promote expectoration; Rhizoma Zingiberis, Herba Asari and

Rhizoma Pinelliae function in warming the lung, eliminating sputum-rheum and lowering the reversed-qi; Flos Farfarae, Radix Asteris and Radix Glycyrrhizae function in removing sputum and relieving cough; Fructus Schisandrae is used to arrest dissipation of lung-qi, Rhizoma Ziziphi Jujubae is used to normalize function of the stomach and spleen. In case of abundant sputum, dyspnea and inabilty to lie flat, Sanzi Yang Qin Decoction is used in combination; or Semen Lepidii seu Descurainiae is added to purge lung-heat, lower qi and remove sputum. In case of coexistence of dominant exterior cold and interior fluid-retention syndrome, Xiao Qinglong Decoction is used in combination with Semen Armeniacae, Fuctus Perillae, Semen Sinapis Albae, Pericarpium Citri Reticulatae, etc. for getting rid of sputum and regulating qi. In severe wheezing patients with definite old cold-evil and obstinate sputum, treatment is given by oral administration of drugs containing white arsenic as Zijin Dan etc. for dispelling sputum and arresting panting under careful observation. White arsenic may cause hydrargyrism, thus, its application should be very careful at small dose and within 5 to 7 days. If cold type wheezing attacks frequently and lasts for a long time, both deficiency- and excess-syndrome or excess in the upper and deficiency in the lower exit at the same time, manifested by wheezing sound in the throat due to sputum like snoring, weak voice, shortness of breath, clear sputum, pale complexion, sweating, cold limbs, bulgy white tongue with white coating, deep thready pulse, it is treated by employing Suzi Jiangqi Decoction combined with Radix Codonopsis Pilosulae, Semen Juglandis, Fluorite, Lignum Aquilariae, Fructus Chebulae, etc. to warm yang, reinforce deficiency, lower qi and resolve sputum. For deficiency of kidney-yang type wheezing, Radix Aconiti Praeparata, Fructus Psoraleae, Stalactite, etc. are employed in combination.

Recipe example:

Rhizoma Belamcandae 10g, Herba Ephedrae 5g, Semen Armeniacae 10g, Fuctus Perillae 1g, Pericarpium Citri Reticulatae 10g, Rhizoma Pinelliae 10g, Herba Asari 3g, Semen Lepidii seu Descurainiae 10g, Radix Asteris 10g, Flos Farfarae 10g and Radix Glycyrrhizae 5g.

(2) Heat type wheezing

Main symptoms: Dyspnea, tachypnea, louder wheezing sound like roaring, strong chest movement, coarse voice, paroxysmal cough, thick, yellow and greasy sputum being difficult to be expectorated, irritability, choking sensation in the chest, restlessness, sweating, flushed face, bitter taste, thirst, preference to water.

Concurrent symptoms: Headache, fever, slight aversion to wind.

Tongue picture and pulse condition: Red tongue with yellow greasy coating, slippery rapid pulse or taut slippery pulse.

Analysis: In addition to latent sputum and accumulation of heat, the lung is also attacked by exogenous evils, leading to failure of the lung to purify, stagnated sputum-heat in lung, reverse up-flow of lung-qi and fighting between sputum and qi. As a result, dyspnea, tachypnea, loud wheezing sound as roaring, strong chest movement, coarse breathing and paroxysmal cough appear. Mutual combination of sputum and heat contributes to formation of greasy, thick, turbid sputum with difficult expectoration. Abundant sputum plus fumigation of stagnated heat leads to irritability, stuffy chest, spontaneous sweating, flushed face and bitter taste. This type of wheezing is induced by invasion of heat-evil, combined with consumption of body fluid by heat, manifesting as thirst, preference to water, and no aversion to cold. Both yellow greasy tongue coating and slippery rapid pulse are signs of hyperactivity of sputum-heat in the interior. Accumulated sputum-heat in the interior plus heat-transformation of exogenous evils result in appearance of a series of symptoms of wind-heat exterior syndrome.

Therapeutic principles: Clearing away heat, ventilating lung, resolving sputum and lowering reverse flow of qi.

Recipes and drugs: Modified Ding Chuan Decoction. In this recipe, Herba Ephedrae is used to relieve panting; Radix Scutellariae and Cortex Mori Radicis are employed to clear away lung-heat; Exocarpium Citri Reticulatae, Rhizoma Pinellae, Flos Farfarae and Fructus Perillae function in resolving sputum and lowering adverse flow of qi; Semen Ginkgo serves for an astringent to arrest dissipation of lung-qi; Radix Glycyrrhizae serves to normalize functions of the stomach and spleen. If cold-evil invades the exterior of the body and lung-heat is exuberant in the interior, Semen Ginkgo is excluded instead of Gypsum Fibrosum for dispelling pathogenic factors from the superficial muscles and reducing interior heat. For severe exterior-cold syndrome, Ramulus Cinnamomi and Rhizoma Zingiberis Recens are supplemented or Modified Da Qinglong Decoction is used. For severer stagnation of lung-qi, dyspnea with wheezing sound due to sputum and inability to lie flat, Semen Lepidii seu Descurainiae and Lumbricus are supplemented. In case of severe accumulation of heat and sputum, obstruction of airway, extremely rapid and short breathing (nearly going to death), the above recipe (Ding Chuan

Decoction) is used in combination with oral administration of Calculus Macacae Powder. In case of accumulation of exuberant interior heat, fumigation of sputum-fire and dry, yellow tongue coating, Radix et Rhizoma Rhei and Natrii Sulfas are added, or Xuan Bai Chengqi Decoction plus Mengshi Guntan Pill are used to promote bowel movement and regulate lung-qi. For patients with yellow, sticky sputum with difficult expectoration, Rhizoma Anemarrhenae, Concha Meretricis seu Cyclinae powder, Rhizoma Belamcandae, Herba Houttuyniae, Succus Bambosae, etc are supplemented, or in combination with Qianjin Weijing Decoction and Xiao Xian Xiong Decoction for getting rid of sputum-heat. In case of chronic wheezing with yin-impairment due to exuberant heat, coexistence of deficiency and excess, respiratory distress, cough, night sweating, less amount of sputum being sticky in texture, tiredness, dry throat, irritability, flushed cheeks, red tongue with less coating, thready, rapid pulse, Mai Men Dong Decoction plus Radix Glehnia, Fructus Schisandrae and Bulbus Fritillariae Cirrhosae are used to nourish yin, clear away heat, moisten the lung and resolve sputum. For reversed flow of qi due to deficiency of the kidney, Redix Rehmanniae Preparata, Radix Angelicae Sinensis, Fructus Corni, Fluorite, Fructus Chebulae, etc. are selected to tonify the kidney for improving respiration.

Recipe example

Prepared Herba Ephedrae 5g, Semen Armeniacae 10g, Radix Scutellariae 10g, Rhizoma Pinelliae 6g, Fructus Trichosanthis 15g, Gypsum Fibrosum 20g (decocted first), Radix Glycyrrhizae 5g, Semen Lepidii seu Descurainiae 10g, Lumbricus 10g, Bulbus Fritillarae Cirrhosae 10g.

(3) Wind type wheezing

Main symptoms: (Sudden onset of asthma due to a certain factor, such as mental distress or inhaling peculiar smell, etc, generally, the predisposing factors are clear), dry wheezing, no sputum, or less amount of sputum with difficult expectoration, fullness and stuffiness sensations in the chest.

Concurrent symptoms: Dryness in the throat and mouth, flushed face or sallow, dim complexion, loose stool.

Tongue picture and pulse condition: Red tongue with less moisture, no or less fur, taut thready pulse.

Analysis: Wind-evil is apt to change. Exogenous wind often first invades the lung while internal wind-evil results from the liver. In case of weak acquired constitution and unconsolidated superficial defensive function, the exogenous wind pathogen is readily to enter the human body from the lung, resulting in failure of the lung to disperse and purify; in case of usual deficiency of yin and blood, the liver-wind is apt to stir in the interior; or in case of stagnation of the liver-qi, the depressed liver causes fire - and wind-syndrome, resulting in disorder of the liver- and lung-qi in ascending and descending and, inability of the lung in purifying. Both the exogenous and endogenous wind-evils may lead to disorder of the lung-qi, up-going of sputum and obstruction of qi flow. The resultant fighting between sputum and qi causes wheezing sound, dyspnea and tachypnea. Disorder of qi-flow leads to stuffiness and fullness feeling in the chest, even distending pain in the chest and at the hypochondrium. Insufficiency of yin and blood results in shallow and dim complexion. Due to depletion of body fluid, dryness in throat and mouth, less amount of sputum and difficult expectoration happen. Because of flaring-up of deficiency type fire, flushed face is thus seen. Red tongue with less moisture, no or less fur and taut, thready pulse all are signs of yin - and blood-deficiency.

Therapeutic principles: Nourishing the liver, dispelling wind-evil and regulating the lung.

Recipes and drugs: Modified Guo Min Jian. In this recipe, Radix Bupleuri functions in nourishing the liver and regulating circulation of qi; Radix Ledebouriellae serves to dispel the exogenous and endogenous wind-evils; Fructus Mume, Fructus Schisandrae and Radix Glycyrrhizae, sour and sweet herbs for producing yin-fluid, are used to replenish yin and nourish the liver and arrest endogenous wind-evil; Semen Armeniacae serves to ventilate lung-qi; Caulis Perillae and Fructus Perillae function in regulating qi, lowering reverse flow of qi and arresting asthma; Lumbricus is salt in flavor and cool in nature and functions in dredging meridians and calming the endopathic wind; in case of significant stagnation of liver-qi, Fructus Aurantii and Radix Paconiae Rubra are added, which are used by adopting the usage of Si Ni Powder for strengthening effects of relieving the depressed liver and regulating disorder of qi. If the predisposing factors are clear, the onset of wheezing is sudden and urgent, and the syndrome belongs to heat in nature, Bombyx Batryticatus and Periostracum Cicadae are supplemented to relieve spasm of trachea, tranquilize the endogenous wind and dredge meridians; or Yang Lishan's "Sheng Jiang Powder" is used in combination to normalize the ascending and descending functions of qi, calm the endopathic wind and dredge meridians. In case of cold-predominance type wheezing, Scorpio and Rhizoma

Ligustici Chuanxion are added to relieve spasm, calm the endopathic wind and dredge meridians; in case of severer stuffy chest, wheezing sound and coarse breathing, Herba Ephedrae and Semen Lepidii seu Descurainiae are added to ventilate the lung, lower adverse flow of qi and arrest asthma, which is used by learning from the usage of San Ao Decoction plus Tingli Dazhao Xiefei Decoction. In case of coexistence of exterior-cold and interior-heat, i. e. "cold wrapping fire syndrome", Herba Ephedrae and crude Gypsum Fibrosum are supplimented to ventilate the lung, clear away heat and relieve asthma, which are employed by adopting the meaning of Ma Xing Shi Gan Decoction. If roundworms hide in the interior of the body, Wu Mei Decoction is used first to expel the worms, then, Modified Guo Min Jian Decoction is prescribed to the patients.

Recipe example:

Radix Bupleuri 10g, Radix Ledebouriellae 10g, Fructus Mume 8g, Fructus Schisandrae 6g, Radix Glycyrrhizae 5g, Semen Armeniacae 10g, Caulis Perillae 10g, Fructus Perillae 10g and Lumbricus 10g.

(4) Blood-stasis type wheezing

Main symptoms: Chronic lingering asthma, attacking repeatedly, chest stuffiness and hypochondrium pain, cyanosis of finger nails, and dim complexion

Concurrent symptoms: Bitter taste, dryness of throat, constipation, abdominal distension, or frequent menoxenia in women, or slight edema.

Tongue picture and pulse condition: Purplish tongue or with ecchymosis, deep, uneven pulse.

Analysis: Protracted wheezing results in disorder of lung-qi, disturbance of flow of liver-qi and lung-qi and derangement of qi and blood. Stagnation of qi induces blood stasis. Because of the resultant blood stasis stays in the interior, dyspnea occurs, characterized by cyanosis of finger nails, dim complexion, purplish tongue with ecchymosis, uneven pulse, menstrual disorder in women, etc. Obstruction of blood stasis in the interior brings about functional disorder of Shaoyang Meridians, in addition, the exogenous pathogenic factors also invades the human body, which combine together to be liable to form a coexistence syndrome of excess-heat and blood stasis in Shaoyang and Yangming Meridians, marked by bitter taste, constipation, abdominal distension, etc.

Therapeutic principles: Promoting blood circulation to remove blood stasis, lowering adverse flow of qi to relieve dyspnea.

Recipes and drugs: Modified Xuefu Zhuyu Decoction. In the present recipe,

Si Ni Powder, a sub-recipe, composed of Radix Bupleuri, , Fructus Aurantii, Radix Paeoniae Rubra and Radix Glycyrrhizae is used to regulate flow of qi; Taohong Siwu Decoction, another sub-recipe, serves to promote blood circulation and dredge meridians; Radix Platycodi and Radix Achyranthis Bidentatae are used to accelerate flow of qi and blood. In case of insufficiency of liver blood, internal stagnation of dampness caused by spleen-deficiency and mutual combination of turbid sputum and blood stasis, Danggui Shaoyao Powder supplemented with drugs for ventilating the lung to lower qi as Caulis Perillae, Fructus Perillae, Semen Armeniacae, Lumbricus and Herba Ephedrae. If symptoms of coexistence of excess-heat and blood stasis of Shaoyang and Yangming Meridians appear, Da Chaihu Decoction combined with Modified Guizhi Fuling Pill is employed to accelerate flow of qi and blood of Shaoyang and Yangming and to make lung-qi unimpeded.

Recipe example:

Radix Angelicae Sinensis 10g, Rhizoma Ligustici Chuanxiong 10g, Radix Paeoniae Rubra 10g, Poria 12g, Radix Bupleuri 10g, Radix Scutellariae 10g, Fructus Aurantii 10g, Rhizoma Pinelliae 10g, wine-fried Radix et Rhizoma Rhei 4g, Fructus Perillae 10g and Semen Armeniacae 10g.

Cold-type wheezing and heat-type wheezing are classified according to the nature of sputum. Although, wind type wheezing results from wind-evil, in fact, it is characterized mainly by yin-deficiency and qi-stagnation. Blood stasis type wheezing is manifested by internal obstruction by blood stasis, blood stasis induced qi-stagnation, and dysfunction of the Lung Meridian. In clinic, the aforementioned four types of wheezing syndrome have their own chief symptoms and should be identified carefully. Because wind-evil, turbid sputum, qi-stagnation and blood stasis are often combined together to cause this disease, thus, when they are treated, therapeutic principles, recipes and drugs selected should be chiefly aimed at eliminating the leading pathogenic factors which induce main symptoms; certainly, the concomitant symptoms are also treated at the same time by choosing some auxiliary drugs.

3. Stage of intermission

1) Deficiency of the lung

Main symptoms: Spontaneous sweating, aversion to wind, frequent common cold due to abnormal changes of climate, manifesting as sneezing, nasal stuffiness, clear nasal discharge, pale complexion, thin white expectoration

Concurrent symptoms: Shortness of breath, lower voice, or mild wheezing sound in the throat.

Tongue picture and pulse condition: Pale tongue with thin white coating, thready weak or deficient large pulse.

Analysis: Weakness of wei-qi leads to unconsolidated superficial defensive function. The body is liable to be attacked by exogenous pathogenic factors, resulting in spontaneous sweating, aversion to wind and frequent common cold. It is often induced by abnormal changes of climate, with some prodromal symptoms of nasal stuffiness, nasal discharge, sneezing, etc. Due to hypofunction, the lung can not dominate qi, and the qi fails to transform body fluid, leading to accumulation of sputum-rheum in the lung. As a result, symptoms of short breathing, lower voice,, cough with thin white sputum, pale complexion, etc and other. manifestations of deficiency of lung-qi are seen.

Therapeutic principles: Reinforcing the lung to consolidate the Wei-system.

Recipes and drugs: Supplemented Yu Ping Feng Powder. Ingredient Radix Astragali seu Hedysari serves to replenish qi for consolidating the superficial defensive function; Rhizoma Atractylodis Macrocephalae and Radix Glycyrrhizae are used to invigorate the spleen and tonify the lung; Radix Ledebouriellae functions in dispelling wind-evil and helping Radix Astragali seu Hedysari to consolidate the body surface and raise the defensive function. In case of obvious aversion to cold and wind, Guizhi Decoction containing Ramulus Cinnamomi, Radix Paeoniae Alba, Rhizoma Zingiberis Recens and Rhizoma Ziziphi Jujubae, etc is used in combination for regulating Ying and Wei. In patients with deficiency of both lung-qi and lung-yin, paroxysmal cough, less, greasy sputum, dryness in the mouth and throat, reddish tongue, etc., Sheng Mai Powder is employed in combination with Radix Glehnia, Rhizoma Polygonati Odorati, Radix Astragali seu Hedysari, etc. for replenishing qi and nourishing yin; or Bu Fei Decoction is prescribed to the patient. In this recipe, Radix Ginseng and Radix Astragali seu Hedysari are used to invigorate qi; Radix Rehmanniae Praeparata and Fructus Schisandrae function in nourishing yin; Radix Asteris and Cortex Mori Radicis function in resolving sputum, lowering qi and relieving cough.

Recipe example:

Dried Radix Astragali seu Hedysari 12g, Radix Ledebouriellae 8g, Rhizoma

Atractylodis Macrocephalae 6g, prepared Radix Glycyrrhizae 5g, Radix Codonopsis 10g, Radix Ophiopogonis 10g, Fructus Schisandrae 10g and Cordyceps 10g.

2) Deficiency of spleen

Main symptoms: Usual less food intake, epigastric stuffiness and loose stool in daily life (which are liable to attack due to improper diet), lassitude and short breathing.

Concurrent symptoms: Frequent diarrhea due to having greasy food, feeble speech.

Tongue picture and pulse condition: Pale tongue with thin greasy or white slippery coating, thready, weak, soft pulse.

Analysis: Due to deficiency, the spleen is unable to function normally in transportation, thus, less food intake, epigastric stuffiness and loose stool happen frequently due to improper diet. Insufficiency of qi in middle-jiao results in lassitude and feeble speech. Pale tongue with thin greasy or white slippery coating, thready, weak, soft pulse are all signs of deficiency of spleen-qi.

Therapeutic principle: Strengthening the spleen and resolving phlegm.

Recipes and drugs: Modified Liu Junzi Decoction. Radix Codonopisis Pilosulae, Rhizoma Atractylodis Macrocephalae, Poria and Radix Glycyrrhizae serve to invigorate the spleen and replenish qi; Pericarpium Citri Reticulatae and Rhizoma Pinelliae function in regulating qi and resolving phlegm. In case of insufficiency of spleen-yang, marked by cold limbs, loose stool, white thin sputum, etc., Ramulus Cinnamomi and Rhizoma Zingiberis are supplemented to warm the spleen and remove fluid-retension.

Recipe example: Radix Codonopisis Pilosulae 15g, Rhizoma Atractylodis Macrocephalae 10g, Poria 10g, Pericarpium Citri Reticulatae 10g, Rhizoma Pinelliae 10g and Radix Glycyrrhizae.

3) Deficiency of the kidney

Main symptoms: Usual short rapid breaking in daily life, worsening while making exertion, dyspnea, soreness and weakness of the waist and legs, dyspnea being liable to attack after overstrain.

Concurrent symptoms: Aversion to cold, cold limbs, pale complexion and spontaneous sweating are often seen in patients with predominant yang-deficiency; while in those with dominance of yin-deficiency, flushed cheeks, dysphoria with smothery sensation and night sweating often seen.

Tongue picture and pulse condition: Bulge tender tongue with white coatingand deep thready pulse seen in cases with yang-deficiency, while red tongue with less coating, thready rapid pulse seen in cases with yin-deficiency.

Analysis: Chronic disease results in deficiency of the kidney, the kidney falls into disorder in accepting the inhaled qi, thus, leading to short breathing, even worsening in making physical exertion and difficult breathing. Insufficiency of essence and qi brings about weakness of the waist and knees, which is readily to occur if the patient gets tired. Because of yang-deficiency, symptoms of exterior-cold syndrome are often seen, while in case of yin-deficiency, internal-heat syndrome happens.

Therapeutic principle: Tonifying the kidney to accept qi normally.

Recipes and Drugs: Jingui Shenqi Pill or Mai Wei Dihuang Pill is used on the basis of differentiation of yin- or yang-syndrome. The former recipe mainly functions in warming the kidney to help yang and the latter mainly in tonifying the kidney to accept qi. If yang-deficiency is dominant, Fructus Psoraleae, Herba Epimedii, sliced Cornu Cervi or Cola Cornus Cervi are added; if yin-deficiency is dominant, tonics warm in nature are excluded, a larger dose of dried Radix Rehmanniae, Radix Angelicae Sinensis, Fructus Ligustri Lucidi, Colla Corii Asini, Colla Plastron Testudinis, etc are supplemented. In case of evident kidney-deficiency and inability of the kidney to accept qi, the above two recipes are used in combination with Semen Juglandis, Cordyceps, Fluorite; or Shen Ga Powder and Placenta Hominis are prescribed to the patients for frequent oral administration.

Recipe example:

Dried Radix Rehmanniae 12g, Radix Rehmanniae Praeparata 12g, Fructus Corni 10g, Poria 12g, Radix Angelicae Sinensis 10g, Fructus Psoraleae 10g, Fructus Ligustri Lucidi 10g, Pericarpium Citri Reticulatae 10g, Fructus Schisandrae 8g and Fructus Perillae 10g.

Lung-deficiency, spleen-deficiency and kidney-deficiency have their own characters, but in clinic, coexistence of two or all of them is often seen, so, in treatment, the principal and secondary aspects should be distinguished first and all aspects should also be taken into consideration at the same time. If the principal and secondary aspects are difficult to be distinguished, all the three zang-organs are reinforced uniformly. Besides, whatever cold type or heat-type wheezing, if it develops continuously and attacks repeatedly, concurrent blood stasis syndrome is often seen. Under the circumstances, Semen Persicae, Rhizoma Ligustici Chuanxiong, Radix Angelicae Sinensis, Radix Salviae Miltiorrhizae, etc. are added and the above-mentioned recipes can be used in combination. In addition to oral administration, external application of mounting method, Chinese herbs-processed aerosol, acupuncture, moxibustion, cutting therapy, catgut embedding therapy, finger-pressure method, simple recipes, proved recipes, etc may also be used on the basis of differentiation of syndromes.

4. Crisis of wheezing syndrome-abrupt collapse of yang-qi, mental confusion due to phlegm-stagnation

Symptoms and pulse condition: In the process of onset of wheezing, symptoms of vomiting, diarrhea, muscular twitching and cramp, purplish complexion, lassitude, or irritability, vague mind, greasy sweating, cold limbs, faint pulse, cyan-purple tongue with slippery greasy coating happen at any time.

Analysis: Protracted wheezing results in progressing weakness of the vital energy day by day. Under this condition, additional sudden invasion of exogenous pathogenic factors leads to obstruction of lung-qi, mutual fighting between yin and yang, causing sudden exhaustion of yang-qi, stagnation of sputum and loss of consciousness.

Therapeutic principles: Restoring yang from collapse, resolving sputum and removing blood stasis.

Recipes and drugs: Modified Siwei Huiyang Decoction. Radix Aconiti Praeparata and Rhizoma Zingiberis are used to eliminate turbid-yin and recuperate depleted yang; Radix Ginseng and Radix Glycyrrhizae serve to replenish qi and relive collapse. In case of cyan-purple complexion, purplish tongue, Semen Persicae and Flos Carthami are supplemented to promote blood circulation and eliminate blood stasis; in case of vague mind, Rhizoma Acori Tatarinowii, Radix Curcumae and a bit of Moschus are used in combination to restore consciousness; in case of collapse of yang-qi and body fluid, Radix Panacis Quinquefolii is added or Fructus Corni, Radix Ophiopogonis and Fructus Schisandrae are added.

〔Measures for Prevention and Nursing〕

1) Keep the air fresh and sunlight full in the room. It is advisable for patients with cold type wheezing that more attention is paid particularly to avoid affection by exogenous wind-cold evils, and the room temperature should be kept slightly

higher. In heat-type wheezing patients with fever, consumption of body fluid and qi should be prevented, the room temperature should be kept lower and the room air and moisture kept suitable; in wind type and blood-stasis type wheezing patients, the state of disease is liable to change. If dyspnea with mouth open and shoulder lifted, restlessness, cyan-purplish complexion and lips, sweating, cold limbs, floating, large and rootless pulse, or knotted uneven pulse — a crisis sign of asthma-collapse of deficiency of both heart and kidney appear, emergency measures should be given immediately.

2) Ask the patient to have light food, avoid eating too salty, too sour, hot or irritable food, keep away cigarettes and wine; be careful about peculiar smell, dust, sea food, etc so as to try one's best to put an end to the source of production of sputum. Avoid overstrain and extreme mental stress.

3) During clinical observation, try to understand the predisposing factors, onset time, duration of wheezing, concurrent symptoms, body temperature, pulse rate, sputum-fluid, etc.

4) If wheezing attacks periodically, ask the patient to take drugs about 1 to 2 hours before onset. In the stage of attack, the patient should lie in bed and take a half lying position. When necessary, give the patient with oxygen inhalation measure. Keep the patient's respiratory tract unobstructed. For patients with profuse sputum, try to eliminate sputum in time.

5) When asthma attacks violently, try to relieve it by using the following methods:

(1) Inhaling flos daturae vapor.

(2) Puncturing Tiantu (RN 22), Shanzhong (RN 17), Qihai (RN 6), etc. combined with moxibustion for cold type wheezing.

(3) Oral administration of aminophylline, isoprenaline, etc., be cautious of application of antitussives and sedatives.

6) In the stage of intermission of wheezing, guide the patient to do physical exercise to strengthen his or her constitution.

〔Analysis of Typical Case〕

Chen ××male, aged 15 years.

Her first visit was on July 12, 1976. When being 3 years old, she began to suffering from asthma. At the beginning, asthma attacked mildly, gradually, more and more frequently especially during spring and summer. If it attacked, she had dyspnea, tachypnea with wheezing sound in the throat, could not lie flat, and had a poor appetite. She often took antitussives and antiasthmatics as aminophylline, ephedrine, etc. and antibiotics such as penicillin, etc. only in this way, could asthma be relieved. Day after day, due to affection by wind-cold evils, her asthma attacked again. Examination showed that the patient experienced rapid breathing, dyspnea with mouth open and shoulders lifted, wheezing sound, scattered dry and damp rale in the bilateral lung, thick profuse sputum, pale complexion, red tongue with yellow greasy coating and thready taunt pulse.

Differentiation of syndromes:

Latent sputum accumulates in the interior for a long time to induce pathogenic heat. The resultant heat and the invaded exogenous cold-evil attract each other to evoke onset of asthma, suggesting cold in the lung and heat below the diaphragm, weakness of the body resistance and excess of the pathogenic factors.

Treatment principles: Ventilating the lung, clearing away heat, relieving cough and arresting asthma (meaning that in emergency cases, treat the acute symptoms first).

Recipe (first recipe) and drugs: Modified Ding Chuan Decoction. Herba Ephedrae 10g, Semen Ginkgo 3g, Radix Scutellariae 10g, Fructus Perillae 10g, Lumbricus 15g, Semen Armeniacae 12g, Flos Farfarae 10g, Rhizoma Ligustici Chuanxiong 10g, Scorpio 5g (6 dose).

Second visit on August 13: After first treatment, her asthma was relieved significantly. During the past month, her asthma attacked only once or twice and was lighter in comparison with pre – treatment. When attacking, it was relieved immediately after administration of Modified Ding Chuan Decoction. But she still experienced dyspnea and hyperhidrosis if making exertion and had no desire to have food. According to the principle that treating the fundamental cause, when acute symptoms being relieved, it was treated by replenishing the kidney to accept qi, nourishing the lung, resolving sputum and relieving asthma.

Radix Rehmanniae Praeparata 2g, Fructus Schisandrae 5g, Cordyceps10g, Placenta Hominis 5g, Radix Glycyrrhizae 5g, Lignum Aquilariae Resinatum1g (taken by pouring hot decoction over it and stirring later), Fructus Perillae 5g, Bulbus Fritillariae Cirrhosae 3g, Radix Codonopsis 5g, Radix Ophiopogonis 3g and Concha Ostreae 12g. (second recipe, 6 doses)

Third visit on September 6, 1977: She told me that when asthma attacked, she used the first recipe and during intermittent period, used the second recipe; in this way and alternately, she insisted on taking Chinese drugs for more than a year (sometimes one dose every day, sometimes suspending for a period of time). Her asthma was under controlled basically. Currently, she had no much expectoration, but underwent light shortness of breath with wheezing sound if making exertion. In the past year, her asthma had no grand mal all along, and she could engage in common daily activities. She was then treated with the second recipe for consolidating the therapeutic effect (with the dose doubled and drugs processed into pills).

Note: The present case belongs to the stage of attack, marked by lung-cold and diaphragm-heat, deficiency in origin and excess in superficiality, which reults from mutual attraction of newly-invaded exogenous cold and interior heat induced by heat-transformation of the protracted accumulation of latent old sputum in the interior. So, it is treated mainly by using Modified Ding Chuan Decoction to ventilate the lung, clear away heat, and relieve cough and asthma for dealing with the superficiality. In Ding Chuan Decoction, Lumbricus, Rhizoma Ligustici Chuanxiong and Scorpio are added instead of Radix Glycyrrhizae, Cortex Mori Radicis and Rhizoma Pinelliae for arresting asthma and relieving spasm. The whole recipe can function both in clearing away lung-heat, lowering reverse flow of qi, resolving sputum and eliminate latent sputum-retention. In the stage of intermission, the fundamental cause of disease is treated, so, Radix Rehmanniae Praeparata, Fructus Schisandrae, Placenta Hominis and Cordyceps are used to replenish the kidney; Radix Codonopsis Pilosulae, Radix Ophiopogonis, Bulbus Fritillariae Cirrhosae, Lignum Aquilariae Resinatum, Fructus Perillae, and Radix Glycyrrhizae serve to nourish the lung, promote flow of qi and remove sputum, combined with Concha Ostreae for arresting sweating. In this way, principles for treatment of both superficiality and origin, chronic and acute symptoms are used alternately to accelerate recovery of functions of the lung and kidney.

Wheezing syndrome is a paroxysmal bronchial disease characterized by rapid breathing, dyspnea, wheezing sound in the throat. Sputum latent originally in the lung is its principal pathogenic factor, when the patient is attacked additionally by exogenous factors, wheezing syndrome may happen immediately. During attack, the respiratory tract is obstructed by sputum, the lung-qi fails in cleaning the inspired air and in lowering downwards, manifested by excess of pathogenic factors. If wheezing attacked repeatedly and develops for a long period of time, serious consumption of qi and yin, and gradual deficiency of the lung, spleen and kidney happen successively. In the stage of intermission, it is mainly manifested by deficiency of the vital energy, and during grand mal, deficiency of the vital energy and excess of evils exist simultaneously. Treatment is given according to differentiation of syndromes (deficiency- or excess-syndrome) and different stages of the disease as stage of attack and intermittent stage. In the stage of attack, excess of pathogenic factors is dominant, so, treatment should be aimed at eliminating pathogenic factors to deal with the superficiality. After distinguishing cold and heat, therapeutic principles of warming and ventilating the lung or clearing away lung-heat are adopted. In treatment of patients with chronic wheezing syndrome accompanied with acute attack which manifests coexistence of deficiency and excess, both the acute symptoms and fundamental cause are considered at the same time. In the stage of intermission, treatment is aimed at strengthening the body resistance to deal with the fundamental cause. After examining the state of yin and yang, reinforcing the lung, invigorating the spleen or nourishing the kidney is adopted respectively.

In short, regarding treatment of wheezing syndrome, situations of coexistence of cold and heat, cold wrapping fire syndrome, heat-transformation of cold-sputum, cold-transformation of heat syndrome, deficiency of vital energy, or excess of pathogenic factors, or coexistence of both, etc. should be understood thoroughly. Generally, in wheezing-syndrome patients with shorter duration of disease and in the stage of attack, excess of evils is dominant; in those with chronic disease and during intermission, weakness of body resistance is predominant. Therefore, the above mentioned situations, including acute and chronic symptoms, excess or deficiency, predominance of symptoms of the lung, spleen and kidney, etc. should be considered comprehensively. On the basis of grasping the focal point, the secondary aspect is also taken into consideration at the same time. The kidney is the origin of the congenital constitution and the root of the five zang-organs. Thus, tonifying the kidney is very important. Only when the essence and qi are sufficient, can the body resistance is consolidated at last.

Questions for Review

1. What are the key points for differentiation of wheezing syndrome ? How to differentiate and treat different types of wheezing syndrome in the acute stage?
2. How to identify wheezing syndrome and panting syndrome?

3. What is the significance of tonifying kidney in the stage of intermission of wheezing syndrome?

Panting Syndrome

〔General Description〕

Panting syndrome is one of the respiratory disease characterized by rapid breathing even with mouth open and shoulders elevated, flaring of nares, dyspnea, worsening while making exertion. If the situation is serious and develops progressively, it may results in prostration syndrome. Panting syndrome may be also seen in the developing process of many acute and chronic diseases.

In the ancient documents, there are abundant descriptions on panting syndrome. Following the usage of Chapter, Panting in the medical book《Jing Yue Quan Shu》(Complete Works of Zhang Jing Yue), panting syndrome is divided into two major categories, i. e. deficiency- and excess-pattern in modern clinic of traditional Chinese medicine. They are different in property. When treated, they should be distinguished strictly first by combining the history and cause of disease, clinical manifestations and signs with necessary physical and laboratory examinations.

In treatment of many respiratory diseases in modern medicine, such as asthmatic bronchial bronchitis, pneumonia, pulmonary emphysema, pulmonary tuberculosis, pneumoconiosis, pulmonary abscess, chronic pulmonary heart disease, and other system-induced respiratory distress syndrome, cardiac asthma, rapid breathing and dyspnea brought about by hysteria, etc., all the contents of differentiation of syndromes and therapeutic methods described in this chapter can be used for reference.

〔Cause of Disease and Pathogenesis〕

In spit of many pathogenic factors, panting syndrome has only two major categories, i. e. exopathy and internal impairment. The former is referred to invasion of six external etiological factors and the internal impairment is referred to injury caused by improper diet, seven emotions, over-strain, etc. The focus is located chiefly in the lung and kidney and also associated with the liver and spleen and heart. The property of disease contains deficiency and excess two patterns. The excess type results from attack of exogenous pathogenic factors, causing failure of the lung to disperse and descend due to accumulated pathogenic factors. Deficiency type panting is induced by inability of the lung to dominate qi or failure of the kidney in accepting qi rather by attack of the pathogenic factors.

1. Attack of exogenous pathogenic factors

In regard to exogenous pathogenic factors responsible for panting syndrome, wind-cold and wind-heat are more often seen in clinic. Because of invasion of wind-cold, the lung-qi is suppressed in the interior and the skin and interstitial space tightened in the exterior. The lung and wei-system are thus injured, inducing disorder of the lung-qi in dispersing and descending functions. In case of attack of the lung by wind-heat, the lung-qi stagnates, even inducing formation of phlegm due to consumption of the body fluid by heat. As a result, the lung is unable to function normally in purifying and descending, inducing reverse flow of lung-qi and panting. Or, there is latent heat in the lung originally, and wind-cold evils tighten the exterior additionally. The exterior cold is not dispelled in time and transforms into heat instead. The heat is obstructed by cold-evil and thus can not disperse, resulting in adverse flow of lung-qi and panting.

2. Abundant sputum

Improper diet, clinging to greasy, sweet, raw and cool food, or addiction to wine all may injury the middle -jiao, leading to dysfunction of the spleen in transportation and transformation of food essence. The resultant accumulation of dampness brings about generation of sputum. Or the patient originally has a constitution of predominance of sputum-dampness. All of these are the internal factors responsible for occurrence of panting. The spleen is the origin of generation of sputum while the lung is an organ for storing sputum. The resultant turbid sputum accumulates gradually and goes up to interfere in the functional activity of the lung. The lung-qi is thus obstructed and falls into disorder in ascending and descending, followed by rapid breathing and onset of panting. In case of heat-transformation of sputum-dampness due to protracted accumulation, or original hyperactivity of lung-fire, the sputum is steamed, leading to wreak havoc of sputum-fire. So, the lung fails in purifying and descending abilities, causing adverse flow of lung-qi and panting. If panting occurs due to sputum and additional affection by exogenous pathogenic factors, a complicated situation of coexistence of turbid sputum, wind-cold, pathogenic heat appear at the same time.

3. Injury by emotions

Mental stress, excessive worry and pensiveness can bring about stagnation of qi which impedes the normal and regular flow of lung-qi; or grief and anger impair the liver, the liver-qi goes up adversely to interfere in the lung, which give rise to panting because of inability of lung-qi in purifying and descending, or more reversed upward flow and less lowering.

4. Hypofunction of the lung and kidney

Chronic cough can impair the lung and chronic disease may also cause hypofunction of the lung. Under the circumstances, insufficiency of lung-qi and lung-yin, shortness of breath and panting will occur due to inability of qi to function normally. If the situations develop continuously for a long time, the lingering lung disease will bring calamity to the kidney. Overstrain and excessive sexual intercourse often impair the kidney, the vital essence and energy are suppressed in the interior. It means that depleted lung-qi and lung-yin are incapable of nourishing the kidney in the lower and the genuine primordial qi of the kidney is injured additionally, inducing unconsolidated foundation of the body. As a result, air-reception is out of order, more expiration and less inspiration, reverse up-flow of qi and panting happen successively. In case of extreme deficiency or exhaustion of the kidney-yang, the water in the body falls into disturbance in metabolism, interferes in the lung and attacks the heart, resulting in panting because of reversed flow of lung-qi and advanced hypofunction of the heart, which belongs to coexistence of deficiency - and excess-syndrome. Moreover, in case of weakness of the middle-jiao, the lung-qi loses normal supplement and nourishment, i. e., the Earth is incapable of producing Gold, panting will also occur due to deficiency of qi and powerless respiration.

To sum up, excess type panting results from disorder of lung-qi in dispersing and descending due to obstruction of the lung by exogenous evils, turbid sputum, reverse flow of the stagnated liver-qi, or blockage of meridians by blood stasis, etc.; while deficiency type panting is induced by insufficiency of essence-qi and disorder of the lung and kidney in regulating respiration. The focus of panting is located mainly in the lung and kidney, and also associated with the liver and spleen. In severe cases, the heart is also involved. Because the lung dominates qi and is in charge of respiration, associated with the skin and hairs in the interior, and compared to a canopy of the five zang-organs, when exogenous evils invade the human body, or pathogenic qi from the other diseased zang-organs attacks it, the lung-qi will lose its function in dispersing and descending, leading to panting due to reverse flow of qi. In addition, if turbid sputum of the Spleen Meridian interferes in the lung, or liver-qi attacks the lung or the qi of the middle-jiao is extremely weak, panting may also happens.

In the severe stage of the developing course of panting, not only extreme weakness of both the lung and kidney presents, but also the heart-yang is involved simultaneously. The cardiac vessels communicate with the lung, and the lung-qi functions normally in regulating circulation of the heart blood. The pectoral qi runs through the heart and lung and performs respiration. A collateral branch of the Kidney Meridian goes out from the lung and connects with the heart. The heart and kidney have mutual helping and checking relations in functional activities. The fire of the life gate is the root of the heart-yang, so, sufficiency or insufficiency of the heart-yang, the congenital kidney-qi and the acquired inhaled and exhaled air all have close relation. Once both the lung and kidney are weak seriously, the heart-yang and heart-qi are also feeble. As a result, normal performance of blood circulation has no enough driving force, tachycardia, blood stasis, cyan-purple complexion, lips, tongue and finger-nails appear subsequently. In case of insufficiency of the heart-qi, the fluid of the heart is out of control, so, profuse sweating and panting present, even causing prostration, exhaustion of yin and yang.

〔Differentiation of Syndromes and Treatment〕

1. Key points for differentiation

1) Differentiation of deficiency - and excess-syndrome

Differentiation of deficiency - and excess-syndrome is most important. If mistakenly running counter to the therapeutic commandments of deficiency and excess syndromes, the state of disease is very readily to get worse. Excess type panting is characterized by deep and long respiration, feeling comfortable when exhaling, coarse respiration, louder voice, rapid and forceful pulse. If panting onset is due to exopathy, it is marked by sudden and acute attack, shorter duration of disease, and a series of symptoms of exterior syndrome in most cases. If panting results from internal injury, it is characterized by longer duration of disease, repeated attack, some manifestations of profuse sputum or hyperactivity of sputum-heat, such as fullness and stuffiness in the chest, etc. but no symptoms of exterior syndrome in most cases. In case of impairment of the liver by great anger, it manifests as dyspnea and tachypnea and a groups of symptoms of abnormal mental activity. The deficiency type panting is marked by rapid breathing, dyspnea, comfort if having a deep inspiration, lower voice, feeble pulse or floating, large, hollow pulse, or longer duration of disease, slow onset, severe or light condition from time to time, and worsening when getting tired. The lung-deficiency type panting is manifested by dyspnea, shortness of breathing, spontaneous sweating and aversion to wind which worsening when having over-exertion, etc. The kidney-deficiency type panting is marked by dyspnea and tachypnea under resting condition, if moving about slightly, these situations worsen immediately, combined with more expiration and less inspiration. Panting patients of deficiency type of heart-qi is marked by continuous gasped breathing.

Schematic Diagram of Causes and Pathogenesis of Panting Syndrome

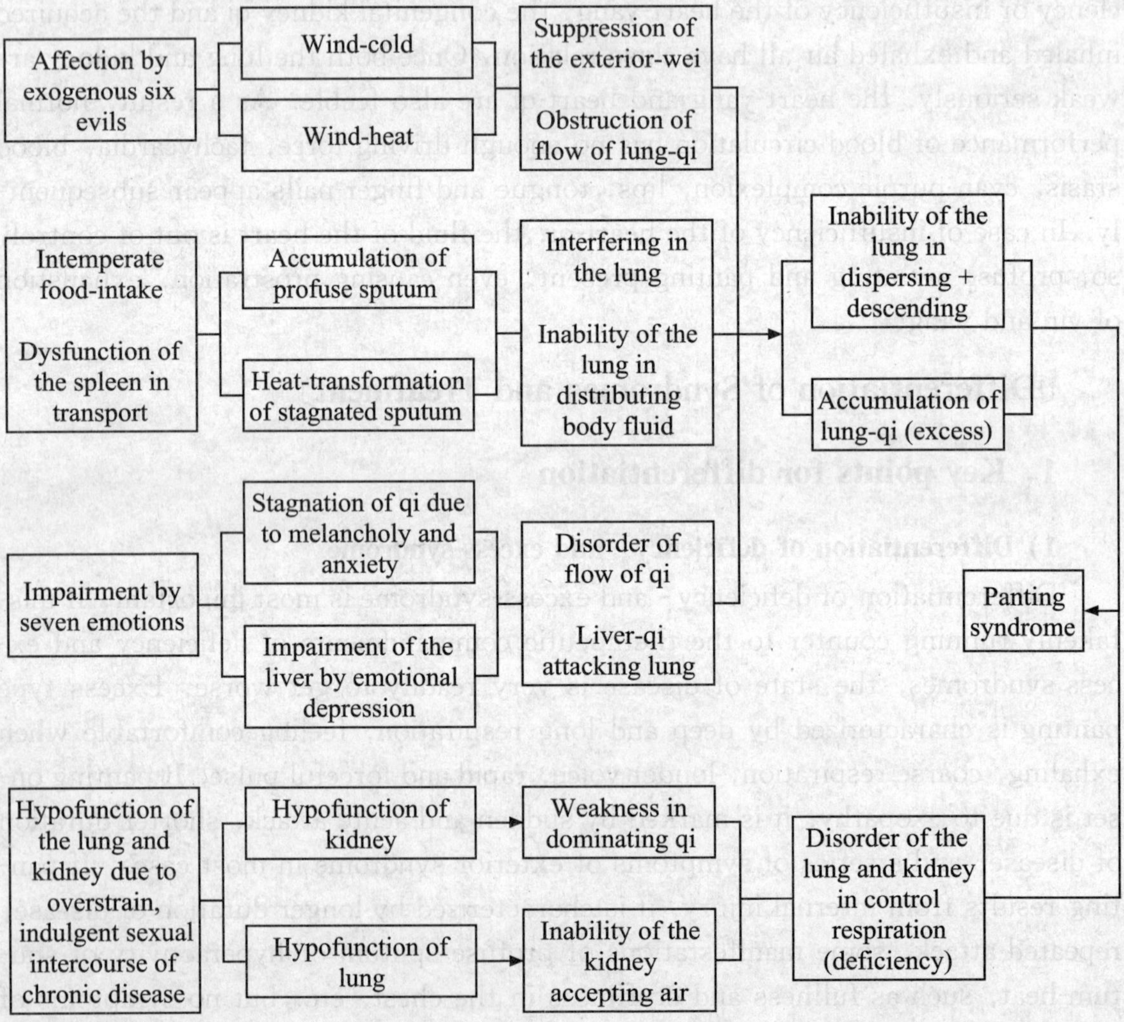

2) Differentiation of cold and heat

Red tongue, rapid pulse and conditions of urine are not enough for identifying cold - or heat-type panting syndrome, only the color of tongue coating and sputum are the key points. Cold type panting is characterized by clear, thin and water-like sputum, or white foamy sputum, dim bluish complexion, no thirst or thirst with preference of hot drink, white slippery tongue coating, floating tense or taunt slow pulse. The heat type panting is marked by yellow, thick, sticky sputum, or white sticky sputum with difficult expectoration, flushed face, thirst with preference of cool drink, red tongue with yellow greasy coating or yellow dry coating, slippery rapid pulse.

3) Differentiation of panting-syndrome, shortness of breath and wheezing-syndrome

(1) Panting-syndrome and shortness of breath

Both panting-syndrome and shortness of breath are abnormal breathing. But, the former is characterized by dyspnea with mouth open and shoulder lifting or even being unable to lie flat, and contains deficiency and excess types; and the later means insufficiency of qi (which is often seen in various acute and chronic diseases), has no excess type and manifests mainly as feeble breathing, being out of breath when speaking or doing light physical labor, lassitude, being reluctant to speak, and weak pulse which result from insufficiency of qi of the middle-jiao, or deficiency of both the lung and kidney. Serious shortness of breath may lead to deficiency type gasp. Generally, shortness of breath may be patient's own feeling while panting syndrome should have external signs and symptoms.

(2) Differentiation of panting- and wheezing-syndrome

Differentiation of panting- and wheezing-syndrome has been discussed in aforementioned Chapter of wheezing syndrome.

2. Typing and treatment

Panting syndrome is made up of deficiency, excess, cold and heat types. For excess type panting, treatment is given to aim mainly at the lung, the general therapeutic principles are removing evils and regulating qi. After differentiation of the cold or heat property of sputum, it is treated by using warming and ventilating the lung, clearing away lung-heat and resolving sputum methods, etc. For deficiency type panting, treatment is conducted to aim at the kidney and lung, particularly at the kidney by reinforcing the kidney-qi to strengthen air-accepting function. According to the concrete pathologic changes of different zang-organs, lung-reinforcing, kidney-invigorating, qi-replenishing or yin-nourishing method is adopted respectively. For coexistence of deficiency and excess or upper excess and lower deficiency, the principal and secondary aspects of the disease, or the superficiality and origin should be distinguished clearly, the proper measures are employed.

1) Excess type panting

(1) Wind-cold attacking the lung

Main symptoms: Gasping for breath, cough, rapid breathing, distending and choking feeling in the chest, abundant white thin sputum.

Concomitant symptoms: Aversion to cold, fever, headache, anhidrosis, absence of thirst, and general aching.

Tongue picture and pulse condition (title): White, thin and slippery tongue coating, floating, tense pulse.

Analysis: The lung is in charge of respiration, and is related to the skin and hairs in the exterior. When wind-cold evils invade the human body, the skin and hairs as well as the lung are attacked first, resulting in accumulation of qi, inability of lung-qi in dispersing. Therefore, gasping, coughing, choking and distending sensation in the chest occur. Cold-evil attacks the lung, the fluid accumulates to become sputum, thus, the sputum is profuse, white and thin. Wind-cold tightens the exterior of the body, the superficial defensive system is suppressed, so, aversion to cold, headache, fever, anhidrosis, etc. are often seen. White, thin, slippery fur and floating, tense pulse are also the signs of wind-cold exterior syndrome.

Therapeutic principle: Ventilating the lung and dispelling cold

Recipe and drugs: Modified Mahuang Decoction is used. In this recipe, Herba Ephedrae and Ramulus Cinnamomi function in ventilating the lung, dispelling cold to remove the exterior syndrome; Semen Armeniacae and Radix Glycyrrhizae are used to resolve sputum and regulate qi. For cold-sputum obstructing lung, Rhizoma Pinelliae, Exocarpium Citri Reticulatae, Fructus Perillae, Radix Cynanchi Stauntonii, etc. serve to resolve sputum and regulate qi. If panting is not relieved after diaphoresis, Guizhi Plus Houpo Xingzi Decoction is used for regulating ying-wei and ventilating lung-qi.

Besides, in case of panting due to coexistence of exterior cold and internal fluid-retention, if belonging to the situation of latent excessive fluid in the hypochondrium and epigastrium combined with additional affection by exogenous cold, manifested by cold back, bluish complexion, clear, thin and foamy sputum, Xiao Qinglong Decoction is used to dispel the exterior cold and warm the interior.

Recipe example:

Herba Ephedrae 6g, Semen Armeniacae 10g, Ramulus Cinnamomi 6g, Radix Glycyrrhizae 5g, Exocarpium Citri Reticulatae 10g, Rhizoma Pinelliae, 8g, Fructus Perillae 10g, Poria 10g and Radix Cynanchi Stauntonii 10g.

(2) Wind-heat attacking lung

Main symptoms: Gasping, rapid breathing, even with flaring of nares, yellow, sticky and thick sputum difficult to be expectorated.

Concomitant symptoms: Chest pain, irritability, headache, fever, sweating, thirst, constipation, brown urine.

Tongue picture and pulse condition: Thin white or yellowish tongue coating, floating or slippery rapid pulse.

Analysis: In case of attack of the lung by wind-heat evils, hyperactivity of heat and accumulation of qi happen, the lung loses its abilities in dispersing and descending and the lung-qi runs urgently, as a result, panting, rapid breathing even with flaring of nares appear. Heat consuming body fluid contributes to generation of sputum, thus, the sputum is yellow, sticky, thick and difficult to be expectorated. Excessive heat consumes body fluid to lead to thirst. Sputum-heat accumulates in the chest, so, there exist irritability, choking or pain sensation in the chest. Fever, sweating and headache suggest excessive heat in the interior accompanied by exterior syndrome. Thin, yellow fur and floating, rapid pulse are due to wind-heat in the lung and exterior.

Therapeutic principles: Clearing away heat from the exterior, ventilating the lung to relieve panting.

Recipes and drugs: Supplemented Ma Xing Shi Gan Decoction is used. In this recipe, Gypsum Fibrosum is used in a larger dose for clearing away lung-heat; Herba Ephedrae serves to ventilate the lung and arrest panting; Semen Armeniacae serves to eliminate lung-heat and lower adverse flow of qi. For severe lung-heat, Radix Scutellariae, Rhizoma Anemarrhenaeand Herba Houttuyniae or a large dose of Gypsum Fibrosum are supplemented. For interior-excess syndrome with accumulation of heat and constipation, Liang Ge Powder or Xuan Bai Chengqi Decoction is used to get rid of fire and lung-heat. For severe exterior syndrome due to attack by wind-heat, Flos Lonicerae and Fructus Forsythiae are added for removing heat pathogen from the exterior. For abundant sputum and serious panting, Semen Lepidii seu Descurainiae and Rhizoma Belamcandae are added for clearing away lung-heat and arresting panting. For cough with yellow, thick sputum, Fructus Trichosanthis and Bulbus Fritillariae Cirrhosae are added to eliminate lung-heat.

Appendix: In case of coexistence of heat in the interior and cold in the exterior, i. e., accumulation of heat in the lung and wind-cold pathogen tightening the lung, or the exterior-cold syndrome being still existing while heat-transformation being developing in the interior, the resultant heat accumulates in the lung to cause the lung-qi to flow adverse, so, panting, coarse breathing, flaring of nares, distending pain sensation in the chest, yellow, sticky and thick sputum occur. It is treated still by using Supplemented Ma Xing Shi Gan Decoction. If there exists sweating, Gypsum Fibrosum is used in a larger dose; and if there is no sweating, Herba Ephedrae is used in a larger dose.

Recipe example:

Herba Ephedrae 6g, Semen Armeniacae 10g, Gypsum Fibrosum (decocted first), Radix Glycyrrhizae 5g, Radix Scutellariae 10g, Fructus Trichosanthis 15g, Fructus Forsythiae 10g, Radix Rhapontici seu Echinopsis 10g and Radix Platycodi 6g.

(3) Accumulation of turbid phlegm in the lung

Main symptoms: Panting, cough, profuse, white and sticky phlegm, fullness and choking sensation in the chest.

Concomitant symptoms: Poor appetite, stickiness in the mouth, no thirst, nausea or vomiting in severe cases.

Tongue picture and pulse condition: Thick, greasy, white tongue coating, slippery pulse.

Analysis: In case of dysfunction of the spleen in transportation, dampness gathers together to become sputum and stagnate in the lung, the lung-qi fails in descending, thus, panting, stuffiness in the chest, dyspnea, profuse, sticky, white sputum appear. In case of accumulation of sputum-dampness in the middle-jiao, the spleen and stomach can not function cooperatively, thus, nausea, poor appetite, stickiness in the mouth, thick, greasy tongue coating and slippery pulse happen.

Therapeutic principle: Resolving sputum and lowering the reversed flow of qi

Recipe and drugs: Er Chen Decoction is used in combination with Modified San Zi Yang Qin Decoction. In this recipe, Rhizoma Pinelliae, Pericarpium Citri Reticulatae and Poria are used to strengthen the spleen, eliminate dampness and resolve sputum; Fructus Perillae, Semen Sinapis Albae and Semen Raphani serve to regulate qi, lower adverse flow of qi and resolve sputum. For excessive sputum-dampness, marked by stuffiness of chest and poor appetite, Rhizoma Atractylodis and Cortex Magnoliae are supplemented for eliminating dampness, enlivening the spleen and promoting flow of qi.

Recipe example:

Pericarpium Citri Reticulatae 10g, Rhizoma Pinelliae 10g, Poria 12g, Radix Glycyrrhizae 5g, parched Fructus Perillae 10g, parched Semen Sinapis Albae 6g, parched Semen Raphani 10g, Cortex Magnoliae 8g and Semen Armeniacae 10g.

(4) Accumulation of sputum-heat in the lung

Main symptoms: Panting, cough, dyspnea, irritable feverish sensation and distending pain in the chest, profuse, yellow, sticky and thick sputum.

Concomitant symptoms: Thirst, preference to cold drinks, flushed face, dryness in the throat, brown urine, constipation or bloody sputum.

Tongue picture and pulse condition: Yellow greasy tongue coating, slippery, rapid pulse.

Analysis: In case of accumulated heat originally in the spleen and stomach due to sustained intake of rich fatty diet or heat-transformation from chronically gathered sputum-dampness or from the entered exterior-pathogens, the resultant sputum-heat stagnates in the lung to obstruct the air passage, so, panting, cough and dyspnea occur. In case of accumulation and steaming of sputum-heat, irritable feverish sensation in the chest, thirst, preference to cold drinks, yellow, sticky, thick sputum, dryness in the throat, flush face, yellow, greasy tongue coating, slippery rapid pulse are seen. Impairment of blood vessels by heat is responsible for bloody sputum.

Therapeutic principles: Eliminating lung-heat and resolving sputum.

Recipe and drugs: Modified Shang Bai Pi Decoction. In this recipe, Cortex Mori Radicis, Rhizoma Coptidis, Radix Scutellariae and Fructus Gardeniae are used to eliminate lung-heat; Bulbus Fritillariae Cirrhosae, Semen Armeniacae, Fructus Perillae and Rhizoma Pinelliae serve to descend qi and resolve sputum;

for patients with fever, Gypsum Fibrosum and Rhizoma Anemerrhenae are used in combination; for abundant, sticky and thick sputum, Concha Meretricis seu Cyclinae or Dai Ge Powder is added; for panting, inability to lie flat, profuse sputum and constipation, Semen Lepidii seu Descurainiae, Radix et Rhizoma RheiNatrii Sulfas Exsiccatus are added. If the sputum is stinking, Herba Houttuyniae, Semen Coicis, Semen Benincasae and Rhizoma Phragmitis are supplemented.

Recipe example:

Fructus Trichosanthis 18g, Bulbus Fritillariae Cirrhosae 10g, Herba Houttuyniae 5g, Radix Scutellariae 10g, Semen Lepidii seu Descurainiae 10g, parched Semen Raphani 10g, Cortex Mori Radicis 10g, Semen Coicis 10g, Semen Benincasae 10g and charred Fructus Gardeniae 10g.

(5) Impairment of the lung by stagnated qi

Main symptoms: Short and rapid breathing, panting, choking sensation in the chest, a feeling of obstruction in the throat, which are evoked usually by mental stress.

Concomitant symptoms: Frequent insomnia, palpitation, chest stuffiness, chest pain, etc.

Tongue picture and pulse condition: Thin tongue coating, taut pulse.

Analysis: In case of impairment of the liver due to great anger, the liver-qi flows adversely to attack the lung, inducing failure of lung-qi to descend. As a result, panting, dyspneic respiration as being blocked in the throat, stuffiness and pain in the chest because of incoordination between the liver and collateral-qi of the Lung Meridian occur. Due to stagnation of the heart-qi and liver-qi, insomnia, palpitation and taut pulse happen.

Therapeutic principle: Alleviating the mental depression, descending adverse flow of lung-qi to relieve panting.

Recipes and drugs: Modified Wu Mo Decoction. In this recipe, aromatics, Lignum Aquilariae, Radix Aucklandiae, Semen Arecae, Radix Linderae and Fructus Aurantii are used to alleviate mental depression and lower qi. For panting patients with palpitation and insomnia, Bulbus Lilii, Flos Albiziae, Semen Ziziphi Spinosae and Radix Polygalae are added to tranquilize the mind; for stuffy chest with distending pain, Flos Inulae and Rhizoma Cpperi are supplemented. For supporting the treatment, console and help the patient to get over his or her worries. For panting patients with mental depression, up-disturbing of accumulated pathogenic fire and qi and irritability, Dan Zhi Xiao Yao Decoction is used in combination with Radix Curcumae but discarding Rhizoma Macrocephalae. In case of qi stagnation and blood stasis, panting, cough, stuffiness and stabbing pain in the chest, worsening on exertion, hypochondriac lump, cyan-purplish complexion, lips and finger nails, less sputum, no thirst, purplish tongue with ecchymosis and taunt, hesitant or taunt, thready pulse, Modified Xuefu Zhuyu Decoction is used. In this recipe, Si Ni Powder (sub-recipe) is used to relieve the depressed liver, and Tao Hong Si Wu Decoction (another sub-recipe) is used to nourish blood and to promote blood circulation; Radix Platycodi and Radix Achyranthis Bidentatae are used for taking their lifting and lowering effects.

Recipe example:

Radix Bupleuri 8g, Fructus Aurantii 10g, Radix Paeoniae Alba 10g, Radix Glycyrrhizae 5g, charred Semen Arecae 8g, Rhizoma Cpperi 10g, Fructus Perillae 10g, Caulis Perillae 10g and Flos Albiziae 10g.

2) Deficiency type panting

(1) Qi-deficiency type panting (deficiency of lung-qi and spleen-qi)

Main symptoms: Dyspnea, tachypnea, short breath, low and weak voice, lower cough sound, thin sputum, spontaneous sweating and aversion to wind.

Concomitant symptoms: Pale complexion, shortness of breath, lassitude, epigastric distension and loose stool after meal, or defecation soon after meal.

Tongue picture and pulse condition: Thin and white or thin, white and greasy tongue coating, enlarged tongue with teeth print at its border, thready and weak pulse.

Analysis: The lung is in charge of qi. If the lung-qi is insufficient, panting, tachypnea, shortness of breath, low and weak voice, lower cough sound appear. The lung is associated with the skin and hairs, so, when the lung-qi is insufficient and weak, the body's superficial regulation and defensive system is in hypofunction, thus, spontaneous sweating and aversion to wind happen. Deficiency-cold of the spleen contributes to thin sputum. Deficiency of both the lung and spleen is responsible for poor appetite, lassitude, epigastric distension and loose stool after meal, or defecation soon after meal, enlarged tongue with thin tongue coating and weak pulse.

Therapeutic principles: Strengthening the spleen and nourishing the lung.

Recipes and drugs: Yu Ping Feng Powder combined with Modified Liu Jun Zi Decoction. In this recipe, Radix Codonopsis, Rhizoma Atractylodis Macrocephalae and Radix Astragali seu Hedysari serve to nourish the lung and strengthen the spleen; Pericarpium Citri Reticulatae, Poria and Rhizoma Pinelliae are used to strengthen the spleen and resolve sputum; Radix Astragali seu Hedysari combined with Radix Ledebouriellae is used to nourish qi and consolidate the superficial resistance. In case of cough with thin sputum, and frequent feeling of cold, which suggest cold in the interior and deficiency of the lung, Rhizoma Zingiberis is added to warm the middle-jiao; for loose stool, Sheng Ling Bai Zu Powder is used; in case of defecation soon after meal, loose stool with tenesmus feeling, which suggest sinking of qi of the middle-jiao, Modified Bu Zhong Yi Qi Decoction is supplemented to elevate the spleen-qi.

Recipe example:

Dried Radix Astragali seu Hedysari 15g, Radix Ledebouriellae 10g, Rhizoma Atractylodis Macrocephalae 10g, Radix Codonopsis 10g, Pericarpium Citri Reticulatae 10g, Poria 10g, Rhizoma Pinelliae 10g, Radix Platycodi 6g and Radix Glycyrrhizae 5g.

(2) Yin-deficiency type panting (deficiency of both lung-yin and kidney-yin)

Main symptoms: Panting and short breath worsening on exertion, dryness in the mouth and throat, tidal fever, night sweating, sticky sputum with less amount and difficulty to be expectorated.

Concomitant symptoms: Flushed face, irritability, feverish sensation in palms and soles, soreness of waist and tinnitus.

Tongue picture and pulse condition: Red tongue with thin yellow coating, thready, rapid pulse.

Analysis: In case of deficiency of both lung-yin and kidney-yin, lung-qi and kidney-qi lose their ability to accept air, so, panting and short breath worsening on exertion happen. Because of yin-deficiency and hyperactivity of fire, flushed face, irritability, feverish sensation in palms and soles appear. Due to losing nourishment of body fluid, dryness in the mouth and throat presents. Due to consumption of body fluid by deficiency-fire, so, sputum is less in amount and difficult to be spitted out. The waist is the house of kidney and the kidney has its specific orifice in the ear, therefore, when kidney-yin is insufficient, soreness of waist and tinnitus occur. Red tongue with thin yellow coating, thready and rapid pulse all are signs of deficiency of both lung-yin and kidney-yin.

Therapeutic principles: Nourishing the kidney and lung.

Recipes and drugs: Sheng Mai Powder combined with Modified Liu Wei

Dihuang Pill. The sub-recipe, Sheng Mai Powder functions in tonifying qi and nourishing yin. Liu Wei Dihuang Pill plus Fructus Schisandrae is called as Du Qi Pill and functions in nourishing the kidney for restoring its action of accepting air. In case of dryness in the mouth and throat, flushed face and irritability due to dominant insufficiency of lung-yin, Bulbus Lilii, Radix Glehnia, Radix Adenophorae and Rhizoma Polygonati Odorati serve to nourish yin and clear away lung-heat; in case of feverish sensation in the palms and soles, tidal fever and night sweating due to dominant deficiency of kidney-yin, dried Concha Ostreae is added to check yang and excessive sweating and eliminate deficiency-heat. In case of panting, rapid breath, flushed face, dryness in the throat, irritability, greasy sweating, red tongue with less moisture and thready, rapid pulse which ared termed as "floating yang" and result from inability of the depleted real yin to check the hyperactive yang, and failure of lung-and kidney-qi in accepting air, Fructus Corni is used in a larger dose and combined with drugs for subduing yang and tranquilizing the mind, such as dried Os Draconis, Concha Ostreae, Fluorite, etc.

Recipe example:

Radix Codonopsis Pilosulae 10g, Radix Asparagi 10g, Radix Ophioponis 10g, Fructus Schisandrae 6g, dried Radic Rehmanniae 12g, Fructus Ligustri Lucidi 10g, Fructus Corni 10g, Bulbus Lilii 10g, Magnetitum 20g (decocted first) and Pericarpium Citri Reticulatae 10g.

(3) Yang-deficiency type panting (deficiency of both spleen-yang and kidney-yang)

Main symptoms: Chronic panting, more expiration and less inspiration, gasp worsening while making exertion, shortness of breath, sweating, cold limbs, edema of face and legs, profuse, clear thin sputum and cyan-purple face and lips.

Concomitant symptoms: Soreness of waist, low-spiritedness, pale or darkish complexion, frequent urination and polyuria during night.

Tongue picture and pulse condition: Pale and enlarged tongue, deep, thready and weak pulse or taunt, large and rootless pulse.

Analysis: In case of insufficiency of kidney-yang, the kidney-qi loses its ability to accept air, so, panting and short breath worsening while making exertion happen. Due to yang-deficiency, yin-cold is predominant in the interior, the body is short of warming, as a result, cold limbs, low-spiritedness, bluish complexion, etc. appear. Because of yang-deficiency, the superficial-qi is weak, so, spontaneous sweating happens. Because of yang-deficiency, the kidney can not perform its functions in qi transformation and water metabolism normally, so, edema in the face and legs appears. Profuse, clear, thin sputum, enlarged pale tongue and deep thready pulse suggest weakness of yang-qi. Taunt, large, rootless pulse is a sign of outward going of yang in deficiency condition.

Therapeutic principles: Warming yang, reinforcing the kidney to accept air.

Recipes and drugs: Jin Gui Shenqi Pill and Modified Shen Ge Powder. The former recipe is used to warm and recuperate kidney-yang and the later employed to promote the inhaled qi to attribute to the kidney. In case of up-adverse flow of qi from the lower abdomen and abnormal movement of qi around the umbilicus, Fluorite, Magnetitum, Lignum Aquilariae, etc. are added to send qi downwards. For patients with panting, cough, palpitation, or edema of legs, oliguria, enlarged pale tongue and deep thready pulse because of yang-deficiency-induced fluid-retention, and attack of the heart and lung by retained fluid, Zhen Wu Decoction is used in combination with Ramulus Cinnamomi, Radix Astragali seu Hedysari, Radix Stephaniae Tetrandrae, Semen Lepidii seu Descuraniniae and Rhizoma Rohdeae Japonicae for warming the kidney, supplementing qi and promoting water metabolism. In case of "excess in the upper and deficiency in the lower", i. e., accumulation of sputum and qi in the upper part of the body and deficiency of kidney-qi in the lower part which manifest as panting, cough, profuse sputum and chest distress worsening while making exertion, soreness of waist, cold limbs, sweating, palpitation, frequent urination, greasy tongue coating, deep, thready pulse or soft, slippery pulse, Modified Suzi Jiang Qi Decoction is employed to resolve sputum, lower qi, warm the kidney to accept inhaled qi.

Recipe example:

Sliced Radix Aconiti Praeparata 6 ~ 10g, Rhizoma Zingiberis 6g, Semen Ginkgo 6g, Fructus Schisandrae 6g, Fructus Psoraleae 10g, Poria 12g, Radix Codonopsis Pilosulae 10g and Fructus Perillae 10g.

3) Crisis of panting syndrome

In case of severe panting with the mouth open and shoulders elevated, flaring of nares, rapid breath, sitting position and inability to lie flat, palpitation, restlessness, cyan-purple complexion, profuse sweating, cold limbs, floating, large, rootless pulse or knotted, faint pulse, which suggest a crisis sign of panting prostration due to confronted exhaustion of all the heart-yang, kidney-yang and lung-qi, it should be treated by taking He Xi Powder, Ge Jie Powder with decocted fluid of Radix Genseng and Radix Aconiti Praeparata for restoring yang from collapse, tranquilizing and subduing the kidney-qi. In case of dryness-heat, flushed cheeks and greasy sweating which suggest exhaustion of qi and yin, Radix Panacis Quinquefolii, Radix Ophiopogonis and Fructus Schisandrae are added instead of Radix Aconiti Praeparata. for replenishing qi and nourishing yin. For hyperhidrosis, Os Draconis Ustum and Concha Ostreae are supplemented to arrest sweating and strengthen the superficial resistance.

〔Measures for Prevention and Nursing〕

1) Keep the air fresh, sunlight full, temperature and humidity suitable in the room. Smoking is prohibited in the room, and the panting patient should give up smoking if he or she smokes. At the same time, ask the patients to have a regular daily life and try their best to avoid attack of six evils.

2) Ask the patient to have light food, avoid eating too salty, too sour, hot or irritable food, keep away wine.

3) During clinical observation, pay attention to the time and duration of onset of panting, try to understand the predisposing factors, concurrent symptoms, body temperature, pulse rate, state of sputum-fluid, etc.

4) In the stage of attack, the panting patient should lie in bed and take a half lying position. When necessary, give the patient with oxygen inhalation measure. Keep the patient's respiratory tract unobstructed. For patients with profuse sputum, try to help him or her eliminate sputum in time. When necessary, help the patient absorb sputum.

5) When asthma attacks violently, try to relieve it by using the following methods:

(1) Inhaling flos daturae vapor.

(2) Puncturing Tiantu (RN 22), Shanzhong (RN 17), Qihai (RN 6), etc..

(3) Oral administration of aminophylline, isoprenaline, etc., be cautious of application of antitussives and sedatives.

6) In the stage of intermission of panting, if the patient can move about for some time, ask him or her to do physical exercise for strengthening his or her constitution.

〔Analysis of Typical Case〕

Zhao ××, female, aged 56 years. Her first visit was on June 15, 1972. She had suffered from cough and panting for many years at that time of treatment. During attack, she could neither lie flat nor fall asleep, had wheezing sound in the throat. Her cough and panting were serious particularly in the morning and night and attacked in recent several days. She also experienced light edema. It was diagnosed as acute attack of chronic asthmatic bronchitis by modern medicine. Examination showed thin yellow tongue coating, slippery, rapid pulse.

Differentiation of syndromes: Accumulation of sputum-heat in the lung, failure of lung-qi to disperse

Drugs: Herba Ephedrae 15g, Semen Armeniacae 15g, Radix Scutellariae 12g, Lumbricus 12g, Rhizoma Ligustici Chuanxiong 5g, Scorpio 3g. 3 doses.

Second visit on June 19: After taking the above-mentioned drugs, her cough and panting were relieved considerably, she could lie flat, sleep well during night, and her edema abated gradually. Then, the above recipe was prescribed to her again but the dose of the first two ingredients decreased: Herba Ephedrae 12g, Semen Armeniacae 12g, Radix Scutellariae 12g, Lumbricus 12g, Rhizoma Ligustici Chuanxiong 5g, Scorpio 3g. After administration of another 3 doses more, her cough and panting were under control and her edema abated completely.

Note: The present case is an excess type panting, or heat type panting with cough due to sputum-heat attacking the lung and failure of lung-qi to disperse. Treatment should be at ventilating the lung and clearing away sputum-heat. In the recipe, Herba Ephedrae and Semen Armeniacae serve to ventilate the lung and arrest panting; for eliminating heat, Radix Scutellariae (with bitter taste and cool property) is used instead of Gypsum Fibrosum pungent in flavor and cool in property for eliminating excess-fire of the upper-jiao and lung-heat. Lumbricus is added to arrest gasp; Rhizoma Ligustici Chuanxiong and Scorpio are of dredging meridians and relieving spasm.

Panting syndrome is a disease manifested by dyspnea with mouth open and shoulders elevated, flaring nares, inability to lie flat, etc. In severe cases, prostration syndrome of panting may happen. It results from affection by exogenous six evils, or internal impairment by improper diet, mental stress, or chronic disease-induced weak constitution. The focus is located mainly at the lung and kidney and is also associated with the liver and spleen. Panting syndrome can be divided into deficiency type and excess type. Excess type panting results from inability of lung-qi to disperse and descend due to accumulation of pathogenic factors in the lung, and is thus treated by dispelling pathogens and regulating qi, aiming chiefly at treating the lung. Deficiency type panting results from insufficiency of the vital energy and disorder of the lung and kidney in dominating respiration and is thus treated by reinforcing and nourishing both lung and kidney, particularly aiming at the kidney. When making differentiation of syndromes for determining a corresponding treatment approach, the cold or heat property of excess type panting and the yin or yang predominance of the deficiency type panting should be identified first. Besides, mutual transformation or coexistence of deficiency and excess, as well as cold and heat may be seen. For crisis syndrome of panting, urgent treatment should be given immediately.

Questions for Review

1. How to differentiate deficiency type and excess type panting ? Try to narrate the differentiation of syndromes and treatment of different types of panting syndrome.
2. How to differentiate and treat cold wrapping fire type, upper-excess and lower-deficiency type and prostration type of panting syndrome ?
3. How to explain: "the excess type panting is due to the lung, while the deficiency type panting results from the kidney" ?

Lung Distension

〔General Description〕

Lung distension is a chronic disease resulted from gradual development of repeatedly attacked, lingering multiple pulmonary diseases which lead to dysfunction of the stagnated lung-qi in dispersing and descending due to deficiency-impairment of the lung, spleen and kidney. In clinic, it manifests as thoracic bulge, gasping respiration, cough, dyspnea, worsening on exertion, chest stuffiness and fullness, or profuse sputum, palpitation, irritability, or dim complexion, cyan-purplish lips and tongue, epigastric and abdominal distension, edema of face and four limbs, or appearance of some crises as panting-prostration syndrome etc. in severe cases. It is lingering and protracted in the course of disease, bettering or worsening from time to time.

In regard to differentiation of syndromes of lung distension, deficiency or excess of the superficiality and origin should be distinguished first, followed by identifying the severity of the disease and understanding the difference and interrelation between lung distension and panting or bronchial wheezing or hypochondriac and epigastric fluid retention. When treated, it can be divided into 5 patterns including accumulation of turbid sputum in the lung, obstruction of the lung by sputum-heat, deficiency of both lung-qi and kidney-qi, edema due to yang insufficiency, mental confusion caused by phlegm. In particular, more attention should be paid to the prevention and treatment of critical syndromes as panting prostration, coma, etc.

In treatment of multiple pulmonary diseases of modern medicine, including chronic disease with combined pneumonectomy, chronic pulmonary heart disease, senile pneumonectomy, etc., contents of syndrome-differentiation and treatment of lung distention in the present chapter can be used for reference. As to pulmonary encephalopathy, its emergency treatment may be conducted in the light of differentiation and treatment of crisis type lung-distention.

〔Etiology and Pathology〕

1. Etiology of lung distention

The basic causes of lung distention are 1) deficiency of the lung induced by chronic disease; and 2) affection by exogenous pathogens. Deficiency of the lung induced by chronic disease mostly results from chronic pulmonary diseases, such as chronic cough due to internal impairment, fluid-retention in the hyochondrium and epigastrium, asthma, impairment of the lung due to overstrain, etc. These diseases are lingering and attack repeatedly, leading to stagnation of turbid sputum and gradual onset of lung distention. Due to deficiency of the lung and unconsolidated superficial defensive function, the human body is readily to be attacked repeatedly by exogenous pathogens, as a result, lung distention occurs step by step.

2. Pathology of lung distention

The pathological characters of lung distention are weakness of body resistance while pathogenic factors prevailing, and coexistence of deficiency and excess.

1) Weakness of body resistance is referred to deficiency and impairment of

the lung, spleen and kidney. The lung is a tender organ and is easy to be injured by exogenous pathogenic factors. It is associated with the skin and hairs and opens into the nose. If the lung is attacked repeatedly by exogenous pathogenic factors, cough and panting will occur due to failure of the lung to disperse and descend. If other chronic pulmonary diseases as chronic cough, fluid retention in the hypochondrium and epigastrium, asthma, consumption of the lung, etc. are lingering or not treated in time or treated improperly, lung-deficiency will happen. When pulmonary diseases develop continuously for a long time, son (lung) consumes mother(spleen)-qi, the spleen can not function normally in transportation, as a result, deficiency of both the lung and spleen appears at last. If the spleen is unable to function normally in transportation first, the resultant sputum stagnates in the lung, it will lead to failure of the lung in dispersing and descending. In patients with chronic lung disease, deficiency of both the lung and spleen is likely to appear more easily. Qi is dominated by the lung and originates from the kidney. Metal and Water have a relationship of interpromotion, if the lung-deficiency lasts for a long period of time, it will bring disaster to thoracic diseases.

2) In treatment of fluid retention, a reasonable measure should be given in accordance with the state of body resistance and pathogenic factors, greater or lesser urgency of the disease, differences of the deficiency and excess of the exterior - or interior-syndrome. For tense water retention, dispelling pathogen method is given to treat the superficiality; for exhaustion of yang and deficiency of qi, warming yang method is adopted to treat the origin. For exterior-syndrome, treatment is performed by using warming, dispelling and sweating methods. For interior-syndrome, treatment is conducted by employing warming, dispelling and diuresis-inducing methods. For weak body resistance, reinforcing method is taken; for excess of pathogens, purging method is taken; for coexistence of excess of pathogens and weakness of body resistance, both climinating and reinforcing methods are employed at the same time; and for coexistence of fluid retention and heat syndromes, warming and cooling methods are taken simultaneously.

3) In one chapter of the medical book《Principle and Prohibition for Medical Profession》, methods for separate treatment of deficiency and excess syndromes are put forward and can be used as the essentials for differentiation of syndromes and treatment of fluid retention. For excess of fluid retention pathogen, eliminating, diuresis-inducing and sweating for removing fluid retention are taken separately in light ofpathogenic factors.

Turbid sputum, water fluid, qi-stagnation and blood stasis often affect each other to induce lung distension. Turbid sputum may results from dysfunction of the lung in dispersing, inability of the spleen in transportation or failure of the kidney in qi-transforming ability. In case of further affection by wind-cold, the sputum syndrome may turn into a syndrome of coexistence of exterior-cold and interior-water fluid. Affection by wind-heat and heat-transformation of accumulated sputum may attribute to sputum-heat syndrome. Internal accumulation of sputum-heat or heat-induced wind-stirring may also cause a series of symptoms of up-stirring of liver. Heat toxin entering the blood is responsible for hemorrhage. In case of obstruction of airway due to abundant sputum, or inability of the lung in exhaling turbid air and inhaling clear air due to deficiency of lung-qi, irritability, drowsiness, coma, etc. may appear because of invasion of sputum to the heart.

Sputum, fluid and water have a same origin and all result from accumulation of body fluid and can transform each other. For example, in case of deficiency of yang and hyperactivity of yin, qi loses its function in transformation of body fluid, as a result, sputum turns into fluid- or water-retention. If the resultant fluid-retention stagnates in the upper-jiao to attack the lung, cough and adverse flow of qi will appear; if it attacks the heart, palpitation, short breath, etc. will appear; if sputum-rheum stagnates in the middle-jiao, poor appetite, vomiting or nausea, abdominal distension and loose stool will happen; and if the fluid-retention spreads in the muscle and subcutaneous tissues, edema and oliguria appear. That fluid-retention is stagnant in the chest and hypochondrium is called as pleural effusion.

In case of accumulation of lung-qi or chronic-disease-induced lung-deficiency, the circulation of heart blood is out of regulation and both heart-qi and heart-yang are weak, so, blood circulation loses driving force, leading to palpitation, uneven pulse, cyan-purplish lips and finger-nails, significant carotid beating (jugular venous engorgement) due to impeded blood flow and stagnation of heart blood. The heart is in discharge of blood and the liver stores blood, so, if the heart blood is out of order or the liver can not function normally in regulation of qi and blood stagnates in the hypochondrium, hemoptysis, spitting blood and hematochezia will be seen because of mass in the abdomen, deficiency of lung-qi and spleen-qi and inability of qi to control blood.

In short, the focus of lung distension is located at the lung and this disease is also closely associated with the spleen and kidney. In the later stage, it may involve the heart and liver. In pathology, it mostly belongs to weakness of body resistance and excess of evils. Weakness of body resistance is referred to hypofunction of the lung, spleen and kidney, or predominant deficiency of both lung-qi and spleen-qi or deficiency of both qi and yin. When developing continuously, it may lead to deficiency of lung-, kidney-, spleen- and heart-yang, or deficiency of both yin and yang. Excess of evils is referred to turbid sputum, water-retention, qi stagnation and blood stasis which are often affected and transformed into each other, even appearing simultaneous coexistence of some of them. In addition, weakness of body resistance and excess of evils may be the cause and sequence mutually. If yang-qi is insufficient, the human body is readily affected by exogenous pathogenic factors and the sputum-rheum is difficult to be eliminated. In patients with internal heat due to yin-deficiency, the invaded exogenous evils and turbid sputum are easy to follow heat-transformation. Therefore, deficiency syndrome and excess syndrome often present at the same time and attack more and more frequently, even resulting in sustaining cough, asthma, stuffy chest, etc.

〔Differentiation of Syndromes and Treatment〕

Schematic Diagram of Causes and Pathogenesis of Lung Distension

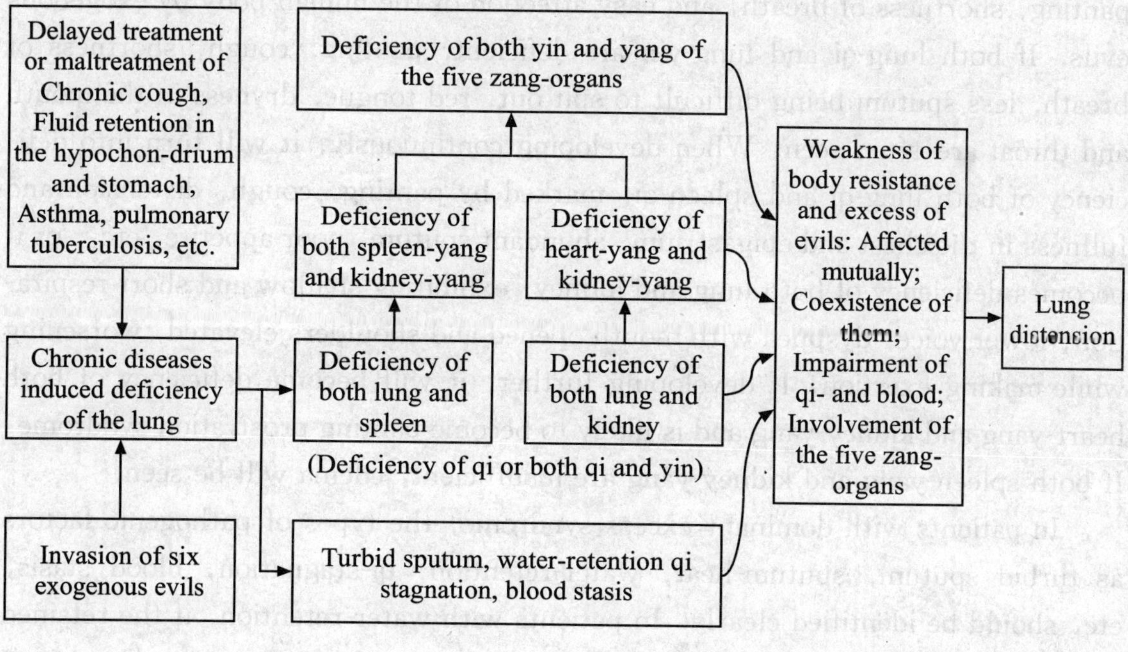

1. Key Points for Differentiation of Syndromes

Lung-distention results from development of multiple chronic pulmonary diseases and is characterized as thoracic bulge and fullness, cough, panting with reversed flow of qi, worsening while making exertion, stuffy chest and abundant sputum. Thus, it is not difficult to be diagnosed by combining carefully questioning the history of disease, detailed observation of vitality, color, figure and posture of patient's body with clinical manifestations. When making a differentiation of syndromes, the following key points should be mastered.

1) Differentiation of deficiency, excess, superficiality and origin

Lung distention always belongs to the syndrome of weakness of body resistance and excess of pathogenic factors, but still has predominant deficiency and predominant excess two types. In treatment of lung-distention patients with predominant deficiency, the focus location should be identified first, among the five zang-organs, which one is chiefly injured and which organs are involved at the same time. When analyzing the nature of deficiency of the lung, it should make clear which one of qi, both qi and yin and yang is dominant. Generally, newly-attacked disease mostly belongs to deficiency of lung-qi, manifested by cough and panting, shortness of breath, and easy affection of the human body by exogenous evils. If both lung-qi and lung-yin are deficient, panting, cough, shortness of breath, less sputum being difficult to spit out, red tongue, dryness in the mouth and throat are often seen. When developing continuously, it will turn into deficiency of both lung-qi and spleen-qi, marked by panting, cough, distension and fullness in the chest and epigastrium, abundant sputum, poor appetite, etc.; or it becomes deficiency of both lung and kidney, exhibiting shallow and short respiration, lower voice, dyspnea with mouth opened and shoulders elevated, worsening while making exertion. If developing further, it will become deficiency of both heart-yang and kidney-yang and is likely to become panting prostration syndrome. If both spleen-yang and kidney-yang are insufficient, edema will be seen.

In patients with dominant excess syndrome, the types of pathogenic factors as turbid sputum, sputum-heat, water-retention, qi-stagnation, blood stasis, etc. should be identified clearly. In patients with water-retention, if the retained fluid flows reversely, palpitation, dropsy, dyspnea, edema, extreme distension, etc. are often seen. In patients with concomitant turbid sputum, if stagnating for some time, the sputum is sticky and difficult to spit out. In patients with concurrent stagnation of qi, when qi stagnates in the chest, the state of distension and fullness is even worse. In patients with accompanied blood stasis, dim complexion, dark purplish lips and tongue, cyan-purple finger nails are often seen. Moreover, it should also make clear that whether there exists exopathy, if so, cold or heat type exterior syndrome is sure to be seen and a series of symptoms of lung distention will be worsened correspondingly. Only by clearly discriminating the principal or secondary aspect of weakness of body resistance or excess of evils, superficiality and origin, can an effective treatment be given.

2) Differentiation of severity of lung distention syndrome

If lung distention patients have no concurrent invasion of exogenous evils, only panting, cough, dyspnea, chest stuffiness, distension and fullness which are worsening while exertion are seen, the state of disease is stable and relatively milder. In case of nose flaring of nares, rapid respiration, dyspnea with mouth opened and shoulders elevated, extreme distention of eyes, dysphoria, profuse sputum being difficult to be expectorated, it suggests worsening of the state of disease and needs paying attention to that if there exists cold or heat type exterior syndrome or coexistence of them. In patients with critical severe lung distention syndrome, palpitation, cyanosis of face and lips, edema of limbs, haematemesis, hematochezia, delirium, somnolence, coma, clonic convulsion, cold limbs and prostration syndrome are often seen, if so, it should be treated urgently.

3) Correlation between lung distension and panting, bronchial wheezing or fluid-retention in the hypochondrium

Lung distention, bronchial wheezing and panting syndromes all manifest chiefly as cough, dyspnea, asthma and chest fullness, but lung distention results from long-term gradual worsening of multiple kinds of chronic pulmonary diseases; bronchial wheezing syndrome is an independent disease with repeated attack, characterized by wheezing sound in the throat during gasp. Panting syndrome is a symptom of multiple acute and chronic lung diseases. Speaking from the mutual relations among the three syndromes, bronchial wheezing syndrome attacks repeatedly, is lingering, and may turn into lung distention, if developing further and constantly; while panting syndrome uncertainly becomes lung distention; but lung distention can be attributed to the category of panting syndrome. Moreover, when attacking due to invasion of exogenous pathogenic factors or worsening in the state of disease, lung distention may exhibit hypochondric and epigastric fluid-retention syndrome which belongs to sputum retention. All these aspects mentioned above should be considered together, and their different and common points should be also understood thoroughly for giving a reasonable differentiation and correct treatment.

2. Therapeutic principles

The general therapeutic principle is divided into two aspects: superficiality and origin. For excess in superficiality, methods of removing evils to ventilate the lung (choosing drugs pungent in flavor and warm or cool in property), lowering the reversed flow of qi and resolving sputum (using drugs for clearing away heat and resolving or warming the cold sputum), or warming yang to promote diuresis (using drugs for activating yang or those bland in property for inducing diuresis), in severe cases, causing resuscitation, calming endogenous wind or hemostasis, etc. are adopted. For deficiency in origin, methods of replenishing the spleen and lung, nourishing the heart and lung, tonifying the kidney and strengthening the spleen are used predominantly, in combination with supplementing qi and nourishing yin, or with tonifying both yin and yang at the same time. For imminent prostration of vital energy, it is treated by strengthening body resistance to arrest collapse, and nourishing yin to restore yang.

3. Typing and Treatment

1) Accumulation of turbid sputum in the lung

Main symptoms: Cough, panting, profuse, white, sticky and foamy sputum.

Concurrent symptoms: Shortness of breath, gasp, worsening on exertion, frequent sweating, cold limbs and aversion to wind, fullness in the stomach, poor appetite, listlessness and weakness.

Tongue picture and pulse condition: Light pale tongue with thin greasy or curdy greasy fur, small, taut and slippery pulse.

Analysis: In case of hypofunction of the lung and spleen, turbid sputum generates and goes to the lung aversely, inducing cough, and the sputum is profuse, white, sticky and greasy. When turning into fluid retention following cold evil, the sputum is foamy. In case of weakness of lung-qi, the lung is unable to function normally in dispersing and descending, if combined with additional mutual obstruction of qi and sputum, short respiration and gasp, worsening on mild exertion will happen. Because of deficiency of the lung, the superficial defensive system of the body is weak, thus, aversion to wind and frequent sweating occur. When lung disease affects the spleen, the spleen falls into hypofunction in transportation and transformation of food, so, fullness in the stomach, poor appetite, fatigue, weakness are seen. Pale tongue with thin greasy fur, small, taut and slippery pulse all are signs of deficiency of both spleen-qi and lung-qi and accumulation of turbid sputum in the interior.

Therapeutic principles: Resolving sputum, lowering qi, strengthening the spleen and nourishing the lung.

Recipes and drugs: Suzi Jiang Qi Decoction, San Zi Yang Qin Decoction and Modified Liu Junzi Decoction are used. The former two recipes can function in lowering reverse flow of qi, resolving sputum and arresting panting, but Suzi Jiang Qi Decoction is predominantly warm in property and used suitably for treatment of excessive sputum-dampness, insufficiency of the kidney-qi, coexistence of upper-excess and lower-deficiency, cold-sputum type cough and panting. San Zi Yang Qin Decoction serves to lower reversed qi, resolve sputum, help food digestion, and is fit to treat lung-excess type panting, fullness in the chest, poor appetite, profuse, greasy and sticky sputum. Liu Junzi Decoction, a dominantly-tonifying recipe, is used to strengthen the spleen, remove dampness and resolve sputum, thus it is fit to treat hypofunction of the spleen accompanied with sputum-dampness and may be also used as a modulation recipe during the stable stage of lung distention syndrome.

Addition and subtraction: For profuse sputum, fullness in the chest, dyspnea, inability to lie flat, Semen Lepidii seu Descurainiae is supplemented to clear away lung-heat and sputum and arrest panting. If sputum turns into fluid retention due to cold and additional affection by wind-cold, panting, cough, profuse sticky and foamy sputum, i.e., exterior-cold and internal fluid-retention syndrome is often seen; under such circumstances, Xiao Qing Long Decoction is used instead for relieving exterior syndrome and eliminating fluid retention. If the stagnated fluid retention transforms heat, irritability, panting, floating pulse, etc., Xiao Qing Long Decoction is used in combination with Shi Gao Decoction for eliminating accumulated heat simultaneously.

Recipe example:

Baked Herba Ephedrae 4g, Semen Armeniacae 10g, Exocarpium Citri Reticulatae 10g, Poria 10g, Rhizoma Pinelliae 10g, Fructus Perillae 10g, Semen Sinapis Albae 3g, fried Semen Raphani 10g and dried Radix Glycyrrhizae 5g.

2) Accumulation of sputum-heat in the lung

Main symptoms: Cough, asthmatic breathing, coarse voice, yellowish and sticky-white sputum being difficult to spit out.

Concurrent symptoms: Irritability, fullness in the chest, or fever, slight aversion to cold, sweating or anhidrosis, brown urine, constipation and thirst.

Tongue picture and pulse condition: Red tongue, thin, yellow or yellow-greasy fur, rapid or slippery-rapid pulse.

Analysis: Because of heat-transformation of accumulated turbid sputum in the interior, and accumulation of sputum-heat in the lung, the sputum is yellow and greasy and difficult to spit out. When pathogenic heat accumulates in the lung, the lung can not function normally in dispersing and purifying and the lung-qi flows adversely, thus, asthma, cough, dyspnea and coarse breathing appear. Mutual obstruction between sputum and pathogenic heat in the chest may contribute to irritability and fullness in the chest; invasion of pathogenic heat in the large intestine is responsible for constipation and brown urine. In case of subsequent affection by exogenous evils, as wind-heat attacking the lung, fever, mild aversion to cold, slight sweating, a series symptoms of exterior syndrome, are seen. Thirst, red tongue, yellow greasy fur, slippery rapid pulse all are signs of accumulation of sputum in the interior.

Therapeutic principles: Eliminating lung-heat, resolving sputum, arresting asthma.

Recipes and drugs: Yue Bi Jia Ban Xia Decoction plus Banxia, Modified Sang Bai Pi Decoction. The former recipe can function in ventilating the lung and clearing away lung-heat, and is used to treat accumulation of fluid-retention heat in the lung and concomitant exterior syndrome which are manifested as gasp, cough, dyspnea, bulged eyes, fever, floating large pulse, etc.; the later recipe functions in eliminating lung-heat and resolving sputum and is used to treat accumulation of sputum-heat in the lung which is marked by panting, rapid respiration, fullness in the chest, yellow sputum, or sticky, thick white sputum.

Addition and subtraction: For hyperactivity of sputum-heat in the interior and sticky sputum being difficult to be expectorated, Herba Houttuyniae,

Pericarpium Trichosanthis, Concha Meretricis seu Cyclinae, etc. are added to eliminate lung-heat and resolve sputum. For adverse flow of lung-qi and severe mutual obstruction between sputum and qi which manifests as asthmatic breathing, rattles in the throat and inability to lie flat, Rhizoma Belamcandae, Semen Lepidii seu Descurainiae, etc. are supplemented to clear away lung-heat and arrest gasp. For consumption of body fluid by sputum-heat, dryness in the mouth and tongue, Radix Trichosanthis, Rhizoma Anemarrhenae, Rhizoma Phragmitis, etc. are supplemented to promote generation of body fluid and moisten the mouth and tongue. In treatment of impairment of yin with less sputum, drugs bitter in flavor and cold in property are removed and Radix Glehnia, Radix Ophiopogonis, Radix Scrophulariae, etc. are added to nourish yin.

Recipe example:

Baked Herba Ephedrae 3g, Semen Armeniacae 10g, Gypsum Fibrosum 30g (decocted first), dried Radix Glycyrrhizae 5g, Rhizoma Pinelliae 6g, Radix Scutellariae 10g, Fructus Trichosanthis 30g (decocted first), Cortex Mori Radicis 10g and Bulbus fritillariae Cirrhosae 10g.

3) Deficiency of both lung-qi and kidney-qi

Main symptoms: Rapid shallow respiration, dyspnea, panting worsening on exertion.

Concurrent symptoms: Gasp for breath even with mouth opened and shoulders elevated, inability to lie flat, lower voice, shortness of breath, cough, white foamy sputum being difficult to spit out, stuffy chest, palpitation, cold limbs and sweating.

Tongue picture and pulse condition: Pale, purplish tongue or pale tongue with ecchymosis, deep, thready, rapid and weak pulse, or uneven pulse.

Analysis: The lung is in charge of qi and the kidney is the root of qi. So, if both lung-qi and kidney-qi are insufficient, these two zang-organs can not function normally in dominating and accepting qi, followed by appearance of shallow rapid respiration, dyspnea with mouth opened and shoulders elevated, inability to lie flat, lower voice, shortness of breath. If cold fluid retention stagnates in the lung and deficiency of kidney induces edema, cough, white, foamy sputum being difficult to be expectorated will happen. When lung disease involves the heart, the heart-qi is weak, so, palpitation, cold limbs, sweating, etc. will present. In case of maltreatment of pulmonary diseases, failure of qi to control blood, or stagnation of qi and blood stasis, pale or deep purple tongue with ecchymosis, deep, thready, weak, rapid pulse or uneven pulse will appear.

Therapeutic principles: Reinforcing the lung, tonifying the kidney, lowering qi and arresting panting.

Recipe and drugs: Ping Chuan Gu Ben Decoction and Modified Bu Fei Decoction. The former recipe functions in reinforcing the lung and kidney, lowering qi and resolving sputum, and is thus used to treat asthma and cough with sputum because of deficiency of both lung-qi and kidney-qi; the later recipe functions in reinforcing and restoring lung-qi and is used to treat panting, cough, shortness of breath due to deficiency of lung-qi. Radix Codonopsis Pilosulae (or Radix Ginseng), Radix Astragali seu Hedysari, stir-baked Radix Glycyrrhizae are used to reinforce the lung; Cordyceps, Radix Rehmanniae Praeparata, Semen Juglandis and Placenta Hominis are used to tonify the kidney; Fructus Schisandrae serves to astringe lung-qi; magnetitium and Lignum Aquilariae Resinatum are employed to improve inspiration; and Radix Asteris, Flos Farfarae, Fructus Perillae, Rhizoma Pinelliae and Exocarpium Citri Rubrum are employed to resolve sputum and lower reversed flow of qi.

Addition and subtraction: For deficiency of the lung with cold, aversion to cold and pale tongue, Cortex Cinnamomi, Rhizoma Zingiberis and Stalactite are used in combination to warm and reinforce the lung-qi; for lower fever, red tongue with less fur due to impairment of yin, Radix Ophiopogonis, Rhizoma Polygonati Odorati and dried Radix Rehmanniae are added to nourish lung-yin and kidney-yin. In treatment of cough, asthma, profuse sputum, vomiting or nausea due to deficiency of both lung-yin and kidney-yin, hyperactivity of sputum-dampness in the interior, Modified Jin Shui Liu Jun Decoction is employed. In this recipe, Radix Angelicae Sinensis and Radix Rehmanniae are used to nourish yin, Er Chen Decoction (sub-recipe) serves to resolve sputum. In case of cyan-purple lips and finger-tips, jugular venous engorgement, etc. due to deficiency of qi and blood stasis, Radix Salviae Miltiorrhizae, Angelicae Sinensis, Ramulus Cinnamomi, Flos Carthami, Lignum Sappan, etc. are used to promote blood circulation and dredge meridians.

If crises of panting prostration as sweating, cold limbs, palpitation, rapid respiration, or irritability, feeble pulse being about to disappear, dyspnea, inability to lie flat, with mouth opened and shoulders elevated, flapping of alae nasi appear, emergency treatment by administration of Concha Meretricis seu Cyclinae or

Heixi (Black Tin) Pill with Shen Fu Decoction is given to the patient for reinforcing the kidney to accept air, restoring yang from collapse. When the state of the disease gets stable, ask the patient to take Zhou Fei Pill frequently.

Recipe example:

Radix Codonopsis Pilosulae 10g, Radix Ophiopogonis 10g, Radix Astragali seu Hedysari 12g, Fructus Psoraleae 10g, Radix Rehmanniae Preparae 12g, Pericarpium Citri Reticulatae 10g, Angelicae Sinensis 10g, Radix Asteris 10g and Flos Farfarae 10g.

4) Edema due to Yang-deficiency

Main symptoms: Asthma, cough, dyspnea, edema in face, eye-lipids and lower limbs or even in the whole body.

Concurrent symptoms: Clear thin sputum, fullness in the stomach, poor appetite, oliguria, aversion to cold, palpitation, abdominal distension and fullness or ascites, cyan-purple face and lips.

Tongue picture and pulse condition: White slippery fur, dim enlarged tongue, deep thready pulse.

Analysis: In case of extreme weakness of lung-qi, spleen-yang and kidney-yang, the lung is incapable of performing dispersing and descending functions, the spleen loses its action in transportation and the kidney fails in qi-transformation, leading to edema in the face, eye-lipid, and limbs due to inability of qi to transforming water, accumulation of water fluid and even formation of phlegm-rheum and fluid retention. Water evil attacking the heart and lung results in palpitation, gasping respiration, cough with clear thin sputum; accumulation of water fluid in the interior contributes to fullness in the stomach, abdominal distention and poor appetite; suppression of heart-yang, insufficiency of yang and blood stasis are responsible for cyan-purple face and lips and dim tongue. Insufficiency of kidney-yang and dysfunction of the urinary bladder in qi-transformation contribute to oliguria and aversion to cold. Enlargement of the tongue, white slippery fur, deep thready pulse all are signs of stagnation of water due to yang-deficiency.

Therapeutic principles: Warming the kidney, strengthening the spleen, removing water and fluid retention.

Recipes and drugs: Zhen Wu Decoction combined with Modified Wu Ling Powder. The former recipe functions in warming yang to induce diuresis and is used to treat edema caused by deficiency of both spleen-yang and kidney-yang; the later recipe functions in activating yang and promoting diuresis, if used in combination with Zhen Wu Decoction, the effect of edema-alleviation by promoting diuresis can be enhanced further. Radix Aconiti Praeparata and Ramulus Cinnamomi are used to activate kidney-yang; Poria, Rhizoma Atractylodis Macrocephalae, Polypourus, Rhizoma Alismatis and Rhizoma Zingiberis Recens serve to strengthen the spleen to induce diuresis; and Radix Paeoniae Rubra is able to enter yin to remove accumulation of pathogens when used in combination with Radix Aconiti praeparata.

Addition and subtraction: For severer edema, dyspnea and tachypnea, Semen Lepidii seu Descurainiae, Lignum Aquilariae Resinatum and Herba Rohdeae Japonicae are added for purging lung-heat to arrest asthma, strengthening the heart to induce diuresis. For apparent cyanosis due to severer blood stasis, Herba Lycopi, Flos Carthami, Semen Persicae and Herba Leonuri are supplemented to promote blood circulation, remove blood stasis and induce diuresis.

Recipe example:

Sliced Radix Aconiti Praeparata 10g, Rhizoma Atractylodis Macrocephalae 10g, Ramulus Cinnamomi 10g, Poria30g, Polypourus 15g, Rhizoma Alismatis 15g, Radix Codonopsis 10g, Semen Lepidii seu Descurainiae 10g, Herba Leonuri 15g and Rhizoma Zingiberis Recens 3 pieces.

5) Mental confusion due to phlegm

Main symptoms: Cough, dyspnea, tachypnea and vague mind.

Concurrent symptoms: Delirium, irritability, floccilation, apathy, drowsiness, coma, or muscular twitching and cramp of the limbs, clonic convulsion, cough with difficult expectoration.

Tongue picture and pulse condition: White greasy fur or yellow greasy fur, dull red tongue or light purple or bright red tongue, thready, rapid slippery pulse.

Analysis: In case of confusion due to invasion of phlegm to the heart, vague mind, delirium, irritability, aimless and incessant grasping about in the air with thumbs and forefingers as if twisting thread, drowsiness and coma happen; in case of up-stirring of liver, muscular twitching and cramp of the limbs and convulsion appear. When the lung falls into hypofunction and sputum evil accumulates in the lung, cough, dyspnea, and difficult expectoration are seen. White greasy or light, yellowish greasy tongue coating, thready, slippery rapid pulse all are signs of accumulation of turbid sputum in the interior; dim red or light purple tongue suggests stagnation of the heart blood and bright red tongue indicates accumulated heat in the blood.

Therapeutic principles: Removing phlegm and causing resuscitation, calming the liver to stop the wind.

Recipes and drugs: Modified Di Tan Decoction is used in combination with oral administration of An Gong Niuhuang Pill or Zhi Bao Bolus. In Di Tan Decoction, Rhizoma Pinelliae, Poria, Exocarpium Citri and Arisaema cum Bile are used to remove phlegm for stopping the wind; Caulis Bambusae in Taeniam and Fructus Aurantii Immaturus serve to clear away heat from the chest and resolve phlegm; Rhizoma Acori Graminei functions in causing resuscitation and resolving phlegm; in case of hyperactivity of sputum evil and non-weakness of the vital energy, Radix Ginseng and Radix Glycyrrhizae of this recipe may be excluded. The whole recipe can function in removing phlegm, causing resuscitation, relieving convulsion and spasm and is fit to treat mental confusion due to phlegm, hyperactivity of wind-sputum in the interior, coma, drowsiness, profuse sputum and muscular twitching and spasm of the limbs. Zhi Bao Bolus and An Gong Niuhuang Pill are employed to eliminate heart-heat and induce resuscitation.

Addition and subtraction: In patients with excessive sputum-heat in the interior, fever, irritability, delibrium, coma, constipation and yellow greasy tongue coating, Liang Ge Powder is used in combination with Concretio Silicea Bambusae, Succus Bambosae, etc for clearing away sputum-heat. Radix et Rhizoma Rhei and unprocessed Natrii Sulfas from the recipe can function in removing dryness-heat; Fructus Gardeniae and Radix Scutellariae serve to eliminate heat and purge fire; Fructus Forsythiae in large dose is used to clear away heat and toxic materials; Herba Menthae and Herba Lophatheri are used to eliminate heat in the lung, stomach, heart and chest; and white honey and Radix Glycyrrhizae are used to moisten the lung and lubricate the intestine. In short, the whole recipe functions in clearing away heat by purgation. In order to reserve body fluid, Liang Ge Powder is used in combination with Zheng Ye Decoction for relaxing the bowels, purging away heat and lowering lung-qi.

In case of up-stirring of liver and convulsion, Ramulus Uncariae cum Uncis, Scorpio and Cornu Saigae Tataricae powder are added to calm the liver and stop the wind. In case of cyan-purple lips and fingernails due to severe blood stasis, Radix Salviae Miltiorrhizae, Flos Carthami, Semen Persicae, etc. are supplemented to promote blood circulation and remove obstruction in meridians. In case of mucocutaneous hemorrhage, hemoptysis and hemafecia, drugs for eliminating pathogenic heat from blood and stopping bleeding as Cornu Bubali, dried Radix Rehmanniae, Cortex Moutan Radicis, Radix Arnebiae seu Lithospermi, etc. are added.

Recipe example:

Exocarpium Citri 10g, Rhizoma Pinelliae 10g, Poria 12g, Arisaema cum Bile 8g, Rhizoma Acori Graminei 10g, Radix Curcumae 10g, Fructus Forsythiae 10g, Radix Salviae Miltiorrhizae 15g, Fructus Aurantii Immaturus 10g and Succus Bambosae fluid 10g (added in the decocted drug fluid directly).

The prognosis and changes of lung distention are closely related to patient's physique, age, duration of disease and timely treatment. Generally speaking, this disease does not solely involve one zang-organ and is complicated in pathology. It mostly results from gradual development of chronic diseases, is lingering in the course of disease, attacks repeatedly and is difficult to be controlled permanently. In clinic, particularly in treatment of senile patients, if the state of disease is not controlled in time, it is very easy to produce abnormal changes. In case of mal-treatment of pulmonary diseases, stagnation of the heart blood, palpitation, rapid, uneven pulse; cough with foaming bloody sputum, or hemoptysis and hemafecia due to failure of qi to control blood; or delirium, drowsiness and coma due to mental confusion by sputum, or tremor and convulsion caused by up-stirring of liver; or panting and edema, or panting collapse crises are seen.

〔Prevention and Measures for Nursing〕

In regard to prevention of lung distention, it is mainly referred to prevention and complete treatment of the primary disease. Therefore, strengthening body's constitution and disease-resistant capability is the fundamental method for prevention and treatment of lung distention. During attack of lung distention, its symptoms should be controlled in time for avoiding worsening; in the remission stage, methods for restoring normal functioning of the body to consolidate the constitution are employed. In treatment of lung distention patients, pay attention to heat preservation in autumn and winter and particularly pay attention to avoid affection by exogenous pathogens. Once the disease happens, immediate treatment is given to avoid worsening. In addition, the patients themselves should make respiration exercise, practice shadow boxing, walking exercise, etc. to enhance body resistance, give up smoking and stop drinking or eating pungent, hot, raw, cool, salty or sweet food. Patients with edema should have food with less salt or no salt.

〔Analysis of Typical Case〕

Lou X, male, aged 61 years, was admitted on December 1, 1972 due to cough and asthma for more than 10 years and worsening for one month.

Current history of disease: He had suffered from cough and asthma for more than 10 years, worsening in winter and bettering in summer. His disease attacked repeatedly, especially when he had cold drinks or met summer heat. At the beginning, treatment with penicillin, streptomycin, prednisolone, benadryl, ephedrine, etc. worked temporarily. Gradually, the therapeutic effect was poor in spit of using larger doses. Recently (at the time of treatment), his state of disease got worse because of cold weather and he was admitted on December 1st due to cough, asthma and edema in the limbs. Fluoroscopy showed pulmonary markings being coarse on the bilateral sides, enhancement of diaphaneity, enlargement of the right heart and lowering of the diaphragm. It was diagnosed as chronic bronchitis, pneumonectasis, cor pulmonale with combined right-heart failure. Treatment with the above-mentioned western medicines had no any effect, so he tried treatment with Chinese medicinal herbs.

Current symptoms: Orthopnea, cough, asthma with mouth opened and shoulders elevated, vague mind, dark red cheeks, jugular venous engorgement, cyanosis of lips, wheezing sound in the throat, cold sweat of the whole body, edema in the lower limbs, being difficult in food intake, etc. Examination showed enlarged liver with the lower edge being 9 cm below the xiphoid process, dark purple tongue with thin, white, light greasy coating, weak, large, rapid pulse. It was diagnosed as lung distention, panting syndrome of the type of exhaustion of kidney-yang and retained fluid attacking the lung and heart and treated with Modified Yang He Decoction for tonifying the kidney to improve respiration, recuperating depleted yang and rescuing the patient from collapse. Ingredients: Herba Ephedrae 3g, Radix Rehmanniae Praeparata 18g, Cornu Cervi Degelatinatum 12g, Cortex Cinnamomi 10g, Radix Aconiti Praeparata 10g, Fructus Corni 15g, Sulfur 2g, Stalactite 12g, Lignum Aquilariae Resinatum 10g, Os Draconis ustum 12g, Concha Ostreae Usta 12g, Radix Ginseng 6g, Rhizoma Dioscoreae 12g, Fructus Schisandrae 15g, one dose, decocted in water and taken orally.

Second treatment (December 2nd): After first treatment, the patient could lie flat, got better in asthma and had no cold sweat again. He had a little porridge and his limbs turned warm, but the rest symptoms, tongue picture and pulse condition still had no any apparent changes. Treatment with two doses of the aforementioned recipe was given to him continuously, with the dosage of Radix Ginseng being increased by 3g (9g /dose).

Third treatment (December 4th): The patient's spirit turned to normal, his asthma was relieved, his cyanosis of lips, jugular venous engorgement, dark purple tongue and enlargement of liver and his pulse condition were all improved. He was treated continuously with six doses of the above-mentioned recipe.

Fourth treatment (December 11th): The patient's asthma stopped, his appetite bettered considerably, the limb edema subsided, his physical power recovered and he could get off the bed and walk about. His lip cyanosis disappeared and had light red tongue with thin white coating, peaceful pulse at the six portions of bilateral sides, his liver reduced in size about the transverse width of a finger below the xiphoid process. His symptoms vanished basically. Considering the patient' weak constitution due to longer duration of disease, treatment with the same recipe at a double dose (processed into pills with honey, 9g/pill, one pill once, twice a day) was given to him continuously for 2 months for consolidating the therapeutic effect. After these treatments, he could take part in light physical labour. Afterwards, in every winter of 9 years, his symptoms were mild, though he had cough and expectoration.

Note: This disease is attributed to acute lung distention syndrome of the type of exhaustion of lung-qi and kidney-qi and imminent collapse of heart-yang. Despite this patient has a set of complicated symptoms as cough, gasping breathing, edema, etc., emergency treatment by warming and strengthening the kidney-yang, replenishing qi and rescuing the patient from collapse should be conducted first. Thus, Radix Ginseng, sweet in taste and warmth in property and a powerful tonic is used to supplement the premordial qi of the heart, spleen and kidney to consolidate the acquired essence; Radix Aconiti Pareparata, Sulfur, Stalactite and Cortex Cinnamomi, components being highly pungent in flavor and very hot in property are used in combination for warming and invigorating the kidney-yang; Lignum Aquilariae Resinatum serves to improve function of the kidney in accepting air and conduct qi back to its origin; Os Draconis ustum, Concha Ostreae Usta and Fructus Schisandrae are used to astringe the floating yang; particularly, large dose of Radix Rehmanniae Praeparata is used in combination with many warm and hot ingredients, which means supplementing yang by nourishing yin in accordance with the principle of inter-dependence between yin and yang. Herba Ephedrae pungent in flavor and warmth in property is used to ventilate the lung to arrest panting for treating the superficiality, while its dose used should be smaller. All the drugs are used together to tonify the heart and lung in the upper part of the body, strengthen the spleen-earth in the middle part and also reinforce the kidney and the gate of life in the lower part, eliminating edema without diuretics and relieving asthma without use of antitussives at last. The present recipe is not solely used to invigorate yang, but also used to strengthen the spleen and stomach for arresting panting, cough and old sputum. Thus, it is a well-considered effective recipe. (selected from the Chapter Asthma of《Collection of Experience of Well-known and Old TCM Practitioners of Henan Province》)

Lung distention results from changes of multiple chronic pulmonary diseases in the advanced stage which attack repeatedly and is lingering, manifested mainly as gasping respiration, cough, dyspnea worsening on exertion, stuffiness and fullness in the chest. If lung distention develops further or the lung distention patient gets an additional exopathic disease, the disease will worsen greatly, marked by dark purple lips and face, edema, or coma and convulsion. In severe cases, a series of symptoms of panting collapse, will happen. In the light of clinical manifestations, it is associated with cough, panting syndrome, sputum-rheum, palpitation, edema, panting syncope, or panting collapse, etc.

Lung distention is a chronic disease and manifests mainly as deficiency of the lung. It presents a progressive worsening in the state of disease. Its focus is located at the lung and is also closely related to the spleen and kidney, and in the later stage, it may involve the heart and liver. In pathology, it develops gradually from qi-deficiency or deficiency of both qi and yin to yang-deficiency, or gradually generates turbid sputum, water retention, qi stagnation, blood stasis, etc. on the basis of deficiency of the origin. Weakness of the body resistance and hyperactivity of pathogens may exist independently or simultaneously and affect each other. At last, they will result in various pathological changes, even jeopardizing patients' life.

Regarding differentiating syndromes of lung distention, deficiency or excess of the superficiality and origin should be identified first, followed by clarifying the severity of the disease, and the interrelation between lung distention and panting syndrome or wheezing syndrome, or excessive fluid retention in the chest and stomach, etc should also be distinguished. In regard to treatment of lung distention, the state of both superficiality and origin should be considered together. In case of affection by pathogenic factors, excess of pathogens is dominant and in the remission stage, weakness of body resistance is predominant. Thus, treatment is conducted by laying particular emphasis on strengthening body resistance or dispelling pathogenic factors respectively.

In clinic, the above-mentioned five types of syndrome including accumulation of turbid sputum in the lung, accumulation of sputum-heat in the lung, deficiency of both lung-qi and kidney-qi, edema due to yang deficiency and mental confusion caused by turbid phlegm are often seen, and can transform each other or appear simultaneously. When treated, characters of different syndromes and possible coexistence of some of them should be understood completely and flexible measures are adopted correspondingly. Among them, deficiency of both lung-qi and kidney-qi, mental confusion caused by sputum and edema due to yang-deficiency are particularly critical and serious. If emergency treatment is not given immediately to control the state of disease, the prognosis is unfavorable.

In the aged patients or those with weak body resistance due to chronic disease (in the advanced stage), when the state of disease worsens because of additional exopathy, signs derived from struggle between vital energy of the body and pathogens are not apparent due to that human body is extremely weak in resistance and has no power to combat with the pathogens. Therefore, if cough and asthma get worsening in recent period, the sputum becomes yellow in color and the tongue turns to red, existence of exogenous pathogens should be taken into consideration even though no fever or aversion to cold, etc. (manifestations of exterior syndrome). Additionally, changes of the color, texture and amount of sputum and patient's general condition should be understood completely and analyzed comprehensively for giving a timely and effectively treatment.

Questions for Review

1. Try to narrate the concept of lung distention.
2. Try to narrate the basis of onset and pathological mechanisms of lung distention. How to understand the two aspects of deficiency of origin and excess of superficiality?
3. What are the five types of syndrome of lung distention? How to differentiate different syndromes and treat lung distention ? Which types of lung distention

have an unfavorable prognosis?

Sputum Retention

〔General Description〕

Sputum retention is referred to a category of disease caused by abnormal stagnation of water fluid in a certain part of the body because of disorder of its distribution, transformation and transportation. It results mostly from dysfunction of the lung, spleen and kidney, particularly dysfunction of the spleen-yang in transportation, due to affection of the body by exogenous cold-dampness evils, improper diet, yang deficiency, etc. Sputum retention may stay in any part of the body. So, if moving in the intestines, it can generate sound; if staying in the hypochondrium, it may cause referred pain on coughing or spitting; if spreading unchecked in the four limbs, it will induce sore and heavy sensations in the four limbs; and if attacking the lung, it will result in cough, dyspnea, shortness of breath, orthopnea, etc.

Both sputum and fluid retention are products of disorders of the water fluid in transportation and transformation, but, sputum is thick and sticky, fluid retention is clear and thin. and accumulation of fluid can generate sputum. Thus, they are different in property and also interrelated each other. Sputum and fluid retention, despite termed in parallel, in fact, are referred to the same fluid retention syndrome. It has broad sense and narrow sense in concept. Broadly speaking, sputum retention is a general term of all kinds of fluid retention, including the four kinds of fluid retention: sputum retention, pleural effusion, anasarca, and fluid retention in the hypochondrium and epigastrium described in medical classics 《Synopsis of Prescription of the Golden Chamber》. In the narrow sense, sputum retention is a symptom of the four kinds of fluid retention. As to prolonged fluid retention and recurrent fluid retention, they are so named because the former evil stays protractedly in the body and the later evil hides in the interior, and they are included in the four kinds of fluid retention.

Early in the medical classics 《The Yellow Emperor's Internal Classic》, there are terms of "fluid retention" and prolonged fluid retention and a description of that "excessive water-dampness and dysfunction of the spleen-yang in transportation are the principal causes of sputum retention". Zhang Zhongjing, a famous physician in Han Dynasty first put forward the name of "sputum retention"and made a detailed description on the classification, clinical manifestations, treatment methods, recipes and drugs by listing special chapters which become an important basis for differentiating syndromes to treat sputum retention for the medical practitioners in later generations. Particularly, the major therapeutic method that "for treatment of patients with sputum retention, it is mediated with drugs warm in property" has been all along considered as a criteria for treatment of could sputum and water retention. It is sure that the medical practitioners of the later generations have incessantly elaborated, enriched and developed the theory and treatment methods of sputum retention.

The key pathogenesis of fluid retention syndrome is dysfunction of the lung, spleen and kidney in qi-transformation. In property, it is always attributed to yang deficiency and yin excessiveness, and the resultant excess is induced also by deficiency. Its pathological basis is usual hypofunction of spleen-yang and insufficiency of qi of the middle-jiao. In regard to differentiation of syndromes, the locations, deficiency, excess, concurrent syndrome and coexistence of deficiency and excess or cold and heat should be identified and the differences and associations of sputum, fluid retention, water and dampness, differences between anasarca and wind-water, interrelations among fluid retention in the hypochondrium and epigastrium, recurrent fluid retention and lung distention, wheezing syndrome and panting syndrome should also be understood thoroughly. A corresponding treatment is given always by using warming and resolving methods on the basis of distinguishing the state of pressing or otherwise, deficiency or excess of the superficiality (pathogens) and origin (body resistance), the exterior and interior syndromes.

In treatment of chronic bronchitis, bronchial asthma, exudative pleurisy, disorders of the stomach and intestines, incomplete pylorochesis, intestinal obstruction, etc. of the modern medicine, the contents of the differentiation of syndromes and treatment in the present chapter can be used as reference, if the clinical manifestations are similar to those of sputum retention in a certain stage of the disease.

〔Cause of Disease and Pathogenesis〕

The onset of fluid retention syndrome is due to affection of the body by exogenous cold and dampness, improper diet or internal impairment caused by overstrain or sexual indulgence. These three aspects are affected mutually to produce dysfunction of the lung, spleen and kidney which leads to sputum retention due to accumulation of water-dampness due to dysfunction of the triple-jiao, and failure of water and food-stuff to be transformed into essence and to be distributed over the whole body.

1. Affection by exogenous cold and dampness

In case of meeting a cold-damp weather, wading across a river, braving the storm, frequently sitting or lying on a damp ground, the human body will be injured by invasion of pathogenic water-dampness, leading to impairment of wei-yang, inability of lung-qi to disperse and dampness evil spreading in the muscles, which result in formation of fluid retention due to stagnation of water dampness caused by suppression of the spleen and stomach in qi-transformation function from the exterior to the interior of the body.

2. Internal impairment by improper diet

The stomach is the house of water and food-stuff and the spleen is in charge of transportation and transformation. In case of intake of an excessive amount of water or tea at a time; or indulging in having cold water, raw and cold food in hot seasons or after drink, the middle-yang is suppressed abruptly and the spleen fails to transport because of injury by cold pathogen in hot circumstances and mutual combination of cold and heat, resulting in fluid retention.

3. Impairment by overstrain or sexual indulgence

Water fluid belongs to yin and depends on yang-qi to be transported and transformed. In case of overstrain, or sexual indulgence, or weak physique due to chronic disease or deficiency of qi because of senile, both the spleen-yang and kidney-yang are insufficient, water fluid fails in transportation and transformation and thus becomes fluid retention. Once the body is injured by pathogenic water-dampness, sputum retention will be easier to produce.

Under normal physiological conditions, transportation, transformation and excretion of water fluid mainly depend on the qi-transformation function of the lung, spleen and kidney. The lung is in the upper-jiao and functions in dispersing and distribution and dredging flow of water fluid. The spleen is in the middle-jiao and governs transportation and transformation of essential substances of foodstuff. The kidney locates in the lower-jiao and·functions in warming, transforming and distilling water fluid, raising the clear part and excreting the waste part. In this way, the whole process of absorption, transportation and excretion of water fluid is fulfilled inside the human body jointly by the lung, spleen and kidney. In one chapter of 《Plain Questions of the Yellow Emperor's Internal Classic》, it says that "water and foodstuff enter the stomach to be processed into essences which are transported to the spleen and then distributed and transported to the lung by spleen-qi; the lung regulates the water passage and the waste fluids are infused downwards to the bladder. The essential substances and water are thus distributed to every part of the body by way of meridians." That is to say, in the process of water metabolism, the lung, spleen and kidney are three inseparable links. If anyone of the three zang-organs falls into dysfunction, i.e., inability of the lung to dredge and regulate water pathway, failure of the spleen in transportation or disorder of the kidney in distilling ability, they will be affected each other to generate fluid retention due to accumulation of water fluid. Among the three zang-organs, dysfunction of the spleen in transportation is principal. Once the spleen-yang is weak, the spleen is unable to transport essential substances upward to nourish the lung, foodstuff becomes sputum to attack the lung instead of becoming essence normally; and in the lower part of the body, the weakened spleen yang can not help the kidney to mediate water metabolism, conversely, cold and water pathogens impair kidney-yang, leading to stagnation of water fluid in the middle-jiao, or involving the five zang-organs, or giving rise to edema in any part of the body.

The triple-jiao is the pathway for circulation of water fluid, connects with the body surface and the internal organs and runs through the interior, exterior, upper and lower parts of the body. Distribution of essential substances of food-stuff in the whole body must go through the triple-jiao. Therefore, when the three zang-organs function normally in qi-transformation, the triple-jiao is unobstructed, otherwise, if qi of the triple-jiao does not flow smoothly, the water passage is blocked, there will also be fluid retention due to stagnation of water. It is recorded in the chapter, General Considerations on Sputum Retention of the medical book《General Collection for Holy Relief》that "the triple-jiao is the pathway of food-stuff and is also the origin and the ending place of qi. If the triple-jiao functions normally, qi flows smoothly and the pulse condition is even, there will be normal metabolism. When water fluid enters vessels, it becomes one part of the blood and circulates in the whole body. If qi stagnates in triple-jiao, the vessels are blocked, there will be accumulation of water fluid and appearance of sputum retention".

In short, out of the various endogenous and exogenous pathogenic factors, dysfunction of the lung, spleen and kidney in qi transformation is the key cause for generation of fluid retention. If the lung, spleen and kidney can not function normally in qi-transformation, the water passage of the triple-jiao is blocked and water accumulates to become fluid retention.

Schematic Diagram of Causes and Pathogenesis of Sputum Retention Syndrome

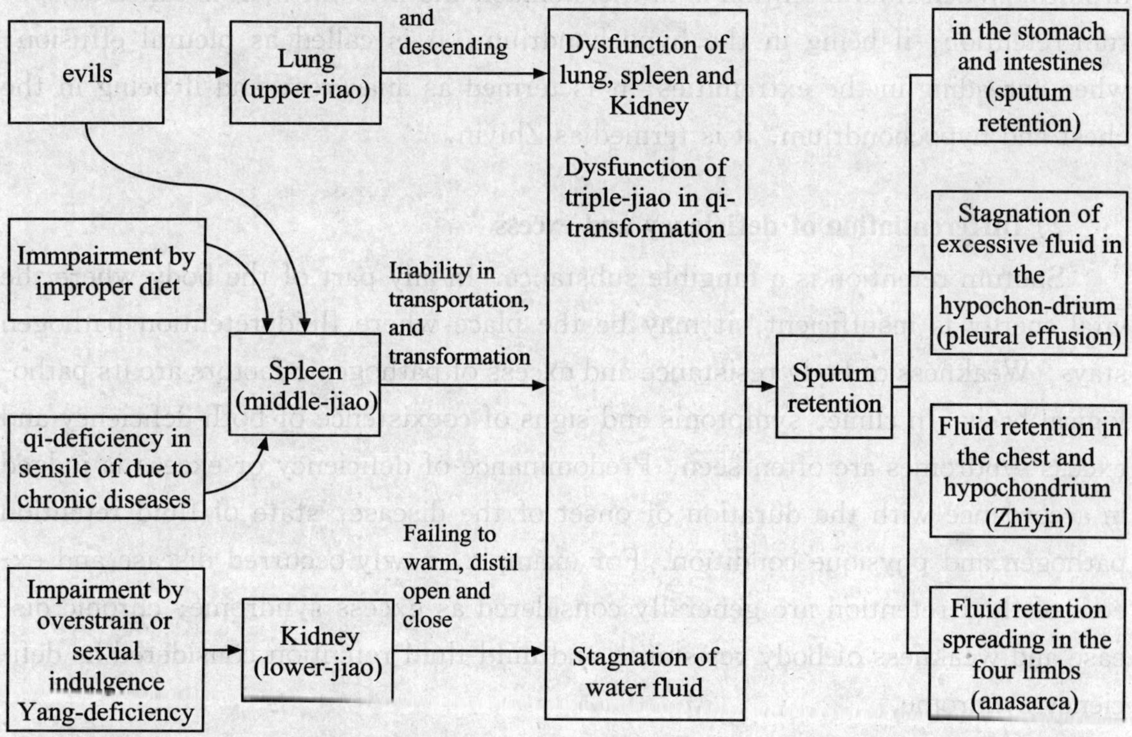

In the property, fluid retention syndrome is always attributed to yang deficiency and yin excessiveness and results from disorder of transportation and transformation of water fluid. It is an excess syndrome due to deficiency of body resistance and stagnation and accumulation of water fluid. Water belongs to the category of yin and can not be transformed into clear component without yang. So, if yang-qi is very weak, qi fails to transform body fluid, there will be predominance of yin-pathogen, and cold fluid retention in the interior. Thus, usual deficiency of yang of the middle-jiao is the intrinsic pathological basis of fluid retention. Fluid retention predominantly belongs to cold syndrome, sometimes or occasionally presents coexistence of cold and heat syndromes because of mutual fighting between seasonal pathogens and internal fluid retention, or heat-transformation of fluid retention due to prolonged accumulation.

〔Differentiation of Syndromes and Treatment〕

1. Key points for differentiation of syndromes

1) Differentiation of locations

Identify the location where fluid retention is, i. e. distinguish various syndromes. When fluid retention is in the stomach and intestines, it is called as sputum retention; if being in the hypochondrium, it is called as pleural effusion; when spreading in the extremities, it is termed as anasarca; and if being in the chest and hypochondrium, it is termed as Zhiyin.

2) Differentiation of deficiency and excess

Sputum retention is a tangible substance. In any part of the body where the vital energy is insufficient, it may be the place where fluid retention pathogen stays. Weakness of body resistance and excess of pathogenic factors are its pathological basis. In clinic, symptoms and signs of coexistence of both deficiency and excess syndromes are often seen. Predominance of deficiency or excess is judged in accordance with the duration of onset of the disease, state of fluid retention pathogen and physique condition. For example, newly-occurred disease and excess of fluid retention are generally considered as excess syndrome; chronic disease and weakness of body resistance and mild fluid retention considered as deficiency syndrome.

3) Differentiation of coexistence of two or more syndromes

Sputum retention is a yin syndrome and mostly belongs to cold syndrome, but when lasting for a long period of time, it may also transform into heat which is judged by considering that whether there is thirst, the state of urine and stool, tongue picture and pulse condition together. At the beginning of onset of sputum retention, if there exist chills, fever, etc., it indicates coexistence of exterior syndrome and sputum retention, then, exterior cold or exterior heat syndrome is further distinguished. If sputum retention does not change, rising and lowering functions of qi are suppressed, it suggests coexistence of sputum retention and stagnation of qi. If sputum retention stays for a long time, qi-stagnation and blood stasis or qi-deficiency and blood stasis are often seen at the same time.

2. Diagnosis

1) Difference and interrelation of dampness, water, fluid retention and sputum

Dampness, water, fluid-retention and sputum are derived from the same origin, and formed by abnormal accumulation of body fluid. Speaking separately, they have their own characters. In regard to the texture and property, fluid retention is thin; sputum is thick and turbid; water belongs to clear fluid; and dampness is sticky and has no fixed shape. Speaking from the focus, fluid retention often appears in the topical part of the body, such as stomach, intestines, chest, hypochondrium, four limbs, etc. sputum and dampness may stay everywhere in the body and is changeable. Water retention may spread within the muscles and skin of the whole body, mostly accumulates in the lower part and the flaccid part of the body. With respect to the property of the disease, fluid retention results from accumulation of body fluid due to yang deficiency and yin-cold; sputum contains cold and heat types, the cold type sputum is similar to water fluid while heat type sputum is derived from heat-consuming-body fluid; water belongs to yin category and can be subdivided into yang-water and yin-water types depending on the pathogenic factors. Dampness is a yin pathogen and has various transformed-types including cold, heat, exterior and interior types. Thus, in clinic, there are cold-damp and damp-heat types; when dampness pathogen invades the exterior of the body, it may injure the skin, and when it invades the interior, it will injure qi, blood, zang- or fu-organs.

In brief, the four pathogens are from the same one origin and can be transformed into each other under certain conditions. In regard to their treatment, water fluid is treated by warming and removing methods; as to coexistence of two or more pathogens, its treatment is not discussed here. Concerning the treatment of sputum and dampness, after distinguishing cold or heat type, warming and resolving, or dispelling and reducing methods are used. They are shown as the following diagrams.

2) Relationship between anasarca and wind-water

Anasarca is also attributed to the category of edema, as recorded in one chapter of the book《The Golden Mirror of Medicine》that "anasarca… is referred to edema caused by wind pathogen". But in patients with anasarca which water evil spreads in muscles and skin of the extremities, soreness and heaviness sensations often appear at the same time, edema in the four limbs is significant, other manifestations of fluid retention attacking the lung, such as normal urination, aversion to cold, anhidrosis, cough, asthma often with foamy sputum, chest stuffiness, etc. are seen. If there exist accumulation of heat in the interior and cold-evil tightening the exterior, cough, panting, fever and irritability will accompany simultaneously. If wind-water pathogens spread unchecked, puffy eye-lipid is seen first, followed by edema involving the four limbs and the whole body, difficult urination, and some possible symptoms of exterior-cold, exterior-heat or exterior-deficiency syndrome.

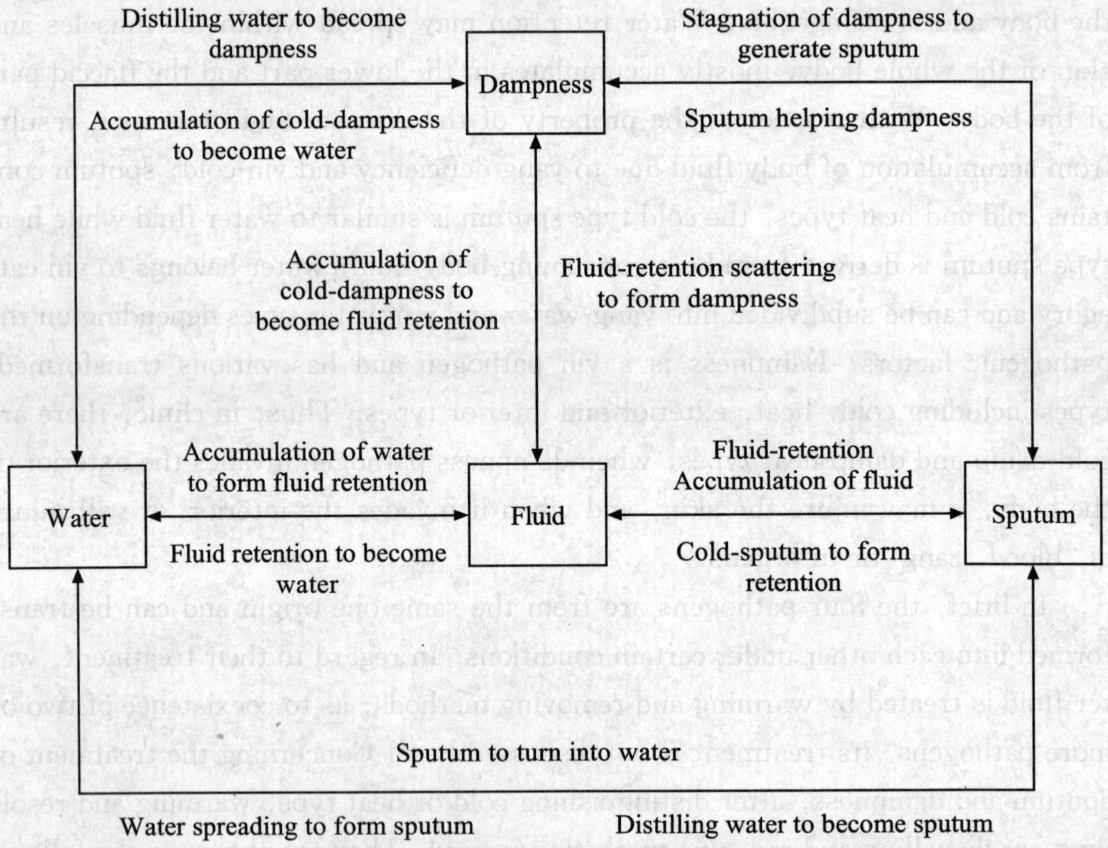

3) Relationship between Zhiyin or pleural effusion and lung distention, bronchial wheezing or panting syndrome

Lung distention in the beginning stage may presents symptoms of Zhiyin-syndrome. Lung-cold and turbid sputum types of panting syndrome are often of some characters of Zhiyin-syndrome. Symptoms of wheezing-syndrome in the attack stage are basically similar to those of pleural effusion. Just as Chen Xouyuan said that "pleural effusion above the diaphragm is conventionally termed as asthma". Zhiyin and pleural effusion are named according to the pathological changes while lung distention, wheezing and panting named based on the characteristics of their own symptoms. Zhiyin or pleural effusion is a symptom of lung distention, bronchial wheezing or panting syndrome or appears in a certain stage of the disease. Lung distention results from gradual development of multiple pulmonary diseases, panting syndrome may be seen in the process of multiple chronic diseases, and bronchial wheezing syndrome is marked by repeatedly attack. During attack of bronchial wheezing, panting-syndrome and lung distention, fluid retention pathogen may also happens.

3. Key Points of the Therapeutic Principles

1) Fluid retention syndrome is always attributed to exhaustion of yang and hyperactivity of yin, weakness of body resistance and excess of pathogenic factors and is treated always by warming and reducing. Fluid retention is considered as yin-pathogen, accumulates when meeting cold-pathogen and flows when warmed. So, warming and reducing principles should be given not only for patients with yang-deficiency and mild fluid retention pathogen but also for those with excess or hyperactivity of fluid retention by combining with drugs warming in property when using recipes for dispelling fluid retention, inducing diuresis and diaphoresis.

2) In treatment of fluid retention, a reasonable measure should be given in accordance with the state of body resistance and pathogenic factors, greater or lesser urgency of the disease, differences of the deficiency and excess of the exterior- or interior-syndrome. For tense water retention, dispelling pathogen method is given to treat the superficiality; for exhaustion of yang and deficiency of qi, warming yang method is adopted to treat the origin. For exterior-syndrome,

treatment is performed by using warming, dispelling and sweating methods. For interior-syndrome, treatment is conducted by employing warming, dispelling and diuresis-inducing methods. For weak body resistance, reinforcing method is taken; for excess of pathogens, purging method is taken; for coexistence of excess of pathogens and weakness of body resistance, both eliminating and reinforcing methods are employed at the same time; and for coexistence of fluid retention and heat syndromes, warming and cooling methods are taken simultaneously.

3) In one chapter of the medical book《Principle and Prohibition for Medical Profession》, methods for separate treatment of deficiency and excess syndromes are put forward and can be used as the essentials for differentiation of syndromes and treatment of fluid retention. For excess of fluid retention pathogen, eliminating, diuresis-inducing and sweating for removing fluid retention are taken separately in light of the location of the pathogen. For exhaustion of yang and mild fluid retention, treatment is given by strengthening the spleen and warming the kidney. When yang-qi is invigorated, the fluid retention pathogen is eliminated spontaneously. Even for excess syndrome, when fluid retention pathogen is removed basically and the body resistance is still weak, drugs for strengthening the spleen and warming the kidney are also needed for consolidating the origin. If accumulating in the interior for a longer period of time, fluid retention pathogen is readily to transform into heat, accompanied with qi-stagnation and blood stasis, which is treated with warming in combination with drugs for clearing away heat, regulating qi, promoting blood circulation to remove blood stasis. When fluid retention hides in the interior of the body, exopathy happens frequently. Under the circumstances, treatment is given by supplementing warm and cold-dispelling drugs for relieving exterior cold syndrome, or adding heat-clearing drugs for relieving exterior-heat syndrome after differentiating the concurrent syndromes.

4. Typing and Treatment

1) Excess syndrome

(1) Sputum retention Sputum retention often results from usual hypofunction of the spleen in transportation and transformation and additional improper diet or exogenous dampness-induced fluid retention in the stomach and intestines.

a) Fluid retention in the stomach without heat-transformation

Main symptoms: Chest fullness, epigastric stuffiness, water-shaking sound in the epigastric part, cold sensation on the back being about a palm size, thirst with intense desire for drinking water, or being readily to vomit on drinking water, throwing up clear water or thin saliva.

Concomitant symptoms: Emaciation, less food intake, or vertigo.

Tongue picture and pulse condition: White and slippery tongue coating, taut slippery or deep, taut and forceful pulse.

Analysis: When the fluid retention occurs in the middle-jiao, qi can not flow normally, thus, water-shaking sound happens in the stomach. The back of the body belongs to yang, in case of hyperactivity of yin-cold in the interior, yang-qi can not reach the exterior part of the body, so, cold feeling appears on the back. In case of fluid retention hiding in the interior, exhaustion of yang and excess of yin, the body fluid is incapable of nourishing the upper part of the body, thus, the patient is thirsty but has no desire for drinking water, is easily to vomit clear water or thin sputum and saliva on intake of water. In case of formation of water retention instead of normal transformation of food-stuff into essences, the body has no sufficient essential substances to nourish and thus becomes thinner and thinner. Retention of fluid in the interior is responsible for less food intake. Failure of the lucid yang to rise and up-stirring of turbid sputum contribute to vertigo. White greasy fur and taut slippery pulse are also signs of cold fluid retention.

Therapeutic principles: Warming yang to induce diuresis.

Recipes and drugs: Supplemented Ling Gui Zhu Gan Decoction. Ramulus Cinnamomi, Radix Glycyrrhizae and Rhizoma Atractylodis Macrocephalae are used to invigorate yang and strengthen the spleen; Poria, a mild-flavoured diuretic serves to remove dampness.

Addition and subtraction: For vomiting, Rhizoma Pinelliae and Rhizoma Zingiberis Recens are added to regulate the stomach and lower the reversed flow of qi. For vertigo, Zhe Xie Decoction is used together for eliminating dampness and raising lucid yang. For unbearable stuffiness in the chest and epigastrium, Zhi Zhu Pill is used together to lower qi and remove stuffiness or Ping Wei Powder used together to regulate qi, remove dampness and modulate the stomach.

Recipe example:

Poria 20g, Ramulus Cinnamomi 10g, Rhizoma Atractylodis 10g, dried Radix Glycyrrhizae 6g, Rhizoma Pinelliae 10g, Pericarpium Citri Reticulatae 10g and

Rhizoma Zingiberis Recens 3 slices.

b) Fluid retention in the stomach and intestines with additional heat-transformation

Main symptoms: Rigidity, fullness and pain sensations in the epigastrium and abdomen, sustained rigidity and fullness in the epigastrium despite having a normal urination, or water moving sound in the intestines, abdominal fullness, constipation, dry mouth and tongue.

Concomitant symptoms: In mild cases, all the symptoms mentioned above can be seen.

Tongue picture and pulse condition: Greasy, or white or yellow tongue coating, deep taut or deep-sited pulse.

Analysis: In case of fluid retention in the stomach and intestines and excess of fluid retention pathogen, epigastric and abdominal rigidity and fullness and pain may happen. In spit of having micturation, new fluid retention generates afterwards, the situation of fluid retention has no any changes. As a result, the epigastric rigidity and fullness are still same. When fluid retention pathogen flows from the stomach to the intestines, its moving sound could be heard. If the accumulated fluid transforms into heat and the large intestine is obstructed, there will be abdominal fullness, constipation, dry mouth and tongue with yellow coating, indicating hyperactivity of fluid retention pathogen.

Therapeutic principle: Purging water retention.

Recipes and drugs: Gan Sui Ban Xia Decoction or Ji Jiao Li Huang Pill is used to treat the origin. The former recipe has both offensive and defensive functions and is used to treat water retention in the stomach. In this recipe, Radix Euphorbiae Kansui and Rhizoma Pinelliae serve to eliminate fluid retention and lower reversed flow of qi; Radix Paeoniae Alba and honey sour and sweet in taste are used to regulate the middle-jiao and to avoid injuring the vital energy. By using the antagonism and mutual activating action, the fluid retention is eliminated. The later recipe with pungent flavor and bitter taste and functioning in purgation is used to eliminate the pathogen separately from the urination and defecation for treatment of water retention in the intestines with heat-transformation of accumulated fluid pathogen. In this recipe, Radix et Rhizoma Rhei and Semen Lepidii seu Descurainiae serve to soften the rigidity and eliminate water retention; Radix Stephaniae Tetrandrae and Pericarpium Zanthoxyli with pungent flavor for dispersion and bitter taste for purgation are used to remove water by diuresis.

Addition and subtraction: For severe distention and fullness in the epigastrium and abdomen, Fructus Aurantii Immaturus and Cortex Magnoliae Officinalis are added to alleviate the fullness. But, it should be noted that despite of excess of fluid retention pathogen, too fast and drastic purgation should not be adopted for avoiding injuring the vital energy.

Recipe example:

For water retention in the stomach: Radix Euphorbiae Kansui powder 1～2g (taken with warm decoction), Rhizoma Pinelliae 10g, Radix Paeoniae Alba 10g, honey 10g (mixed with the hot decoction) and Radix Glycyrrhizae 5g.

For water retention in the intestines with heat-transformation: Radix Stephaniae Tetrandrae 12g, Pericarpium Zanthoxyli 5g, Semen Lepidii seu Descurainiae 10g, dried Radix et Rhizoma Rhei 3～5g, Fructus Aurantii Immaturus 6g and Cortex Magnoliae Officinalis 6g.

(2) Pleural effusion

Pleural effusion, i.e. fluid retention in the hypochondrium often results from deficiency of lung-defensive system and subsequent seasonal pathogens invasion-induced obstruction of the lung due to weak physique or other chronic diseases.

Main symptoms: Distending pain in the hypochondrium, worsening while spitting, coughing, even breathing or turning round body, fullness in the hypochondrium on the affected side.

Concomitant symptoms: Alternate attacks of chills and fever in most cases, or tidal fever in the afternoon, bitter taste, dry throat, etc., chest discomfort and stuffiness, obstructed respiration, or dull coughing, etc. due to water retention. If it lasts longer, dry mouth and throat, tidal fever, night sweating, flushed cheeks, dysphoria, feverish sensation in palms and soles will be seen.

Tongue picture and pulse condition: White or yellowish tongue coating and taut rapid pulse in the early stage; reddish or dim tongue with less fur, small rapid pulse in the late stage.

Analysis: In case of attack of the hypochondrium by pathogens, fluid retention will appear due to stagnation of lung-qi and failure of qi to distribute body fluid. The hypochondrium is the passage where qi rises and lowers. So, if the meridians are blocked, there will be chest and hypochondriac distending pain and referred pain on coughing or spitting, obstructed respiration or dull cough which are manifestations of dysfunction of the collateral branches of meridians. The lung lies in the chest and the bilateral hypochondria are the places where Shaoyang Meridian distributes and passes through. If pathogens attack the hypochondria, there will be dysfunction of the Shaoyang, manifested as alternate fever and chills, bitter taste, dry throat, afternoon tidal fever, etc. If the accumulated fluid transforms into heat, lung-yin will be injured and a series of symptoms of dry mouth and throat, tidal fever, night sweating, flushed cheeks, dysphoria are seen. The above-mentioned tongue picture and pulse condition are also signs of water retention, stagnation of qi, obstruction of the collateral branches of meridians or impairment of yin by fluid retention.

Therapeutic principles: Purging heat from the lung, lowering qi, and removing water retention.

Recipes and drugs: Modified Jiaomu Gualou Decoction combined with Shi Zao Decoction or Kong Xian Pill. In the former recipe, Semen Lepidii seu Descurainiae and Cortex Mori Radicis are used to purge lung-heat and eliminate fluid retention; Fructus Perillae, Pericarpium Trichosanthis, Paericarpium Citri Reticulatae and Rhizoma Pinelliae serve to lower qi and resolve sputum; Pericarpium Zanthoxyli, Poria and Corex Zingiberis are used to remove water retention; Fructus Tribuli is used to guide drug to reach the bilateral hypochondria, to calm the liver and help the lung lower qi. Shi Zao Decoction and Kong Xian Pill are recipes for purging water retention. Shi Zao Decoction has a powerful action and is used to treat patients with excess syndrome, larger amount of fluid retention, better physique and without exhaustion of the vital energy. Radix Euphorbiae Kansui, Radix Knoxiae and Flos Genkwa are processed into powder and taken with decocted Fructus Ziziphi Jujubae fluid at a draught and under fasting. Kong Xian Pill has a weaker power and is made up of Shi Zao Decoction plus Semen Sinapis Albae instead of Flos Genkwa. It is good at clearing away sputum-water in the subcutaneous tissues and at the outside of the membrane and functions in ventilating the lung and regulating qi. The later two recipes are used in smaller dosage at the beginning of treatment and then increased gradually in dosage, taken continuously for 3～5 days, suspended for 2～3 days and then taken again. If vomiting, abdominal pain and over-frequent diarrhea occur, they are taken in smaller dosage or suspended.

Addition and subtraction: In case of severer sputum-rheum, chest fullness and turbid greasy fur, Bulbus Allii Macrostemi and Semen Armeniacae are supplemented to resolve sputum and remove water retention. If the long-term stagnated water fluid is difficult to be removed, and the patient also has fullness in the chest and hypochondrium, weak constitution and less food intake, Ling Gui Zhu Gan Decoction is added for invigirating yang, strengthening the spleen and removing fluid retention. Under the circumstances, drastic purgation is definitely not recommendable. In case of weak body resistance and excess of pathogens, except purging water retention, Tingli Dazao Xiefei Decoction combined with Modified San Zi Yang Qin Decoction may also be used to lower qi and eliminate fluid retention.

At the early stage of pleural effusion, alternate chills and fever, symptoms of dysfunction of the Shaoyang Meridian are often seen, Modified Cai Zhi Banxia Decoction can be used to remove sputum, relieve the stagnation and reduce fever by reconciliation. Radix Bupleuri and Radix Scutellariae are used to reduce fever by mediation; Fructus Trichosanthis, Rhizoma Pinelliae and Semen Armeniacae are used to resolve sputum; Fructus Aurantii, Radix Platycodi and Radix Paeoniae Rubra serve to regulate qi and dredge collateral branches of meridians, and Radix Glycyrrhizae functions in mediating actions of all the drugs.

When fluid retention lasts for a long time, it will lead to disorder of flow of qi and dysfunction of collateral branches of meridians and stabbing pain in the chest and hypochondrium, which is treated with Xiangfu Xuanfuhua Decoction. The present recipe functions in mediating qi, resolving sputum and regulating the collateral branches of the meridian. Flos Inulae, Fructus Perillae, Semen Armeniacae, Rhizoma Pinelliae, Semen Coicis and Poria are used to lower qi and resolve sputum, Rhizoma Cyperi and Pericarpium Citri Reticulatae are used to regulate qi and relieve depression. For severe stabbing pain, Radix Angelicae Sinensis, Radix Paeoniae Rubra, Semen Persicae, Flos Carthami, Olibanum, Myrrha are supplemented; for failure of water retention to lower, Medulla Tetrapanacis, Fructus Liquidambaris, Exocarpium Benincasae, etc. are used together.

When fluid retention stays for a long time, the stagnated qi will transform into heat to consume yin, appearing a group of symptoms of hyperactivity of internal heat due to yin deficiency which is treated with Xiebai Powder combined with Sashen Maidong Decoction. Cortex Mori Radicis and Cortex Lycii Radicis are used to remove pathogenic fire from the lung; Radix Glehniae, Radix Ophiopogonis,

Rhizoma Polygonati Odorati, Radix Trichosanthis, etc., serve to nourish yin and promote secretion of body fluid. For tidal fever, Carapax Trionycis and Caulis Mahoniae are added; for cough, Radix Stemonae and Bulbus Fritillariae are used together; for severe stuffiness and pain in the chest, Fructus Trichosanthis, Fructus Aurantii, Radix Curcumae, Retinervus and Luffae Fructus are supplemented: for remained fluid retention, Concha Ostreae and Rhizoma Alismatis are added; and for qi-deficiency and fatigue, Radix Pseudostellariae, Radix Astragali seu Hedysari and Fructus Schisandrae are supplemented.

Recipe example:

Pericarpium Zanthoxyli 50 grains, Fructus Trichosanthis 15g, Cortex Mori Radicis 10g, Semen Lepidii seu Descurainiae 10g, Fructus Perillae 5g, Rhizoma Pinelliae 5g, Poria 12g, Exocarpium Citri Reticulatae 5g, Fructus Tribuli 10g and Rhizoma Zingiberis Recens 3 slices.

(3) Fluid retention in the chest and hypochondrium

When the body is affected by cold pathogen, chronic cough happens, gradually leading to asthma. When asthma develops continuously and injuries the lung repeatedly, the lung-qi is very weak and can not distribute body fluid normally, as a result, fluid retention appears in the chest and hypocondrium.

Main symptoms: Cough, dyspnea, orthopnea, and profuse white foamy sputum, etc. which last all the year round and worsen if affected by cold pathogen in cold seasons.

Concomitant symptoms: Puffiness in the face and ankle part in severe cases, if induced by cold attack, cold or heat type exterior syndrome may be seen.

Tongue picture and pulse condition: White greasy tongue coating and taut tense pulse.

Analysis: When fluid retention rises reversely to attack the lung, the lung-qi is not able to lower normally, so, cough, dyspnea, orthopnea, profuse foamy sputum, etc. are seen. Fluid retention pathogen has a stronger passion with the lung, thus, it lasts long and is difficult to be cured. Fluid retention is a yin-pathogen, hence, its attack is readily evoked when the human body is affected by cold. When spreading unchecked in muscles and skin, water retention will lead to dropsy in the face and four limbs. The recurrent fluid retention is evoked due to new invasion of cold, so, exterior-cold syndrome is seen. White greasy or white slippery tongue coating and taut tense pulse suggest hyperactivity of cold fluid retention in the interior.

Therapeutic principles: Warming the lung and removing fluid retention.

Recipes and drugs: Modified Xiao Qing Long Decoction. This recipe can function in warming the interior and dispelling pathogens from the superficial part of the body and is used to treat combined syndrome of internal fluid retention and exterior cold. In this recipe, Herba Ephedrae, Ramulus Cinnamomi, Rhizoma Zingiberis and Herba Asari serve to warm the lung, remove cold; Rhizoma Pinelliae and Radix Glycyrrhizae are used to resolve sputum and regulate qi, combined with Fructus Schisandrae and Radix Paeoniae Alba which means inducing astringency while dispersing pathogens.

Addition and subtraction: For patients with weak body resistance and mild exterior syndrome, Ling Gan Wu Wei Jiang Xin Decoction is used instead. For patients who have more fluid retention, less cold and no exterior syndrome, but experience dyspnea, cough, profuse sputum and inability to lie flat, Tingli Dazao Xiefei Decoction is used. In case of profuse sticky sputum, chest fullness and dyspnea, Semen Raphani and Semen Sinapis Albae are supplemented to lower qi and get rid of sputum; or Sang Su Gui Ling Decoction is used to lower qi and resolve sputum. For warming yang to dispel fluid retention, Cortex Mori Radicis, Fructus Perillae, Rhizoma Pinelliae, Pericarpium Arecae and Semen Armeniacae are employed to lower qi, Ramulus Cinnamomi and Pericarpium Citri Reticulatae used to warm yang and regulate qi and, Polyporus, Poria and Rhizoma Alismatis used to eliminate water retention.

In case of asthma, chest fullness, epigastric rigidity, polydipsia, darkish complexion, yellow greasy tongue coating and deep tense pulse due to heat-transformation of the accumulated fluid pathogen, weakness of the body resistance and excess of pathogens and suppression of the yang by yin pathogen, Mufangji Decoction is employed to induce diuresis, dissolve rigidity, supplement deficiency and clear away heat pathogen. For rigid accumulation of water pathogen, this recipe is used in combination with Poria and Natrii Sulphas instead of Gypsum Fibrosum.

Recipe example:

Herba Ephedrae 4g, Semen Persicae 10g, Semen Armeniacae 10g, Cortex Mori Radicis 10g, Fructus Perillae 10g, Ramulus Cinnamomi 3g, Polyporus 10g, Poria 10g, Rhizoma Pinelliae 8g and dried Radix Glycyrrhizae 4g.

(4) Anasarca

Anasarca is often caused by spreading of water retention in the four limbs due to failure of the lung and spleen to disperse and transport resulted from affection by exogenous wind-cold pathogens and obstruction of sweat pores.

Main symptoms: Arthralgia, heaviness sensation and edema in the four limbs.

Concomitant symptoms: Chills and anhidrosis seen in most cases, or gasping breath, cough, foamy sputum, chest stuffiness and no thirst.

Tongue picture and pulse condition: White tongue and taut tense pulse.

Analysis: When water retention spreads unchecked in the four limbs and body surface, it would cause arthralgia, heaviness sensation and edema in the body. Wind-cold tightening the superficial part is responsible for chills and anhidrosis. If cold fluid retention stays in the interior and goes up reversely to attack the lung, it can lead to gasping breath, cough, foamy sputum, chest stuffiness and no thirst. White tongue coating and taut tense pulse are manifestations of combined exterior- and interior-cold syndromes.

Therapeutic methods: Relieving exterior-syndrome by diaphoresis and removing fluid retention.

Recipes and drugs: Xiao Qing Long Decoction or Modified Ma Xing Yi Gan Decoction. The former recipe functions in relieving exterior-syndrome by means of diaphoresis and warming the interior and the later recipe is capable of dispelling exogenous pathogens and eliminating dampness and fluid retention. Moreover, Mahuang Jia Zhu Decoction may also be used to dispel exopathogens, strengthen the spleen and get rid of water retention.

Addition and subtraction: For treatment of anasarca patients with oliguria, Polyporus, Poria and Rhizoma Alismatis are added to eliminate water retention; If fever, irritability and white and yellowish tongue coating appear together, it indicates exogenous cold pathogen tightening the body surface and accumulated pathogenic heat in the interior. Under the circumstances, Gypsum Fibrosum is added to clear away heat. If manifestations of cold syndrome are not significant, Rhizoma Zingiberis and Herba Asari are not used and treatment is given by employing Da Qinglong Decoction or Yue Bi Jia Zhu Decoction instead for expelling exopathogens and removing pathogenic heat from the interior. If the anasarca patient has no apparent exterior syndrome but has significant melalgia, chest stuffiness and poor appetite, it can be treated with Shen Zhu Powder for dispelling dampness, removing fluid retention and regulating the stomach.

Recipe example:

Ramulus Cinnamomi 6g, Polyporus 10g, Poria 10g, Rhizoma Atractylodis 10g, Rhizoma Atractylodis Macrocephalae 10g, Semen Coicis 20g, Semen Armeniacae 10g, Rhizoma Zingiberis Recens 3 slices, Rhizoma Alismatis 10g and Herba Ephedrae 6g.

2) Deficiency syndrome

(1) Weakness of spleen-yang

Weakness of spleen-yang is often referred to hypofunction of the spleen in transportation and transformation due to attack of the exogenous dampness pathogen or improper diet. It is also referred to the stage which the fluid retention pathogen is eliminated basically after treatment while the body resistance is also weak considerably.

Main symptoms: Feeling of fullness and discomfort in the chest and hypochondrium, being comfortable if having a long sigh or the abdomen pressed, frequently vomiting thin fluid or thin sputum, palpitation, shortness of breath and dizziness.

Concomitant symptoms: Cold feeling on the back, water shaking sound in the stomach, nausea, gasping breath, dyspnea, or eyelid puffiness after getting up in the morning, and lower limb edema in the afternoon.

Tongue picture and pulse condition: Enlarged tongue with white slippery fur, taut, thready and slippery pulse.

Analysis: In case of hypofunction of the spleen in transportation, water fluid can not be distributed normally. If staying in the chest and lung, it will lead to fullness feeling and discomfort in the chest and hypochondrium; if staying in the stomach and intestines, it will induce shaking sound there and vomiting of thin fluid. Water retention attacking the heart and lung contributes to palpitation and shortness of breath. When invading the openings of the head, it will cause dizziness. White slippery fur, enlarged tongue, and taut, thready and slippery pulse all suggest water retention in the interior of the body, weakness of the spleen-qi and spleen-yang.

Therapeutic principles: Warming and reinforcing the spleen to remove fluid retention

Recipes and drugs: Supplemented Li Zhong Pill. For yang-deficiency and yin-hyperactivity, Radix Aconiti Praeparata, Fructus Euodiae and Cortex Cinnamomi are added to warm yang and dispel cold. In case of severer sialemesis, Wu Ling Powder is used in combination for warming yang to remove fluid retention, and in case of predominance of spleen-deficiency and no striking fluid retention, Xiang Sha Liujunzi Decoction may be used instead.

Recipe example:

Radix Ginseng powder 3g (taken after being infused in hot decocted drug fluid), Poria 10g, Ramulus Cinnamomi 10g, Rhizoma Atractylodis Macrocephalae 10g, Radix Glycyrrhizae Praeparata 6g, Rhizoma Pinelliae Praeparata10g, Exocarpium Citri Reticulatae 10g, Cortex Cinnamomi 5g, Rhizoma Zingiberis 6g and Rhizoma Zingiberis Recens 3 slices.

(2) Weakness of kidney-yang

Weakness of kidney-yang is often seen in the aged people and patients with impairment of the kidney due to chronic disease.

Main symptoms: Chills, cold limbs, cramping and numbness sensations or tremor in the lower abdomen, rapid breathing, shortness of breath, gasp-worsening on exertion, vomiting, fright due to qi-deficiency, oliguria and ankle edema.

Concomitant symptoms: Vomiting of foamy fluid, dizziness.

Tongue picture and pulse condition: White, greasy and moist or white slippery tongue coating, enlarged tongue and deep, thready and slippery pulse.

Analysis: When injured due to chronic diseases, the kidney can not accept air normally, leading to dyspnea, tachypnea, shortness of breath and worsening on exertion. In case of deficiency of both spleen-qi and lung-qi and excessive fluid retention in the interior, vomiting, fright due to qi-deficiency, profuse sputum, chest stuffiness and poor appetite are often seen. If the deficient yang can not warm the body, it would cause chills and cold limbs. When kidney-qi is weak and can not function in qi-transformation, water retention occurs in the lower-jiao to cause oliguria, cramping sensation and numbness or tremor in the lower abdomen. When fluid retention spread unchecked in the muscles and skin, it will lead to edema; if fluid retention goes up reversely, it will cause sialemesis and dizziness. Enlarged tongue, white fur and deep, thready, slippery pulse also suggest deficiency of yang and fluid retention.

Therapeutic principles: Warming the kidney to remove fluid retention.

Recipes and drugs: Zhen Wu Decoction is used in combination with Modified Jin Gui Shen Qi Pill. The two recipes both can function in warming yang to eliminate fluid retention. The former recipe serves to warm both spleen and kidney and the later recipe functions predominantly in warming the kidney and is slow in action. Sliced Radix Aconiti Praeparata, Cortex Cinnamomi and Rhizoma Zingiberis Recens are used to warm yang to eliminate fluid retention; Rhizoma Dioscoreae, Rhizoma Atractylodis Macrocephalae and Radix Glycyrrhizae are used to reinforce qi and strengthen the spleen; Poria and Rhizoma Alismatis serve to remove fluid retention by inducing diuresis; and Radix Rehmanniae Praeparata and Fructus Corni are employed to tonify the kidney to improve respiration.

Addition and subtraction: For less food intake, Pericarpium Citri Reticulatae and Rhizoma Pinelliae are supplemented. For tremor in the lower abdomen, sialemesis and dizziness which suggest up-flow of fluid retention, it can be treated with Wu Ling Powder for relieving the exterior syndrome and removing water retention.

Recipe example:

Cortex Cinnamomi 6g, Sliced Radix Aconiti Praeparata 6g, Radix Rehmanniae Praeparata 10g, Poria 10g, Rhizoma Alismatis 15g, Rhizoma Atractylodis Macrocephalae 10g, Rhizoma Zingiberis 6g and Fructus Corni 10g.

In the light of records in the book 《Synopsis of Prescriptions of the Golden Chamber》, the prognosis of sputum retention is deduced according to the pulse condition. It is held that in patients with long duration of disease and weak pulse, if the pulse condition and the syndrome tally with each other, it is curable; if the pulse condition is forceful and large instead, it indicates weakness of body resistance and excess of pathogenic factors and belongs to crisis. Taunt rapid pulse also suggests a refractory disease, because fluid retention is attributed to yin-pathogen, deep taunt pulse should be seen, while taunt rapid pulse is just contrary to the syndrome. All these can be used as a reference in clinic.

〔Analysis on Typical Cases〕

Case 1. Deng X, female, aged 48 years, married, was admitted to our hospital on June 15, 1963 due to edema and shortness of breath for half a year and worsening for a week.

In January of 1961, she caught a cold and began to have cough with white sputum, shortness of breath, edema in the lower limbs, epigastric fullness and oliguria. She has had chronic cough for 8 years at that time. Examination showed taunt thready rapid pulse, white tongue coating and purple lips. It was diagnosed as chronic pulmonary heart disease by modern medicine.

Differentiation of syndromes: Deficiency of heart-yang and kidney-yang, water retention in the interior, obstruction of sputum-dampness, Stagnation of lung-qi.

Therapeutic principles: Clearing away lung-heat, ventilate the lung, lowering qi, resolving sputum, warming yang and eliminate dampness.

Recipes and drugs: Yue Bi Decoction combined with Modified Zhen Wu Decoction. Gypsum Fibrosum 12g, Herba Ephedrae 3g, Radix Glycyrrhizae 9g, Poria 12g, Rhizoma Atractylodis Macrocephalae 9g, Radix Paeoniae Alba 9g, Radix Aconiti Praeparata 6g, Rhizoma Zingiberis Recens 9g, Fructus Ziziphi Jujubae 5 pieces, Semen Plantaginis 15g, Rhizoma Imperatae 30g and Semen Armeniacae 9g.

After taking 3 doses, her urine amount increased to 1500～1900ml/day, and her lower-limb edema reduced considerably. After taking 5 doses, her edema was not apparent, her enlarged liver reduced and her cough was relieved. After taking the above recipe combined with Cortex Magnoliae Officinalis 6g and and Percarpium Citri Reticulatae 6g, her gasping breathing was relieved but had chest stuffiness instead. So, Rhizoma Imperatae, Semen Plantaginis and Cortex Magnoliae Officinalis were dismissed from this recipe while Fructus Perillae was supplemented. After taking 5 doses more, her cough still existed due to inability of lung-qi to disperse. Then, she was treated with soothing the chest oppression, regulating qi and removing lung-heat methods by using Modified Houpu Mahuang Decoction.

Cortex Magnoliae Officinalis 6g, Herba Ephedrae 3g, Rhizoma Pinelliae 9g, Semen Armeniacae 9g, Radix Glycyrrhizae 9g, Radix Glehniae 18g, Fructus Tritici 30g, Poria 9g, Herba Asari 3g, Fructus Schisandrae 6g and Rhizoma Zingiberis Recens 4.5g.

After administration of this decoction, her symptoms were relieved considerably, ... and her conditions were stable. (selected from 《Collections of Zhao Xiwu's Clinical Experience》)

Note: Cough, shortness of breath, edema, oliguria, epigastric fullness, white sputum, white tongue, purple lips of this case resulted from water retention in the interior and accumulation of sputum-dampness in the lung due to long-term stagnated pathogenic factors' injury-induced hypofunction of the lung, spleen and kidney, particularly deficiency of the lung and kidney-yang. It was thus treated predominantly by warming yang to remove dampness, ventilating the lung and inducing diuresis. Yue Bi Decoction combined with Zhen Wu Decoction plus Semen Plantaginis, Rhizoma Imperatae and Semen Armeniacae. were used to restore the dispersing and lowering functions of the lung, and warming yang to induce diuresis. After treatment, the amount of urine increased significantly and the edema abated strikingly. She was then treated with Supplemented Houpo Mahuang Decoction which functions in relieving chest stuffiness by regulating qi and clearing away lung-heat, predominantly in lowering qi and resolving sputum. Chinese predecessors pointed out that accumulation of water becomes fluid retention and the fluid retention condenses to turn to sputum. Fluid retention is easy to be removed while sputum is difficult to be resolved. The present case is treated with the easier way first then with the relatively more difficult method, i. e., removing the fluid retention first followed by resolving sputum which suits the pathological characters of this disease.

Case 2. Wang ××, male, aged 45 years, suffered from cough, chest pain, dyspnea, inability to lie flat due to sputum retention and obstruction of lung-qi caused by affection by exogenous wind-cold pathogens. Examination showed thin greasy tongue coating and slippery forceful pulse. Fluoroscopy suggested exudative pleurisy. According to the theory of traditional Chinese medicine, it was attributed to fluid retention in the chest and hypochondrium and was treated by using dispelling wind, ventilating the lung and purging water retention methods and with drugs as follows.

Caulis Perillae 10g, Semen Lepidii seu Descurainiae 15g, fried Radix Asteris 5g, Fructus Perillae 10g, Radix Platycodi 5g, Semen Armeniacae 9g, Caulis Bambusae in Taeniam 10g, Pericarpium Citri Reticulatae 6g, preprepared Rhizoma Pinelliae 10g, Poria 12g, Fructus Euodiae 1. 5g, Fructus Trichosanthis 10g, Concha Meretricis seu Cyclinae 30g, 10g, Radix Curcumae 10g and Kong Xian Pill 2g (wrraped with a piece of cloth).

After taking 3 doses, her gasping breathing was relieved but occurred again.

Treatment with the same recipe worked well. (《Collections of Huang Yifeng's Medical Records And Talks》)

Note: This case belongs to fluid retention in the chest and hypochodrium, manifesting as chest pain, distention feeling in the hypochodrium, worsening on coughing, dyspnea, inability to lie flat, thin greasy tongue coating and slippery replete pulse which are caused by exopathic wind-cold invasion-induced stirring of sputum retention and obstruction of lung-qi. It is treated with both decoction (She Shi Zao Decoction) and drug pills (Kong Xian Pill) for dispelling wind, ventilating lung and purging water retention which are treated by using methods for dispelling wind, ventilating the lung and removing sputum retention and Kong Xian Pill for purging water retention instead of Shi Zao Decoction. The treatment of this case given follows the therapeutic way of Shi Zao Decoction rather than employment of the recipe itself, imitates its formation but is less strong in purgative action and is especially effective in removing sputum retention.

Sputum retention is a major disease in the department of medicine and is caused by disorder of water metabolism and retention of fluid in some parts of the body due to dysfunction of the lung, spleen and kidney which results from weakness of yang-qi because of affection of the body by cold-dampness, improper diet or overstrain or sexual indulgence. The fluid retention occurs in the middle-jiao and may stay in any part of the body. If moving in the intestines, it will become sputum-retention; if staying in the hypochondrium, it will form pleural effusion; if attacking the lung, it will form zhiyin, and if spreading the four limbs, it will become anasarca.

With respect to clinical differentiation of syndromes, the location of fluid retention, predominance of excess of pathogens or weakness of body resistance and coexistence of both should be identified. Because sputum retention always belongs to yang-deficiency, hyperactivity of yin, weakness of body resistance and excess of pathogenic factors, it is treated with yang-warming and pathogen-removing methods. In case of hyperactivity of sputum retention belonging to excess syndrome, it is treated with retention-purging, qi-regulating, separate eliminating methods for getting rid of pathogens, followed by strengthening the spleen and kidney for treating its fundamental cause. As to mild fluid retention due to deficiency of both spleen-yang and kidney-yang, drugs for strengthening body resistance are used first in combination with a few of drugs for eliminating fluid retention. If fluid retention lasts for a long time, it is often accompanied by other syndromes including sputum, heat, qi-stagnation, blood stasis, exopathy, etc. If so, after differentiation of syndromes, a reasonable treatment is given respectively.

Regarding to changes of sputum retention, it results first from hypofunction of the lung and spleen, if developing continuously for a long time, it will gradually involve the kidney. When the kidney-yang is insufficient, its opening and closing functions are out of order. The resultant water retention may attack the heart, lung or spleen. On the other hand, sputum retention is mostly attributed to a chronic disease, lingering, and is often accompanied with changes of cold, heat, deficiency or excess. Moreover, accumulation of fluid may generate sputum, sputum and blood stasis often combine together. If so, it is more difficult to be cured rapidly. Thus, it should be treated in time.

Questions for Review

1. Try to narrate the concept of sputum retention; How to distinguish sputum and fluid retention?
2. How to understand and master that "in treatment of patients with sputum retention, it should be mediated with drugs warm in property"?
3. How to differentiate various syndromes of pleural effusion and treat them ? What are the principles for forming Gualou Jiaomu Decoction ?
4. What are the differences between Xiao Banxia plus Fuling Decoction and Ling Gui Zhu Gan Decoction, between Ganshui Babxia Decoction and Ji Jiao Li Huang decoction? What are their clinical indications?

Spontaneous Perspiration and Night Sweat

〔Introduction〕

Spontaneous perspiration and night sweat are the diseases marked by abnormal hidrosis in TCM. They are caused by imbalance of yin and yang, disharmony between ying and wei, or dysfunction of connecting tissues. If one perspires awake, and the perspiration become heavily after activity, he suffers from spontaneous perspiration. If the perspiration only appears at the head, hand, foot or half of the body, he suffers from sweating locally. If one sweats in sleep, and the sweat is stopped as soon as awake, he suffers from night sweat. In clinical, a patient may suffer from both spontaneous perspiration and night sweat at the same time.

Spontaneous perspiration and night sweat can be not only a single syndrome, but also can accompanied with other diseases. In this chapter, the diseases whose main syndromes are spontaneous perspiration or night sweat will be discussed.

As to the western medical diseases, such as vegetative nerve functional disturbance, hyperthyroidism tuberculosis, paroxysmal hypoglycemosis, collapse, shock, and some infectious disease, manifested mainly as spontaneous perspiration or night sweat, the determination of treatment and differentiation showed in this chapter can be referred to.

〔Etiology and pathogenesis〕

"Yang adding to yin" and "connecting tissues failing to protect the body", as "*Huang Di Nei Jing*" said, are the primary pathogenic changes of sweat syndrome. Sweat syndrome was expounded as heat disease due to exopathogen, miscellaneous disease due to internal injury, spontaneous perspiration and night sweat, respectively. Now the summing up of the pathogenesis of sweat syndrome is disharmony between ying and wei, hyperactivity of fire due to yin deficiency and stagnant pathogenic heat evaporating the body fluid. They will be expounded as follows:

1. Disharmony between ying and wei

Wei qi, which is governed by the lung, plays the role in keeping body fluid from hidrosis. If the lung qi is too deficient and the connecting tissue is too loose to strengthen the exterior wei, the patient will suffer from sweating. If pathogenic wind attack the superficial asthenia body, or pathogenic dampness stay in the muscle and skin, it will lead to disharmony between Ying and wei failing to control the exterior wei. Then the manifestation will be sweating and aversion to wind.

If yang deficiency occurs in a part of the body, it will also lead to dysfunction of exterior wei. Then the manifestation will be marked by sweat locally.

2. Hyperactivity of fire due to yin deficiency

The heart governs the blood circulation and the kidneys store the life essence. Over wrought, sexual strain, hemorrhage or over consuming of the essence will lead to deficiency of blood and essence, fire of deficient type generated inside, and disturbance of Yin body fluid. Thus body fluid gets out of the body and becomes sweat.

If a patient has suffered from insomnia for a long time, his heart-blood will be consumed and his mind will be disturbed. Those will result in failure of Yin and Yang to counteract with each other. Once the patient is irritated, Yang disturbs Yin and makes body fluid get out of the body to become sweat.

3. Stagnant pathogenic heat evaporating the body fluid

If wind-cold invades the interior and then transformed into heat, or if the patient is affected by wind-warm or summer-heat, the heat will accumulate in the lung and stomach and evaporate the body fluid to get out of the body. Then the manifestation will be profuse sweating. If the patient is affected by the pathogenic dampness, or has improper diet, the damp-turbid will be transformed into heat. The latter evaporates the body fluid, then it will marked as sweat locally or yellowish sweat. Those pathogenic changes may appear alone, at same time, or transform into each other to form complicated syndromes.

〔Treatment according to differentiation of syndromes〕

Sweating is a physiological phenomenon. Many causes, such as dressing too much, staying in the heat, drinking hot spoil working, running, or taking drugs for inducing diaphoresis, can lead to sweating slightly. The normal sweating will not make the person uncomfortable. Inducing sweat is a treatment to dispel the pathogen out of the body. Because sweat is derived from heart blood, which comes from the essence, sweating too much is not permitted. Otherwise, it will result in the impairment of vital energy and the illness of body.

1. Differentiation of similar syndromes

In clinical, besides the normal sweat syndromes of spontaneous perspiration and night sweat, there are sweating in shock, sweating after shivering and tawny sweat. All of them have different manifestation, treatment and prognosis. Not to delay the disease, we should distinguish them carefully.

(1) Sweating in shock

Sweating in shock also pertains to spontaneous perspiration. Its features are profuse sweating all over the body or greasy sweating accompanied with cold limbs, vague pulse, weak respiration, and obtuse reaction in urgency. It is also called "jue han" by ancient medicine. Compared to spontaneous perspiration, they are the signs of yin and yang exhaustion and their nature are serious.

(2) Sweating after shivering

Sweating after shivering only appears in the course of the valetudinarian's exogenous disease, which is marked by sweating after rigor. It's the sign of vital qi striving against the pathogenic factor out of the body.

If the vital qi is sufficient, the manifestation will be sweating after shivering, calm pulse and no fever. In this case, the disease is tends to cure. Otherwise, in the case of shivering without sweat or shivering with sweat but without quiet pulse, the prognosis is unfavourable. Over sweating will even turn into sweating in shock.

(3) Tawny sweat

The feature of tawny sweat is yellow sweat capable of staining the undergarment, often accompanied with heaviness sensation, dropy in limbs like wind edema, thirsty but not tending to drink, greasy yellow tongue fur, and deep smooth pulse. The pathogenesis is damp-heat evaporating body fluid or pathogenic dampness stagnating on the surface of the muscle.

Illustratin of etiology and pathology of spontaneous perspiration and night sweat

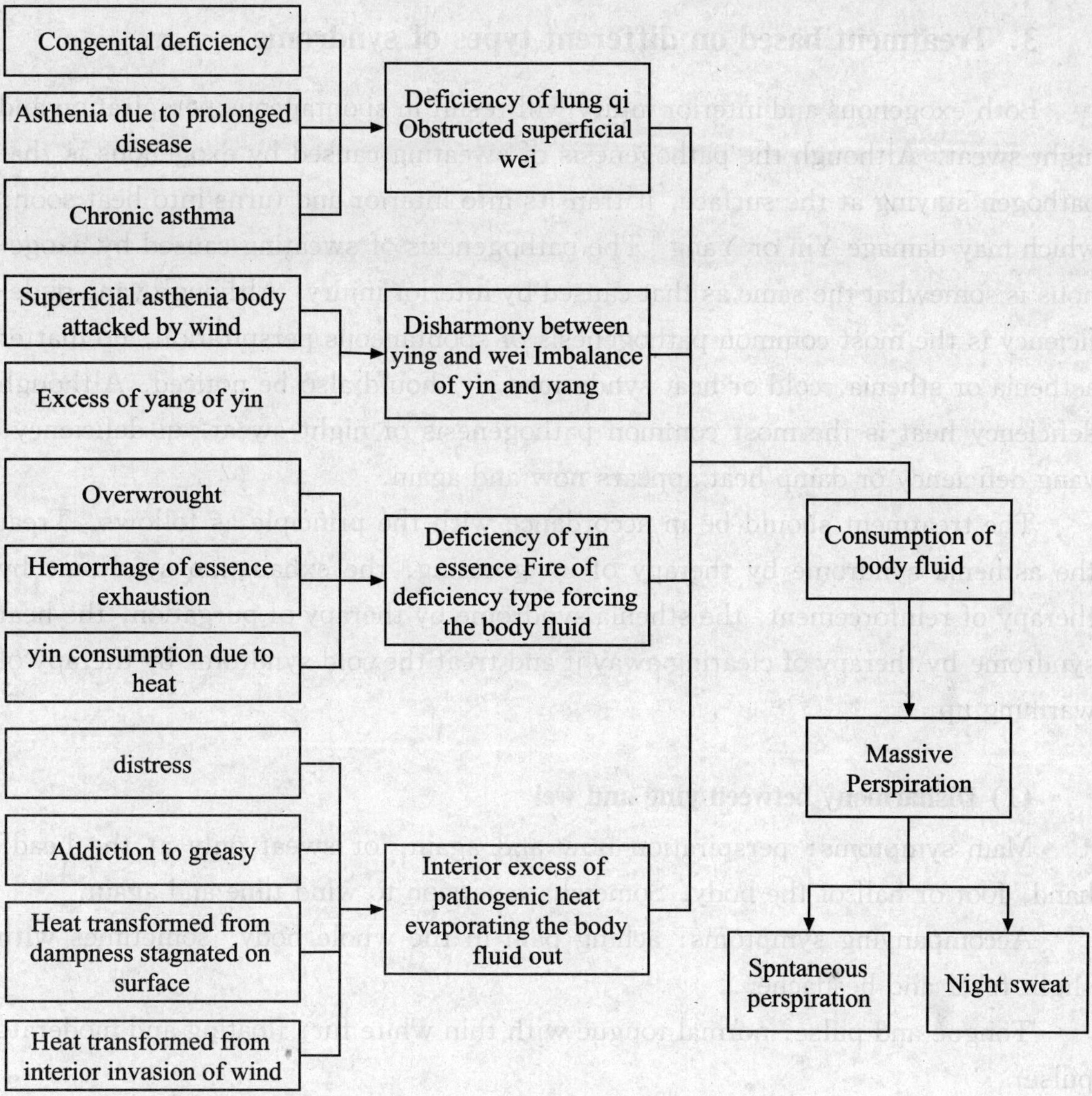

2. Main points of differentiating the syndromes

As to sweating, we should distinguish not only between asthenia syndrome and sthenia syndrome, but also between cold syndrome and hot syndrome. As to differentiation of asthenia and sthenia, we should consider both vital qi and pathogenesis. In most cases, excess of pathogen means sthenia, it may be on surface or in interior, and may be cold or hot. While exhaustion of vital qi means asthenia, which may be deficiency of qi, blood, yin or yang. If excess of pathogen and exhaustion of vital qi exist at the same time, asthenia and sthenia will complicate with each other. As to differentiation of cold and heat, exhaustion of yang results in cold, and excess of yang results in heat.

3. Treatment based on different types of syndrome

Both exogenous and interior injury will result in spontaneous perspiration and night sweat. Although the pathogenesis of sweating caused by exogenous is that pathogen staying at the surface, it transits into interior and turns into heat soon, which may damage Yin or Yang. The pathogenesis of sweating caused by exogenous is somewhat the same as that caused by interior injury. Although yang qi deficiency is the most common pathogenesis of spontaneous perspiration, no matter asthenia or sthenia, cold or heat syndromes, it should also be noticed. Although deficiency heat is the most common pathogenesis of night sweat, qi deficiency, yang deficiency or damp heat appears now and again.

The treatment should be in accordance with the principle as follows. Treat the asthenia syndrome by therapy of invigorating, the exhaustion syndrome by therapy of reinforcement, the sthenia syndrome by therapy of purgation, the heat syndrome by therapy of clearing away it and treat the cold syndrome by therapy of warming up.

(1) Disharmony between ying and wei

Main symptoms: perspiration now and again, or sweat only at the head, hand, foot or half of the body. Somewhat aversion to wind time and again.

Accompanying symptoms: aching pain in the whole body, sometimes with slight fever and headache.

Tongue and pulse: normal tongue with thin white fur, floating and moderate pulse.

Analysis: Asthenia body attacked by pathogenic wind, disharmony between ying and wei and irresistibility of striae of skin lead to sweating with aversion to wind and aching pain in the whole body. The vigor qi fighting against the pathogen results in fever and headache. Floating and moderate pulse and thin white fur of tongue are the signs of pathogenic wind staying on the surface of the body.

Treatment: dispelling wind to relieving exterior syndrome, regulating ying and wei.

Prescription: The main prescription is Gui Zhi Decoction. Of the ingredients in the recipe, cinnamon twig relieves exterior syndromes by expelling pathogenic factors from the muscles; white peony root regulates ying and astringes yin. The combination of cinnamon twig and white peony root resuls in the role of regulating ying and wei and consolidating the connecting tissue. Ginger, Chinese date and liquorice roots are used as adjuvant drugs to coordinate the effective of the above drugs in the recipe. Massive sweating, heaviness sensation in the body with white greasy tongue fur are the signs of dampness. In this case, ledebouriela root and sprouted black soybean, which clear away wind and eliminate dampness, should be added to activate yang and consolidate superficial resistance. If the case is marked by fever, perspiration, throat-ache and cough, which result from disharmony between the lung and wei due to wind-heat attacking the lung, treatment should be aimed at clearing away wind-heat with drugs pungent in flavor and cool in property. The advisable prescription is Sang Ju Decoction, which is modified by scrophularia root and honeysuckle flower. If the case is marked by perspiration and thirsty due to summer-heat injuring qi, pungent, cool and drastic prescription, such as Bai Hu Decoction modified by fresh lotus leaf and water melon peel, should be used to clear away the pathogenic summer-heat.

Besides, in clinical, it is very common for a patient with asomnia to be marked by spontaneous perspiration in the case of being irritated. Those symptoms result from imbalance between heart-yin and heart-yang.

The treatment should be according to the item, "for those whose heart is damaged, regulate ying and wei," which is recorded in Nei Jing, to regulate yin and yang. The prescription is Gui Zhi Jia Long Gu Mu Li Decoction

Prescription for example: Cinnamon twig 10g, White peony root 10g, Ginger 3 pieces, Chinese date 7g, Prepared liquorice 6g, Ledebouriella root 6g, Sprouted black soybean 10g, Big head atractylodes 10g.

(2) Failure of lung qi to protect the body against disease

Main symptoms: The valetudinarianism due to chronic cough, vomit or diarrhea, suffers from sweating now and again, and sweating even more after activity.

Accompanying symptoms: Pale and sallow complexion, anorexia, lassitude and tending to have a cold.

Tongue and pulse: Reddish tongue with thin whitish fur, thready and weak pulse.

Analysis: The lung is in charge of the skin to govern wei. It has the function of protecting the body against exterior pathogen. If the patient suffered from chronic cough and dyspnea, the lung qi will be impaired, the superficial muscle, skin and fur will be not consistent enough, and connective tissue will be loose. Therefore, perspiration occurs after activity and movement will consume qi. The impaired qi can't govern the body fluid so that the patient sweating even more. Illness of the child organ may involve the mother organ. Deficiency of lung qi and spleen qi results in pale and sallow complexion, anorexia and lassitude. Failure of the deficient lung qi to protect the body results in tending to common cold. Pale tongue with thin whitish fur, thready and weak pulse are the signs of qi deficiency.

Treatment: Invigorating qi to consolidate superficial resistance.

Prescription: Modified Yu Ping Feng Powder. In the recipe, astragalus root was used rawly to invigorate qi, consolidate superficial resistance and arrest sweating. Bighead atractylodes rhizome invigorates the spleen, eliminates dampness to consolidate superficial resistance. Ledebouriella root acts on surface to assistant the superficial resistance consolidating function of astragalus and the eliminating dampness function of atractylodes. If the patient suffered from sweating, ephedra root, light wheat, glutinous rice root, cyster shell, dragon's bone and dried peach can be added to arrest sweating and astringe yin. For those due to deficient qi, dangshen, siberian solomonseal rhizome and schisandra fruit can be use to replenish qi and control the hidrosis. For those sweating at hand or foot locally, since the pathogenesis it that the spleen dominates the limbs, deficient qi can't reach the limbs and can't govern yin, Hung Qi Jan Zhong Decoction should be used to warm the middle, tonify the asthenia and consolidate superficial resistance to arrest sweating.

Prescription for example: Astragalus root 30g, Bighead atractylodes 12g, Ledebouriella root 6g, Ephedra root 10g, Glutinous rice root 10g, Calcined cyster shell 30g(be decocted first), Calcined dragon's bone 30g(be decocted first), Dangshen 10g, Liquorice 6g.

(3) Hyperactivity of fire due to yin deficiency

Main symptoms: Sweating during sleeping, or continuous sweating in the day.

Accompanying syndromes: Insomnia due to vexation, mainly appear in the chronic cough and dyspnea patients, marasmus, hectic fever due to yin deficiency, dysphoria with feverish sensation in the chest, palms and sales, irregular menstruation or nocturnal emission.

Tongue and pulse: Reddish tongue with little fur, thready taut pulse.

Analysis: Chronic cough due to pulmonary tuberculosis or sexual overstrain, hemorrhage, emission, and consumption of yin blood will lead to interior flaring of fire of deficiency type. If the fire make body fluid out of the body, the manifestation will be sweating during sleeping or continuous sweating in the day, marasmus, hectic fever and hot sensation in the heart, palms and soles. If heat disturbs the mental, the manifestation will be insomnia and vexation. Hyperactivity of fire and ministerial fire due to yin deficiency leads to irregular menstruation with menorrhage in female or nocturnal emission in male. Thready taut pulse and red tongue with little fur are the signs of exhaustion of yin essence due to hyperactivity of fire.

Treatment: Nourishing yin to lower the fire, preserving yin with astringent

Prescriptions: As to sweating slightly, the prescription should be modified Dang Gui Liu Huang Decoction. In the recipe, red sage root, which is replaced with Chinese angelica root, combining with dried root and prepared rhizome of rehmannia, has the effect of nourishing yin and blood. And the dose of rehmannia is increased to restrict the kidney yang, phellodendron and coptis root clear away the fire in the heart and lung. For those due to fire of hyperactivity type, the doses of these two drugs should be limited, because they are bitter and dry in taste. Phellodendron purge away the ministerial fire to fortify yin. Astragalus, whose qi scatters on skin following with hidrosis, replenishes qi to consolidate the surface. For those suffered from prolonged disease due to yin exhaustion of the lung and kidney, Mai Wei Di Hang Pill adding dragon's bone, cyster shell and glutinous rice toot can be employed to nourish yin and astringe sweating. For those suffered from hectic fever, anemarrhena rhizome, sweat wormwood, tortoise, and freshwater turtle shell can be used to nourish yin and remove heat.

Prescription for example: Astragalus root 15g, Dried root and Prepared rhizome of rehmannia 10g respectively, Phello dendron 10g, Red sage root 20g, Coptis root 5g, Scutellaria root 10g, Schisandra fruit 10g, Light wheat 30g, Calcined cyster shell and Dragon's bone each 30g respectively, Dogwood fruit 10g.

(4) Interior excess of heat

Main symptoms: Restlessness and hot sensation in the chest, continuous profuse perspiration. Sometimes sweating only at head, or at hands and feet.

Accompanying syndromes: Thirsty or mucosity in mouth, tending to drink the cold, fever, restlessness and constipation.

Tongue and pulse: Red tongue with thick yellow fur and little saliva, or with yellow greasy fur, slippery and rapid pulse or great and full pulse.

Analysis: Heat can be transformed from interior invasion of pathogenic factor, from stagnated dampness, from stagnated liver-qi or due to overtaking greasy and sweet food. If the heat accumulates in the spleen and stomach and evaporates the body fluid, the manifestation will be profuse sweat, restlessness and hot sensation in the chest, sweating at head, at hands or at feet. If heat consumes the body fluid, it will be marked by thirsty and tending to drink the cold. If damp-heat fumigates the body fluid, it will be marked by mucosity sensation in mouth, drinking the cold but not tending to swallow. If heat disturbs the mind, it will be marked by restlessness. If superficial pathogenic factor hasn't been expelled, it will be marked by fever. Sthenia syndrome of fu- organ due to accumulation of heat will result in constipation with dry stool. Red tongue with thick yellow fur and little saliva, great and full pulse are the signs of body fluid consumption due to heat. Red tongue with yellow greasy fur and slippery rapid pulse are the signs of accumulation of damp-heat.

Treatment: Clearing away stomach heat, or eliminating damp-heat.

Prescription: The main prescription is Bai Hu Decoction. In the recipe, gypsum clears away heat to relieve restlessness. Anemarrhena rhizome clears away heat to protect yin, adjavanting with Polished round-grained nonglutinous rice, liquorice to nourish the stomach and regulate the middle. For those marked by sweating and thirsty, the drugs for clearing away heat and promoting salivation such as fresh reed rhizome, trichosanthes root and dendrolium should be added. For those marked by constipation due to heat accumulation, the treatment should focus on removing burnning wood from under the boiler. Xiao Cheng Qi Decoction can be employed. To clear away heat and eliminate damp, Long Dan Xie Gan Decoction or Si Miao Pill should be used. In the former recipe, gentian root, scutellaria root, capejasmine seed and bupleurum root clear away liver heat. Oriental water plantain rhizome, manshurian aristolochia stem and plantain seed clear away heat and promote diuresis. Chinese angelia and dried rehmannia rhizome nourish yin and blood and regulate ying. The main function of the latter recipe is clearing away and eliminating damp-heat in lower Jiao by phellodendron, atractylodes rhizome and capejasmine seed. Thus it is particularly adapted for those who suffered from massive sweating at lower limb and perineum. Achyranthes root can be added to ensure proper down ward flow of those drugs. For those marked by stuffiness and tightness sensation in the chest with sweating, which are due to damp-heat obstructed in the middle. Coptis root and magnolia bark can be added to clear away and eliminate damp-heat.

Prescription for example: Gypsum 30g (decocted first), Anemarrhema rhizome 10g, Fresh reed rhizome 30g, Trichosanthes root 10g, Scrophularia root 10g, Capejasmine seed 10g, Dried peach 10g, Liquorice 6g.

〔Prevention and nursing methods〕

1. The temperature of circumstanc is very important for the sweating patients. Patients with excess Yang syndromes should reside in a cooler place, while with excess Yin syndromes in a warmer place.
2. The patients should keep a calm emotion and never be irritated. For those who suffers from serious insomnia, he should exercise Nei Yang Gong, get rid of any idea, and have a good sleep.
3. Light food. The greasy and strongly flavored food should be limited.
4. The weak person should do more exercises to improve the condition of the body. Pay attention to the whether when it changes.
5. Those who sweated too much should be protected from wind and cold to prevent getting a cold. Change clothes and quilts frequently. Clean the body with warm water after sweating or pat the body with the powder for stringing sweat. Have a rest in the quiet place. Drink water or water with a little salt after sweating.
6. If the sweat is in great amount, we should prevent it changing into sweating inshock. Taking Sheng Mai Powder or Shen Fu Fluid in time is useful.

〔Typical cases analysis〕

Case 1, Yu ××, female, 72 years old.

Paroxysmal hot sensation in stomach, the heat tending to be outwards, then massive sweating occurs and the underclothes are wet. The manifestation occurs several times during a day, particularly at the just before wake. After sweating, the symptoms are aversion to cold, thirsty but not tending to drink, slight cough, normal diet, urine and stool. The sweating syndromes succeeded to pneuminia. Now the fluoroscopy of chest has been normal, but the sweating syndromes remain. It was not effective by treating with the drugs such as ginseng, lilyturf root, schisandra, dragon's bone, cyster shell and Yu Ping Feng Powder by the former doctor. Deep and thready pulse at Cun and Chi, full and rapid pulse at Guan, Red tongue with yellow greasy fur. The pathogenesis is that damp-heat are stagnated in the lung and stomach without being removed away. It is advisable to follow the therapeutic principle of clearing away the stagnated heat in the lung and stomach. Recipe:

Waxgourd seed 9g, Coix seed 12g, Apricot kernel 6g, Reed rhizome 18g, Lophatherum 6g, Calcined gypsum 9g, Anemarrhena 3g, Loquat leaf (prepared) 6g, Lotus leaf 6g, Polished round-grained nonglutinous rice 12g. Two doses.

The second visit: After taking the decoction, the patient felt that the hot gas ran downward to the legs with formication. Sweating is deduced. There is no massive sweating found when the patient awaked. Dry and thirsty sweat tastes remain. There is somewhat stuffy sensation in the chest and tunt or slippery pulse with interval. Red tongue and yellow greasy are relieved. Those magnifications result from downward transiting of damp-heat and disharmony between the lung and the stomach. The therapeutic principle is clearing away heat and ventilating the lung, which are guided adroitly according to circumstances. Recipe:

Waxgourd seed 9g, Coix seed 12g, Apricot kernel 6g, Reed rhizome 12g, Lophatherum 6g, Crude gypsm 9g, Oriental warmwood 6g, Sprouted black soybean 9g, Tetrandra root 5g, Turmeria 5g, Recipaper pich 3g. Three doses.

The third visit: After taking the decoction, the patient's sweat was arrested and the heat was removed, thirsty sensation was relieved. Diet, stool and urine became normal. The pulse of left hand is tunt, rapid and strong, while that of right hand is moderate. Normal tongue remains thin, greasy and yellow fur, which are the signs that surplus heat has not been removed. The treatment should be regulating the lung and stomach to go on clearing away dampness heat. Recipe:

Poria peel 9g, Coix seed 6g, Mulberry bark 6g, Sprouted black soybean 9g, Scutellaria root 3g, oriental warmwood 9g, Turmeria 3g, talc 9g, Recipaper pich 3g, Coix seed 12g. After taking 3 doses continuously, all the symptoms of the patient were relieved.

Note: The pathogenesis of the case is that the residual dampness heat stagnated in the lung and stomach without dispersing forces the sweat to be formed. Mr. Pu employed the lophatherum and gypsum to clear away the latent heat in Yang Ming Channel, combined with Wei Jing decoction, replaced apricot kernel with peach kernel to disperse the lung qi, added lotus leaf to ventilate the lung and increase appetite. After taking two dosages of decoction, the patient's sweat was reduced, hot qi ran downward with formication in the legs. In Mr. Pu's opinion, the prepared gypsum had the potential function of clearing away interior heat but without the function of pungent flavour to induce perspiration, the stagnated heat tended to run downward interiorly, in the second diagnosis it was replaced by crude gypsum, adding oriental warmwood, sprouted black soybean, tetrandra root and recipaper pich to clear away heat and dampness according to circumstance. After two decoctions, the heat is removed and sweat is astringed. It can be concluded from this case that treatment must search for the primary causes of diseases. The hidroschesis drugs such as ginseng, lilyturf root and schisandra fruit had no use for arresting sweat. We concluded that the drugs were not suitable for the syndromes. However, the latter treatment of clearing away heat and dry had the functions of removing pathogenic factors to arrest sweating. Thus we are more sure the importance of differential diagnosis aiming at the etiology (The cases above are selected from *Pu Fu Zhou Yi An*).

Spontaneous perspiration and night sweat are the diseases marked as abnormalhidrosis in TCM. They are caused by imbalance of yin and yang, disharmony between ying and wei, or dysfunction of connecting tissues. They are very common in clinical. Although the pathogenesis of spontaneous perspiration is deficiency of yang qi and that of night sweat is interior heat due to yin deficiency, they are not always true. Treatment based on the differential diagnosis is very important to use the right drugs to cure the disease. As to excess syndrome, liver fire, interior heat and dampness heat are common. As to deficiency syndrome, disharmony between ying and wei, body fluid exhaustion due to yin deficiency, hyperactivity of fire due to yin deficiency, deficiency of lung qi are very common. The therapeutic principles are regulating ying and wei, clearing away the heat, purging fire, eliminating damp, supplementing qi to strengthen superficial to arresting sweating. Sweat is the fluid of impairment of vital qi. To cure the sweating disease, we should grasp the pathogenesis, administrate positive measurement, therapy both interior and exterior, regulate yin and yang of the organism, remove the pathogenic factor.

Questions for Reviews

1. What's the conception of spontaneous perspiration and night sweat?

2. Try to describe the etiopathology of spontaneous perspiration and night sweat.
3. What's the therapeutic principle of the diseases based on different diagnosis.
4. How to take care of the sweating patients?

Blood Syndrome

〔Introduction〕

The Blood syndrome has two implications, the broad sense and the narrowsense. The broad sense of blood syndrome refers to all diseases about blood, such as deficiency of blood, blood stasis, and bleeding. While, the narrow sense of blood syndrome, a collective term of all bleeding disease, is generally used. Bleeding, which is also called blood syndrome, refers to the diseases that the blood dose not follow normally within its vessels, but bleed from the muscle or skin. It is caused by interior pathological. The blood syndrome has many names in accordance with the bleeding sites and the symptoms. In internal medicine, it is commonly named as hemoplysis, hematemesis, epistaxis, gingival hemorrhage, bleeding from muscle (also called "*ziban*"), hematuria, hemafecia, etc.

Huang Di Nei Jing has make a deep understanding of the physiology and pathology of blood. In some chapters of this book, the disease, such as epistaxis, hemoptysis, hematermesis, hematuria and hemaxchezia were recorded. The cause of bleeding, and the prognosis of some blood syndrome were expounded. The prescriptions for hematemesis and hemafecia, such as Xie Xin Decoction, Bai Ye Decoction, Huang Tu Decoction and Chi Xiao Dou Dang Gui Powder are recorded in Jin Gui Yao Lue. The prescription for blood syndrome, Xi Jiao Di Huang Decoction recorded in Bei Ji Qian Jin Yao Fang has been used up to today. The cause and the pathology of blood syndrome have been expounded in Zhu Bing Yuan Hou Lun, Ji Sheng Fang and Ping Zhi Hui Cui. It is very brilliant that Jing Yue Quan Shu summarized the pathogenesis of blood syndrome as excess of fire and impairment of Qi. Xue Zheng Lun is a special book on blood syndrome, in which, the discussion about the etiopathology and treatment based on the differentiation of blood in the book is very comprehensive. The therapeutic principle of arresting bleeding, eliminating blood stasis, calming blood and replenishing deficiency in the book, have become the therapeutic principle of blood syndrome.

Blood syndrome includes a large range of disease. In modern medicine, the bleeding may be caused not only by many acute or chronic diseases, such as all kinds of acute or chronic hematopathy; but also by viscera infectious, tuberculosis and tumor, or by hepatopathy, gastropathy, nephrosis, pulmonary disease and angiocardiopathy. Sometimes, blood syndrome may be acute symptom in internal medicine. Hemorrhage will lead to syncope (asphyxia) and prostraition syndrome (shock). We should pay more attention to it.

〔Etiology and pathology〕

Blood is transformed by the spleen, stored in the liver, governed by the heart, disseminated by the lung and transformed into life essence by the kidney. Generating, regulating and disseminating of the blood all over the body depend on the function of five viscera. qi and blood relying on each other, circling continuously in the vessels to nourish viscera-fu, limbs and skeletons, and keeping the normal activity of life. If the vessels are injured or the blood don't follows its normal way, which may be caused by pathogenic factor in environment, overdrinking alcohol, over feeding hot or pungent food, emotional stimuli, overstrain and deficiency, the bleeding syndrome will occur. Most bleeding syndrome pertains to heat syndrome. The location of disease should be decided according to the bleeding site, characters and related Zang and Fu organs. Now, it will be discussed in brief as follows:

1. Infection by extronous pathogenic factor

Bleeding may be caused by extronous pathgenic factors attacking the body, injury of blood vessels and pathogenic heat. The pathogenic factors of wind heat dryness and fire, which belong to Yang, are common. Sometimes, the affected wind-cold penetrates from superficial to interior and transformed into heat. If heat attacks lung, it will injure pulmonary vessels, make blood run upward, then lead to hemoptysis and epistaxis. If pathogenic factor of warm heat and infectious toxin consume the blood and make the blood not to follow the circulation, bleeding from the nose, gums or muscles may occur. Dampness heat attacking intestine will lead to hemafecia.

2. Improper diet

Over drinking alcohol, over feeding the hot or pungent food, emotional stimuli will lead to damp heat accumulating in the stomach and intestine. The heat fumigates and burns the blood vessels, and forces the blood disorder, then epistaxis, hematemesis and hemafecia take place. Improper diet injures the spleen and stomach, results in dysfunction of the spleen and stomach to transport the food and govern the blood, then instead of following the circulation and the blood flows out of the vessel to form hematemesis, hemafecia, epistaxis and hematuria.

3. Five emotions in excess

Five emotions in excess produce endogeous fire. The fire stirring inside and upward reversed flow of qi result in blood disorder to form blood syndrome. If depression or angry injures the liver, liver qi is stagnated. The excessive dispersing activity of the liver attacks the stomach and injures the gastral vessel so as to hematemesis. Stagnated qi transforms into fire, liver fire attacks the lung. and blood rises following with the up-flairing of fire. Therefore hematemesis and epistaxis occur. If grief or thinking too much disturbs the heart, heart fire burns inside and transit down to the small intestine or to the bladder, hematuria occurs.

4. Overstrain

Mental overstrains hurts the heart because spirit is stored in the heart. Physical overstrains hurts the spleen because the spleen nourishes the muscles. Sexual overstrains hurts the kidney. Overstrain injures qi and Yin of the heart, the spleen and the kidney. Damage of qi leads to failure of qi to keep blood flowing within the vessels. Then hematemesis, hemaxchezia and epistaxis occur. Impairment of Yin leads to hyperactivity of fire due to Yin deficiency. Deficiency fire burns the vessels and makes the blood not following its vessels. Then bleeding syndromes such as bleeding from the nose, gums or muscles occurs.

5. After febrile disease of prolonged illness

The pathogenic of bleeding due to febrile disease prolonged illness have three aspects. First, they impair Yin fluid and Yin blood, which results in hyperactivity of fire failing to keep the blood following its normal circulation. Then bleeding occurs. Secondly, they consume the principal qi. If Qi fails to keep blood flowing within the vessels, bleeding occurs. Thirdly, according to the theory of "at the beginning, the location of the disease is qi fen, while that of the prolonged illness is xue fen.". If pathogenic Qi transmits into the vessels and blocks the vessels, the blood circulation will be hampered, and the blood can't follow its vessels. Then bleeding occurs.

In short, in the case of affection by exopathic factor, the cause of bleeding syndrome is dampness, heat, noxious factor or the heat transformed from the pathogenic Yin, which has invaded into the body, as well as pathogenic Yang, such as wind, heat, dryness and fire attacking the body. While, in the case of internal injury, the bleeding is caused by improper diet, emotional strain exhaustion, or after febrile of prolonged illness. The main pathogenesis of bleeding syndrome is hyperactivity of fire, damage of Qi and blood stasis. In the cases of hyperactivity of fire, fire-heat burns and injuries the vessels, or made the blood not flow within its vessels. In the case of qi impairment, qi will fail in keeping the normal circulation of blood. In the case of blood stasis, the vessels are blocked and the blood escape from the vessels and channels. Hyperactivity of fire is divided into excess type and deficiency type. Exogenous pathogenic factor of wind heat, dryness and fire, retention of damp-heat in interior and fire transformed from stagnated qi all belong to fire of excess type. While, the hyperactivity fire due to yin deficiency belongs to fire of deficiency type. Qi-impairment includes deficiency of qi only or deficiency of yang-qi due to qi impairment. Blood stasis results from qi deficiency, qi stagnation, accumulation of pathogenic coldness and heat, and traumatic injuries. Blood stasis is a pathogenic product since it comes from the blood out of vessels. It can worsen bleeding. During the process of disease, There are not only differentiation and combination, but also transforming among pathogenic fire, qi-impairment and blood stasis. The nature of bleeding syndrome includes sthenic and asthenic. The bleeding syndromes caused by exogenous ingenous fire or other pathogenic factor pertains to sthenic syndrome. The bleeding syndromes caused by blood stasis, which due to qi stagnation, coldness accumulation and heat accumulation, also pertain to sthenic syndrome. While, the bleeding syndromes caused by hyperactivity of fire due to yin deficiency, blood disorder due to deficiency of qi, and deficiency of vital-qi pertain to asthenic syndrome. Although the etiopathology of sthenic syndrome and asthenic syndrome are different, sthenic syndrome often transforms into asthenic syndrome during the course of the disease. For example, if at the beginning of the disease the pathogenesis is excess of fire and reversed flow of qi failing in governing the blood, after bleeding again and again the pathogenesis will be deficiency of yin blood and interior deficiency fire producing. For another example, bleeding too much will lead to Qi-impairment due to deficiency of blood, yang exhausted due to qi deficiency, and the body will be too asthenic to keep normal circulation; then the diseases changes from sthenic syndrome to asthenic syndrome step by step. Thus, hyperactivity of fire due to deficiency of Yin and failure of Qi to keep the blood within its vessels are not only the results of bleeding, but also the pathogenesis of continuous bleeding. For instant, after bleeding, the blood, which bleeds out of the vessels, will accumulate in the body to form stasis blood. If the stasis blood can not be cleared away, it will hamper the generation of new blood, affect the normal running of qi and blood, then worsen bleeding or lead to bleeding repeatedly. Thus the disease may be transformed from sthenic syndrome to asthenic syndrome or asthenic syndrome complicated with sthenic syndrome. As to the location of bleeding, they are different according to the bleeding site, clinical features and medical history. Even bleeding at the same site, the impaired viscera is different according to different syndromes. In general opinion, as to bleeding due to excess fire, the main locations are the lung, stomach, heart, liver or bladder; as to bleeding due to deficiency fire, the main locations are the liver, kidney, and sometimes are the lung or stomach. As to bleeding due to qi deficiency, the main locations are the spleen and kidney.

〔Treatment according to differentiation of syndrome〕

Main points of differentiation

As to bleeding syndromes, we should differentiate the bleeding sites and the location of related viscera first. For instant, the ill viscera of epistaxis may be lung, stomach and liver. We should differentiate it according to the medical history, clinical feature and the relationship among Zang-fu viscera, meridians and collaterals. Next, we should make clear that whether the syndromes are sthenic or asthenic, whether the disease is chronic or acute, urgency or severity. It will not be very difficult to differentiate according to the analysis of the bleeding sites, color, quantity, and tongue, pulse and symptoms manifested in clinic.

Principle of treatment

The treatment of bleeding syndromes should be aimed at the cause of bleeding and the damaged viscera. The differentiation should be based on the justification that whether the syndromes are sthenia or asthenia, and whether the disease condition is urgent or sevious. We should administrate the principle of treatment, which are arresting bleeding, treating the disease from cause, consolidating the "root" freely. To choose the prescription and drugs of the bleeding syndrome, the methods of treating blood, treating Qi, and treating fire are to be considered first. Then the major method and miner method should be determined. Stopping bleeding means applying the proper hemostatics and the proper dozes according to the patient's condition. It is not only the aim of treatment but also the method of treating symptoms in emergency cases. This principle is often selected first in the case of acute vital bleeding. Searching for primary cause of disease in treatment means treatment aiming at the cause of bleeding. It is a method of treating the "root". It includes treating the asthenia syndrome with tonifying method, sthenia syndrome with purgation method, blood stasis syndromes with the method of promoting blood circulation, and heat syndromes with the method of removing the heat. Consolidating the root means recover. Use the tonifying method according to the deficiency. Because Qi and blood is deficient after bleeding, the method of tonifying as well as the treatment of stopping bleeding and treating from the cause should be used. The treatment method of tonifying can be applied to attend and cure not only the required root such as invigorating the middle to benefit Qi, but also the innateness, such nourishing the liver and the kidney. It is a method of reconstruction.

Treating blood constists of stopping bleeding and treating the root. For example, to stop bleeding, the treatment of clearing away heat, cooling the blood, using astringe drugs, and promoting blood circulation may be used. To therapy the bleeding syndromes, the drugs for cooling the blood to stop bleeding are usually used, since most bleeding are caused by invasion of blood by noxious heat. Treating fire and treating Qi belong to the treatment of treating the root. As to treating fire, for the fire of excess type, the heat clearing and fire purging herbs should be used; for the fire of deficiency type, the drugs of pourishing Yin to lower the fire should be used. As to treating Qi, for a sthenia syndrome, the drugs for clearing Qi and lowering the rebellious Qi should be used; for asthenia syndrome, the drugs for invigorating and nourishing Qi should be used.

Treatment by differentiation of the type of the syndrome

1. Epistaxis

Epistaxis means nasal bleeding, which is the commonest syndrome in bleeding disease. Most cases of epistaxis are caused by invasion of blood by fire heat, especially lung heat, stomach heat and liver heat. It belongs to sthenic syndrome. A few cases of epistaxis are caused by failure of deficient qi and blood to keep the blood flowing normally. It belongs to asthenic syndromes.

Illustratin of etiology and pathology of Blood syndrome

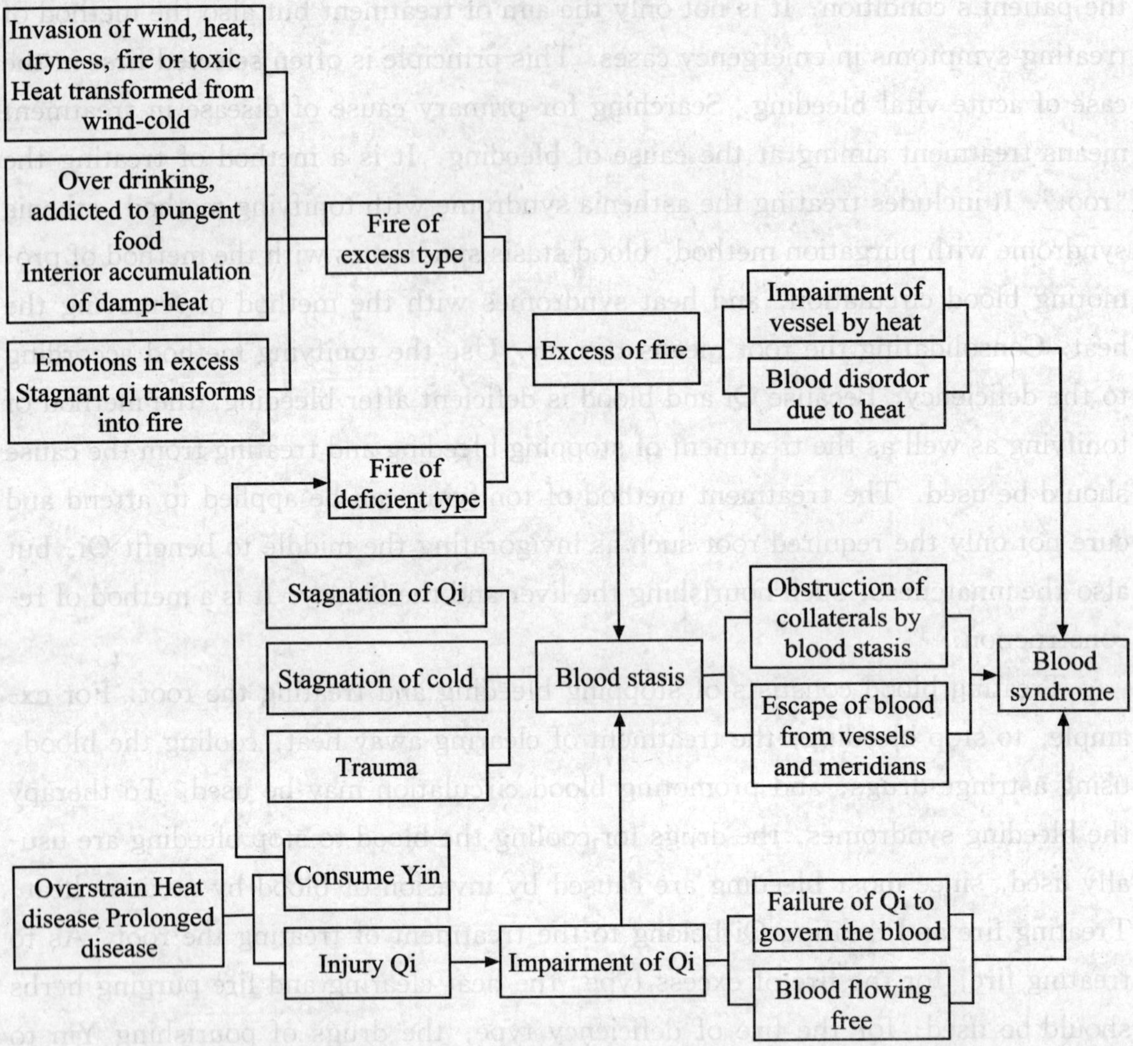

(1) Pathogenic heat attacking the lung

Main symptoms: Dryness of nasal cavity and bleeding from the nose.

Accompany symptoms: fever, dry mouth and throat, cough with little sputum.

Tongue and pulse: Red tongue with thin yellowish fur, rapid pulse.

Analysis: Nose is the special opening of the lung. If wind heat attacking the lung or retention heat in the lung consumes the lung Yin, it will make the blood not follow its normal circulation but flow along the orifice and lead to bleeding from the nose dryness of nasal cavity. If wind heat attacks the head, superficial Wei will be in trouble. The symptoms will be characterized as fever, sore throat, caught with little sputum. Dryness, red tongue and rapid pulse are the signs of body fluid impairment due to heat.

Therapeutic principles: clearing away lung heat, cooling the blood to stop bleeding.

Prescription: Modified Sang Ju Yin Decoction, which has the mild functions of facilitating the lung, cooling the blood and expelling the superficial pathogenic factor. In the recipe, Mulberry leaf, Chrysan themum flower, Peppermint and Forsythia fruit are pungent in flavor and cool in property, relieving the exterior syndrome and dispelling wind-heat. Platycilon root, Bitter apricot kernel, Licorcc root promote the disbursing function of lung, benefit the throat and relieve cough. Reed rhizome has the effect of clearing away heat and promoting the production of body fluid to quench thirst. Moutan Bark, Cogongrass rhizome, Chinese arborvitae can be employed to cool the blood and stop bleeding.

In the case of epistaxis due to excess lung heat but without superficial syndromes, Peppermint and Platycodon should be replaced by Scutellaria root and Capejasmine fruit to clear away the lung heat. In the case of epistaxis due to heavy impairment of Yin, which characterized by dry mouth, nose and throat, Figwort root, Lilyturf root and dried rehmannia should be used to nourish Yin and clear away heat. For epistaxis with constipation, Trichosanthes fruit and Rhuborb should be added. For epistaxis with red throat and yellow sputum, Actium fruit and Honcysuckle flower can be added to disperse wind and clear away heat.

Prescription for example: Mulberry leaf 10g, Chrysan themum flower10g, Platycodin root 10g, Liquorice 10g, Cogongrass rhizome 30g, Reed stem 15g, Scutellarid root 10g, Scrophularia root 15g, Arborvitae tops 10g, Mullerry bark 10g.

(2) Excess of stomach heat

Main symptoms: Epistaxis with scarlet blood, dryness of nasal cavity.

Accompany symptoms: Sometimes accompanied with bleeding from gums, dryness of mouth, foul breath, restlessness, constipation or swelling and soreness of the gums.

Tongue and pulse: Red tongue with yellowish fur, rapid pulse.

Analysis: The Stomach Channel of Foot Yang Ming runs across the gums. Epistaxis due to up flaring of stomach fire, the syndromes will be manifested as dryness of mouth and nose, foul breath, swelling and soreness of the gums. If heat injury the vessels too much to keep the blood following its normal circulation, it will be marked by bleeding from the nose and gums with scarlet blood. If epistaxis is cause by stomach heat consuming the body fluid, it will be marked by dryness of mouth and nose, thirsty tending to drink and constipation. For epistaxis due to stomach heat disturbing the heart, the accompanying symptoms will be restlessness. Red tongue, yellowish fur and rapid pulse are the signs of excess heat in the stomach.

Therapeutic principles: clearing away stomach fire, cooling the blood to stop bleeding.

Prescription: Modified Yu Nu Jian Decoction, The prescription has the function of clearing away stomach heat and nourishing Yin. In the recipe, Gypsum is used to clear away stomach fire. Anemarrhena rhizome, Ophiopgon roots and rehmannia roots have the effect of nourishing Yin and clearing away heat. Achyanthes and cyathula root is used to induce bloods downward. In the original prescription, prepared rehmannia, which nourishes Yin but impedes the stomach qi, was replaced by dried rehmannia, which share the role of cooling the blood to stop bleeding. Congograss rhizome, Japanese thistle herb, field thistle, node of lotus rhizome and Chinese arborvitae tops and twig can be employed to enhance the function of stopping bleeding. For epistaxis due to excess heat, Capejasmine fruit, Moutan bark and Scutellarid root should be used to clear away heat and fire. Epitaxis with constipation due to excess heat, dried rhubarb can be used to clear away heat with purgatives. Epistaxis due to consumption of Yin, accompanied with thirsty, red tongue with little fur and rapid thready pulse, Trichosanthes root, Fragrant solomonseal rhizome and Pendrobium stem should be used to nourish the stomach and promote the production of body fluid. In the case of excess stomach fire without consumption of body fluid, modified San Huang Shi Gao Decoction could be used.

Prescription for example: Gypsum 30g (To be decocted first), Coptis root 6g, Scutellarid root 10g, Anemarrhena rhizome 10g, Moutan bark 10g, Dried rehmannia root 10g, Congograss rhizome 30g, Achyanthes and cyathula root 10g, Ophiopgon root 10g.

(3) Up firing of liver fire

Main symptoms: Epistaxis, headache, blurred vision and bitter taste.

Accompany symptoms: Conjunctival congestion, tinnitus, irritability and tendency to anger.

Tongue and pulse: Red tongue with thin yellowish fur, taut and rapid pulse.

Analysis: If fire transformed from depressed liver Qi, driving blood up to lucid orifices, it will be marked by epistaxis. The liver fire up stirring lucid orifices, it will be marked by headache, blurred vision, tinnitus and bitter taste. The eye is the orifice to the liver. Liver fire upward attack, results in blood-shot eyes. Red tongue with thin yellowish fur and taut rapid pulse are the signs of interior excess liver fire.

Therapeutic principles: Clearing away liver fire, cooling the blood to stop bleeding.

Prescription: Modified Long Dan Xie Gan Decoction, which has the function of purging excess fire from the liver and gallbladder and removing damp heat from the three Jiao. In the recipe, Gentian root, Scutellarid root and Capejasmine fruit, are chiefly used to purge excess fire in the liver. Oriental water plantain, Caulis Aristolochiae and Plantain seed are used to remove heat and induce diuresis to dispel damp heat. Bupleurum root has the effect of relieving the depressed liver. Chinese angelica root, Dried rehmannia root and Liquorice root have the effect of nourishing Yin and blood, and regulating the middle. Combining of all the drugs has the function of purging fire and removing damp without consuming yin-blood, by the method of invigorating during purging and nourishing during clearing. To cool the blood and stop bleeding, Congograss rhizome, Cat-tail pollen, Japanese thistle herb, field thistle, Montan bark and Node of lotus rhizome can be used according to the disease condition. Epistaxis due to excess liver fire manifested as tinnitus and irritability, Common selfheal fruit wpike and Natural indigo can be added to cool the blood by clearing away liver heat. Epistaxis due to consumption of Yin fluid is marked by dryness of mouth and nose, red tongue with little saliva and rapid thready pulse. To nourish Yin and clear away heat, Plantain seed, Orential waterplantain rhizome and Chinese angelica root should be replaced by Figwort root, Lilyturf root, Glossy privet fruit and Yerbadetajo herb.

(4) Deficiency of Qi and blood

Main symptoms: Epistaxis with light red color, sometimes accompanied with bleeding from the gums, muscles.

Accompany symptoms: Pale complexion, amnesia, mental fatigue, lassitude, dizziness and palpitation.

Tongue and pulse: Pale tongue, thready weak pulse or hollow pulse.

Analysis: If Qi is too deficient to keep the blood flowing within the vessels, bleeding from the nose or even from the gums or muscles will occur. Deficiency of Qi and blood will fail to nourish the viscera. If the brain without nourishing, it will be marked by dizziness and tinnitus; the heart without nourishing, palpitation and asomnia; Limbs and skeleton without nourishing, mental fatigue and lassitude. If the blood is too deficient to upward nourishing the face, it will be marked by pale complexion. If Qi and blood is so deficient that the vessels is not full, it will be marked by bleeding with light red blood, pale tongue, thready weak pulse or hollow pulse.

Therapeutic principles: Replenishing Qi to govern the blood.

Prescription: Modified Gui Pi Decoction. This prescription has the function of replenishing Qi, nourishing the blood, governing the blood and tonifying both the heart and the spleen. The components of the recipe are Si Jun Zi Decoction and Dang Gui Bu Xue Decoction adding Longan aril, Wild spony jujuba sead, Polygala root, Aucklandia root, ginger and Chinese date. The intention of the recipe is replenishing Qi to produce the blood and govern the blood. It is a common prescription for spleen failing to govern the blood due to deficiency of the heart and spleen, and deficiency of Qi and blood. To increase the hemostasis effect, Hairy vein agrimony, Dankey-hide gelatin and India madder root can be used.

Prescription for example: Dangshen 10g, White Atractylodes Rhizome 10g, Astragalus root 15g, Poria 10g, Chinese angelica 10g, Polygala root 10g, Wild spony jujuba seed 10g, Dankey hide gelatin 10g(to be melted), Liquorice 10g, Aucklandia root 6g, Hairy vein agrimony 12g.

As to all types of epistaxis above, when epistaxis occurs, besides taking in the decoction, the drugs for external application should be used locally to stop bleeding in time. The drugs for external application can be chosen as follows:

a. Yun Nan Bai Yao applied to the bleeding site.

b. Fill the cotton with Natural Indigo Powder in the nasal cavity to stop bleeding.

c. Damp cotton with Sai Bi powder (mixed dried alum 60g, dragon's bone 15g and hedychiumopicatum 15g together for pounding carefully) into nasal cavity to stop bleeding.

d. Have fresh Firstle hurb washed and make it paste, fill in nasal cavity.

e. Plug the cotton with Carbonized hair into nasal cavity.

2. Gingival bleeding

Bleeding from the gums terms gingival bleeding, also called "chi nu", "ya xuan" and "ya nu" in TCM. The Large Intestine channel of Hand-Yang Ming enters into the lower gum. The Stomach Channel of Foot- Yang Ming enters into the upper gum. The kidney dominates bones. The teeth are the surplus of the bone. According to the theory above, gingival bleeding has main bearing on the pathological changes of the stomach, intestine and kidney. It is mainly caused by flaring of stomach fire, hyperactivity of fire due to yin deficiency. The former belongs to the heat of excess type and the latter belongs to the fire of deficient type.

(1) Flaring of stomach fire

Main symptoms: bleeding from gum with scarlet blood, reddish swelling and pain at the gum.

Accompanying symptoms: headache, foul breath and constipation.

Tongue and pulse: red tongue with yellow fur, full and rapid pulse.

Analysis: Flaring of stomach fire fume the gum upward along the Channel of Yang Ming so as to reddish swelling and pain occurring at the gum. If the vessels is impaired and the blood flows out of the vessels, bleeding occurs. Upward evaporating of stomach heat results in headache and foul breath. heat accumulating in the Yang Ming results constipation. Yellow fur, full and rapid pulses are the signs of the excess heat in Yang Ming Channel.

Therapeutic principle: clearing away stomach fire, cooling the blood to stop bleeding.

Prescriptions: Modified Qing Wei Powder and Xie Xin Decoction. Qing Wei Powder has the function of clearing away stomach heat, lowering the fire and cooling the blood to stop bleeding. In the recipe, Dried rehmannia root, Moutan bark and rhinoceros horn (be placed by buffalo harn), clear away heat to cool the blood. Coptis root and Forsythia fruit clear away heat and purge fire. Cimicifuga rhizome induces channel clear away heat, and removes toxic substance. Chinese angelica root and Liquorice nourish the blood to regulate the middle. Combining with Xie Xin Decoction can increase the function of clearing away stomach fire. To cool the blood and stop bleeding, Cogongrass rhizome, Japanese thistle hurb, Field thistle and Node of locus rhizome can be employed. For the case of pus, Honeysuckle flower, Dandelion herb and Viola herb can be added to increase the effect of clearing away heat and removing toxic substance. If gingival bleeding accompanied by thirsty tending to drink, which results from excess of stomach heat, Gypsum and Anemarrhena rhizome, which are sweat in taste and cold in nature, can be used to clear Qi.

Prescription for example: Dried rehmannia root 12g, Moutan bark 10g, Gypsum 30g(to be decocted first), Anemarrhena rhizome 10g, Scutellaria root 10g, Coptis root 6g, Rhubarb 5g, cimicifuga rhizome 6g, Liquorice 6g, Forsythia fruit 10g.

(2) Hyperactivity of fire due to Yin deficiency

Main symptoms: bleeding from gum with light red blood, swelling of gums, and odontoseisis.

Accompanying symptoms: Bleeding from the gums repeatedly, induced by pathogenic heat or fatigue, sometimes accompanied with hot sensations in the palms and soles.

Tongue and pulse: red tongue with little fur, rapid thready pulse.

Analysis: The kidney dominates the bone. The teeth are the surplus of the bone. If Yin deficiency of the liver and kidney, If heat from upward floating of ministerial fire makes the blood upward flow, gingival bleeding with odontoseisis will occur. Because attacked by the heat or fatigue will increase deficiency of Yin, they are easy to induce gingival bleeding. Hot sensation in palms and soles, red tongue with little fur, and rapid thready pulse are the signs of hyperactivity of fire due to Yin deficiency.

Therapeutic principle: Nourishing Yin to lower the fire, cooling the blood to stop bleeding.

Prescription: Modified Zi Shui Qing Gan Yin and Qian Gen Powder. The former is derived modified Liu Wei Di Huang Pill and Dan Zhi Xiao Yao Powder. Its effect is mainly in tonifying the liver and kidney, nourishing Yin to lower the fire. There are three tonics and three purgative drugs in Liu Wei Di Huang Pill, which treat the three Yin viscera, especially tonify the liver and kidney. In the prescription of Dan Zhi Xiao Yao Powder, White atractylodes rhizome, baked ginger, peppermint are replaced by Wild jujube seed, aiming at nourishing the liver, cooling the blood and clearing away heat. In the prescription of Qian Gen Powder, Stutellaria root and liquorice remove the heat and regulate the middle. Burnet root and arborvitae tops cool the blood to stop bleeding, Dried rehmannia root and dankey-hide gelatin nourishing yin, replenishing the blood and cooling the blood to stop bleeding. The combined prescription has the function of nourishing Yin to lower the fire and cooling the blood to stop bleeding. As to cases marked by tidal fever and lassitude in waist, due to deficiency of the kidney Yin, the prescription of Er Zhi Pill can be added to increase the effect of nourishing and reinforcing the liver and kidney.

Prescription for example: Dried rehmannia 15g, Dogwood fruit 10g, Chinese yams 10g, Moutan bark 10g, Oriental water plantain rhizome 10g, Glossy privet fruit 10g, Eclipta 12g, Biota tops 12g, Rubia root 12g, Dankey-hide gelatin 10g (To be melted).

3. Purpuras (Bleeding from muscle)

The disease that bleeding from the muscle and skin, accompanied by purple spot and plague in skin is called purpuras, also called "ji nu", or "zi ban" in TCM. Purpuras due to invasion of yin blood by heat and blood disorder due to heat belongs to sthenia. Purpuras due to hyperactivity of fire due to yin deficiency impairing the vessels, or due to failure of deficient qi to govern the blood to follow the circulation, belongs to asthenia.

(1) Bleeding due to blood-heat

Main symptoms: The onset of disease is sudden, manifested as purple spots or plague in skin.

Accompanying symptoms: Gingival bleeding, epistaxis, hemaxchezia or hematuria. Sometimes accompanied with fever, thirsty and constipation.

Tongue and pulse: Red tongue with yellowish fur, taut and rapid pulse.

Analysis: Excess of heat-toxin transits into ying blood, results in blood disorder and bleeding from muscle striae. The manifestation is purple spot and plague. If heat-toxin injuries the vessels of nose, gums, intestine and stomach, it will be accompanied with epistaxis, gingival bleeding, hemaxchezia, hematuria. Evaporation of stagnant interior heat gives rise in fever. Consumption of body fluid due to excess heat results in thirty and constipation. Red tongue with yellowish fur, taut and rapid pulse are the signs of excess of heat.

Therapeutic principle: Clearing away heat and toxic material, cooling the blood to stop bleeding.

Prescriptions: Modified Xi Jiao Di Huang Decoction. It has the function of clearing away heat, cooling blood and removing blood stasis. In the recipe, rhinoceros horn (placed by buffalo horn) and rehmannia clear away heat and toxic material, nourish blood and cool blood. Peony root and Moutan bark clear away heat to cool blood, promote blood circulation to remove stasis. It is a common and effective prescription for the blood syndrome due to heat in the xue fen and due to blood disorder. To cool the blood and stop bleeding, Shi Hui Powder can be added. For those marked by fever and thirsty due to excessive heat-toxin, Gpysm, Anemarrhemna rhizome and Capejasmine or Zi Xue Dan Pill (infusion) can be added to enhance the effect of clearing away heat. For those marked by abdominal pain and hemaxchezia, which are caused by heat accumulated in the stomach and intestine and stagnation of qi and blood, White poney root, Liqourice, Nutgrass, Sanguisorba root and Sophora flower should be added to relieve spasm and pain, stop bleeding by cooling the blood. For those marked by constipation, Rhubarb, Trichosanthes fruit should be used. As to the case marked by artyroncus and arthralyia, which is due to obstacle of meridian and collateral by pathogenic heat, Large leaf gentian root, Mullbery tigs, Chaenomeles fruit and Honeysuckle should be added to clearing and activating the channels and collaterals.

Prescription for example: Bufflo horn 30g, Dried rehmannia 12g, Red moutan bark 10g, Gympsy 30g (To be decocted first), Anemarrhena rhizome 10g, Capejasmine 10g, Biota tops 10g, Lipourice 6g.

(2) Hyperactivity of fire due to yin deficiency

Main symptoms: Purple spots or plague in skin appears from time to time.

Accompanying symptoms: Gingival bleeding, epistaxis. Profuse menstruation, flush cheek, restless, hot sensation in the palms and soles, thirsty, hectic fever, night sweat.

Tongue and pulse: Red tongue with little fur, thready and rapid pulse.

Analysis: Hyperactivity of fire is due to yin deficiency, and leads to yin consumption reversely. Impairment of vessels due to deficient fire gives rise in bleeding from the muscle under skin or other places. Purpuras appeas from time to time, because it is induced by lassitude of heat. If exhaustion of kidney water fails in coordinate the heart fire, and it was stirred, it will be marked by restlessness. Interior evaporation of deficient fire result in restlessnes of heart, soles and palms, hectic fever and flushed cheeks. Deficient fire forcing the body fluid to release results in night sweat. Deficiency of Yin fluid lead to thirsty and dry throat.

Red tongue with little fur, thready and rapid pulse are the signs of hyperactivity of fire due to yin deficiency.

Therapeutic principle: Nourishing yin to lower the fire, calming the vessels to arrest bleeding.

Prescription: Modified Qian Gen Powder. The prescription has the function of nourishing yin to clear away heat, cooling the blood to stop bleeding. For the case marked by the syndromes due to Yin deficiency, Tortoise plastrion, Scrophularia root, Glossy privet fruit and Eclipta can be added to nourish yin and clear away heat. Fatigue in waist and kneen, dizziness, lassitude, hot sensation in the palms and soles, red tongue with little fur, thready and deep rapid pulse are the syndromes of deficiency in kidney yin with little fire heat. Liu Wei Di Huang Pill combining with Rubia root, Purple gromwell root, Biota tops and Hairy vein acrimony are selected to nourish kidney yin.

Prescription for example: Dried rehmannia 12g, Dogwood fruit 10g, Glossy privet fruit 10g, Eclipta 10g, Moutan bark 10g, Oriental water plantain rhizome 10g, Rubia root 12g, Biota tops 12g, Anemarrhena rhizome 10g.

(3) Failure of deficient qi to govern the blood

Main symptoms: Chronic purple spots or plague in skin with dark color, appears from time to time.

Accompanying symptoms: Dizziness, poor appetite, mental and physical lassitude, pale or sallow complexion.

Tongue and pulse: Fat, light color tongue with thin white fur, thready weak pulse.

Analysis: Failure of deficient qi to govern the blood results in bleeding from time to time without cure. Dysfunction of deficient qi to guide the blood circulation results in blood stasis marked by bleeding with dark light blood, tendon vessels and skeleton with being nourished due to consumption of qi and blood results in mental and physical lassitude, dizziness, dim complexion. Dysfunction of spleen qi in transporting results in anorexia. Fat, light color tongue with thin white fur, thready weak pulse are the signs of deficiency of qi and blood.

Therapeutic principle: Replenishing qi to govern the blood.

Prescription: Modified Gui Pi Decoction, the prescription has the function of invigorating the heart and spleen, replenishing qi to govern the blood. According to the symptom, the astringent such as Hairy vein acrimony, Carbonized palmae bark, Notoginseng Cat tail pollen, Rubia root and Carboniazed hair can be selected to stop bleeding and remove stasis. For the case of loose stool due to failure of the spleen to distinguish clear from turbid, Chinese Yam, Locus receptacle and Gordon euryale seed can be added to invigorate the spleen and relieve diarrhea. For those accompanied with lassitude in waist and knees due to deficiency of kidney qi, Doder weed, Dogwood fruit, Dipsacus root can be added to replenish kidney qi. For the cases marked by aversion to cold, Curculigo, Cinnamon bark can be used to warm kidney yang.

Prescription for example: Dang shen 10g, Astragalus 15g, White atracylode rhizome 10g, Chinese angelica root 10g, Poria 10g, Hairy vein acrimony 20g, Notoginseng powder 3g (taken with water), Carbonized palmae bark 10g.

Epstaxis, gingival bleeding and purple dot, above all belong to "nuxue" in TCM. Spontaneous bleeding terms "nu". Nuxue generally means bleeding from the locations such as nose, gums, ear, muscle and skin. The name is different based on various bleeding sites. Notes that NuXue recorded in some medical books sometimes means epistaxis only.

Although the main etiopathogenesis of epistaxis, gingival bleeding or "Ji Nu" is the heat making the blood not to flow its circulation, the etiopathogenesis, such as deficiency of Qi and blood, and Qi failing to govern the blood are also very common. We should distinguish the syndromes between excess and deficient. As to bleeding due to heat, excess heat often results from lung heat, liver fire, stomach fire and heat transmitting into Ying blood; deficient heat often results from Yin deficiency. As to bleeding due to deficiency, at the beginning of the disease, the pathogenesis is deficiency of Qi and blood; gradually, the spleen and kidney become deficient.

As to bleeding due to lung heat, the manifestation is often accompanied with dryness in the nose and throat, and cough. The principle of the treatment should be clearing away lung heat and cooling the blood to stop bleeding. The prescription usually is modified Sang Ju Yin. As to bleeding due to stomach fire, the manifestation is often accompanied with thirsty, foul breath, yellow tongue fur, rapid and full pulse. The principle of the treatment should be purging the fire, removing stomach heat and cooling the blood to stop bleeding. The prescription usually is modified Yu Nu Jian and San Huang Shi Gao Decoction. As to bleeding due to liver fire, the manifestation is often accompanied with dizziness, distention sensation in the head, bitter taste and irritability. The principle of the treatment should be removing liver fire and cooling the blood to stop bleeding. The prescription usually is modified Long Dan Xie Gan Decoction. As to bleeding due to heat transmitting into Ying blood, there are multiple bleeding sites. The manifestation is sometimes accompanied with fever. The principle of the treatment should be removing heat and toxic substance, cooling the blood to stop bleeding. The prescription usually is modified Xi Jiao Di Huang Decoction. As to bleeding resulted from hyperactivity of fire due to Yin deficiency, the manifestation is often accompanied with hot sensation in the palms, soles and heart, dizziness, tinnitus, tidal fever and night sweat. The principle of the treatment should be nourishing Yin to lower the fire and cooling the blood to stop bleeding. The prescription can be modified Zi Shui Qing Gan Yin combined with Qian Gen Powder Decoction. As to bleeding due to deficiency of Qi failing to govern the blood, the manifestation is often accompanied with mental and physical fatigue, palpitation, short in breath and loss of appetite. The principle of the treatment should be replenishing Qi to govern the blood. The prescription usually is modified Gui Pi Decoction. Besides, epistaxis and gingival bleeding can be treated with external drugs locally.

4. Hemoptysis

The disease characterized by blood coming from the respiratory system, getting out of the respiratory tract with cough is called hemoptysis. It refers to cough with blood. It is also called "kexue", "souxue" or "kaxue". The manifestation is marked by phlegm with blood or shredded blood, or scarlet blood with foam-like phlegm.

Generally, hemoptysis is caused by impairment of pulmonary vessels. Being a delicate organ, the lung resists neither cold nor heat. Its location is above all of the viscera. Its function is dispersing and descending. The lung prefers to be moistened rather than be dried, and prefers to clear rather than turbid. It is easy to be attacked by pathogenic factor. If lung qi fails in descending due to pathogenic factor, cough will occur. If the pulmonary vessels are impaired so that blood flows out of the vessels, hemoptysis will occur. The location of the disease is mainly lung, as well as liver and kidney.

In clinical, the syndromes of hemoptysis are divided into impairment of lung by dryness heat, liver-heat attacking lung and lung-heat due to Yin deficiency. The therapeutic principles are clearing heat, moistening lung, keeping the normal circulation to stop bleeding; or purging the fire of liver and lung, cooling the blood to stop bleeding; or nourishing pulmonary Yin and keeping the normal circulation to stop bleeding, respectively.

(1) Impairment of lung by dryness-heat

Main symptoms: Itching of throat, cough, phlegm with a little fresh blood.

Accompanying symptoms: dryness of mouth and nose, or accompanied by fever, light aversion to wind and cold, stuffy nose and headache.

Tongue and pulse: Red tongue with little saliva and thin yellowish fur, rapid pulse.

Analysis: Impairment of lung caused by the external invasion of pathogenic wind, heat and dryness not only results in failure of the lung to disperse and descend but also in impairment of pulmonary vessels. Its manifestations are characterized by itching of throat, cough, and phlegm with scarlet blood. If it is caused by consumption of body fluid due to dryness heat, they are characterized by dryness of mouth and nose. If it is caused by disorder of superficial Wei due to external invasion of wind, heat and dryness, they will be marked by fever and slight aversion to wind, which are the syndromes of superficial heat. The manifestations such as red tongue with little saliva and thin yellowish fur, and rapid pulse are all the signs of impairment of body fluid by dryness heat.

Therapeutic principle: clearing away the lung- heat and moistening the lung, keeping the normal circulation to stop bleeding.

Prescriptions: Modified Sang Xing Decoction can be used. Its function is clearing away lung-heat, ventilating and moistening the lung, and cooling the blood. In the recipe, Mulberry leaf, Capejasmine fruit and prepared soybean are combined to clear away and ventilate the lung-heat; Ladybell root and Pear peel nourish yin and clear away heat; while Bitter apricot root and Fritiallary bulb moisten the lung, resolve phlegm and relieve cough. To cool the blood and stop bleeding, Cogongrass rhizome, Biota tops, India madder root, and Node of lotus rhizome can be used. As to accompanied by fever, headache, cough, sore throat and rapid floating pulse, drugs of diaphoretic, pungent in flavour and cool in property, such as Honeysuckle flower, Forsythia fruit, Arctium fruit and Chrysanthemum flower can be used to clear away heat and relieve sore throat. For cases with cough, yellow phlegm and lots of blood due to interior excess heat of lung, the drugs such as Gypsum, Scutellarea root, Mulberry bark and Wind-wead rhipome can be used. For the cases due to impairment of body fluid by dryness-heat, the drugs such as Ophiopogon root, Figwort root, Trichosanthes root powder and Reed rhizome can be used to nourish Yin and moisten the lung.

Prescription for example: Mulberry leaf 10g, Bitter apricot seed 10g, Ladybell root 15g, Anemarrhena rhizome 10g, Fritillary bulb 10g, Scutellaria10g, Capejasmine fruit 10g, Mulberry bark 10g, Chinese arborvitae leaf and twig 12g, Cogongrass rhizome 30g.

(2) Liver-heat attacking lung

Main symptoms: Paroxysmal cough with scarlet blood, or phlegm with blood.

Accompanying symptoms: The symptoms are restlessness, irritability, bitter taste, dryness in throat, distending pain in the chest and hypochondriums, which are changed in accordance with mood.

Tongue and pulse: Red tongue with thin yellowish fur, rapid taut pulse.

Analysis: If one feels depressed or angry, stagnated liver-qi will transform into fire, which runs up to attack the lung. Because of impairment of purifying and descending function of lung and impairment of pulmonary vessels, it is manifested as cough and hemoptysis, which are changed in accordance with mood. Hepatic channels are distributed throughout the hypochondriums and the ribs. Because of excess of liver-fire and stagnation of hepatic channels, it is manifested as distending pain in the chest and hypochondriums. Because of up flaring of liver-fire, it is manifested as bitter taste, restlessness and irritability. Red tongue with thin yellowish fur and rapid taut pulse are the manifestation of excess liver-fire.

Therapeutic principle: Purging the fire of liver and lung, cooling the blood to stop bleeding.

Prescriptions: Modified Xie Bai Powder and Dai Ge Powder. Xie Bai Powder has the function of purging the lung heat and relieving cough and asthma. Dai Ge powder has the function of purging the fire of liver and lung, cooling the blood to resolve phlegm. In the recipe, Muberry bark and Wolfberry bark purge lung-heat, conchae clears away lung-heat to resolve phlegm, Natural indigo clears away liver-heat to cool the blood, Liquorice and Polished round-grained nonglutinous rice nourish the stomach and regulate the middle. To cool the blood and stopping bleeding, Dried rehmannia root, Yerbadetaji herb and Congonfrass rhizome, Japanese thistle herb, Field thirstle and Node of lotus rhizome should be used. For cases with dizziness, blood-shot eye, restlessness and irritability, which are due to excess of liver-fire, Moutan bark, Capejasmine fruit and Scutellaria root can be used. As to hemoptysis with a lot of scarlet blood, Xi Jiao Di Huang Decoction added Notoginseng powder, Mulberry bark powder and Rhubarb powder should be employed to purge the heat and fire, and cool the blood to stop bleeding.

Prescription for example: Muberry bark 10g, Wolfberry bark 10g, Dai Ge Powder 12g (To de decocted in pack), Scutellaria root 10g, Moutan bark 10g, Node of lotus rhizome 10g, Baked capejasmine fruit 10g, Congonfrass rhizome 30g.

(3) Lung-heat due to Yin deficiency

Main symptoms: Cough with little phlegm, phlegm with blood or hemoptysis repeatly with scarlet blood.

Accompanying symptoms: Dryness of mouth and throat, flush cheek, hectic fever and night sweating.

Tongue and pulse: Red and thin tongue with thin yellowish fur, rapid thready pulse.

Analysis: If interior burning of deficiency fire due to deficiency of lung-Yin and kidney-Yin results in impairment of purifying and descending function of lung, it will be manifested as cough with little phlegm, or short dry cough. Because fire-heat burning the lung results in impairment of pulmonary vessels and phlegm is caused by deficient fire burning the body fluid, the manifestation is marked by little but viscous phlegm with blood, or hemoptysis repeatedly with scarlet blood. If body fluid is too deficient to moisten the throat, which is caused by Yin deficiency, hemoptysis will be accompanied with dryness of mouth and throat. If hyperactivity of fire due to Yin deficiency, hemoptysis will be accompanied with flush cheek, hectic fever, night sweating, red and thin tongue with thin yellowish fur and rapid thready pulse.

Therapeutic principle: Nourishing and moistening pulmonary Yin and keeping the normal circulation to stop bleeding.

Prescriptions: Modified Bai He Gu Jin Pill. Its function is nourishing and moistening pulmonary Yin, harmonizing both lung and kidney. In the recipe, Lily bulb, Lilyturf root, Figwort root; Dried and prepared rehmannia have the effect of nourishing Yin to purge heat and moistening lung to produce fluid; Chinese angelica root and White peony root, moister in nature, nourishing Yin; Bulb fritillary and Liquorice resolving phlegm to relieve cough. It is advisable to remove Root of Balloon flower, which has the function of ascending in the original recipe, and has no benefit to reliving hemoptysis. Usually the drugs such as Arborvitae tops, Node of lotus rhizome, Cogongrass rhizome and Hyacinth blrtilla, sometimes Shi Hui Powder are added. Those drugs can arrest bleeding by cooling the blood or by astringency to. For cases with hemoptysis repeatly or with profuse blood, Dankey-hide gelatin, Tortoiseplastron and Notoginseng powder can be added to nourish blood and stop bleeding. For the case with hectic fever and flush cheek that is caused by interior heat due to Yin deficiency, Sweet wormwond, Fresh-water turtle shell, Wolfberry bark and swallowwort can be used to clear the heat of deficient type. For cases with heavy night sweat, Glutinous rice root, Light wheat, Schisandra fruit and Oyster shell should used to arrest sweat.

Prescription for example: Lily bulb 20g, Dried rehmannia 12g, Lilyturf root 10g, Figwort root 10g, White peony root 10g, Wolfberry bark10g, Bulb fritillary10g, Chinese arborvitae leaf and twig 12g, Cogongrass rhizome 20g, Hyacinth bletille tuber 10g.

5. Hematemesis

Hematemesis, also called "tu xue"or "ou xue" in TCM, refers to the disease of vomiting blood, which is scarlet or dark red, and often mixes with residues of food. The blood comes from digestive system. Yi Bian-Tu Xue recorded that "Tuxue is the same as Ouxue. In the past, tu xue means vomiting blood without nausea, while ouxue means vomiting blood with nausea.

Since both cases of hematemesis and hemoptysis, blood gets out from mouth, we should differentiate them, the color is fresh red carefully. Generally the blood due to hemoptysis hemoptysis comes from the respiratory system, the color is fresh red often mixes with foam like phlegm. Before hemoptysis, it is often accompanied by cough. After serious hemoptysis, the blood can be formed in the phlegm for a few days. The blood due to hematemesis comes from digestive system. It is scarlet or dark red, and often mixes with residues of food. Before hematemesis, it is accompanied by discomfort, pain in stomach, and nausea. After hematemesis, it is often accompanied by black stool, but no blood in the phlegm.

Hemeatasis is mainly caused by stagnated heat in the liver and stomach leading to disorder of blood circulation, sometimes caused by failure of qi governing the blood due to deficiency and coldness of the spleen and stomach. Syndrome of asthenia and coldness type is the root, while that of sthenia and heat is a incidental. Only a few hematemesis belong to asthemic syndrome and cold syndromes. In clinical, according to the pathogenesis, it can be divided into three types. They are excess stomach-heat, liver-fire attacking the stomach, bleeding due to qi deficiency. The principles of treatment are clearing away stomach heat, removing blood stasis to stop bleeding; purging liver-fire, clearing away stomach heat, cooling the blood to stop bleeding; or invigorating the spleen and replenishing qi to govern the blood and arrest bleeding, respectively.

(1) Excess stomach fire

Main symptoms: Distension or even pain in stomach and abdomen, the blood due to hematemesis is scarlet or dark red, and often mixes with residues of food.

Accompanying symptoms: foul breath, constipation or black stool.

Tongue and pulse: Red tongue with yellow greasy fur, rapid slippery pulse.

Analysis: Stomach is the reservoir of water and food. It is abundant in qi and blood. Its function is to receive, digest and transform water and food. It is normal for stomach-qi to descend. If stagnated stomach-qi fails in descending heat, or disharmony between qi and blood due to improper diet or drinking, it will be marked by distension and pain in the stomach, or in the abdomen. Disorder of circulation due to impairment of gastral vessels by heat will results in hematemesis with scarlet or dark purplish blood, which is due to stasis for a long time. If the stomach-qi up rises, it will be marked by hematemesis with residues of food. If accumulated food is corrupt, hematemesis will be accompanied with foul breath. If stomach-heat consumes body fluid, it will be accompanied with constipation. If blood get out of the body with stool, it will be accompanied with black stool. Red tongue with yellow greasy fur, rapid slippery pulse are the signs of interior stagnation of heat.

Therapeutic principle: Clearing away stomach heat, removing blood stasis to stop bleeding.

Prescriptions: Modified Xie Xin Decoction and Shi Hui Powder. Xie Xin Decoction, bitter in flavor and cold in property, has the function of clearing away stomach heat. As Xue Zheng Lun-Hematemesis said, although the prescription is named as "XieXin", which means purging heart fire, its real function is purging the stomach-fire. It is consists of Scrtellarid root, Coptis root and Rhubarb. Shi

Hui Powder not only can cool the blood to stop bleeding, but also can remove blood stasis. Rhubarb, bitter in flavor, cold in property, lowering and sinking in action, has the function of purging excess heat potently to clear the intestine and stomach. It is the main drug for hematemesis due to excess heat in the stomach. Hyacinthe bletilla tuber, bitter, sweat and astringent in flavor, slightly cold in property, has the function of stopping bleeding by astringing, subduing swelling and promoting granulation. It is a common drug for hemoptysis and hematemesis. These drugs can be used in compatibility, or used alone after ground into powder. If vomiting and nausea is due to up rising of stomach-qi, Inulla flower, Red ochre and Bamboo shavings can be used to regulate stomach-qi and lower the reversal flow of stomach qi.

If distent pain in abdomen and stomach is due to dysfunction of stomach to lower qi, Fruit of citron of trifoliate orange, Tangerine peel or Sichuan chinaberry and Figwort root can be added to regulate stomach qi and relieve pain.

Prescription for example: Coptis root 6g, Scutellaria root 10g, Arborvitue tops 12g, Lous leaf 12g, Fruit of citron or trifoliate orange 10g, Bamboo shavings 10g, Jiao San Xian 10g, Rhubab powder 3g (To be taken with water), Hyacinth bletilla powder 6g (To be taken with water) and Notoginseng powder 3g (To be taken with water).

(2) Liver-fire attacking the stomach

Main symptoms: Hematemesis with scarlet or dull-purple blood.

Accompanying symptoms: Restlessness, irritability, insomnia, dreaminess, bitter taste and hypochondriac pain.

Tongue and pulse: Deep red tongue and rapid taut pulse.

Analysis: If gastral vessels are impaired by the reversal flow of liver fire, which is transmitted from depressed qi, it will be marked by hematemesis with red or dull-purple blood. Uprising of liver fire will result in irritability, bitter taste and hypochondriac pain. If liver-fire disturbing the heart so as to dysphoria, it will be marked by restlessness, insomnia and dreaminess. Deep red tongue and rapid taut pulse are the signs of consumption of stomach-yin by excess liver fire.

Therapeutic principle: Clearing away stomach heat, cooling the blood to stop bleeding.

Prescriptions: Modified Long Dan Xie Gan Decoction for removing the damp-heat from the liver and gallbladder. In this case, the recipe must be modified in accordance with the symptoms. To cool the blood and stop bleeding, Cogongrass rhizome, Node of lotus rhizome, Yerbadetajo herb, India madder root and Hyacinth bletilla, sometimes along with Shi Hui Powder are added. In the case of massive bleeding, Xi Jiao Di Huang Decoction added Notoginseng powder, Hyacinth bletilla powder and Rhubarb powder can be given to clear away heat, cool the blood, remove blood stasis and stop bleeding.

Prescription for example: Gentiana root 6g, Scutellaria root 10g, Baked Capejasmine fruit 10g, Moutan bark 10g, Cogongrass rhizome 30g, Japanese thistle hurb 10g, Field Thistle 10g, Notoginseng powder 10g (To be taken with water), Hyacinth bletilla powder 6g (To be taken with water) and Yerbadetajo herb 12g.

(3) Bleeding due to deficiency of qi

Main symptoms: Chronic hematemesis with dark and light color blood, sometime mild, sometime serious.

Accompanying symptoms: Pale complexion, palpitation, shortness of breath, fatigue and weakness.

Tongue and pulse: Pale tongue, thready and weak pulse.

Analysis: The main symptoms result from bleeding out of the vessels, which is due to failure of deficient spleen-qi to keep the normal circulation. If hemorrhage follows with spleen-qi deficiency and exhaustion of qi results from bleeding, the syndromes of deficiency of qi and blood appears. If they are too deficient to nourish the heart, the manifestation will be marked by palpitation and shortness of breath; as to face, pale complexion; as to extremities and muscles, fatigue and weakness. Pale tongue, thready and weak pulses are the signs of deficiency of qi and blood.

Therapeutic principle: Invigorating the spleen and replenishing qi to govern the blood and arrest bleeding.

Prescriptions: Modified Gui Pi Decoction. Drugs for arresting bleeding by inducing astringency, reinforcing and warming the meridian, such as Cuttle bone, Hairy vein agrimony, Hyacinth bletilla and Baked ginger can be added in accordance with the syndromes. Both deficient qi affecting yang and interior deficient cold of the spleen and stomach lead to cold limbs, aversion to cold, and loose stool. In this case, Jin Gui Bai Ye Decoction and Li Zhong Pill should replace the prescription. In the recipe, Dangshen, Astragalus and Liquorice strengthen the spleen and replenish qi to govern the blood. Anyi wormwood leaves and Baked ginger warm the meridian to stop bleeding. Arborbvitae tops clear the heat, cool and lower the blood to diminish the tending of upwards reversing. Urine of boy under, which substitute for Dark plum juice in the ancient prescription, has the function of removing the blood stasis to stop bleeding. The combined prescription has the function of replenishing qi to govern the blood and warming the meridian to stop bleeding. In the case of hemorrhage so as to exhaustion of qi, and marked by pale complexion, sweating and weak pulse, the patient should take Du Shen Decoction immediately. "Since the blood can't be produced rapidly, we should strength qi immediately". If the manifestation is marked by sweating and cold limbs, which is results from exhaustion of qi and Yang, Prepared aconite root can be added into Du Shen Decoction, namely Shen Fu Decoction, to recuperate depleted Yang and rescue the patient from danger.

Prescription for example: Dangshen 10g, White atracylide rhizome 10g, Astragalus 15g, Chinese argelica root 6g, Liquorice 6g, Poria 10g, Baked ginger 10g, Cuttle bone 12g, Hyacinth bletilla powder 5g (To be taken with water).

6. Hemaxchezia

Blood passing from the anus, before or after defecation, mixed with or without stool, are all called hemaxchezia, also called bianxue, xiaxue, xiexue in TCM. They are divided into yuan xue, jin xue, changfeng and zangdu by the doctors in past dynasties. Yuanxue refers to hemafecia after defecation. The location of the disease is commonly at small intestine and stomach, far from the anus. Jinxue refers to hemafecia before defecation. The location of the disease is commonly at colon, rectum or anus, near to anus. Changfeng refers to hemafecia with clear blood and bright red color. Zangdu refers to hemafecia with turbid blood and dull red color. In clinical, it is not reliable to distinguish Jinxue from yuanxue in the light of blood coming before or after defecation. In most cases the blood mixes with stool so that we are not sure which passing from the anus first. While the color of the blood can be referred to diagnosis the location of hemaxchezia. Usually, if hemaxchezia with bright blood, the bleeding is near to the anus; if hemaxchezia with purplish red blood, the bleeding is far from the anus. Hemafecia is different from dysentery with blood stool, the former is marked by bloody stool without abdominal pain and tenesmus; the latter is marked by purulent bloody stool, red moucs, abdominal pain and rectal tenesmus.

Usually, hematochezia results from impairment of gastral vessels and intestinal vessels. In clinical, it is divided into damp-heat in the intestine and asthenia cold in the spleen and stomach. The therapeutic principles of these syndromes are removing heat and dampness, cooling the blood to stop bleeding; or invigorating the spleen, warming the middle Jiao and nourishing the blood to stop bleeding.

(1) Damp heat in the intestine

Main symptoms: Hematochezia with bright red blood.

Accompanying symptoms: Dyschesia or loose stool; sometimes accompanied by burning sensation in the anus.

Tongue and pulse: Yellow and greasy tongue coat, rapid soft or slippery pulse.

Analysis: Hemaxchezia results from intestinal vessels burned by damp heat, which is accumulated in the intestine. If the function of digestion and elimination of the intestine are disorder, it will be marked by hemaxchezia. If functional activities of intestine qi are disorder, it will be marked by abdominal pain. If damp heat upward flows, it will be marked by bitter taste. If damp heat downward flows, it will be marked by burning sensation in the anus. Yellow and greasy tongue coat, rapid soft or slippery pulses are the signs of interior accumulation of damp heat.

Therapeutic principle: Removing heat and dampness, cooling the blood to stop bleeding.

Prescriptions: Modified Di Yu Powder and Huai Jiao Pill. Both prescriptions have the function of removing heat and dampness, cooling the blood and astringe bleeding. The former is much better in removing heat and dampness; besides above functions, the latter can also nourish blood and promote the circulation of qi and blood. In the recipe of DiYu Powder, sanguisorba root and rubia root are combined to cool the bloods to stop bleeding. Scutellara root, coptis root and capejasmine fruit have the effect of clearing heat, eliminating dampness, purging the fire and removing toxic substance. The bland drug, poria, induces diuresis. In the recipe of Huai Jiao Pill, Japanese sophora fruit and garden burne root are combined to cool the blood and stop bleeding. Scutellarea root clears away heat. Ledebouriella root, immature bitter orange peel and Chinese angelica roots have the effect of dispelling wind, promoting diureses, nourishing blood and promoting circulation. In clinical, if hematochezia is with massive blood, based on the condition, hyacinth bletilla tuber, notoginseng and arborvitae tops can be used to cool the blood and stop bleeding. If the patient has been suffered from hematochezia for a long time, and over hemorrhage, Ying Yin fluid and twig has been consumed, while damp-heat hasn't been cleared away. The symptoms will be marked by restlessness, red tongue with yellow fur, rapid thready pulse. In this case, white peony root, dunkey-hide gelatin and dried rehmannia root can be added to nourish blood, astringe Yin fluid, regulate the nutrient system and clear away heat.

Prescription for example: Garden bernet root 15g, sophora fruit 10g, rubia root 10g, baked capejasmine fruit 10g, poria 10g, coptis root 6g, scutellaria root 6g, hyacinth bletilla tuber powder 5g, notoginseng powder 3g.

(2) Deficient cold in the spleen and stomach

Main signs and symptoms: Bloody stool with purplish red blood, even tarry stool.

Accompanying symptoms: Dull pain in abdomen, the pain relieved after heated, dim complexion, mental fatigue, hypologia and loose stool.

Tongue and pulse: Tongue lighter in color than the normal one. thready and weak pulse.

Analysis: Hemafecia is caused by insufficiency of spleen Yang, deficiency of qi in middle-energizor, failure to keep blood flowing within the vessels, overflow of blood into intestines and excretion with feces. The manifestation will be characterized as bloody stool with purplish red blood, even tarry stool. If qi disorder due to deficient cold in middle Jiao and qi stagnation due to cold, it will be marked by dull pain in abdomen and the pain will be relieved after heated. If dysfunction of spleen in transport failing to produce qi and blood, it will be marked by dim complexion, mental fatigue, hypologia, tongue light in color, thready and weak pulse.

Therapeutic principle: Invigorating the spleen, warming the middle Jiao and nourishing the blood to stop bleeding.

Prescriptions: Modified Huang Tu Decoction. The recipe has the function of invigorating the spleen, warming the middle Jiao, nourishing the blood and stopping bleeding. In the recipe, baked yellow earth, warms the middle Jiao and stops bleeding, exerting a role of principle drug. Bighead atractylodes rhizome and prepared aconite root, invigorating the spleen Yang, act as assistant drug. Dried rehmannia root and dankey-hide gelatin, not only nourish blood to stop bleeding, but also restrict the warm and dry nature of bighead atractylodes rhizome and prepared aconite root, acting as adjuvant drugs. Scutellaria root, bitter in taste and cold in nature, as an adjuvant to regulate the middle. Combination of all the drugs, couples hardness with softness, warms yang and arrests bleeding without yin consumption, nourishes yin and blood without impeding the spleen qi. When the prescription is employed in clinical, prepared aconite root, a drug with great pungent and great heat, moving qi without stopping, can be replaced by baked ginger. Baked ginger is not tending to move qi and has the effect of warming the middle and stopping bleeding as well as purgation. Based on different situation, hyacinth bletilla and cuttle bone can be used to arrest bleeding by astringency, notoginseng and ophicalcite to arrest bleeding by promoting blood circulation. For the deficiency of yang, antler extract, baked ginger and Chinese mugwort leaf can be added to stop bleeding by warming yang.

Prescription for example: Baked yellow earth 30～60g (packeted), baked ginger 10g, bighead atractylodes rhizome 10g, Dried rehmannia root 10g, donkey-hide gelatin (To be taken with water)10g, Scutellaria root 10g, Astragalus 15g, Chinese angelica root 10g, prepared liquorice 6g, cuttle bone 12g, hyacinth bletille tuber 10g.

7. Hematuria

Urine with blood or even blood clot terms hematuria, also called "sou xue" and "niao xue" in TCM. The urine appears light red, bright red or brown color, based on the quantity of blood.

Urine with blood can be devided into hematuria and gonorrhoea. Urination without pain or without obvious pain terms hematuria. Painful and dribbling urination with bloody urine terms "xue lin" in TCM. The pathogenesis of the disease is impairment of vessels by heat and dysfunction of spleen and kidney. The heat of the former pathogenesis can be divided into excess type and deficient type. For those patients whose syndromes belong to sthenia heat, the principle of treatment is clearing away fire heat and cooling the blood to stop bleeding. For the patient whose syndrome belongs to asthenia heat, the principle of treatment is nourishing Yin to lower the fire, keep the normal circulation to stop bleeding. The latter pathogenesis can be divided into spleen deficiency and kidney deficiency, the treatment should focus on replenishing spleen and kidney qi and stopping bleeding with astringents.

(1) Excess heat accumulating in lower Jiao

Main symptoms: Dark urine, burning sensation during urination, blood with bright red color.

Accompanying symptoms: Restlessness, thirsty, flush face, oral ulceration and insomnia.

Tongue and pulse: Red tongue and rapid pulse.

Analysis: If excess heat accumulates in lower Jiao, it will manifest as dark urine and burning sensation during urination. If heat injures the vessels, the blood will bleed out of the vessels and flow into the bladder, it will manifest as hematuria with bright red color. If heat disturbs the mental, it will manifest as restlessness and insomnia. Consumption of body fluid due to heat gives rise to thirsty. Red tongue and rapid pulse are the signs of excess heat.

Therapeutic principle: Clearing away fire heat, cooling the blood to stop bleeding.

Prescriptions: Modified Xiao Ji Yin Zi Decoction. The recipe has the function of clearing away fire heat, inducing urine, cooling the blood and stopping bleeding. In the recipe, field thistle and dried rehmannia, as principal drugs, clear away heat and cool the blood to stop bleeding. Cattail pollen and node of lotus rhizome, as assistant drugs, stop bleeding by removing stasis. Talcum powder, Rece paper pith and Lophatherum, as adjuvant drugs, clear away heat and induce urine. Chinese angelica promotes blood circulation and regulates Ying. Liquorice, as a guiding drug, regulates the middle and relieves spasm. If heat resulting from flaring heart-fire transsits into small intestine and bladder, and the manifestation marked by burning sensation during urination, restlessness and thirsty, Manshurian aristolochia stem, coptis root or phellodedron bark, which is bitter in flavour and cold in property, will be used to purge the fire. If the patient suffered from insomnia, amber powder (1～2g) can be used to tranquilize the mind through sedation and promoting blood circulation to remove stasis.

Prescription for example: Dried rehmannia12g, Japanese thistle herb 12g, Capejasmine 10g, Field thistle 12g, Manshurian aristolochia stem 6g, Lophatherum 10g, Liquorice 6g, Cogograss rhizome 30g, Baked cattail pollen 6g.

(2) Hyperactivity of fire due to kidney deficiency

Main symptoms: Scanty dark urine.

Accompanying symptoms: Dizziness, tinnitus, thin, fatigue, flushed cheeks, hectic fever and lassitude in loin and legs.

Tongue and pulse: Red tongue and rapid thready pulse.

Analysis: If interior burning of deficiency fire, which is due to kidney deficiency, in juries the vessels, it will be marked by scanty dark urine. If deficiency of the reservoir of marrow due to deficiency of kidney Yin, it will be marked by dizziness and tinnitus. If deficiency of kidney due to being malnourished, it will be marked by lassitude in loin and legs. If hyperactivity of fire due to Yin deficiency and up- flaring of deficiency fire, it will be marked by flushed cheeks and hectic fever. Red tongue and rapid thready pulse are the signs of hyperactivity of fire due to Yin deficiency.

Therapeutic principle: nourishing Yin to lower the fire, cooling the blood to stop bleeding.

Prescriptions: Modified Zhi Bai Di Huang Pill. The recipe has the function of nourishing Yin to lower the fire. In the recipe, Liu Wei Di Huang Pill replenishes the kidney Yin and strengthens the governor of water to restrain hyperactivity of Yang. Anemarrhena rhizome and phellodedron bark have the effect of nourishing Yin and purging fire. Eclipta and tortoise plastron can be added to nourish Yin and stop bleeding. To stop bleeding by cooling blood drugs such as Japanese thistle herb, field thistle, garden burnet root, cattail pollen and node of lotus rhizome can be added.

Prescription for example: Dried rehmannia 15g, Evodia fruit 10g, Eclipta 30g, Glossy privet fruit 10g, Mutan bark 10g, Oriental water plantain rhizome 10g, Anemarrhena rhizome 10g, Phellodedron bark 6g, Japanese thistle herb 10g, Field thistle 10g, Cogograss rhizome 30g.

(3) Failure of the spleen to keep the blood flowing within the vessels

Main signs and symptoms: Chronic hematuria with light color blood.

Accompanying symptoms: Dim complexion, physical fatigue, shortness of breath, weak voice, often accompanied by other bleeding syndromes, such as bleeding from gums, muscles and nose.

Tongue and pulse: Bulgy tongue with light color compared with normal tongue. thready weak pulse.

Analysis: If spleen Qi is too deficient to govern the blood, so that the blood bleeding out of the vessel, it will be marked by hematuria with light color blood, even accompanied with bleeding from gums, muscles and nose.

If dysfunction of spleen in transporting the essence results in little origins to form the Qi and blood, it will be marked by loss of appetite, mental or physical fatigue, shortness of breath and weak voice. Bulgy tongue with light color compared with normal tongue and thready weak pulse are the signs of deficiency of Qi and blood.

Therapeutic principle: Tonifying the spleen to govern the blood.

Prescription: Modified Gui Pi Decoction. Prepared rehmannia, Dankey-hide gelatin, and hairy vein agrimony can be added to nourish the blood and stop bleeding. If accompanied loose stool, abdominal distent tenesmus, shotness of breath and not tending to talk, which results from collapse due to deficiency of Qi, Modified Bu Zhong Yi Qi Decoction should be used to tonify the spleen, replenish Qi and rise Yang.

Prescription for example: Dangshen 12g, Astragalus root 15g, Chinese angelica root 10g, Bighead atractylodes 10g, Poria 10g, Tangerine peel 10g, Hairy vein atrimony 15g, Prepared licorice root 6g, Placenta hominis 3g(to be taken with water).

(4) Unconsolidation of the kidney qi

Main symptoms: Chronic hematuria with light color blood, frequency of micturition.

Accompanying symptoms: Dizziness, tinnitus, mental fatigue, lassitude and pain in loin and legs, frequent and massive micturition in night.

Tongue and pulse: Light color tongue, weak deep pulse.

Analysis: Impairment of kidney due to lassitude or prolonged illness, unconsolidationof the kidney qi and dysfunction of kidney to store essence result in bleeding accompanying with urine. Therefore, the blood of hematuria due to prolonged illness is bleeding with light red blood. The kidneys control the two private parts. It has function of warming up. Deficiency and dysfunction of kidney qi result in frequency of micturition. Waist is charged by kidney. The brain is the reservoir ofmarrow. If the kidney is too deficient to nourish the relating organs, the manifestation will be dizziness, tinnitus, mental fatigue, lassitude and pain in loin and leg. Light color tongue, weak deep pulse are the signs of dysfunction of kidney qi.

Therapeutic principle: Replenishing the kidney qi and governing the blood to stop bleeding.

Prescription: Modified Wu Bi Shan Yao Pill. It has the function of tonifying and reinforcing the kidney to govern the blood. In the recipe, Prepared rehmannia, ChineseYam, Dogword fruit and Achyranthes root tonify the kidney and replenish the essence; Desertliving cistanche, Podder seed, Eucommia bark and Medicinal indionmulberry root warm and reinforce the kidney Yang; Poria invigorate the spleen; Schisandra fruit, Red halloysite have the effect of replenishing qi, inducing astringe. To stop bleeding, the astringent drugs and circulation promoting drugs such as Hairy vein agrimony, Arborviatae tops, Cattail pollen and Garden burnet root can be used. If emission or spermatorrhoea due to failure of deficient kidney to store essence, Cherokee rose fruit, Oyster shell and Gordon euryale can be used to induce astringency. As to the case marked by lassitude and pain in loin and legs, cold sensation in limbs and aversion to cold, Venison, Scythian lamb rhizome and Psoralea fruit can be used to warm and tonify the Du channel and Kidney Channel.

Prescription for example: Prepared rehmannia 15g, ChineseYam 12g, Dogword fruit 10g, Psoralea fruit 10g, Podder seed 12g, Medicinal indionmulberry root 10g, Eucommia bark 10g, Poria 10g, Hairy vein agrimony 15g, Notoginseng 3g(to be taken with water).

〔Method for precaution and nursing〕

Prevention of the blood should be determined according to the constitution, the inducing factors, the location of bleeding and the character of syndromes. For those due to blood disorder by heat, the food of activating fire, such as pungency, smoke and alcohol should be forbidden. To prevent interior firing liver fire, keep calm and pleasing emotion. To prevent invasion of yin blood by heat, cure the disease caused by expatogen in time. For those resulting from hyperactivity of fire due to yin deficiency, the patient should pay attention to regular life and proper activity to prevent yin of live and kidney from consuming. For those resulting from failure of deficient qi to govern the blood, prevent cold particularly, increase nourishment and make sure the function of spleen and stomach being in order. Distress, overthought, angry and lassitude should be avoided.

The nursing of blood syndrome is advised as follows:

1. To observe the location, nature and condition of blood syndrome, pay attention to the site, amount and color of the blood, and pay attention to the tongue, pulse, spirit, complexion, sweating or not, temperature of the limbs.

2. Bleeding with massive blood in urgency or with unstable quantity for a long time, accompanied with pale complexion, mental fatigue or vague mind, cold limbs with sweating are the signs of blood exhaustion. In this case, we should stop bleeding by taking emergency treatment.

3. As to bleeding from up orifices, such as hemoptysis, hematemesis, epistaxis, we should calm the patient and make the patient have a proper posture to let the blood flow out. Supine position, rising the head of fill in the blood way with a towel should be avoided. Or the blood stasis will obstruct the airway and result in asplyxia and syncope. If the blood obstruct in the airway, pat the back or induce vomiting to get rid of the blood.

4. To prevent exterior affection, keep fresh air, proper temper of the room. Take simple and light diet. If qi and blood as well as spleen and kidney have been deficient, the patient should increase nourishment. Care after the spirit and regular life.

5. According to different blood syndrome, nurse the patient basing on differentiation of the disease as well as the syndromes.

〔Typical cases analysis〕

Case 1: Hematuria

Zhan * *, male, 35 years old, cadre, Hunan province.

First visit: Janu 9th, in 1980.

Hematuria for a month caused by fatigue during a business trip. NO abnormal phenomenon was found by the examination of X ray photograph, cystoscopy, intravenous pyelography and bacterial culture. Because western medicine was invalid for hematuria, the patient asked for traditional medicine.

The symptoms are: hematuria still, burning got sensation in the waist, mental and physical fatigue, restlessness, thirst tending to drink without edema, frequency of micturition, urgency of urination, urodynia, or interruption of urination, red tongue with yellowish thin fur, thready and taut pulse. The result of urine examination, red blood cells ++++; leukocyte count 0—1; protein, micro quantity. Hematuria mostly results from heat, which accumulates at the lower

Jiao forcing the blood to flow abnormally. In this case, however, both qi and yin of the patient have been impaired. Thus the therapeutic principle should be replenishing qi, nourishing blood, clearing away heat to cool the blood, removing stasis to arrest bleeding and treat the primary and secondary symptoms simultaneously. The prescription is Modified Xiao JI Yin Zi. Recipe:

Astragalus root 15g, white peony root 10g, field thistle 10g, dried rehmannia 20g, manshurian aristolochia stem10g, Chinese angelica root10g, capejasmine seed10g, Cat-tail pollen 10g(in pack), poria 12g, cogongrass 15g, baked node of lotus rhizme 10g, carbonized hair 5g, liquorice 5g. Five doses.

The second visit: Janu 14th, 1980.

After taking the decoction, the patient's hematuria is reduced. The result of urine examination is Red blood cells 0—3. The symptoms are the same as that of last week. Continue to take the former decoction for another 5 doses.

The third visit: Janu 20th, 1980.

Hematuria has been disappear, the results of urine examination has turned into normal. The symptoms only remain pain in the left waist with burning hot sensation which becomes sever after activity, tends to fatigue, urine with deep color. The tongue and pulse are the same as that in last week. Those signs indicate that qi and yin should be recover. The therapeutic principle are replenishing qi and nourishing yin. Recipe:

Astralus 15g, anemarrhena rhizome 10g, dried rehmannia 20g, moutan bark 10g, phelldendrow bark 10g, oriental water plantain rhizome 10g, Chinese yam 15g, dogwood fruit 6g, poria 12g, cogongrass rhizome 15g himalayan teasel root 12g, walnut kernel 15g. After taking 5 doses, the disease is cured.

According to the SuWen-Qi Jue Lun, if heat in the uterus transits into the urinary bladder, it will result in dysuria, frequent micturition or hematuria. Jin Gui Yao Lue said, heat in the lower Jiao results in hematuria. It is concluded that damp heat in lower Jiao is a common cause, which is categorized as sthenia syndromes. But in this case, according to the mass quantity and prolonged time of hematuria without urethral irritant syndromes, we concluded that the syndromes is due to impairment of both qi and yin, which is different from that due to pure damp-heat. It's categorized as the syndromes due to deficiency complicated with excess. The principle is treating the principal and secondary symptoms simultaneously. The prescription is Xiao Ji Yin Zi without talc and lophetherum, which are sweet, cold and slippery, adding cogograss and carbonized hair to stop bleeding by clearing away heat cooling blood and removing stasis, adding astralus rhizome and Chinese angelica root to replenish qi and nourish yin. The drug of dried rehmannia is used in great doses, whose function is not only to cool the blood and stop bleeding, but also to nourish yin and blood. The whole prescription has the function of removing heat and stasis, replenishing qi and nourishing yin (Selected from Yi Nan Bing Zhong Yi Zhi Liao).

Cases 2: Hematochezia

Mao * *, male, 18 years old, pain in the stomach for 10 years., which occurs in every winter and spring. In the latest week, pain in the stomach particularly at night with sour regurgitation and nausea, tarry stool, pale tongue with white fur, thready pulse. The deficient spleen will generate cold and not govern the blood. The deficient liver will generate heat and not store the blood. Dysfunction in governing and storing blood will result in the blood not following its normal way but running downwords to big intestine to form hemetochzia. Huang Tu Decoction in Jin Gui, which is a prescription with the nature of hardness, softness, warming and clearing, will be used to regulate the liver and the spleen and to stop bleeding.

dangshen 12g, large headed atractylodes 9g, prepared aconite root 9g (to be decocted first), prepared renmannia root 12g, scutellaria root 10g, dankey-hide gelatin 9g (To be melted) hairy vein agrimony 30g, baked yellow earth 30g(in pack). After taking four doses, the occult blood in stool is negative.

Note: Hematochezia, the bleeding site may be near to the anus, or far from the anus, and the syndrome may be heat or cold. The patient has been suffered from stomach pain for 7 years. Hematochezia with black stool and heavier pain at night indicates a syndrome due to deficient coldness in the spleen and stomach. Regurgitation and nausea frequently are the symptoms of the liver heat. Since the syndrome is deficient cold complicated with heat, and the cold syndrome is more serious than heat syndrome, Jin Gui Huang Tu Decoction was selected to couple hardness with softness and clear away heat during warming up. The prescription has the character of warming yang with out consume Yin (Selected from Zhang Bo Yu Yi An).

Case 3: Chen * *, male, 42 years old, farmer, Junu 29th, 1977.

The patient has chronic cough for 10 years, hemoptysis discontinuely several times, and massive hemorrhage was added up to 5 times, 100～200ml each times. According to the results of bronchial iodized oilroentgenograph by Wen Zhou * * hospital, the disease was right pulmonary extensive cylindrical bronchiectous. Because it is no use to taking the antibiotic, the drugs for eliminating phelegm and for arresting bleeding for a long time, and because the patient is not adapt for the surgery therapy, he visit our hospital. Recently, the patient suffered from hemoptysis after drinking alcohol, having been hemotysis with fresh blood for continuous five day, stuffy in the chest, paroxysmal cough, dry mouth and bitter taste, sweating, constipation like goat's stool, red tongue with yellow greasy and rough fur, taut and rapid pulse. According to pulse as well as the syndromes, hemoptysis results from heat accumulating in the intestine and stomach, qi and fire flaring upwards along airway and making ying-blood running abnormally. The therapeutic principle should be clearing away heat and fire ing stomach, lowering qi to stop bleeding. Recipe:

Baked camejasmine 9g, Mulberry bark 9g, Biota tops 9g, Scutellatea root 8g, Huacinth bletilla 10g, Rhubarb 10g (to be decocted later), Cogongrass rhizome 30g (to be decocted first), Red oche 30g (to be decocted first).

After taking the prescription for three doses, hemoptysis is eliminated; stool became normal, the pulse is taut and moderate. Because the fu-viscera has run downward, and hyperactivity of liver fire has been calmed. The drugs for clearing away lung heat and replenishing yin, protecting the lung and calming the vessels, was employed to regulate the body. The disease hasn't break out till now.

Note: Zhang Jin Yue said, it's only fire and qi that can promote blood. Tang Rong Chuan said, Qi is the governor of blood, while blood circles following with qi. The syndromes of hemoptysis due to reversed flow of qi are mainly categorized as heat. Yang Ming Stomach is a organ full go qi and blood, and the six fu-viscera prefers to smooth, qi and blood prefer to be descended. In this case, accumulated heat in the stomach due to drinking alcohol, lead to up-flaring of qi and fire, then result in blood bleeding out of the vessels. Thus, to suppress the reversed flow of qi and enhance the lowering effect, rhubarb must be combined with red ache. If blood runs down wards following qi, it will not bleeding out of the vessel. (Selected from XinZhong Yi 1986, 3)

Cases 4: Epistaxis

Shi Ming Yu, the son of Mr. Ma, suffered from profuse epistaxis like blood column. Any treatment for stopping epistaxis had no use for it. Because his symptoms and signs are vague, big and moderate pulse, fat face with sallow complexion, lassitude of the whole body, myasthenia of limbs, disinclination to talk or move but to sleeping has appeared for a long time. It is true. The epistaxis took place on his way home from Zhong Xi, when he is operating a boat against wind. Now epistaxis has lasted for 4 days. In my opinion, the patient not only suffered from failure of impaired qi to govern blood, but also impairment of stomach vessel due to lassitude. The stomach vessel belongs to the vessel of yang type. Impairment yang vessel will lead to bleeding from the up orifice. Since stomach channel connects with the nose, blood bleeds out of the nose. Taking Bu Zhong Yi Qi Decoction and baked black dry ginger for one dose arrested the epistaxis. Then go on taking the former prescription, in which the dried ginger is replaced by while peony root and sdhisandra fruit, and the symptoms of lassitude, disinclination to talk but to sleeping are relieved gradurally (Qian Cun Yi An).

Note: Most of bleeding due to excess heat. In this case, epistaxis is like a column. It's invalid that the former doctor treated the disease with routine drugs for clearing away heat and cooling blood. Zhang Shi Yi Tong recorded that as to epistaxis, the patient whose pulse is big but vague, the pathogenesis is failure of deficient spleen to govern the blood. In this case, the patient suffered from lassitude and addicted to lie for a long time. It indicated that the epistaxis resulted from constitution of spleen deficiency and lassitude. The latter doctor differentiated and analysis the disease thoroughly symptoms of sallow complexion, lassitute, fat and big tongue, moderate but feeble pulse, determined that the pathogenesis of syndromes was due to failure of impaired middle qi to govern blood and the blood bleeding out of nasal orifice to become epistaxis. Treated with the method of replenish the middle qi, Epistaxis was stopped.

Cases 5: Hematemesis

Yang * *, male, 28 years old, appetite to alcohol, having insomnia history. More insomnia leads to more drinking. One day, he felt stuffy sensation in midriff, the gas rush upward to throat. Soon, hematemesis occurred without stopping, accompanying with pale complexion, mental fatigue, taut big and rapid pulse and yellowish tongue coating. The blood comes from Yang Ming Stomach vessel. Impairment of yang channel leads to upward bleeding. Since the patient has been overdrinking alcohol, damp-heat has impaired the stomach, stomach qi is tending to lowering. The nature of alcohol is hot and noxious. Its qi and taste all belong to Yang. Impairment by alcohol too much, dampness in the stomach along with qi in Chong Channel loads the blood run upward, Chong channel is the reservoir of-blood, it is more bright than Yang Ming. The method should be clearing away stomach lowering the Chong channel, Inducing purgation to remove alcohol.

After taking two doses a day for continuous two days, hematemesis is cured. Spontaneous perspiratin, anenmia, somewhat floating and hollow pulse remain. They resulted from innourishment of the heart ad spleen due to blood exhaustion. The treatment is called Gui Pi Method, which make blood normal circulation and the heart well nourished.

Note: In this case, hematemesis is in urgency with massive quantity. After the treatment of clearing the stomach heat, lowering the qi of Chong channel and stopping bleeding rapidly and immediately. The syndrome due to blood deficiency in heart and spleen appeared. Thus relieving the secondary symptoms is urgent which relieving the first symptoms should also be important. Otherwise, primordial qi will be exhausted following with blood exhaustion. How to understand adding 1gram ginger in Gui Pi Decoction? The reason is that after the exhaustion of yin blood, there is no yin for deficient yang to astringe. It is manifested by taut, big and rapid pulse changing into floating and hollow pulse. Using a little baked ginger can transmit pungent and hot decoction into bitter and warm decoction, which has the rapid effect of taking in the efficient yang. Drinking alcohol is forbidden after vomiting, or consumptive disease will be formed. (Li Cong Pu Yi An)

In general, blood syndrome results from many causes such as affection by exopathogen and internal injury. In conclusion, its principal pathogenesis are burning and fumigating by fire heat, failure of qi to govern the blood and blood stasis obstructing the vessel. The fire can be divided into excess type and deficient type. In most cases, the fire of excess type includes lung heat, stomach heat, liver fire and heart fire, damp-heat in the intestine and heat burning in blood. The fire of deficient type includes hyperactivity of fire due to yin deficiency in the liver and kidney, or due to yin impairment in the lung or stomach. As to deficiency of qi, we should distinguish qi deficiency from yang deficiency due to qi deficiency. Deficiency of qi mainly includes deficiency of lung qi, spleen qi or kidney qi. Deficiency of yang mainly includes deficiency of spleen yang deficiency of both of spleen yang and or kidney yang. Blood stasis mainly results from stagnation of qi, deficiency of qi, retention of cold, accumulation of heat and the blood out of vessels. Excess syndromes and deficiency syndromes are the two aspects of blood syndrome. In most cases, excess syndrome results from excess of fire heat, deficiency syndrome results from hyperactivity of fire due to yin deficiency and failure of deficient qi to control the blood. To cure the blood syndrome, we should grasp the principle of stopping bleeding, treating the cause and consolidating the root, with the treatment of treating blood, qi and fire. To cure excess fire, clear away heat and purge fire. To cure deficient fire, nourish yin and lower fire. To cure sthenia qi, clear and low it. To cure deficient qi, reinforce it. Treating blood should aim at the symptoms of bleeding, combining he drugs for stop bleeding by astringent, cooling the blood, warm meridian or remove stasis, according to cause and nature of the disease. In the case of profuse hemorrhage, lower the fire directly or consolidate the exhaustion immediately. It is critical to decide whether the treatment focuses on symptom or the cause. The prognosis of blood syndrome has relation with three factors. The first factor is the cause of blood syndrome,. In most cases, blood syndrome caused by exopathogen and disease breaking out recently is easy to be cured; while caused by interior injury and prolong disease is difficult to be cured. The second factor is the amount of blood and whether the hemorrhage is acute or chronic. Hemorrhage with little blood and slow speed is slight, while with massive blood and in urgency is serious. We should pay attention to critical cases of exhaustion of qi following with blood due to profuse bleeding. The third factor is the accompanying symptom and the pulse. Hemorrhage accompanying with fever, dyspnea, restlessness, sweating, coldness in limbs and full, great or rapid pulse are in danger. After bleeding the patient will suffer from general debility. The treatment should be according to the various cases to deficiency of qi, yin and blood. Pay attention to the regular life, diet and emotion to prevent the relapse.

Questions for Review

1. What's the etiopathology and pathogenesis of blood syndrome?
2. Try to expound the key point of differentiation and treatment of blood syndrome.
3. How to treat the different types of epistaxis, hemoptysis, hematemesis, hematochezia and hematuria?
4. To cure the blood syndrome, how to select the prescription of Xie Xin Decoction, Yu Nu Decoction, Xi Jiao Di Huang Decoction, Xiao JI Yin Zi Decoction

and Di Yu Decoction?

5. As to cure the liver, the stomach and the spleen, try to expound the clinical symptom character of hematemesis.
6. How to differentiate the hematochezia due to deficiency of spleen and stomach and accumulated damp-heat? Expound their treatment and prescription, respectively.

Palpitation

〔Introduction〕

Palpitation involves pavor and severe palpitation which denote the subjective symptoms of the patients: pulsation, terror and unease, even involuntary feeling. Or concurrently, symptoms of corresponding changes of pulse condition, such as fast, rapid, running, knotted and infrequent pulses, appeared singly or simultaneously. It is usually paroxysmal in clinical practice and often caused by emotional stress or over-exertion. However, some of the patients are attacked persistently.

The symptoms of pavor and severe palpitation are either different or having inter-relations. In clinical practice, they may be differentiated by the cause and condition of illness, principal symptom and sign, and we can find their close relations by mutual transformation and influences.

The main symptoms and signs of palpitation are the subjective feelings of pulmus, pavor, unrest and inability of autonomy. The disease may simultaneously hold other symptoms as insomnia, dreaminess, dizziness, chest distress and asthma, precordial pain, infrequent, rapid or knotted pulse. The focus of the disease is at the heart, but it may affected the spleen, kidney, liver and lung. The pathogenesis is mostly deficiency in origin and excess in superficiality. The deficiency in origin manifested as insufficiency of qi, blood, yin and yang, and the excess syndrome includes the blockade of qi, stasis, phlegm and fluid in the circulation. The condition of illness is severe in general, but it may be manifested as prostration syndrome including cold limbs, sweating, weak pulse, unconsciousness and exhaustion of heat-yang.

In modern medicine, the arrhythmia caused by various causes, such as tachycardia, bradycardia, cardiataxia, auricular fibrillation and flutter, atrioventricular block, bundle-branch block (BBB), sick sinus syndrome (SSS), pre-excitation syndrome, heart failure, myocarditis, pericarditis and part neuroses may be treated on the basis of differentiation of symptoms and signs of traditional Chinese medicine.

〔Pathogenesis and Pathology〕

The formation of palpitation is related to the mental state, constitution and turbid pathogenic factors. The mental state includes pavor, depression and fury. The constitution factors include deficiency of heart-blood, kidney-yin, insufficiency of yang. The turbid pathogenic factors involve phlegm, fire, dampness, fluid, blood stasis and stagnancy of qi. The palpitation is caused by influencing each other and interacting of the three kinds of pathogenic factors.

The following are the common pathogenesis and pharmacology of palpitation in clinical practice.

Ⅰ. Lacking of self-confidence and timid: To those who are congenitally deficient and diffident and afraid of loud noise, strange things and dangerous situations, the disease is often occurred. In addition, the disease may also be induced by anger affected liver, great fright impaired kidney energy, because anger causes reversed flow of qi, terror leads to disorder of vital essence, thereby yin being deficient and fire flaring up and affecting the mental condition. Other pathogenic factors causing this disease involve accumulation of phlegm and heat plus anger, failure of descending of the stomach-qi and the combination of phlegm and fire to attack mind upwards.

Ⅱ. Insufficiency of heart-blood: The heart governs the blood circulation, and both the circulation of blood and nourishing the whole body depend upon the heart qi. Because of the spirit stored in the heart, the mind is arranged in order if the heart blood is abundant and the heart is nourished, otherwise the pavor and severe palpitation will occur. If there are congenital defects, deficiency in viscera, or lack of good care during convalescence, or anxiety impairing the heart and spleen, or weakness of the spleen and stomach, dysfunction of qi and blood, or excessive blood loss, these may lead to deficiency of heart-blood, failure to nourish the heart, disable to store the spirit, thus eventually to palpitation.

Ⅲ. Hyperactivity of fire caused by yin deficiency: Weakness and deficiency due to protracted illness, or intemperance in sexual life, or frequent emission, excessive pregnancy inducing deficiency of kidney-yin, discordance between water and fire, flaring-up of fire of deficiency type to disturb mind, all these lead to palpitation.

Ⅳ. Insufficiency of the heart-yang: The heart yang has the functions of maintaining normal physiological activities of the heart, promoting blood circulation, and assisting the spleen- and kidney-yang. The blood circulation would fail to act normally and the heart could not be nourished if the heart-yang and heart-qi are insufficient. Then the palpitation occurs.

Ⅴ. The excessive fluid invades the heart: The deficient spleen- and kidney-yang is unable to evaporate the fluid. The accumulation of water results in excessive fluid which will invade upwards, then the heart-yang will be inhibited. Or, owing to the insufficiency of heart-yang, the evaporation is blocked, the fluid is unable to move downwards and staying beneath the heart, hence resulting in palpitation. So as it said in the book "Shang Han Ming Li Lun. Ji", "Because of the water accumulated beneath the heart, the fire arose and avoided water, thereby leading to the retention of fluid, Since the retention of fluid has happened, the mind is no longer tranquil. Thus palpitation occurred."

Ⅵ. Blood stasis blocked channels: There are two causes of palpitation due to blockade of heart channel by blood stasis: first, heart channel blocked by obstruction of blood circulation, second, long-standing stagnation-syndrome of qi and blood develops to palpitation. The combating between wind-cold and dampness pathogens in the blood vessels attacked heart, the resulted obstruction led to the stagnation of blood channels, then causing palpitation. It said in the book "Su Wen. Bi Lun", "The continuous stagnation of channels and being infected by pathogenic factors invade the heart" and "The so called stagnation is caused by obstruction of blood vessels, and restlessness causes heart beating. It was explained in"Yi Zong Bi Du. Ji "that" the heart beating is like beating drums.

To sum up, the location of palpitation is in the heart and is closely related to spleen, kidney, liver and lung. The characteristics of its pathogenesis is perturbed feeling. The causes of pathogenesis involve two aspects, deficiency and excess. The "deficiency" denotes vital-qi, i. e., deficiency in yin yang, qi and blood. These led to the loss of nourishment of the heart and the functions of circulating and mental governing. The "excess" denotes the blockade of heart channel by the accumulation of qi, phlegm and fluid, and blood stasis thus the heart-qi is inhibited and the circulation obstructed. The deficiency and excess can be both in acting of transform each other. If the excess syndrome prolonged, vital-qi will be deficient and yin, yang, qi and blood all entering into insufficient states. The deficiency syndrome is often mixed up with phlegm-heat. The deficiency of yang and retention of water induce the accumulation of phlegm retention, then the fluid retention attacks the heart. So the deficiency of yang is often mixed up with phlegm retention. The deficiency of qi and the blood brings about obstruction of the circulation hence inducing blood stasis. The interior accumulation of phlegm-fire which burns the fluid to impair yin will result in yin deficiency and accumulation of water. The abundant accumulation of coldness of the genitals impairs the yang to bring about yang deficiency. The attention should be paid to the regulations of the mixing and transforming each other of deficiency and excess syndromes during the process of diagnosis and treatment based on overall analysis of symptoms and signs.

〔Diagnosis and Treatment by Differentiation of Syndromes〕

Ⅰ. Key points of the differentiation

1. Differentiation of the deficiency or excess of the superficiality and origin In the case deficiency of origin, the heart-qi, -blood, -yin and -yang should be carefully observed to see which is the most important. If the disease showed excess of superficiality, we should observe which of the phlegm, fluid, water, fire, blood stasis and pathogenic factors is the principal thing. It is important to differentiate comprehensive characteristics of palpitation and both pulse condition and syndromes.

(1) Characteristics of palpitation: In the case of deficiency of heart-qi and heart-yang, the syndromes are pavor, shortness of breath, exacerbated after exercise. If it deficiency of heart-blood and heart-yin, the syndromes are fidgeting with pavor, exacerbated when over depressed. Common heat syndromes of the excess type manifested as mental disturbance due to phlegm-fire includes palpitation, restlessness, dysphoria in the chest, sleeplessness and dreaminess. In the case of phlegm moving upwards, it showed liable to anger, frightened, distension and discomfort in chest and hypochondrium. The palpitation caused by upward attacking of the pathogenic fluid showed dizziness, frightening, discomfort in chest, asthma and/or edema. The palpitation caused by blood stasis manifested as pavor mostly with precordial pain, obstruction of qi in the chest, dark purple lips

and tongue proper, or sometimes ecchymosis.

(2) Comprehensive analysis of both pulse condition and pulse syndromes The pulses of accumulation of phlegm-fire involve rapid and strong slippery, and that of hyperactivity of fire due to yin deficiency are thread, rapid and weak. Infrequent pulse denotes cold syndrome and that of weak deep infrequent and weak means yang deficiency and interior cold.

Knotted and intermittent pulse: The so called knotted and intermittent pulse is the joint name of running, knotted and intermittent, appeared singularly or in combination. The pulse is occasionally occurred in healthy people when they are in low spirit or sorrowful situation. In this circumstances the pulse condition will disappear in a short time. If the patient with palpitation shows knotted and intermittent pulse, it may be caused by insufficiency of qi and blood and obstruction of heart-blood. In case of this symptom occurred in patients with severe palpitation, it means the exhaustion of heart-qi. When knotted and intermittent recovered gradually to normal state, it means the heart-qi is recovering. When knotted and intermittent pulse exacerbated and stop beating gradually and appeared coma and convulsion, that means the critical and dangerous state of heart failure approaching.

In the differentiation of palpitation, attention must be paid to the combination or mixing of deficiency and excess syndromes, because in many of the syndromes, deficiency in origin often mixed up with excessive superficiality. For examples, the deficiency of heart-qi is often concomitant with blood stasis and excessive fluid, the deficiency of heart and blood and of heart-yin is often mixed up with heat of deficiency type and phlegm-fire.

2. Differentiation of mild, serious and critical palpitation If the disease is caused by exogenous factors and paroxysmal with short duration and spontaneous remission, it is confirmed as mild disease. If it is not induced by exogenous factors and the palpitation is persistent and accompanying with asthma, edema, precordial pain, cold feeling of extremities and dizziness, it can be confirmed as serious disease. If the symptoms and signs manifested as excessive perspiration, cold limbs dark purple lips, weak respiration and pulse, even vague mind, it is confirmed as critical or dangerous disease of almost cutting off of heart-yang.

3. Differentiation the differences and interrelations of pavor and severe palpitation

(1) Differences: Pavor and severe palpitation are of the same category of diseases but they are different in some aspects. In general, savere palpitation is caused by endogenous factors rather than exogenous terror. The patient is vigilant. The disease is attacking after light labor or exercise and manifested as general asthenia and relatively serious condition. On the contrary, pavor is usually caused by exogenous stimulation, frightening or anger. The disease is manifested as palpitation, occurred intermittently. Though the attacking of the disease is fast, the general condition is good and the illness is mild and transient.

(2) Interrelations: On the one hand, the pavor may be developed into severe palpitation with the passing time, and on the other hand, the patients with severe palpitation are liable to be attacked by exogenous frightful things, hence exacerbating the illness.

Ⅱ. Treatment by differentiation of types and syndromes

The location of palpitation is in the heart and the characteristics of the syndrome is mixed deficiency and excess with deficiency as the principle aspect. Therefore, invigorating qi is the main principle of treatment. Therapeutic methods of supplementing qi, nourishing blood, nourishing yin and warming yang should be employed according to the difference of the conditions of qi, blood, yin yang and deficiency, so as to subdue yang hyperactivity and promote the circulation of qi and blood. The commonly encountered pathogenic factors of the disease are phlegm-fire, fluid and blood stasis. So the therapeutic methods employed may be resolving phlegm and purging fire, resolving phlegm and removing fluid, promoting blood circulation to remove blood stasis, respectively. To those cases of mixed deficiency and excess with complex conditions, the treatment should be based on the differentiation of the important from the less important syndromes, and the urgent from the less urgent conditions, so as we can treat with the method of both invigorating qi and eliminating pathogenic factors, or lay particular emphasis on one or another. Since the palpitation and restlessness are the main clinical symptoms of the disease, we often use drugs or prescriptions of relieving palpitation, tranquilization and nourishing heart in addition to the methods of invigorating qi and eliminating pathogenic factors.

Diagram of the Causes and Pathogenesis

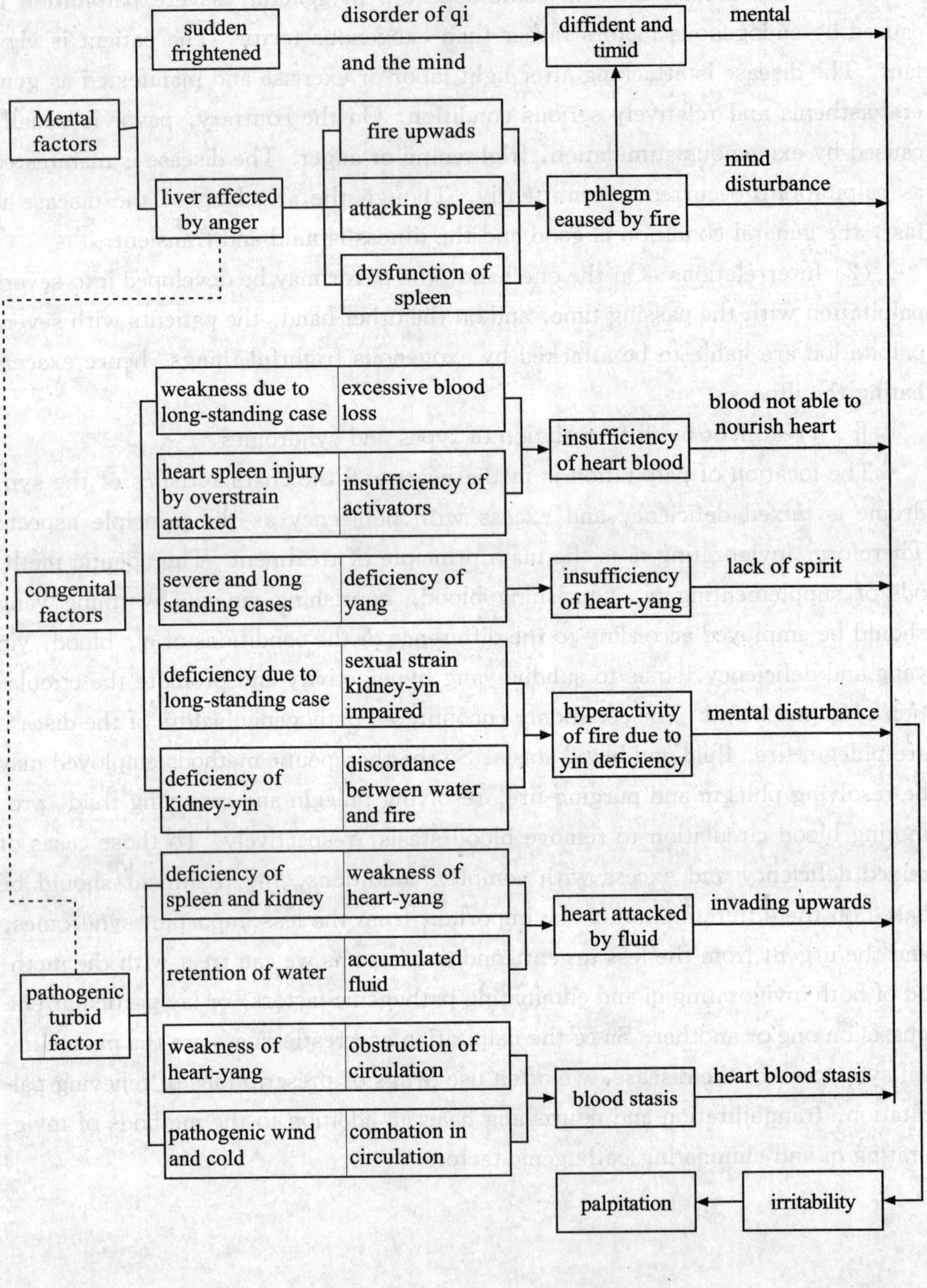

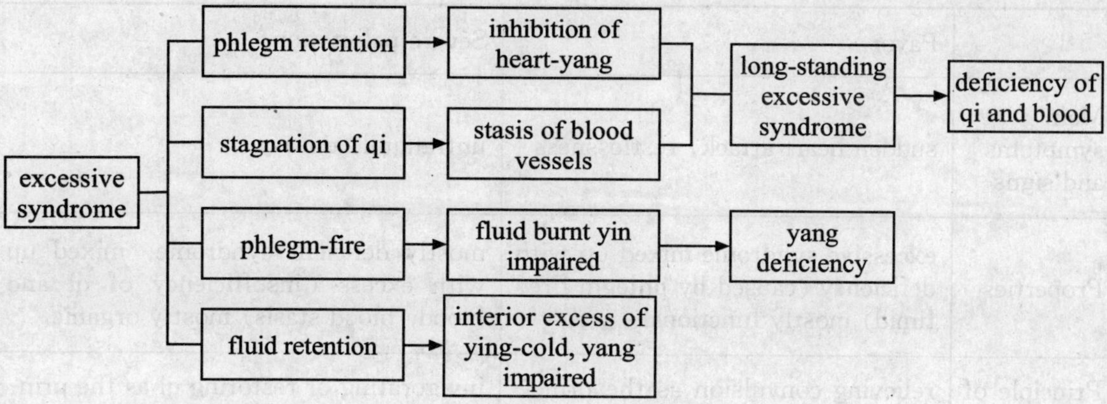

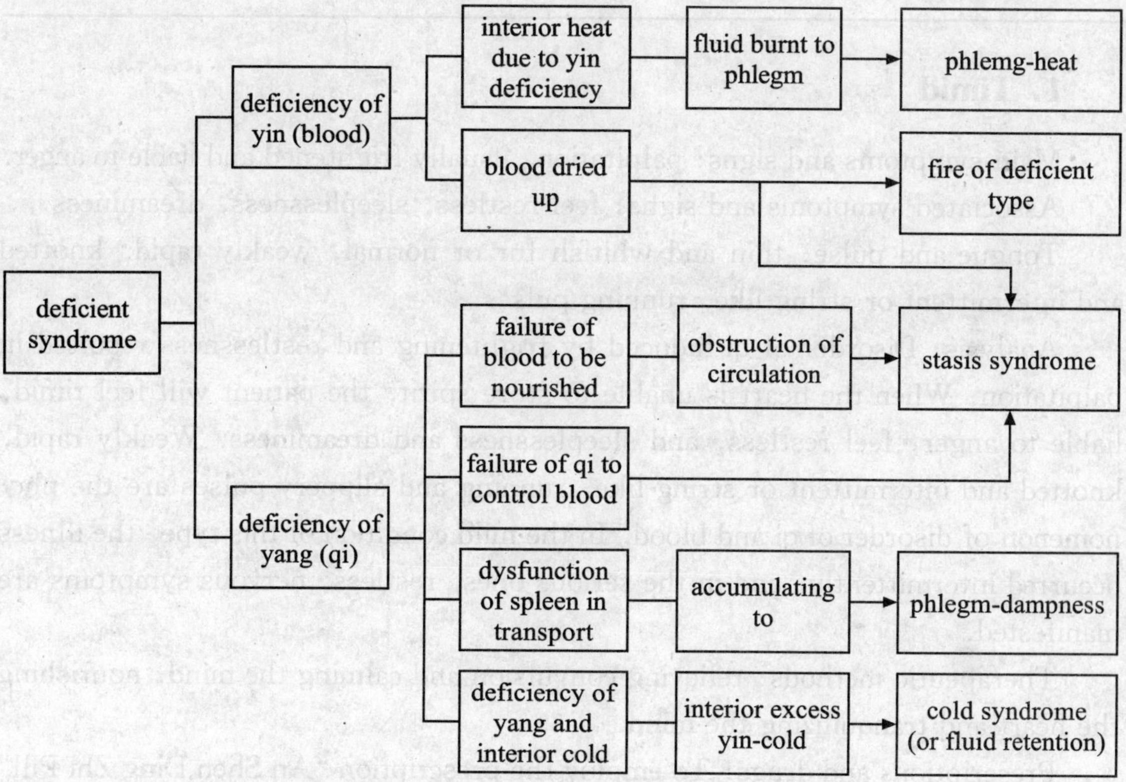

Differentiation of Pavor and Severe Palpitation

	Pavor	Severe palpitation
Causes	attacking mostly by exogenous factors (frighten, anger) (usually timid)	attacking mostly by endogenous factors (usually deficiency in viscera) long-standing cases, labor and exercise)
Condition	mild, good therapeutic efficacy, spontaneous remission	relatively poor therapeutic efficacy, attacking persistently

	Pavor	Severe palpitation
Main symptoms and signs	sudden heart attack, restlessness	untranquil, uneasy
Properties	excessive syndrome mixed up with deficiency (caused by phlegm-fire, timid) mostly functional	mostly deficient syndrome, mixed up with excess (insufficiency of qi and blood, blood stasis) mostly organic
Principle of treatment	relieving convulsion as the principle	invigorating or restoring qi as the principle

1. Timid

Main symptoms and signs: palpitation, usually frightened and liable to anger.

Associated symptoms and signs: feel restless, sleeplessness, dreaminess.

Tongue and pulse: thin and whitish fur or normal, weakly rapid, knotted and intermittent or string-like, running pulses.

Analysis: Disorder of qi induced by frightening and restlessness resulted in palpitation. When the heart is unable to store spirit, the patient will feel timid, liable to anger, feel restless, and sleeplessness and dreaminess. Weakly rapid, knotted and intermittent or string-like, running and slippery pulses are the phenomenon of disorder of qi and blood. In the mild condition of this type, the illness occurred intermittently, and in the serious ones, restless, nervous symptoms are manifested.

Therapeutic methods: relieving convulsion and calming the mind, nourishing the heart and tranquilizing the mind.

Prescriptions and drugs: To employ the prescription "An Shen Ding Zhi Pill" compound with amber, magnetite and cinnabar. Use dragon's teeth, amber and magnetite to relieve convulsion and mental stress. Use cinnabar mixing poria with hostwood, grassleaved sweetflag rhizome and polygala root to tranquil mind, and ginseng (or pilose asiabell root) to nourish the heart qi. Ginseng will not be used if deficiency of qi is not apparent. In the case of restless and timid symptoms, add prepared licorice root to nourish heart-qi. If heart-yin is insufficient, add arborvitae seed, schisandra fruit and wild jujuba seed to nourish heart, tranquilize and restrain the mind. If the patient feels restless and unduly rapid action of the heart, and shows the symptoms as: frighten, excessive sputum, poor appetite, nausea, yellow and greasy tongue fur, rapid pulse, the symptoms are caused by phlegm inward invading, failure of descending of the stomach-qi, and restlessness. In this case, the prescription "Huang Lian Wen Dan Decoction" is used to reduce phlegm-heat, normalize the functions of stomach and spleen, and send down the turbid pathogen. The heart is tranquilized as a matter of course after the phlegm eliminated. Adding jujuba seed and polygala root in the prescription is helpful for tranquilizing and normalizing the heart.

Example of prescriptions: magnetite (pre-decocted) 30g, grassleaved sweetflag rhizome 10g, polygala root 10g, poria with hostwood 10g, red sage root 10g, pseudostellaria root 12g, prepared licoric root 8g, crude dragon's bone and oyster shell shell 15g (pre-decocted), cinnabar (mixed).

2. Insufficiency of heart blood

Main symptoms and signs: palpitation, dizziness, asthenia.

Associated symptoms and signs: dim complexion, tiredness, fatigue.

Tongue and pulse: light red tongue proper, thin and weak pulse.

Analysis: Insufficiency of heart blood and failure to nourish the heart lead to palpitation. Owing to the deficiency of heart blood, the brain could not be nourished, thus resulting in dizziness. The heart is in charge of the blood circulation, and the complexion reflects the condition of the heart. So, deficiency of blood leading to dim complexion and deficiency of blood and weak qi result in fatigue and tiredness. The tongue is as the sprout of the heart and the heart governs the blood circulation, thus when heart blood is insufficient the tongue proper will be light red and the pulse thin and weak.

Therapeutic methods: enriching blood and nourishing heart, invigorating qi and tranquilizing the mind.

Prescriptions and drugs: "Modified Gui Pi Decoction" is recommended. Chinese angelia root and longan aril in the prescription have the functions of invigorating qi and enriching blood. The actions of ginseng, astragalus root, white atractylodes rhizome and prepared licorice involve replenishing qi to invigorate the spleen thereby promoting generation of the blood. The functions of wild jujuba seed, poria with hostwood and polygala root involve tranquilizing and calming the mind. If the prescription is supplemented with aucklandia root that promotes the the flow of qi, it will have the function of replenishment without obstruction.

Modification: In treating the palpitation with knotted and intermittent pulse that is caused by deficiency of qi, lack of blood and failure of blood to replenish the heart, "Zhi Gan Cao Decoction" is used to invigorate qi and enrich blood, nourish yin and restore pulse.

In this prescription, prepared licorice of warm property possesses the functions of restoring pulse, promoting heart-qi. Ginseng and date have the functions of reinforcing the stomach, cinnamon twig and fresh ginger of pungent flavor and warm property, activating yang; rehmannia root, donkey-hide gelatin, ophipogon root and hemp seed, nourishing yin and enriching blood, thereby replenishing the vital essence. The compatibility of these drugs results in the activities of supplying qi and blood, thus curing the palpitation and the symptoms of knotted and intermittent pulse. In the later stage (anaphase) of febrile disease caused by impaired heart-yin, the prescription "Sheng Mai Powder" may be used. In this prescription, the functions of invigorating the premordial energy of ginseng, nourishing yin of ophiopogon root and astringing the dispersed lung-qi, make it has the activities of supplementing qi and nourishing yin.

Example of prescription: pilose asiabell root 10g, prepared astragalus root 12g, white atractylodes rhizome 8g, poria with hostwood 10g, polygala root 10g, ophiopogon root 10g, schisandra fruit 8g, prepared licorice 20g.

3. Hyperactivity of fire due to yin deficiency

Tongue and Pulse: Red tongue with less coating or no coating, thin and rapid pulse.

Main symptoms and signs: palpitation, unease, vexation, sleeplessness

Associated symptoms and signs: feverish sensation in the palms and soles, soreness of waist, tinnitus, dizziness, and thin.

Analysis: The symptoms of palpitation, vexation and sleeplessness are caused by insufficiency of kidney-yin, incoordinate between water and fire hence heart-fire flammed and the mind disturbed. Deficiency of yin in the lower part of the body induces soreness of waist and the disturbance of yang in the upper part of the body results in dizziness, tinnitus and feverish sensation in the palms and soles. The syndrome of yin deficiency and hyperactivity of fire is manifested as red tongue proper and thin rapid pulse.

Therapeutic method: nourishing yin and purging fire, nourishing yin and tranquilizing the mind.

Prescriptions and drugs: "Modified Tian Wang Bu Xin Pill" and "Modified

Zhu Sha An Shen pill" are used because they both have the functions of nourishing yin, enriching blood, clearing away heat-fire and tranquilizing the mind. The former prescription is applied to the patients with deficiency of yin and minor fire invasion. In the prescription drugs as dried rehmannia root, figwort root, ophipogon root and astragalus root have the functions of nourishing yin and clearing away heat, red sage root and Chinese angelica root enriching blood and nourishing heart; ginseng nourishing the heart-qi; cinnabar, poria with hostwood, polygala root, jujuba seed and aborvitae seed nourishing heart and tranquilizing the mind; schisandra fruit restraining heart-qi; platycodon root guiding upward flow of the drugs to activate the heart-qi. The prescription "Zhu Sha An Shen Pill" is suitable for treating the patients with heat symptoms of fidgeting, dry throat, bitter taste in the mouth. The Chinese angelia root and fresh rehmannia root in the prescription posses the functions of nourishing the blood and yin, rhubarb tranquilizing the mind by clearing away heart-fire. The compatibility of these drugs makes the prescription has the activities of purging the heart-fire, nourishing heart-yin, heart blood and calming the mind. The prescription is commonly used for treating the symptoms of restlessness and vexation.

Modification: In the case of hyperactivity of fire due to yin deficiency mixed up with dysphoria with feverish sensation in chest, palms and soles, nocturnal emission and soreness of waist cause by deficiency of yin and hyperactivity of the ministerial fire, the prescription "Zhi Bai Di Huang Pill" may be used to nourish yin and removing fire.

Example of prescriptions: ophiopogon root 10g, schisandra fruit 10g, fresh rehmannia 12g, adenophora root 12g, figwort root 12g, red sage root 12g, pseudostellaria root 10g, flavescent sophora root 10g, prepared licorice root 8g.

4. Insufficiency of heart-yang

Main symptoms and signs: palpitation, restlessness, oppressed feeling in chest, short-breathing.

Associated symptoms and signs: pale complexion, cold limbs.

Tongue and pulse: light whitish tongue proper, weak or deep thin or deep, infrequent, knotted or intermittent pulse.

Analysis: The heart-yang is impaired by prolonged illness, failure of heart to be nourished. The symptoms of oppressed feeling in chest and short breathing are caused by insufficiency of yang in the chest. The insufficiency of heart yang, slow moving of the blood circulation and the extremities not being warmed lead to the cold limbs and pale complexion. All of the symptoms of light whitish tongue proper, or feeble thin and weak pulse are the syndromes of insufficiency of heart-yang and lack of energy activation.

Therapeutic methods: warming the heart-yang, tranquilizing the mind and arresting palpitation.

Prescriptions and drugs: "Modified Gui Zhi Gan Cao Long Gu Mu Li Decoction" is used. Cinnamon twig and licorice root activate the heart-yang for their warm nature. Dragon's bone and oyster shell tranquilize the mind and arrest palpitation. Addition of ginseng and prepared aconite root in the prescription is helpful to warm the yang and invigorate qi.

Modification: If the disease condition of the patient is severe and manifested as perspiration, cold limbs, dark complexion, purple lips, and asthma being too rapid to lie down, put ginseng and prepared aconite root in large amount and add "Heo Xi Pill" to recuperate the depleted yang and rescue the patient from collapse. If the patient shows the syndrome of nearly exhaustion of heart-yang, unease, palpitating, deep infrequent pulse, serios cold limbs, the condition being deficiency of both heart, kidney and yang, excessive cold of yin type. In this circumstance, "Ma Huang Fu Zi Xi Xin Decoction" with pilose asiabell root and prepared licorice root should be used for the treatment.

Example of prescription: prepared aconite root 6g, cinnomon twig 10g, astragalus root 12g, Siberian slolomonseal rhizome 12g, prepared licorice 10g, dragon's bone and oyster shell 15g each, ginseng powder 3g (mixing) (or pilose asiabell root 10g), Chinese angelica root 10g, dried ginger 6g.

5. Attacking of heart by excessive fluid

Main symptoms and signs: palpitating, oppressed feeling in the chest, dyspnea, edema.

Associated symptoms and signs: dizziness, cold limbs, feeling of stuffiness and fullness in the chest, oliguria, thirst, nausea and vomiting of water fluid.

Tongue and pulse: whitish and slippery tongue fur, taut and slippery pulse.

Analysis: Water and fluid are yin pathogens and can be only removed by yang-qi. Owing to the failure of deficient yang to remove water, the fluid is accumulated within the body, then attacking upwards the heart thus palpitation occurred. And, the oppressed feeling in chest is due to the substitution of yin pathogen for yang. Asthma and cough are caused by attacking of the heart and lung by fluid. The disturbance of qi transformation and retention of water within the body lead to thirst, oliguria or edema in legs. When the yang-qi could not circulate through the limbs and attain the skin, the patient feels cold in limbs. Dizziness is caused by the obstruction of fluid and failure of the lucid yang to rise. The disorder of qi leads to the feeling of stuffiness and fullness in the chest. The whitish and slippery tongue fur and taut, slippery pulse denote the retention of water as well.

Therapeutic methods: activating the heart-yang, promoting the circulation of qi to induce diuresis.

Prescriptions and drugs: "Modified Ling Gui Zhu Gan Decoction" is used. The functions of the drugs in the prescription are as follows: poria cocos as a bland drug, inducing diuresis; cinnamon twig and licorice root, activating yang and promoting the circulation of qi: and white atractylodes rhizome, invigorating the spleen and removing dampness.

Modifications: Addition of pinellia tuber, tangerine peel and fresh ginger is used for treating the patient with adverse rising of fluid, nausea and vomiting. In the case of deficiency of kidney-yang, attacking of heart by fluid, and severe symptoms of palpitating and asthma, oliguria and severe edema, "Modified Zhen Wu Decoction" should be used to warm the yang and promote the water circulation. The prescription "Modified Chun Ze Decoction" can be used to treat the symptoms of deficiency of spleen-qi, retention of excessive fluid, syndrome of attacking of heart by retained water, palpitating, edema, fatigue and asthenia. This prescription is a modification of "Wu Ling Powder" by adding ginseng, hence possessing the functions of replenishing qi and invigorating spleen, promoting the circulation of qi and inducing diuresis.

Example of prescription: pilose asiabell root 12g, prepared aconite root 6g, cinnomon twig 10g, poria cocos 12g, umbellate pore fungus 15g, alisma orientale 12g, white atractylodes rhizome 10g, prepared licorice root 5g, perilla fruit 6g, fresh ginger 3 pieces.

6. Stagnation of the heart blood

Main symptoms and signs: palpitaitng, restlessness, paroxysmal precordial pain.

Associated symptoms and signs: oppressed feeling in chest, unease, dark purple lips and nails.

Tongue and pulse: dark purple tongue proper, or ecchymosis, knotted, intermittent or uneven pulse.

Analysis: Since the heart is in charge of blood circulation, the obstruction of circulation and failure of heart to be nourished will lead to palpitation. The stuffiness feeling in chest is caused by blood stasis, stagnation of qi and restraining of heart-yang. The stagnation of blood vessels and subjective sensation of contraction result in precordial pain. When the vessels and channels have been stagnated, dark purple lips, nails and tongue proper, ecchymosis, uneven, knotted, intermittent pulse occurred. All these are belonging to the syndromes of accumulation of blood stasis and obstruction of heart-yang.

Therapeutic methods: removing blood stasis by promoting blood circulation.

Prescriptions and drugs: "Modified Tao Ren Hong Hua Decoction" is used. In the prescription, peach kernel, safflower, red sage root, red peony root and chuanxiong rhizome have functions of removing blood stasis and promoting blood circulation; corydalis tuber cyperus tuber and green tangerine orange peel promoting the circulation of qi and blood; dried rehmnnia root, Chinese angelica root enriching blood and promoting the blood circulation.

Modifications: Addition of cinnamon twig and licorice root to the prescription is helpful to activate yang-qi. Add dragon's bone and oyster shell to tranquilize the mind. All these drugs used in combination make the blood circulation unobstructed and the palpitation and pain cured. In the case of stagnancy of phlegm dampness associated with the symptoms of excessive phlegm, nausea, loss of appetite, mass in the abdomen, thick greasy tongue fur and slippery pulse, this prescription may be used in combination with the prescription "Gua Lou Xie Bai Ban Xia Decoction" to soothe the chest oppression and resolve sputum.

Example of prescription: red sage root 15g, red peony root 10g, Chuanxiong rhizome 10g, safflower 10g, trichosanthes fruit 20g, macrostem onion 6g, pinellia tuber 10g, pilose asiabell root 10g, curcuma root 10g, corydalis tuber 10g.

In summary, the palpitation is a disease which manifested as self-conscious palpitating involuntarily. The disease may be differentiated into two types: pavor and severe palpitation. In clinical, six syndromes of it have been observed, i. e., diffident and timid, insufficiency of heart-fire, deficiency of yin and hyperactivity of fire, insufficiency of heart-yang, excessive fluid attacking the heart and stagnation of the heart blood. Each syndrome has its own characteristics. In clinical practice, the disease is treated and diagnosed by differentiating the syndromes carefully, so as to attain proper curative effect.

〔Measures of Prevention and Nursing〕

1. Keep the mind in a cheerful state and avoid sick at heart. pavor is often caused by mind injury and being frightened. Keeping one's mind in a happy mood regularly will avoid the injury of the mind and prevent the onset of the disease.

2. Being moderate in eating and drinking and lead a regular daily life. Don't eat and drink too much at a meal. Eat less pungent, spicy and greasy food. Keep a regular life. Ensure regular rest and sleep and strike a proper balance between work and rest.

3. Pay attention to the changes of cold and hot weather to avoid the attacking of exogenous pathogenic factors. Avoid the attack or exacerbation of the palpitation induced by exogenous pathogenic factors, such as wind, cold, dampness and heat.

4. To those patients with mild illness, proper exercise is necessary. Avoid strenuous exercise, physical exertion. Don't be overworked. To those patients with severe illness conditions, as usually palpitating, short breath, even edema of face and limbs, the bed rest is necessary.

5. Therapy with drugs is very important for the patients. During the treatment, the patients have to take medicines persistently and continue medication after the remission of the illness condition follow the doctor's advice or medical order.

〔Analysis of Typical Cases〕

Case 1. Chen, male, age 50. suffered from hypertension for twenty years, dizziness and light headedness in recent five to six years, restlessness exacerbated. Examination: heart rate 58/min., blood pressure 170/100mmHg, obesity, purple lips, lung(—), apex beat, 1.5cm beyond midclavicular line, having apex impules, absolute arrhythmia, systolic numbling murmur heard at apex, miosphygmia, Diagnosis of western medicine: ① phase Ⅲ hypertension; ②hypertensive cardiopathy; ③ coronary heart disease complicated with atrial fibrillation; ④ heart failure Ⅱ°, treated by western medicine for a long time, no significant improvement, later onset of serious condition after exercise: stuffiness in chest, short breath, mouth breathing, dizziness, frontal hidrorrhea, after the emergency treatment of western medicine, the condition is still dangerous. Later, Doctor Xiao was invited to treat the patient. Syndromes: palpitating, restlessness, dizziness, fatigue and rest on bed, low and timid speech, pale complexion, dry lips, sleepless, infrequent, knotted and intermittent pulse. Differentiation of the syndromes: insufficiency of heart-yang, deficiency of both qi and yin. Treatment principles: warming and activating the heart-yang, invigorating qi and nourishing yin. Prescribe: prepared aconite root 9g, cinnamon bark 4g, ophiopogon root 12g, pilose asiabell root 20g, schisandra fruit 9g, prepared Siberian solomonseal rhizome 15g. The prescription was modified during the treatment and the illness condition has abated on return visit, early heart beat and diffident syndromes disappeared, state of mind improved, able to walk a short distance. ("Jiangxi Zhong Yi Yao", 1983:2)

Comment: The syndrome of the case belongs to the palpitation with deficiency of both yin and yang. The syndromes of heart-yin deficiency, failure of heart to be enriched cause nervous, dizziness, insufficiency of heart-yang, so appeared the stuffiness in chest, palpitating and infrequent, knotted and intermittent pulse. Use pilose asiabell root, schisandra fruit and ophiopogon root in the prescription to invigorate qi and nourish yin, promote the production of body fluid and restore pulse, prepared aconite root and cinnamon bark of pungent and heat nature to supplement the fire from the gate of life and heart-yang; Siberian solomonseal rhizome of sweet taste to nourish spleen-yin, invigorate the qi of middle energizer, moisten the viscera. The drug Siberian solomonseal rhizome is an excellent drug for nourishing yin and invigorating qi. The whole prescription has the functions of warming yang and promoting qi without impairing yin, replenishing yang and enriching heart without injuring the stomach. The compatibility of the prescription possesses the features of strictness, efficacy and containing only few drugs within it.

The palpitation is the disease that manifested as self-conscious diffident and heart beating involuntarily. It is differentiated into two syndromes: pavor and severe palpitation. The main causes of the illness include deficiency of qi, blood, yin and yang or inherent defect, or dysfunctioning of viscera due to prolonged illness, mind impaired and invading of exogenous pathogenic factors. These three causes influence each other and have reciprocal causation on the other hand. There is relationship between the principal and subcordinate syndromes, and the root cause being the constitution factor (health). The location of the disease is at the heart but often in close relation to other viscera. The pharmacological changes involve nothing more than deficiency and excess. The deficiency syndrome manifested as failure of heart to be nourished due to deficiency of qi, blood, yin and yang. The excess syndrome manifested as the stagnation of vessels and channels by blood stasis which causes obstruction of circulation and restlessness. One of the two syndromes is often mingled with the other, or vice versa. The deficiency syndrome is often associated with stagnation of phlegm, excessive fluid or blood stasis. The excess syndrome is often mixed up with the deficiency of viscera. The relation of the two syndromes changes along with the changes of the illness condition and they can transform mutually.

The syndrome differentiation of the palpitation should first differentiate deficiency or excess in origin and superficiality according to the features of palpitation and pulse, the second differentiate the illness condition, mild, severe or dangerous, and the third, differentiate the difference and relationship of pavor and severe palpitation.

The syndrome of the palpitation can be divided clinically into six types, i. e., diffident and timid, insufficiency of heart-blood, hyperactivity of fire due to yin deficiency, insufficiency of heart-yang, excessive fluid invading the heart, and stagnation of the heart blood. The therapeutic methods include nothing more than tranquilizing, nourishing, relieving and warming. Diffident and timid syndrome should be treated with the method of nourishing heart and tranquilizing the mind; insufficiency of heart blood, with enriching blood and nourishing the heart, invigorating qi and tranquilizing the mind; hyperactivity of fire due to yin deficiency, with nourishing yin to reduce pathogenic fire and nourishing heart and tranquilizing; insufficiency of heart-yang, with warming and recuperating the heart-yang, tranquilizing mind and relieving convulsion; excessive fluid invading heart, with activating heart-yang, promoting qi and diuresis; the stagnation of the heart blood, with removing blood stasis to promote blood circulation, regulating the flow of qi and removing obstruction in the channels. Since the main symptoms is palpitating and unease, the prescription and drugs used should contain those for nourishing heart, calming mind or tranquilization with heavy materials. The heavy materials for tranquilization can not be used for long time.

In the initial stage of palpitation, the treatment is easy for the illness condition is mild and the deficiency syndrome is not serious. If the disease prolonged, been not treated or mistreated, viscera will be attacked. In the case of body resistance weakened while pathogenic factors prevailing and the illness condition is serious, the cure will be difficult. If prostration or exhaustion of heart- and kidney-yang appeared, prompt rescue treatment is needed.

Questions for Review

1. Describe the causes and pathogenesis of the palpitation.
2. Describe the differences and relations between pavor and severe palpitation.
3. What are the six types of palpitation commonly encountered in clinical practice? How to treat them according to the diagnosis and differentiation of the syndromes?

Pectoral pain and Stuffiness

(Obstruction of qi and blood in the chest)

〔Introduction〕

Pectoral pain and stuffiness is the disease caused by stagnation of qi and blood in the chest. The main symptoms of the disease manifested as chest and back pain, short breathing, asthma, even disabling to lie down when it is in serious condition. In the cases of mild illness condition, the patient feels chest pain and breathe with difficulty. Chest pain and palpitating occur in serious cases and precordial pain, back pain, cold feeling in limbs in more serious cases.

Pectoral pain and stuffiness is different from stomach-ache and chest pain. They may be differentiated by the site of pain, associated symptoms, electrocardiogram, x-ray and other physical and chemical examinations.

The site of pectoral pain and stuffiness is at the heart and lung and the onset of the disease is related to liver, spleen and kidney. The causes of it are mainly the impairment or attack by exogenous pathogenic cold and heat, emotions, diet, over-exertion, bleeding and emission. The characteristics of the pathogenesis of pectoral pain and stuffiness is deficiency in origin and excess in superficiality. The manifestation of deficiency of origin is the deficiency of qi, blood, yin and yang of the viscera, and of the excess of superficiality, stagnation of qi and blood, accumulation of phlegm, and excessive cold and heat stagnation. The basic pathogenesis is the stagnation of qi and blood caused by insufficiency or obstruction of the heart, vessels and channels. Along with the development of the illness condition, the crisis as cardialgia, exhaustion, palpitation, asthma and cough, edema of limbs occurred.

The precordial pain induced by coronary atherosclerotic cardiopathy, angina pectoris, myocardiac infarction and pericarditis in western medicine can be diagnosed and treated in the light of the disease described in this chapter.

〔Pathogenesis and Pathology〕

The site of the pectoral pain and stuffiness is in the heart and lung. The chest is the "dwelling place" of heart and lung. The heart governs the blood circulation and the lung is in charge of qi. Provided that the heart acts in coordination with the lung, the qi and blood will normally circulate. The onset of the disease is closely related to health conditions of kidney, liver and spleen. The pectoral pain and stuffiness will be attacked by the following pathogenic conditions: insufficiency of chest-yang, dysfunction in viscera, failing of yin, yang, qi and blood to coordinate, infection of exogenous pathogenic factors, excessive eating, drinking and contemplation, stagnation of phlegm-dampness, and the vessels and channels being not in harmony. The pathogenesis and pathology are summarized as follows:

Ⅰ. Attacking of heart by heat and cold pathogenic factors: The pectoral pain and stuffiness may be caused by congenital insufficiency of heart-qi, and heart-yang, and later invading of cold pathogen which then accumulated in chest, resulting in insufficiency of heart-yang and stagnation of vessels and channels. Therefore the disease is often occurred when the weather is suddenly changing to cold. The yang insufficiency in origin involves deficiency of heart-qi, heart-yang and of the spleen and kidney. The superficiality is excessive cold. As for the origin and superficiality, we must differentiate carefully which is the primary from which is the secondary. In addition, invading of heart by extreme hot weather, then exhaustion of heart-qi also induce cardialgia due to the obstruction of blood circulation.

Ⅱ. Impairing of the seven emotions: Anxiety and anger often cause the stagnation of qi, and the obstructions of qi and blood circulation results in cardialgia. The fluid may accumulated and burnt into phlegm, or prolonged stagnation of qi changed to fire which will burn the fluid into phlegm. All of the stagnation of phlegm in vessels and channels, accumulation and obstruction of qi and blood, insufficiency of chest-yang will result in pectoral pain and stuffiness.

Ⅲ. Excessive eating and drinking: Excessive eating of fat, sweet and greasy food, or pungent and spicy foodstuff, or having an addiction to wine will cause the impairment and dysfunction of the spleen and stomach. The indigestion of foodstuff induce the formation of phlegm which blocked the vessels and channels, thus the condition of the stagnation of qi and blood stasis and the obstruction of vessels and channels result in pectoral pain and stuffiness.

Ⅳ. Insufficiency of qi and blood: The syndrome manifested as anxiety and over-exertion impairing the heart and spleen, vital qi not been restored during the convalescence of serious illness, dysfunction of the spleen and stomach, lacking of the source to generate qi and blood. The deficiency of qi and blood causes the heart failing to be nourished. When a patient has a great blood loss, his heart will not be nourished and the blood circulation obstructed, thus occurred the pectoral pain and stuffiness. Insufficiency of qi and blood in the heart and not been restored for a long time will cause insufficiency of heart-yang. The situation of deactivation of lucid yang and slow flow of the blood will eventually result in cardialgia. If the insufficiency of qi and blood in heart could not be recovered for a long time, it will cause deficiency of yin and blood, thus the blood vessels are disable to be nourished and manifested as contracture and pain.

Ⅴ. Deficiency of liver and kidney: Multiple pregnancy and emission can cause impairment of kidney-qi, ages over 50 will gradually induce weakening of sexual function of both sexes. Owing to the liver and kidney having a common source, insufficiency of yin and essence of life will not nourish the viscera-yin, hence resulting in deficiency of heart-yin, pectoral pain and stuffiness and cardialgaia. If there is hyperactivity of fire due to yin deficiency and the fire of deficiency type flaring up, the heart-yin may also be burnt and lead to the exhaustion of blood vessels and cardialgia.

In summary, in the development of pectoral pain and stuffiness, the main syndrome is deficiency in origin and excess in superficiality. The manifestation of excess in superficiality are stagnation of qi, blood stasis, accumulation of phlegm, excessive cold and heat stagnation. The deficiency syndrome in origin may be differentiated into deficiency of heart-qi, deficiency of heart blood, deficiency of heart-yang, deficiency of liver- and kidney-yin, deficiency of spleen- and kidney-yang and deficiency of lung-qi. The pectoral pain and stuffiness may be caused by one or more of these pathological changes.

The further development of the pectoral pain and stuffiness may lead to many other diseases. If the heart and vessels are stagnated by blood stasis, excess of yin leading to prostration of yang, a sudden severe and persistent pain occurs in the chest and heart, so developing into genuine cardialgia. If the heart vessels are obstructed, and yin yang exhausted, the prostration syndrome occurs. If there is deficiency of qi and blood in the heart and the heart is failing to be nourished, may appear severe palpitation, knotted and intermittent pulse. If the accumulated fluid invade upwards the heart and lung, cough, asthma and edema in limbs may occur.

〔Diagnosis and Treatment by Differentiation of Syndromes〕

Ⅰ. Main points of the differentiation

1. Differentiation of deficiency and excess, and primary from secondary: Most of the syndromes of pectoral pain and stuffiness are deficiency in origin and excess in superficiality. The deficiency syndromes in origin may be divided into several types: deficiency of heart-qi (including of lung-qi), deficiency of heart blood, deficiency of heart-yang, deficiency of spleen- and kidney-yang and deficiency of liver- and kidney-yin. The excess syndromes in superficiality include stagnation of qi, blood stasis, accumulation of phlegm, excessive cold, accumulation of heat. If the pectoral pain and stuffiness manifested primarily as deficiency syndrome and feeble pulse, the origin should be treated. If it manifested mainly as excess syndrome and replete pulse, the superficiality should be treated.

2. Differentiation of the properties of pain: There are several kinds of cardialgia in pectoral pain and stuffiness in clinical practice, namely oppressive pain, stabbing pain, burning pain, colicky pain and vague pain.

Oppressive pain: paroxysmal, heavy sensation of oppression with light pain. Most of the cases of qi stagnation are related to emotional changes. If the patients have the sensation of oppression and pain simultaneously, obesity, abundant sputum, greasy tongue fur, it may be caused by accumulation of phlegm. The insufficiency of heart-qi manifested as feelings of oppression and a dull pain, exacerbated after light exercise, short breathing, asthma and perspiration. The symptoms manifested as oppressive pain in chest, bleeding or onset postmenstruation, palpitating and sleeplessness, pale tongue, it belongs to deficiency syndrome of heart blood.

Stabbing pain: The symptoms of this type belong to blood stasis that involve pain feeling as stabbing, fixed location without moving, dark purple tongue proper with or without ecchymosis, or dark purple sublingual muscles. The blood stasis may be induced by various causes, so it must be diagnosed in the light of the comprehensive analysis of illness conditions.

Burning pain: The symptom is always caused by fire-heat and divided into two types of excess and deficiency. The syndrome of fire excess type involves burning pain feeling in chest, restlessness, dysphoria, sleeplessness, and dry mouth with bitter taste. The phlegm-fire syndrome manifested as oppressed feeling with burning pain in chest, thick yellow sputum and yellow greasy tongue fur. Most of the syndrome of fire of yin deficiency manifested as light burning pain in chest, dysphoria with feverish sensation in chest, palms and soles, dizziness, palpitating, red and thin tongue proper, and less tongue fur.

Colicky pain: The syndrome of accumulation of cold pathogens in heart channels manifested as colicky or twisting pain, onset suddenly or induced by cold pathogen, exacerbated when attacked by cold, aversion to cold, cold feeling in limbs, oppressed feeling in chest as being suffocated. The syndrome of yang deficiency and interior cold involves the symptoms of yang deficiency, aversion to cold, lying with bending gesture, pale and thick tongue proper. In addition, the violent cardialgia of this type are often caused by over exertion, emotional changes and excessive eating and drinking. Therefore in the diagnosis of this disease should inspected in accordance with the syndrome and not to be limited to "cold".

Vague pain: Most of the syndromes of dull pain feeling, onset after exercise, short breathing and tiredness are belonging to deficiency of qi or yang. If the syndromes are vague pain in chest, dysphoria, dizziness and tinnitus, it belongs to deficiency of yang.

3. Differentiation of mild from severe, and positive from negative illness conditions

(1) Differentiation of mild and severe illness conditions: In general, pain is the indication of mild and severe conditions. The judgement may adhere to the followings:

a. Frequency of its onset: attacking frequently, severe; occasionally, mild.

b. Duration of each onset: The mild cases cured in a twinkling. The persistent cases are serious and the more serious one continued for several hours.

c. Fixed or unfixed locations of its onset: If the location of pain is fixed, the condition is severe, and the mild one is on the contrary.

d. Deficiency or excess of the pain: mild condition, excessive syndrome and pulse; severe condition, deficient syndrome and pulse.

e. Course of the disease: In general, the incipient and short-term cases are mild, and the severe cases are on the contrary.

Diagram of the causes and pathogenesis

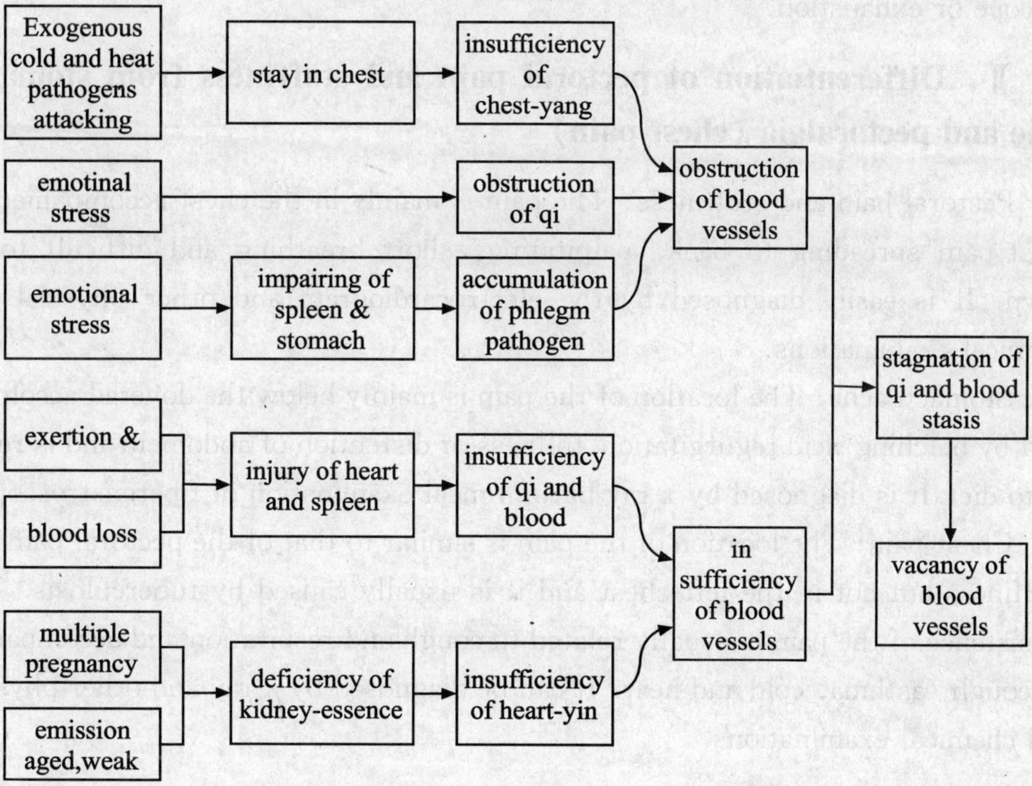

In summary, in the judgement of the illness condition of pectoral pain and stuffiness, a comprehensive analysis of the regional and systemic conditions is necessary for obtaining correct conclusions.

(2) Differentiation of positive from negative conditions of cardialgia: The genuine cardialgia is the serious state of pectoral pain and stuffiness. Because the serious cardialgia may endanger one's life, it is important to observe the positive and the negative conditions. The differentiation is generally started with the symptoms of emotion, breathing, perspiration, warm or cold in palms and soles, tongue and pulse. If the spirit of the patient is normal, breath evenly, normal sweating, mild condition and short duration, warm palms and soles, normal tongue proper and slow pulse, the state is defined as positive. If the patient is in low spirit and has the symptoms of dysphoria, short breathing or asthma, spontaneous perspiration or greasy sweating, palpitating, nervous, nausea and vomiting, cold or purple limbs, violent and persistent cardialgia without resolving, pain spreading to shoulder, back, left forearm, throat, stomach and abdomen, purple tongue proper, infrequent or rapid, knotted and intermittent pulse, the

situation is defined as negative. This condition must be watched closely to prevent syncope or exhaustion.

Ⅱ. Differentiation of pectoral pain and stuffiness from stomach-ache and pectoralgia (chest pain)

Pectoral pain and stuffiness: The pain is mainly in the chest accompanied by chest pain spreading to back, palpitating, short breathing and difficult to lie down. It is easily diagnosed by the electrocardiogram and other physical and chemical examinations.

Stomach-ache: The location of the pain is mainly below the dovetail accompanied by belching, acid regurgitation, fullness or distention of abdomen, and is related to diet. It is diagnosed by x-ray barium meal examination of fibergastroscopy.

Chest pain: The location of the pain is similar to that of the pectoral pain and stuffiness but not in the left chest and it is usually caused by tuberculosis. The persistence of the pain is usually related to cough and respiration and accompanied by cough, asthma, cold and heat. It can be diagnosed by x-ray and other physical and chemical examinations.

Ⅲ. Key points of therapeutic principles

The therapeutic principle of pectoral pain and stuffiness being: treating the superficiality first and the origin second, that is starting the treatment with eliminating the pathogenic factors and then strengthening the body resistance. If the superficiality is not severe, and the origin has been deficient already, the disease should be treated by the combination of reinforcement and resolving, and give consideration to both superficiality and origin. If the vital-qi is beginning to decline, the treatment should be strengthening the body resistance. The methods of eliminating pathogenic factors or treating superficiality mainly involve removing blood stasis and promoting blood circulation, activating yang with drugs pungent in flavor and warm in property, purging turbid pathogens and eliminating phlegm, regulating the flow of qi and soothing the chest oppression, or clearing away heat and promoting the functions of viscera. The therapeutic principle of strengthening body resistance and restoring normal functions of the body to consolidate the constitution commonly employ the methods of warming the middle energizer to assist yang, invigorating qi to nourish yin, nourishing qi and blood, and nourishing the liver and kidney.

Ⅳ. Treatment by differentiation of types and syndromes

1. Stagnation of the heart blood

Maim symptoms and signs: stabbing pain in the chest, location of the pain fixed, exacerbated at the nightfall.

Associated symptoms and signs: Palpitating, restlessness, usually feeling oppression in the chest, remission after massage.

Tongue and pulse: dark purple tongue proper, or having ecchymosis, or dark purple sublingual muscles, deep and uneven pulse.

Analysis: The stabbing pain is formed by prolonged stagnation of qi, accumulation of blood stasis, and obstruction in vessels. Owing to the obstruction of blood vessels, the site of the pain is fixed. The blood is classified with yin, and so is the night. So the disease is exacerbated at nightfall. Palpitation and restlessness are caused by blood stasis and failing of the heart to be nourished. When qi and blood are accumulated in the chest, the patient feels fullness and stuffiness in the chest. To massage with hands is helpful to blood circulation, so the patient feels relieved. All of the symptoms mentioned above of dark purple tongue proper, or ecchymosis, or dark purple sublingual muscles, deep and uneven pulse are the expression of the accumulation of stagnated blood.

Therapeutic methods: promoting blood circulation to remove blood stasis, removing obstructions in the channels to relieve pain.

Prescriptions and drugs: "Modified Xue Fu Zhu Yu Decoction" is used. In the prescription, Chinese angelica root, chuanxiong rhizome, peach kernel, and safflower promote blood circulation to remove blood stasis, bupleurum root soothe the liver, and the immature bitter orange regulate the flow of qi. Their main functions involve regulating the flow of qi. Since qi is the commander of blood, the latter will circulate normally when qi is in motion. In the cases of severe chest pain, add dalbergia wood, notoginseng, curcuma root and corydalis tuber to promote blood circulation, regulate the flow of qi and alleviate pain. If the oppressed feeling is obvious in the chest, add inula flower, trichosanthes peel, corydallis tuber and green tangerine orange peel for soothing the chest oppression and regulating the flow of qi. If the disease manifested as severe palpitating and restlessness, dragon's bone, oyster and red ochre can be used to relieve palpitation and tranquilize the mind.

In the case of mild blood stasis, "Dan Shen Decoction" may be used as the substitute. Red sage root in the prescription promote blood circulation to remove blood stasis and can cure the pain caused by blood stasis; sandalwood warm the middle energizer and regulate the flow of qi and cure cardialgia and stomach-ache.

Example of prescription: Chinese angelica root 10g, red peony root 12g, chuanxiong rhizome 10g, red sage root 20g, notoginseng powder 3g (mixed), parched bitter orange 10g, dalbergia woof 6g, trichosanthes peel 15g, red ochre 20g (pre-decocted).

2. Accumulation of the pathogenic phlegm

Main symptoms and signs: oppressed and asphyxia feeling and pain in chest, or the pain spreading to shoulder and back.

Associated symptoms and signs: obesity, excessive sputum, fullness feeling in stomach.

Tongue and pulse: mucous and greasy fur, slippery pulse.

Analysis: The oppressed and asphyxia feeling and pain in the chest is caused by the accumulation of phlegm in the lung which induces the deactivation of chest-yang. Owing to the pathogenic phlegm obstructs the vessels and channels, the pain spreads to the shoulders and back. The spleen is in charge of muscles and extremities. When the spleen is afflicted by pathogenic phlegm, the spleen-qi functioned abnormally hence inducing obesity, excessive sputum, fullness in stomach and sense of heaviness in extremities. Short breathing and asthma are caused by the stagnation of phlegm in the lung thus inducing the obstruction of the flow of qi. Mucous and greasy tongue fur and slippery pulse are also the expressions of the accumulation of phlegm.

Therapeutic methods: activating yang and purging away the turbid pathogens, eliminating phlegm and relieving stagnation.

Prescriptions and drugs: Modified "Gua Lou Xie Bai Ban Xia Decoction" is used. Trichosanthes in the prescription has the functions of relieving the accumulation of phlegm in chest; pinellia tuber resolving phlegm and descending the adverse flow of qi; macrostem onion (pungent in flavor and heat in property) activating yang, eliminating phlegm and descending the flow of qi. The addition of perillla fruit, perilla stem, immature bitter orange, tangerine peel, round cardamon seed, and poria cocos to the prescription will strengthen the functions of regulating the flow of qi, eliminating phlegm, activating yang and dispersing the phlegm accumulation.

If the symptoms manifested as fullness in the stomach, nausea, loss of appetite, mouth mucus and bitter taste, greasy and yellow tongue fur, it showed that the middle energizer is obstructed by the dampness-heat and adverse flow of stomach-qi. In this case, "Xiao Xian Xiong Decoction" or "Huang Lian Wen Dan Decoction" may be used to clearing away the dampness-heat. Treatment of both heart and stomach symptoms simultaneously could also be effective.

If both the accumulation of phlegm and blood stasis appeared at the same time, and the symptoms manifested as greasy fur, dark tongue proper or having ecchymosis, the disease should be treated with both the methods of activating yang to eliminate phlegm, and promoting blood circulation to remove blood stasis. The two therapeutic methods may be used according to the diagnosis with particular emphasis laid on one or another prescription.

Example of prescription: Whole trichosanthes 30g, macrostem onion 10g, pinella tuber 10g, parched tangerine peel 10g, poria cocos 15g, perilla stem 10g, parched immature bitter orange 10g, round cardamon seed 6g, chuanxiong rhizome 10g, safflower 10g, dalbergia wood 6g.

3. Accumulation of severe pathogenic cold

Main symptoms and signs: chest pain spreading to back, back pain to the heart, exacerbated by cold, sudden onset after infected by cold.

Associated symptoms and signs: oppressed feeling in chest, short breathing, palpitating, asthma in severe cases, disable to lie down, pale complexion, cold in limbs.

Tongue and pulse: normal tongue proper with whitish fur, deep, thready and tense pulse.

Analysis: The flow of qi from chest to the back is obstructed by pathogenic cold and then accumulated in the chest hence resulting in loosing of vitality of yang-qi, obstruction of qi and chest pain spreading to back. The more the cold is the more the pain feeling. The disease is often attacked by cold and onset suddenly. The symptoms of oppressed feeling in chest, short breathing, palpitating even asthma are caused by obstruction of chest-yang and the flow of qi. Insufficiency of yang-qi causes pale complexion, cold limbs, whitish tongue fur, deep and thready pulse. All of these are the expressions of the accumulation of severe pathogenic cold and lack of vitality of yang to circulate normally.

Therapeutic methods: activating yang with drugs pungent in flavor and warm in property, relieving numbness and expelling cold.

Prescriptions and drugs: "Gua Lou Xie Bai Bai Jiu Decoction" modified by addition of immature bitter orange, cinnamon twig, prepared aconite root, red sage root and sandalwood is used. In the prescription, cinnamon twig, prepared aconite root and macrostem onion activate yang, relieve numbness and dispel cold, trichosanthes and immature bitter orange eliminate phlegm, remove obstruction, resolve fullness and descend the adverse flow of qi; sandalwood regulate the flow of qi and warm the middle energizer; and red sage root promote blood circulation and remove obstruction in the channels.

If the symptoms manifested as cardialgia spreading to back, pain feeling to the heart, ceaseless pain, cold feeling in the body and limbs, asthma, deep and tense pulse, the disease is in the severe condition of excess yin-cold. It should be treated with the prescription "Wu Tou Chi Shi Zhi Pill" plus "Su He Xiang Pill" to warm channels and alleviate pain by aromatic drugs. Sichuan prickly ash and dried ginger in the prescription warm the middle energizer and dispel cold, prepared aconite root and Sichuan aconite root cure cardialgia and cold limbs. The red halloysite in the prescription is used to nourish heart-qi, and warm the channels to alleviate pain in combination with the prescription "Su He Xiang Pill". In clinical practice, prepared aconite root (lateral root of common monkshood) is seldom used in combination with Sichuan aconite root (mother root of common monkshood), so the effect will be better by cinnamon bark as substitute for Sichuan aconite root. The commonly used "Guan Xin Su He Pill" is the modification of the prescription "Su He Xiang Pill".

Example of prescription: Whole trichosanthes 30g, macrostem onion 10g, cinnamon twig 10g, vinegar 20g (separately mixed), fresh ginger 5 pieces, parched tangerine peel 10g, parched immature bitter orange 10g, red sage root 30g, sandalwood 6g, amomum fruit 5g, prepared aconite root 6g.

4. Deficiency of heart- and kidney-yin

Main symptoms and signs: dull burning pain in chest, paroxysmal attacking.

Associated symptoms and signs: palpitating, night sweating, restlessness, sleeplessness, soreness of waist, disorder of knee-joint, dizziness, tinnitus.

Tongue and pulse: red tongue proper, thin, or having ecchymosis, taut and thready or thready and rapid pulse.

Analysis: The prolonged illness makes the yin-blood exhausted, blood vessels obstructed thereby inducing dull pain in chest. Because the hyperactivity of fire is induced by yin deficiency, the fire of the deficiency type then attacked the interior, so appeared the burning pain in the chest. The pain thus formed is not serious than that caused by the fire of excess type. The fire of deficiency type invades the heart, so inducing paroxysmal palpitation, restlessness and sleeplessness. When yin could not restrain yang, or the fire of deficiency type forces the fluid excreted, so appeared the night sweating. The soreness in waist and the knee joint is caused by deficiency of kidney-yin and the muscles are disable to be nourished. Dizziness and tinnitus are caused by hyperactivity of yang due to yin deficiency. All of the symptoms of red tongue proper, thin, or ecchymosis, thready and taut or thready and rapid pulse are caused by deficiency of yin-blood, obstruction of heart vessels and the heart not been nourished.

Therapeutic methods: nourishing yin and tonifying the kidney, nourishing the heart to calm the mind.

Prescriptions and drugs: Modified "Zuo Gui Decoction" is used. In the prescription, prepared rehmannia root, dogwood fruit and wolfberry fruit nourish yin and kidney; Chinese yam, poria cocos and licorice root strengthen the apleen to invigorate the functions of spleen in transporting and transforming food essence. In the case of palpitation, night sweat, restlessness and sleeplessness caused by deficiency of heart-yin, add ophiopogon root, schisandra fruit, aborvitae seed and wild jujuba seed to nourish heart and calm the mind, in which the ophiopogon root may be used in larger dosage. If the patient feels oppression and pain in the chest, add Chinese angelica root, red sage root, chuanxiong rhizome and curcuma root to nourish heart and remove obstructions in the channels. If the syndrome manifested as hyperactivity of yang due to yin deficiency with the symptoms as dizziness, numbness feeling in tongue and limbs and flushed face, add prepared fleece flower root, glossy privet fruit, uncaria stem with hooks, crude abalone shell, crude oyster and turtle shell to nourish yin and suppress hyperactive yang.

Example of prescription: fresh and prepared rehmannia root 10g each, dogwood fruit 10g, alisma orientale 10g, poria cocos 15g, asparagus root 10g, ophiopogon root 10g, red sage root 20g, schisandra fruit 6g, glossy privet fruit 10g, eclipta 10g, notoginseng powde 3g (mix).

5. Deficiency of both qi and yin

Main symptoms and signs: paroxysmal oppressed feeling and dull pain in chest.

Associated symptoms and signs: palpitating, short breathing, lassitude, lazy to speak, dim complexion, dizziness, exacerbated after labor, constipation or loose stool.

Tongue and pulse: light red tongue with or without teeth print, thready and weak, or knotted and intermittent pulse.

Analysis: Prolonged illness of pectoral pain and stuffiness and deficiency of both qi and yin cause the obstruction of vessels and channels, and of blood circulation, accumulation of qi and blood thereby inducing oppressed and dull pain in the chest. Palpitating is caused by deficiency of both qi and yin and failing of the heart to be nourished. The deficiency of qi also manifested as sluggish, lazy to speak and dim complexion. The hyperactivity of yang due to yin deficiency causes dizziness. The patient with deficient syndrome is liable to be attacked by overwork which will exacerbate the disease. If deficiency of qi is superior in the deficiency of both qi and yin, the functions of digestion will be impaired hence inducing loose stool; if yin deficiency is superior, then causing constipation. Light red tongue proper, with or without teeth prints, thready and weak, or knotted and intermittent pulse are the expressions of the syndrome of deficiency of both qi and yin.

Therapeutic methods: invigorating qi and nourishing yin, promoting blood circulation and removing obstruction in the channels.

Prescriptions and drugs: Modification of the prescription "Sheng Mai Powder" plus "Ren Shen Yang Ying Decoction" is used. In the prescription, ginseng, astragalus root, white atractylodes rhizome, poria cocos and licorice root reinforce the spleen and activate qi to promote digestion; ophiopogon root, rehmannia root, Chinese angelica root and white atractylodes rhizome nourish yin and blood; polygala root and schisandra fruit nourish the heart and calm the mind. If the symptoms manifested as knotted and intermittent pulse, palpitating caused by insufficiency of qi and blood and heart not been nourished, "Zhi Gan Cao Decoction" can be used in combination to activate qi and enrich blood, nourish yin and restore pulse. If the deficiency of heart-yin is serious, the symptoms manifested as burning pain in chest, palpitating, restlessness, sleeplessness, night sweat, flushed face, constipation, red tongue proper with less fur, thready and rapid or knotted and intermittent pulse, the modified prescription "Tian Wang Bu Xin Pill" with the functions of nourishing yin, enriching blood, promoting blood circulation and purging heat is used. In this prescription, fresh rehmannia root, scrophularia root, asparagus root and ophiopogon root nourish yin and purge fire of deficiency type; ginseng, prepared licorice root and poria cocos invigorate heart-qi. Their actions imply the meaning of inducing yin from yang. Aborvitae seed, jujuba seed, polygala root and schisandra fruit activate qi and clam mind, disperse yin and arrest sweating; red sage root and Chinese angelica root nourish heart, promote blood circulation; platycodon root and cinnabar are the drugs for leading the guide drug. The whole prescription has the functions of restoring heart-yin, inhibiting the fire of deficiency type, removing obstructions in blood vessels to relieve the burning pain an the heart and chest. If there is excessive burning pain in heart and chest, drugs with cool and slight cold in property, such as tree peony bark, red peony root, Chinese trumpetcreeper and curcuma root should be used. In the case of oppressed feeling in chest and chest pain, add red sage root, notoginseng, motherwort, curcuma root, trogapterus dung and dalbergia wood to promote blood circulation and remove obstructions in the channels.

Example of prescription: ginseng powder 3g (mix), ophiopogon root 10g, schisandra fruit 10g, red sage root 20g, white and red peony root 10g each, prepared astragalus root 15g, Chinese angelica root 10g, prepared rehmannia root 10g, notoginseng powder 3g (mix), crude dragon's bone 30g, crude oyster 30g, poria cocos 15g, tree peony bark 10g.

6. Deficiency of yang-qi

Main symptoms and signs: oppressed feeling and dull pain in chest, occasionally colicky pain, spreading to back when exacerbated, exacerbated by cold attack.

Associated symptoms and signs: palpitating, short breathing, perspiration and asthenia, cold, cold limbs, pain feeling in waist and knee joint, pale complexion, light whitish or dark purple lips and nails.

Tongue and pulse: light whitish or dark purple tongue proper, deep and thready or deep and indistinct pulse.

Analysis: The oppressed feeling and dull pain in the chest are caused by deficiency of yang-qi, loss of vitality of chest-yang and obstructions in the circulation of blood and the flow of qi. Deficiency of yin brings about the interior cold which accumulated within blood vessels. Owing to the pain is caused by obstruction of cold, the cardialgia exacerbated by cold attack, even spreading to the back. Loss of vitality of heart-yang causes palpitating and short breathing. In the case of yang deficiency, the superficial-qi is failing to protect the body against diseases, hence resulting in perspiration and asthenia. Deficiency of spleen- and kidney-yang causes the symptoms of aversion to cold, cold limbs, cold and pain in waist and knee joint, pale complexion, light whitish or dark purple lips and nails. All of the light whitish or dark purple tongue proper, deep thready or deep indistinct pulse are the expressions of deficiency of yang-qi and obstruction due to blood stasis.

Therapeutic methods: activating qi and warming yang, promoting blood circulation and dispersing the channels.

Prescriptions and drugs: Modified "Shen Fu Decoction" and "You Gui Decoction" is used. In the prescription, ginseng invigorate the primordial qi; prepared aconite root and cinnamon bark warm the kidney to reinforce yang; prepared rehmannia root, dogwood fruit, wolfberry fruit and eucommia bark reinforce kidney to arrest spontaneous emission. If the symptoms manifested as dark purple lips, profuse sweating, cold limbs, deep and indistinct pulse, it shows the heart-yang is almost exhausted and should be treated with larger dosage of red ginseng, prepared aconite root and in combination with dragon's bone and oyster to recuperate the depleted yang and rescue the patient from collapse. In the case of deficiency of both yin and yang due to the impairing of yin and yang, add ophiopogon root and schisandra fruit to warm yang and nourish yin. In the case of kidney-yang deficiency syndrome manifested as palpitating, asthma, disable to lie down, less urine, edema in limbs, the prescription "Zhen Wu Decoction" modified by addition of tetranda root, umbellate pore fungus and plantain seed is used to warm yang and promote diuresis.

Example of prescription: ginseng powder 3g (mix), prepared aconite root 6g, cinnamon bark powder (mix), poris cocos 15g, crude dragon's bone 30g (predecocted), white atractylodes rhizome 10g, red and white peony root 10g each, notoginseng powder 3g (mix), epimedium 10g.

〔Measures of Prevention and Nursing〕

Ⅰ. Prevention

1. Pay attention to keep up the spirits avoiding depression. The emotional changes, such as melancholy and anxiety will induce the obstruction of blood vessels and the flow of qi, and finally resulting in precordial pain. Therefore, to keep the spirit in a cheerful frame, avoid exciting and melancholy is very important for prevention the attack of precordial pain.

2. Pay attention to the daily life and the weather. The changes in weather (cold, hot, fine, rain) have significant effect on the attack of precordial pain. When one is infected by pathogenic cold which obstruct the chest-yang, or infected by pathogenic heat which invade the heart, the precordial pain may be occur. Therefore pay attention to the daily life and take note to the changes of the weather are very important to prevent the attack of precordial pain.

3. Pay attention to the diet, avoid fat and greasy food and partiality for a particular kind of food. In the theory of traditional Chinese medicine, eating excessive fat, sweet and greasy food is liable to form phlegm which will block the channels, induce accumulation of phlegm, obstruction of the flow of qi, and finally result in precordial pain. The results of investigations carried out in recent years revealed that the incidence of the disease in those who are fond of sweet and greasy food is higher than that of ordinary person. Similarly, the person who has food preference is liable to be attacked by the disease. Therefore, it is important to balance the diet at ordinary times. In addition, the irritant agents such as wine and cigarettes should be prohibited because they also affect the normal functions of the viscera.

4. Pay attention to strike a proper balance between work and rest, and persist in proper physical exercises. Overworking is liable to impair the state of qi, blood, yin and yang of the heart and other internal organs. The habit of loving ease and hating work will result in the obstruction of the flow of qi and blood. It is important to strike a proper balance between work and rest and persist in proper physical exercises, so as to prevent or reduce the attacking of precordial pain.

Ⅱ. Nursing

1. Make the patients in cheerful spirit and build up their confidence in

overcoming the disease, free their mind of misgivings, alleviate undue nervousness, so as to benefit the normal functioning of the blood circulation and the flow of qi, and the coordination of the internal organs.

2. Lead the patients to have proper exercise follow in order and advance step by step, for example, take a walk, play shadow boxing (Chinese Taiji) thereby restoring to health.

3. Avoid eating excessive fat and sweet food, prohibit alcoholic drinks, and have more meals a day with less food at each.

4. When the precordial pain has attacked, keep calm, don't be frightened and take quick-acting analgesic to prevent the exacerbation of the illness condition.

5. Don't eat excessive food and don't be overworked after remission of the disease.

〔Analysis of Typical Cases〕

Case 1. Jiang, male, age 48. suffered from numbness of the left chest for 4～5 years, confirmed as coronary heart disease by a hospital, coronary insufficiency, abnormal electrocardiogram in several examinations, dark purple lips and tongue, dark complexion, restlessness, sleeplessness, arrhythmic, partly released or complete rest for three years, dry mouth and drink less for a long time, diagnosis: the syndrome of stagnation of blood vessels, and treated with the modified prescription "Xuan Fu Hua Decoction": inula flower 15g (packed), rubia root 9g, safflower 9g, Chinese green onion 15g, trichosanthes seed 12g, red sage root 15g, red peony root 15g, chuanxiong rhizome 9g, dalbergia wood 9g, amber powder 1.5g (take predormitally).

Oppressed feeling and pain alleviated after taking five dosages, continuously taking the above prescription for more than three months, symptoms disappeared, then take the pill manufactured based on the original prescription for more than one year, electrocardiogram turned normal, gone to work nowadays, no relapse in the later three to four years ("Zhong Yi Nei Ke Yin Lun").

Comment: In this case, the symptoms of face, tongue and pulse were caused by blood stasis. Restlessness and sleeplessness were caused by the obstruction in heart vessels and the failure of heart and mind to be nourished. Dry mouth and drink less are the syndrome of so called "desire to drink but hate to swallow". This is because that the blood has stagnated and not transported upwards, thus inducing dry mouth. The blood stasis belongs to yin. Its excessively accumulation induces the symptoms of drink less. The constipation was caused by the stagnation of qi and the blockade of the transport activity of the large intestine. The prescription "Xuan Fu Hua Decoction" in the classic work "Jin Gui" is composed of inula flower, dalbergia wood and Chinese green onion. The physician Ye Tianshi of Qing Dynasty often employ this prescription to treat the hypochondriac pain caused by prolonged illness and attain better curative effect. In this case, the "Xuan Fu Hua Decoction" is modified. In addition to drugs for promoting blood circulation and removing blood stasis, inula flower, Chinese green onion, trichosanthes seed and dalbergia wood have the functions of promoting the dispersing function of the lung and relaxing bowels. The drug with pungent and aromatic flavor promote the flow of qi, hence promoting the circulation. The prescription is helpful for removing the obstructions in heart channels.

The pectoral pain and stuffiness is one of the commonly and frequently encountered diseases. The clinical symptoms are manifested as dull pain in chest, short breathing, asthma and disable to lie down. The causes of the disease include attacking by exogenous cold and heat pathogenic factors which accumulated in the chest, improper diet, emotional stress, anxiety and overworked, multiple pregnancy and spontaneous emission, blood loss, aged and weakness and deficiency of vital-qi caused by severe or prolonged illness. The pathogenesis belongs to deficiency in origin and excess in superficiality, in which the deficiency of origin manifested as deficiency of yin, yang, qi and blood; while excess in superficiality as yin-cold (cold sensation of the genitalia), accumulation of phlegm and blood stasis. The disease is caused by the two aspects alternatively. In clinical practice, the disease should be differentiated from stomach-ache and chest pain. The contents of the differentiation involves differentiation of deficiency vs. excess, primary vs. secondary, nature of the precordial pain, and mild vs. severe, positive vs. negative of the illness condition. The syndromes of the disease can be roughly classified into six types, i.e., stagnation of heart-blood, accumulation of phlegm, accumulation of yin-cold, deficiency of heart- and kidney-yin, deficiency of both qi and yin, and deficiency of yang-qi. They are falling in two categories: excess and deficiency syndromes. For excess syndrome, the therapeutic methods may be promoting blood circulation by removing blood stasis, activating yang with drugs pungent in flavor and warm in nature, eliminating phlegm and purging turbid pathogens with the treatment of the superficiality as the primary method. The therapeutic method for deficiency syndrome should be primarily nourishing and strengthening the body resistance. They include replenishing vital essence and tonifying the kidney, activating qi and nourishing yin, nourishing yang and invigorating qi. Generally the excess and deficiency syndromes are mixed up and transform mutually. Therefore in the treatment one must differentiate the syndrome is primary or secondary, greater or lesser urgency, then treat the disease with the consideration of both excess and deficiency. The disease may be treated in combination with effective patent drugs to attain curative effect. The key in the treatment of genuine cardialgia is to prevent exhaustion and collapse and take care of the slight changes of the illness condition so as to treat with drugs properly and promptly. The prognosis and the change of the disease in most cases can be controlled and remitted so long as prompt therapy and nursing are provided. The prevention measures of the disease involve providing mental relaxation, regulating daily life, being abstemious in eating and drinking, and striking a balance between work and rest and practicing these perseveringly.

Questions for Review

1. What is the concept of pectoral pain and stuffiness?
2. How to know well the contents and interrelations of the superficiality and the origin in the pathological changes of pectoral pain and stuffiness?
3. In treating pectoral pain and stuffiness, how to know well the principles and methods of the treatments for superficiality and the origin?
4. How to differentiate the mild from severe, positive from negative pectoral pain and stuffiness?
5. Which patent drugs of Chinese materia medica can be used for treating pectoral pain and stuffiness?

Insomnia

〔Introduction〕

Insomnia is generally called "sleeplessness". The name of the disease "no sleep" was first appeared in an ancient book "Nan Jing". The disease is characterized by the patient usually being unable to get to normal sleep. The manifestations of the disease involve the following types according to the illness condition. First, the patient has no sleepiness in the initial stage after getting in bed, the condition is called "difficult to sleep". Second, the patient is liable to wake up in the sleep, and then doesn't go to sleep again, called "early awake". Third, the patient is in a state between sleep and wake and could not get a deep sleep, or having a nightmare, called "light sleep". Fourth, the patient lies awake all through the night, called "awake all night". If the sleeplessness is caused by temporary causes, such as exciting, terror, anxiety, grief, or by environmental factors, such as noise, bright lamp light, and there is no other associated symptoms, it will take a turn for the better after these factors been removed. If the sleeplessness is caused other illness, such as fever, cough, pain, these causes should be treated first. The sleeplessness will be on the mend. Don't attend to trifles to the neglect of essentials. The sleep time of the people is different from one to another. If one who takes a short sleep everyday, but in a cheerful spirit, the situation is normal and should not be recognized as morbid state. The insomnia may onset singly or complicated by headache, dizziness, palpitation and amnesia. In clinical practice, it is treated in the light of related diseases.

Insomnia is different from the illness that the patient is unable to lie down or go to sleep by other diseases.

The prognosis of insomnia is good for most of the patients. Only for those who has severe insomnia with amentia, necessary measures should be employed to avoid accidents.

The diseases in western medicine, such as neurosis, hypertension, cerebral arteriosclerosis, anemia, hepatitis, menopausal syndrome and several mental diseases which have the symptoms of sleeplessness can be treated in the light of the disease mentioned in this chapter.

〔Causes and Pathogenesis〕

The causes of insomnia is related to the factors of emotional stress, imbalance between work and leisure, excessive eating and drinking, and usually weak constitution, or prolonged illness not been recovered. The main pathogenesis involves the followings: anxiety and tiredness, heart and spleen impairing, thus yang could not be entering yin, causing breakdown of the normal physiological coordination between the heart and kidney; stagnation of qi transforms into fire, then the liver-yang is disturbed; deficiency of heart-qi causes restlessness; indigestion and phlegm-heat causes disorder of the stomach-qi. All of these will disturb the mind and result in insomnia. The clinical syndromes involve both deficiency and excess which may transform mutually or mixed up with each other.

1. Emotional stress: Anxiety and anger impair the normal functions of the

liver, hence making the liver-qi stagnated. The stagnated qi transforms into fire which attacks the mind due to its tendency of flaring up. The irritability of disturbed mind results in sleeplessness. The fire may also be formed by overacting of five emotions. The flame of the heart-fire causes the breakdown of the normal physiological coordination between the heart and the kidney. So the heart-fire is flaring and disturbing the mental activity, and finally resulting sleeplessness. Violent terror may cause emotional stress which gradually makes the patient be timid and restless, and results in sleeplessness finally. Or, the excessive anxiety impairs the heart and spleen. The impaired heart causes the yin-blood consumed and mental deranged. The impairment of the spleen causes loss of appetite, insufficiency of the sources of growth and development, deficiency of yin-blood and the heart not be nourished, and inducing sleeplessness finally.

2. Immoderate diet: Addiction of pungent, spicy, fried, fat and greasy food, or eating and drinking too much at one meal, and immoderate diet result in impairment of the intestine and stomach. Retention of food brings about phlegm-heat which accumulated in the middle energizer and then causes the disorder of stomach-qi. The phlegm-heat disturbs upwards inducing sleeplessness.

3. Weak constitution, prolonged illness or during the convalescence of serious diseases: Insufficiency in natural endowment, aged, weakness and not been recovered all bring about impairment of the kidney. The depleted kidney-yin could not nourish the heart and the discordance between water and fire all cause the hyperactivity of heart-yang and mental derangement. The insomnia caused by this pathogenesis is of the breakdown of normal physiological coordination between the heart and kidney. In addition, the weak and aged person who had undergone illness, post-delivery or blood loss, may suffer from insufficiency of heart-blood and failure of heart to be nourished and finally be filling ill at ease. This is another cause of insomnia. If a weak and timid person is frightened suddenly, his heart-qi will be more deficient and his mind is in unease state, the insomnia occurs. Therefore, frightening and deficiency may be reciprocally causation, and all can cause insomnia.

4. Imbalance between work and leisure: Overwork induce consumption of qi and undue easy and leisure causes dysfunction of the spleen. Thus the spleen could not transport the essentials from foodstuff and transform them into qi and blood, so the deficiency of blood makes the failure of heart to be nourished and insomnia occurred. Or, intemperance in sexual life and sexual indulgence will be

causing hyperactivity of liver-qi and accumulation of qi in the chest and diaphragm. The blood is going upwards along with the ascending qi, thus causing dizziness, even being faint. The disease is also alleviated when qi and blood restored to normal state. The disease is also related to mental disorder and so belonging to the syndrome of liver stagnancy. The stagnation enters the blood from qi system, thus forming dim complexion and purple lips. Therefore the disease is treated with the prescriptions of soothing liver, alleviating depression, activating qi and promoting blood circulation. If the tongue proper is bulgy with teeth prints on its border, it indicates the spleen is deficient, then the astragalus root should be added to invigorate the spleen functions.

Diagram of the Causes and Pathogenesis of Insomnia

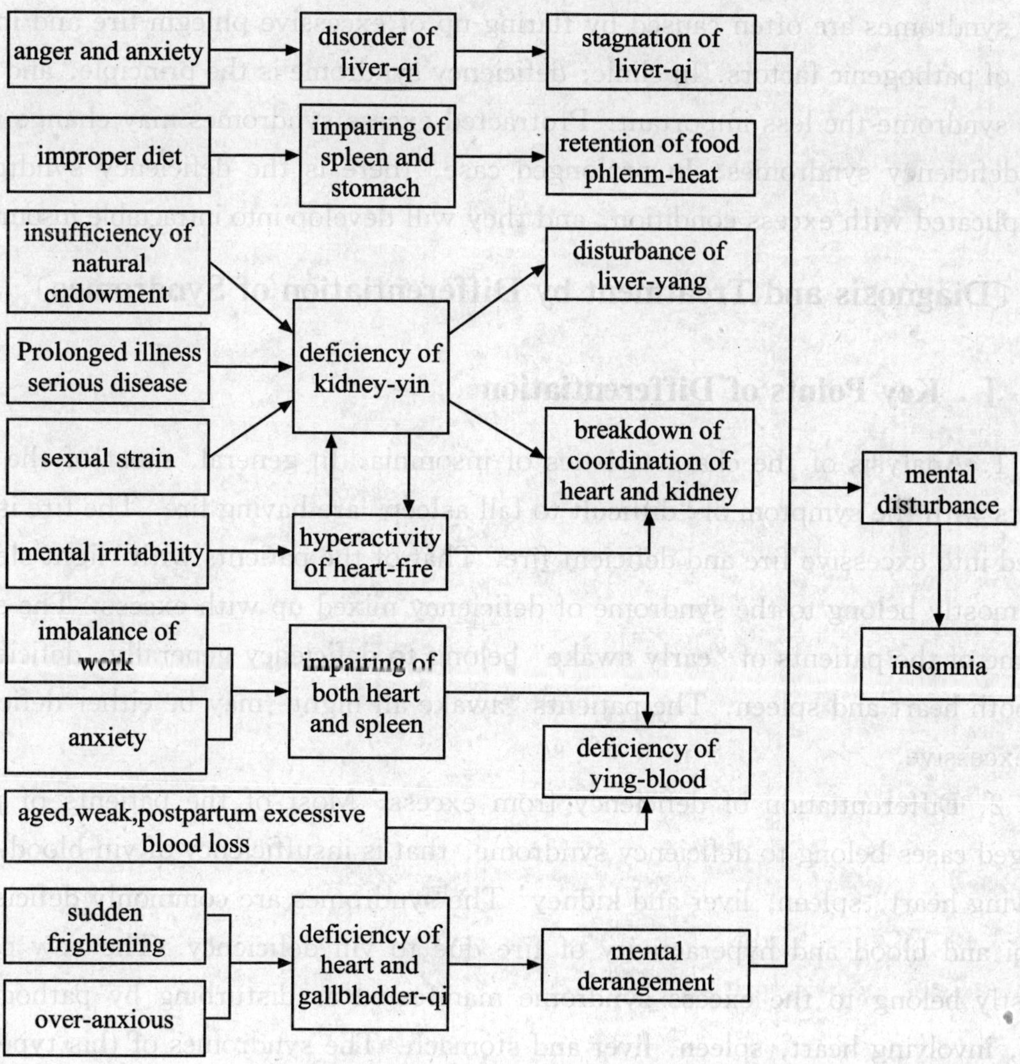

In summary, there are many causes of insomnia, but most of them can be classified into two categories: weak congenital constitution and postnatal emotional stress and immoderate diet. Its pathological changes include the dysfunction of Zang and Fu-organ, disorder of qi and blood, and imbalance of yin and yang, then leading to hyperactivity of heart and liver fire, upward disturbance of phlegm-fire, disharmony between heart and kidney, insufficiency of yin-blood, and deficiency of heart-qi and gallbladder-qi. The basic pathogenesis is disharmony between hyperactivity yang and insufficiency yin and disturbance of mental activity. Insomnia is closely related to the dysfunction of heart, spleen, liver, kidney, also involving gallbladder and stomach. Insomnia has the deficiency and excess syndromes. Deficiency syndromes usually result from insufficiency of yin and blood, consumption of essence and blood, and Qi deficiency of heart and gallbladder. Excess syndromes are often caused by flaring-up of excessive phlegm-fire and invasion of pathogenic factors. In clinic, deficiency syndrome is the principle, and excess syndrome the less important. Protracted excess syndromes may change into the deficiency syndromes. In prolonged case, there is the deficiency syndrome complicated with excess condition, and they will develop into intractable insomnia.

〔Diagnosis and Treatment by Differentiation of Syndromes〕

Ⅰ. Key Points of Differentiation

1. Analysis of the characteristics of insomnia: In general, most of the patients with the symptom of "difficult to fall asleep" are having fire. The fire is divided into excessive fire and deficient fire. That of the patients with "light sleep" are mostly belong to the syndrome of deficiency mixed up with excess. The syndrome of the patients of "early awake" belong to deficiency generally, deficiency of both heart and spleen. The patients "awake all night" may be either deficient or excessive.

2. Differentiation of deficiency from excess: Most of the patients of prolonged cases belong to deficiency syndrome, that is insufficiency of yin-blood, involving heart, spleen, liver and kidney. The syndromes are commonly deficiency of qi and blood and hyperactivity of fire due to yin deficiency. The new cases mostly belong to the excess syndrome manifested as disturbing by pathogenic fire, involving heart, spleen, liver and stomach. The syndromes of this type are

stagnation of liver transforms to fire, retention of food causing phlegm-heat and dysfunction of the stomach. If the syndrome is persisted for a long time, the qi and blood are exhausted, it may be transformed into deficiency. In the meantime, the deficiency syndrome may also mix the excess, hence forming the syndrome of mixed deficiency and excess.

3. The principles of the treatment should be regulation of yin yang by reinforcing deficiency and reducing excess. To those patients belonging to deficiency syndrome, treat with supplementing qi and nourishing blood, and invigorating both the liver and kidney. Patients with excess syndrome, may be treated by reducing the excess, removing food retention to regulate the stomach, and clearing away phlegm-heat. patients with mixed syndromes may be treated by both methods of reinforcing and reducing. Furthermore, in order to improve the curative efficacy, the drugs for nourishing heart and tranquilizing mind can also be used in addition to the therapy of syndromes.

Ⅱ. Treatment by Differentiation of Types and Syndromes

1. Excess syndrome

(1) Fire syndrome caused by hyperactivity of liver-qi (the stagnated liver-qi turning into fire)

Main symptoms and signs: no sleep, difficult to fall asleep, dreaminess.

Associated symptoms and signs: impatient, liable to be angry, conjunctival congestion and bitter taste in mouth, thirst, loss of appetite, dark urine and constipation.

Tongue and pulse: red tongue proper, yellow fur, taut and rapid pulse.

Analysis: The insomnia is caused by depression, anger injuring mind, disorder of the liver, stagnated qi turning into fire which invades upwards The fire belongs to pathogenic yang. If the fire is flaming within the body so that yang couldn't enter yin, to fall asleep must be difficult until midnight. At that time, yin is abundant and then yang begin to enter yin. Owing to the mind is disturbed by hyperactivity of liver-fire now and then, the patient suffers from dreaminess. The activity of liver-fire causes the symptoms of impatience, liable to be angry, conjunctival congestion and bitter taste in the mouth. Invading of stomach by liver-qi induces the loss of appetite and thirst. Dark urine, constipation, red tongue proper, yellow fur, taut and rapid pulse are all the expressions of heat syndrome. Excessive heat and impaired yin cause red tongue proper and heat in stomach induce yellow tongue fur. The taut and rapid pulse is caused by hyperactivity of liver-fire.

Therapeutic methods: soothing the liver and purging heat together with tranquilizing the mind.

Prescriptions and drugs: Modified "Long Dan Xie Gan Decoction" is used. In the prescription, gentian root, scutellaria root and pittosporm root purge the liver-fire; arisma orientale, manshuvian aristolochia stem and plantain seed remove the dampness-heat in the liver channel; bupleurum root disperse the liver and gallbladder-qi; and being the medicinal guide as well; Chinese angelica root and fresh rehmannia enrich blood and nourish yin to soothe the liver. Compatibility of Chinese angelica root and fresh rehmannia with drugs of clearing away heat bring about a good prescription that has the functions of supplementing implying purging, relieving implying nourishing, either preventing the impairing of yin by drugs of purging fire or preventing the burning of yin fluid by hyperactivity of liver- and gallbladder-fire. Licorice root regulates the stomach and relieve spasm, and can nourish yin to suppress hyperactive yang, tranquilization by addition of the drugs as magnetite, dragon's teeth and pearl oyster. In the case of stuffiness and distention in chest and hypochondrium, add curcuma root, cyperus tuber and white peony root to soothe the liver and regulate the flow of qi. In the case of loosing appetite and stuffiness in gastric cavity, belching and nausea, add red ochre, finger citron, citron fruit and immature bitter orange to soother the liver and regulate the stomach-qi.

Example of prescription: gentian root 9g, scutellaria root 10g, bupleurum root 10g, white peony root 10g, pittosporm root 9g, curcuma root 10g, cyperus tuber 10g, tangerine peel 10g, pearl oyster (pre-decoctied) 30g, crude dragon's bone and oyster (pre-decocted) 30g each, fresh rehmannia root 10g.

(2) Disturbance of phlegm-heat

Main symptoms and signs: no sleep, difficult to fall asleep, often caused by improper diet.

Associated symptoms and signs: heaviness in the head, dizziness, abundant expectoration, loss of appetite, belching, vexation and heartburn.

Tongue and pulse: yellow and greasy fur, slippery and rapid pulse.

Analysis: Most of the cases of this type are caused by improper diet, retention of food in stomach, spleen impaired, dysfunction of transporting and transforming food essentials, accumulation of dampness to produce phlegm, then the stagnated phlegm forming heat. Thus the retention of food and phlegm-heat obstruct the middle energizer and then cause abundant expectoration and stuffiness in chest. The disturbance of phlegm-heat causes restlessness, vexation and heartburn, difficult to fall asleep or light sleep, and further exacerbated by improper diet. The obstruction of phlegm-heat attacks the lucid yang, causing the symptoms of heaviness in head, dizziness, retention of food and phlegm, obstruction of the flow of qi. The failure of stomach to descend stomach-qi causes loss of appetite, belching, acid regurgitation and vomiting. Yellow greasy fur, rapid and slippery pulse are expressions of the syndrome retention of food.

Therapeutic methods: eliminating phlegm and clearing away heat, regulating stomach and tranquilizing the mind.

Prescriptions and drugs: The prescription "Wen Dan Decoction" is used in combination with coptis root and pittosporm root. "Wen Dan Decoction" is composed of "Er Chen Decoction" plus bamboo shavings, immature bitter orange, fresh ginger and dates. The functions of the prescription involve removing dampness from the gallbladder, regulating the stomach, reducing phlegm and arresting vomiting. In the prescription, pinellia tuber, tangerine peel, poria cocos, and immature bitter orange regulate qi and eliminating phlegm; coptis root, pittosporm root and bamboo shavings clear away the heart-fire. Poris cocos tranquilize the mind as well. In the case of retention of food and accumulation of phlegm and the upset stomach, use the prescription "Ban Xia Shu Mi Decoctiion", or "Bao He Pill" or "Zhi Shi Dao Zhi Pill" in combination to remove food retention and regulate stomach-qi. Among them, "Ban Xia Shu Mi Decoction" can nourish yin, regulate stomach-qi and tranquilize mind. "Bao He Pill" or "Zhi Shi Dao Zhi Pill" can remove food retention, regulate stomach-qi, and eliminate dampness-heat. In the case of evident food retention and dyspepsia, add areca seed, charred malt, millet sprout and medicated leaven, radish seed and membrane of chicken gizzard to promote digestion and eliminate phlegm. In the case of serious phlegm-heat and retention of feces, use the prescription "Meng Shi Gun Tan Pill" in combination with rhubarb and trichosanthes to purge fire and heat, eliminate phlegm and tranquilize the mind. If the symptoms manifested as palpitating, restless, add pearl oyster, dragon's teeth, dragon's bone and magnetite to relieve convulsion and calm the mind.

Example of prescription: Poria cocos 15g, red tangerine peel 10g, pinellia tuber 10g, bamboo shavings 10g, immature biter orange 10g, rhubarb 6g, pittosporm root 12g, hucked sorghum 10g, charred malt, millet sprout and medicated leaven 10g each, trichosanthes 20g.

2. Deficiency syndrome

(1) Hyperactivity of fire due to yin deficiency

Main symptoms and signs: restlessness, sleeplessness, difficult to fall asleep.

Associated symptoms and signs: Palpitating, unease, dysphoria with feverish sensation in chest, palms and soles, dizziness, tinnitus, soreness of waist and knees, amnesia, nocturnal emission, dry mouth, less fluid.

Tongue and pulse: red tongue proper, thready and rapid pulse.

Analysis: The heart is one of the viscera belonging to yang, lodged in the upper energizer, with fire in nature. The kidney belongs to viscera of yin type, lodged in the lower energizer, with water in nature. If the heart and the kidney are in normal coordination, the kidney-yin (kidney-water) should not be cold, and inversely, the kidney-yin gives assistance to the heart upwards, so as the heart shall not be hyperactive. The situation is called "water and fire coordinated". If the kidney-yin is insufficient and could not assist upwards the heart-yang, the heart- and liver-fire will be hyperactive, thus the fire of deficiency type disturbs the mind causing vexation, sleeplessness, palpitating and unease. Dizziness, tinnitus and amnesia are caused by consumption of the kidney essence and the hollow reservoir of marrow. The deficiency of kidney causes the failure of the waist lodgment to be nourished, thus causing soreness in waist and knees. The nocturnal emission is caused by the breakdown of normal physiological coordination between the heart and the kidney. The dysphoria with feverish sensation in chest, palms and soles, dry mouth, less fluid, red tongue proper and thready and rapid pulse are all the expressions of hyperactivity of fire due to yin deficiency.

Therapeutic methods: nourishing yin, removing fire, nourishing heart and tranquilizing the mind.

Prescriptions and drugs: The prescription of "Huang Lian E Jiao Decoction", "Zhu Sha An She Pill" and "Tian Wang Bu Xin Pill" can be selected for treatment according to the clinical syndromes. All of the functions of these three prescriptions are clearing away heat and tranquilizing mind. The main functions of "Huang Lian E Jiao Decoction" and "Zhu Sha An Shen Pill" are nourishing yin and removing fire. The functions of "Tian Wang Bu Xin Pill" are mainly nourishing yin and blood, and clearing away heat concurrently. In the prescription

"Huang Lian E Jiao Decoction", coptis root and scutellaria root purge the heart-fire and remove dysphoria with smothery sensation; donkey-hide gelatin, white peony root and egg yolk nourish yin and blood, and tranquilize the mind. Acting of both purging and nourishing functions simultaneously make the heart and the kidney coordinated, "water and fire coordinated", thereby the vexation and restlessness recovered as a matter of course. The drug cinnabar in the prescription "Zhu Sha An Shen Pill" possesses the property of slight cold, "weight sedative", thus being used as the main constituent to clear away heat, relieve palpitating and tranquilize mind; coptis root remove heart-fire, Chinese angelica root and rehmannia root nourish yin and blood as the assistants; prepared licorice root as the guide to nourish and regulate the stomach, coordinate the actions of other drugs in the prescription, and remove heart-fire and tranquilize the mind. The principles of the above two prescriptions are similar. "Zhu Sha An Shen Pill" may be made into bolus which is easier to take. Since the main constituent of cinnabar is mercury sulfide, the prescription is unsuitable for protracted use and taking a large amount, so as to prevent mercurialism. In the prescription "Tian Wang Bu Xin Pill", main drugs are fresh rehmannia root and figwort root which nourih yin and clear away heat, red sage root and Chinese angelica root as complement to enrich blood and nourish heart, pilose asiabell root and poria cocos invigorate heart-qi, aborvitae seed and polygala root tranquilize the mind; astragalus root and ophiopogon root as assistants nourish yin and clear away heat, schisandra fruit and wild jujuba seed restrain heart-qi; and platycodon root as guide transport other drugs upwards; and cinnabar tranquilize mind. All these drugs in the prescription act together to nourish yin and tranquilize the mind. The prescription is used in combination with oyster shell, magnetite, pearl oyster, the drugs for nourishing yin and tranquilizing the mind, for the treatment when the syndromes manifested as deficiency of yin and less blood and the activity of fire is not very vigorous, thus restraining the rise of yang. When yang enters into yin, the disease recovered. The prescription "Liu Wei Di Huang Pill" or "Mai Wei Di Huang Pill" in combination with "Jiao Tai Pill" are used. The former two have the functions of nourishing kidney-yin or reinforcing heart and kidney and the latter conducting the fire back to its origin.

Example of prescription: coptis root 6g, scutellaria root 10g, donkey-hide gelatin (melted) 10g, white peony root 12g, fresh rehmannia root 12g, ophiopogon root 12g, schisandra fruit 6g, lotus plumule 3g, crude oyster shell (pre-decocted) 30g, crude licorice root 6g.

(2) Deficiency of both the heart and the spleen

Main symptoms and signs: dreaminess, liable to awake, light sleep.

Associated symptoms and signs: palpitating, amnesia, dizziness, low spirit, tiredness, loss of appetite, pale complexion.

Tongue and pulse: light tongue proper, thin and whitish fur, thready and weak pulse.

Analysis: The heart governs the blood circulation and stores the spirit within it. The spleen has the function to transport and transform nutrients and is the source of blood generation. So, undue anxiety, imbalance between work and rest cause the impairment of both heart and spleen, hence inducing insufficiency of ying-blood, and failure of the heart to be nourished and finally palpitating and amnesia. If yin couldn't restrain yang and the mental derangement appeared, it shall result in light sleep. Anxiety and labor not only consume the blood but also impair the heart- and spleen-qi, hence resulting in deficiency of yang-qi. So the patient often awake after midnight when yang-qi is rising. Therefore the features of this syndrome are: going to bed and fall asleep at first without difficulty, having dreams in sleep and being easy to awake. When insufficient blood is unable to nourish the brain, weak lucid yang is unable to ascend, dizziness occurred. Pale complexion and light red tongue proper are caused by deficiency of blood that couldn't nourish the face. Deficiency of both qi and blood causes low spirit, tiredness and weak or feeble pulse.

Therapeutic methods: nourishing heart and invigorating spleen to generate qi and blood.

Prescriptions and drugs: Modified "Gui Pi Decoction" is used. The prescription has the functions of activating the flow of qi, invigorating spleen, nourishing blood and relieving mental stress. In the prescription, the functions of ginseng, white atractylodes rhizome, astragalus root and licorice root are mainly replenishing qi and invigorating spleen, so as to make the spleen and stomach healthy and qi and blood generated spontaneously. Chinese angelica root as assistant nourish yin and blood. Plenty of blood makes the mental stress relieved. Poria with hostwood, Chinese date seed, longan aril and polygala root nourish heart and invigorate spleen, tranquilize mind; aucklandia root regulate the flow of qi and enliven the spleen so the spleen is supplemented without obstruction. Ginger and Chinese date as guides regulate the function among the viscera. The combination of these drugs has the functions of replenishing qi and generating the blood, nourishing heart and tranquilizing the mind. If the palpitating and short breathing are serious, add prepared rehmannia root, white peony root and donkey-hide gelatin to nourish heart and blood. If sleeplessness and dreaminess are serious, add schisandra fruit, aborvitae seed to nourish heart and tranquilize mind. Addition of dragon's teeth, dragon's bone, oyster shell and pearl oyster will give the functions of tranquilization. If the symptoms manifested as water retention due to dysfunction of the spleen, stuffiness in stomach, loss of appetite, abdominal distention and loose stool, slippery and greasy fur, add poria cocos, pinellia tuber, tangerine peel and magnolia bark to invigorate spleen, regulate the flow of qi and eliminate dampness. If the deficiency of heart, spleen, qi and blood is excessive, the prescription "Yang Xin Decoction" may be used in combination. In the latter, schisandra fruit, aborvitae seed can enhance the functions of nourishing heart and tranquilizing mind. Besides, these two drugs also function as drugs for nourishing blood and qi in combination with few cinnamon bark to give the functions of warming yang-qi, promoting the generation of qi and blood.

Example of prescription: pilose asiabell root 10g, white atractylodes rhizome 10g, prepared astragalus root 12g, Chinese angelica root 10g, poria with hostwood 10g, aucklandia root 6g, prepared date seed 15g, polygala root 10g, fleeceflower stem 30g, prepared licorice root 6g, longan aril 10g, tangerine peel 10g.

(3) Deficiency of both heart- and gallbladder-qi

Main symptoms and signs: sleeplessness, dreaminess, liable to awake.

Associated symptoms and signs: timid, palpitating, frightened easily, low spirit and tiredness, spontaneous perspiration, short breathing.

Tongue and pulse: light tongue proper, taut and thready or thready and weak pulse.

Analysis: The relation between the liver and the heart is that of mother and child organs. they influence each other. The liver is appended to the gallbladder and reciprocal interior and exterior. Frightening injures the gallbladder and causes deficiency of gallbladder-qi. The impaired gallbladder attacks the heart, and then induces deficiency of heart-qi, which in turn causes deficiency of gallbladder-qi. The condition of deficiency of gallbladder-qi is liable to be frightened and deficiency of heart causes palpitating and sleeplessness. Therefore the patient with deficiency of both heart- and gallbladder-qi is often sleepless and dreamy, liable to awake and vigilant after wake. Low spirit, tiredness and spontaneous perspiration are all the expressions of qi deficiency. Light tongue proper, taut and thready, or thready and weak pulse are the symptoms caused by insufficiency of qi and blood. In summary, insomnia caused by both heart- and gallbladder-qi can be divide into two types: frightening due to deficiency and deficiency due to frightening. They have reciprocal causation and should be given consideration to both of them in the treatment.

Therapeutic methods: replenishing qi, relieving convulsion, tranquilizing and calming mind.

Prescriptions and drugs: Modified "An Shen Ding Zhi Pill" is used. In the prescription, ginseng replenish qi and dragon's teeth relieve convulsion as the main drugs; poria cocos, poria with hostwood, grassleaved sweetflag rhizome, polygala root as assistants for replenishing qi, reinforcing gallbladder and relieving mental stress. In the case of deficiency of both heart-qi and heart-yang, add cinnamon twig and licorice root to replenish heart-qi and warm the heart-yang. If the symptoms manifested as fidgeting, sleeplessness and deficiency of blood, the prescription "Suan Zao Ren Decoction" is used to replenish heart and tranquilize the mind, clear away heat and relieve restlessness. In this prescription, wild jujuba seed nourish liver-blood and tranquilize mind; chuanxiong rhizome regulate the flow of qi and blood and soothe liver-qi; poria cocos and licorice root relieve mental stress; anemarrhena rhizome remove heat and relieve restlessness. To those patients of this type with severe deficiency of qi and blood, the prescription of "An Shen Ding Zhi Pill" combined with "Gui Zhi Gan Cao Decoction" or "Suan Zao Ren Decoction" is used according to the different conditions between qi and blood deficiency.

Example of prescription: pilose asiabell root 10g, poria with hostwood 10g, crude dragon's teeth (pre-decocted) 30g, grassleaved aweetflag rhizome 10g, cinnamon twig 6g, prepared licorice root 6g, parched date seed 15g, polygala root 10g, anemarrhena rhizome 10g.

In addition, in the case with restlessness and sleeplessness, pale complexion, low spirit, tiredness, light tongue proper, thready and weak pulse after sickness, or the patient is aged and weak, "early to awake" without fidgeting, the treatments should be nourishing blood and tranquilizing mind because of their insufficiency of qi and blood. The prescription used may be "Gui Pi Decoction". If sleeplessness with deficiency of blood and liver-heat after sickness, "Hu Bo Duo Mei Pill" or "Suan Zao Ren Decoction" is used in combination with crude abalone shell, dragon's teeth, or oyster shell and the like for the treatment. If the syndrome manifested as breakdown of normal physiological coordination between the heart and the kidney, yang of the deficiency type attacking upwards, the prescription "Jiao Tai Pill" should be used. In this prescription, rhubarb clear away fire as its main activity, associated with cinnamon twig to warm the kidney and conduct fire back to its origin for it is warm in nature. To treat the symptoms of general sleeplessness, dreaminess, palpitating and restlessness by differentiation method, drugs for expectorant treatment may be used to calm the mind, such as dragon's bone, dragon's teeth, magnetite and pearl oyster for calming the liver and suppressing hyperactive yang of the liver, relieving convulsion and calming the mind, and cinnabar for relieving mental stress; wild jujuba seed, aborvitae seed and fleece-flower stem for nourishing heart and tranquilizing mind.

〔Measures of Prevention and Nursing〕

Since insomnia is a disease occurred in the heart, the prevention of it should take care of the state of mind. Be moderate in changing moods and have easy of mind. After the patient has suffered from the disease, pay attention to the spirit state of the patient, and speak comfort to him (her) and free his (her) mind of apprehensions and misgivings. Lessen or avoid irritation. Don't drink wine, strong tea and smoke before going to bed. Wash feet with warm water. The environment noise often influence the patient's sleep. Try to find a way to reduce the noise.

The patient with insomnia is better to take proper exercise every day. The exercise will improve the patient's constitution and health. Keep in a regular daily life. Work and rest according to schedule. Form a good habit of sleep.

As for the nursing of the patient, the administration of the drug is important. In order to achieve good result, advise the patient not to take the drugs in the morning or forenoon. Only take medicines once in the afternoon or before afternoon nap and once in the evening just before going to bed. To those who suffered from severe insomnia or even with mental symptom concurrently, take note to safety, thereby avoiding accident.

〔Analysis of Typical Cases〕

Case 1. Xu, young. Because of working hard and anxiety, being mentally and physically exhausted with the passing of time, often awake all the night. taking medicines of western medicine can sleep for a few hours, dreamy during sleep, feel fatigue after wake up. Since summer of this year, the sleeplessness became more serious, fail to respond to all previous treatments, no sleep for three nights from 14th to 16th, August, muddleheaded, loss of appetite. pale complexion but glowing with health, going on talking and laughing as if nothing had happened. light conjunctival congestion, taut and long guan pulse, dark lines on tongue edge. Drugs used in prescription: peach kernel 12g, safflower 9g, Chinese angelica root 9g, chuanxiong rhizome 9g, achyranthes root 9g, notoginseng 9g, rehmannia root 9g, bupleurum root 6g, red peony root 9g, parched immature bitter orange 6g, prepared licorice root 3g.

The patient fell asleep easily after one dosage, no relapse after been administered fifteen dosages. The patient asked for help two months later, complaining no sleep again. The illness condition was milder than before. taut guan pulse, showing excess syndrome, prescribed "Long Dan Xie Gan Decoction" because the symptoms manifested as head-ache, conjunctival congestion and flaming-up of the liver-fire. Drugs used in prescription:

Scutellaria root 9g, gentian root 4.5g, crude rehmannia root 9g, alisma orientale 9g, plantain seed 9g, crude licorice root 3g, bupleurum root 6g, pittosporm root 9g, Chinese angelica root 6g, manshurian aristolochia stem 9g.

The disease was fully recovered after taking five dosages of the above prescription, the symptoms of flaring-up of liver-fire eliminated entirely (from the medical records of Dr. Fan Wenhu, "Zhong Yi Za Zhi", 7,15,1963.).

Comment: The patient has been overworked and was anxious excessively. The disease was caused by the stagnation of qi for a long time and obstruction of blood circulation. The obstructed blood circulation then turn into heat which invades the heart. The blood stasis affects the liver causing light conjunctival congestion, taut and long guan pulse and dark lines on the tongue edge. Therefore the insomnia was cured by treatment with the prescription "Xue Fu Zhu Yu Decoction" in combination with notoginseng that has the functions of promoting blood circulation and removing blood stasis. In the patient's return visit, the syndrome manifested as flaming-up of liver-fire, as said Dr. Ke Yunbo "the hyperactive liver-fire attacking upwards causing no sleep". The treatment was changed according to the syndrome to use the prescription "Long Dan Xie Gan Decoction" for eliminating liver-fire. Since the prescription was tally with the syndrome, the therapeutic effect was obvious.

Insomnia, the sleeplessness is caused mostly by impairing of mental state, immoderate diet, imbalance between work and rest or weakness during convalescence. The disease can be classified into five types according their pathogenesis, i. e., stagnation of liver turning fire, disturbance of phlegm-heat, hyperactivity of fire due to yin deficiency, deficiency of both heart and spleen, and deficiency of both heart- and gallbladder-qi. The site of the disease is in the heart, involving liver, gallbladder, spleen, stomach and kidney. The basic pathogenesis are excess of yang and deficiency of yin, imbalance of yin and yang and the disturbance of the mental activity. Since the causes of mental stress can be differentiated as weakness of body resistance and prevailing of pathogenic factors, the differentiation of insomnia must be starting with the differentiation of excess and deficiency. The deficiency is manifested as insufficiency of qi and blood, and the excess as hyperactivity of phlegm-heat and retention of food. Most of the disease are of the deficiency type, some of them are coexisted. The principle of the treatment should be reinforcing the deficiency and reducing the excess and regulating the relation of yin and yang. The therapeutic methods may be as follows at doctor's discretion: soothing liver and removing heat, nourishing yin to reduce pathogenic fire, coordinating between the functions of the heart and the kidney, supplementing the heart and spleen, replenishing qi and relieving convulsion, and resolving phlegm to purge heat.

Questions for Review

1. Describe the causes and the pathogenesis of insomnia.
2. Describe the main symptoms and signs, therapeutic method and prescriptions and drugs used of insomnia caused by hyperactivity of fire due to yin deficiency or accumulation of phlegm invading upwards, respectively.

Mclancholia

〔Introduction〕

The melancholia is the general name of the diseases caused by emotional stress and stagnation of functional activities of qi. The so called stagnation means blockade, obstruction or not smooth. It contains either the causes or the pathogenesis of the disease. Melancholia is a concept of its pathogenesis and pathology, and a syndrome complex as well. The clinical manifestation of the disease is very complicated. Broadly speaking, all the symptoms manifested as dysfunction of viscera and obstruction of the flow of qi, blood and fluid caused by affection of the six external etiological factors, internal injury by the seven emotions, and the symptoms of accumulation of the pathologic products of qi, blood, phlegm, fire, dampness, food, are called melancholia. The definition of melancholia in narrow sense refers to a complicated syndromes manifested as depression, moodiness, sorrow, susceptible to cry, distention and pain in chest and hypochondrium, foreign body sensation in throat caused by emotional discomfort and stagnation of qi.

Early in an ancient book "Nei Jing·Liu Yuan Zheng Ji Da Lun" appeared the concept of "five kinds of stagnation" and its therapeutic principles. The principles read, "To treat wood stagnation by extending, fire stagnation by dispersing, earth stagnation by taking away, metal stagnation by purging, water stagnation by subduing". The author holds that all the disease are caused by qi, it may occur in all five solid organs (viscera), and considers that the emotional discomfort is one of the important causes of the disease. In the classics "Jin Gui Yao Lue" recorded various clinical manifestations and effective therapeutic measures. Chen Yan of North Song Dynasty in his book "San Yin Fang" put forward the theory of the etiology of seven emotions and laid a foundation of the theory that "stagnation is caused by nothing more than seven emotions".

Zhu Danxi of Yuan Dynasty first proposed the theory of "six kinds of stagnancy", namely, qi, blood, phlegm, heat, dampness and food, in which the qi stagnancy is the most important. He first set up the prescription "Yue Ju Pill" for treating melancholia. In the prescription, the drug cyperus tuber for relieving stagnation is the main constituent. Zhang Jingyue, the famous physician of Ming Dynasty considered in a broad sense that sometimes "disease causes stagnation" and sometimes "stagnation causes disease". The understanding was more profoundly than before. In Qing Dynasty, Ye Tianshi emphasized that "the stagnation of seven emotions is in the majority" and the lesions involve liver, gallbladder, heart and spleen. In the treatment, the disease should first be differentiated the causes or condition of qi, blood, initial or protracted. The drugs used may be that bitter and pungent in flavor, cool and moist in property and possess the dispersing function. It is not practicable to relieve the stagnation of qi with potent drugs pungent in flavor in the treatment. Care should be devoted to the regulation of mental activity. So far these suggestions still have directive function.

All the diseases in western medicine, such as neurosis, hysteria, menopausal syndrome, that possess the symptoms of melancholia can be differentiated and treated in the light of what described in this chapter.

〔Pathogenesis and Pathology〕

Melancholia is caused mostly by emotional stress, such as failing in an attempt, depression, stagnation of qi and pent-up vexation that induce the stagnation of liver-qi. The disorder of liver-qi further causes the disturbance of visceral functions. The site of the lesions mainly in the liver, spleen and heart. The main pathology being derangement of qi and blood.

Ⅰ. Smoldering discontent causes the disorder of liver-qi. The stagnated qi results in the stagnation of liver-qi. The stagnation will turn into fire for it could not be relieved in course of time. The prolonged stagnation of qi causes the obstruction of blood circulation, thus bringing about blood stasis. If the stagnation or vexation injure the spleen, the transporting function of the spleen will be deactivated. The accumulation causes phlegm, which in turn integrates with qi to form the stagnation of qi and phlegm. Then the stagnation of dampness occurred because of the obstruction of the flow of qi and intensifying of pathogenic dampness. The retention of food thus formed due to dyspepsia. Thus the stagnation of qi, dampness, phlegm and retention of food all occurred and turn into heat with the passing of time. If the stagnated heat can no be relieved, the heat stagnation formed finally.

Ⅱ. Depression and discontent cause stagnation of liver and inhibit the spleen functions. The dysfunction of the spleen in transporting, loss of appetite and lack of source of growth and development cause insufficiency of qi and blood, deficiency of both the heart and spleen, and finally the failure of the heart to be nourished. On the other hand, the deficient heart and spleen turn into fire with the passing of time which burn the yin-blood and involve in the kidney thereby causing hyperactivity of fire and deficiency of yin, then developing into various deficiency syndromes.

In summary, the main causes of melancholia involve the emotions of indignation, pent-up vexation, anxiety and grief. These induce the failure of dispersing of liver-qi, dysfunction of the spleen in transporting nutrients, mental stress and incoordinate of viscera, yin, yang, qi and blood. At the initial stage of the disease, the flow of qi is obstructed, the blocked qi then influence the blood and viscera. The obstruction of qi and blood further causes the stagnation of dampness, phlegm, heat and retention of food successively. The syndromes are mainly belonging to the excess type. These stagnancies in turn exacerbate the stagnation of the activity of qi. Prolonged stagnation of qi impairs the qi-blood and transform the syndrome from excess to deficiency. At this time, deficiency of both the heart and spleen, hyperactivity of fire and deficiency of yin appeared and these may even developed into consumptive disease.

〔Diagnosis and Treatment by Differentiation of Syndromes〕

Ⅰ. Key points of differentiation

1. Since melancholia is caused by mental stress and the obstruction of functional activities of qi, the general causes of the disease are mental stimulation and impairing of seven emotions. Most of the diseases are caused by smoldering or pent-up fury, others by melancholy, anxiety, grief and fear emotions.

2. Determination of the main symptoms and differentiation between the syndromes of excess and deficiency. In the initial stage of melancholia, the syndrome is mainly belonging to excess manifested as stagnation of liver-qi or mixed up with phlegm-dampness, retention of food and heat stagnancy. In protracted cases, the disease is developing from to the blood system, from excess to deficiency. Most of the diseases in clinical practice are of the mixing type. The differentiation should further apply to other aspects: initial or protracted, in qi or blood system, single or multiple stagnancy.

3. Clinical features of melancholia: The principal feature is the symptoms of stagnation of liver-qi because the disease is beginning from the qi system. The manifestations are complicated, changeable, obscure or delayed to occur. Sometimes the patients complains to the doctor of his sufferings that cannot be described, but there are no subjective symptoms under examination. Sometimes complicated diseases may occur owing to misdiagnosis or improper medication. If the patient could not be recovered promptly, it finally became the so-called "difficult and complicated cases". In clinical practice, the symptoms must be traced to its source or origin.

Diagram of the Causes and Pathogenesis of Melancholia

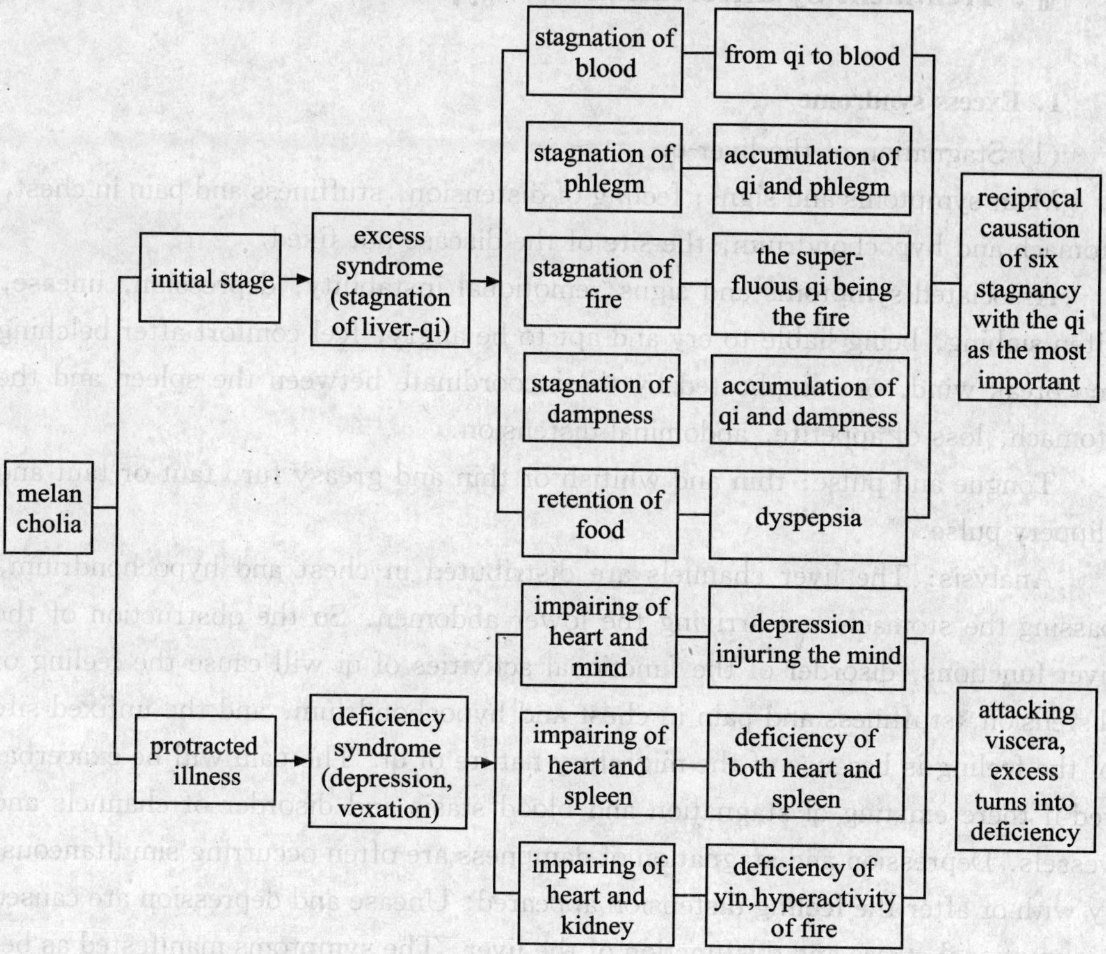

Ⅱ. Principles of the treatment

The general principle of the treatment is regulating the circulation of qi, that is so-called wood stagnancy by extending. It is important to regulate the circulation of qi in the initial stage of the disease, so as to prevent the occurring of other diseases. To those patients with excess syndrome, the treatments may be soothing the depressed liver and regulating the circulation of qi, and with the prescriptions that have the functions of promoting the circulation of blood, resolving phlegm, removing dampness, clearing away heat and promoting digestion. To those with deficiency syndrome, treat them by the therapeutic methods of supplementing qi and enriching blood, and with the drugs that nourish yin and the heart, and strengthen the body resistance.

Ⅲ. Treatment by differentiation of types and syndromes

1. Excess syndrome

(1) Stagnation of the liver-qi

Main symptoms and signs: feeling of distension, stuffiness and pain in chest, stomach and hypochondrium, the site of the disease not fixed.

Associated symptoms and signs: emotional instability, depression, unease, often sighing, being liable to cry and apt to be angry, feel comfort after belching and break wind, or complicated by the incoordinate between the spleen and the stomach, loss of appetite, abdominal distension.

Tongue and pulse: thin and whitish or thin and greasy fur, taut or taut and slippery pulse.

Analysis: The liver channels are distributed in chest and hypochondrium, passing the stomach and arriving the lower abdomen. So the obstruction of the liver functions, disorder of the functional activities of qi will cause the feeling of distension, stuffiness and pain in chest and hypochondrium, and the unfixed site of the feeling is because of the migratory nature of qi. The pain will be exacerbated if there existing qi stagnation and blood stasis and disorder of channels and vessels. Depression and stagnation of dampness are often occurring simultaneously with or after the feeling distension appeared. Unease and depression are caused by emotional stress and dysfunction of the liver. The symptoms manifested as being liable to cry and apt to be angry, feel comfort after belching and break wing are the result of the relaxation of qi stagnation. The impairing if the stomach and spleen, causes the failing of descending of the stomach-qi and dysfunction of the spleen in transporting, thereby appearing the symptoms of loss of appetite, abdominal distension, nausea, vomiting and irregular bowel movement. If the stagnation of qi attacks the blood which then causes the qi stagnancy and blood stasis and debility of Chong and Ren channels, the irregular menstruation occurs. Taut pulse, thin and whitish tongue fur are caused by stagnation of liver-qi, and when the latter combined with stagnation of dampness, it will cause taut and slippery pulse and whitish greasy tongue fur.

Therapeutic methods: soothing the liver, alleviating of mental depression.

Prescriptions and drugs: Modified "Chai Hu Shu Gan Powder" is used. The prescription has the functions of regulating qi by alleviation of mental depression, and promoting blood circulation and assuaging pain. In the prescription, bupleurum root, immature bitter orange and cyperus tuber soothe the liver and activate the flow of qi, and alleviate mental depression. Chuanxiong rhizome, peony root and licorice root promote blood circulation and alleviate pain. Bupleurum root combining with peony regulate the functional activities of qi for the arrangement of their functions: one dispersing and the other restraining. Bupleurum root, bitter in taste and mild in nature, is acting on the liver by alleviating mental depression in the qi system. White peony root, sour and bitter in taste, slightly cold in nature is also acting on the liver. It soothes and relieves spasm in the blood system. Bupleurum root and white peony root as drug pair has given consideration to both qi and blood systems, and complemented each other. Addition of curcuma root, green tangerine orange peel, finger citron and citron fruit enhances the activity of alleviating depression. In the case of belching frequently, feeling of fullness and stuffiness in chest and stomach, add inula flower, red ochre, perilla stem and tangerine peel to calm the liver, normalize the stomach, lower the adverse flow of qi and arrest vomiting. If the symptoms manifested as retention of food, abdominal distension and fullness, loss of appetite and stuffiness in stomach, add medicated leaven, hawthorn fruit, malt, radish seed and membrane of chicken gizzard to promote digestion and remove food stagnation. In the case of abdominal distension and loose stool, thin greasy or thin whitish tongue fur, add atractylodes rhizome, poria cocos and magnolia bark to invigorate spleen and eliminate dampness. If the symptoms manifested as fixed feeling of distension and pain in chest and hypochondrium, or irregular menstruation, taut and uneven pulse, add Chinese angelica root, motherwort, red sage root, peach kernel and safflower to promote blood circulation and remove blood stasis.

Since the qi stagnancy is the principal cause of the six kinds of stagnancy, the prescription "Yue Ju Pill" is used or used in combination with other drugs in the treatment of melancholia to promote the flow of qi and alleviate depression. The main function of the prescription is treating the qi stagnancy, and in the same time relieving the stagnancy of blood, phlegm, dampness, food and fire. So it is a prescription that relieve all of the six kinds of stagnancy.

In treating the stagnation of liver-qi, first to determine the degree of qi stagnancy on the basis of the degree of distension and pain, the location of the illness, and then choose drugs for soothing the liver and regulating qi. In the case of slight distension, use citron fruit, finger citron and mume flower to regulate qi. If the distension is not very serious, use cyperus tuber, tangerine peel, curcuma root, Sichuan chinaberry, immature bitter orange, green tangerine orange peel, magnolia bark and aucklandia root to promote and regulate the flow of qi. If the distension and pain is serious, use immature bitter orange, eagle wood, sandalwood, dalbergia wood, safflower and red sage root to promote the flow of qi, relieve the qi stagnancy, and then promote the blood circulation. Since most of the drugs for regulating qi are pungent and aromatic in flavor, warm and dryness in nature, and the accumulated qi stagnancy would turn into fire with the passing of time, the drugs used in clinical practice are usually citron fruit, finger citron and oroxylum seed that are pungent in flavor, mild in nature, or, use the drugs bitter in flavor, cold in nature, such as curcuma root, Sichuan chinaberry, corydalis tuber and areca seed. The prescription may be modified in the light of associate symptoms and signs.

Example of prescription: bupleurm root 10g, white peony root 10g, immature bitter orange 10g, cyperus tuber 10g, curcuma root 10g, chuanxiong rhizome 6g, finger citron 10g, atractylodes rhizome 9g, charred malt, millet sprout and medicated leaven, 10g each.

(2) Stagnation of qi turning into fire

Tongue and pulse: red tongue with thin yellow coating, taut rapid pulse.

Main symptoms and signs: feeling of distension, stuffiness and pain in chest and hypochondrium, irritable, be liable to be angry.

Associated symptoms and signs: head-ache, tinnitus, flushed face, conjunctival congestion, or dry and bitter taste in mouth, gastric discomfort with acid regurgitation, constipation.

Analysis: The stagnation of liver-qi and blood stasis cause the feeling of fullness, stuffiness and pain in chest and hypochondrium because of the theory "obstruction causing pain". The irritable emotion, head-ache, tinnitus, flushed face and ears are caused by the stagnated qi turning into fire and the flaming-up of the liver-fire. The attacking of the stomach by liver-fire causes dry and bitter taste in mouth, gastric discomfort with acid regurgitation and constipation. Red tongue proper, thin yellow fur, taut rapid pulse are all the expressions of the superfluous liver-fire.

Therapeutic methods: purging the liver of pathogenic fire, alleviating mental depression and regulating the stomach function.

Prescriptions and drugs: The prescription "Dan Zhi Xiao Yao Powder" is used in combination with "Zuo Jin Pill". "Dan Zhi Xiao Yao Powder" is composed of "Xiao Yao Powder" and red sage root and capejasmine fruit. The compound prescription has the functions of soothing liver, alleviating depression, clearing away heat, strengthening spleen and nourishing blood. "Zuo Jin Pill" has the functions of removing fire from liver and regulating the stomach function. In the prescription "Xiao Yao Powder", bupleurum root, white peony root and peppermint soothe liver and alleviate depression; white peony root and Chinese angelica root nourish blood and soothe liver; white atractylodes rhizome, poria cocos, licorice root and roasted ginger strengthen the spleen and regulate the middle energizer, and add red sage root and capejasmine fruit to purge liver-fire and remove heat from blood. In the prescription "Zuo Jin Pill", coptis root is used to purge the heart- and stomach-fire according to the principle "treating the excess syndrome (of the mother organ) by reducing the son organ", and evodia fruit as assistant to alleviate depression and regulate the stomach. If the symptoms manifested as bitter taste in mouth, yellow tongue fur, constipation, add gentian root and rhubarb to purge fire and relax the bowels. In the case of hyperactivity of liver-fire, feeling of fullness and pain in the head, anxiety and anger, and constipation, use "Dan Zhi Xiao Yao Powder" plus "Dang Gui Long Hui pill" for the treatment.

Example of prescritpion: bupleurum root 9g, white peony root 12g, peppermint 6g (decocted later), Chinese angelica root 10g, poria cocos 12g, tree peony bark 9g, capejasmine fruit 9g, coptis root 6g, evodia fruit 2g, curcuma root 10g.

(3) Stagnation of qi and accumulation of phlegm

Main symptoms and signs: discomfort in the throat, having foreign body sensation which could not be either expectorated or swallowed, stuffiness feeling in chest.

Associated symptoms and signs: feeling of distension, stuffiness and pain in chest and hypochondrium.

Tongue and pulse: whitish and greasy fur, taut and slippery pulse.

Analysis: The liver stagnancy attacks the spleen when one is in low spirits. The foreign body sensation in throat, so called "globus hystericus" is caused by the symptoms manifested as failing of the spleen to transport nutrients, accumulation of phlegm-dampness, integration of phlegm and qi in the chest and throat. The symptoms are exacerbated or alleviated along with the emotional changes. Stuffiness in chest, distension and pain in chest and hypochondrium are caused by disorder of the liver function and obstruction of the flow of qi. Whitish and greasy tongue fur and taut and slippery pulse are the expressions of integration of phlegm and qi.

Therapeutic methods: resolving phlegm, promoting flow of qi, alleviating depression.

Prescriptions and drugs: Modified "Ban Xia Hou Pu Decoction" is used. The prescription has the functions of alleviating depression, lowering the adverse of qi, resolving phlegm and dispersing accumulation. In the prescription, use pinellia tuber, magnolia bark, and fresh ginger to disperse accumulation of for they are pungent in flavor, and lower the adverse flow of qi for they are bitter in taste. Poria cocos is used in combination to invigorate spleen and resolve phlegm, and perilla leaf to alleviate depression and regulate the blood. Add cyperus tuber, immature bitter orange, finger citron and citron fruit to regulate the flow of qi and alleviate depression. Add perilla stem, perilla fruit, inula flower and red ochre to resolve phlegm and lower the adverse flow of qi. If the symptoms associated with dry and bitter taste in mouth, vomiting and restlessness, yellow and greasy tongue fur, the prescription "Wen Dan Decoction" should be used in combination with scutellaria root, fritillary bulb, trichosanthes peel, cyperus tuber, curcuma root and perilla stem to resolve phlegm, clearing away heat, and regulate the functional activities of qi.

Example of prescription: Inula flower 15g (parched separately), perilla stem 10g, cyperus tuber 10g, scutellaria root 10g, poria cocos 15g, red ochre 30g (predecocted), pinellia tuber 10g, magnolia bark 9g, immature bitter orange 9g, tangerine peel 10g.

2. Deficiency syndrome

(1) Depression impairing the mental activity

Main symptoms and signs: grief, depression, be liable to cry, sometimes loudly, sometimes weep in silence.

Associated symptoms and signs: absentminded, feel uneasy or perturbed

Tongue and pulse: light tongue proper, thin and whitish fur, taut and thready pulse.

Analysis: The absentminded and uneasy mood is caused by excessive depression and melancholy which exhaust the heart-qi and consume the ying-blood. The patients often show amentia, unease, grief and cry involuntarily, frequent yawning, or other uncommon behaviors. This is what called "Zang Zao (hysteria)" in the classics "Jin Gui Yao Lue" which is often occurs in women. The light tongue proper, thin and whitish tongue fur, taut and thready pulse are all the expressions of qi stagnancy and insufficiency of blood.

Therapeutic methods: nourishing the heart to calm the mind.

Prescriptions and drugs: Modified "Gan Mai Da Zao Decoction" is used. In the prescription, licorice root regulate the stomach, nourish qi and relieve spasm, wheat of sweet in flavor and slightly cold in nature nourish the heart-qi and tranquilize the mind. Chinese date of sweet in flavor, mild in nature and moist in property, replenish the spleen and moisturize the dryness. These three drugs in combination possess the functions of relieving spasm, nourishing heart and calm the mind. Addition of aborvitae seed, wild jujuba seed, poria with hostwood and albizia flower enhance the actions of other drugs. For the symptoms manifested as palpitating, unease, dysphoria with feverish sensation in chest, palms and soles and sleeplessness, add donkey-hide gelatin, dragon's teeth, oyster shell, nacre, pig iron cinder to nourish the heart- and liver-yin and tranquilize with heavy materials. The symptoms may also be treated by modified "Gan Mai Da Zao Decoction", i.e., by adding peony root and amethyst to the prescription. The prescription is originated from the book "Fu Ke Ji Yao" in which the peony root and licorice root of the sweet flavor and sour taste nourish yin and the amethyst relieve palpitating and tranquilize the mind. If the patient is impatient, apt to be angry, dizzy with tinnitus, add crude abalone shell, red ochre, tribulus fruit to clam the liver and check exuberance of yang.

Example of prescription: Prepared licorice root 12g, light wheat 30g, Chinese date 7 pieces, parched jujuba seed 20g, poria with hostwood 15g, white peony root 10g, albizia flower 10g, crude dragon's teeth 30g (pre-decocted), crude oyster shell 30g (pre-decocted).

(2) Deficiency of both the heart and the spleen

Main symptoms and signs: over-deliberated, palpitating and timid.

Associated symptoms and signs: short of sleep, amnesia, pale complexion, dizziness, loss of appetite.

Tongue and pulse: light tongue proper, thready and weak pulse.

Analysis: Over-deliberation impairs the heart and spleen, hence causing deficiency of both qi and the blood. When the heart is failing to be nourished, gallbladder-qi deprived, and the mental activity deranged, the palpitation, timid, sleeplessness and amnesia appear. Loss of appetite and pale complexion are caused by dysfunction of the spleen, incoordinate between the spleen and the stomach and lack of the source of nutrients to nourish qi and blood. Light tongue proper, thready and weak pulse are the expressions of dizziness and mental fatigue.

Therapeutic methods: invigorating spleen, nourishing heart, replenishing qi and enriching blood.

Prescriptions and drugs: Modified "Gui Pi Decoction" is used. The prescription is composed of "Si Jun Zi Decoction", "Dang Gui Bu Xue Decoction" and drugs of longan aril, wild jujuba seed, aucklandia root, polygala root, fresh ginger and Chinese dates. The prescription possesses the functions of invigorating spleen, nourishing heart, activating qi and enriching blood, hence being the prescription commonly used for treating deficiency of both the heart and the spleen. The purpose of the prescription is to invigorate spleen and replenish qi for generating blood. The normalization of the functions of qi and blood will bring about the heart to be nourished. The drugs for alleviating depression and causing tranquilization, such as curcuma root, cyperus tuber and albizia flower may be added. And, the drugs for soothing liver and normalizing stomach may also be added, such as citron fruit and finger citron and mume flower.

Example of prescription: Pseudostellaria root 15g, astragalus root 10g, parched white atractylodes rhizome 10g, poria with hostwood 15g, Chinese angelica root 10g, parched jujuba seed 15g, longan aril10g, aucklandia root 4g, prepared licorice root 6g, curcuma root 10g, finger citron 10g, Chinese date 5 pieces.

(3) Hyperactivity of fire due to yin deficiency

Main symptoms and signs: dizziness, tinnitus, dysphoria, be apt to be angry, palpitating, short of sleep.

Associated symptoms and signs: sourness of waist, emission, or irregular menstruation.

Tongue and pulse: red tongue proper, taut, thready and rapid pulse.

Analysis: Stagnation of liver-qi or usually yin deficiency will turn into fire that cause the impairing of yin fluid. Then insufficiency of visceral ying-yin and hyperactivity of fire due to yin deficiency cause dizziness, tinnitus, dysphoria and being apt to be angry. The palpitation and short of sleep are caused by the failure of the heart to be nourished due to exhaustion of yin-blood. Insufficiency of kidney-yin and failure of the waist to be nourished cause sourness of waist. The spontaneous emission is caused by the minister fire disturbing the essence lodgment and the fragility of the essence gate. The failure of liver and kidney to be nourished and the debility of Chong and Ren channels cause irregular menstruation. Red tongue proper, taut, thready and rapid pulse are the expressions of hyperactivity of fire and yin deficiency.

Therapeutic methods: nourishing yin, clearing away heat, tranquilizing the mind.

Prescriptions and drugs: The modified prescription "Zi Shui Qing Gań Decoction" is used. The prescription is composed of "Liu Wei Di Huang Pill", and drugs of Chinese angelica root, white atractylodes rhizome, bupleurum root, pittosporm root and wild jujuba seed. The functions of the prescription involve nourishing yin, clearing away heat, soothing the liver and tranquilizing mind. In the prescription, "Liu Wei Di Huang Pill" nourish yin and reinforcing kidney, enriching fluid and restrain fire; bupleurum root, white atractylodes rhizome and Chinese angelica root soothe, replenish and nourish the liver; tree peony bark and pittosporm root purge the liver-fire; wild jujuba seed nourishes the heart and calms the mind. The addition of heavy materials, such as nacre, magnetite, pig iron cinder, crude dragon's teeth and crude oyster shell, take the effects of tranquilization, calming the liver and suppressing yang hyperactivity. If the symptoms manifested as sourness of waist, spontaneous emission, add tortoise plastron, anemarrhena rhizome, gordon euryale seed and cherokee rose-hip to supplement kidney and control nocturnal emission. In the case of irregular menstruation, add cyperus tuber, curcuma root and mothewort to relieve depression and regulate the menstruation.

Example of prescription: Fresh rehmannia root 12g, dogwood fruit 10g, Chinese yam 12g, tree peony bark 9g, glossy privet fruit 10g, eclipta 30g, white peony root 10g, pittosporm root 9g, poria with hostwood 15g, nacre 30g (pre-decocted).

〔Measures of Prevention and Nursing〕

1. In addition of the treatment by medicines (pharmacotherapy), the psycotherapy should be used as well in the therapy of melancholia. The physician should show concern for the sufferings of the patient, free their mind of misgivings. Make the patients be optimistic about the disease, adopt a correct attitude towards the disease. To keep ease of mind is beneficial to the recovery of the disease. The suggestion therapy may also be used when it is necessary.

2. Strengthen physical exercises and practise Qigong and shadow boxing (Taiji) as accessory treatment.

〔Analysis of Typical Cases〕

Case 1. Gao, male, age 40. Four months ago, being angry for something, suddenly felt stuffy and suffocated in chest, dizziness, then fainted, and recovered after a little while. Thereafter feeling of stuffiness and suffocation involving soreness of back occurred frequently. The feeling were often related to emotional changes. It was diagnosed as "suspected coronary heart disease" by doctor of western medicine. Recently occurred again due to anger, onset frequently, feeling of fullness and pain in right hypochondrium, light gloomy complexion, purple lips, light fat tongue proper, and having teeth prints on it, taut pulse. Doctor Fang diagnosed the illness as "chest numbness-like syndrome". The site of the disease is in the liver, belonging to the syndrome complex of stagnation of liver-qi and stasis. To treat by soothing liver, alleviating depression, activating qi, promoting blood circulation. Later, treat with method of invigorating spleen to prevent relapse, prescribed modified "Dan Zhi Xiao Yao Powder":

Red sage root 30g, Chinese angelica root 12g, white and red peony root 12g each, bupleurum root 10g, poria cocos 30g, atractylodes rhizome 10g, licorice root 6g, fresh ginger 6g, peppermint 3g (decocted later), turmeria 10g, curcuma root 10g, chuanxiong rhizome 10g, cyperus tuber 10g, immature bitter orange 10g, tangerine peel 10g.

After administered another two dosages, the greater part of the symptoms of the illness alleviated, occasionally felt stuffy in chest from afternoon till midnight. Prescribed the above prescription by adding pilose asiabell root 15g, astragalus root 30g. The patient recovered after administered four dosages (Wang Keqin, "Liao Ning Zhong Yi Za Zhi" 1985{10}:37).

Comment: The patient suffered from the feeling of stuffiness and suffocation in chest because of anger injuring the liver hence causing hyperactivity of liver-qi and accumulation of qi in the chest and diaphragm. The blood is going upwards along with the ascending qi, thus causing dizziness, even being faint. The disease is also alleviated when qi and blood restored to normal state. The disease is also related to mental disorder and so belonging to the syndrome of liver stagnancy. The stagnation enters the blood from qi system, thus forming dim complexion and purple lips. Therefore the disease is treated with the prescriptions of soothing liver, alleviating depression, activating qi and promoting blood circulation. If the tongue proper is bulgy with teeth prints on its border, it indicates the spleen is deficient, then the astragalus root should be added to invigorate the spleen functions.

Melancholia is a category of diseases that are caused by mental stress and stagnation of functional activities of qi. The causes involve anger, depression, excessive deliberation and melancholy. The pathogenesis of the disease include mental stress, disorder of the spleen function and the stagnation of liver-qi. The initial stage of the disease is of qi stagnancy that causes phlegm stagnancy, dampness stagnancy, food retention, heat stagnancy and blood stasis. Prolonged deficiency of the spleen causes the failure of heart and mental activity to be nourished, insufficiency of kidney-yin, finally bringing about imbalance or disorder of viscera, yin, yang, qi and blood. The syndrome of melancholia may be divided into two categories: excess and deficiency. The initial stage is mostly belonging to excess syndrome. It is treated by soothing liver and alleviating depression as the principal therapy, supported by the methods of clearing away heat, resolving phlegm, eliminating dampness, promoting digestion and blood circulation. Protracted illness is mostly belonging to deficiency syndrome. The principal therapeutic methods involve replenishing qi, enriching blood and nourishing heart, supported by invigorating spleen, nourishing yin and tranquilizing mind. When the drugs for regulating qi are used, attention must be paid to the fact that although these drugs are able to regulate qi and alleviate depression, most of them are aromatic and pungent in flavor, dryness and warm in nature. To those patients with the syndromes as stagnancy turning into fire, or yin impaired due to protracted illness, these drugs should be used cautiously. Drugs as citron fruit, finger citron, oroxylum seed and the like can be used for treating either new or protracted disease, either cold or feverish symptoms because of their mild nature and the properties that regulating qi without impairing yin In diagnosis and differentiation of melancholia, the main symptoms and signs must first be determined, and then differentiate deficiency from excess syndrome, locating in qi or blood system, inclining to cold or heat, relating to which of the viscera, according to its medical history and course. Finally determine the therapeutic methods and prescriptions and drugs. The drugs may be mild, cool and moist in nature, bitter and pungent in flavor for their actions of dispersing. The drugs with heavy, restraining, greasy properties should not be used. The patients are asked to take good care of their mental mood, keep optimistic spirit and set up confidence to overcome the disease.

Questions for Review

1. What is melancholia? What are the clinical features of melancholia?
2. Describe the causes and pathogenesis of melancholia.
3. Describe the relationships of the six kinds of stagnancy and their clinical significance.
4. What are the principles of the treatment of melancholia? How to diagnose and treat melancholia based on overall analysis of symptoms and signs?

Manic and Depressive Psychosis

〔Introduction〕

Both the manic and depressive psychoses are the diseases of mental disorder (amentia). The features of depressive psychosis involve mental depression, apathetic expression, dull-witted, speaking incoherently, silent and be liable to laugh. It is mostly caused by the accumulation of phlegm which covers the mind. The features of manic psychosis involve mental hyperactivity, mania, violent-temper, defacing things and maltreated and be easily in a rage. The latter is caused by the accumulation of phlegm-fire which obstructs the heart channel. In clinical, no hard and fast line can be drawn between the two diseases. since they are able to transform each other, an incorporated name, manic and depressive psychosis is generally used.

The manic and depressive psychosis is corresponding to various mental diseases (psychoses) in modern medicine, including organic and functional psychoses. All these diseases that are manifested as above symptoms can be treated in the light of the methods described in this chapter.

〔Pathogenesis and Pathology〕

The exogenous pathogenic factors of manic and depressive psychosis are mostly the attacking of the six climatic conditions in excess and injuries from falls, fractures, contusions and strains. The endogenous pathogenic factors include internal injury of seven emotions or over-deliberation, desire unsatisfied, or intermingles joy and sorrow, anger or frightening. All these impair the heart, spleen, liver, gallbladder and kidney, which then result in the disorder of viscera and imbalance of yin and yang. These further develop the symptoms of qi stagnancy, accumulation of phlegm, excessive fire, blood stasis. Then the symptoms bring about the failure of the mind to be nourished, emptying of the brain and the spinal cord, and finally the mental disorder occurring. Since manic psychosis belongs to yang, depressive psychosis to yin, their causes and pathogenesis are different. Here, the causes and pathogenesis are analyzed in following aspects: imbalance of yin and yang, depression, phlegm-fire invading upwards, stagnation of qi and blood, infection of six exogenous pathogenic climatic factors and the injuries from falls, fractures, contusions and strains.

Ⅰ. Imbalance of yin and yang

Most of the ancient famous physicians of successive dynasties explained the causes of manic and depressive psychosis by the theory of imbalance, excess and deficiency of yin and yang, such as "yin and yang in equilibrium, mental disorder cured". Only yin and yang coordinated, can the mental activities maintain. If the equilibrium are destroyed, mental disorder occurred. hence causing manic and depressive psychoses. All the factors of six climatic conditions, seven emotions and those other than endogenous and exogenous factors bring about the relative imbalance of yin and yang. In addition of the manic and depressive psychosis that are affected by exogenous pathogens, endogenous infection of seven emotions causes the imbalance and injuries as well.

The syndromes of excess and deficiency of yin yang are different. In general, manic psychosis is partial to excess of yang, and the depressive psychosis to excess of yin. In the book "Mai Jing" recorded "When the yin is attached to yang, madness occurs, and if yang attached to yin, depression occurs." The physician Zhu Danxi claimed that "Depression belongs to yin, madness to yang."

Ⅱ. Endogenous infection of seven emotions

The internal injury of seven emotions is one of the important causes. In the book "Nei Jing", the emotional activities were belonging to five solid organs (viscera) respectively, and the viscera-qi may be injured by emotional hyperactivity thereby causing the disorder of the mental normal physiological activities, and finally manic and depressive psychoses. Owing to the changeable emotional mood, vigorous emotional stimulation or emotional hyperactivity, the five solid organs may be injured. This made the functions of viscera abnormal hence causing various pathological changes, failure of the mind to be nourished and affection by endogenous pathogens. Anger, frightening injure the liver and kidney, and being subject to changing mood and anxiety causes impairing of spleen. These cause the impairing of both the heart and spleen, insufficiency of liver and kidney, consumption of heart-yin, hence inducing the emptying of brain and the cord, failure of the mind to be nourished, look being distraught, emotional change, unusual behaviors, losing memory and failing intelligence. When the heart-yin is insufficient, and the heart-fire is hyperactive, the patient will talk wild language and speak disorderly, ceaseless racket and cursing unceasingly, stark-naked without clothing, climbing wall or jumping roofs. If the patient's desire is not satisfied or over deliberated, the heart and the spleen will be impaired. The impaired heart causes exhaustion of mind and deficiency of spleen causes the failure of qi and blood not to circulate or function normally. These finally cause the deficiency of heart blood, failure of the heart to be nourished and state of utter derangement.

Ⅲ. Mental confusion due to phlegm

Owing to the accumulation of phlegm disturbing upwards the vital organ, the heart channel is covered, mental state confused, and occurring the state of unconsciousness, mania, or being reticent, or dull-witted. It finally bring about manic and depressive psychosis. The traditional Chinese medicine is consistently thinking highly of the important role of phlegm in the onset of manic and depressive psychosis. Sun Simiao held that the disease is related to that "influence of phlegm and heat each other causing wind". During the period of Jin through Yuan Dynasties, Zhang Zihe and Zhu Danxi definitely put forward the pathological actions of phlegm in the onset of manic and depressive psychosis. If the dysfunction of the activities of qi, stagnation of liver involving spleen and dysfunction of the spleen are caused by long-term mental factors, the phlegm and qi stagnancy will produced. If the phlegm is produced by deficiency of spleen, abnormality of the transporting of lucid and turbid pathogens and the accumulation of yin pathogenic factors, the syndrome is recognized as deficiency of qi and accumulation of phlegm. The mental confusion is always occurred due to phlegm, no matter the syndrome is accumulation of phlegm due to qi stagnancy, or qi deficiency. The manic psychosis may be caused by failure of the five emotions to be dispersed which condensed to form phlegm, or the impairing of stomach by wind-fire which stored the body fluid to form phlegm-fire, or prolonged accumulation of phlegm turning into fire. In brief, the manic psychosis is always caused by the upwards disturbing of phlegm-fire, mental confusion and disorder.

Ⅳ. Pathogenic fire subjugating the heart

Most of the manic psychosis are caused by the subjugating of the heart by pathogenic fire. According to the circulation rule of channel and collateral, the stomach collateral extends upwards to the heart causing hyperactivity of heat in yangming channel. The latter disturbs the heart and cause aberration and amentia. In general, the excess fire from stomach, liver and gallbladder which disturb the mind can also cause manic psychosis. If the manic psychosis is protracted, or the phlegm still accumulated after the treatment of purging fire, it may change to depressive psychosis.

Ⅴ. Stagnation of qi and blood

The madness may be caused by the failure of brain- and viscera-qi to be integrated smoothly due to the stagnation of qi and blood. Early in the book "Nei Jing" was recorded the relationship between "blood" and "mind". It said "blood being the qi of mind", and "surplus blood causes anger, insufficient blood causes frighten". This indicated that the blood is related to the mental activities. Li Yuan posed the concept that "blood obsessing mind" causes madness. Wang Qingren of Qing Dynasty posed definitely that manic and depressive psychosis is caused by "stagnation of qi and blood". He in his book "Yi Lin Gai Cuo" recorded the treatment of the disease by prescription "Meng Xing Decoction" formulated by himself. The stagnation of qi and blood causes the failure of brain and the cord to be nourished. Or the stagnation of qi and blood stasis occurred in the brain that causes the failure of the house of mental activity to be nourished by qi and blood generated from viscera. Or, the blockade of the channels and vessels by blood stasis and the failure of qi and blood to nourish the brain and the cord cause amnesia and amentia. All these mentioned above are the causes of manic and depressive psychosis.

To sum up, the main inducing factors of the basic causes and pathogenesis of manic and depressive psychosis involve imbalance of yin and yang, internal injury of seven emotions, phlegm-qi disturbing upwards and stagnation of qi and blood. Unresolved anxiety and undue joy and sorrow cause impairing of the heart, liver, spleen and kidney. The impairing of liver- and kidney-yin causes discordance between water and fire, hyperactivity of heart-fire and the stagnation of liver-fire. The prolonged liver-fire stagnancy turns into fire which disturbs upwards the mind. And, liver stagnancy causes the failure of the spleen to transport nutrients, and unresolved dampness pathogen accumulated to form phlegm. The fire and phlegm integrated and stagnated in chest and diaphragm, which disturbs upwards the mind causing mental disorder. The stagnation of qi and blood, and the failure of heart and vital organ to be nourished cause imbalance of yin and yang, disorder of normal functions. These cause manic and depressive psychosis due to yang hyperactivity, or reticence and dementia due to yin hyperactivity.

Diagram of Causes and Pathogenesis

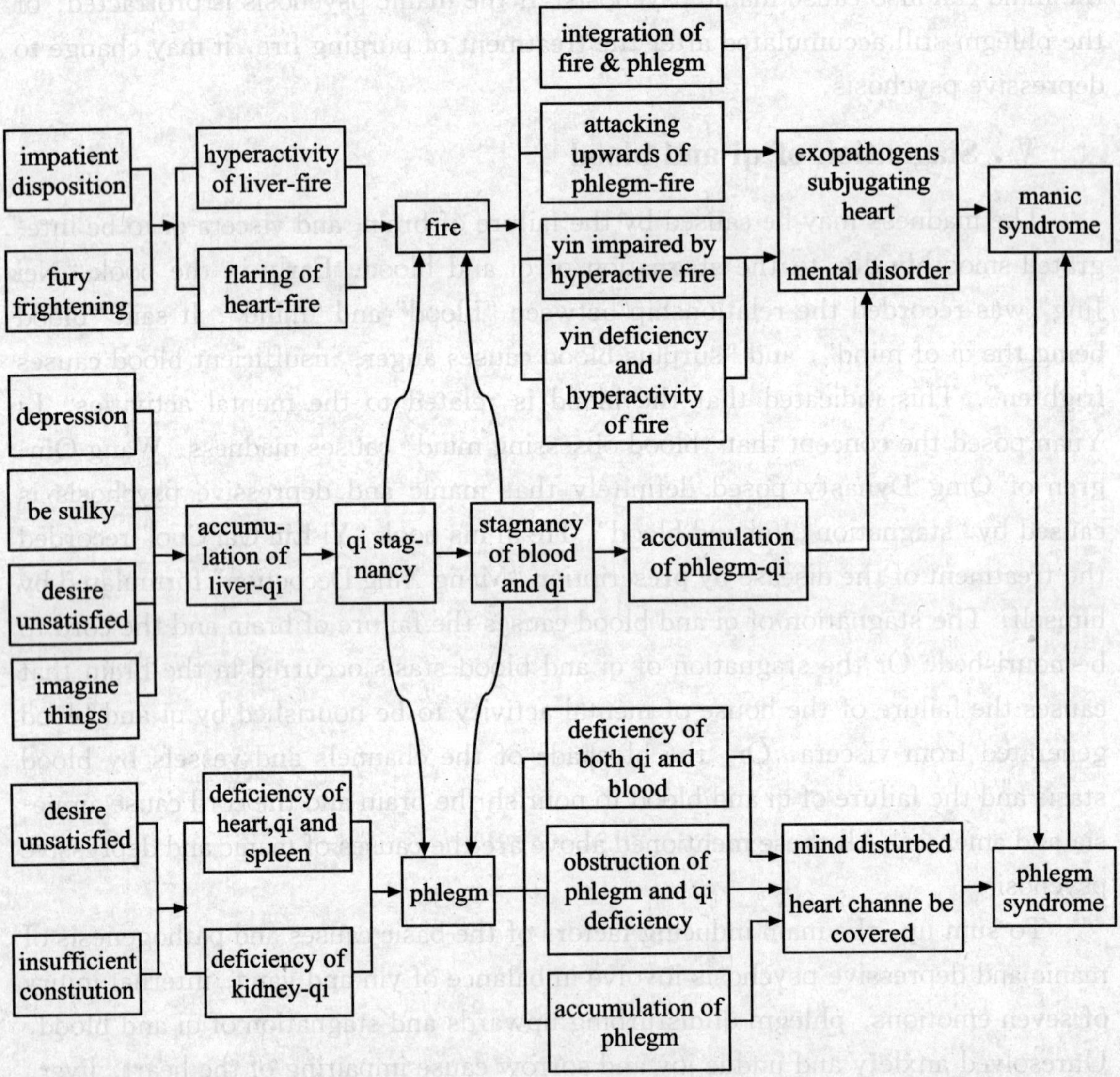

In addition, in Zhang Zhongjing's work "Shang Han Lun", there was the record of "accumulation of blood causing madness". It probably referred to blood stasis. It was stated in the book "Yi Xue Zheng Zhuan" that "the depressive psychosis is due to insufficiency of heart blood". Thus it is clear that deficiency of blood also causes the disease. Further, the outbreak of manic and depressive psychosis is related to congenital constitution. If one has a good constitution with strong physique and balanced yin and yang, the stimulation of seven emotions may be only a transit influence. On the contrary, one may be suffered from the disease by the simulation of grief, frightening, mental stress, imbalance of yin and yang because of insufficient inherent physique. The inherent insufficiency is often having family likeness, so the family members of the patient may often have similar medical history.

It is important to notice that the factors causing the disease are interacting each other even within the same patient.

〔Diagnosis and Treatment by Differentiation of Syndromes〕

The manic and depressive psychosis is as group of diseases that are mainly manifested as mental disorder (insanity) in clinical practice. The mental activities are governed by the heart but closely related to liver and gallbladder, and having internal associations with spleen and kidney as well. If the functions of viscera are in normal state, that means "yin and yang in equilibrium, mind keeping sound." The main causes and pathogenesis are internal injury of seven emotions, obstruction of qi activities, accumulation of phlegm-fire, imbalance of yin and yang. The location of the disease is in the liver, gallbladder, heart and spleen, with heart as the principal. The clinical features are classified into mania and depression because the properties of the pathogens possess the difference of yin and yang, and the constitution of healthy and weak. The key point of the differentiation is to differentiate the depressive and manic syndromes. The features of the depressive syndrome are manifested as mental depression, reticence, dementia, being slow moving and the manic syndrome as racketing, maltreatment, mania, unease and hyperactive behaviors. The clinical features of the two syndromes are different but they have internal relations and no hard and fast lines can be drawn between the two. The protracted depressive psychosis may convert into manic psychosis because of the obstruction of qi activities and endogenous production of phlegm-heat. Similarly, protracted manic psychosis may also convert into depressive psychosis because of violent injury of vital-qi and transforming of pathogens into yin. Sometimes they are complicated by mixing-up each other in clinical practice. In the initial stage of manic and depressive psychosis, the syndrome manifested mostly as excess. If the illness protracted, the vital-qi weakened gradually or the qi and blood being insufficient, or both yin and yang became deficient, the syndrome may become the mixing type of the two. The differentiation of them must be carried out carefully.

The manic and depressive psychosis is usually caused by the internal injury of seven emotions which develops the imbalance of yin and yang or caused by integration of qi and yang. So the principle of the treatment is regulating yin and yang to restore their equilibrium. Most of the depressive psychosis are caused by stagnation of phlegm-qi which obstructs the flow of qi, or they may be caused by deficiency of both the heart and spleen and failure of the heart and mind to be nourished. The therapeutic methods should involve the regulation of qi, relieving stagnation, causing resuscitation and reducing phlegm, nourishing the heart and spleen, enriching blood and tranquilizing mind. The syndromes of manic psychosis involve the upward attacking of phlegm or impairing of yin by hyperactive fire, hence the pathogenic factors are hyper- functioning but the vital-qi is not yet attenuated. The emphasis of the therapeutic methods is eliminating pathogenic factors. The methods of purging fire, reducing phlegm, nourishing yin and removing fire are also commonly used. Most of the drugs used are drastic in property so that to calm the mind of the patients. To those who have the symptoms of blood stasis and interior obstruction, the method of promoting circulation and removing blood stasis should be used. In the cases of protracted manic and depressive psychosis, the methods should be mainly strengthening the body resistance or reinforcing and eliminating in combination because the vital-qi had been injured and the syndrome being mixed deficiency and excess. Special nursing and therapeutic measures should be employed during the convalescence of the disease so as to avoid inducing factors and relapse of the disease.

Most of the depressive psychosis are belonging to deficiency syndrome, the disease of superposed yin. They are mainly caused by qi and phlegm, so the therapeutic methods are relieving stagnation, reducing phlegm, relieving mental stress and nourishing qi and blood. Most of the manic psychosis are belonging to excess syndrome, the disease of superposed yang. They are caused by phlegm-fire and blood stasis, so the therapeutic methods are to wrest the excess first, and then purge fire, or eliminate the phlegm first, and then nourish the heart, liver and yin fluid, so as to clear away the fire of deficiency type. In brief, the manic and depressive psychosis are caused by internal injury of seven emotions, imbalance of yin and yang, incoordinate of deficiency and excess, or integration of qi and yang, or of blood and yin. Therefore the principles of the therapy should be regulating yin and yang so that they can reach an equilibrium.

I. Depressive psychosis

Stagnation of phlegm-qi

Main symptoms and signs: mental depression, apathetic expression, reticent, dull-witted (dementia), or suspicious and over-anxious, subjecting to changing mood, speaking incoherently.

Associated symptoms and signs: muttering to oneself, subjecting to changing mood, loss of appetite.

Tongue and pulse: light tongue proper, whitish and greasy fur, taut and slippery pulse.

Analysis: The over-anxious, desire unsatisfied condition makes the liver-qi be stagnated, obstructed, depressed and finally the formation of pathogenic phlegm. The accumulation of phlegm and the mind been covered cause depression, dull-witted look and talking in a confused manner. Because the phlegm disturbs the mind, the patient became subjecting to changing mood. Loss of appetite is caused by the stagnation of phlegm in the middle energizer. The tongue and pulse are the expressions of stagnation of phlegm.

Therapeutic methods: soothing the liver, relieving stagnation, resolving phlegm and inducing resuscitation.

Prescriptions and drugs: Modified "Xiao Yao Powder" and "Di Tan Decoction" in combination is used. In the former prescription, bupleurum root soothes the liver, alleviates depression, combing with white peony root to enrich blood and soothe the liver; cyperus tuber and curcuma root to enhance the actions of regulating the flow of qi and alleviating depression; poris cocos and white atractylodes rhizome to invigorate the spleen, remove dampness and turbid pathogens. The main functions of the prescription are to soothe liver and alleviate depression. The function of resolving phlegm is relatively weak. So the prescription of eliminating phlegm should be used in combination. The prescription "Di Tan

Decoction" is composed of the prescription "Er Chen Decoction" and five drugs: araesma with bile. immature bitter orange, ginseng, grassleaved sweetflag rhizome and bamboo shavings. "Er Chen Decoction" is the basic prescription for resolving phlegm. The grassleaved sweetflag rhizome is used in combination with curcuma root to induce resuscitation, immature bitter orange with cyperus tuber to regulate the flow of qi. Ginseng here may not be needed.

If the symptoms manifested as mental perplexity, apathetic expression, speaking incoherently, glowering and glaring at things, whitish and greasy tongue fur, the state is recognized as mental disorder. It is treated with the methods of eliminating phlegm and inducing resuscitation. In treatment, use the prescription "Su He Xiang Pill" first to induce resuscitation by aromatics, and then us "Si Qi Decoction" in combination with araesma with bile, grassleaved sweetflagrhizome, polygala root and the like to activate the flow of qi and reduce phlegm.

In the cases of accumulation of phlegm in chest and diaphragm, dull-witted expression, speaking in a confused manner, but the patient is tough and sturdy, with slippery and strong pulse, use the prescription "San Sheng Powder" first to promote expectoration of phlegm. In the prescription, use musk-melon pedicel, ledebouriella root and hellebore root to eliminate phlegm rapidly for the hellebore root possesses vigorous actions though it is toxic. If the patient feels fatigue after vomiting, care and regulate the diet promptly. The purpose of this method is emphasizing on the action of eliminating the pathogenic factors, but it is liable to impair the vital-qi, so it is not recommended to use for a long time. In addition, the prescription "Kong Xian Pill" can also be used to eliminate stubborn phlegm and promote bowel movement for the patients with excessive accumulation of phlegm and a sound body.

If the symptoms are associated with sleeplessness and being subjecting to frightening, dysphoria and unconsciousness, tongue fur turns yellow greasy, tongue proper turns red gradually, the condition showed that the phlegm-qi is accumulated and turning into heat which then integrated with phlegm to disturb the mind. To treat such patient with the prescription "Zhi Bao Pill" which possesses the functions of purging phlegm-heat, clearing away the heart-fire. If the symptoms manifested as hyperactivity of fire and about to be mad, such as ceaseless racket and cursing unceasingly, destroying things and harming others, it is treated by the methods for manic psychosis.

Example of prescriptions: Chinese angelica root 10g, white peony root 10g, poria cocos 30g, curcuma root 10g, bupleurum root 9g, white atractylodes rhizome 12g, pinellia tuber 10g, tangerine peel 9g, arisaema with bile 10g, immature bitter orange 9g, graasleaved sweetflag rhizome 10g, bamboo shavings 6g.

Ⅱ. Deficiency of qi and accumulation of phlegm

Main symptoms and signs: apathetic and indifferent expression, reticent even transfixed, staring like a fool, thinking aloud, lack of initiative, confused mind, presumption, reckless action, blame oneself.

Associated symptoms and signs: sallow complexion, loose stool, clear urine.

Tongue and pulse: light and enlarged tongue proper, whitish and greasy fur, slippery or weak and feeble pulse.

Analysis: When the depressive psychosis is protracted for a long time, the vital-qi must be deficient, the spleen is failing to function transporting and the accumulation of phlegm been more intensified. On the one hand, the accumulation of phlegm intensified gradually and causes the symptoms of apathetic expression, dumb-struck, staring foolishly, or even mental disorder with hallucination. And on the other hand, the yang-qi is gradually exhausted by the pathogenic phlegm and the spleen-qi weakened. These cause the symptoms of sallow complexion, loose stool and clear urine. The abnormal tongue fur and pulse are caused by deficiency of qi and accumulation of phlegm.

If the treatment is prompt and the health care is active, the patient will be recovered after administering the drugs for invigorating qi and eliminating phlegm. These drugs can eliminate the pathogenic phlegm and enable the vital-qi restored. This type of the disease is more easily recur than that caused by accumulation of phlegm-qi. If the disease is protracted and the measures of nursing is improper, the deficiency of qi and the accumulation of phlegm will be more intensified, and thus the disease will be more seriously. The patient may become a disabled person due to the protracted course of the disease and mental disorder.

Therapeutic methods: supplementing qi, invigorating spleen, eliminating phlegm and inducing resuscitation

Prescriptions and drugs: A modification of the prescription "Si Jun Zi Decoction" in combination with "Di Tan Decoction" is used. The "Si Jun Zi Decoction" is composed of pilose asiabell root, poria cocos, white atractylodes rhizome and prepared licorice root. The decoction possesses the functions of supplementing qi, invigorating spleen, strengthening the body resistance and restoring the normal functioning of the body to consolidate the constitution. To use it in combination with pinellia tuber, araesma with bile, red tangerine peel, immature bitter orange, grassleaved sweetflag rhizome and bamboo shavings for eliminating phlegm, and polygala root and curcuma root for regulating qi and relieving phlegm. The addition of grassleaved sweetflag rhizome can enhance the functions of inducing resuscitation of grassleaved sweetflag rhizome. The severe perplexed and dull-witted state is caused by mental confusion due to phlegm. The treatment of it should be eliminating cold-phlegm for resuscitation. Use the prescription "Su He Xiang Pill" to eliminate phlegm and induce resuscitation, one pill, twice a day.

Example of prescriptions: Pilose asiabell root 10g, white atractylodes rhizome 10g, poria cocos 30g, pinellia tuber 10g, tangerine peel 9g, immature bitter orange 10g, glassleaved sweetflag rhizome 12g, bamboo shavings 6g, polygala root 10g, curcuma root 10g.

Deficiency of both heart and spleen

Main symptoms and signs: protracted course of disease, the illness developed slowly, pale complexion, sluggish, too lazy to speak, listlessness, absentminded, palpitating, susceptible to fright and sorrow, presumption, disturbance of thought, talk in a confused manner, demoralized.

Associated symptoms and signs: dreaminess, loss of appetite, loose stool.

Tongue and pulse: light tongue proper, enlarged tongue with teeth prints, thin and whitish fur, weak and feeble pulse.

Analysis: When the disease protracted, qi of the middle energizer weakened and lack of vital source to generate qi and blood, the symptoms will be manifested as pale complexion, fatigue and even extremely tired. The symptoms of absentminded, palpitating, susceptible to fright and despondent are caused by interior deficiency of heart blood and the failure of heart and mind to be nourished. Deficiency of both qi and blood and failure of mental activity to be nourished cause hallucination and presumption. In brief, the disease is usually caused by protracted course, deficiency of both heart and spleen, lack of blood and qi weakness and the failure of mental activity to be nourished. The tongue and pulse express the syndrome of exhaustion of both qi and blood.

Therapeutic methods: strengthening the spleen, replenishing qi, nourishing heart and tranquilizing mind.

Prescriptions and drugs: Modified "Yang Xin Decoction" is employed. In the prescription ginseng, astragalus root and licorice root supplement spleen-qi; Chinese angelica root and chuanxiong rhizome nourish the heart and blood; poria cocos, polygala root, aborvitae seed, wild jujuba seed and schisandra fruit calm the mind, and cinnamon bark introduce the drug into the heart. All these drugs used in combination will take the effects of nourishing heart and tranquilizing mind. If the symptoms associated with aversion to cold, crispation, lie with bending body, clear urine, diarrhea with undigested food in the stool, the syndrome is belonging to insufficiency of kidney-yin. To treat this by adding the drugs that are able to warm kidney-yang, such as psoralea fruit, morinda root, cistanche and so forth, or the modified presription "You Gui Decoction" can be used as well.

Example of presecriptions: Ginseng 6g, astragalus root 20g, prepared licorice root 10g, Chinese angelica root 10g, chuanxiong rhizome 6g, poria cocos 30g, polygala root 10g, aborvitae seed 6g, wild jujuba seed 10g, schisandra fruit 12g, cinnamon bark 3g, curcuma root 10g.

Ⅲ. Manic psychosis

1. Phlegm-fire disturbing heart

Main symptoms and signs: onset suddenly, impetuousness, head-ache, sleeplessness, staring angrily, flushed face and ears, suddenly mad and violent rage, enthusiasm running high, speaking disorderly, climbing walls and roofs, abnormally powerful, making racket and shout in confusion, not caring about various relations, or destroying things and harming others persons, ascending a height and singing, throwing away clothing and running, loving cold drinks, constipation, dark urine.

Associated symptoms and signs: day and night without sleep and eating.

Tongue and pulse: deep red tongue proper, yellow and greasy fur, taut slippery or slippery, rapid and forceful pulse.

Analysis: The violent rage injures the liver causing the hyperactivity of liver-yang. The hyperactivity of fire due to excessive yang-heat activates the yang-ming phlegm-heat which disturb upwards the seven orifices. So the symptoms manifested as impetuousness, head-ache and sleeplessness. When the seven orifices have been covered, the mental activities disordered. Thus the symptoms are expressed as mania, unconsciousness, talking in a confused manner and maltreatment. The limbs are the root of various kinds of yang. When various kinds of yang are hyperactive, the limbs are excessive. The excess of limbs will bring about the symptoms of climbing walls and roofs and exceptional energy. The deep red tongue proper, yellow and greasy fur, and taut, slippery and rapid pulse are all the expressions of the accumulation and hyperactivity of phlegm-fire which is tending to impair yin. The sudden onset and ceaseless madness of the disease is because that the fire belongs to yang and yang has the property of moving about.

Therapeutic methods: purging fire, eliminating phlegm, relieving palpitation and tranquilizing mind.

Prescriptions and drugs: The prescriptions of modified "Xie Xin Decoction" and "Meng Shi Gun Tan Pill" are used. In the prescription rhubarb, coptis root and scutellaria root purge the fire of the heart, liver and stomach channels for their bitter in flavor and cold in nature. The association of anemarrhena rhizome plays the role of maintaining the yin-fluid and pig iron of relieving palpitation and tranquilizing mind. The decoction procedure of the prescription should be as follows: decoct the pig iron first for 20 minutes, then add anemarrhena rhizome, decoct for another 15 minutes, add rhubarb, coptis root and scutellaria root as the drug infusion is still boiling. Continue to boil for 2～3 minutes, filter the extract. The prescription "Meng Shi Gun Tan Pill" is composed of chlorite-schist, eagle wood, rhubarb and mirabilite. The prescription possesses the activities of resolving phlegm and removing fire with vigorous drug property. So the dosage is not allowed to exceed 10g each time. Take drug following its infusion twice a day. After the phlegm-fire is alleviated gradually, the prescription may be decocted with the drugs in a bag and the amount reduced to 3～5g gradually.

If the syndrome is the concentration of heat in yang-ming, the symptoms may be manifested as aberration, delirium, agitation, flushed face, fullness in stomach, constipation, sallow fur with splinter of burned black with breaches, deep red tongue proper, slippery, replete and forceful pulse. Use prescription "Da Cheng Qi Decoction" first to wash away the turbid pathogens, purge excessive fire in stomach and intestines, timely purgation to preserve yin. In the case of extremely thirst, add gypsum and anemarrhena rhizome to clear away heat. For severe cases, use the prescription "Long Hu Pill" that is composed of cow-bezoare, defatted powder of croton seed, cinnabar and arsenolite. The patient may often show the symptoms of vomiting and having diarrhea after taking the prescription. So the prescription is not suitable for protracted use. It is better within the limit that the excess fire is removed. Protracted use will cause the impairing of the stomach and intestines and the consumption of vital-qi.

If the patient is in his (her) right mind, but the phlegm-fire is not entirely removed, and showed restless, sleepless, subjecting to changing mood after treated by the method of purging fire and eliminating phlegm, the prescription "Wen Dan Decoction" may be taking with "Zhu Sha An Shen Pill" to reduce phlegm and tranquilize mind. If the fire is gradually fading and the pathogenic fire is difficult to remove, the patient showed dumb-struck and depressive, it is treated in the light of the methods for treating depressive psychosis.

Example of prescriptions: Chlorite-schist 30g, red ochre 30g, crude gypsum 20g, crude rhubarb 10g (decocted later), scutellaria root 12g, lotus plumule 6g, eagle wood 6g, fleece-flower stem 30g, tree peony bark 12g.

2. Hyperactivity of fire due to yin deficiency

Main symptoms and signs: illness condition alleviated after protracted manic psychosis, be weary in mind, emotional instability, nervous, impatient, palpitating, be susceptible to fright, sometimes mad, restlessness, sleeplessness, dysphoria with feverish sensation in chest, palms and soles.

Associated symptoms and signs: thin body shape, scanty dark urine, constipation.

Tongue and pulse: red tongue proper, less or no fur, thready and rapid or taut and thready pulse.

Analysis: The protracted mania and moving restlessly will certainly cause the injury of both qi and yin. Insufficiency of qi causes weariness in mind, impairing of yin and hyperactivity of fire, which disturb the mental activity. So appeared the symptoms of madness and moving restlessly. The state can not be prolonged for the vital-qi has been impaired. The syndrome is caused mostly by hyperactivity of fire due to yin hurt, and disturbance of mental activity Therefore the symptoms are manifested as anxiety, talk much, susceptible to fright, restlessness, sleeplessness, thin shape and flushed face. Red tongue proper and thready and rapid pulse are the expressions of interior heat due to deficiency of yin.

If the treatment is prompt and proper, the interior heat has cleared away and yin-fluid restored, the illness will be cured. On the contrary, the more yin is deficient, the more the fire is active. The manic symptoms will sometimes appear, sometimes disappear and the illness condition is sometimes mild, sometimes severe. On the other side, according to the theory that the fire and the vital-qi can not coexist, the pathogenic fire not only impairs yin but also exhausts qi. Thus the disease is protracted because of the deficiency of both qi and yin. The disordered mind results in unfavorable prognosis.

Therapeutic methods: nourishing yin and removing fire, tranquilizing mind

Prescriptions and drugs: Take the prescription "Ding Zhi Pill" with the modified prescription "Er Yin Decoction". In the prescription, use rehmannia root, ophiopogon root and scrophularia root to nourish yin and clear away heat; coptis root, manshurain aristolochia stem, lophatherum and rush pith to purge heat, clear away heart-fire and ease the mental activity. Add swallowwort root and wolfberry bark to remove fever of deficiency type; poira with hostwood, parches date seed and licorice root to nourish heart and tranquilizing mind. The prescription "Ding Zhi Pill" is composed of ginseng, poria with hostwood, grassleaved sweetflag rhizome, polygala root and licorice root. The prescription has the functions of invigorating spleen, nourishing heart and tranquilizing mind. It may be taken with the decoction or decocted with the drugs in a bag.

Example of prescriptions: Dried rehmannia root 30g, ophiopogon root 10g, schisandra fruit 12g, scrophularia root 10g, manshurian aristolochia stem 3g, lophatherum 6g, swallowwort root 10g, poria with hostwood 30g (pre-decocted), wolfberry bark 10g, parched date seed 10g, prepared licorice root 10g, crude oyster shell 30g.

3. Stagnation and retention of blood and qi

Main symptoms and signs: dysphoria, fury, talk much, even ascending a height and singing, running and taking off clothing, hallucination, or, dumbstruck, talk less, be in a confused state of mind, often with darkish complexion, stabbing pain and fullness feeling in chest and hypochondrium, palpitating, , or abdominal pain during the menstrual period in women, dark and clot in menstruation, or having injuries from falls, fractures, contusions and strains.

Associated symptoms and signs: head-ache or feeling fullness in the head.

Tongue and pulse: dark purple tongue proper with ecchymosis, thin and whitish or thin and yellow fur, taut and thready or deep and taut pulse.

Analysis: Since qi as the commander of blood, qi activates the blood circulation, qi in motion renders blood circulating normally, and stagnation of qi usually leads to blood stasis. If qi and blood are stagnated, the vital essence and energy could not be supply upwards, thus the heart and mind are failing to be nourished.

The syndrome is formed by the failure of brain-qi and viscera-qi to be linked because of the stagnation of blood and qi. If the stagnation is associated with heat of excess type, yellow tongue fur and taut rapid pulse, the disease is mostly coming on as depressive psychosis. However, the stagnation of qi and blood stasis are the main causes no matter the disease is manic or depressive.

When the patient is treated with the drugs for promoting blood circulation, removing blood stasis and activating the flow of qi, the blood stasis will be alleviated progressively. The patient may be cured and the syndrome improved. If the blood stasis is protracted and causes deficiency, the prognosis will be unfavorable.

Therapeutic methods: promoting blood circulation, removing blood stasis, associated with activating the flow of qi.

Prescriptions and drugs: Take the prescription "Da Huang Zhe Chong Pill" with modified "Dian Kuang Meng Xing Decoction". In the prescription, use peach kernel and red peony root to promote blood circulation and remove stagnation. Add red sage root, safflower and leech to enhance the effect of promoting blood circulation. Bupleuurum root and cyperus tuber regulate qi and alleviate depression. Green tangerine orange peel, shell of areca nut, mulberry bark and perilla fruit activate qi and send down the abnormally ascending qi. Pinellia tuber normalize the function of stomach, licorice root regulate the middle energizer. In the case of protracted stagnation with the accumulation of interior heat, use manshurian aristolochia stem and scutellaria root to remove it. If it is associated with cold, use dried ginger and prepared aconite root to restore yang and warm channels. The prescription "Da Huang Zhe Chong Pill" is composed of rhubarb, scutellaria root, licorice root, peach kernel, peony root, rehmannia root, horsefly, leech, gadfly (tabanus), grub and ground beetle. The functions of the prescription involve eliminating stagnation and promoting generation of vital essence and blood, and eliminating the extravasated blood. It should be taken for a long time, ex. at least for more than half a year. Administer 4g each time, four times a day.

Example of prescriptions: Peach kernel 10g, red peony root 12g, pinellia tuber 6g, red sage root 30g, safflower 6g, curcuma root 10g, cyperus tuber 10g, corydalis tuber 10g, licorice root 6g.

[Measures of Prevention and Nursing]

It is important to look after properly the patients with manic and depressive psychosis except that to treat them actively. The manic and depressive psychosis is one of the diseases that manifested as mental and behavior disorder. Once suffered from the disease, the patients will meet difficulties in daily life, learning and work, and became a burden to their family and the society. The disease is liable to recur. Therefore, to those who suffered from acute illness, emphasis should be laid on nursing after proper treatment has alleviated the patients' conditions so as to prevent its relapse. It is important for the patients to keep cheerful and ease spirit and leave off depressive mood for the better. To keep full of energy and ease of mind will maintain the equilibrium of yin and yang, as it is said in an ancient Chinese medical book, "Yin and yang in equilibrium carrying on the normal life activities". In addition, attention must also be paid to daily life and diet of the patients. Eat less pungent, hot, fat and greasy food can protect the spleen and stomach from impairing and prevent the accumulation of pathogenic dampness hence the production of phlegm. The labor protection is also important to prevent injuries from falls, fractures, contusions and strains which will cause the obstruction of blood circulation.

In the respect of nursing, first to adopt a correct attitude towards various illness expressions of the patients, no jeering, no satirizing. Respect and show loving care for the patients. The psychotherapy may be employed for those patients who yet have part of ability to fit in with the environment. For unreasonable demands of the patients, explain and persuade patiently, and to those reasonable require, satisfy them as far as possible. When the patients with severe disease show the behavior of hitting and swearing at people, self-wounding and destroying things, take appropriate measures to ensure safety and avoid accident. For the patients who refuse to take food, to find out the reason and persuade, supervise and urge them or employ the methods of feeding or nasal feeding so that to ensure sufficient nutrients. Strict measures must be adopted for the patients who have the tendency or actions of suicide and homicide. Send special staff to look after them, and hide all dangerous articles away, such as knives, scissors, strings and drugs. And, notice and wall up such accidents as drawn in river, jumping out from high buildings and touching electricity.

〔Analysis of Typical Cases〕

Case 1. Jiang, female, age 45, usually narrow-minded, oversensitive, overanxious, feeling incompatibility between she and her husband. Her husband stayed at other places for a long period of time, and suspected that she has unfaithful intentions after back home and later beat her. Once after vigorous quarrel, she suddenly look steadily, reticent, refuse to take food and drink, then shouting at the top of her voice, climbing walls and getting on roofs, being subject to changing mood, taking off her clothes in the presence of all, hitting others and destroying things; three or four young men could not check her. When seeking medical advice, most of the above symptoms had alleviated. Her symptoms manifested as flushed face and ears, red tongue proper, yellow fur and constipation. Diagnosed as manic psychosis. It was caused by the stagnation of phlegm-fire which disturbs the mental activities. The doctor gave guidance to the patient and her family patiently, told her family to show every loving care to her, not to add mental burden to her. Prescribed to take "Meng Shi Gun Tan Pill" with the decoction of modified "Dan Zhi Xiao Yao Powder", two pills a day. Constipation alleviated after taking the drug, mental state gradually eased up. The patient was fully recovered after taking some ten dosages.

Comments: The patient aged over 40 was usually incompatible with her husband. This caused depression and disorder of liver-qi. Later, continuous quarrel caused the stagnation of liver turning into fire and the spleen lost the normal activity of transporting. The fire produced by stagnation of fire invades upwards the heart orifice and thus the mental activities disordered hence causing manic symptoms in the heart, liver and spleen. The therapeutic methods thus involve purging fire, eliminating phlegm, invigorating spleen and tranquilizing mind. Use "Dan Zhi Xiao Yao Powder" to regulate liver and spleen functions, remove liver-fire, and "Meng Shi Gun Tan Pill" to purge fire and eliminating phlegm. The two prescriptions used in combination just accord with the pathogenesis of the disease. After administered some ten dosages, phlegm-heat was removed and qi stagnancy relieved. The patient recovered gradually with additional care of her mental activities.

The manic and depressive psychosis are both the diseases of mental disorder. They have different clinical features but they can transform each other, so no hard and fast line can be drawn between them. The features of depressive psychosis are expressed mainly as reticence, deficiency, and stagnation of phlegm qi. The therapeutic methods involve alleviating depression, resolving phlegm, calming and tranquilizing mind, nourishing heart and enriching blood. The commonly used prescriptions are "Xiao Yao Powder" and "Yang Xin Decoction". The features of manic psychosis are expressed mainly as mania, excess, phlegm-fire invading upwards. The therapeutic methods involve removing fire, eliminating phlegm, relieving palpitation tranquilizing mind, and nourishing liver and kidney. The prescriptions commonly used are "Meng Shi Gun Tan Pill", "An Shen Ding Zhi Pill" and "Er Yin Decoction". The diseases of nervous system in modern medicine with similar symptoms may be diagnosed and treated in the light of the descriptions in this chapter.

Questions for Review

1. Is the manic and depressive psychosis a single disease? What are the differences and similarities of the two?
2. What are the basic causes of manic and depressive psychosis?
3. How to treat manic and depressive psychosis? What are the principles of treatment of manic psychosis?
4. How to correctly use the prescriptions and drugs of purgation, eliminating phlegm and inducing vomiting for the treatment of manic and depressive psychosis?

Epilepsy

〔Introduction〕

Epilepsy is one of paroxysmal diseases that are mainly manifested as: suddenly falling on the ground, unconsciousness, spitting saliva, staring upwards, clonic convulsion, or shouting as bleat or pig yell, and regaining consciousness some time later. The epilepsy possesses two particular clinical features: (1) special symptoms as clonic convulsion in an unconscious state, and (2) paroxysmal, attacking suddenly, regaining consciousness some time later, and all as usual after waking, repeated attacking.

〔Causes and Pathogenesis〕

In an ancient medical book "Su Wen", the disease was called "disorder of head". It indicated that the lesion is in the head and the disease is caused by the pathogenic change of the brain and medulla. The syndrome is caused mainly by mental disorder, congenital factors, immoderate eating and drinking, imbalance of work and rest, trauma from falls and restrains, or dysfunction of viscera after suffered from other diseases, disorder of functional activities of qi, accumulation and obstruction of pathogenic phlegm, entanglement of wind and phlegm and stirring up of internal wind. The pathogenic phlegm is the most important among various causes.

Ⅰ. Mental disorder: In the seven emotions, terror is of vital importance to the onset of epilepsy. There exist two conditions in the relations of the onset of epilepsy and terror. First, attacking of violent terror causes irritability and mental disorder. Other inducing factors including stimulation of mind also cause the disease. Second, the viscera-qi may be disturbed by terror which then causes dysfunction of mental activities and impairing of viscera. The injury of liver and kidney is liable to induce the failure of yin to keep yang well. The moving wind from yang impairs the spleen and stomach hence causing the failure of nutrients transportation and accumulation of pathogenic phlegm. In this case, once attacked by certain inducing factors, the pathogenic phlegm follows qi to ascend up, or goes after fire to flare, or follows wind to move, and then they cover and stuff the heart and mind orifices, disturb the channels, obstructs the circulation of qi and blood. The symptoms thus manifested as falling unconsciously on the ground suddenly, coma, spasm of muscles and ceaseless clonic convulsion.

The children are susceptible to fright because their viscera are tender and delicate, vital-qi have not strengthened yet and their mind are timid and weak-willed.

Ⅱ. Congenital factors: The epilepsy is often coming on in childhood because its attack is related to congenital factors. In the classic "Nei Jing", the epilepsy was recognized as congenital disease. In the book "Huo You Xin Fa", the congenital factors were further expounded following the theory of "Nei Jing" that if the mother encountered fright, her baby may suffer from "disorder of head". It says "attacking of the disease of human embryo is because that the mother encountered terror during pregnancy, or the original qi of fetus obstructed by seven emotions. The disease will occur within hundred days after birth". The mother suddenly encountered terror that induce dysfunction of normal activities of qi and the exhaustion of vital essence and energy. These influence the normal development of the fetus and the baby will be susceptible to fright after birth.

Ⅲ. Miscellaneous: The impairing of viscera can be caused by the invading of the six climatic conditions in excess, immoderate eating and drinking, or brain trauma and suffering from other diseases. Thus the phlegm accumulated in internals and it will cause dysfunction of the activities of qi if one took angry, being over-worked of lack of proper adjustment of the daily life. The disorder of the activities of qi promotes the internal phlegm accumulation which disturbs upwards the heart orifice, causing obstruction of mental activity and channels, then epilepsy occurred.

In summary, the onset of epilepsy is mainly caused by the following causes: stagnation of liver-qi, impairing of kidney by terror, or injury of spleen and stomach due to immoderate eating and drinking, or congenital deficiency, and lack of proper health care. The main causes involve accumulation of phlegm, disorder of qi and blood, adverse flow of endogenous wind due to dysfunction of the viscera. The locations of the disease are in liver, spleen and kidney, involving heart vessels and gallbladder channels. The transformation of pathogenesis includes no more than terror, phlegm and fire. If terror injured the liver and kidney, the heat will be produced due to deficiency of liver- and kidney-yin and failure of them to restrain yang and the hyper-activity of heat then strengthen the endogenous wind. And, the pathogenic fire and heat can burn the body fluid to form phlegm. The phlegm may also produced by immoderate eating and drinking, impairing of spleen and stomach, dysfunction in transport hence forming the accumulation of endogenous pathogenic phlegm. In addition, stagnation of qi turning into fire and the fire burns yin. The injury of kidney essence must induce the hyperactivity of liver-wind. All of these are the pathological basis of epilepsy with the internal accumulation of phlegm as the most important cause. If there is no internal accumulation of phlegm, one may be suffering from disease rather than epilepsy, though he(she) has encountered terror or internal wind. If the inducing factors, such as internal accumulation of phlegm, mental depression or tiredness due to over-work, activate the accumulated phlegm and cause disorder of functional activities of qi. The entanglement of wind-yang and phlegm disturbs upwards, obstructs channels and collaterals and block the heart orifice, thereby causing the symptoms of sudden falling on the ground and clonic convulsion. Dr. Ye explained the reasons why the disease is paroxysmal that it attacks when the accumulated phlegm is activated by inducing factors, and it stops attacking when the vital-qi restored. The opinion possesses guiding significance for the treatment and prevention of epilepsy.

〔Diagnosis and Treatment by Differentiation of Syndromes〕

Epilepsy has special pathogenesis and clinical manifestations of its own. However, its symptoms and intermittent features are very complicated because of the differences of the patients' age and constitution, causes, duration of illness course and attacking frequencies. Therefore, in clinical practice one must find out the key points, differentiate the stage of attack from intermittent period, make clear the types of the disease, yang or yin type, and the expressions of tongue picture and pulse.

There are three characteristics involving in the attack of epilepsy: sudden, transient and repeated. In most of the cases, the disease is attacking suddenly and in some of the cases, paroxysmal symptoms of nervousness and disposition appeared several hours or days before its onset. Some of the patients feels dizziness, head-ache, numbness of the extremities, and fullness in chest close to the attack, but the feelings are transient. The duration of epilepsy is relatively short, general several minutes from the attacking to consciousness. In some of the patients, the duration time may only be several seconds. The disease often attacks repeatedly. The intervals between the attacks and onset frequency are different because of the different illness conditions, i.e. mild or severe, and attacking appearance.

Diagram of causes and pathogenesis

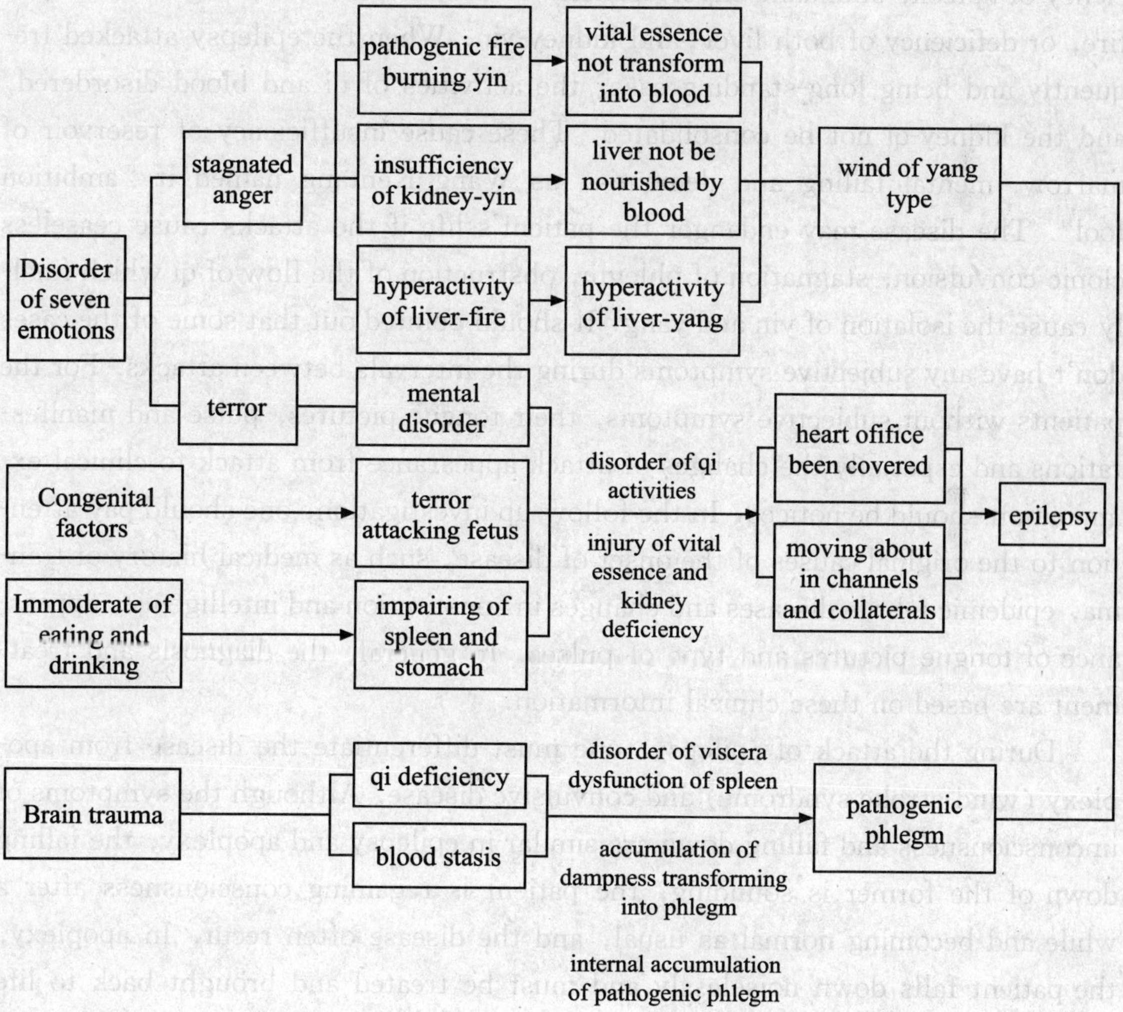

Epilepsy of yang type is the syndrome of excess heat. The patients of this type have generally good constitution, their symptoms are manifested as sudden attack, falling down and shout, clonic convulsion and spitting, lockjaw, looking upwards with taut, rapid or taut, slippery pulse. Epilepsy of yin type is the syndrome of deficient cold. The constitution of the patients are generally not very good, or they suffered from frequent attack of epilepsy. In these patients, the vital-qi is gradually exhausted and the accumulation of phlegm not resolved. The symptoms of attack manifested as pale complexion, dull-witted, unconsciousness, reticent, dumb-struck with deep, taut or deep, slippery pulses. During the stage of attack, the manifestation of symptoms, picture of the tongue are examined so as to differentiate the type of disease and determine the therapeutic principle. The clinical manifestations of epilepsy in intervals between the attacks involve deficiency of spleen, abundant expectoration, or accumulation of phlegm with liver-fire, or deficiency of both liver- and kidney-yin. When the epilepsy attacked frequently and being long-standing case, the activities of qi and blood disordered, and the kidney-qi not be consolidated. These cause insufficiency of reservoir of marrow, mental failing and dementia, as Wang Kentang named it "ambition fool". The disease may endanger the patient's life if the attacks cause ceaseless clonic convulsion, stagnation of phlegm, obstruction of the flow of qi which finally cause the isolation of yin and yang. It should pointed out that some of the cases don't have any subjective symptoms during the intervals between attacks. For the patients without subjective symptoms, their tongue pictures, pulse and manifestations and especially the changes of attack appearance from attack to clinical examination should be noticed. In the follow-up investigation, one should pay attention to the original causes of the onset of disease, such as medical history of trauma, epidemic febrile diseases and changes in constitution and intelligence, appearance of tongue pictures and type of pulses. In general, the diagnosis and treatment are based on these clinical information.

During the attack of epilepsy, one must differentiate the disease from apoplexy (wind-stroke syndrome) and convulsive disease. Although the symptoms of unconsciousness and falling down are similar in epilepsy and apoplexy, the falling down of the former is sounding, the patient is regaining consciousness after a while and becoming normal as usual, and the disease often recur. In apoplexy, the patient falls down noiselessly and must be treated and brought back to life from unconscious state or regained consciousness gradually, and the patient may have the sequela of hemiparalysis, hemianaesthesia, etc. Epilepsy and convulsive disease have similar symptoms of convulsion of the extremities and contracture sensation of contractin, but the patient with epilepsy feels weak and feeble after its onset, regains consciousness a short time later and has no fever. The patient with convulsive disease manifested as rigidity of body, opisthotonus, difficult to regain consciousness and often complicated with fever.

The epilepsy is one of the paroxysmal diseases. It possesses the characteristics of sudden and repeated attack and transience. In the treatment of the disease, the stage of attack and intervals between its onset must be differentiated, so that one can employ different therapeutic methods according different causes and clinical manifestations.

Ⅰ. Syndromes and treatment of the stage of attack

1. Epilepsy of yang type

Main symptoms and signs: head-ache and dizziness, and fullness in chest as premonitory symptoms, then falling down on the ground unconsciously, looking upwards, dark lips, lockjaw, rigidity of neck, clonic convulsion, or rale of sputum in the air passage, or splitting saliva.

Associated symptoms and signs: shouting as bleat or pig yell, even fecal and urinary incontinence, be conscious gradually after the attack stops, daily life goes on as usual except that the patient feels tired.

Tongue and pulse: whitish and greasy or yellow and greasy fur, taut and slippery or taut and rapid pulse.

Analysis: The symptoms of dizziness and head-ache, fullness in chest and being unconsciousness only a while after attacking are all premonitory manifestations of the adverse flow of wind-phlegm. The symptoms of coma and falling down on the ground are caused by the transverse moving of wind-phlegm, adverse flow of qi and blood in chest and the mental activities been obstructed. Dark lips are caused by wind-phlegm and phlegm-heat stuffing in the heart and chest, obstruction of yang-qi and blood circulation. All the manifestations of looking upwards, lockjaw, rigidity of neck, clonic convulsion are caused by the moving wind which disturbs the muscles. During the stage of attack the patient can not help spitting. The saliva spitted is the excessive fluid of the body flowing out accompanying the adverse flow of qi. It is actually not the visible sputum but slobber.

The greasy tongue fur shows excess of dampness, light yellow and greasy tongue fur indicates internal accumulation of phlegm-heat and the pulse is the expression of abundant wind-phlegm. Because of the irregular gathering and dispersing of the wind-phlegm, the disease is attacking frequently and the patient acts as usual after recovery.

Therapeutic methods: removing phlegm-heat, calming the pathogenic wind and arresting convulsion.

Prescriptions and drugs: Take "Ding Xian Pill" with the decoction of the modified prescription "Qing Re Zhen Jing Pill". The prescription is composed of crude abalone shell, amethyst, gentian root, pittosporm root, manshurain aristolochial stem, crude rhubarb, dried ginger, bupleurum root, ophiopogon root, bamboo siliceous concretion, arisaema with bile, polygala root, grasssleaved sweetflag rhizome. gastrodia tuber and uncaria stem with hooks. In the prescription, abalone shell calms the liver to stop the wind, amethyst tranquilizes mind and arrests convulsion, gentian root removes the fire of excess type in liver channel. Use gentian root in combination with pittosporm root and manshurian aristolochia stem has the functions of removing dampness by attaining the three energizers. Use crude rhubarb to purge heat, and regulate the stomach and lower the adverse flow of qi when assisted by dried ginger that is bitter in nature and pungent in flavor. The crude rhubarb also enhances the actions of bamboo siliceous concretion and arisaema with bile which clear away heat and resolve phlegm. Polygala root and grassleaved sweetflag rhizome eliminate phlegm and induce resuscitation. Gastrodia tuber and uncaria stem with hooks stop wind and assuage convulsion. The drug bupleurum root can either be the medicinal guide or regulate qi and alleviate depression. When bupleurum is used in combination with bamboo siliceous concretion and ophiopogon root, the impairing of yin by bitter drug arisaema with bile can be prevented. Bupleurum root can tranquilize mind as well.

Example of prescriptions: crude abalone shell 30g (pre-decocted), amethyst 15g, gentian root 10g, crude rhubarb 6g, arisaema with bile 10g, bamboo siliceous concretion 10g, uncaria stem with hooks 30g, gastrodia tuber 10g, grassleaved sweetflag rhizome 10g, polygala root 9g, bupleurum root 6g, ophiopogon root 10g, pittosporm root 6g, manshurian aristolochia stem 3g.

There are several cases in which the epilepsy did not recur for some ten years if the therapeutic method is adequate and administer pills for several months after the epilepsy resolved. If the measures of nursing are not proper or the patients often encountered terror, or over-worked, immoderate eating and drinking, the epilepsy will recur frequently and may transform into the epilepsy of yin type because of the exhaustion of vital-qi and internal accumulation of phlegm-dampness.

2. Epilepsy of yin type

Main symptoms and signs: dim and sallow complexion, cold limbs, unconsciousness, eyes slightly open, with spasm of muscles, clonic convulsion.

Associated symptoms and signs: generally no shouting or only making a little sound, some transfixed or dumb-struck, looking but seeing not, listening but hearing not, no moving, no speaking, recurring frequently, tired all over after wake, recovered gradually.

Tongue and pulse: light tongue proper, whitish and greasy fur, deep thready or thready slippery pulse.

Analysis: This syndrome is commonly encountered in children. It is mostly caused by phlegm-induced mental confusion. In adults, it is formed by protracted epilepsy of yang type and frequent relapse which cause exhaustion of vital-qi and accumulation of phlegm. The interior epilepsy of yin type belongs to the diseases of viscera. It is caused mainly by both congenital and postnatal impairing, lack of source for generating qi and blood, insufficiency of the fire from life gate (kidney-yang) and the functional activity of qi, and the water-cold overflowing upwards. Thus the patient shows dim and sallow complexion and cold limbs. The symptoms of slightly opened eyes and unconsciousness are caused by accumulated and abundant damp phlegm disturbing mental activity and deficiency and exhaustion of heart- and chest- yang-qi. It says in the medical book "Nei Jing" that "domination of pathogenic wind may disturb the body" and "the extremities are the origin of various yang". It is thus clear that the more the wind-yang is hyperactive, the more the clonic convulsion is intensified. When the blood is failing to nourish muscles, the muscles became dry, don't work smoothly, and only possess wind of deficiency type. Thus the symptoms of lying down, contracture sensation of contraction or clonic convulsion will occur. Spitting saliva indicates that the abundant internal phlegm-dampness wells up followed the adverse qi. If the orifices are obstructed by accumulated phlegm, and the pathogenic factors have not been overcome by vital energy, the symptoms will manifest as no shouting or a little sound heard. The causes of unconsciousness and dumb-struck are in the heart and kidney because that the heart governs the blood and the kidney is in charge of the marrow. So if the heart and blood are not coordinated and the reservoir of marrow is not full, the patient will lose his (her) mental activity due to obstruction of seven orifices by pathogenic phlegm.

Therapeutic methods: warming viscera and eliminating phlegm.

Prescriptions and drugs: Take "Wu Sheng Pill" with the decoction of the prescription "Er Chen Decoction". The prescription of "Wu Sheng Pill" is composed of equal amounts of the drugs arisaema tuber, pinellia tuber, Sichuan aconite root, giant typhoium tuber and black soybean. The paste pills are made with ginger juice and take 6～10g each time. Arisaema tuber, pinellia tuber and giant typhonium tuber in the prescription are all pungent in flavor and warm in nature, and all have the function of eliminating phlegm. Pinellia tuber is acting on the spleen and stomach and can lower the adverse flow of qi and dissolve lumps. Arisaema tuber is acting on the lung, liver and spleen and has the functions of expelling wind and relieving spasm. Giant typhonium tuber is acting on the stomach and can expel wind-phlegm and dispel cold dampness. Sichuan aconite root is heavy pungent in flavor and intense heat in nature, it possesses the activities of warming the spleen and stomach, promoting the qi transformation and dispelling the accumulation and obstructions of cold. The black soybean can tonify kidney and remove dampness. Thus the main functions of the whole prescription "Wu Sheng Pill" are warming viscera and eliminating phlegm. Combine it with modified "Er Chen Decoction" will strengthen the actions of the pill by regulating the flow of qi and phlegm.

Other factors causing epilepsy include wind attacking during sweating, pathogenic wind invading muscular striae, obstruction of ying-wei circulation, pathogenic wind disturbing heart and blood stasis. These make the blood circulation disorder and unease of mind. For these patients, the therapeutic method may be expelling wind and eliminating phlegm. Take the prescription "Hua Hueng Pill (Ding)", 1 or 2 pills each time.

Some of the patients with epilepsy are caused by terror which induced the disorder of qi and mental derangement. The symptoms of these patients are manifested as throwing the tongue out, hurried shouting, whitish and reddish complexion changing abruptly. After the epilepsy has alleviated, the patient is still badly shaken as if he (she) is going to be arrested. The pulse is feeble and taut. To treat with the methods of relieving convulsion and tranquilizing mind and take "Jin Bo Zhen Xin Pill", 1～2 pills each time.

Example of prescriptions: Arisaema with bile 10g, pinellia tuber 10g, red tangerine peel 9g, poria cocos 30g, batryticated silkworm 10g, fresh ginger 10g, giant typhonium tuber 6g.

Although the illness condition of epilepsy of yin type is severe, it can be cured by proper treatment and nursing. After the attack stopped, first to regulate the spleen and stomach, promote qi and blood circulation and nourish brain and marrow. And then combine with the method of reinforcement and elimination in combination to lower the adverse flow of qi, eliminate phlegm, promote blood circulation and remove blood stasis. If it is proved effective, the patients' health will be recuperated gradually and the epilepsy alleviated.

Those patients with frequently attacked epilepsy of yang type manifested as unconsciousness, dementia and amnesia after repeated treatments will not be competent at their former jobs. There are individual cases who have been suffocated when attacking by sputum obstructing the aír passage suddenly, and finally died of the isolation of yin and yang if the emergency treatment was not given in time.

Ⅱ. Syndromes and treatment of the intermittent epilepsy

The syndromes of the intermittent epilepsy may be divided into four types, i. e., deficiency of spleen and abundant expectoration, liver fire and phlegm-heat, deficiency of both liver- and kidney-yin, and liver wind and phlegm, according to their clinical features, tongue pictures and pulse types.

1. Deficiency of spleen and abundant expectoration

Main symptoms and signs: tiredness, asthenia, thin of stature and weakness, frequent dizziness, dim complexion, loss of appetite, loose stool.

Associated symptoms and signs: nausea, vomiting, or feeling of fullness in stomach and stuffiness in hypochondrium, or spitting whitish sputum.

Tongue and pulse: light tongue proper, whitish and greasy fur, soft slippery or thready, taut and slippery pulse.

Analysis: The symptoms of tiredness, asthenia, thin of stature and weakness, dim complexion are caused by the failure of the spleen to transport nutrients due to its deficiency which induces the lack of source for generation and insufficiency of qi and blood. The pathogenic dampness accumulated and then gathered into phlegm. Protracted retention of the accumulated phlegm made the spleen be further injured. The more the spleen is deficient, the more the pathogenic phlegm is intensified. When the middle energizer is obstructed by the pathogenic phlegm, the appetite will be lost. Disturbance in ascending and descending causes nausea and vomiting. Disorder and obstruction of functional activities of qi cause the feeling of fullness and stuffiness in chest and stomach. Loose stool and spitting sputum are the expressions of deficiency of spleen. Light tongue proper is the symptom caused by spleen deficiency and the whitish and greasy tongue fur by phlegm-dampness.

Therapeutic methods: mainly invigorating spleen and eliminating phlegm.

Prescriptions and drugs: Modified prescription "Liu Jun Zi Decoction" is used. In the prescription, pilose asiabell root, poria cocos atractylodes rhizome and licorice root invogorate spleen and supplement qi; pinellia tuber and tangerine peel normalize the functions of stomach and resolve phlegm. In the case of abundant sputum, add arisaema tuber and trichosanthes fruit. For the patients with nausea and vomiting, add bamboo shavings and inula flower. Add coix seed and white hyacinth bean to cure the patients with loose stool. Other drugs, such as grassleaved sweetflag rhizome, polygala root, batryticated silkworm, may also be selected to eliminate pathogenic phlegm and ease mental stress. For the patients with abundant yellow sputum and yellow greasy tongue fur, the modified prescription "Wen Dan Decoction" may be used as a substitute.

Example of prescriptions: Pilose asiabell root 10g, poria cocos 15g, white atractylodes rhizome 10g, prepared licorice root 10g, pinellia tuber 9g, tangerine peel 6g, arisaema tuber 6g, parched coix seed 20g.

2. Liver-wind and pathogenic phlegm

Main symptoms and signs: premonitory symptoms as dizziness, head-ache, fullness feeling in chest, asthenia before onset, no premonitory symptoms in some of the patients, suddenly falling down, unconsciousness, clonic convulsion and spitting saliva when attacking, some of the patients are unconscious for a while, or absentminded without clonic convulsion.

Associated symptoms and signs: maybe screaming when attacking, urinary and fecal incontinence, expectorating.

Tongue and pulse: red or dark red tongue proper, greasy fur, taut and slippery pulse.

Analysis: Frequently dizzy, fullness feeling in chest and asthenia are all premonitory symptoms of upwards invading of wind-phlegm. The unconscious state in sudden attacking is caused by up-stirring of liver-wind, integration of wind and phlegm, wind-phlegm disturbing mental activity, and the heart opening been recovered and stuffed. The up-stirring of liver, failure of spleen to transport and generation of pathogenic phlegm make the phlegm moves follow the wind and surges out from mouth. Greasy tongue fur and taut slippery pulse are the expressions of wind-phlegm.

Therapeutic methods: eliminating phlegm and stopping wind, induce resuscitation and arresting epilepsy.

Prescriptions and drugs: The prescription of modified "Ding Xian Pill" is used. The prescription is composed of gastrodia tuber, Sichuan fritillary bulb, arisaema with bile, pinellia tuber, tangerine peel, poria cocos, poria with hostwood, red sage root, ophiopogon root, polygala root, grassleaved sweetflag rhizome, scorpion, batryticated silkworm, amber and cinnabar. The decoction is condensed with bamboo shavings, licorice root and ginger juice and made it into pills. The pills are coated with cinnabar. Take 1～3 pills each time. In the prescription, gastrodia tuber, scorpion and batryticated silkworm stop the liver -wind so as to arrest convulsion; Sichuan fritillary bulb, arisama with bile, pinellia tuber, bamboo shaivngs and grassleaved sweetflag rhizome resolve phlegm and induce resuscitation to lower the adverse flow of qi; amber, poria with hostwood, polygala root and cinnabar relieve palpitation and tranquilize mind so as to arrest convulsion; poria cocos and tangerine peel invigorate spleen and arrest the flow of qi; red sage root and ophiopogon root treat blood disorders and nourish yin; ginger juice and licorice root can warm the middle energizer and normalize the stomach functions.

Example of prescriptions: Gastrodia tuber 10g, arisaema with bile 10g, pinellia tuber 9g, poria with hostwood 20g, grassleaved sweetflag rhizome 10g, polygala root 10g, batryticated silkworm 9g, scorpion 6g, infusion of bamboo shavings 20ml.

3. Deficiency of both liver - and kidney-yin

Main symptoms and signs: epilepsy frequently attacking, vital-qi greatly exhausted, usually poor memory, absentminded, dim complexion, dizziness, dry and unsmooth eyes.

Associated symptoms and signs: amnesia, sleeplessness, lassitude and soreness in loin and legs, constipation.

Tongue and pulse: red tongue proper, less fur, thready and rapid pulse.

Analysis: In the patients with frequently attacked epilepsy, qi and blood would be deficient first and the protracted illness involved the kidney because that the liver and the kidney have a common source. When the deficiency of blood has been exacerbated gradually, the kidney-essence must be exhausted because that essence and blood have a common source. Insufficiency of kidney-essence and void of marrow reservoir cause dim complexion and amnesia. Because the eyes are the body openings(windows)of the liver, deficiency of blood and dryness of fluid will cause dryness and unsmoothness of eyes. Deficiency of blood and hyperactivity of the liver cause dizziness. Since the kidney has its specific orifice in the ear and is in charge of loins, so deficiency and weakness of kidney will cause the withering of auricles and lassitude and soreness in loin and legs. Those manifestations of tongue proper and pulse are the expressions of insufficiency of essence and blood.

Therapeutic methods: Tonifying liver and kidney, nourishing heart and tranquilizing mind.

Prescriptions and drugs: The modified prescription "Zuo Gui Pill" is used. In the prescription, prepared rehmannia root, Chinese yam, dogwood fruit, tortoise plastron and wolfberry fruit have the functions of tonifying liver and kidney. Add oyster shell and fresh water turtle shell to nourish yin and check exuberant yang. Use aborvitae seed, magnetite and cinnabar to ease mental strain. Add fritillary bulb bamboo siliceous concretion and bamboo shavings to clear away heat and eliminate phlegm. In the case of severe dysphoria with smothery sensation, add lophatherum, pittosporm root and lotus plumule to clear away heart-fire and relieve restlessness. For the patients with constipation, add scrophularia root, Chinese angelica root and hemp seed to enrich fluid and loose the bowel.

Example of prescriptions: Prepared rehmannia root 30g, Chinese yam 10g, dogwood fruit 10g, wolfberry fruit 12g, oyster shell 30g (pre-decocted), aborvitae seed 10g, magnetite 30g (pre-decocted), Sichuan fritillary bulb 10g, bamboo shavings 6g, lotus plumule 3g, pittosporm root 6g.

4. Liver-fire and phlegm-heat

Main symptoms and signs: unconsciousness and falling down on the ground when attacking, clonic convulsion, spitting saliva, sometimes shouting, usually impetuous, be apt to be angry, vexation, dizziness, head-ache.

Associated symptoms and signs: dry and bitter taste in mouth, constipation, hard expectoration.

Tongue and pulse: red tongue proper, yellow greasy fur, taut, slippery and rapid pulse.

Analysis: Dizziness and head-ache are caused by the flaring-up of liver-fire and the disturbance of seven orifices. Impetuousness state is caused by disorder of liver-qi and functional activities of qi. Vexation is caused by fire disturbing mind. The upward moving of fire and wind steams the body fluid to form phlegm. The twine each other of wind and phlegm obstructs the seven orifices thereby causing the symptoms of unconsciousness, falling down on the ground and mental disorder. The moving nature of wind causes clonic convulsion. Red tongue proper, yellow greasy tongue fur, taut slippery pulse are all the expressions of liver-fire and intense phlegm-heat.

Therapeutic methods: purging the liver-fire, eliminating phlegm and inducing resuscitation.

Prescriptions and drugs: The modified prescription "Long Dan Xie Gan Decoction" is used in combination with the prescription "Di Tan Decoction". In the prescription, gentian root, scutellaria root, capejasmine fruit and manshurian aristolochia stem quench the pathogenic fire from liver, and remove dampness as well. Pinellia tuber, red tangerine peel, arisaema with bile and grassleaved sweetflag rhizome resolve phlegm and induce resuscitation. Add abalone shell, uncaria stem with hooks, fresh bamboo shavings, bamboo siliceous concretion and earthworm according to the syndromes to remove heat, stop wind, resolve phlegm, activate the collaterals and relieve spasm. In the case of dysphoria, add lotus plumule. If the phlegm-fire is accumulated and abundant and stool constipated, add rhubarb or use the prescription "Zhu Li Da Tan Pill".

Example of prescriptions: Gentian root 10g, scutellaria root 10g, capejasmine fruit 9g, manshurian aristolochia stem 6g, pinellia tuber 6g, arisaema with bile 10g, grassleaved sweetflag rhizome 10g, uncaria stem with hooks 30g, crude abalone shell 30g (pre-decocted), bamboo siliceous concretion 10g.

In addition, the onset of some of the patients with epilepsy is caused by head trauma. If the epilepsy is protracted, the patients often fall down on the ground suddenly, and the head is thus injured. Some of the patients are attacked frequently and being ceaselessly convulsive. In the above cases, blood stasis is a common symptom. Dizziness, head-ache, numbness in limbs and fullness and stabbing pain in chest bring about dark purple tongue proper or ecchymosis on tongue edge and deep thready pulse. The emphasis of the therapeutic methods should lay upon promoting blood circulation and removing blood stasis. The drugs for lowering adverse qi, resolving phlegm and soothing liver may be used in combination. The modified prescription "Tong Qiao Huo Xue Decoction" is generally selected for the treatment.

〔Measures and Prevention and Nursing〕

There are two aspects in the prevention of epilepsy. First, to prevent the attack of pathogenic and inducing factors and build up the patients' health. It is important to maintain high spirits and optimistic mood. Avoid all moral stimulus to contribute peace of mind. Daily life should be regular and keep normal urination and defecation. Take part in proper recreational activities and physical exercises while avoid overdoing. Have enough sleep. It is also to reinforce the nutrition for those patients with protracted illness and a poor constitution. Second, to strengthen the treatment for the cases during intermittent period to prevent frequent attack of epilepsy. This also an important aspect of prevention.

The nursing of epilepsy is very important. The illness condition and the mental changes must be observed carefully. In addition, attention should be paid to the duration of the disease, manifestation of syndromes, tongue picture, pulse type and urination and defecation, so as to provide reliable information for diagnosis and treatment. For the inpatients with frequently attacked epilepsy, safety device should be installed on the hospital beds so that to avoid falling down of the patients. Take off the false teeth and place a guaze wrapped depressor in the patient's mouth between the motar teeth to prevent injury from biting. For the patient with amentia, the nursing must be tighten up so as to avoid accidents. For the severe and critical patients with protracted and frequently attacked epilepsy, pay special attention to maintain respiratory tract unobstructed when attacking in order to avoid death by suffocation. Put the patients on a light diet and eat more green vegetables. The porridges made by Chinese yam, coix seed, red bean, mung bean and rice may be taken for they have the functions of invigorating spleen and removing dampness.

〔Analysis of Typical Cases〕

Case 1. Li, male, age 14. seeking medical advice on May 6, 1985. suffered from epilepsy as a child, onset at intervals of one or several months, often caused by terror or nervousness, feels fullness in chest and dizziness when attacking, then shouting, falling down on the ground, unconscious, clonic convulsive, lockjaw, even biting the tongue, spitting saliva. attack sustained 5～6 minutes, awake gradually and felt weary. His daily life was as usual after recovery. sought medical advice and medication on many occasions. No curative effects were obtained. In recent years, his memory was failing, school record decreased, felt tired and sluggish. Tongue fur: whitish greasy. pulse: taut, slippery and moderate. Treat with the methods of lowering the adverse flow of qi, resolving phlegm, stopping wind and relieving epilepsy. Prescribed:

Arisaema with bile 10g, bamboo siliceous concretion 10g, polygala root 10g, grassleaved sweetflag rhizome 6g, crude abalone shell 30g (pre-decocted), amethyst 15g, gastrodia tuber 10g, uncaria stem with hooks 30g, poria cocos 30g.

The prescription "Ding Xian Pill" was taken with the above decoction.. Take when attacking.

Treat the intermittent period with the method of invigorating spleen and resolving phlegm. Take the modified prescription "Liu Jun Zi Decoction":

Pseudostellaria root 15g, poria cocos 30g, white atractylodes rhizome 10g, pinellia tuber 6g, crude coix seed 30g, tangerine peel 10g, arisaema tuber 6g, licorice root 6g.

Take "Ding Xian Pill" with the above prescription, one pill each time, two times a day.

After the treatment, the patient was recovered and the disease did not recur in the later two years. He was attacked by the disease again owing to the intense review work during the period of the entrance examination of senior middle school. The duration of its onset was shorter than before, only three minutes before awaking. The therapy was continued and the disease never recur up to now.

Comments: This case of epilepsy was caused by the up-stirring of liver-fire, twine of wind and phlegm, wind-phlegm disturbing heart and the blocking of heart orifice. Owing to the protracted illness, the vital-qi became insufficient, spleen functions were impaired and the expectoration was more abundant. Therefore the main therapeutic method should be resolving phlegm. Treated with stopping wind and relieving epilepsy when it was attacking and invigorating spleen and resolving dampness during the intermittent period, so as to prevent the generation of phlegm and its onset. Since the accumulated phlegm in the body was difficult to clear away, the disease recurred due to inducing factors.

The epilepsy is a transient paroxysmal disease of the brain. There are a lot of expositions on the disease in the medical books of traditional Chinese medicine. Most of the physicians of later generations claimed that the pathogenesis is the internal accumulation phlegm and the disease is attacked by inducing factors such as emotional discontent and overworking. These cause the adverse flow of qi, upwards disturbing of wind-yang with phlegm, blocking of the seven orifices, and finally the onset of the disease. The initial stage of epilepsy is mostly belonging to excess or yang syndrome. It should be treated mainly by stopping wind and eliminating phlegm. The protracted illness is mostly belonging to deficiency or yin syndrome. It should be treated mainly by supplementing qi and nourishing yin and blood. It is treated firstly by relieving epilepsy and merely alleviating the symptoms during its attacking. And, during the convalescent period, the methods of nourishing qi and blood, invigorating spleen and stomach and tonifying the liver and kidney should be taken as the principal things.

Questions for Review

1. What are the clinical features of epilepsy?
2. How to understand the causes and pathogenesis of epilepsy?
3. What are the principles of the therapy of epilepsy? What types of the syndromes of epilepsy are commonly encountered? How to treat them?

Stomachache

(and gastric discomfort with acid regurgitation)

〔**Summary**〕

Pain in the gastric cavity caused by impairment of the spleen and stomach and by derangement of qi and blood is called stomachache or epigastralgia. The gastric cavity, generally divided into upper, middle and lower parts, refers to the trapezoid area from the line connecting the lowest edges of ribs on both sides to the xiphoid process.

In ancient literature, stomachache used to be replaced by cardiac pain. In fact, they are different and should be strictly differentiated. In clinical practice, it is not difficult to distinguish them from cause of illness, clinical manifestations, physical signs and necessary physiochemical examinations. This is extremely important for the treatment and prognosis of stomachache.

The main symptom of stomachache is various kinds of pain in the stomach, often accompanied with fullness and distention in the stomach, eructation, regurgitation of acid and food from the stomach, anorexia, hypochondriac and abdominal distention, and other symptoms. Stomachache frequently relapses. It is difficult for stomachache to be cured by long-term treatment, even with hematemesis, melena, dysuria with incessant vomiting and other symptoms.

Stomachache in acute and chronic gastritis, digestive ulcer, gastroneurosis, carcinoma of stomach as well as some diseases of the liver, gallbladder and pancreas in western medicine can be diagnosed and treated in reference to this disease.

〔Etiology and Pathology〕

Stomachache at its onset largely belongs to excess syndrome with the disease mainly in the stomach and sometimes in the liver. Lingering stomachache often belongs to deficiency syndrome with the disease mainly in the spleen. Sometimes, deficiency syndrome is complicated with excess syndrome with the disease in the spleen and the stomach or in the liver and spleen. Ancient people often said: "Yangming disease occurs in strong persons while Taiyin disease in weak persons." It is the same with stomachache.

The common causes of stomachache can be summarized as invasion of the stomach by exopathogen, improper diet, emotional depression and feeble spleen and stomach. They are described as follows.

1. Invasion of the stomach by exopathgen: Among exopathogens, cold most easily affects the stomach, and summer-heat and dampness can also invade the stomach. Impairment of the stomach-qi due to invasion of the stomach by exopathogen causes qi stagnation in mild cases and failure of the stomach-qi to descend in serious cases, leading to stomachache. Colicky pain is mainly caused by cold stagnation, summer-heat often leads to burning pain, and dampness frequently gives rise to oppressing pain.

2. Improper diet: The stomach receives food with the mouth as its opening. Overeating, excessive starvation, exposure to cold or heat, addiction to wine and cigarette, or overdose of stomach-impairing drugs can make the stomach-qi fail to ascend and descend to cause stomachache. In clinical practice at present, excessively taking fat and sweet food is the commonest cause for stomachache. Fat food, cigarette smoke and wine, damp and hot in nature, staying in the stomach can consume body fluid and impair the spleen.

3. Emotional depression: Emotional depression affecting functions of the

liver and the spleen can also cause stomachache. For example, Depression and anger impairing the liver makes hyperactive liver-qi invade the spleen and stomach to cause incoordination between the liver and the stomach or between the liver and the spleen and stagnation of qi and blood, thus leading to gastropathy. Anxiety impairing the spleen makes it fail to transport and transform nutrients and makes the spleen-qi fail to ascend and descend normally, thus also leading to gastropathy.

Schematic diagram for etiology and pathology of stomachache

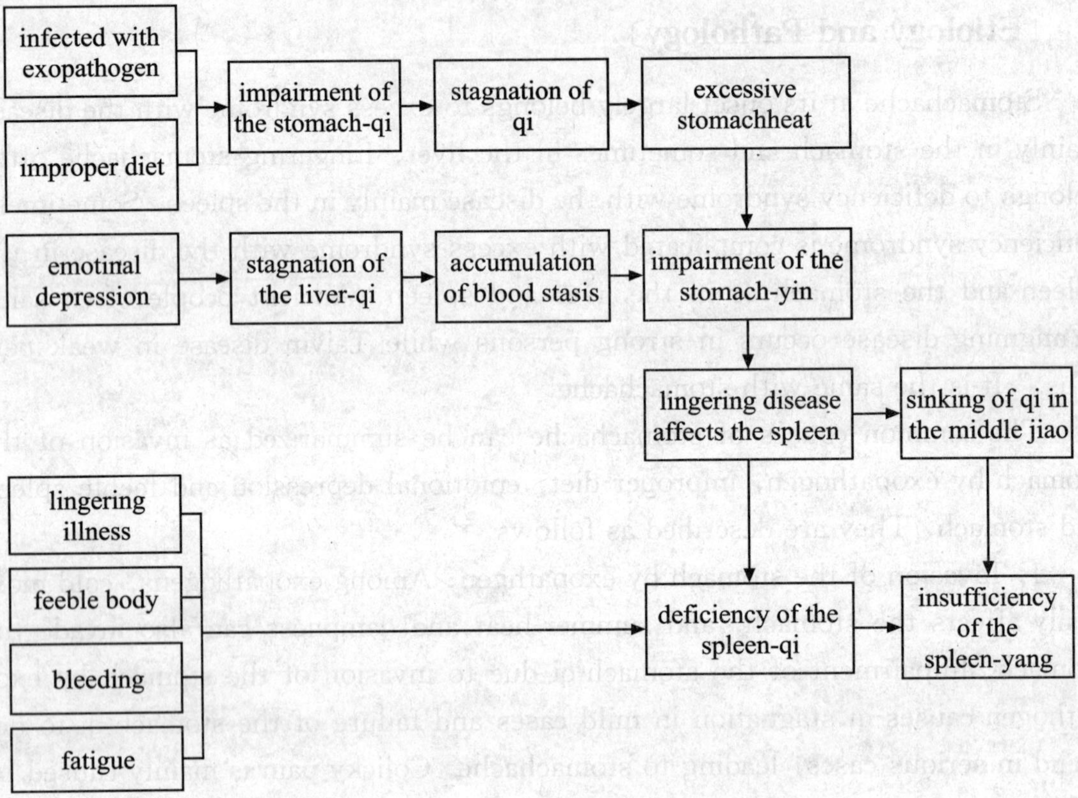

4. Feeble spleen and stomach: Excessive fatigue, too much bleeding or lingering illness without cure can impair the spleen and the stomach. Feeble body, weak spleen and stomach, failure to transport and transform nutrients, disorder of qi in ascending and descending, and qi stagnation can give rise to gastropathy. The illness condition can be further aggravated in those patients with sinking of qi in the middle jiao. Spasmodic stomachache can be caused by yang deficiency of the spleen and the stomach, endogenous yin-cold, and failure to warm and nourish channels and collaterals. In those cases with lingering gastropathy, stomachache can be caused by consumption of yin-fluid, failure to moisten and nourish the

stomach, and disorder of qi.

To sum up the above-mentioned description, stomachache is most closely related to the stomach, liver and spleen. Stomachache at its onset has its source mainly in the stomach, and sometimes in the liver. Lingering stomachache has its source mainly in the spleen and stomach or in the liver and spleen. The stomach corresponds to yang-earth, likes moisture and dislikes dryness. Its function is mainly to receive food and transform food into chyme. It is appropriate for the stomach-qi to descend. When impaired, the stomach-qi can stagnate and adversely rise. This means that stagnation of the stomach-qi can cause stomachache. Stagnation of the stomach-qi can be caused by exopathogen and indigestion and by transverse invasion of the stomach by hyperactive liver-qi. Qi governs blood circulation, so stagnation of qi for a long time can lead to blood stasis. In addition, "excessive qi becomes fire", meaning that long-term disorder of qi can become heat. The fire is in the stomach or in both the liver and stomach. Fire can impair yin-fluid, or blood stasis makes blood not to generate. Deficiency of yin-blood can be caused by deficiency of stomach-yin, or by yin deficiency of the spleen and stomach, or by yin deficiency of the liver and stomach, or by yin deficiency of the liver and spleen. Lingering gastropathy can affect the spleen. The spleen corresponds to yin-earth, prefers dryness, and is averse to dampness. Its function is to transport and transform fluid and nutrients. It is appropriate for the spleen-qi to ascend. Impairment of the spleen-qi causes deficiency of qi in the middle jiao and failure of the spleen to transport and transform nutrients in mild cases, sinking of qi in the middle jiao and disorder of sending up or down essential substances in moderate cases, and yang deficiency of the spleen and stomach, endogenous yin-cold and failure to warm and mourish stomach-collateral in serious cases. In short, in spite of the above-mentioned differences in the causes of stomachache, and despite different syndromes of deficiency, excess, cold, heat, qi system and blood system in its pathology, there is a point in common, which is so-called "stagnation causes pain". No treatment or mistreatment of stomachache impairs blood vessels with hematemesis, hemafecia and other symptoms.

Ⅰ. Main Points of Differentiation of Symptoms

1. Differentiation of Cold and Heat Syndromes: Attack or deterioration due to affection by exopathogenic cold or taking over raw and cold food, colicky pain of the stomach, pain relieving when warming application and taking hot drink,

tastelessness and no thirst, belong to cold syndrome; burning pain in the stomach, the pain relieving when taking cold drink or cold application, dry mouth or bitter taste, belong to heat syndrome.

2. Differentiation of Deficiency and Excess: All sudden and sevious pain and tenderness, pain becoming more severe after meal, repeated pain, belong to excess syndrome; chronic pain or repeated attack, preference for pressing, relieving after meal or deterioration after tiredness, relieving after taking a rest, belong to deficiency syndrome; most diseases in robust or at initial stage belong to excess syndrome, and most diseases in aged patients and refractory diseases belong to deficiency syndrome. The pain that is deteriorated by reinforcement belongs to excess syndrome and by purging method belongs to deficiency syndrome.

3. Differentiation of Qi and Blood: as concerns nature of pain, distending pain is main with belching, belonging to stagnation of Qi; needing-like or cuting-like pain or with hemoptysis, black stool, belongs to blood stasis. As concerns location of pain, moving pain belongs to stagnation of Qi; pain on fixed parts or with mass, belongs to blood stasis. As concerns duration of disease, most diseases at early stage are involved in Qi, and most chronic diseases are involved in blood.

4. Differentiation of Diseases in Stomach, Liver, Spleen: most diseases in the stomach at early stage are involved in the stomach, which are caused often by exopathogenic factors, impairment by overeating, with symptoms such as disteding pain in the chest and abdomen, belching, continuous pain, dyschesia, slippery pulse, and so on.

Most diseases in liver attack repeatedly and are related with mood change, distention pain in the stomach involved in hypochondriac region, moving pain, taut pulse, etc.

Diseases in the spleen are mainly by protracted disease, vague pain in the stomach, pain becoming more severe when hungry and pain relieving after meal. Exterioration at fatigue and alliviating after taking a rest, sallow complexion, fatigue, weakness, loose stool, slow pulse, etc.

Differentiation of Stomachache and Angina Pectoris:

Stomachache: most have history of stomach disease, pain in the stomach part, belching, acid regurgitation, lost appetide, abnormal stool and other symptoms. Most of them can be clearly diagnosed by combination with barium meal examination and gastroscopy of upper digestive tract.

Angina Pectoris: most have history of heart disease, with pain on the scrobiculus cordis, commonly seen in the patient of over mid-ages, often with oppressed feeling in chest, palpitation, dyspnea, dizziness, tinnitus, purple-dim lip and nail, stagnation pulse, etc. Most of them can be clearly diagnosed by combination with elctrocardiogram and biochemical examinations.

Ⅱ. Treatment Based on Classification of Syndromes

Stomachache at the early stage is involved in Qi and most of them belong to excess syndrome. Diseases in the stomach or the liver, affection by cold, summer-heat, accumulation of heat easily injure the stomach, inducing stagnation of food in stomach; mood change induces earsily impairment the liver, stagnation of liver-Qi can injure the stomach, inducing stagnation of Qi of the liver and stomach. Protracted stagnation of Qi can produce pathogenic heat or chronic pain involves the collateralls. If diseases in the stomach do not receive good treatment or receive incorrective treatment, it will invade the spleen. Most diseases in the spleen belong to deficiency syndrome, or excess syndrome with deficiency syndrome. Diseases in the spleen manifest weakenness of spleen-Qi, or sinking of Qi of middle-Jiao, or insufficiency of the spleen-Yang. Therefore, regulating of Qi and regulating stomach are mainly used for treatment of diseases of stomach, and eliminating cold, or removing heat, or promoting digestion, clearing away heat, removing stasis is adopted respectively according to different causes of diseases. Soothing the liver and removing depress are mainly used for treatment of hepatic diseases, clearing the liver should be used for heat-transmission, and activating circulation of blood should be used for that involved in collaterals, nourishing for injury of Yin. Strengthening the spleen and suplpementing Qi are mainly used for treatment of spleen diseases, raising method is used for the patients with sinking of Qi of middle -Jiao, warming and reinforcing methods for the patient with Yang-deficiency. Treatment based on differentiation of symptoms and signs are given for the patients with diseases of the liver and stomach, or the liver and spleen, or the spleen and stomach at the same time, according to severity of the principal and the secondary aspects of the disease.

(Ⅰ) Stagnation of Stomach-Qi

1. Pathogenic Cold Affecting the Stomach

Main Symptoms: sudden attack, colicky pain, pain relieving after warming application or taking hot drink.

Accompanying Symptoms: aversion to cold, pain becoming more severe after cold, no thirst, preference for hot drink.

Tongue and Pulse: normal tongue with thin and white fur, floating and tense or tense pulse.

Analysis: Pathogenic cold attacks middle-Jiao, or by eating over raw and cold food. Pathogenic cold can influence Qi, cold can induce stagnation of Qi, Yang-Qi is depressed, so as to cause colicky pain of stomach. Warming can remove pathogenic cold and dampness, thus, stomachache relieves after hot application or hot drink. Stagnation of Yang-Qi induces aversion to cold, no thirst, preference for hot drink. Thin and white fur on tongue, floating and tense, or tension pulse all are sings of excessive cold.

Therapeutic Principle: Warming middle-Jiao and dispelling cold, regulating stomach and relieving pain.

Prescription: Hot-application can give on the upper abdomen, or taking hot ginger and onion soup, or moxibustion is given at Zhongwan(Ren 12), Zusanli (ST 36) and other points, the pain can be relieved for mild symptom. Modified Liang Fu Pill is used for treatment of severe symptom. In the prescription, galangal rhizome is used for warming middle-Jiao and dispelling cold, nutgrass for promoting flow of Qi and relieving pain; or litse, cinnamom twig, long pepper, fresh ginger, pepertree, etc are added for strengthening the function of dispelling cold and relieving pain. For the patient accompanied with affection by exopathogen, marked by aversion to cold and pain of body, perilla leaf and onion are added for relieving the exterior syndrome with drugs pungent in flavor and warm in property, or are used in combination with Xiang Su Powder for relieving the exterior syndrome, dispelling cold to relieving pain. For stomachache induced by Yin summer-heat in summer, elscholtzia, wrinkled gianthyssop, eupatorium should be added for regulating middle-Jiao.

Example of Prescription: 10g ganangal rhizome, 10g prepared nutgrass, 10g perilloa leaf, 10g fried tangerine peel, 3 pieces of fresh ginger, 10g litse, 10g pinellia tuber, 10g poria.

2. Retention of Food

Main symptoms: fullness and pain in the stomach, with relieving after belching.

Accompanying symptoms: belching with fetid odor, distention of stomach, with slight relieving at hunger and exterioration after meal, vomiting up indigested food, with pain relieving of stomachache after vomiting, or defecation with difficulty.

Tongue and Pulse: white and thick, or greasy fur on the tongue, slippery pusle.

Analysis: Improper diet, injuring stomach-Qi, dysfunction of stomach in receiving and digesting food, anorexia and stagnation of Qi, induce fullness and pain in the starnach; belching promotes functional activities of Qi, vomiting reduces retention of food, resulting in relieving fullness and pain. Retention of food in the stomach, heat-transformation, constipation, induce eructation with fetid odor. White and thick, or greasy fur, slippery pulse all are marks of indigestion.

Therapeutic Principle: Promoting digestion, eliminating indigested food, and regulating function of the stomach and relieving pain.

Prescription: Bao He Pill combined with modified Xiang Su Powder. In Bao He Pill, Er Chen Decoction is used for regulating stomach and desending adverse rising of stomach-Qi, reducing fullness, medicated leaven, germinated barley, hawthorn fruit are combined for promoting digestion. in Xiang Su Powder, perilla stem, tangerine peel, nutgrass flatsedge rhizome for regulating flow of Qi, and regulating stomach and desending adverse rising of stomach-Qi, forsythia fruid is added for clearing away the the heat induced by the indigested food. Fruit of immature citron or trifoliate orange, magnolia bark, radish seed, shell of areca nut, areca seed etc. are added for relieving epigastric distention and reducing the stagnation, and desending the stomach-Qi for the patient with obvious stomachache. Xiao Cheng Qi Decoction is combined for activating function of Fu-organs and removing heat, or Zhi Shi Dao Zhi Pill is used for the patient with stagnation of Qi of Fu-organ-Qi.

Example of prescription: 10g perilla stem, 10g processed nutgrass flatsedge rhizome, 10g fried tangerine peel, 10g fermented pinellia tuber, 10g poria, 10g fried areca, 10g radish seed, and 10g forsythia fruit.

(Ⅱ) Stagnation of Qi of the Liver and Stomach

Main Symptoms: Fullness and pain in the stomach, with hypochondrium involved, with exterioration due to dysthymia.

Accompanying Symptoms: preference for eructation, lost of appetite.

Tongue and pulse: thin and white fur, taut and slippery pulse.

Analysis: Stagnation of the liver-Qi, with the stomach involved, stagnation of the liver and stomach Qi, results in destention and pain in stomach. Most diseases induced by Qi do not have a fixed location, and the costal regions are related with the liver, so stomachache involving the costal regions. Dysfunctional activity of Qi were exacerbated by dysthymia, so sigh can relieve it. Disorder of the stomach-Qi and dysfunction of the stomach to receive food lead to lost of appetite. Thin and white fur, taut and slippery pulse are signs of incoordination between the liver and the stomach.

Therapeutic Principle: soothing the liver and regulating the stamach function, regulating the circulation of Qi and relieving pain.

Prescription: Modified Chai Hu Shu Gan Powder. In the prescription, Si Ni Powder can regulate both Qi and blood, nourish the liver; Chuanxiong rhizome is added for regulation of Qi in blood, nutgrass flatsedge rhizome for regulating blood in Qi; green tangerine orange peel, tangerine peel for regulating function of the liver and the flow of Qi, so as to result in coordination between the liver and stomach, eliminating distention and relieving pain. Curcuma root is added for soothing the liver and relieving the depressed liver. For severe pain, corydalis turber and Sichuan chinaberry are added for regulating circulation of Qi and blood, and relieving pain; for pathogenic heat induced by stagnation of Qi, capejasmine fruit, moutan bark, dandelion herb are added for promoting the flow of Qi and clearing away heat.

Example of Prescription: 10g bupleurum root, 10g fried fruit of citron or trifoliate orange, 10g red peony root, 10g white peony root, 10g processed nutgrass flatsedge rhizome, 6g green tangerine orange peel and 6g tangerine peel, 10g inula flower, 10g curcuma root, 6g Chuanxiong rhizome, 10g corydalis turber, 10g Sichuan chinaberry.

(Ⅲ) Accumulation of Heat in the liver and stomach

Main Symptoms: acute and sudden burnig pain in stomach.

Accompanying Symptoms: acid regurgitation, dry mouth and bitter taste, thirst and preference for cool drink, restlessness.

Tongue and Pulse: reddish tongue with yellowish fur, taut, slippery and rapid pulse.

Analysis: "excessive Qi indicated excess of pathogenic fire". Incoordination between the liver and stomach, protracted dysfunction of Qi can transform pathogenic heat. Accumulation of heat in the middle-Jiao results in acute and sudden burning pain in the stomach. If liver-heat invades the stomach, stomachache, hypochondriac pain, acid regurgitation, restlessness will be induced. Pathogenic heat burns the body fluid, so dry mouth and bitter taste and preference for cool drink appear. Reddish tongue with yellowish fur, and taut, slippery and rapid pulse are signs of accumalation of heat in the liver and stomach.

Therapeutic Principle: dispelling heat of the liver, regulating function of the stomach and relieving pain.

Prescription: Modified Hua Gan Jian is used for the patient with liver heat moving to the stomach. For patients of stomach heat injuring body fluit, modified Bai Hu Decoction is used; For accumulation of heat in the stomach and intestine, and stagnation of Qi of Fu-organs, Xie Xin Decoction is applied.

At present, over smoking and drinking indeed are immportant factors inducing stamachache. Tobacco and alcohol belong fire and heat articles, smoking causing dry-heat and alcohol inducing damp-heat in nature; Over smoking and drinking result in accumulation of heat in the stomach, marked by burning pain in the stomach. Therapeutic principle of clearing away the stomach and promoting production of body fluid or clearing the stomach and removing dampness are adopted for their treatment.

Additionally, accumulation of pathogenic heat for long time produce toxic material, and toxic heat can injure the stomach. It is seen under gastroscope that hyperemia, idema of gastric macosa, even erosion and ulcer of gastric mucosa. Dandelion herb, forsythia fruit, honeysuckle flower, giant knotweed rhizome, fresh coix seed, fritillary bulb, etc. are applied for clearing away heat and toxic material, with positive action for stomach diseases.

Example of prescripton: 10g Sichuan fritillary bulb, 6g green tangerine orange peel, 15g dandelion herb, 10g citron fruit, 10g finger citron, 10g fried chuanxiong rhizome, 5g coptis root, 3g evodia fruit, 10g trichosanthes root.

(Ⅳ) Stasis of Blood

Main Symptoms: Pain in the stomach, like needling or cutting, with fixed position and tenderness.

Accompanying symptoms: Long duration of disease, repeated stomachache, dull complexion and lip; For women, delayed menstrual period with dark menstrual blood.

Tongue and Pulse: dark-purgine tongue with ecchymosis, petechia on the tongue, and taut or uneven pulse.

Analysis: the stomach is a Fu-organ with more Qi and more blood. Qi is charge for blood circulation, flow of Qi promotes normal circulation of blood, stagnation of Qi results in blood stasis. After hematemesis or hematochezia, the blood from the channels accumulates in the stomach, constituting stasis of blood. Stasis of blood in the stomach induces pain like needling or cutting, with fixed position and tenderness. If blood stasis is not cleared away, new blood will not produce, leading to dull complexion, and dark purgine lip. For women, menstrual disorder and delayed menstruation with dark menstrual blood appearing. Purgine tangue proper, or ecchymosis, petechia on the tongue, and taut or uneven pulse are signs of blood stasis.

Therapeutic principle: regulating the flow of Qi, treating blood, removing stasis of blood and relieving pain.

Prescription: Shi Xiao Powder combined with Dan Shen Drink. They are commonly-used prescription for stasis of blood and stomachache. Drugs of regulating flow of Qi are added for blood stasis and obvious stagnation of Qi. Shi Wu Decoction and other drugs of nourishing blood and activating circulation of blood are added for both blood stasis with blood deficiency. Honey-fried astragalus root, dangshen and other drugs of strengthening the spleen and supplementing Qi are added for blood stasis with deficiency of the stomach and spleen, so as to promote circulation of blood. Treatment of chronic stasis of blood should refer to the treatment in the chapter of hematemesis and hemafecia.

Example of prescription: 10g fried trogopterusdung, 10g fresh cat-tail pollen, 20g red sage root, 6g sandalwood, 5g amomumfruit, 10g processed nutgrass flatsedge rhizome, 10g fried tangerine peel, 3g notoginseng powder, 6g corydalis tuber, 6g chuanxiong rhizome.

(Ⅴ) Insufficiency of Stomach-Yin

Main symptoms: vague pain or burning pain in the stomach.

Accompanying Symptoms: gastric discomfort with acid gurgitation, dry mouth and dislike to drink, dry thoat and lip, and dry stool.

Tongue and Pulse: Thin tongue body, reddish tongue with less or no fur, fine and rapid pulse.

Analysis: The stomach belongs earth, likes moisture and dislikes dry, stagnation of Qi transforms pathogenic heat. The heat injuries body fluid, or accumulation of blood stasis, production of no new blood all induce insufficiency of stomach-Yin. Insufficincy of body fluid induces lack of nourishing stomach channel, leading to stomachache. For Yin-deficiency with fire, burning sensation occurs in the stomach. Insuffiency of stomach fluid induces dysfunction of receiving diet. Insufficiency of body fluid induces dry thoat and lip, and insufficiency of Yin fluid causes dryness in the intestine tract, leading to dry stool. Reddish tongue body with less or no fur, and fine and rapid pulse are signs of insufficiency of stomach-Yin with deficiency-fire.

Therapeutic Principle: Nourishing Yin and supplementing the stomach, regulating collaterals and relieving pain.

Prescription: Yang Wei Decoction combined with modified Shao Yao Gan Cao Decoction. Finger citron, citron fruit, rose and bitter orange flower ect. are added for obvious stagnation of Qi; Jin Ling Zi Powder is combined for more severe stomach disease, relieving pain and not producing dryness. Reed rhizome, trichosanthes root and black plum which can produce body fluid are added for the patient with obvious insufficiency of body fluid. Hemp seed, bush-cherry seed, trichosanthes seed which can moisture the intestine are added for patients with dry stool. White peony root, wolfberry fluit, dried rehmannia root which can soothe the liver are added for the patients with deficiency of the liver-Yin, marked by stomachache involving costal regions.

Example of Prescription: 15g adenophora root and 15g red sage root, 10g lucid asparagus root and 10g ophiopogon root, 15g fragrant solomonseal rhizome, 6g fresh liquorice, 10g finger citron, 10g citron fruit, 10g fried sichuan chinaberry, 6g black plum, 15g hemp seed and 6g rose.

(Ⅵ) Yang-deficiency of the spleen and the stomach

Main symptoms; vague pain in the stamach with more severe pain after cold and hunger, and pain relieving after hot application or taking meal, and preference for warmness and pressing.

Accompanying symptoms: dull complexion, mental fatigue, cool extremities, anorexia, loose stool or regurgitation of water from stomach.

Tongue and pulse: pale and enlarged tongue with teeth prints on the margin, and thin and white fur, deep, fine and weak pulse.

Analysis: chronic stomach disease damages the spleen-Yang. Yang-deficiency of the spleen and the stomach induces stomachache, with more severe pain when cold or hungry, relieving after warm application or taking meal, preference for warmness and pressing. The spleen is source of production of Qi and blood, dysfunction of the spleen induces weakness of Qi and blood, lost of nutrition in the body, so dull complexion and mental tiredness appear. The spleen dominates the extremities, Yang-Qi can not reach to the extremites due to deficinecy of Yang-Qi, Yang, leading to cold cxtremities. Failure of the intestine in transform due to deficiency of the spleen produces anorexia and loose stool. Dysfunction of spleen-Yang, production of cold and dampness in interior, pathogenic fluid rising induces regurgitation of water from the stomach. Pale and enlarged tongue with teeth prints on the margin, and thin and white fur, and deep, fine and weak pulse are signs of deficiency of spleen-Yang.

Therapeutic principle: Warming middle-Jiao and strengthening the spleen

Prescription: Modified Huang Qi Jian Zhong Decoction. Da Jian Zhong Decoction can be applied for the patients with severe Yang-deficiency and internal cold, or prepared aconite root, bark of Chinese cassia tree, long pepper, litse, etc. are added for warming middle-Jiao and dispelling cold; evodia fruit fried by juice of coptis root, calcined blood clam sell, cuttle-bone and other drugs of anti-acid can be added for the patient with acid regurgitation. Xiao Ban Xia plus Fu Ling Decoction or combination with Ling Gui Zhu Gan Decoction can be used for treatment regurgitation of water from the stomach.

Xiang Sha Liu Jun Zi Decoction can be used for only weakness of the spleen and the stomach, inobvious Yang-deficiency and internal cold; Gui Qi Jian Zhong Decoction for the patient accompanied with blood deficiency. Bu Zhong Yi Qi decoction for stomachache, belonging to sinking of Qi of middle-Jiao.

Clinically, the cases of strong stomach with weak spleen, and upper heat with lower cold are not less found. Ban Xia Xie Xin Decoction, Lian Li Decoction or Wen Pi Decoction can be used for the treatment.

Example of prescription: 30g honey-fried astragalus root, 10g honey-fried cinnamontwig, 15g fried white peony root, 6g honey-fried liquorice, 3 pieces of fresh ginger, 7 grains of Chinese-date, 30 malt extract (taking with the decoction), 10g litse, 10g Chinese angelica.

Appendix 1: Clinically, acid regurgitation, or acid taste in the mouth has differences of cold and heat, and differences of diseases in the liver and the stmoch. Gao Gu Feng indicated in the book Yi Jia Xin Fa. Tun Suan that acid regurgitation belonged to disease of the liver. Cold inducing stagnation of of Yang-Qi, and stagnation of Qi transforming pathogenic heat, the heat inducing acid; but the no-cold-induced acid is caused by retention of fluid in the body, attacking the spleen, results in acid regurgitation. Also, over eating, fillng in the stomach and dysfunction of the spleen-Qi in transportation also induce acid. So, acid regurtitation is correlated with the liver and the stomach. It should be treated based on the liver.

Heat syndrome: It is caused most by stagnation of the liver-Qi, transverse invading the stomach. It is stated in Nei Jing that acid regurgitation belongs to heat-syndrome. Heat-syndrome manifests as restlessness, dry throat and bitter taste, lost of appetite, red tip and margin of the tongue with yellowish fur, taut and slippery pulse. The therapeutic principle of expelling the pathogenic heat and regulating the stomach, and modified Zuo Jin Pill is used for its treatment.

Example of prescription: 6g coptis root, 3g evodia fruit, 15g calcined blood clam shell, 15g cuttle-bone, 6g sichuan fritillary bulb, 10g capejasmine fruit, 6g green tangerine orange peel, 10g forsythia fruit.

Cold-syndrome: It is caused mostly by deficiency and cold of the spleen and the stomach, manifesting as regurgitation of acid and clear water from the stomach, fullness in the stomach and loss of appetite, more severe after improper diet, relieving by warm application and pressing on the gastric region, cool extremities, tiredness and weakenes, loose stool, pale tangue with white and slippery fur, fine and taut pulse. Therapeutic principle of warming the middle-Jiao and checking hyperfunction of the liver and regulating the stomach is adopted, with combination of Xiang Sha Liu Jun Zi Decoction with Wu Zhu Yu Decoction used.

Example of prescription: 10g dangshen, 15g poria, 12g fried bighead atractylodes rhizome, 6g amomum fruir, 10g aucklandia root, 10g pinellia tuber, 10g fried tangerine peel, 3 pieces fresh ginger, 5g evodia fruit, 10g magnolia bark, 10g agastache.

Appendix 2: gastric discomfort with acid regurgitation has differences of stomach-heat, stomach deficiency and blood deficiency.

Stomach-heat: Symtoms are gastric discomfort with acid regurgitation accompanied by oppressed feeling in chest and more phlegm, vexation, insomnia, dry mouth, preference for cool drink, acid regurgitation, red tongue with yellowish fur, taut and slippery or taut and rapid pulse. Treatment should be clearing heat and regulating the middle-Jiao, with modified Huang Lian Wen Dan Decoction.

Example of prescription; 6g coptis root, 10g pinellia, 10g fried tangerine peel, 15g poria, 6g bamboo, 10g fruit of immature citron or trifoliate orange, 6g dried liquorice, 10g capejasmine fruit.

Stomach deficiency: Stomach-deficiency is marked by gastric discomfort with acid regurgitation, tastelessness, distention of stomach after meal, mental fatigue, pale tongue with thin and white fur, fine and weak pulse. Strengthening the spleen and regulating the stomach are adopted with modified Xiang Sha Liu Jun Zi Decoction used.

Example of prescription: 6g amomum fruit, 10g aucklandia root, 15g dangshen, 15g poria, 10g fried bighead atractylodes rhizome, 10g fermented pinellia tuber, 6g fried tangerine peel, 10g chicken's gizzard-skin, and 10g fruit of immature citron or trifoliate orange.

Blood-deficiency: Gastric discomfort with acid regurgitation, pale complexion, palipitation and dizziness, insomnia and dreamful sleep, pale tongue, fine pulse. Therapeutic principle of supplementing Qi and blood is adopted, with Gui Pi Decoction used.

Example of prescription: 20g honey-fried astragalus root, 15g dangshen, 10g Chinese angelica root, 15g poria, 10g white peony root, 10g bighead atractylodes rhizome, 10g longan aril, 6g honey-fried liquorice, 6g aucklandia root, 10g polygala root, 30g raw dragon's bone, 30g raw oyster shell.

〔Meassures of Prevention and nursing care〕

1. Occurrence of stomachache of excess syndrome is closely related with affection by external pathogenic factors, especially cold, improper diet, mental stress and over smoking and drinking. Thus, in order to prevent it, the patients should keep warmness for avoiding invation of exopathogenic factors; and take light food, half-fluit meal, easily to be digested, no-cold and no-hot food. Occurrence of gastric diseases of deficiency syndrome is closely related with weakness of the body, the spleen and stomach. Therefore, they should strike a proper balance between work and rest, and avoid over tiredness and over deficiency.

2. If stomachache is severe with difficulty to undure, tenderness on the gastric region, or with high fever, pale complexion, cool extreminties, the patient should keep calm, take rest in bed, and report to doctors in time.

3. Stomachache with vomiting, hematochezia, constipation should be treated according to blood syndrome or constipation, after hemorrhage and constipation relieve, the gastric disease is treated, or stomachache will relieve itself.

4. Pay attention to differentiation of gastric disease and angina pectoris. Angina pectoris should be treated according to its law of diagnosis and treatment, for avoidinng incorrective diagnosis.

Analysis of Typical Cases

Cases 1, Tian xx, male, 27-years-old, a worker, had pain in the gastric region with vomiting, hematochezia for 3 days, and was admited to the hospital. He had suffered gastric disease for 6~7 years, with pain in the gastric region, more severe before meal, and slightly relieving after meal, and acid regurgitation. 3 days ago, he took more meat, and stomachache was very severe at night, vomiting undigested food with fresh red or dark red blood clot, once diarrhea with tar-like stool, twice haematemesis, and hematochezia, with large amount of blood. Hematochrome reduced to 6. 9g. He had severe pain, distension and fullness in the gastric region, dry mouth and thirst, nausea, dizziness, palpitation, pale complexion and lip, taut, fine and slippery pulse, enlarged and pale tongue with thin and yellowish fur. Gastricopy found a 1. 8×0. 7cm size ulcer at the back wall of the junction of duodenal bulb and descending part of duedenu. It belonged to long-standing gastric disease, which was insufficiency of spleen-Qi, dysfunction of food transportation, and improper diet, retention offood and stagnation of Qi, transforming pathogenic heat, the heat causing overflow of blood from blood vessels. Hyacinth bletilla powder and rhubarb powder were administrated with boiled water for cooling blood, activating circulation of blood and stopping bleeding. A decoction of prescription was applied for treating both the principal and the secondary aspects of the disease, its symptoms and causes at the same time, which was formulated by 20g honey-fried astragalus root, 12g fried red peony root, 10g whole Chinese angelica, 10g forsythia fruit, 5g dried liquorice, 10g fried trogopterus dung, 10g dried cat-tail pollen, 3g notoginseng powder(taking with the decoction), 15g cuttle-bone, 20g red ochre and 10g dangshen. After taking one dose the pain was relieved. On the next day, three times of defecation a day, tar-like stool in the morning, it became light colour at the noon and yelowish colour in the night. Occult blood of stool turned to negative. Zuo Jin Pill was added for acid regurgitation; donkey-hide gelatin, fleece-flower root and plancenta coating tablete were added for blood deficiency; tangerine peel and pinellia tuber for nausea. After treatment for over two months, gastroocopy found union of duodenal bulbar ulcer, with a small superficial erosion, hematochrome increased to 11. 3g, and then he was discharged from the hospital.

Note: The case of stomachache, had longer duration of disease, state of illness was more complicated, dificiency syndrome with excess, and cold syndrome with heat, for example, more severe pain, distension and fullness in the gastric region, nausea, all belong to deficiency syndrorome of stagnation of Qi and reversed flow of Qi; more severe pain of stomach before meal and relieving after meal, dizziness, palpitation, pale complexion and lip, enlarged and pale tongue belong to deficiency of spleen; dry mouth and thirst, thin and yellowish fur on the tongue belong to heat syndrome; enlarged and pale tongue belong to cold syndrome. Therapeutic principale of reinforcement and elimination in combination, regulation of cold and heat in combination, supplementing Qi and activating blood circulation, removing toxic material are adopted, stomachache relieved, and spitting blood and hematochezia alliviated within 3 days and a large uncer healed after over 2 months. (see Journal of Beijing College of TCM, 85, 4)

Stomachache is in the stomach at early state and chronic pain of stomach is involved in the spleen, also it is closely related with the liver. At the early stage both invasion of exopathogens, improper diet, or stagnation of liver-Qi can injure stomach-Qi. Exopathogen and improper diet can directly injure the stomach, mild lesion can induce stagnation of stomach-Qi, and severe lesion can induce dysfunction of descending to cause reversive rising of flow of Qi; stagnation of liver-Qi, transverce attacking the stomach causes often stagnation of Qi of the liver and stomach. If it is not treated in time or incorrectly, stagnation of Qi will transform heat or protracted disease attacking, collaterals will induce blood stasis. Pathogenic heat injuring body fluid, blood stasis leads to no new blood produced, the disease gradually turns to deficiency, deficiency of stomach-Yin is seen mostly. For chronic gastric disease, the illness transforms to the spleen from the stomach, and to deficiency or deficiency with excess from excess. For deficiency of spleen, there are insuficiency of splee-Qi, sinking of Qi of middle-Jiao Qi, deficiency and cold of the spleen and the stomach, treatment should be given according to the differentiation.

Treatment of stomachache should adopt mainly regulating the flow of Qi, regulating the function of the stomach, and promoting the desending function, removing summer-heat, promoting digestion, clearing away heat, or removing blood stasis are adopted according to causes of disease; for injury of the stomach-yin, promoting production of body fluit and nourishing Yin are used for supplementing the stomach, relieving the depressed liver and promoting the flow of Qi should be mainly used for treating diseases of the liver, with removing heat from the liver for heat-transformation and promoting blood circulation for invasion of collaterals. The diseases of the spleen is treated mainly by strengthening the spleen and supplementing Qi, with ascending Qi as adjuvant method for sinking of Qi of middle-Jiao, and warm reinforcement for cold of deficiency type. Treating both the principal and the secondary aspects of a disease for simultanious occurrence of deficiency and excess syndromes, or cold and heat syndromes.

Acid regurgitation occurs often with stomachache at the same time, if acid regurgitation is major, it should be treated based on differentiation of signs and symptoms of acid regurgitation. There are differences in excessiveness of cold and heat syndromes, and in location of diseases, in the liver or the stomach for acid regurgitation. Heat syndrome is most caused by stagnation of the liver-Qi producing pathogenic heat, and dysfunction of the stomach in descending the flow of stomach-Qi. Purging the liver of pathogenic fire and regulating the function of the stomach should be used for their treatment; Warming the middle-Jiao and regulating the function of the stomach should be adopted because cold syndrome is often the basic cause of deficiency and cold syndrome of the spleen and the stomach.

Gastric discomfort with acid regurgitation, mainly marked by a faint hunger, and discomfort in the stomach, also occurs in tranformation of stomachache. It is often divided into three types, stomach-heat, stomach deficiency and blood deficiency to be treated based on differentiation of symptoms and signs.

Questions for Review

1. Which Zang-organs and Fu-organs are most closely related stomachache? What are Its pathlogical changes?
2. How to differentiate the syndromes and treat for stomachache due to stagnation of stomach-Qi and due to stagnation of Qi of the liver and the stomach?
3. What are the clinical characteristics, therapeutic principle and prescription stomachache turning to deficiency from excess, involving blood from Qi and transformation of cold syndrome and heat syndrome?
4. What are the pathological characteristics of acid regurgitation?
5. How to treat gastric discomfort with acid regurgitation based on differentiation of symptoms and signs?

Vomiting

〔General Survey〕

Dysfunction of the descening of the stomach, reversive flow of Qi inducing the food in the stomach adversely going up, through the mouth going out is called as vomiting. Nausea and vomiting often occur simultaneously and are difficult to be completely differentiated. Additionally, vomiting with sound and no food is called retching and vomiting with no sound and no food is called as nausea. Although they have differences in symptoms, their pathological machanisms are same, only with the differences in seviousness, and their treatment can be referred each other, so they are discussed together.

Sometimes, vomiting is a protective reaction for ejecting harmful substances from the stomach, being a physiological phenomenon. In clinical treatment, it should be clearly differentiated.

In many diseases of western medicine, such as nervious vomiting, acute and chronic gastritis, pyroric spasm or incomplete pyloric obstruction, cholecystitis, acute and chronic pancreatitis, and some chronic renal insufficiency, and so on, with vomiting as main symptoms, can refer to the present syndrome for treatment based on differentiation of symptoms and signs.

〔Causes of Disease and Pathology〕

Vomting is caused by adverse rising of the stomach-Qi. Because the stomach has the function of receiving food, with normal descending of the stomach-Qi, pathogenic Qi attacking the stomach or disorder of the stomach due to deficiency of stomach, inducing reverse rising of the stomach-Qi so vomiting occurs.

The spleen and the stomach are interior-exteriorly related, and the spleen is a hub of ascendintg and descending of the flow of Qi. The spleen has the function to transport and transform nutrients, dysfunction of the spleen in transporting and transforming nutrients, clear Qi is not sended up, influencing normal flow of the stomach-Qi and impairment of descending function, and reversing rising, results in vomiting.

In addition, vomiting also is related with dysfunction of both the liver and the lung. The liver corresponds to spring wool, and is in charge of sending up, the lung corresponds to autumn gold and is in charge of descending function, The Qi of the liver and lung aids function of the spleen and the stomach in sending up and descending of Qi. Stagnation of the liver-Qi and hyperactive liver-Qi attacking the stomach, may induce the reverse rising of the stomach-Qi, leading to vomiting; impairment of the lung in dispersing and descending function, easily inducing asthma and cough, even often influencing descending function of the stomach, the Qi of the lung and the stomach rise reversely simultaneously, resulting in vomiting-asthma and vomiting-cough. Causes of disease and pathology of vomiting are summerized as follows:

1. inversion of exopathogens: the environmental pathogenic factors and abnormal Qi from the mouth and the nose, invades the stomach, inducing not descending of the stomach-Qi, reverse rising, causes vomiting. Additionally, external pathogens attacking the lung, with impairment of dispersing and descending function of the lung, inducing the reverse rising of the stomach-Qi, so as to produce vomiting.

2. Improper diet: Overeating raw, cool, fat, sweet and unclear food injures the stomach-Qi, leading to dyspepsia, failure of descending of the stomach-Qi, even reverse rising, so vomiting occurs. If deficiency of the spleen and the stomach, dysfunction of tranportion and transformation, foodstuff does not transformation into nutrients, forming phlegm retention in the middle-Jiao, dysfunction of sending and descending of Qi, phlegm reversed up, induces vomiting.

3. Emotional disorder: Angry may damage the liver, hyperractive liver-Qi attacking the stomach, upward invasion of the hyperactive stomach-Qi, induces vomiting. Additionally, over thinking damages the spleen, impairing the function of transportation and transformation of the spleen, and failure of descending of the stomach-Qi, causes vomiting.

4. Deficiency of the spleen and the stomach: over tired, protracted disease consumes Qi of middle-Jiao, or due to weakness in aged people, dysfunction of transportation, impairing the function of sending up and descending, reverse rising of Qi, leads to vomiting. In addition, Yin-deficiency of the spleen and stomach, with difficulty in descending of Qi, reverse rising of Qi causes vomiting.

In short, vomiting is a disease in the stomach, adverse rising of the stomach-Qi is the key of the pathogenesis. The six exopathogenic factors, seven emotions, improper diet, over tiredness, and chronic desease, aged, weakness, inducing adverse rising of the stomach-Qi, can induce vomiting. Most of the desease belong to excess syndrome; most of chronic disease belong to deficiency syndrome. There are differences of Yin and Yang; in most of chronic diseases belong to deficiency complicated with excess, cold with heat.

〔Treatment Based on Differentiation of Systems and Signs〕

For vomiting, deficiency or excess should be first differentiated. Generally, excess syndrome is marked by sudden attack, short duration of disease, severe and continuous vomiting, most are induced by exopathogens attacking the stomach, improper diet injuring the stomach, stagnation of the liver-Qi or impairment of dispersing and descending of the lung, inducing averse rising of the stomach-Qi; deficiency syndrome is characterized by slow attack, long duration of disease, repeated attack, mild and discontinuous vomiting, most are caused by deficiency of the spleen and the stomach, and are closely related with failure of the fire of the gate of life.

Vomiting is a disease and symptom, and also is a protective reaction for ejucting harmfull substances from the stomch at a certain state, and also it is a method of treating disease. Clinically, it should be differentiated.

Diagram of Causes of Disease and Pathogensis

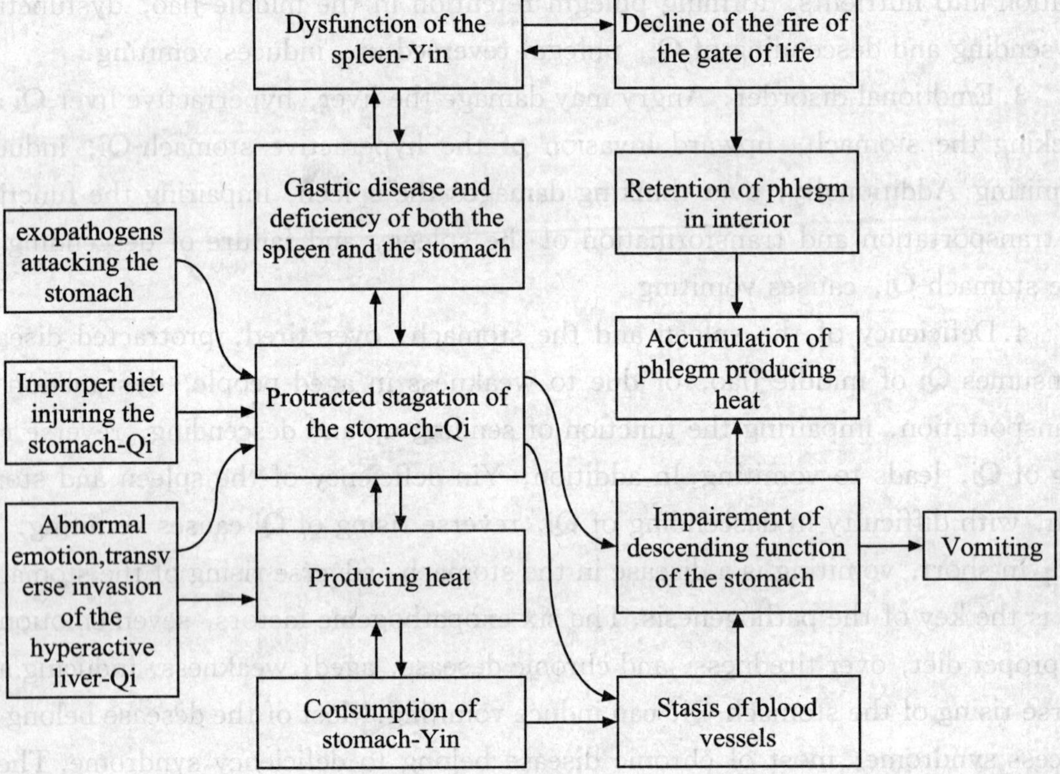

Ⅰ. Excess syndrome

(1) Exopathogens invading the stomach

Main symptoms: sudden vomiting, it is obviously related with exopathgens.

Accompanying symptoms: the patient affected by pathogenic wind and cold manifests severe aversion to cold, mild fever, headache, soreness in the body; that affectd by pathogenic wind and warmness is marked by high fever, mild aversion to wind, throat pain and dry mouth; that affected by summer-dampness manifests dull complexion, weakness of extremities, fullness in the stomach, indigestion, regurgitation of food from the stomach, stick mouth and loose stool, or low fever.

Tongue and Pulse: Normal tongue position, with thin or white fur, or thin and yellowish, or white and greasy fur, foating or tense pulse, foating, slippery and rapid or weak pulse.

Analysis: exopathogenic factors invasing the stomach, stagnation of Qi flow inducing impairment of the flow of Qi, adverse rising of dirty Qi, causes sudden vomiting. It is related obviously with exopathogen. If pathogenic wind and cold attack superfecial muscle, incoordination between Yi and Wei, aversion to cold and fever, headache, pain of the body will be seen; if pathological wind and warmness upwards attack the lung and the stomach, Qi can not be descended, inducing throat pain and dry mouth, fever, aversion to wind; affection by pathogenic summer-heat and dampness, stagnation in the upper and middle-Jiao, dysfunction of the flow of Qi, can induce fullness of the chest and gastric region, lost of appetite, dull complexion and weak extremities, thin and white fur on the tongue, floating and tense pulse are signs of affection by pathogenic wind and cold, and thin and yellowish fur, floating, slippery, rapid pulse are signs of affection by pathogenic wind and warmness, white and greasy fur, weak and slippery pulse are signs of affection by pathogenic summer-dampness.

Therapeutic Principle: removing pathogens and relieving exterior syndrome, dispelling dirty and regulating the function of the stomach.

Prescription: Modified Xiang Su Powder. In the prescription, perilla leaf has functions of relieving exterior syndrome, regulating the function of the stomach, tangerine peel has the function of regulating the flow of Qi and regulating the stomach and adverse rising of Qi; nutgrass flatsedge can regulate flow of Qi and blood in the stomach; liquorice can regulate the middle-Jiao. The four herbs perform commonly functions of relieving exterior syndrome, regulating the middle-Jiao, regulating the flow of Qi and adverse rising of Qi.

Fresh ginger, ledebouriella root are added for the patient with severe wind and cold syndrome; schizonepeta, peppermint, reed rhizome are added for severe wind and heat; fresh agastache, fresh eupatorium, fresh lotus leaf, watermelon peel, Liu Yi Powder are added for the patient injuried by summer-dampness. Xiao Chai Hu Decoction or Hao Qin Qing Dan Decoction are used in combination for pathogens transporting to Shaoyang, reverse asending of Qi of gallbladder and the stomach, marked by restlessness and vomiting; the patient with pathogen invading the Yangming, characterised by dry mouth, bitter taste, preference for cold drink, or vomiting after meal, restlessness, constipation, scanty dark urine, reddish tongue with yellowish fur, should be treated by clearing away the stomach-heat and lowering adverse flow of Qi, using Da Huang Gan Cao Decoction or Xie Xin Decoction; vomiting induced by severe cough with dyspnea belongs failure of descending of adverse rising of the flow of Qi, whole linear stonecrope, loquat leaf are added for simultaneous treatment of diseases of the lung and stomach. Fresh ginger is applied on the face of tongue, or drinking a little juice of fresh ginger, or Yu Shu Dan Ban Ding is grinded and orally administrated with boiled water for the patient with sevious vomiting and unablity to take medicine. In the patient with indigestion and vomiting undigested food with fetid odor, germinated barley and hawthorn fruit are added for promoting digestion.

Example of Prescription: 10g perilla stem and 10g perilla leaf, 10g fried tangerine peel, 10g prepared nutgrass flatsedge rhizome, 10g ginger-prepared pinellia tuber, 15g poria, 3 pieces of fresh ginger, 10g rice spout, 10g germinated barley, 10g fried hawthorn fruit, 10g loquat leaf, 10g fresh agastache, and 10g fresh eupatorium.

(2) Indigestion

Main Symptoms: vomiting indigestive food, more severe after meal, and comfort after vomiting.

Accompanying symptems: distension and fullness in the stomach, eructation and anorexia, tenderness, loose stool or constipation.

Tongue and Pulse: white and thick or greasy fur, slippery pulse.

Analysis: improper diet, retention of food in the stomach transforming heat, failure of descending of the stomach-Qi, vomit acid and indigestive food, comfort after vomiting and severe after meal. Indigestion checkinging functional activity of Qi leads to distention and fullness in the stomach, eructation and anorexia, even pain and tenderness. Retention of food in the stomach, dysfunction of tranportation, induce loose stool or constipation. White and thick, or greasy fur, slipy pulse are signs of indigestion.

Therapeutic Principle: promoting digestion, regulating the stomach and relieving vomiting.

Prescription: Modified Bao He Pill. In the prescription, hawtform fruit, medicated leaven, germinated barley, fried radish seed are used for promoting digestion, regulating the stomach, tangerine peel, pinellia tuber, poria for regulating the flow of Qi and regulating the middle-Jiao, adverse rising of the stomach-Qi, relieving vomiting. Forsythia fruit can remove heat due to retention of food. Hawtform fruit is more used for retention of meat food, rice sprout for retention of rice food, germinated barley and fried radish seed for retention of cooked wheaten food; medicated leaven for retention of indigestive alcohol and food. For yellowish fur and heat-transmission due to food retention, scutellaria root, coptis root or capejasmine fruit are addded for clearing away stomach-heat; areca seed, rhubarb are added for removing food retention and promoting digestion.

For pain in the stomach and vomiting at early stage, which are caused by eating inclean and putrefactive food, should promote vomiting with saline, for vomiting toxic material, and the patient who had taken the food for long time, relaxing the bowels for diarrhea should be adopted for ejecting the toxious substanses.

Example of prescription: 10g fermented pinellia tuber, 10g fried tangerine peel, 15g poria, 3 pieces of fresh ginger, 12g fried hawtform fruit, 10g medicated leaven, 10g rice sprout, 10g fried germinated barley, 10g fried radish seed, 10g forsythia fruit, 10g fried scutellaria root, 15g sword bean.

(3) Retention of phlegm and fluid in the body

Main symptoms: Nausea, vomiting phlegm and clear saliva, or cough with white or yellowish phlegm and saliva.

Accompanying symptoms: fat or thin body, preference for eating fat and sweet food, or discomfort in the stomach after meal, dizziness and palpitation.

Tongue and Pulse: white and greasy fur or moist or yellowish fur, thin and slippery pulse.

Analysis: dysfunction of the spleen in transportation, and failure of foodstuff transformating into nutrients, retention of phlegm in the stomach, failure of descending of the stomach-Qi, inducing neasea, vomiting phlegm and saliva. Food retention induce discomfort in the stomach after meal, comfort after vomiting. Retention of fluid in the stomach induces water sound when motion. Phlegm and fluid upward invasing the upper, leads to dizziness and palpitation. White and greasy, or moist fur, and fine and slippery pulse are signs of retention of pathogenic phlegm in the body. Thin and yellowish fur are seen for the heat-transformation.

Therapeutic Principle: warming and removing retention of phlegm and fluid, regulating function of the stomach and descending reversed flow of the stomach-Qi.

Prescription: Xiao Ban Xia Decoction combined with Ling Gui Zhu Gan Decoction. In the prescription, pinellia tuber, fresh ginger have functions of resolving phlegm and relieving distention, regulating function of the stomach and descending adverse flow of the stomach-Qi. Porica, cinnamon twig, bighead atractylodes rhizome, liquorice have function of warming and resolving retenton of phlegm. Tangerine peel, fruit of citron or trifoliate are added for strengthening the action of promoting the flow of Qi and resolving phlegm. Huang Qin Wen Dan Decoction plus Modified Ze Xie Decoction are used for the patient with nausea, vomiting, dizziness and palpitation for removing the gallbladder-heat and regulating function of the stomach, resolving phlegm, lowering adverse flow of the stomach-Qi, checking vomiting, and perilla fruit, radish seed, inula flower, loquat leaf are added for keeping the adverse Qi of the lung and the stomach downwards. Modified Gan Sui Ban Xia Decoction is adopted for the patient with vomiting yellow and green bitter liquid, dry mouth and disliking to drink, thin and yellowish fur and less fluid.

Example of prescription: 10g pinellia tuber, 3 pieces of fresh ginger, 15g poria, 10g fried tangerine peel, 10g fried bighead atractylodes, 6g cinnamon twig, 6g Prepared liquorice, 10g fried perilla fruit, 15g oriental water plantain rhizome.

(4) Hyperactive liver-Qi attacking the stomach

Main Symptoms: Vomiting acid and bitter substances in taste, frequent belching, comfirt after belching.

Accompanying symptoms: Fullness and pain in the chest and hypochondrium, restlessness, discomfort, indigestion, deterioration at dysthymia.

Tongue and pulse: red margin of tongue, with thin and greasy fur, taut and slippery pulse.

Analysis: Vomiting acid and bitter substancea in taste due to stagnation of the liver-Qi attacking the stomach, upward invasion of the hyperactive liver-Qi with the stomach-Qi. The acid and bitter taste are induced by heat-producing due to stagnation of Qi of the liver and the gallblader. Invasion of the hyperactive Qi of the liver and stomach induce frequent beelching, belching removing the stagnation of Qi, so confirm appears after belching. Stagnation of the liver-Qi, disorder of Qi, incoordination between the channel and the vessel, lead to fullness and pain in the chest and hypochondrium. Prolonged stagnation of Qi transforms pathogenic heat, so restlessnes occurs. The conditions of tongueue and pulse are signs of incoordination between the liver and the stomach, heat-transforming due to stagnation.

Therapeutic principle: soothing the liver and regulating the circulation of Qi, regulating the stomach and lowering the adverse flow of Qi.

Prescription: combination of Si Qi Decoction with Zuo Jin Pill. In the prescription, purple perilla has function of regulating the stomach, lowering the adverse flow of Qi and checking vomiting, magnolia bark has function of regulating the flow of Qi and relieving depression, pinellia tuber, poria, fresh ginger regulating the stomach, lowering the adverse flow of Qi, and relieving vomiting; coptis root, evodia fruit removing bitter taste, simultanious treatment of the liver and the stomach, relieving acid and checking vomiting. Chai Shen Wen Dan Decoction can be used for treatment of obvious vomiting acid and bitter taste. Scutellaria root, bamboo shaving and capejasmine are added for clearing the liver-fire; rhubarb and fruit of citron or trifoliate orange are added for the patient with bitter taste, gastric discomfort with acid regurgitation for removing heat and lowering adverse flow of Qi; red peony root, trogopterus dung, dried cat-tail pollen and other drugs removing stasis are added for dark tongue with ecchymosis.

Example of prescription: 10g whole purple perilla, 10g ginger-prepared pinellia tuber, 6g magnolia bark flower, 10g poria, 12g fried tangerine peel, 10g inula flower, 10g fried scutellaria root, 10g uncaria stem with hooks, 6g coptis root, 3g evodia fruit, 10g fried fruit of immature citron or trifoliate orange.

Ⅱ. Deficiency syndrome

(1) Insufficiency of the spleen-Yang

Main symptoms: protracted vomiting, or repeated vomiting, or nausea and vomiting after over tired or improper diet, or vomiting clear.

Accompanying symptoms: sallow complexion, tiredness, weakness, loose stool, or pale complexion, cool extremities, preference for warmness and aversion to cold.

Tongue and pulse: pale tongue proper with white and thin fur, fine and weak pulse.

Analysis: after protracted disease and severe disease, weakness of the spleen and stomach, even dysfunction of Yang-Qi in the middle-Jiao, and transportation and transformation, impairment of ascending and descending function of Qi, injury again of the spleen and stomach due to over tiredness or improper diet, disorder of the flow of Qi, adverse rising of the flow of Qi induces vomiting. Dysfunction of trasportation and trasformation due to deficiency of the spleen induces retention of excessive fluid in the interior, leading to vomiting clear saliva; protracted disease or repeated attack, insufficiecy of Qi of middle-Jiao, deficiency of Qi and blood, causes sallow complexion, tiredness, weakness; deficiency of middle-Yang and failure of warming Yang-Qi lead to pale complexion, cool extremites, preference for warmness and aversion to cold; insufficiency of the spleen-Yang, dysfunction of transportation and transformation, so loose stool, even watery stool occurs. Conditions of tongue and pulse are signs of Yang-deficiency of the spleen and stomach.

Therapuetic principle: warming the middle-Jiao and strengthening the spleen, regulating function of the stomach and lowering the adverse flow of Qi.

Prescription: Modified Sha Ban Li Zhong Decoction. In the prescription, dangshen, bighead atractylodes rhizome and liquorice have functions of strengthening the spleen and supplementing Qi; dried ginger warming the middle-Jiao and dispelling cold; pinellia tuber and amomum fruit resolving phlegm and regulating the spleen, lowering adverse flow of Qi and relieving vomiting. They perform commonly functions of warming the middle-Jiao, strengthening the spleen, regulating function of the stomach and checking vomiting.

Fresh ginger and evodia fruit are added for the patient with continuous vomiting clear water for warming the middle Jiao, dispelling cold and removing retention of excessive fluid in interior; inula flower and red ochre are added for the patient with continuous vomiting and repeated attack belching for strengtheninig action of lowering adverse flow of Qi and relieving vomiting. For protracted vomiting, with enlarged and pale tongue, and deep and slow pulse, belonging to severe dificiency of the spleen and stomach, earth in the cooking stove and nutmeg should be added for warming the middle-Jiao, strengthening the spleen and relieving vomiting; vomiting, marked by with thin and white tongue fur, vague pain of stomach and loose stool, fine and slippery pulse are signs of incoordination between the spleen and the stomach, and heat in the upper and cold in the lower, Ban Xia Xie Xin Decoction can be used for its treatment, for regulating the spleen and stomach, treating both cold and heat. Protracted vomiting, except the syndromes of Yang-deficiency of the spleen, with cold pain of loin and knee, damp and cool scrotum, fine, deep and slow pulse, belonging Yang deficiency of the spleen and kidney, prepared aconite root, bark of Chinese cassia tree, eagle wood, cloves should be added for warming, reinforcing the spleen and kidney, and relieving vomiting; repeated nausea and vomiting, yellowish, thick and greasy fur on the tongue, fine and weak pulse, belonging to Yang-deficiency of the spleen and kidney, failure of water-transformation due to accumulation of water in interior, production of heat being the sign of deficiency in origin and excess in superficiality, Wen Pi Decoction should be used for treating both the principal and the secondary aspects, with both reinforcing and reducing methods adopted.

Example of prescription: 5g amomum fruit, 10g ginger-prepared pinellia tuber, 15g dangshen, 12g fried bighead atractylodes rhizome, 10g dried ginger, 10g liquorice, 10g fried tangerine peel, 15g poria, 30g earth in cooking stove.

(2) Insufficiency of the stomach-Yin

Main symptoms: repeated vomiting, or occasional retching.

Accompanying symptoms: gastric discomfort with acid regurgitation, hunger-like and anorexia, dry mouth and throat, dislike drink.

Tongue and pulse: reddish tongue proper with less fluid, or no fur, fine and slightly rapid pulse.

Analysis: the stomach is Yang-earth, preference for moisture and aversion to dry. After febrile disease, or stagnation of Qi producing fire, or over eating food warm and dry in nature, inducing consultation of body fluid, failure of the stomach nourishing moisture, impairement of lowering adverse flow of Qi, and adverse rising of Qi induces vomiting, with repeated attack or occational retching. Yin-deficiency and excess of fire invade the stomach, inducing gastric discomfort, and lost of appetite. Insuficiency of the stomach-Yin, body fluid can not supply the upper, leading to dry mouth and throat. Reddish tongue with less saliva and no fur, fine and slight rapid pulse also are signs of production of deficiency-heat due to injury of Yin-fluid in the stomach.

Therapeutic principle: nourishing the stomach-Yin, lowering the adverse flow of Qi and relieving vomiting.

Prescription: Modified Mai Men Dong Decoction, In the prescription, ginseng ophiopogon root, polished round-grained mongloutinous rice, liquorice are used for nourising the stomach-Yin, pinellia tuber, bamboo shavings for lowering adverse flow of Qi and relieving vomiting. Fresh reed rhizome, forsythia fruit, peppermint for clearing away heat and promoting production of body fluid. Dendrobium, dried rehmannia root, adenophora root and other drugs of nourishing Yin, with sweet in favor and cold in nature are added for severe deficiency of the stomach-Yin with reddish tangue proper. Loquat leaf, inula flower are added for simultanious treatment of diseases of the lung and stomach. In the patient with impairment of Yin and dry intestine, marked by dry stool, hemp seed and Mongolian snakegourd fruit are added for relieving constipation.

Example of prescription: 15g adenophora root, 10g ophiopogon root, 10g dendrobium, 10g pinellia tuber, 6g bamboo shavings, 30 fresh reed rhizome, 12g loguat leaf, 15g sword bean, 10g finger citron.

Measures of Prevention and Pursing Care

1. For mild vomiting, after properly controling diet and eliminating causes of disease, it can be relieved; for severe vomiting, diagnosis and treatment should be carefully made for preveting accident.

2. During vomiting, generally, the patient should keep calm, tranquilization, and severe patients should take bed rest. At vomiting, the head of the patient should lower or turn to one side for preventing inhalation of vomiting substance into the trachea.

3. After vomiting relieving, take blank food of proper temperature, and do not take raw, cold and greasy food. Fluid diet or half fluid diet is better, meal of more times with less amount are more proper.

4. Decoction of Chinese drugs for relieving vomiting should be taken more times with less volume, for avoiding vomiting when taking drugs.

5. For severe vomiting, with high fever, severe headache; restlessness or lethargy, coma; vomiting substance with large amount of blood; pain in the stomach with tenderness, without stool or wind from bowels, primary disease should be diagnosed and treated.

6. For severe vomiting with dry tongue and mouth, dry skin with reduction of spring, mental fatigue, supplement of fluid should be given in time.

7. Acupuncture can be used in combination for preventing vomiting.

Analysis of Typical Case

Case 1: Zhang xx, male, 35 years old, a techear, had had gastric disease for over 4 years. In recent 2 months, the gastric disease had frequently attacked, more severe after meal, with distention of stomach, more severe in the evening, relieving after vomiting all food. He had been diagnosed as Yang-deficiency of the spleen and stomach, and he had taken Li Zhong Decoction and Da Ban Xia Decoction for over one month with no effect before. Physical examination found water-flow sound in the stomach, pale tongue, thin and white fur, taut pulse. He was diagnosed as duodenal bulbar ulcer and incomplete pylorochesis by barium meal examination. This is caused by stagnation of qi and stasis of blood, disorder of functional activity of Qi, adverse flow of the stomach-Qi. The therapeutic priciple of regulating flow of Qi and regulating the Yin, and relieving vomiting. The prescription, 6g chuanxiong rhizome, 9g Chinese angelica root, 20g peony and 6g liquorice were taken, after taking two doses, vomiting relieved and after 3 doses the symptoms disapeared completely.

Note: The patient belongs to deficiency and cold of the spleen and stomach, which is caused by weakness of warming and transportation. The previous treatment with warming method was ineffective because the patient had false deficiency and cold, but in fact he had stasis of blood in the hypoabdomen, and dysfunction of Yang-Qi, so chuanxiong rhizome, Chinese angelica root were used for regulating circulation of blood, and removing stasis of blood; normal circulation of blood inducing normal flow of Qi, and then liquorice was used for regulating the middle-Jiao, protecting the stomach-Qi. Because circulation of Qi and blood normarised, and normal rising and descending of Qi, so vomiting relieved and disease disappeared(See Journal of Traditional Chinese Medicine, 1990; No. 6).

Vomiting is caused by adverse rising of the stomach-Qi. Therapeutic principle of regulating the stomach and lowering adverse flow of the stomach-Qi is adopted. For vomiting of excess syndrome, marked by short duration of disease, continuous and severe vomiting, often has superficial syndrome after external pathogens attacking the stomach; retention of food induces vomiting acid and indigesive food, odor mouth, anorexia; stagnation of the liver-Qi invading the stomach induces vomiting substances of acid and bitter taste, distention and pain in the stomach with hypochondriac region involved; retention of phlegm in the body induces vomiting phlegm, saliva and clear water or thick phlegm In vomiting of deficiency syndrome, with longer duration of disease and repeated attack, improper diet or slight tiredness often induce attack, it is often found in the persons after disease or weakness; occasional and intermitent and in severe vomiting is found in weakened body resistance, for example, vomiting due to the spleen deficiency induces sallow complexion, mental fatigue and weakness; vomiting of Yang-deficiency causes pale complexion, aversion to cold and cool extremities; for vomiting of Yin-deficiency, restlesness caused by deficiency and gastric discomfort with acid regurgitation. In treatment, for vomiting of escess syndrome, removing pathgenic factors should be adopted as main method, after removing pathogenic factors, vomiting may relieve; for vomiting of deficiency syndrome, strengthening resistance of body should be applied as main method.

Questions for Review

1. How to consider that vomiting should be controled or should not be controled?
2. Try to describe pathological changes of vomiting. And how to recognized relations of vomiting with the stomach, spleen, lung, liver and kidney?
3. How to diffrentiate vomiting of retention of phlegm in the body and deficiency and cold type of the spleen and stomach?
4. How to treat based on differentiation of symptoms and signs for commonly-seen syndrome types of vomitting?

Diarrhea

〔General Introduction〕

Diarrhea is referred to increase of defecation times, with clear and dilute stool, even watery stool, or undigested stool and most seen in the summer.

Diarrhea syndrome is firstly seen in Nei Jing. It is caused by pathogenic wind, dampness, cold, or heat. In Yi Zong Bi Du, treatment of diarrhea is summarised as 9 methods. In Jing Yue Quan Shu, diarrhea was classified as spouting diarrhea and protracted diarrhea and it was held that diarrhea was caused by water, fire and earth, basic causes of diarrhea were related to the spleen and stomach, which are of important directive significance for syndrome differentiation and treatment of diarrhea.

In the western medicine, all diarrhea induced by functional or organic pathological changes of the stomach, intestine, liver, gallbladder, pancrease and other digestive organs, such as diarrhea caused by acute, chronic colitis, irritable colon, intestinal tuberculosis, etc. and some pathological changes of other systems, all refer to this syndrome for treatment based on diferentiation of symptoms and signs.

〔Causes of Disease and Pathology〕

Main pathologic changes of diarrhea are located in the spleen, stomach, and large and small intestine, mainly being in the spleen. For the causes of disease, affection by exopathogenic factors, injury by improper diet, stagnation of the liver-Qi attacking the spleen, weakeness deficiency and weakness of the spleen and stomach and deficiency of the kidney-Yang, and its main pathogenes is disorder of the functions of the spleen and stomach, and main causes of disease are pathogenic dampness, including cold-dampness, damp-heat, often with wind, summer-heat, food retention. Disfunction of the spleen and stomach is indued by many causes, such as effect of exopathogens, weakness of the spleen and stomach, incoordination between the liver and spleen and insufficiency of the kidney-Yang, all can lead to disorder of transportation and tranformation function, inducing diarrhea.

1. Affection by exopathogens: external causes inducing diarrhea have pathogenic wind, cold, summer-heat, damp, heat, with dampness as main. The spleen preferences for dryness with aversion to dampness. Dampness can often induce diarrhea. Exopathogen also can directly attack the stomach and intestine, leading to disturbance of transporting and transforming function of the spleen and stomach. Food stuff can not transform nutrition and become pathogenic dampness, and flow downwards into the intestine, producing diarrhea. Clinically, pathogenic dampness often with pathogenic wind, cold, summer-heat, heat injure the stomach and intestine. Due to different constituttion of patients and different pathogenic factors, different pathological changes produce, pathogenic dampness with wind, cold invading the body, most turns to cold-dampness; pathogenic dampness with summer-heat invading the body, heat turns easily to damp-heat.

2. Injury by diet: In summer, over eating raw and cold, or unclean food, impairing the spleen and stomach; overeating induces retention of food; or eating over fat and sweet foot, insufficient transportation and transformation, retention in the stomach and stagnation in the spleen, injuring the spleen and stomach. Lesion of the spleen and stomach leads to dysfunction of the stomach in tranportation, disorder of ascending and desending, induce diarrhea. Deficiency of the spleen and stomach induces impairment of function to transport and transform nutrients, improper diet produces more easily diarrhea.

3. Stagnation of the liver-Qi attacking the spleen: disorder of the liver-Qi and disorder of Qi, influence most easily transporting and transforming functions of the spleeen and stomach, dysfunction of the spleen in transportation, failure of food transforming nutrients, forming pathogenic dampness and lowering to form diarrhea. Stagnation of the liver-Qi due to deficiency of the spleen and stomach,

and grief, anger and mental tension transverse attacking the spleen, disorder of transportation and transformation, lead to diarrhea.

4. Weakness of the spleen and stomach: the spleen has the function to transpot and transform nutrients, and to receive food, if improper diet, internal injury caused by overtiredness, protracted disease, weakness, injury of vital Qi by protracted diarrhea, all can induce deficiency of the spleen and stomach, disorder of transport and transformation, unable to receive digested food and transport and transform nutrients, water from pathogenic dampness, retention of digested food forms diarrhea.

5. Deficiency and weakness of the kidney-Yang: the spleen in transport and transformation completely depends on warmness of the kidney-Yang; and the kidney is in charge of urination and defecation. Protracted disease and weakness due to aging and bleeding, Yang-deficiency, emission, over production all cause deficiency and weakness of kidney-Yang, dysfunction of the spleen in transportating and transforming nutrients, Yin-cold produces in the body, clear Qi lowers and water and dampness pure down, leading to diarrhea.

To sum up, deficiency of spleen and over dampness are main cause of this syndrome. Pathogenic dampness is most important factor in external causes, invasion of pathogenic dampness, stagnation of Yang of the middle-Jiao, injury of the spleen and stomach, dysfunction in transport and transformation, so undigested food lower to form diarrhea. Deficiency of the spleen is most important factor of internal causes, deficiency of spleen induces dysfunction to transport and transform nutrients, digested food can not become nutrients and clear Qi fails to ascending, undigested food lowers to form diarhea. Diarrhea due to other diseases produce often on basis of deficiency of spleen. Dysfunction of transportation due to deficiency of spleen induces excess of dampness, and excess of dampness can influence transportation and transformation of the spleen, so interraction of spleen deficiency and excessive dampness are basic causes for occurrence, development and difficult cure of diarrhea. Hyperactive liver-Qi attacking the spleen or deficiency of the spleen involving the kidney, at once kidney deficiency exacerbates further functions of transporting and transforming nutriets, diarrhea is difficult to be cured.

〔Treatment Based on Differentiation of Symptoms and Signs〕

Ⅰ. Main points of differentiation of syndromes and signs

Clinically, differentiation of symptoms and signs is made based on fulminant diarrhea and protracted diarrhea, and deficiency, excess, cold and heat. Excess syndrome includes three types, cold-dampness, dampness-heat, impairment by over eating; deficiency syndrome includes spleen deficiency and kidney deficiency; deficiency complicated with excess is more seen in the hyperactive liver-Qi attacking the spleen.

(Ⅰ) Differentiation of deficiency and excess: sudden attacking, short duration of disease, frequent diarrea, abdominal pain with tenderness, pain relieving after diarrhea, belong excess syndrome; slowly attack, long duration of disease, intermittent diarrhea, abdominal pain with preference for pressing, pain exacerbation after defecation, belong deficiency syntrome.

(Ⅱ) Differentiation of cold and heat: See the following table.

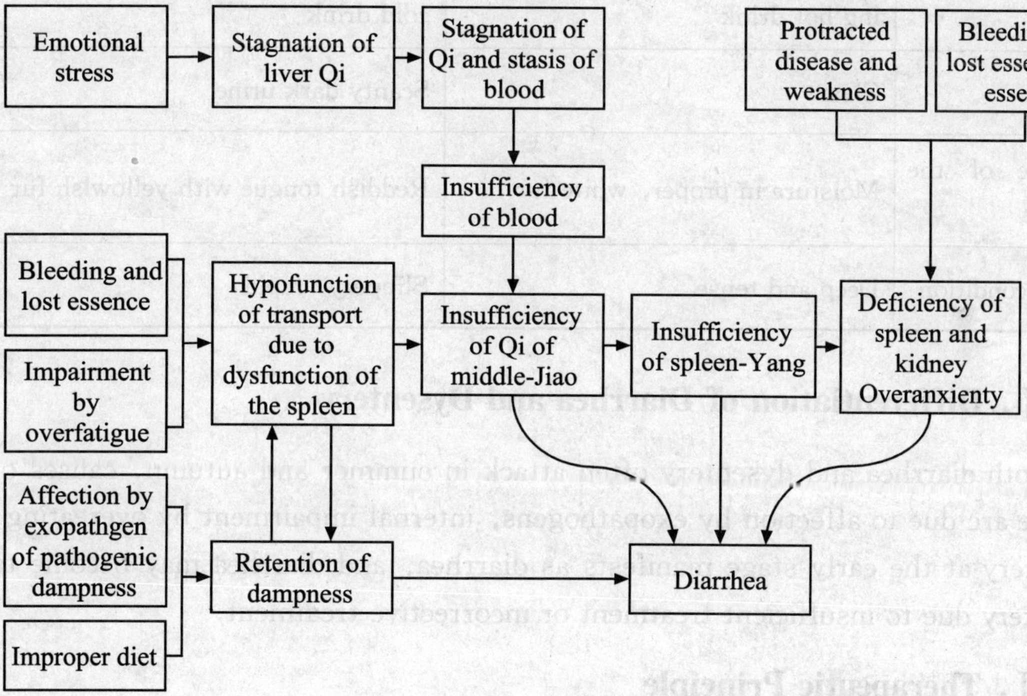

(Ⅲ) Differentiation of colour and property of stool: yellow and brown, viscous stool with odor, feeling of burning heat in the anus, most belong damp-heat; green-gray or green-black stool, clear, dilute or watery stool, not obvious odor, most belong cold-dampness; loose stool, viscous and odor stool with undigested food, most belong impairment by overeating; loose stool with normal colour, occational attack, and attack due to emothional factors, more belong hyperactive liver-Qi invading the spleen; loose stool with undigested food, deterioration after tiredness or meal, belong deficiency of spleen; white and clear stool, even indigested food, and more accurrence of diarrhea before dawn, belong kidney deficiency.

	Cold syndrome	Heat syndrome
Property and shape of stool	loose, clear, cool, or watery, even indigested food	sudden, ropy and yellow stool, burning in the anus
Abdominal Pain	Gurgling sound and cutting pain in the abdomen, relieving after heat application	Burning pain in the abdomen, paroxysmal dairrhea and pain
Thirst	No thirst. pain relieving after taking hot drink	Excessive thirst and preference for cold drink
Urine	Clear	Scanty dark urine
Picture of the tangue	Moisture in proper, white fur	Reddish tongue with yellowish fur
Pulse condition	Deep and tense.	Slippery, rapid

Ⅱ. Differentiation of Diarrhea and Dysentery

Both diarrhea and dysentery often attack in summer and autumn, causes of disease are due to affection by exopathogens, internal impairment by overeating; dysentery at the early stage manifests as diarrhea, and diarrhea may become to dysentery due to insufficient treatment or incorrective treatment.

Ⅲ. Therapeutic Principle

For fulminant diarrhea with excessive pathogen as main, first should eliminate pathogens, and dispel dampness and dry the spleen. For the patient with superficial syndrome, should relieve exterior syndrome; for with heat, should clear away heat, for dyspepsia, should promote digestion; for protracted diarrhea, often seen deficiency of vital essense, should firstly strengthen resistance of the body, and then adopt the therapeutic principle of strengthening the spleen and warming Yang, and regulating the liver and the kidney. For deficiency complicated with excess, and cold with heat, should treat both the principal and the secondary aspects of the disease, regulate both cold and heat. Additionally, reinforcing method and astringing intestine method can not be together used for acute diarrhea, in order to avoid inducing chronic diarrhea; for chronic diarrhea, should not adopt over clearing and removing methods, for avoiding injury of vital Qi and Yin, inducing difficulty in treat.

differen-tiation / name of the disease	Parts of disease	Hema-tochezia with pura	Defeca-tion	Abdom-inal pain	Rotine exami-nation WBC + RBC	Pathology	Crisis
Diarrhea	Spleen (middle-Jiao)	No	free	Abdom-inal pain with bowel sound	<15	Over damp-ness and spleen defi-ciency	less
Dysentery	Intes-tine (Lower-Jiao)	yes	Patho-gen at-tacking Diarrhea with discom-fort, difficulty in dis-charge, rectal tenesmus	intestine, incoor-dination Severe abnormi-nal pain, pain at-tacking with dysen-tery	>15	between Qi and blood, forming pura Pathogen at-tacking in-testine, in-coordination between qi and blood, forming pura	more

Ⅳ. Treatment based on classification

(Ⅰ) Fulminant Diarrhea

1. Diarrhea of cold-damp type or diarrhea of wind-cold type

Main symptoms: acute and fulminant attack, clear and dilute, even watery stool, paroxysmal pain and diarrhea with bowel sound.

Accompanying symptoms: often seen exterior syndrome of wind-cold with dampness, such as aversion to cold, fever, heavy head and tiredness, general sureness, fullness in the stomach, anorexia, no thirst or viscous mouth with discomfort.

Tongue and pulse: thin and white or white greasy fur, weak and slow or floating and tense pulse.

Analysis: affection by exopathogenic wind-cold, or cold-dampness, retaining in the intestine and the stomach, or overeating raw, cool, viscous, greasy and unclean food, injuring the stomach and intestine, disturbance in ascending and descending, pathogenic dampness pour down, forming clear and dilute, even watery stool, with acute and fulminat attack. Cold causes contraction, dampness induces moisture, retention of cold and dampness pathogens, and stagnation of Qi, so paroxysmal pain and diarrhea produce, water and dampness pour down, inducing bowel sound. Wind and cold with dampness attacking the muscle and skin, Wei-Yang is dispressed, so fever, aversion to cold, heavyness in head, and general pain. Retention of dampness in the middle-Jiao induces fullness in the stomach and loss of appetite, no thirst, or discomfort in the mouth with viscous. Affection by pathogenic wind-cold leads to thin and white fur, floating and tense pulse. If cold-dampness attacks the middle-Jiao, white and thin fur, and weak and slow pulse will be seen.

Therapeutic principle: Relieving exterior syndrome to dispel cold, turbid-transmission and removing dampness by diuresis.

Prescription: Wei Ling Decoction combined with modified Huo Xiang Zheng Qi Powder.

Huo Xiang Zheng Qi Powder is specially used for treatment of stagnation of dampness-turbid Qi in the intestine and stomach. In the prescription agastach is used as main drug pungent in flavor and warm in property for dispelling cold, and eliminating dampness with aromatics; atractylodes rhizome and poria for strengthening the spleen and eliminating dampness; magnolia bark and shell of areca nut for promoting the flow of Qi and resolving the fullness, promoting functional activity of Qi. Purple perilla and dahurrian angelica root for relieving exterior syndrome and dispeling cold. Ping Wei Powder is a good prescription for removing dampness and regulating the middle-Jiao. Wu Ling Powder for removing dampness and promoting diuresis, removing pathogenic dampness and turbid from urine; dampness is a Yin pathogen, when cold-damp is obvious, in the prescription cinnamon twig can remove dampness by warming Yang Qi. Wind-cold retains in the stomach, with obvious abdominal pain, can be treated by Zheng Qi Tian Xiang Powder combined with Wei Ling Decoction.

Prepared soybean and ledebouriella root are added for more severe wind-cold for strengthening power of dispelling wind-cold by warming; and chicken's gizzard-membrane for promoting digestion; for watery diarrhea with severe abdominal pain and frequent defecation, Zhou's Hui Sheng Dan can be administered, twice each day, 10 pieces each session.

Example of prescription: 10g agastach, 10g perilla leaf, 10g atractylodes rhizome, 5g round cardamon seed, 10g tangerine peel, 10g pinellia tuber, 10g magnolia bark, 12g shell of areca nut, 5g fresh ginger, one pack of Wu Ling Powder.

2. Diarrhea of Damp-heat Type or Diarhhea of Summer-heat and Dampness Type

Main symptoms: immediate diarrhea after abdominal pain, acute and sudden diarrhea or discomfort in diarrhea, yellow -brown and viscous stool with odor.

Accompanying symptoms: feeling of burning heat in the anus, restlessness, thirst, short and scanty dark urine.

Tongue and pulse: reddish tongue with yellowish and greasy fur, slippery and rapid, or weak and rapid pulse.

Analysis: more excessive summer-dampness in the summer and autumn, because of overeating fat, sweet food, retention of damp-heat injuring the intestine and stomach, disorder of transportation, diarrhea appears. Dampness lowering downward and heat excesses, damp-heat pours down, abdominal pain with sudden diarrhea produces. Moisture with viscous and greasy property easily checkes the functional activity of Qi, so diarrhea with discomfort. Excessive damp-heat, pathogenic dampness pours down, forming yellow-brown stool with odor, feeling of burning heat in the anus. Protractive damp-heat induces restlessness and thirst, short and scanty dark urine. Yellowish and greasy fur, and weak and rapid or slippery and rapid pulse are signs of excessive damp-heat pathogen in the body.

Therapeutic principle: Clearing heat and removing dampness.

Prescription: Modified Ge Gen Qin Lian Decoction.

In the prescription, pueraria root is used for resolving muscular pain and clearing away heat, raising and relieving diarrhea; scutellaria root and coptis have bitter taste with cold in property, having functions of clearing away heat and dry-transformation by removing dampness and being good at relieving diarrhea. Fresh liquorice has mild sweet taste and has the function of regulating the middle-Jiao,

tale and Liu Yi Powder for removing summer-heat and relieving restlessness. Coix, poria, Caulis aristolochiae or Clematidis Armandii are added for the patient with serious dampness for promoting removing dampness by diuresis, removing damp-heat pathogen; flower, forsythia fruit, rhubarb are added for excess of heat pathogen for removing toxic substances; medicated leaven, germinated barley, hawthorn fruit are added for patients of indigestion for promoting digestion; agastach, eupatorium, fresh lotus leaf and hyacinth-bean flower are added for patients with ovbious signs of summer-heat for relieving summer-heat and clearing away heat.

For treatment of diarrhea of damp-heat type, should differentiate more damp pathogen or more heat pathogen. For more dampness, more drugs for removing dampness and diuresis are used, and for more heat, more drugs for clearing away heat are used.

When disease attacks in the hot days, for the patients of rice shoup -like diarrhea, extreme thirst, reddish urine, thin and yellowish fur on the tongue, weak and rapid pulse, therapeutic principle of clearing away summer-heat and removing dampness are atopted, and the prescription, Xing Jia Xiang Ru Decoction combined with Liu Yi Powder or Xiang Lian Pill.

Example of Prescription: 10g pueratia root, 12g fried scutellaria root, 6g coptis root, 6g dried liquorice, 10g tale, 15g dried coix seed, 10g ricepaper pith, 20g plantain herb, 10g aucklandia root.

3. Diarrhea due to impairment of overeating

Main symptoms: immediate diarrhea after abdominal pain, odor stool, pain relieving after diarrhea.

Accompanying symptoms: Fullness in the stomach, loss of appetite.

Tongue and pulse: Thick and greasy fur on the tongue, slippery pulse.

Analysis: improper diet, retenton of food in the intestine and stomach, disorder of transportation, induce abdominal pain and diarrhea. Indigetion, adverse rising of the dirty Qi inducing regurgitation of undigested food, pouring down, forming odor stool, turbit Qi flowing downwards, so pain relieves after diarrhea. Retention of food in the middle-Jiao, disorder of functional activity of qi, inducing fullness in the stomach, and abdominal pain; failure of descending of the stomach-Qi, and dysfunction of the spleen in transport, so loss of appetite appears. Thick and greasy fur, and slippery pulse are signs of dyspepsia.

Therapeutic Principle: removing food retention and promoting digestion.

Prescription: Modified Bao He Pill.

This is an important prescription treating food retention, removing stagnated food and promoting digestion, and regulating the middle-Jiao and removing dampness. In the prescription, medicated leaven, germinated barley, hawthorn fruit, radish seed have functions of promoting digestion, sending Qi down and removing food retention, tangerine peel and pinellia tuber regulating the stomach and lowering adverse rising flow of the stomach-Qi; poria regulating the spleen and eliminating dampness; forsythia fruit with bitter taste and slight cold in property, is good at clearing away pathogenic heat produced by protracted food stagnation.

Scutellaria root and coptis root are added for clearing away heat and eliminating dampness in the patient who takes over pungent flavor, sweet and fried food, marked with yellowish fur and slippery pulse. Ping Wei Powder is added for strengthing power of eliminating dampnes in the patient who eats over cold food, marked by white fur and slow pulse. Zhi Shi Dao Zhi Pill is uaed for severe retention of food, fullness in the stomach, and diarrhea with discomfort, in the prescription rhubarb and fruit of immature citron or trifoliate orange are main.

Example of prescription: 10g fermented pinellia tuber leaven, 10g fried tangerine peel, 15g poria, 10g medicated leaven, 10g fried germinated barley, 10g hawthorn fruit, 10g fried radish seed, 10g forsythia fruit, 10g fried bighead atractylodes rhizome, 10g aucklandia root.

(Ⅱ) Chronic diarrhea

1. Diarrhea of the spleen deficieny type

Main symptoms: loose stool, watery stool or diarrhea, times of defecation increases after eating a little fat or tiredness, even with undigested foot.

Accompanying symptoms: sallow complexion, fatigue and weakness of extremities, or thin in the body, loss of appetite, fullness in the stomach, bowel sound.

Tongue and pulse: pale tongue, enlarged tongue with thin and white fur, fine and weak pulse.

Analysis: chronic injury of the spleen and stomach, deficiency and weakness of the middle-Qi, dysfunction of the spleen in transport, sinking of clear Qi, indigestion, dispepsia, undigested food pours down, loose stool and bowel sound appear. A little fat or overwork injure the spleen-Qi, so diarrhea deteriorates with increase of defecation times and with undigested food. Deficiency of both the spleen and stomach, dysfunction of digestion, insufficiency of Qi and blood, so sallow complexion appears, with tiredness and weakness of extremities and thin body. Deficiency and weakness of the spleen and stomach, leading to slower digestion, loss of appetite occurs, slower flow due to weakness of Qi, inducing fullness in the stomach; pale and enlarged tongue with thin and white fur, and fine weak pulse are signs of deficiency and weakness of the spleen and stomach.

Therapeutic principle: Strengthening the spleen and supplementing qi.

Prescription: Modified Shen Ling Bai Zhu Powder.

Si Jun Zi Decoction is the basis of this prescription, supplementing Qi and strengthening the spleen, hyacinth bean, Chinese yam, lotus seed, fried coix seed are used for eliminating dampness and regulating the spleen; amomum fruit is added for promoting the functional activity of the spleen and stomach, tangerine peel for activating flow of Qi and regulating the middle-Jiao; root of balloomflower for raising the sinked clear Qi. This is a commonly-used prescription for treating diarrhea due to hypofunction of the spleen.

Bu Zhong Yi Qi Decoction may be used for supplementing Qi and strengthening the spleen and relieving diarrhea in the patient of chronic diarrhea with proctoptosis due to sinking of Qi of middle-Jiao; pomegranate rind, Chinese gall and ha wthorn fruit are added for the patient of chronic diarrhea with injury of both Qi and Yin, and reddish and thin tongue, and thin, yellowish and greasy fur. It should be paid attention to that drugs for warming and drying do not used for strengthening the spleen and supplementing Qi, greasy not for supplementing the stomach and nourishing Yin, bitter taste and cold in nature not for clearing away heat and eliminating dampness, not inducing over diuresis with bland drugs, that is, nourishing Yin with no increasing dampness, eliminating dampness with no injury of Yin, clearing away heat without injury of the middle-Jiao. Flavescent sophora root, phellodendron bark and other drugs are added for clearing away heat and eliminating dampness are added in the patient of chronic diarrhea with deficiency of the spleen, retention of dampness and heat-transmission. Fu Zi Li Zhong Decoction plus evodia fruit and bark of Chinese cassia tree are used for warming the middle-Jiao and dispelling cold in the patient with failure of the splees-Yang, excessive Yin and cold in the body, cool pain in the stomach and bowel sound, cool extreminties.

Example of prescription: 10g dangshen, 15g poria, 12g fried bighead atractylodes rhizome, 15g fried hyacinth bean, 10g Chinese yam rhizome, 10g fried tangerine peel, 10g cooked aucklandia root, 15g fried coix sead, 3g root of ballonflower, amomum fruit, 10g lotus seed.

2. The hyperactive liver-Qi attacking the spleen

Main symptoms: Abdominal pain and diarrhea after emotional disorder, and slight relieving of abdominal pain after defecation, and diarrhea again after abdominal pain.

Accompanying symptoms: fullness in the chest and hypochondrium, belching, loss of appetite, bitter mouth and acid regurgitation, sallow complexion, tiredness and weakness.

Tongue and pulse: reddish tongue with thin and white or thin and yellowish fur, taut and fine pulse.

Analysis: Emotional disorder induces stagnation of the liver-Qi, transverse attacking the spleen. Disease of the spleen induces dysfunction of the spleen in transporting and transforming nutrients, and ascending and descending, undigested food pours down, so abdominal pain appears with diarrhea; temperally the dipressed hyperactive liver-Qi, slightly quickening flow of stomach-Qi after diarrhea, so pain relieves, renewing stagnation of hyperactive the liver-Qi and then abdominal pain appears again, and then diarrhea appears; chronic diarrhea injuring the spleen, insufficiency of Qi and blood, so lead to thin in the body and sallow complexion, mental tiredness and weakness. Failure of nourishing the liver and disorder of flow of Qi, easily induce stagnation of the liver-Qi, in an anxious state of mind, fullness in the chest and hypochondrium with discomfort. The hyperactive liver-Qi attacking the stomach induces belching and anorexsia, bitter mouth and acid regurgltaion. reddish tongue, taut and fine pulse are signs of hyperactive liver-Qi and deficiency of the spleen.

Therapeutic principle: Depressing the hyperactive liver-Qi and supporting the spleen.

Prescription: Modified Tong Xie Yao Fang.

In the prescription, white peony root is used for nourishing the liver; ledebouriella root can dispel the hyperactive liver-Qi and regulate the spleen and eliminate dampness; bighead atractylodes rhizome can strengthen the spleen to eliminate dampness and relieve diarrhea; tangerine peel can promote functional activity of Qi, and regulate the middle-Jiao. Combination of the four herbs can regulate hyperactive liver-Qi, promote functional activity of the spleen, commonly performing the action of depressing the liver-Qi and supporting the spleen.

Schisandra fruit, Chinese gall and chaenomeles fruit are added for insufficiency of the liver-Yin; poria, hyacinth bean and Chinese yam are added for supplementing Qi and strengthening the spleen for the patient with dysfunction of the spleen; white mume flower, curcuma root, albizia flower, fresh dragon's bone and oyster shell for regulating Qi by alleviation of mental depression, transquillixation in the patient with emmotional disorder.

Example of prescription: 12g fried white peony root, 6g ledebouriella root, 10g fried bighead atractylodes rhizome, 10g fried tangerine peel, 15g fried hawthorn fruit, 5g black plum, 5g liquorice, 15g poria, 15g fried hyacinth bean, 10g Chinese yam, 10g white mume flower.

3. Deficiency of the kidney-Yang

Main symptoms: Diarrhea before dawn, loose stool, even with undigested food, and comfort after diarrhea.

Accompanying symptoms: vague pain in the navel-abdomin, aversion to cold, bowel sound, cool body and extremities, soreness and cold pain in the loin, impotence, damp and cool scrotum in male, and delayed menstrual cycle with oligomenorrhea in female.

Tongue and pulse: enlarged and pale tongue, with white, moist and slippery fur, and deep and slow pulse.

Analysis: Lack of nourishing in Chronic disease, deficiency of the kidney-Yang, can not warm the spleen to promote the function of the spleen in transporting and transforing nutrients, and before dawn extreme excess of Yin and cold, so diarrhea before dawn appears, even with undigested food, comfort after diarrhea. Yang-deficiency of the spleen and kidney, dysfunction of Yang-Qi can not warm and nourish the internal organs, so induce aversion to cold and pain in the navel-abdomin, bowel sound; failure of warming and nourishing the channels and blood vessels, so cause cool pain in the loin and knee, impotence and cool and damp in scrotum in male, and deficiency and cold in Ren Channel in female, leading to delayed menstrual cycle with oligomenorrhea. The enlarged and pale tongue with white and watery slippery fur, and deep and slow pulse are signs of Yang-deficiency and excess of Yin.

Therapeutic principle: warming the kidney and strengthening the spleen.

Prescription: Modified Si Shen Pill.

In the prescription, psoralea fruit can warm and supplement fire of the life gate to relieve diarrhea, nutmeg and can warm the spleen and dispel cold, schisandra fruit can astring to arrest diarrhea, ginger and jujube can strength the spleen and regulate the middle-Jiao.

Combination with Fu Zi Li Zhong Decoction for stengthening power of warming and reinforcing the spleen and kidney in the patient of obvious dysfunction of the spleen-Yang. Morinda root, cardamon, bark of Chinese cassia tree are added for warming the kidney in the patient of obvious deficiency of fire of the life gate. Bu Zhong Yi Qi Decoction is combined for raising clear Yang in the aging patient, weakness, chronic diarrhea induces sinking of of Qi of the middle-Jiao; Tao Hua Decoction is added for arresting diarrhea in the patient with chronic diarrhea and fecal incontinence; For the patient of chronic dirrhea with Yang-deficiency of the spleen and kidney, dysfunction of circulation of Qi and blood, marked by signs of Yang deficiency and blood stasis, Shao Fu Zhu Yi Decoction can be used in combination for treatment.

Example of prescription: 10g psoralea fruit, 10g nutmeg, 5g evodia fruit, 10g schisandra fruit, 15g dangshen, 15g poria, 6g prepared aconite root, 6g baked ginger, 12g fried bighead atractylodes rhizome, 6g roasted aucklandia root, 10g lindera root.

〔Messures of Prevention and Nursing Care〕

1. Pay attention to alimentary hygience, do not eat putrid and degenerative food.

2. Do not drink unboiled water and eat unclean melon and fruit, wash hand before meal.

3. The patient of diarrhea should take fluid and semi-fluid meal, and do not eat purgent, fried, fat and sweet food. In the patient who suffers from diarrhea with injury of the stomach-Qi, blank salt water, boiled rice liquid, and rice gruel are given for nourishing the stomach-Qi; in the patient with diarrhea of deficiency-cold type, blank ginger tea is administrated for activating the spleen-Yang to regulate the stomach-Qi. The patient of chronic diarrhea, should avoid overwork and mental stimulation, and keep warmness and prevent from affection by cold.

4. Gruel with drugs.

〔Analysis of Typical Case〕

Case 1, Liu Huafu treated by Xue Lizhai, Liu had retention of food and abdominal pain, diarrhea with yellow stool, vomiting phlegm, after took tangerine peel, pinellia tuber, capejasmine fruit, coptis root, fruit of immature citron or trifoliate orange herbs, the symptoms relieved. Taut and tense pulse on the left Guan and taut and long pulse on the right Guan, caused by the liver-Qi attacking the spleen, Liu Jun Zi Decoction combined with aucklandia were administrated with cure. If food has been digested and diarrhea is not cured, Yi Gong Powder will be used for reinforcing the spleen, or Bu Zhong Yi Qi Decoction is used for activating Yang-Qi. The Bu Zhong Yi Qi Decoction should be used in combination with aucklandia root and galangal fruit for warming and reinfocing in the patient with yellow dysentery, deficiency of the spleen, and sinking of the spleen-Qi. If it is ineffective, Ba Wei Pill will be used.

Note: The drugs of tangerine peel, pinellia tuber, capejasmine fruit, coptis root, etc. have good effects for this syndrome, retention of food and abdominal pain, and diarrhea with yellow stool and vomiting phlegm, appear to be accumulation of phlegm and heat with no excess. This is due to deficiency of the spleen and stomach, deficiency of the spleen and hyperfunction of the liver, i, e. the liver (wood) restricts the spleen(earth). The treatment should give mainly for reinforcing the spleen, hyperfunction of the spleen is not easily affected by pathogens. "Liu Jun" can be used for supplementing the spleen, and aucklandia root is added for promoting the flow of the Qi and relieving pain, warming the middle-Jiao and regulating the stomach.

Diarrhea is marked by increase of defecation times, clear and dilute stool, even watery stool. It is caused by pathogenic dampness, and the key of atttack is deficiency of the spleen and excessive dampness. Pathogenic dampness is caused by excessive dampless of environment and dysfunction of the spleen in transport, the both influence each other.

Pathological changes of diarrhea are mainly in the spleen, stomach, large intestine and small intestine, also are related with the liver and kidney. In differentiation of symptoms and signs, firstly should differentiate deficiency, excess, cold and heat. Acute and fulminant diarrhea belongs often heat syndrome or excess syndrome; chronic and protracted diarrhea often belong deficiency syndrome or cold syndrome; hyperactive liver-Qi attacking the spleen belongs often deficiency syndrome with excess syndrome. Therapeutic principle of promoting function of the spleen and eliminating dampness always is used with flexibly working out a therapy based on differentiation of fulminant diarrhea, protracted diarrhea and cold, heat, deficiency and excess. In addition, in the process of treatment should pay attention to diet, emotiom, keeping warmness, taking rest and other measures of nursing care.

Questions for Review

1. How to comprehend the important significance of deficiency of the spleen and excessive dampness in attack of diarrhea?
2. How many kinds of types for diarrhea are there ? How to differentiate their syndromes and treat them?
3. How to differentiate diarrhea and dysentery?
4. How to differentiate and treat chronic diarrhea injuring the spleen-Yang, and chronic diarrhea injuring the spleen-Yin?
5. Which should be pay attention to in treatment of chronic diarrhea injuring both Qi and Yin with dampness and heat removed incompletely?
6. How to use the drugs inducing astringency and the drugs of sour flavor inducing astringing to arrest diarrhea in treatment of diarrhea?
7. How to understand and treat indigestion in fulminant diarrhea and chronic diarrhea?
8. How to differentiate and treat uninjury and injury of the liver-Yin in diarrhea due to hyperactive the liver-Qi attacking the spleen?

Dysentery

〔General Introduction〕

Dysentery is characterized by abdominal pain, rectal tenesmus, with red, white and pus and blood stool, often seen in the summer and autumn seasons.

Dysentery was recorted in Nei Jing, Nan Jing, Shang Han Lun, Zhu Bing Yuan Hou Lun and Qian Jin Fang, etc. In the Jin and Yuan Dynasties it was aknowledged that dysentery had infectiivity.

In western medicine, acute and chronic bacterial dysentery, amebic dysentery and some pathologic changes of colon, marked mainly by mucus and bloody stool, can refer to the treatment of this disease based on differentiation of symptoms and signs.

〔Causes of the Disease and Pathology〕

This disease is caused often by affection of external dampness-heat, and epidemic pathogenic factors, and internal impairment of raw and cold diet, injuring the spleen, stomach and intestine.

1. Affection by exopathogens: in the summer and autumn, summer-heat, dampness and epidemic pathogenic factors retain in the stomach and intestine, accumulation of dampness and steaming if heat, stagnation of Qi and blood, putrescence transforms pus, defecating red, white and mucus and bloody stool, forming damp-heat dysentery or epidemic dysentery. In addition, pathogenic cold-dampness invading the stomach and intestine, or chronic dysentery, injury of both the spleen and stomach, disorder of transporting and transforming nutrients, pathogenic dampness produces in the body, becoming cold from Yin, interaction between Qi and blood, forming cold-damp dysentery. Generally, it is considered that lesion of Qi system forms white dysentery, lesion of blood system forms red dysentery and lesion of both Qi and blood forms red-white dysentery.

2. Internal impairment of diet: improper diet, overeating fat, sweet food, or eating unclean food injure the intestine and stomach, producing damp-heat, accumulation of dampness and steaming of heat, stagnation of Qi and blood, forming pus-blood, i.e. damp-heat dysentey; stagnation of damp-heat injuring Yin-blood, forming Yin-deficiency dysentery; overeating raw and cold melon and fruit, injuring the intestine and stomach, retention of dampness in the body, inducing retention of cold, dampness and food in the intestine, impairment of functional activity of Qi, stagnation of Qi and stasis of blood, which are interacted with undigested food in the intestine, producing pus-blood, forming cold-damp dysentery. In the patient with deficiency of the spleen and stomach, repeated affection by pathogenic cold-dampness, or for the patient with hot-dysentery takes over drugs cold and cool in nature, it will become cold-dysentery.

Although the above-mentioned causes of disease are divided into affection by exopathogen and improper diet, they are interacted each other, affection by internal and external pathogensinduces attack of the disease.

This disease occurs in the intestine, but it is correlated with the stomach, such as damp-heat, epidemic pathogenic factors attacking up the stomach, or chronic dysentery injuring vital Qi, deficiency of the stomach and adverse rising of the stomach-Qi, induce vomiting with no eating and drinking, forming fasting dysentery. Protracted dysentery, deficiency of vital Qi and retention of pathogens form chronic dysentery. Chronic dysentery, or repeated attack of dysentery, the spleen, even the kidney are involved. Lesion of both the spleen and kidney causes discontinuous dysentery.

In short, occurrence of this disease is related with affection by exopathogenic factors and improper diet, and the disease is in the intestine. Damp-heat, epidemic pathgenic factors, cold-dampness, indigestion, and retention of undigested food in the intestine, interaction between Qi and blood, induce dysfunction of the intestinal tract in transport, injury of channels and colleterals, stagnation of Qi and blood, forming pus and blood, so red and white dysentery appears; impairment of functional activity of Qi, stagnation of Qi of Fu-organs induce abdominal pain, rectal tenesmus.

〔Treatment Based on Differentiation of Symptoms and Signs〕

Generally speaking, dysentery at early state is often excess syndrome, should be treated with promoting digestion and removing food retention; chronic dysentery often is deficiency syndrome, or deficiency with excess, should be treated with reinforcement and astringency, or reinforcement and elimination in combination. The pathologic change is in the blood system for dysentery with bloody stool, it should be treated by means of removing heat from blood and regulating blood, using more drugs for blood; dysentery with mucus or purulent discharge, should improve flow of Qi and eliminate dampness in treatment, using more drugs for Qi. In the treatment of various types of dysentery, drugs for promoting digestion and removing food retention, regulating functional activity of Qi, and regulating blood should be added on the basis of treatment based on differentiation of symptoms and signs. At first stage of dysentery, most have damp-heat; at chronic stage, Qi of spleen is gradually injured, easily inducing cold-transmission, should solidate and protect stomach-Qi.

(Ⅰ) Dysentery due to damp-heat pathogen

Main symptoms: dysentery with bloody stool and mucus or purulent discharge, main bloody stool, feeling of burning heat in the anus, abdominal pain and rectal tenesmus.

Accompanying symptoms: fullness in the stomach, indigestion, viscous mouth and acid regurgitation, scanty dark urine.

Tongue and pulse, reddish tongue with yellowish and greasy fur, slippery and rapid pulse.

Analasis: Stagnation of damp-heat pathogens in the intestine, injuring channels and colletarals, and interaction with Qi and blood, produce pus and blood, forming dysentery with bloody stool or mucus discharge; lesion of blood vessels, forming dysentery with bloody stool as main. Stagnation of Qi induces abdominal pain. Damp-heat pathogen with food retention induces rectal tenesmus. Failure of descending of the stomach-Qi induces fullness in the stomach and indigestion, mucous mouth, nausea. damp-heat pathogen pours down induces feeling of burning heat in the anus, scanty dark urine. Tongue and pulse are signs of accumulation of damp-heat pathogen in the body.

Diagram of Causes of Disease and Pathology

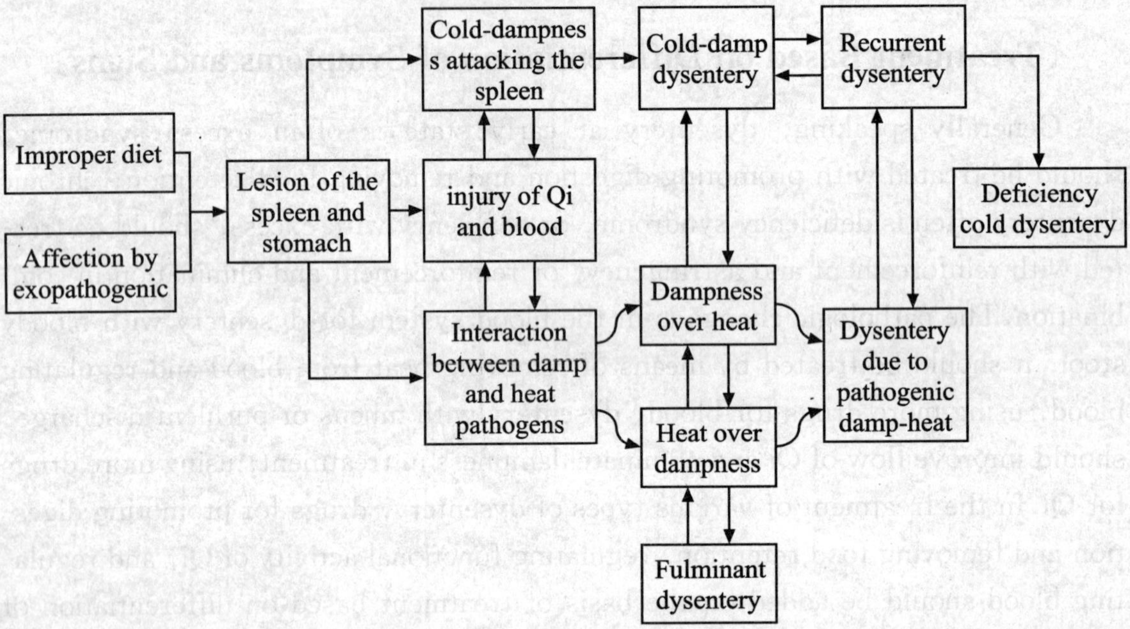

Therapeutic principle: Clearing away heat, eliminating dampness, removing toxic substances, and regulating activity of Qi and promoting circulation of blood, and removing food retention, promoting digestion.

Prescription: Modified Shao Yao Decoction. In the prescription, scutellaria root and coptis root can clear away heat and eliminate dampness to remove toxic substances; peony root, Chinese angelica root, liquorice can promote circulation of blood, regulate Ying and relieve pain; aucklandia root and betel nut can promote flow of Qi and promote digestion and remove food retention. Small amount of bark of Chinese cassia tree can strengthen the power of promoting circulation of blood and regulating Ying. Rhubarb can purge excessive heat, remove food retention and clear away heat from Ying-blood.

Hawthorn fruit and medicated leaven and fruit of immature citron or trifoliate are added in the patient with food retention, for promoting digestion and removing food retention. For the patient with more serious exterior syndrome, schizonepeta, peppermint, perilla leaf, agastach, eupatorium can be added for relieving exterior syndrome according to different pathogenic factors affected. For the patient in whom exterior pathogen does not relieve and has excessive internal heat, Ge Gen Qin Lian Decoction is added for expelling pathogenic factors from muscles and skin and clearing away heat, and Xiang Lian Pill is used for treatment of the patient in whom exterior pathogen has dispelled, but dysentery has not relieved.

For the patient with more serious heat syndrome, dysentery with more bloody and less mucus stool, or only bloody discharge, higher fever, thirst and preference for cool drink, reddish tongue with yellowish fur, slippery and rapid pulse, Bai Tou Weng Decoction plus drugs of clearing away heat and removing toxic substances, such as honeysuckle flower, dandelion herb, portulaca, red peony root and liquorice can be used for removing toxic substances, regulating Ying, promoting flow of Qi and removing food retention.

Example of prescription: 15g fried white peony root, 10g whole Chinese angelica root, 5g dried rhubarb, 5g coptis root, 10g fried scutellaria root, 10g aucklandia, 10g betel nut, 10g fried hawthorn fruit and 6g dried liquorice.

(Ⅱ) Fulminant dysentery

Main symptoms: acute and sudden attack, high fever and restlessness, dysentery with fresh and purple mucus and bloody stool, colicky in the abdomen, rectal tenesmus.

Accompanying symptoms: Thirst and preference for cool drink, headache, even coma and convulsion.

Tongue and pulse: dark red tongue with yellowish and dry fur, slippery and rapid pulse.

Analysis: Affection by exterior epidemic pathogenic factors, excessive pathogen, sudden attack, heat with no cold; heat pathogen invading the intestine, injuring Qi and blood, induce fresh and purple mucus and bloody stool; disturbance of function of the intestinal tract, induce colicky pain in the abdomen with intolerable tenesmus. Excessive heat injuring body fluid induces thirst and preference for cool drink, and heat pathogen upwards attacking the head, so headache appears; heat pathogen attacking the heart causes restlessness, heat pathogen invading the seven orifices induces unconsciousness and coma; occurrence of wind syndrome in case of extreme heat brings about convulsion. Tongue and pulse are signs of excessive heat pathogen.

Therapeutic principle: Clearing away heat, removing heat from blood, removing toxic substances.

Prescription: Modified Bai Tou Weng Decoction. In the prescription, pulsatilla root can clear heat and removing heat from blood and it is an important drug. Coptis root and phellodendron bark can clear away heat and remove toxic substances, arrest dysentery; ash bark can clear away heat and eliminate dampness. Honeysuckle flower, forsythia fruit, red peony root, moudan bark, sanguisorba root can be added for strengthening power of removinig toxic substance, removing heat from blood and arresting dysentery. 30～60g buffalo horn is added for the patient with coma due to high fever, i, e. heat pathogen attacking Ying-blood; Zi Xue Pill or An Gong Niu Huang Pill is added for clearing Ying and removing heat from blood, inducing resuscitation. Uncaria stem with hooks, powder of antelope's horn, scorpion and centipede are added for tranquilizing liver-wind in the patient with convulsion.

The patient with pale complexion, extreme cool extremities, sweating and short breath, fine and weak pulse, Shen Fu Decoction should immediately take by oral administration for recuperating depleted Yang and rescuing the patient from collapse, or by nasal feeding and in combination with acupuncture and moxibustion treatment. After prostration syntrome relieves, treatment can be given according to original synrdome. Critical patients should recieve emergency treatment by combination of Chinese and western medicine.

Example of prescription: 10g pulsatilla root, 6g coptis root, 10 fried scutellaria root, 10g ash bark, 10g honeysuckle flower, 10g forsythia fruit, 15g fried hawthorn fruit, 10g sanguisorba root, 15g portulaca.

(Ⅲ) Dysentery of cold-damp type

Main symptoms: Dysentery with bloody and mucus discharge, more mucus and less bloody discharge, or complete mucus discharge, abdominal pain, rectal tenesmus.

Accompanying symptoms: heaviness in the head and body, fullness in the stomach, tastelessness in diet.

Tongue and pulse: normal or slight pale tongue with white fur, weak and slow pulse.

Analysis: retention of cold-dampness pathogen in the intestine injures the membrance, forming dysentery with bloody and mucus discharge, more mucus and less bloody, or complete mucus. Incoordination between Qi of Fu-organs, dysfunction of transport, induce abdominal pain with rectal tenesmus. Accumulation of cold and dampnees in the middle-Jiao, dysfunction of transporting and transforming nutrients induce heaviness in the head and body, fullness in the stomach, tastelessness in diet. White and greasy fur, and weak and slow pulse are signs of cold and dampness.

Therapeutic principle: Warming and dispelling cold and dampness, promoting flow of Qi as adjuvant method.

Prescription: Modified Wei Ling Decoction. In the prescription, atractylodes rhizome, magnolia bark, tangerine peel can elimilate dampness, activate function of the spleen, promoting flow of Qi and resolve fullness; Wu Ling Powder can warm and eliminate cold and dampness. Chinese angelica root is added for regulating blood, aucklandia root and betel nut for promoting flow of Qi, eliminating cold and relieving pain. In the patient with external dampness, heaviness in the head, notopterygium root and ledebouriella are added for dispelling wind and eliminating dampness; In the patient with excessive cold and dampness, baked ginger is added for strengthening power of dispelling cold, or poria and plantain seed and other drugs of eliminating dampness are added. For protracted accumulation of cold and dampness, injuring the spleen-Yang, modified Li Zhong Decoction is used for warming the middle-Jiao and strengthening the spleen.

Example of prescription: 10g atractylodes rhizome, 10g magnolia bark, 6g dried ginger, 3g lindera root, 10g aucklandia root, 10g betel nut, 10g whole Chinese angelica root, 15g fried hawthorn fruit, 10g fried tangerine peel, 6g dried liquorice, 6g Wu Ling Power.

(Ⅳ) Dysentery of Deficiency-cold type

Main symptoms: Protracted dysentery with lingering diarrhea, dysentery with watery and more mucus in stool, difficulty in discharge, even incontinence of feces and prolapse of anus following prolonged dysentery, dull abdominal pain with preference for warmth and pressure, slight tenesmus.

Accompanying symptoms: Lassitude and weakness, aversion to cold, cold limbs, poor appetite, tastelessness with no thirst.

Tongue and pulse: Pale tongue with thin and white coating, deep, weak and slow pulse.

Analysis: In prolonged case marked by deficiency of both spleen and kidney results in lingering chronic dysentery with watery and more mucus in stool. The sinking of spleen qi leads to incontinence of feces and prolapse of anus following prolonged dysentery. Dysfunction of spleen in transportation and transformation and retained cold-dampness in the intestine block the flow of Qi, giving rising to dysentery with difficulty in discharge, dull abdominal pain and slight tenesmus. Splenic yang deficiency which causes the failure of warming function induces lassitude, weakness, aversion to cold, cold limbs, poor appetite, tastelessness with no thirst. Pale tongue with thin and white coating, deep, weak and slow pulse indicate the yang deficiency of spleen and kidney.

Therapeutic principle: Warming and tonifying spleen and kidney, inducing the astringency and arresting dysentery.

Prescription: Modified Zhen Ren Yang Zang Decoction.

In the prescription, dangshen acts as strengthening the spleen and replenishing qi.

Nutmeg, dried ginger, and bark of Chinese cassia tree share the efforts of warming the spleen and kidney. Myrobalan fruit and poppy capsule are used as arresting diarrhea with its astringency. Aucklandia root regulates qi to remove stagnancy and arrest abdominal pain. White peony root, combined with prepared licorice root, can be selected to relieve spasm and pain.

Aucklandia root can be reduced for patient with the sinking of the middle-qi, also astragalus root and cimicifuga rhizome can be added to improve the tone of qi and elevate it. If the patient with obvious aversion to cold, cold extremities, evodia fruit and prepared aconite root are used for warming the interior and expelling cold. For the patient with retention of food, less amount stool and difficulty in diarrhea, myrobalan fruit and poppy capsule should be removed; hawthorn fruit as well as areca seed are employed to remove food stagnation.

Example of prescription: 10g dangshen, 10g fried bighead atractylodes rhizome, 10g roasted galangal fruit, 6g bakedginger, 3g bark of Chinese cassia tree, 10g white peony root, 10g aucklandia root, 6g chebula fruit, 15g fried hawthorn fruit, 6g liquorice, 30g earth in cooking stove.

(Ⅴ) Chronic dysentery with frequent relapse (Recurrent dysentery)

Main symptoms: recurrent dysentery, protracted chronic dysentery, dysentery with mucus and bloody discharge, abdominal pain and rectal tenesmus.

Accompanying symptoms: Anorexia, tiredness and weakness, thin body.

Tongue and pulse: Pale tongue with greasy fur, weak pulse.

Analysis: Deficiency of vital-Qi due to chronic disease, weakness of the spleen and stomach, stagnation of damp-heat pathogen, it is induced by improper diet or affection by cool. When vital-Qi restores, dysentery relieves. Insufficiency of spleen-Qi induces anorexia, tiredness and weakness; dysfunction of the spleen in transforming nutriens, brings about deficiency of Qi and blood, so thin body appears. Excessive damp-heat pathogens form dysentery with mucus and bloody discharge, abdominal pain, rectal tenesmus. Tongue and pulse are signs of deficiency of vital-Qi and stagnation of dampness pathogen.

Therapeutic principle: Strengthening the spleen and supplementing Qi alternate with clearing away heat and eliminating dampness.

Prescription: at attack, modified Lian Li Decoction; at ordinary times, modified Liu Jun Zi Decoction; Li Zhong Decoction can warm the middle-Jiao and strengthen the spleen; coptis root can eliminate damp-heat in the intestine; Chinese angelica root, red peony root and sanguisorba root are properly added for regulating Ying; aucklandia root can regulate the flow of Qi. Modified Shao Yao Decoction can be used for more severe damp-heat. After relief of dysentery, Liu Jun Zi Decoction in normal times may be taken for strengthening the spleen and regulating the stomach; coptis root is added for clearing away leaved heat to consolidate therapeutic effects.

Modified Wen Pi Decoction can be used for warming middle-Jiao and dispelling cold, and removing foot retention and promoting digestion in the patient with dysfuction of the spleen-Yang, accumulation of cold pathogen in the intestine, dysentery with mucus discharge, tiredness, anorexia, and pale tongue with white fur, deep pulse.

Example of prescription: 10g dangshen, 10 baked ginger, 12g fried bighead atractylodes rhizome, 6g prepared liquorice, 5g coptis root, 12g Chinese angelica root, 9g aucklandia root, 15g fried hawthorn fruit.

(Ⅵ) Dysentery of Yin-deficiency type

Main symptoms: dysentery with bloody and mucus discharge, less amount and difficulty in discharge, acute pain in the navel.

Accompanying symptoms: Restlessness, dry mouth, afternoon low fever, mental tiredness and weakness.

Tongue and pulse: Reddish tongue with less fluid, less fur or lingua geographica, fine and rapid pulse.

Analysis: Protracted dysentery, damp-heat injuring Yin induce dysentery of Yin-deficiency type, deficiency of blood, stagnation of damp-heat, forming stool with mucus and bloody discharge; consumption of body fluid induces restlessness, dry mouth, low fever; deficiency of the spleen and weakness of Qi induce mental tiredness and weakness. Reddish tongue with less fur, and rapid pulse are signs of Yin-deficiency.

Therapeutic principle: Nourishing Yin, clearing away heat and arresting dysentery.

Prescription: Modified Zhu Che Pill.

In the prescription, coptis root can clear away heat and arrest dysentery, Chinese angelica and donkey-hide gelatin can nourish Yin and regulate Ying; baked ginger can be reduced for the patient with obvious heat; white peony root, liquorice and black plum charcoal are added for regulating Ying and relieving pain in the patient with severe injury of Yin, or prepared rehmannia root and ophiopogon root are added for nourishing Yin and promoting production of body fluid; moudan bark charcoal and sanguisorba root are added for removing heat from blood and stopping bleeding in the patient of dysentery with more blood; for the patient of protracted dysentery, with lingering diarrhea, pomegranate rind and chebula fruit are added for astringing to arrest dysentery; for Yin-deficiency complicated by damp-heat, nourishing Yin can arrest eliminating dampness, eliminating dampness can injure Yin-blood, clearing away heat and drugs bitter in flavour and cold in nature have disadvantages of impairment of function of the stomach and dry-transmission. It is difficult to be treated. In the treatment, Li Zhongzi's acid-astriction method, with berbs such as Chinese gall, pomegranate rind, phellodendron bark, etc. used for treatment of both the principal and the secondary aspects of disease.

In addition, for the patient of dysentery who can not eat, or can not vomit, which is called fasting dysentery. The syndrome should be differentiated deficiency and excess. Exess syndrome is often caused by accumulation of damp-heat and epidepic pathogenic factors in the intestine, attacking upwards the stomach, leading to failure of descending of the stomach-Qi, marked by fullness in the chest, regugitation of food from the stomach, indigestion, yellowish and greasy fur on the tongue. Treatment should adopt the therapeutic principle of descending the stomach-Qi, removing heat and regulating the stomach with drugs of bitter taste and pungent flavor, using modified Kai Jin Powder for removing toxic substance and adverse rising of the flow of Qi, or first taking a small amount of Yu Shu Dan juice. For the patient with frequent vomiting, dark red and dry tongue, fine and rapid pulse, which are caused by more severe consumption of the stomach-Qi Yin, ginseng, ophiopogon root, adenophora root, schisandra fruit, etc. can be added for supplementing Qi and nourishing Yin. Deficiency syndrome is induced often by deficiency and weakness of the spleen and stomach, or deficiency due to chronic dysentery, adverse rising of the stomach-Qi, marked by vomiting and nausea with no eating, or vomiting after meal, no thirst, pale tongue and weak pulse, treatment should mainly adopt the therapeutic principle of strengthening the spleen and regulating the stomach, with Liu Jun Zi Decoction plus amomum fruit, grassleaved sweetflag rhizome, fresh ginger juice used for activating the spleen-Qi and inducing appetite and digestion.

〔Meassures of Prevention and Nursing Care〕

1. Pay attention to dietary hygiene, do not eat raw and cold, greasy, unclean and degenerative food.

2. Enjoying cool or keeping warm should be proper according to changes of weather; be in a good mood.

3. In the summer, often eating raw gailic can prevent from dysentery.

4. Pay attention to balanced or regular diet.

〔Analysis of Typical Case〕

Case 1: Xi xx, female, 46 years old, a peasant, presented herself on July 2, 1970, complaining that at yesterday noon she had aversion to cold with fever, and in this morning nausea and vomiting, abdominal pain with fullness in the hypoabdomen, with bloody, mucus discharge, rectal tenesmus, defecation of more than 10 times a day, fullness in the stomach, thirst, sourness and aching pain in extremintes; white, yellowish and greasy fur on the tongue, slippery and rapid pulse, 39.2℃ body temperature. Routine examination of stool: pus cells (++), red blood cell(+++), twice culture of stool found production of Bacillus Dysenteriae. In syndrome differentiation of traditional Chinese medicine, it belongs affection by exopathogenic wind and heat, accumulation of damp-heat in the body, dysfunction of the intestine in transport, which is regarded as fulminant dysentery. Jiu Jue Shen Dian is selected for the treatment, which consists of 30g Chinese angelica root, 30g white peony root, 30g tale, 5g dried liquorice, 10g betel nut, 10g fried radish seed, 6g fried friut of citron or trifoliate orange, 3g aucklandia root, 10g onion bulb. After taking one dose, fever reduced and dysentery relieved, and after taking 3 doses he was cured. Bacteria culture for three times show negative. (Shanghai Jounal of Traditional Chinese Medicine and Pharmacy, 1989; (3): 34)

Note: Ancient prescription Jiu Jue Shen Dan is used for treatment of dysentery in modern times with better therapeutic effects. It has functions of regulating blood and Qi, eliminating dampness, removing toxic substances and it can be used for treating dysentery due to damp-heat in the intestine, no serious heat pathogen, incoordination between Qi and blood, obstruction of water and dampness. Doctor Pu Fu Zhou indicated that the ancient prescription Jiu Jue Shen Dan treated recurrent dysentery with better results. The prescription is fomulated by Chinese angelica root, and peony root as main drugs, betel nut, aucklandia root, radish seed and fruit of citron or trifoliate orange as adjuvant, liquorice for regulating the midle-Jiao and removing toxic substances as adjuvant drug, onion bulb for activatng diurisis as conductant drug, tale for eliminating pathogenic factors. In the patient with deficiency of both Qi and blood due to great damage of primordial Qi, sweating, impairment of the spleen and stomach, more Chinese angelica root and white peony root are used for regulating the liver and spleen, liquorice for regulating the middle-Jiao and detoxisation. Dysentery is characterized by abdominal pain, rectal tenesmus, bloody and mucus discharge. Pathogenic machanisms: interaction between pathogen and Qi and blood in the intestine leading to damage of intestinal membrance and blood vessels in the intestine, forming pus and bloody or bloody and mucus stool. Cause of disease is affection by exopathogenic dampness, epidemic, internal impairment by eating raw and cold food, injuring the spleen, stomach and intestine. It attacks more in summer and autumn.

In differentiation of symptoms and signs, dysentery has differences of cold and heat, deficiency and excess. Generally speaking, sudden dysentery is more excess, chronic dysentery more deficiency. Excess syndrome has differences of dysentery due to damp-heat and dysentery due to cold-dampness, and dysentery due to damp-heat pathogen is more seen. Fulminant dysentery attacks suddenly, with severe state of disease, should be early treated. For deficiency syndrome, there are dysentery of Yin-deficiency type and dysentery of deficiency-cold type. Fasting dysentery is caused by damp-heat pathogen attacking upwards or reversed flow of Qi due to deficiency of the stomach. Recurrent dysentery is marked by frequent relapse.

Treatment of the disease should depend on cold, heat, deficiency or excess of the syndrome. Generally, first affecting fulminant dysentery is more heat syndrome, excess syndrome, should adopt the therapeutic principle of removing pathogenic factor as main; dysentery due to damp-heat pathogen should be treated by clearing heat and eliminating dampness, and regulating Qi to promote circulation of blood; fulminant dysentery should be treated by clearing away heat, removing heat from blood and removing toxic substances as adjuvant method; for the patient with coma, removing heat from the heart to restore to consciousness should be used in combination; for the patient with convulsion, the drugs of removing heat from blood and calming the endopathic wind should be added; dysentery due to cold-damp pathogen should be treated by means of eliminating cold-dampness by warming. Chronic dysentery is often deficiency syndrome and cold syndrome, treatment, firstly should strength resistance of the body, and nourish Yin and clear the intestine in chronic dysentery with impairment of Yin-blood; for deficiency-cold of the spleen and kidney, should warming and reinforcing the spleen and kidney, with arresting discharge as adjuvant method; for fasting dysentery should warming the middle-Jiao and clearing the intestine, with regulating Qi and removing stagnation as adjuvant method. But for both deficiency syndrome and excess syndrome, drugs of regulating Qi and blood can be used as adjuvant method and for the patient complicated with food retention, should remove food retention and promote digestion. In addition, should prevent the stomach qi in treatment of dysentery.

Questions for Review

1. How to aknowledge the source of dysentery?
2. What are main causes of disease for dysentery? Why do hold that accumulation and retention in the intenstine are the key of attack of desentery?
3. What are characteritics of dysentery? In which conditions Ni Liu Wan Zhou method is applied?
4. What is the relationship between dysentery due to damp-heat pathogen and fulminant dysentery? How to treat it ?
5. How to treat chronic dysentery with incompletely cleared damp-heat and injury of Yin blood? Which points should be paid attention to?
6. What is the relation between chronic dysentery and blood stasis?
7. How to use astringents in treatment of dysentery?

Constipation

〔General Introduction〕

Constiption includes three aspects, i, e. dry stool, prolonged duration of defecation, or dyschesia with no dry stool.

In western medicine, habitual constipation, intestinal neurosis, and constipation induced by inflammation in the colon, rectum and anus, and other disease, conspitation induced by weakness to defecate in the aged and persons of debility, constipation induced by drugs, and constipation often seen in other various acute and chronic diseases, all can be treated by refenrece to the chapter.

〔Causes of Disease and Pathogenesis〕

After food gets into the stomach, receiving and digestion in the stomach, and transportation and transformation of the spleen, absorpting neutrents, and leaving waste matter, and then is transmitted out, forming defecation. Constipation is caused mainly by dysfunction of the large intestine intransport, stool retention in the intestine for over long time, water being absorbed, leading to stool over dry, firm. Commonly-seen causes of disease and pathology of constipation are: accumulation of dry-heat pathogen in the body, insufficiency of body fluid; emotional fluctuation, stagnation of Qi; internal damage due to tiredness, insufficiency of Qi and blood; weakness in the aged, accumulation of severe pathogenic cold, etc. all can induce dysfunction of the stomach and intestine, disturbance of transport, leading to constipation.

1. Accumulation of heat in the intestine and stomach, all excessive Yang, or preference for drinking, eating over pungent, hot and greasy food, or drugs of pungent in flaver, heat, warming and reinforcing in property, leading to stagnation of heat pathogen. Also, after fever diseases, pathogenic heat is not completely removed and retains in the intestine and stomach, consuming body fluid, resulting in dry-heat in the intestine; in addition, dry pathogen and heat pathogen of the lung move down to the large intestine, causing dry-heat of the intestine and damaging body fluid, induces dry, astringency, stagnation in the intestinal tract, forming constipation due to heat pathogen.

2. Stagnation of Qi: Melancholy, anxiety, unhappies, or sitting for long

time and less motion often induce stagnation of Qi, also adhension after surgical operation, or traumatic injury bring about impairment of function of the stomach and intestine, or dysfunction of the lung in purifying and descending, dysfunction of the large intestine, all may cause dysfunction of the stomach and intestine in descending and transportation, leading to retention of waster matter, so appearence of constipation.

3. Deficiency of Qi and blood: Tiredness, internal impairment of the spleen and stomach by improper died, in digestion, deficiency of Qi and blood; or severe disease, protracted disease, after birth and the aged with weakness, deficiency of both Qi and blood; Also, using over diaphoretic and drying prescription, consuming body fluid; or hemorrhage, intemperance, injuring Qi and blood. Qi-deficiency induces dysfunction of the large intestine in transportation; deficiency of blood, less body fluid, essence exhaustion induce inability to moisten the large intestine, drying intestine, difficulty in stool transportation. If injuring of Yin affecting Yang, deficiency of both Yin and Yang induces indigestion, inability to produce body fluid, and failure of moisture of the intestinal tract, all can cause difficulty in defecation, forming constipation.

4. Accumulation and stagnation of severe pathogenic cold: the aged with weakness, or chronic disease, Yang-deficiency, imparment of functional activity of Yang-Qi, inducing accumulation and stagnation of Yin pathogen; also in the person with deficiency of the spleen who eats raw and cold food for long time, or eats over reagents of bitter taste and cold in nature property, injuring Yang-Qi, leading to Yang-deficiency of the spleen and kidney, inability to warming, accumulation of Yin-cold in the body. Accumulation of cold induces stagnation of Qi, weakness of the intestinal tract in transporting stool, that is constipation due to accumulation of cold pathogen, or is called as constipation of cold type.

In short, although constipation belongs dysfunction of the large intestine in transportation, it is very closely related with the lung, spleen and kidney. The lung and the large intestine are interior-exteriorly related. The lung has functions of regulating the flow of Qi. Impairment of dispersing and disecending function of the lung induces often disorder of the large intestine in transport, leading to constipation; the spleen has the function to transport, transform and absorb nutrients, so disease of the spleen results in lack of resource of Qi and blood, dysfunction of transportion, retention of waste matter in the interior, inducing constipation; the kidney controls normal urination and defecation, so deficiency of the kidney or Yin-deficiency induces dryness of the intestine, or Yang-deficiency induces accumulation of pathogenic cold, dysfunction of the intestine in transportation, forming costipation.

〔Treatment Based on Differentiation of Symptoms and Signs〕

Constipation manifests clinically as dryness of stool, prolongation of interval of defecation, often one defecation each 3～5, or 7～8 days, even longer in individual personal patient, or although times of defecation do not reduce, it is difficult to defecate with dryness and firmness of stool; or often has desire to defecate, but stool can be not discharged completely. Protracted constipation often causes other symptoms, such as distention and fullness of the abdomen, even abdominal pain, nausea, belching, anorexia, dizziness, restlessness.

Ⅰ. Main points of differentiation of symptoms and signs

(Ⅰ) Differentiation of deficiency and excess syndromes: Constipation is divided into constipation due to dxficiency syndrome and constipation due to excess syndrome, according to causes of disease and clinical manifestion. Generally, constipation due to excess syndrome attackes suddenly, with short duration of disease, although it has severe symptoms, therapeutic effects are better; Constipation due to deficiency syndrome attackes slowly, with longer duration of disease, although it has mild symptoms, therapeutic effects are worse. Constipation due to excess syndrome has dryness-heat type and Qi-stagnation type; constipation due to deficiency syndrome has differences of Qi-deficiency, blood-deficiency and Yang-deficiency. Constipation due to heat pathogen is marked by dry stool, longer interval of defecation and difficulty in defecation; Constipation due to Qi is characterised by dry stool or no dry stool, difficulty in defecation; constipation due to Qi-deficiency is marked by having desire to defecate, with difficulty in defecation; constipation due to blood deficiency is characterised by normal defecation times, with ball-like dry stool, and difficulty in defecation; constipation due to Yang-deficiency is marked by dry or not dry stool, and difficulty in defecation.

(Ⅱ) Differentiation of benign and malignant constipation: Pathological changes of constipation have functional and organic, which, generally, can be differentiated by means of inspection, questioning, pulse-feeling and palpation, etc. Clinically, they are easily confirmed by barium mean examination, sigmoidoscopy or fibergastroscopy. In organic pathological changes, it is more neccessary to differentiate benign and maligant pathological changes. Benign pathologic changes most produce in younger patients, with shorter duration of disease and no severe constipation, no general weakness and no obvious symptoms of dysfunction of Zang-and Fu-organs, and malignant pathological changes most occur in older patients with longer duration of disease and severe constipation, general weakness and more obvious symptoms of dysfunction of Zang-and Fu-organs. Physical and chemical examinations are benifit to their differentiation. Differentiation of benign and malignant pathological changes is closely related to therapeutic effects and prognosis.

Ⅱ. Main points of therapeutic principle

Relaxing the bowels is a commonly-used method for treatment of constipation, but different methods should be adopted in concreat application according to deficiency syndrome or excess syndrome. Therapeutic principle of clearing away heat and relaxing the bowels, or promoting the flow of Qi and removing food retention is used for excess syndrome, and supplementing Qi and nourishing blood, or promoting production of body fluid and moistening, or warmly relaxing the bowel for deficiency syndrome.

Ⅲ. Treatment based on classification of syndromes

(Ⅰ) Constipation due to excess syndrome

1. Constipation due to pathogenic heat

Main symptoms: Dry stool, difficulty in defecation, longer interval of defecation, once 3～5 days or 7～8 days.

Accompanying symptoms: mild fever, foul breath and bitter taste, aphthae, flushed face, conjunctival congestion, restlessness, abdominal distention, indigestion, scanty dark urine.

Tongue and pulse: Reddish tongue with yellowish or yellowish-dry fur, slippery, intermittent, and rapid pulse.

Analysis: Accumulation of excessive heat in the body, excessive heat burning body fluid, less fluid in the intestine, so dry stool and difficulty in defecation appear. Excessive heat in the interior, stagnation of Qi of Fu-organs, induce abdominal distention and indigestion, foul breath and bitter taste, aphthae, flushed face and conjunctival congestion, restlessness; heat pathogen is not removed completely, so mild fever occurs; heat pathogen moves to the urine bladder, producing scanty dark urine. Reddish tongue with yellowish or yellowish-dry fur, and slippery, intermittent and rapid pulse all are signs of accumulation of pathogenic heat in the intestine and stomach.

Diagram of Causes of Disease and Pathology of Constipation

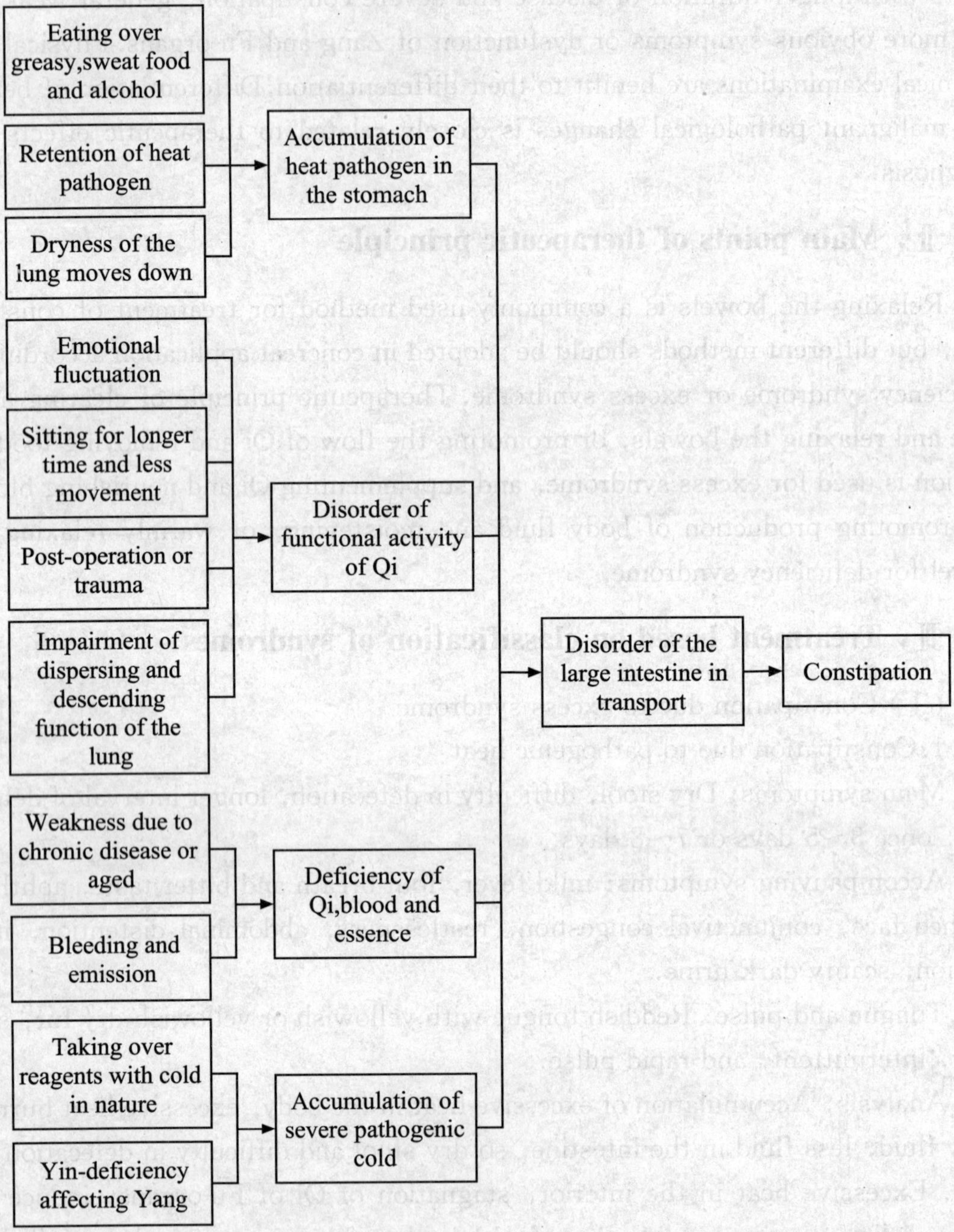

Therapeutic principle: expelling the pathogenic heat to loosen the bowel, or clearing away heat and moistening the intestine.

Prescription: Tiao Wei Cheng Qi Decoction is used for expelling the pathogenic heat to loosen the bowel, and the Ma Zi Ren Pill for clearing away heat and moistening the intestine. In the former, rhubarb can expel pathogenic heat to loosen the bowels; mirabilite can soften and resolve hard mass, and move down stool; liquorice can regulate the middle-Jiao and coordinate the actions of various ingredients in the prescription. In the latter, rhubarb also is used for expelling pathogenic heat to loosen the bowel; fruit of immature citron or trifoliate orange, magnolia bark for keeping the adverse Qi flowing downward and relieving fullness; hemp seed, bitter apricot seed, white honey for sending down abnormal ascending Qi and loosening bowels; white peony root for nourishing Yin and supplementing blood; scrophularia root, dendrobium, ophiopogon root, and dried rehmannia root and other drugs of promoting production of body fluid are added in the patient with excessive heat impairing body fluid and obvious dry mouth and tongue; sanguisorba root, sophora flower and other drugs of removing heat from the blood and stopping bleeding are added for dry stool, anal fissure and bleeding; shell of areca nut and Jiao Si Xian for promoting digestion and removing food retention in the patient with abdominal distention and indigestion; for the constipation due to pathogenic heat of the liver moving down to the stomach and intestine, with conjunctival congestion and bitter taste, taut and slippery pulse, Geng Yi Pill or Dang Gui Lu Hui Pill may be selected or used in combination for clearing away heat in the liver and relaxing the bowels. For the costipation due to dry-heat in the lung moving down to the large intestine, with dry mouth and nose, dry cough and less phlegm, the drugs for promoting the production of body fluid to moistening and loosening bowels should be used in combination, such as trichosanthes fruit and pittosporm root etc, with better therapeutic effects.

Expelling pathogenic heat and relaxing bowels are a commonly-used method for treatment of constipation due to heat, but over use or use for long time is forbitened, otherwise injury of the stomach by bitter taste and cold in nature is often seen, thus it is used until the disease relieves, and then the prescription for nourishing Yin and loosening the bowels is adopted for recuperation.

Example of prescription: 9g prepared rhubarb, 10g hemp seed, 10g bitter apricot seed, 10g fruit of immature citron or trifoliate orange, 10g shell of areca nut, 10g Jiao Si Xian each, 6g dried liquorice, 30g honey, 10 green pinellia tuber, 10g fried tangerine peel.

2. Constipation due to Qi

Main symptoms: dry or not dry stool, difficulty in defecation, constipation exacerbating after emotional fluctuation.

Accompanying symptoms: frequent belching, fullness in the chest and hypochondrium, abdominal distention and pain, preference for sighing, or slight comfort after intestine flatus from anus.

Tongue and pulse: reddish tongue with thin, white and greasy fur, taut pulse.

Analysis: the lung and liver is the way of ascending and descending of the flow of Qi, and invasion of the lung by pathogens induces blockage of Qi and failure of dispelling and descending function, and injury of the liver by emotion causes stagnation of Qi and failure of soothing the liver and regulating the circulation of Qi. Depression and stagnation of Qi, failure of the large intestine controling transportation, so difficulty in defecation appears; incoordination between the lung and the liver, so fullness in the hypochondrium and frequent attack of belching, and abdominal distention and pain appear; thin, white and greasy fur on the tongue, and taut pulse are signs of depression and stagnation of Qi; when heat produces, the fur on the tongue will turn to yellowish.

Therapeutic principle: Checking upward adverse flow of the lung or the stomach-Qi, promoting circulation of Qi.

Prescription: Liu Mo Decoction as main prescription. In the prescription, fruit of immature citron or trifoliate orangecan keep the adverse Qi flowing downward and soothing the chest oppression, promoting the lung-Qi flowing downward; aucklandia root can regulate Qi of the middle-Jiao; lindera root can promote circulation of Qi to relieve fullness in the abdomen, treating the middle-Jiao and the lower-Jiao; eagle wood can keep the adverse Qi flowing downward; betel nut can send the Qi down and relieve fullness; rhubarb can expel pathogenic heat and relax bowels. Chai Hu Shu Gan Powder may be used for the patient with gradually flowing of the Qi of Fu-organs and unsoothing of the liver-Qi. In the patient with stagnation of Qi producing heat, marked by bitter taste and dry thoat, yellowish fur on the tongue, rapid pulse, aloes, scutellaria root, capejasmine fruit, etc. are added for purging the liver of pathogenic fire, and relaxing bowels. Bitter apricot seed, trichosanthes peell epidium seed and other medicines of purging the lung of pathogenic fire can be added for the patient with blockage of the lung-Qi. Peach kernel, safflower, red peony root, notoginseng, etc. Medicines of activating blood circulation to remove blood stasis are added for regulating blood for the constipation due to oparation or trauma; Sou Feng Shun Pill can be used for the patient of apoplexy, hemiplesia with constipation.

Example of prescription: 10g fried fruit of immature citron or trifoliate orange, 10g aucklandia root, 12g lindera root, 3g eagle wood powder, 5g prepared rhubarb, 10g betel nut, 10g bitter apricot seed, 10g bupleurum root, 10g red peony root, 6g green tangerine orange peel, 6g tangerine peel.

(Ⅱ) Constipation of deficiency type

1. Deficiency of qi

Main symptoms: Difficulty in defecation with desire to defecate, and generally, stool is not dry.

Accompanying symptoms: emaciation with sallow complexion, mental tiredness, short breath, and more severe after defecation in the aged, weakness or chronic patients.

Tongue and pulse: pale tongue with thin and white fur, fine and weak pulse.

Analysis: In the patient of deficiency of the lung and spleen-Qi, because the lung is in charge of Qi, and the lung and the large intestine are interior-exteriorly related, deficiency of the lung-Qi induces weakness of the large intestine in transportation, so difficulty in defecation occurs with stool incompletely ejected. Deficiency of the lung-Qi induces failure of superfical-Qi to protect the body against disease, connecting tissue looses, so sweating and short breath appear due to defecation with force. The spleen is in charge of transportion and transformation, and it is resource of acquired essence, dysfunction of the spleen in transportation, lack of resource of Qi and blood, leads to emaciation with sallow complexion, mental tiredness. After defecation, Qi dispels with the stool, so the symptoms of short breath and mental tiredness deteriorate. Pale tongue with thin and white fur, fine and weak pulse are signs of deficiency of the lung and spleen-Qi.

Therapeutic principle: Strengthening the spleen and supplementing Qi.

Prescription: Huang Qi Decoction is used as main prescription for supplementing Qi and promoting transportation. In the prescription, astragalus root is an important herb for strengthening the spleen and supplementing Qi; liquorice for reinforcing the middle-Jiao and increasing power of supplementing Qi of astragalus root; tangerine peel for regulating Qi and the function of the stomach; hemp seed and white honey for moistening the intestine and relaxing the bowels. Dangshen and siberian solomonseal rhizome are added for supplementing Qi;

Cimicifuga rhizome and bupleurum root are added for rising clear Qi and descending turbit in the patient with sinking due to Qi-deficiency; Sheng Mai Powder or Shen Ha Powder is used in combination for the patient with obvious deficiency of the lung-Qi, marked by chronic cough and asthma; modified Da Bu Yuan Jian can be used for treatment of the kidney in the patient with deficiency of Qi and protracted constipation, because the kidney is resource of Qi.

Example of prescription: 30g astragalus root, 10g dangshen, 30g siberian solomonseal rhizome, 10g fried tangerine peel, 15g hemp seed, 30g white honey, 6g prepared liquorice, 10g fruit of immature citron or trifoliate orange, 10g lindera root and 10g aucklandia root.

2. Deficiency of blood

Main symptoms: ball-like dry stool, normal defecation times with difficult in defecation.

Accompanying symptoms: dizziness, palpitation, insomnia and dreamful sleep, pale complexion and lip and nail.

Tongue and pulse: pale tongue with thin and white fur, fine and weak pulse.

Analysis: Deficiency of blood and less body fluid, failure of moistening the intestinal tract, so induces ball-like stool and difficulty in defecation; deficiency of blood induces lack of nourishing in the head, so dizziness occurs; failure of blood nourishing the heart, irritability, results in palpitation and insomnia and dreamful sleep; insuficiency of blood in blood vessels, leads to pale complexion, lip and nail. Pale tongue with thin and white fur, fine and weak pulse all are signs of deficiency of blood and lack of blood in blood vessels.

Therapeutic principle: enriching the blood and moistening dryness.

Prescription: Run Chang Pill is used as main prescription. In the prescription, Chinese angelica root and dried rehmannia root are used for supplementing blood and nourishing Yin; peach hernel and hemp seed for moistening dryness and promoting free movement of bowels; fruit of immature citron or trifoliate orange for relieving the stagnation of Qi and promoting the Qi flowing downdard, the five herbs perform commonly the actions of supplementing blood and moistening the dryness in the intestine. For deficiency of blood, marked by dysphoria with feverish sensation in chest, palms and soles, and dry mouth, reddish tongue without fur or lingua geographica, should mainly adopt therapeutic principle of nourishing Yin to increase body fluid, with scrophularia root, ophiopogon root, and fleeceflower root, etc. added; For deficiency complicated by stasis, marked by pale and dark tongue or with petechiae, Tong You Decoction can be used for nourishing blood and promoting circulation of blood, moistening dryness and relaxing the bowels. For the patient complicated with lassitude in loin and spinal column, scanty menstruation with light colour, prepared fleece-flower root, desertliving cistanche, walnut kernel, etc. herbs of supplementing the kidney and nourishing Yin can be added. For frequent constipation of dryness type, Wu Ren Pill can be often taken for moistening the intestine and relaxing the bowels.

Example of prescription: 10g Chinese angelica root, 10g dried rehmannia root, 10g prepared rehmannia root, 10g peach kernel, 3g amomum fruit, 10g hemp seed, 10g fried fruit of immature citron or trifoliate orange, 10 fleece-flower root, 10g walnut kernel, 10g red peony root, 6g dried liquorice.

3. Constipation of cold type

Main symptoms: Difficulty in defecation with dry or not dry stool.

Accompanying symptoms: pale complexion, aversion to cold, cool extremeties, abdominal pain due to cold Qi in the abdomen, bowel sound, or cold pain along the spinal cord, clear and more urine.

Tongue and pulse: Pale and enlarged tongue with white and moist fur, deep, slow and weak pulse.

Analysis: Yang-deficiency of the spleen and kidney, production of severe pathogenic cold in the interior and retention in the intestine, stagnation of Yin-Qi and disorder of Yang-Qi in transport, lead to weakness of the intestine in transport and difficulty in defecation. Deficiency of Yang-Qi. Qi can not reach the extremities, pale complexion and aversion to cold, cool extremities, or cold pain along the spinal cord appear; stagnation of pathogenic cold in the abdomen, so brings about abdominal pain, sound bowel; insufficiency of Yang-Qi, hypofunction of the urinary bladder with cold syndrome, failure of water producing Qi induces clear and more urine. Pale and enlarged tongue, with white and moit fur, and deep, slow and weak pulse are signs of deficiency of Yang and excess of Yin.

Therapeutic princple: relaxing the bowels with drugs warm in nature.

Prescription: Ji Chuan Jian is used as main prescription. In the prescription, Chinese angelica root, desertliving cistanche, achyranthes root can nourish essence and blood, moisten the intestine and relax the bowels; cimicifuga rhizome can rise clear Qi and descend turbit Qi; fruit of citron or trifoliate orange can keep the adverse Qi flowing downward and remove stagnation; bark of Chinese cassia tree and lindera root can be added for promoting functional activity of Qi with drugs warm in nature; oriental water plantain rhizome is reduced; or walnut kernel, fleece-flower root are added for supplementing the kidney, nourishing blood and moistening the intestine; Ban Liu Pill can be used in combination for the patient with more excessive pathogenic cold, 6g each time, twice a day, for strengthing the power of removing cold stagnation by drugs warm in nature. You Gui Pill or Jin Kui Shen Qi Pill can be often taken for warming and recuperating the kidney-Yang, relaxing the bowels with drugs warm in nature.

Example of prescription: 10g whole Chinese angelica root, 15g desertliving-cistanche, 10g walnut kernel, 10g fleece-flower root, 6g bark of Chinese cassia tree, 10g lindera root, 10g fruit of immature citron or trifoliate orange, 12g achyranthes root, 5g cimicifuga rhizome, 9g Ban Liu Pill.

In treatment of constipation, besides internal administration of Chinese herbs, drug application on the navel, and other therapies, such as acupuncture and moxibustion, massage etc. can be used in combination, simple recipe and proved recipe attain often better results, such as senna leaf, cassia seed, dried bighead atractylodes rhizome, radish seed, etc. In addition, diet therapy also can be used, such as sesame seed, walnut kernel, pine seed, etc in equal mount are grinded into powder and a little white honey is added, taking with hot decoction, with effective for constipation due to insuficiency of Yin-blood. In addition, for habitual constipation, keeping happy, slight exercise and diet regulation and defecation at regular intervals, all are benefit for treatment of constipation. In the patients after febrile disease, or other diseases, constipation due to taking less food, do not hurry to relax the bowel, only it is necessary to supplement the stomach-Qi, gradually increasing diet, normal defecation occurs.

〔Meassures of Prevention and Nursing Care〕

1. Keeping a regular life and the habit of defecation on time each day.

2. Proper diet, and eat more vegetable and coarse food grain, without pungent and stimulative food.

3. The patient of deficiency syndrome, should strengthen functional exercice of the abdomen for helping to defecate.

〔Analysis of Typical Case〕

Case 1: Lin xx, female, 29 years old, presented herself on September 13, 1984.

She suferred constipation from last September, and took rhubarb with effect. Examination showed old anal fissure.

Anorexia, belching after meal, dry stool, failure of defecation for 3 days with desire to defecate, night sweat, dry mouth and throat, reddish tongue with lingua geographica, taut, fine and slight rapid pulse.

Diagnosis of traditional Chinese medicine: constipation.

Syndrome: Deficiency of Yin and lack of body fluid, stagnation of Qi in the large intestine.

Therapeutic principle: nourishing Yin and moistening dryness, removing stagnation and relaxing the bowels.

Prescription: Combination of Zeng Ye Decoction with Liu Mo Decoction.

18g dried rehmannia root, 12g scrophularia root, 12g ophiopogon root, 1. 5g eagle wood (taking with the Decoction), 6g lindera, 6g aucklandia root, 9g betel nut, 9g prepared rhubarb, 10g fruit of citron or trifoliate orange, 20g cassia seed.

After taking 2 doses, on the next day she had 5 times of free defecation, belching reduced and appetite increased, and other symptoms improved. After taking 3 doses, defecation tended to normal and then the herbs for nourishing Yin and moistening dryness were used for consolidating therapeutic effect.

Note: The patient had emotional disorder, incoordination between the liver and the spleen, stagnation of Qi for long time producing fire, injuring Yin, and leads to constipation. Dried rehmannia, ophiopogon root and scrophularia root were used for nourishing Yin and moistening dryness; aucklandia, lindera and eagle wood for regulating functional activity of Qi; rhubarb, betel nut and fruit of citron or trifoliate orange for keeping adverse Qi flowing downward; cassia seed for promoting stool moving down. (Chi ShengYe; Constipation, New Traditional Chinese Medicine, 1987;(1):18)

Clinically, constipation is a commonly-seen disease and induced by many causes. Clinically, it should be treated based on differentiation of deficiency and excess syndromes according to cause of disease and clinical manifestion. Constipation of excess syndrome type includes constipation due to heat and constipation due to Qi, and constipation of deficiency syndrome type includes constipation of Qi deficiency type, blood deficiency type and cold type. Treatment should be given based on differentiation of syndromes, constipation due to heat should be treated by dispelling heat and relaxing the bowels or clearing away heat and moistening the intestine; constipation due to Qi should be treated by promoting the flow of Qi and removing stagnation, based on diseases of the liver and the lung; constipation due to Qi deficiency should be treated by supplementing Qi and moistening the intestine; constipation due to blood deficiency shoulld be treated by nourishing blood and moistening dryness, and constipation due to blood deficiency complicated with Yin deficiency should be treated by nourishing blood to moistening the intestine; constipation due to pathogenic cold should be treated by warming Yang and relaxing the bowels. Above-mentioned constipation is seen singly or complicatedly, so different therapeutic methods should be adopted according to differences of syndrome, for example, production of heat caused by protracted constipation due to Qi, constipaton due to Qi complicated with constipation due to heat, in treatment, removing stagnation and dispelling heat should be adopted simultaneously; lack of treatment and incorrect treatment for constipation due to Qi-deficiency often induce Yang-deficiency, and Yang-deficiency of the spleen and the kidney, in treatment, supplementing Qi and warming Yang should be simultaneously adopted, and so on. Therefore, except the above-mentioned therapies, other therapeutic methods such herbs application on the navel, acupuncture and moxibution, massage, etc. can be also used in combination for strengthening therapeutic effects.

Questions for Review

1. What are pathological changes of constipation?
2. Which types are constipation divided commonly into? How to grasp the law of the treatment based on differentiation of symptoms and signs?
3. Which are main points of differentiation of symptoms and signs for constipation? How to differentiate characteristics of malignant pathologic changes of constipation?
4. Which convenient therapeutic methods are there for costipation?

Hypochondriac Pain

〔General Introduction〕

All the diseases and syndromes induced by lesion of the liver and gallbladder, and incoordination between Qi and blood, marked mainly by pain in hypochondiac region on one or both sides, are called as hypochondriac pain. Clinically, it is often accompanied by distending pain in the stomach, mass of hypochondrium.

In western medicine, deseases of the liver and the gallblader, such as acute and chronic hepatitis, cirrhosis of liver, infection of biliary tract, cholecystitis, gallstones, dry or exudative pleurisy, intercostal neuralgia, costal perichondritis, etc. marked mainly by hypochondriac pain, can refere to the treatment of this disease based on differentiation of symptoms and signs.

〔Causes of Disease and Pathogenesis〕

The liver is located in the hypochondrium, and its channel and collateral distribute on hypochondrium of both sides, and the gallblader attaches to the liver and its channel and collateral travel along the hypocondrium, so hypochondriac pain is caused mainly by the diseases of the liver and the gallblader. Because blood stores in the liver, the liver is in charge of soothing and regulating the circulation of Qi, and likes soothing. Bile stores in the gallblader and it flows with the liver-Qi, so emotional disorder, stagnation of the liver-Qi in the interior, or protracted stagnation of Qi, stagnation of Qi and blood stasis; or consumption of essence and blood, insufficiency of liver-Yin, lack of nourishing channels and collaterals, or dysfunction of the spleen in transport and transformation, accumulation of dampness and heat pathogens in the interior, and hypofunction of dispelling, all can induce hypochondiac pain. The causes of disease and pathogenesis are described in the following.

1. Stagnation of the liver-Qi: mental depression, or violent anger injuring the liver, disorder of the liver-Qi, hypofunction of dispelling, obstruction of collaterals by stagnation of Qi induces hypochondriac pain.

2. Blood stasis: protracted stagnation of Qi, failure in free circulation of blood, blood stasis, failure in free flow of Qi in the collaterals on hypochondrium, hypochoidriac pain appears, or strong load, sudden trauma, lesion of hypochondiac collaterals, stasis of blood, obstruction of hypochondriac collaterals, leads to hypochondriac pain.

3. Dampness and heat in the liver and the gallbladder: external dampness pathogen invading the interior, or impairment by overeating, dysfunction of the spleen in transport, stagnation of phlegm in the middle-Jiao, stagnation of Qi producing heat, stagnation of dampness and heat in the liver, gallblader, spleen and stomach, failure of the liver and the gallblader in soothing, lead to hypochondriac

pain.

4. Insufficiency of the liver-Yin: Chronic disease with weakness, or over work, consumption of essence and blood, insufficiency of the liver-Yin, and unability to nourish the liver due to deficiency of blood, inducing lack of nourishing collateral-vessels, also can cause hypochondriac pain.

5. Fluid retention in hypochondium: Fluid retention in chest and hypochondrium, obstruction in channels and blood vessels, hypofunction of ascending and descending of Qi of the liver and lung, leads to hypochondriac pain.

6. Stagnation of pathogens in a half exterior and a half interior: Exopathogenic factors can not be removed and be stagnated in a half exterior and a half interior, hypofunction of Shao-Yang gallbladder-Qi, results in hypochondriac pain.

Diagram of causes of disease and pathogenesis of hypochon

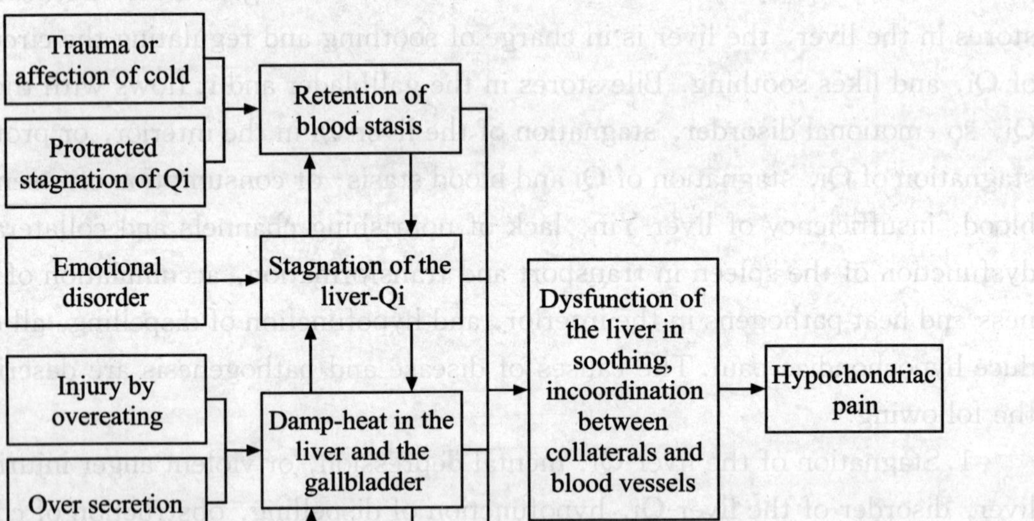

In short, pathological change of hypochondial pain is mainly in the liver and the gallbladder, both internal injury and affection by exopathogenic factors can cause hypochondriac pain, and its causes of disease and pathgenesis are related with the spleen, stomach, lung and kidney. Because failure of free flow of Qi of the liver and gallblader, not only attacking the spleen and the stomach, also invading the lung along channels, leading to disorder of the liver and the lung in ascending and descending, and because the liver and the kidney have same resource, insufficiency of the kidney-Yin can not nourish the liver, resulting in hypochondriac pain due to deficiency of the liver. In the chapter, former four kinds of hypochondriac pain are mainly discussed. Hypochondriac pain has deficiency syndrome and excess syndrome, with excess syndrome often seen. Excess syndrome has mainly stagnation of Qi, blood stasis and damp-heat, with stagnation of Qi being main; deficiency syndrome, in most cases, belongs to deficiency of Qi and blood; in addition, injury of Yin by production of heat due to protracted excess syndrome can induce Yin-deficiency of the liver and kidney, deficiency syndrome accompanied by excess syndrome is also seen.

〔Treatment Based on Differentiation of Symptoms and Signs〕

Ⅰ. Main points of differentiation of symptoms and signs

1. Differentiation of exterior and interior syndrome: i, e. internal injury and affection by exopathogenic factors, hypochondriac pain due to affection by exopathogens attackes more suddenly, and most of them are caused by damp-heat pathogen attacking the liver and the gallbladder, clinically having often exterior syndrome, marked by fever, aversion to cold, accompanied by vomiting, jaundice, etc., floating and rapid or taut and rapid pulse, reddish tongue with greasy, yellowish or white fur; hypochondriac pain due to internal injury attackes slowly, without appearence of cold and fever. There are more interior syndrome and less exterior syndrome for hypochondriac pain.

2. Differentiation of cold and heat syndromes: Hypochondriac pain is marked by weakness, cold, tastlessness in mouth, pale tongue with thin fur, preference for warmness, pain relieving after warming and deteriorating after cold, taut, slow, deep and uneven pulse, belonging to cold syndrome. Flushed face, strong constitution, bitter taste in mouth, reddish tongue with yellowish or yellowish and greasy fur, preference for cool, pain becomes more severe after heating on the affected part and taut, full and rapid pulse, belong to heat syndrome.

3. Differentiation of Qi and blood: acute disease is often caused by Qi, and chronic disease damages blood, pain is not fixed on a part. Distending pain is caused mainly by stagnation of Qi. Pain located on a fixed part, exacerbating afternoon or at night, the patient with ecchymosis on the lip and the tongue belongs

to blood stasis, more pain with less distention or only pain with no distention, stabbing pain with a fixed part or having history of trauma also belongs to blood stasis.

4. Differentiation of deficiency and excess syndromes: acute disease and severe pain, strong constitution, full and forceful pulse, tenderness, belong to excess syndrome; chronic disease, weakness, vague pain, thin, deep and weak pulse, prerefence for pressing, belong deficiency syndrome. Clinically, deficiency syndrome is accompanied often by excess syndrome, damp-heat with deficiency of blood or with retention of blood stasis in the interior. Therefore, treatment should be given based on the principal and the secondary, mild and severe aspects of disease.

Ⅱ. Differential diagnosis

For pain syndrome, hypochondriac pain should be differentiated with epigastralgia, obstruction of Qi in the chest. Generally, they are differentiated with no difficulty from the parts of pain. Hypochondriac pain is mainly located on both hypochondrium, with differences of distending pain, stabbing pain, burning pain, vague pain, or with touch-able mass in the abdomin, or having had over drinking, pain being related with taking greasy food, at severe pain, the patient likes to change body position. Epigastragia has obvious pain on the topographical region below the xiphoid process, pain of deficiency type, preference for warmness and pressing, and pain of excess syndrome type has tenderness, often with acid regurgitation; pain due to obstruction of Qi in the chest is located on the chest, even on the back, occasionally on the left hypochondrium, mainly being vague pain, often accompanied by palpitation and short breath, etc.

Differentiation of hypochondriac pain, epigastragia and obstruction of Qi in the chest

Name of the disease / differentiation	Hypochondriac	Epigastralgia	Obstruction of Qi in the chest
Parts	hypochondrium on one or two sides	Gastric cavity	Behind the sternum or left-anterior of the chest, or involving left hypochondrium and left shoulder and arm

Name of the disease / differentiation	Hypochondriac	Epigastralgia	Obstruction of Qi in the chest
Specificities	Distending pain, stabbing pain, vague pain, burning pain and colic pain often seen, with preference for changing body position at severe pain	Distention and fullness, stabbing pain, mass in the abdomin often seen, for pain of deficiency type, preference for pressing, and tenderness for pain of excess type	Fullness-pain as main, dislike to change body position at pain
Accompanying symptoms	Mass in the hypochondrium, or having had fluid retention in the hypochondrium-xuan Yin	Often accompanied by vomiting, nausea, acid regurgitation	Often accompanied by short breathing, oppressed feeling in chest, cool palpitation, etc.
Causes	Affection by exopathogen, diet, seven emotional factors	Diet, emotion, affection by cold	Overeating, emotional fluctuation
History of disease	Diseases of the liver and the gallbladder	Diseases of the spleen and the stomach	Diseases of the heart
Radiating parts	Right shoulder and back	The back	Left shoulder and back

Ⅲ. Main points of therapeutic principle

Soothing the liver, purging the liver of pathogenic fire and nourishing the liver are flexibly applied for relieving the depressed liver and regulating the circulation of Qi, dredging the liver collaterals and clearing away damp-heat in the liver channel, sufficincy of the liver-Yin and receiving nourishing in the liver collaterals, naturally leads to disappearence of hypochondiac pain.

Ⅳ. Treatment based on syndrome types

(Ⅰ) Stagnation of the liver-Qi

Main symptoms: Distending pain is main for hypochondriac pain, with no fixed part, releiving or exacerbation of pain due to emotional fluctuation.

Accompanying symptoms: often complicated by distention and fullness in the stomach, oppressed feeling in chest, frequent belching.

Tongue and pulse: thin fur on the tongue, taut palse.

Analysis: failure of normal circulation of the liver-Qi, and stagnation of the liver-Qi in the collaterals in the hypochondium, so result in distenting pain in the hypochondrium. Qi is flowing, so pain does not fix on a part, wandering pain. Emotional changes are related closely with stagnation of Qi, so pain is related to emotional changes. Failure of free flow of Qi induces opperessed feeling in chest, and transverse inversion of the hyperactive liver-Qi, often attacking the spleen and stomach, cause anorexia and belching, and distention and fullness in the stomach. Taut pulse is a sign of stagnation of the liver-Qi.

Therapeutic principle: Soothing the liver and regulating the circulation of Qi.

Prescription: Modified Chai Hu Shu Gan Powder. In the prescription, bupleurum root can soothe the liver; fruit of immature citron or trifoliate orange, nutgrass flatsedge and tangerine peel can regulate the flow of Qi; chuanxiong rhizome can promote circulation of blood; peony root and liquorice can relieve pain; green tangerine orange peel, Sichuan chinaberry, curcuma root and corydalis tuber are added for severe hypochondriac pain for strengthening the action of regulating the flow of Qi and relieving pain; For stagnation of Qi producing fire, marked by hypocondriac pain, restlessness, dry mouth and bitter taste, yellowish urine and constipation, reddish tongue with yellowish fur, taut and rapid pulse, chuangxiong rhizome is reduced and moutan bark, capejasmine fruit, coptis root, Sichuan chinaberry, corydalis tuber, etc. are added for clearing the liver and regulating the flow of Qi, activating the circulation to relieve pain; for stagnation of Qi producing fire and injuring Yin, marked by discontinuous vague pain, more severe pain induced by overwork, dizziness, restlessness, insomnia, reddish tongue with yellowish fur and less fluid, fine and taut pulse, chuanxiong rhizome can be reduced and red sage root, fleece-flower root, wolfberry fruit, moutan bark, capejasmine fruit, chrysanthemum flower, etc are added for nourishing Yin and clearing away heat, and regulating the hyperactive liver-Qi; for the transverse inversion of the hyperactive liver-Qi, and hypofunction of the spleen in transport, marked by hypochondriac pain with bowel sound and diarrhea, bighead atractylodes rhizome, poria, coix seed and hyacinth bean are added for strengthening the spleen and arresting diarrhea, and for complication by failure of descending of the stomsch-Qi, marked by nausea and vomiting, inula flower, red ochre, pinellia tuber, fresh ginger are added for regulating the stomasch and arresting vomiting.

Example of prescription: 10g bupleurum root, 10g fried fruit of citron or trifoliate orange, 10g fried red peony root, 6g liquorice, 6g green tangerine orange peel, 10g tangerine peel, 10g chuanxiong rhizome, 10g prepared nutgrass flatsedge, 12g curcuma root, 6g corydalis tuber, 10g Sichuan chinaberry.

(Ⅱ) Blood stasis

Main symptoms: stabbing pain in hypochondrium with a fixed part, and more severe in night.

Accompanying symptoms: mass in hypochondrium.

Tongue and pulse purplish dark tongue, or with ecchymosis, deep and uneven pulse.

Analysis: protracted stagnation of the liver-qi, stagnation of qi and blood stasis, or trauma induce stasis of blood, obstruction of collaterals in the hypochondrium, so stabbing pain occurs with a fixed part and more severe pain in night. Accumulation of stagnation, protracted accumalation gradually form mass. Purplish dark tongue, ecchymosis, and deep and uneven pulse are signs of blood stasis.

Therapeutic principle: Removing stasis and dredging collaterals.

Prescription: Modified Xuan Fu Hua Decoction. In the prescription, rubia root is used for activating the circulation of blood and dredging the collaterals, inula flower can regulate the flow of Qi and relieve pain, curcuma root, peach kernel, tail of Chinese angelica root, corydalis tuber etc. can strengthen power of regulating Qi and promoting the circulation of blood. Xue Fu Zhu Yu Decoction also can be used. Fu Yuan Hou Xue Decoction can be used for more severe stasis of blood, or induced by trauma for activating the circulation of blood to remove stasis of blood, soothing the liver and dreging the collaterals, and in the prescription, rhubarb, peach kernel, safflower, pangolin scales can remove stasis and stagnation, and Chinese angelica root can nourish blood and remove stasis of blood, bupleurum root can regulating the flow of Qi and resolving mass, conducting the drugs to the hypochondrium; burreed tuber, zedoary, earthworm and other drugs of removing blood stasis and resolving mass are added for mass in the hypochomdium, and no deficiency of vital Qi, and Bie Jia Jian Pill can be orally administrated.

Example of prescription: 10g bupleurum root, 10g red peony root, 10g white peony root, 10g tail of Chinese angelica root, 10g peach kernel, 10g safflower, 10g pangolin scales, 6g zedoary, chuangxiong rhizome, 12g curcuma root, 6g corydalis tuber, 3g powder of notoginseng(taking with the decoction).

(Ⅲ) Dampness and heat in the liver and the gallbladder

Main symptoms: tightening and fullness pain in hypochondrium.

Accompanying symptoms: oppressed feeling in chest and hypochondrium, anorexia, nausea and vomiting; yellowish eyes and body, or with cold and fever, difficulty in micturition, or vomiting roundworm.

Tongue and pulse: yellowish and greasy fur on the tongue, taut and rapid pulse.

Analysis: stagnation of dampness and heat in the liver and gallbladder, incoordination between the liver collaterals, dysfunction of the gallbladder, so hypochondiac pain and bitter taste in the mouth, stagnation of dampness and heat in middle-Jia lead to fullness and oppressed feeling in chest and stomach, anorexia, nausea and vomiting. The liver has its specific body opening in the eye, flaming-up of the liver-fire, so appearence of conjunctival congestion appears. Relation between dampness and heat pathogens, bile goes out without circulation in normal tract, inducing yellowish eyes and the body. Dampness and heat flow downward into the gallbladder, leading to yelowish urine, or difficulty in micturition. Stagnation of dampness and heat pathogens in the liver and the gallbladder, incoordination between Shao Yang, bring about cold and fever; yellowish and greasy fur on the tongue, taut and rapid pulse are signs of dampness and heat in the liver and the gallbladder.

Therapeutic principle: Clearing away heat and eliminating dampness.

Prescription: Modified Long Dan Xie Gan Decoction. in the prescription, gentian root is used for removing dampness and heat in the liver and gallbladder; bupleurum root for regulating the liver-Qi; scutellaria root and capejasmine fruit for clearing away heat and eliminating fire; oriental water plantain rhizome, five-leaf akebia stem and plantain seed for eliminating damp-heat. Jin Ling Zi Powder, green tangerine peel, curcuma root and pinellia tuber can be added for severe hypochondriac pain for soothing the liver and regulating the stomach, regulating Qi to relieve pain. In the patient with fever and jaundice, oriental wormwood, phellodendron bark are added for removing damp-heat and eliminating jaundice. For the patient who has exacerbation of pain and vomits roundworm, firstly Wu Mei Pill is used for removing roundworm. lysimachia, climbing fern spore, curcuma root and niter and alum are added for accumalation of damp-heat into stone obstructing the bile tract, marked by hypochondriac pain involving the shoulder and the back, for normalizing the secretion of bile and removing gallstone. Rhubarb and mirabilite are added for excessive heat damaging body fluid, dry stool, fullness in the abdomen, for eliminating heat and relaxing the bowels.

Example of Prescription: 10g bupleurum root, 10g gentian root, 10g scutellaria root, 10g capejasmine fruit, 12g curcuma root, 30g lysimachia, 12g red peony root, 5g fiveleaf akebia, 30g poria, 10g pinellia tuber, 10g green tangerine peel.

(Ⅳ) Insufficiency of Liver-Yin

Main symptoms: Vague pain in hypochondrium.

Accompanying symptoms: Dry mouth and throat, dysphoria with smothery sensation, dizziness, tidal fever, night sweat, dysphoria with feverish sensation in chest, palms and soles, soreness and weakness of waist.

Tongue and pulse: Reddish tongue with less fur, fine, taut and rapid pulse.

Analysis: Fire-syndrome caused by protracted stagnation of the liver-Qi, impairing liver-Yin, or failure of nourishing the liver collaterals due to the impaired essence and blood induced by chronic disease with weakness, cause vague pain in hypochondrium. Yin-deficiency is in charge of internal heat, so dry mouth and throat with dysphoria, soreness and weakness of waist, even tidal fever and night sweat, inability of nourishing upwards due to impaired essence and blood, lack of nutrient in senven orifices, give rise to dizziness. Reddish tongue with less fur, and fine, taut and rapid pulse are signs of internal heat due to Yin-deficiency.

Therapeutic principle: nourishing Yin and the liver.

Prescription: Modified Yi Guan Jian. In the prescription, dried remannia root and wolfbery fruit are used for nourishing the liver and the kidney; root of straight ladybell, ophiopogon root and Chinese angelica root for nourishing Yin and the liver; Sichuan chinaberry for soothing the liver and regulation Qi and relieving pain; albizia flower, rose and tribulus fruit are added for soothing the liver and regulating Qi; wild or spiny jujuba seed and fried capejasmine are added for dysphoria with smothery sensation, for clearing away heat and tranquilization; siberian solomonseal rhizome, glossy privet fruit, and chrysanthemum flower are added for dizziness, for nourishing the kidney and clearing away heat from the liver.

Example of priscription: 15g root of straght ladybell, 30g red sage root, 10g ophiopogon root, 10g dried rehmannia root, 10g wolberry fruit, 10g fried sichuan chinaberry, 6g corydalis tuber, 10g white mume flower, 10g dried white peony root, 6g prepared liquorice, 10g rose.

〔Measures for Prevention and Nursing Care〕

1. Keep happy, and avoid restlessness and depression.

2. Proper diet, eat less pungent, greasy and sea foot, do not drink wine.

3. Lead a regular life, pay attention to own hygiene, preventing from affection by exopathogen.

4. Finger-needling and massage are used in combination.

5. Properly do exercise, promoting the circulation of Qi and blood.

〔Analysis of Typical Case〕

Case 1: Feng xx, male, 54 years, a cadre.

Main complaints: Hypochondriac pain had repeatedly attacked for 3 years.

History of disease: He had hepatitis in 1960. After treatment he was cured basically, but hypochondriac pain often attacked at the situation of overwork, abnormal weather or emotional fluctuation. In recent 3 years, hypochondriac pain has attacked more frequently, even influencing normal work and sleeping, and he had taken Chinese drugss for liver-pretection and soothing the liver and regulating Qi with on effect, and pain exacerbates graduelly, with anorexia and thin body.

Examinaton showed dry skin, dull and dark complexion, thin body, anorexia, dry mouth with bitter taste, dry stool, hypochondriac pain, reddish tongue with thin and yellowish fur, taut and fine pulse.

Diagnosis of traditional Chinese medicine: Hypochondriac pain (stagnation of the liver-Qi and Yin-deficiency.

Therapeutic principle: Nourishing Yin and soothing the liver.

Prescription: Yi Guan Jian.

10g Chinese angelica root, 10g white peony root, 10g wolfberry fruit, 10g dried rehmannia root, 10g curcuma root, 10g sichuan chinaberry, 10g tribulus fruit, 15g glehnia root, 15g ophiopogon root, 15g prepared lindera root, 15g glossy privet fruit, 15g eclipta.

After he took 5 doses, hypochondriac pain relieved obviously, appetite increased, and after other 5 doses were taken, hypochondriac pain relieved completely with normal appetite.

Note: the patient had stagnation of the liver-Qi, injury of Yin due to fire-pathogen caused by stagnation of the liver-Qi, and the drugs for regulating Qi and warmness and dryness in property he took impaired more severely Yin, so in the treatment both nourishing Yin and soothing the liver were adopted at same time. Chinese angelica, white peony root, wolfberry fruit, dried rehmannia root, tribulus fruit, glehnia root, ophiopogon root, prepared lindera root, glossy privet fruit and eclipta were used for reinforcing blood, nourishing Yin of the liver and the kidney to regulate the liver, and curcuma root and sichuan chinaberry were added for soothing the liver without injury of Yin. [Zhang Zhen Ru, Treatment of hypochondriac pain due to Yin-deficiency with Modified Yi Guan Jia, New Treaditional Chinese Medicine, 1984;(2):25]

Hypochondriac pain is a commonly-seen disease, the disease is to be mainly in the liver and the gallbladder and it is caused by internal injury and affection by exopathogen. Clinically differentiation of syndrome should combine with accompanying symptoms, and differentiate internal injury, affection by exopathogen, in Qi, in blood, and deficiency, excess, heat and cold syndromes. Hypochondriac pain caused by stagnation of Qi, blood stasis and damp-heat belongs often excess syndrome, and that due to insufficiency of the liver-Yin belongs often deficiency syndrome. Deficiency and excess syndromes can change. For example, the disease attackes mainly due to stagnation of Qi, after long time it can induce blood stasis, blood stasis or damp-heat as main, accompanied by stagnation of Qi. Excess syndrome producing heat and impairing Yin, or deficiency syndrome with stagnation of Qi, or deficiency syndrome with excess syndrome is often seen. Therefore, analysis should be made in an all-round way in differentiation of syndromes.

In treatment, regulating Qi, removing stasis, clearing away heat, eliminating dampness and other therapeutic principle are used for excess syndrome, and nourishing Yin and the liver for deficiency syndrome. At the same time, the drugs for regulating Qi should be added, but the drugs over pungent in flavor and dryness in property do not used in regulating Qi, for avoid of further injury of Yin.

Questions for Review

1. How to grasp pathological characteristics of hypochondriac pain? How to differentiate syndromes of Qi and blood, deficiency and excess?
2. Try to describe differentiation of syndromes and treatment for hypochondriac pain due to stagnation of the liver-Qi, blood stasis, damp-heat of the liver and the gallbladder and insufficiency of the liver-Yin.

3. How to comprehend that free circulation of Qi and blood can relieve pain in treatment of hypochondriac pain?

Jaundice

〔General Introduction〕

Jaundice is a disease and syndrome, marked mainly by yellow in eyes, the body and urine. Generally, it is divided into 3 kinds, Yang jaundice, Yin jaunndice and acute jaundice. Yang jaundice is more often seen and a part of them is of infectivity.

Jaundice in traditional Chinese medicine and western medicine has same meaning, so jaundice in infectious hepatitis, cholecystitis, diseases of biliary tract, cirrhosis, hemolysis, acute or subacute yellow atrophy of liver, leptospirosis etc. all can refere the treatment based on differentiation of symptoms and signs in the chapter.

〔Causes of Disease and Pathogenesis〕

Causes of disease of jaundice have internal cause and exopathic cause. The exopathic cause is mainly affection by exopathogenic factors or improper diet and the internal cause is more related with deficiency-cold of the spleen and stomach, and internal injury. The internal and external causes are correlated often. They are discussed respectively in the following.

Ⅰ. Affection by external pathogens: Affection by damp-heat, fulminant pathogens, from surface to interior, stagnation in the middle-Jia, dysfunction of the spleen and stomach in transport and transformation, accumulation of dampness and heat pathogens in the liver and gallbladder, induce impairment of dispelling function of the liver, bile overflowing and infusing into the muscle and skin, flowing down to the urine bladder, so yellow body, eyes and urine appear. Invasion of excessive dampness, heat and epidemic pathogens with acute or infectivity very quickly manifests as serious phenomenon of invading the Yin-blood, which is called as acute jaundice.

Ⅱ. Impairment due to improper diet: Improper diet, often hunger or full, or over drinking, over eating fat, sweet, greasy food, all can impaire the spleen and stomach, even lead to dysfunction of transportation and transformation, accumulation of dampness pathogen in the body. Excessive Yang-Qi in the interior, damp-heat is formed due to dampness easily producing heat, and attacking the liver and gallbladder, bile does not circulate in bile tract, infusing into the muscle and skin, so Yang jaundice appears; improper diet, over cold and cool impairing Yang-Qi of the spleen and stomach, or deficiency-cold in the spleen and stomach, dysfunction of the spleen in transport, so dampness pathogen easily poroduces from cold, and stagnation of cold-dampness in the middle-Jiao, stagnation of bile, failure of normal circulation, flowing into the muscle and skin to induce Yin jaundice.

Diagram of Causes of Disease and Pathogenesis of Jaundice

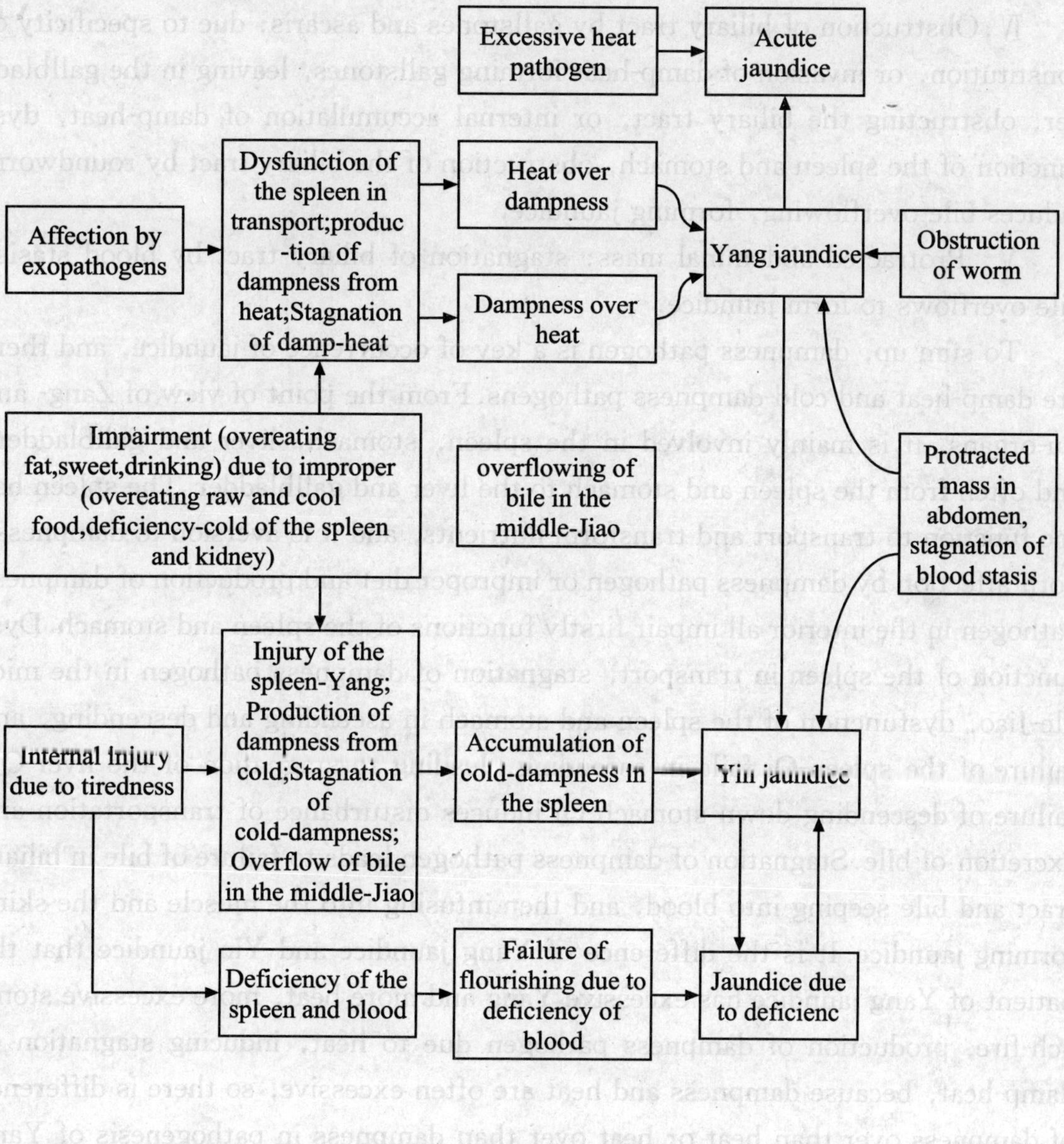

Ⅲ. Internal injury due to tiredness: Overwork, weakness of the spleen and stomach can induce jaundice. It is mainly divided into two aspects: Firstly, injury of the spleen-Yang or deficiency-cold of the spleen and stomach, failure of transport of water and dampness, dampness produces from cold, leading to stagnation of cold-dampness in the middle-Jiao, blockade of bile excretion, flowing into the muscle and skin to form Yin jaundice. This also is caused by deficiency of the spleen and internal excess of cold-damp pathogens; Secondly, failure of producing Qi and blood due to deficiency of the spleen, deficiency of Qi and blood, so results in jaundice. This jaundice is also caused by deficiency, so it is called as jaundice due to deficiency.

Ⅳ. Obstruction of biliary tract by gallstones and ascaris: due to specificity of constitution, or invasion of damp-heat forming gallstones, leaving in the gallbladder, obstructing the biliary tract, or internal accumulation of damp-heat, dysfunction of the spleen and stomach, obstruction of the biliary tract by roundworm induces bile overflowing, forming jaundice.

Ⅴ. Protracted abdominal mass: stagnation of biliary tract by blood stasis, bile overflows to form jaundice.

To sum up, dampness pathogen is a key of occurrence of jaundice, and there are damp-heat and cold-dampness pathogens. From the point of view of Zang- and Fu-organs, it is mainly involved in the spleen, stomach, liver and gallbladder, and often from the spleen and stomach to the liver and gallbladder. The spleen has the function to transport and transform nutrients, and it is aversion to dampness, both affection by dampness pathogen or improper diet and production of dampness pathogen in the interior all impair firstly functions of the spleen and stomach. Dysfunction of the spleen in transport, stagnation of dampness pathogen in the middle-Jiao, dysfunction of the spleen and stomach in ascending and descending, and failure of the spleen-Qi fails in ascending, leading to stagnation of the liver-Qi, failure of descending down stomach-Qi induces disturbance of transportation and excretion of bile. Stagnation of dampness pathogen leads to failure of bile in biliary tract and bile seeping into blood, and then infusing into the muscle and the skin, forming jaundice. It is the difference of Yang jaundice and Yin jaundice that the patient of Yang jaundice has excessive Yang and more heat, more excessive stomach-fire, production of dampness pathogen due to heat, inducing stagnation of damp-heat, because dampness and heat are often excessive, so there is difference of dampness over than heat or heat over than dampness in pathogenesis of Yang jaundice. Extremely excessive fire-heat is called as toxin, as excess of heat toxin, the pathogenic factor attacking Ying-blood, and invading pericardium, often forming acute jaundice. The patient of Yin jaundice has excessive Yin and severe cold, insufficiency of the spleen-Yang, dampness pathogen is caused by cold, forming cold-dampness; and protracted Yang jaundice, or over taking drugs of cold in nature, damaging the spleen-Yang, dampness produces from cold pathogen, also forming Yin jaundice. In addition, at once the jaundice caused by obstruction the biliary tract by gallstones and roundworn, symptoms of the liver and gallbladder will be seen, manifesting often heat as main, belongs Yang jaundice. In the patient of the jaundice caused by protracted abdominal mass, stagnation of blood stasis in the biliary tract, Yin jaundice or Yang jaundice is formed often due to consititution of cold and heat.

〔Treatment Based on Differentiation of Symptoms and Signs〕

Ⅰ. Main points of differentiation of syndrome and signs

(Ⅰ) Firstly, confirm whether it is jaundice. Yellow conjunctivas are an important basis for diagnosis of jaundice, so clinically should observe colour of the conjunctiva, skin and urine.

(Ⅱ) Differentiation of jaundice property:

1. Differentiation from time of attack and duration of disease: Yang jaundice attackes suddenly, with short duraton of disease; Yin jaundice attackes slowly with long duration; Acute jaundice attackes suddenly and changes quickly.

2. Differentiation from colour of jaundice: Yang jaundice is of fresh yellow colour, belonging to heat syndrome and excess syndrome; Yin jaundice is of dull or dim, belonging to deficiency syndrome and cold syndrome; Aute jaundice is of yellow body like gold colour, belonging excessive heat pathogen, and deficiency syndrome complicated by excess syndrome may appear due to exhausion of Qi-Ying at late stage.

(Ⅲ) Differentiation of state of illness: Mainly observe colour of jaundice.

That colour of jaundice darkens gradually suggestes exacerbation of the disease; That Jaundice becomes gradually light indicates improvement of state of illness; Fresh colour for jaundice and consciousness indicate favorable case, mild state of disease; Dull colour and restlessness indicate a deteriorating case, sevious state of disease.

Main points of differentiation of Yang jaundice and Yin jaundice

	Yang jaundice	Yin jaundice
Causes of disease pathogenesis	Affection by damp-heat, often by exopathogens	Stagnation of cold-dampness. often with deficiency of Qi of the spleen and stomach-Qi
Specificity of yellow	Fresh yellow like orange	Dark like smoking
Specificity of syndrome	Excess syndrome, heat syndrome	Deficiency syndrome, cold syndrome or deficiency syndrome complicated with excess syndrome
Duration of disease	Short	Long
State of illness	Generally, mild in most cases except acute jaundice	Severe in most cases
Treatment	Clearing away heat and eliminating dampness as main methods, clearing away heat and detoxicating and removing heat from blood for acute jaundice	Strengthening the spleen and warming and dispelling cold-dampness as main methods, strengthening the spleen, nourishing Qi and blood for jaundice due to deficiency

Ⅱ. Differentiative diagnosis

Jaundice should be differentiated with Wei-jaundice

(Ⅰ) Causes of disease and pathogenesis: Causes of disease of jaundice are affection by exopathogens, impairment due to improper diet, deficiency and cold in the spleen and stomach, and turning of mass in abdomen, and its pathogenesis is stagnation of dampness pathogen in the middle -JIao, failure of the liver and gallbladder in excretion, or obstruction of biliary tract by blood stasis, roundworm and gallstones, etc. leading to failure of bile to circulate in normal tract, flowing into the muscle and skin to produce yellow; or due to deficiency of the spleen and lochioschesis, and unability to flourih due to retention of lochioschesisin the body lead to appearence of yellow. Wei-jaundice is caused by retention of worm and food, inducing deficiency of the spleen, failure of food to transform into neutrients and to produce Qi and blood, or bleeding, deficiency of Qi and blood after illness, insufficiency of Qi and blood, yellow appears in the muscle and skin.

(Ⅱ) Main syndromes: Yellow eyes, body and urine are main syndromes for jaundice, and with different pathogenesis of damp-heat, cold-dampness and stagnation of blood stasis in the interior, the yellow may show the differences of fresh yellow and dark yellow.

Main symptoms of Wei-jaundice are: the muscle and skin show light yellow, dry and no gloss, but without yellow in eyes and urine, often accompanied by dizziness, tinnitus, palpitation, insomina and other symptoms.

Ⅲ. Main points of therapeutic principle

Because jaundice is caused by dampness pathogen, eliminating dampness and diuresis are basical principle for treatment of jaundice. The method of eliminating dampness includes mainly inducing diuresis with bland drugs, clearing away heat and promoting diuresis, warming Yang for diuresis. In treatment of jaundice, eliminating dampness, resolving dampness and dispelling dampness are often used for removing dampness and resolving yellow. Resolving dampness, i, e. warming Yang for diuresis, clearing away heat and eliminating dampness, eliminating dampness with aromatics, removes dampness pathogen from the middle-Jiao; dispelling dampness, i. e. relaxing the bowels to eliminating dampness, removing stagnation to dispel dampness, eliminate dampness pathogen from stool. Clinically, different methods of eliminating dampness are respectively used for jaundice of different properties. For Yang jaundice, clearing away heat and eliminating dampness method is mainly used, and if it is necessary, relaxing the bowels is combined; Yin jaundice adopts mainly warming Yang for removing dampness, and its combination with nourishing Qi and blood, or soothing the liver and promoting flow of blood; acute jaundice belongs Yang jaundice, and it is caused by excessive heat pathogen, pathogen invading Ying-blood, so clearing away heat and toxic material, and removing heat from Ying and inducing resuscitation methods should adopted.

Ⅳ. Treatment based on classifications of jaundice

(Ⅰ) Yang jaundice

Yang jaundice has mainly three types, always with damp-heat.

1. Heat over dampness

Main symptoms: Yellow body and eyes, orang-like fresh yellow, with brightness, and scanty dark urine.

Accompanying symptoms: often fever and thirst, restlessness, fullness of abdomen, nausea and desire to vomit, dry mouth and bitter taste, constipation.

Tongue and pulse: yellowish and greasy fur on the tongue, taut and rapid pulse.

Analysis: Accumulation of damp-heat, bile flowing into the muscle and skin, heat is yang pathogen, so fresh yellow appears. Excess of damp-heat in the interior, over heat pathogen, heat consumes of body fluid, so fever and thirst occur. Damp-heat interfering the gallbladder, hypofunction of Qi-transmission induces scaty dark urine. Excessive heat in Yangming causes constipation, and failure of the flow of Fu-organ-Qi results in distention and fullness of abdomen; accumulation of damp-heat, turbit of the stomach and bile adversely flow up, causing restlessness, nausea and desire to vomit, dry mouth and bitter taste. Yellowish and greasy fur, and taut and rapid pulse are signs of excessive damp-heat of the liver, gallbladder, spleen and stomach in the interior.

Therapeutic principle: Clearing away heat and eliminating dampness.

Prescription: Modified Yin Chen Hao Decoction. In the prescription, oriental wormwood is an important drug for clearing away heat, eliminating dampness and removing jaundice, using a large dose, 30～50g; capejasmine fruit can cearing away damp-heat in the three-Jiao; rhubarb can eliminate accumulation of heat. Combination of oriental wormwood and capejasmine fruit eliminate damp-heat from urine; combination of oriental wormwood and rhubarb can eliminate heat from stool. Umbellate pore fungus, plantain seed, tale and other herbs for excreting dampness can be properly added for eliminating dampness and heat pathogens from stool and urine. In the patient with nausea, desire to vomit and restlessness, coptis, bamboo shavings and tangerine peel etc. are added, which can remove fire, descend the adverse rising of Qi, arrest vomiting. In the patient with more severe pain in right hypochondium, bupleurum root, curcuma root, sichuan chinaberry, corydalis tuber, etc. can be added, which can soothe the liver, regulate Qi and relieve pain. Smallamount of fruit of citron or trifoliate orange, magnolia bark or agastach and eupatorium can be added for distention and fullness of abdomen.

For obstruction of biliary tract by gallstones, marked by pain in the right hypochondrium, involving the shoulder and the back, or aversion to cold, and fever, and pale and gray stool, Da Chai Hu Decoction plus oriental wormwood, curcuma root, climbing fern spore, chicken's gizzard-skin and lysimachia are used for normalizing functioning of the gallbladder and removing gallstones, clearing away heat and resolving jaundice.

For obstruction of worm in the biliary tract, marked by sudden occurrence of jaundice, with cold or fever, and pain attacking or relieving, vomiting roundworm, Wu Mei Pill and oriental wormwood, capejasmine fruit are used in combination for relieving pain and normarizing functions of the gallbladder and resolving jaundice. For the patient with more manifestation of heat syndrome, prepared aconite root and cinnamon twig can be subtracted, and less sichuan chinaberry and dried ginger can be used, and more coptis root, phellodendron bark can be used, and dangshen and Chinse angelica root are subtracted for the patient with no deficiency syndrome, and generally, sichuan chinaberry, betel nut and quisqualis fruit can be added for expelling worms, promoting flow of Qi and relieving pain.

Example of prescription: 30g wormwood, 10g capejasmine fruit, 6g dried rhubarb, 15g isatis root, 10g large-leaf gentian root, 15g umbellate pore fungus, 15g oriental water plantain rhizome, 6g dried liquorice, 15g dandelion herb, 10g tangerine peel and 10g pinellia tuber.

2. Dampness over heat

Main symptoms: Yellow body and eyes, with no so bright yellow as that in more heat syndrome.

Accompanying symptoms: No high fever, heaviness of head, tastelessness with no thirst, fullness in the chest and the stomach, anorexia, distention in abdomen, aversion to greasy food, nausea and desire to vomit, loose stool.

Tongue and pulse: Thick, greasy and yellowish fur on the tongue, taut and slippery, or weak and slow pulse.

Analysis: Retention of dampness and heat, failure of bile to circulate in normal tract, flowing into muscle and skin and inducing yellow body and conjunctivas. Because of dampness over heat, and dampness is Yin pathogen, so the yellow is not so bright as that in more heat. No high fever occurs due to excessive dampness. Retention of damp-heat in interior, clear Yang can not be dispeled, so haviness of the head appears. Tastelessness with no thirst, fullness in the chest and stomach, anorexia, nausea and desire to vomit, distention in abdomen all are caused by retention of dampness in the spleen, and dysfunction of the spleen and stomach. Thick, greasy and yellowish fur, and taut and slipery or weak and slow pulse are signs of more dampness syndrome with less heat syndrome.

Therapeutic principle: Eliminating dampness and turbit-transmission, clearing away heat as adjuvant method.

Prescription: Modified Yin Chen Wu Ling Powder. In the prescription, oriental wormwood is a main drug for clearing away heat, eliminating dampness and resolving jaundice, Wu Ling Powder are combined for warming Yang, Qi-transmission and eliminating dampness, removing dampness from urine; for same severe of dampness and heat syndromes, Gan Lu Xiao Du Pill can be used, in which scutellaria root, fiveleaf akebia stem, tale and other drugs bitter in taste and cold in nature can clear away heat and eliminate dampness; agastach and round cardamon seed for promoting the function of Qi to removing dampness pathogen. For vomiting, tangerine peel and pinellia are added for removing dampness, regulating the function of the stomach and adverse rising the flow of the stomach-Qi; for distention in abdomen, aucklandia root, shell of areca nut, etc are added for keeping Qi flowing downward and eliminating the distention in abdomen.

Yang jaundice with exterior syndrome at initial stage, firstly, should use Ma Huang Lian Qiao Chi Xiao Dou Decoction for relieving exterior syndrome, clearing away heat and removing dampness. For failure of damp-heat in dispelling and un-resolving of fever, Zhi Zi Bai Pi Decoction can be added for strengthening the action of clearing away heat and eliminating dampness. For Yang jaundice with excessive heat in Yangming, burning injury of body fluid, mass in the abdomen, constipation in the course of disease, should use Da Huang Xiao Shi Decoction for removing heat and resolving the mass.

Example of prescription: 30g oriental wormwood, 15g umbellate pore fungus, 15g poria, 10g bighead atractylodes rhizome, 10g oriental water plantain, 10g pinellia tuber, 10g tangerine peel, 10g bamboo shavings, 6g round cardamon seed, 10g agastach, 10g shell of areca nut.

3. Excessive noxious heat type(acute jaundice)

Main symptoms: Sudden and acute attack, jaundice rapidly becomes darkness, gold-like colour.

Accompanying symptoms: High fever and excessive thirst, hypochondrial pain and abdominal fullness, coma and delirium, or epistaxis, hemafecia, or ecchymosis on the skin, bright red tongue.

Tongue and pulse: Bright red tongue with yellowish and dry fur, taut, slippery and rapid or fine and rapid pulse.

Analysis: Damp-heat with noxious pathogen, excessive noxious heat, induce rapid attack; high fever and thirst, noxious heat inducing bile flowing into the muscle and skin, so jaundice rapidly becomes dark with yellow body and conjunctias, like gold colour. Excessive noxious heat in interior, disorder of activity of Qi induces hypochondrial pain and abdominal fullness; noxious heat causes failure of blood to circulate in blood vessels, so epistaxis and hemafecia appear, or ecchymosis occurs on the skin. Bright red tongue, yellowish and dry fur, and taut, slippery, rapid or fine, rapid pulse are signs of excessive nocxious heat in the liver and gallbladder.

Therapeutic principle: Clearing away heat and toxic material, removing heat from blood and inducing resuscitation.

Prescription: Modified Xi Jiao Powder. In the prescription, rhinoceros horn is an important drug for clearing away noxious material and removing heat from blood and its combination with coptis root, capejasmine fruit, cimicifuga rhizome has stronger action of clearing away heat and noxious material. Oriental wormwood can removing heat and eliminating jaundice, isatis leaf, honeysuckle flower, forsythia fruit can be added, which can cleare away heat and remove toxious material, and dried rehmannia root, moutan bark, scrophularia root, dendrobium are added for increasing action of clearing away heat and removing heat from blood.

An Gong Niu Huang Pill can be used in combination for coma and delirium, or Zhi Bao Pill is combined for removing heat from blood and inducing resuscitation; For the patient with epistaxis, femafecia or severe ecchymosis on the skin, the drugs for removing heat from blood and arresting bleeding, such as sanguisorba root charcoal, biota tops charcoal can be added. For the patient with oliguria, or ascites, the drugs for clearing away heat and diuresis, such as fiveleaf akebia stem, cogongrass rhizome, plantain herb, shell of areca nut can be added.

Example of prescription: 1.5g powder of rhinoceros horn (taking with the decoction) or 10g rhinoceros horn, 6g coptis root, 10g capejasmine fruit, 45g oriental wormwood, 10g isatis leaf, 10g honeysuckle flower, 15g forsythia fruit, 15g dried rehmannia root, 10g moutan bark, 15g scrophularia root.

(Ⅱ) Yin jaundice

1. Retention of cold-damp pathogen

Main symptoms: Dark yellow, like smoking.

Accompanying symptoms: Mental tiredness and aversion to cold, anorexia and indigestion, fullness in the stomach, loose stool, tastelessness and no thirst.

Tongue and pulse: Pale tongue with white and greasy fur, weak and slow or deep and rapid pulse.

Analysis: retention of cold-damp pathogen in the spleen and stomach, hypofuction of Yang-Qi, bile overflowing, and cold -dampness is Yin pathogen, so dark yellow skin appears like smoking; retention of dampness in the spleen, hypofunction of the spleen-Yang, disorder of transporting and transforming nutrients, lead to anorexia, fullness in the stomach, loose stool, tastelessness, no thirst and other symptoms. Insufficiency of Yang, deficiency of Qi and blood induce aversion to cold and mental tiredness. Pale tongue with greasy fur, weak and slow or deep and slow pulse are often signs of Yang-deficiency and unability to remove dampness, and retention of cold-dampness in Yin system.

Therapeutic principle: Strengthening the spleen and regulating the stomach, warming and removing cold-dampness.

Prescription: Modified Yin Chen Zhu Fu Decoction. In the prescription, oriental wormwood and prepared aconite root are used for warming and removing cold and dampness and eliminating jaundice. Bighead atractylodes rhizome, dried ginger and liquorice for strengthening the spleen and warming the middle-Jiao, and drugs for promoting flow of Qi and eliminating dampness, such as curcuma root, magnolia bark, poria, and oriental water plantain can be added.

For the patient with abdominal distention and thick fur on the tongue, bighead atractylodes rhizome and liquorice are subtracted, and atractylodes rhizome and magnolia bark are added for eliminating dampness and resolving distention; and for the patient with cutaneous pruritus, large-leaf gentian root and broom cypress fruit are added for expelling wind to relieve itching.

Example of prescription: 30g oriental wormwood, 6g prepared aconite root, 10g bighead atractylodes rhizome, 10g fried ginger, 10g pinellia tuber, 10g tangerine peel, 15g poria, 10g magnolia bark, 10g aucklandia root, 6g round cardamon seed, 10g atractylodes rhizome.

2. Retention of blood stasis

Main symptoms: Dark yellow body and eyes.

Accompanying symptoms: vascular spider in the skin, darkish complexion, mass in hypochondrium with fixed pain, black stool.

Tongue and pulse: green and purple tongue or with ecchymosis, taut and uneven or fine and uneven pulse.

Analysis: Retention of blood stasis, checking of the flow of bile result in yellow body and eyes; retention of blood stasis in interior, new blood can not supply to the face, so dimmish and blackish complexion appears; retention of blood stasis in the hypochondium, ckecking of circulation of Qi and blood bring about mass in the hypochondium with pain. And vascular spider in the skin, dark stool and changes of tongue and pulse are signs of blood stasis.

Therapeutic principle: Activating circulation of blood, removing blood stasis and eliminating jaundice.

Prescription: Modified Ge Xia Zhu Yu Decoction. In the prescription, peach kernel, safflower, moutan bark, trogopterus dund are used for activating circulation of blood and removing blood stasis; Chinese angelica root and chuanxiong rhizome for nourishing blood and promoting circulation of blood; corydalis tuber, lindera root, nutgrass flatsedge rhizome for promoting circulation of Qi and blood to relieve pain, and oriental wormwood can be added for eliminating jaundice. Or Xiao Shi Fan Shi Powder are used for turbit-transmission, removing blood stasis and softening hard masses, and Xiao Yao Powder can be combined for soothing the liver and suporting the spleen. For the patient with obvious deficiency of spleen, Xiang Sha Liu Jun zhi Decoction can be combined for strengthening the spleen and regulating the stomach. For the patient with protracted jaundice and obvious mass in hypochondrium, retention of dampness pathogen may form masses or tympanites.

Example of prescription: 10g whole Chinese angelica root, 10g chuanxiong rhizome, 10 red peony root, 10g white peony root, 10g peach kernel, 6g safflower, 10g moumtan bark, 10g rubia root, 30g oriental wormwood, 10g cat-tail pollen, 10g prepared nutgrass flatsedge rhizome, 15g curcuma root.

3. Deficiency of the spleen and blood(Jandice of deficiency type)

Main symptoms: yellow eyes and skin, pale and dim complexion, dark urine, or obvious in night.

Accompanying symptoms: mental tiredness and weakness, lassitude in limbs, palpitation and shortness of breath, anorexia and loose stool, restlessness in night.

Tongue and pulse: Pale tongue with thin and white fur, fine and weak pulse.

Analysis: Deficiency of the spleen and stomach, dysfunction of transporting and transforming nutrients, insufficiency of resource of Qi and blood, poor blood supplying to the face and the body, so appearence of yellow face and skin, pale and dim complexion, dark urine, or being obvious in night. Insufficiency of the spleen-Qi induces mental tiredness and weakness, lassitude in limbs, shortness of breath and dislike to speak. Deficiency of blood is inable to nurish the heart, irritability induces palipitation and restlessness in night. Hypofunction of transport due to deficiency of the spleen, leading to anorexia and loose stool. Pale tongue with thin and white fur, and fine and weak pulse are signs of deficiency of the spleen and blood.

Therapeutic principle: strengthening the spleen and warming the middle-Jiao, supplementing and nourishing Qi and blood.

Prescription: Modified Xiao Jian Zhong Decoction. In the prescription, cinnamon twig should be fried with honey for strengthening the spleen and warming the middle-Jiao, and its combination with ginger and Chinese-date of sweet taste and pungent flaver for producing Yang; white peony root is used for nourishing blood, and its combination with liquorice with sour and sweet taste for Yin-transmission. Cinnamon twig and white peony root can regulate Yin and Yang. Malt extract can strengthen the spleen. Thus, strength of the spleen and stomach promotes production of Qi and blood, jaundice is eliminated. For the patient with obvious deficiency of Qi, astragalus root and dangshen can be added; for obvious deficiency of blood, Chinese angelica root, rehmannia root, donkey-hide, eclipta, etc can be added; for obvious deficiency of Yang, bark of Chinese cassia tree is used instead of cinnamon twig, and dried ginger can be added.

Example of prescription: 10g cinnamon twig fried with huney, 12g white peony root, 10g liquorice fried with huney, 3 pieces of fresh ginger, 7 grains of Chinese-date, 30g malt extract(taking with the decoction), 20g astragalus root, 10g whole Chinese angelica root, 10g donkey-hide, 10g eclipta, 10g dangshen.

Appendix: Obstructive jaundice.

Wei- jaundice has some differences with jaundice, its main symptoms are no yellow in both eyes, light yellow in muscle and skin in whole body, dry skin with no gross, free urination with no yellow, tiredness and weakness, dizziness and tinnitus, palpitation and insomnia, loose stool, pale tongue with thin fur, weak and fine pulse.

In the disease, retention of worm and food induce deficiency of the spleen and stomach, failure of food in transforming nutrients to produce Qi and blood, and deficiency of Qi and blood can not nourish the skin and muscle, and viscera, leading to yellow muscle and skin with no gross. In addition, loss of blood, or after servere disease, exhaustion of Qi and blood induces insufficiency of Qi and blood, leading to attack of this disease, which is commonly-seen clinically.

For treatment of the disease, regulating the spleen and stomach, nourishing Qi and supplementing blood should mainly adopted, with Huang Qi Jian Zhong Decoction or Ren Shen Yang Ying Decoction selected. For the disease caused by hookworm, antiscolic therapy should be adopted.

〔Measures of Prevention and Nursing Care〕

1. Pay attention to take rest, bed rest is a main when jaundice has not been eliminated.

2. Proper diet, avoid fat, oil, greasy, sea food and purgent food, and fornbid drinking.

3. For the patients with infectivity, should take isolation for prevention from transport of noxious pathogens.

4. Keep optimistic and stable emotion, actively coorperate for treatment.

〔Analysis of Typical Case〕

Case 1: Lei XX, female, 20 years old, a worker.

4 months ago, he had fever and aversion to cold, nausea and vomiting, anorexia, bitter taste and dry mouth, gradual appearence of yellow in the body and eyes, yellow urine like orange colour. She was diagnosed as acute and infectious hepatitis. She was admitted to the hospital for 4 months, and administered capejasmine fruit, phellodendron bark, gentian root and other herbs of bitter taste and cold in nature, jaundice eliminated slightly, but with abdominal distention, weakness, and thin body. Then she was treated in outpatient department.

Examination showed shallow complexion, thin body, mentional tiredness and aversion to cold, distending pain in hypochondrium, fullness of the stomach, yellowish eyes, loose stool, white and greasy fur on the tongue, taut and full pulse on the left Guan and deep, slow and weak pulse on the right Guan.

Physical and chemical examinations: thymol turbidity test(TTT) 15u, thymol flocculation test(TFT) +++, glutamic-pyruvic transaminase(GPT), 300u.

Diagnosis of traditional Chinese medicine: Jaundice (the liver-Qi invading the spleen, retention of cold and dampness pathogens).

Thrapeutic principle: strengthening the spleen and soothing the liver, warming the middle-Jiao and regulating the stomach, and removing dampness as adjuvant method.

Prescription: 12g dangshen, 12g bighead atractylodes rhizome, 12g poria, 9g tangerine peel, 9g galangal rhizome, 12g fresh Chinese yam, 6g amomum fruit, 10g oriental wormwood, 9g orage leaf, 12g white peony root, 12g corydilis tuber, 5g liquorice.

Second visit: after took over 10 doses of the above mentioned prescription, the symptoms relieved markedly, with disappearence of jaundice. Afterwards, the methods of strengthening the spleen, regulating the stomach and soothing the liver were used for 3 months, and then reexamination of hepatic function for 4 times indicated gradual normarization each time.

Note: The disease is caused by protracted injury of the spleen-Yang due to taking over drugs of bitter taste and cold in nature in the patient with Yang jaundice. Differentiation of syndrome showed Yin-jaundice due to the liver-Qi invading the spleen, retention of cold-dampness. Treatment should adopt strengthening the spleen, soothing the liver, warming the middle-Jiao, regulating the stomach, and removing dampness as adjuvant method, and oriental wormwood was used for eliminating jaundice and removing dampness, galangal rhizome and amomum fruit for warming the middle-Jiao, expelling cold, white peony root, corydalis tuber, orage leaf for soothing the liver, regulating Qi and relieving pain, combination of the drugs can exert commonly the action of strengthening the spleen, soothing the liver, warming the middle-Jiao, regulating the stomach and removing dampness, so as to relieve the symptoms. After elimination of jaundice, the methods of strengthening the spleen, regulating the stomach, soothing the liver were continuously used for 3 months, and then she was cured. (Cases Treated by Xu Yu Shan).

Jaundice is marked by yellow conjunctivas, body and urine. Yellow conjunctivas is a key for diagnosis of the disease. Its attack is always related with affection by exopathogens, improper diet, deficiency and cold of the spleen and stomach, blood stasis, obstruction of gallstones and worm in biliary tract, and injury of internal organs, but it is mainly caused by dampness pathogen, most invading the liver, gallblader, spleen and stomach.

Clinically, should differentiate Yang jaundice and Yin jaundice, jaundice due to deficiency and Wei- jaundice. Both Yang jaundice and Yin jaundice are caused by dampness pathogen, and Yang jaundice belongs to excess syndrome, heat syndrome, and Yin jaundice belongs to deficiency syndrome, cold syndome or deficiency syndrome accompanied by excess syndrome. The differences of Yang jaundice and Yin jaundice are not absolute, they can transform each other. Both Jaundice due to deficiency and wei- jaundice belong to deficiency syndrome, jaundice due to deficiency is marked by yellow conjunctiva, body and urine as main symptoms, and wei- jaundice does not have yellow conjunctiva and urine, which can be used for their differentiation.

Removing dampness from urine is an important therapeutic principle for treatment of jaundice. The drugs of cleraing or warming, and expelling dampness from stool, and strengthening the spleen and nourishing blood, activating circulation of blood, etc. can be combined according to property of jaundice. The patient who at initial stage receives in time proper treatment, has favourable prognosis. In the patient with protracted disease, repeated attack, stagnation of Qi and blood stasis, mass in the hypocondrium, body resistance weakened while pathogenic factors prevailing, is often difficult to be cured. Acute jaundice is a crisis of jaundice, it should actively receive emergence treatment. After elimination of jaundice, medication can not be suddenly stopped and should properly administer drugs of regulating the spleen and stomach according to differences of syndromes.

Questions for Review

1. What is the conception of jaundice? which symptom is main characteritics of jaundice?
2. How to classify jaundice clinically at present?
3. How to differentiate jaundice due to deficiency and wei- jaundice?
4. Which kinds of pathogenic factor are closely related with pathological changes of jaundice? and which Zang- and Fu-organs are related with pathological changes of jaundice?
5. Try to describe the laws of differentiation of syndromes and treatment of Yang jaundice, acute jaundice and Yin jaundice.

Accumulation and Aggregation

〔General Introduction〕

Accumulation and aggregation are a disease and syndrome of mass in the abdomen, with distention or pain. Accumulation and aggregation have some differences in serious extents of disease and pathologic changes. Accumulation has a form and fixed parts of distention and pain. It belongs to a disease of blood system, and it is a disease of Zang-organs; aggregation does not have a form, without fixed parts of distention and pain. It belongs to a disease of Qi system and it is a disease of fu-organs.

Generally, aggregation disease is milder, with shorter duration of disease, so it is easily to be cured. Accumulation disease is more severe, with longer duration of disease, accumulating as mass, so it is difficult to be cured.

In western medicine, gastrointestinal dysfunction, incomplete intestinal obstruction, pyloric obstruction, hepatosplenomegaly, visceroptosis, intestinal tuberculosis, abdominal swelling and pain, etc all can be treated based on differentiation of symptoms and signs referencing this syndrome.

〔Causes of Disease and Pathogenesis〕

Occurrence of accumulation and aggregation have a process of gradual production and development. emotional disturbance, impairment of improper diet, attack of excess of Qi and weakness after illness, or lack of treatment and delayed treatment of jaundice, hypochondial pain, malaria lead to protracted illness and injury of the liver and spleen, incoordination between viscera, stagnation of Qi, blood stasis in the interior, or with stagnation of phlegm and dampness forming accumulation and aggregation. Occurence of accumulation and aggregation is related mainly with the liver and spleen. Generally speaking, aggregation syndrome is caused mainly by stagnation of Qi, and accumulation syndrome by retention of blood stasis, but the both may be accompanied by phlegm and dampness. Because Qi and blood are correlated each other, protracted stagnation of Qi can induce blood stasis, and failure of removing blood stasis also can cause stagnation of Qi, so, accumulation and aggregation have differences and correlation in pathogenesis. Protracted aggregation syndrome induces often accumulation syndrome; unability to remove accumulation syndrome often occurs distending pain. In addition, protracted accumulation and aggregation can induce dysfunction of the liver and spleen, leading to deficiency of vital Qi. Therefore, this syndrome is often excess syndrome at inlitial stage, and often deficiency syndrome at chronic stage, or deficiency with excess. Causes of disease and pathogenesis of accumulation and aggregation syndromes are discussed in the following.

Ⅰ. Emotional disturbance, stagnation of Qi and blood stasis: melancholy and over thinking impair the liver and spleen. Injury of the liver induces stagnation of Qi. Qi is the commander of blood, protracted stagnation of Qi can induce blood stasis. After prolonged stagnation of Qi and blood stasis can form accumulation and aggregation; injury of the spleen causes dysfunction in transporting and transforming nutrients, failure of food producing nutrients forms phlegm pathogen, obstruction of blood vessels by phlegm pathogen results in unfree flow of blood, stasis of phlegm and blood leads to accumulation and aggregation in the Abdomen.

Ⅱ. Improper diet, production of phlegm pathogen: over drinking, or eating over fat, sweet, fried, pungent and hot food; or improper diet, over hungry or full, inregular daily life induce injury of the spleen and stomach, dysfuction in transporting and transforming nutriets, leading to production of dampness pathogen in body and coagulation of phlegm, and phlegm causing stagnation of Qi. Incoordination between Qi and blood, and interraction of Qi, blood and phlegm form accumulation and aggregation in the abdomen.

Ⅲ. Attack of pathogenic factors, and retention of pathogenic factors: Cold pathogen or damp-heat pathogen and other exopathogens invade the body, retenting in the abdomen and forming aggregation after long time, and then causing accumulation.

Ⅳ. Jaundice, hypochondial pain, malaria, infection by blood fluke, etc.: Stagnation of dampness pathogen, incoordination between Qi and blood induce incoordination between the liver and spleen, and interraction of stagnation of Qi and blood stasis and phlegm pathogens forms accumulation and aggregation in the abdomen.

To sum up, this disease and syndrome have many causes of disease, but the part of disease is mainly in the liver and spleen, and its pathlogical changes are closely related with stagnation of Qi, blood stasis and coagulation of phlegm. Formation of the syndrome also is closely related to strength and weakness of vital Qi. Generally, at initial stage, it is often caused by stagnation of Qi, retention of dampness and blood stasis; at chronic stage, it is often caused by interaction of phlegm retention and blood stasis, and deficiency of vital Qi. Dysfunction of the liver and spleen, or burning injury of blood vessels by heat retention may induce bleeding; retention of damp-heat in the middle-Jiao invades the liver and gallbladder, jaundice may occur; retention of water and dampness may induce fullness and swelling in the abdomen, and other syndromes.

Diagram of Causes of Disease and Pathogenesis of Mass in the abdomen

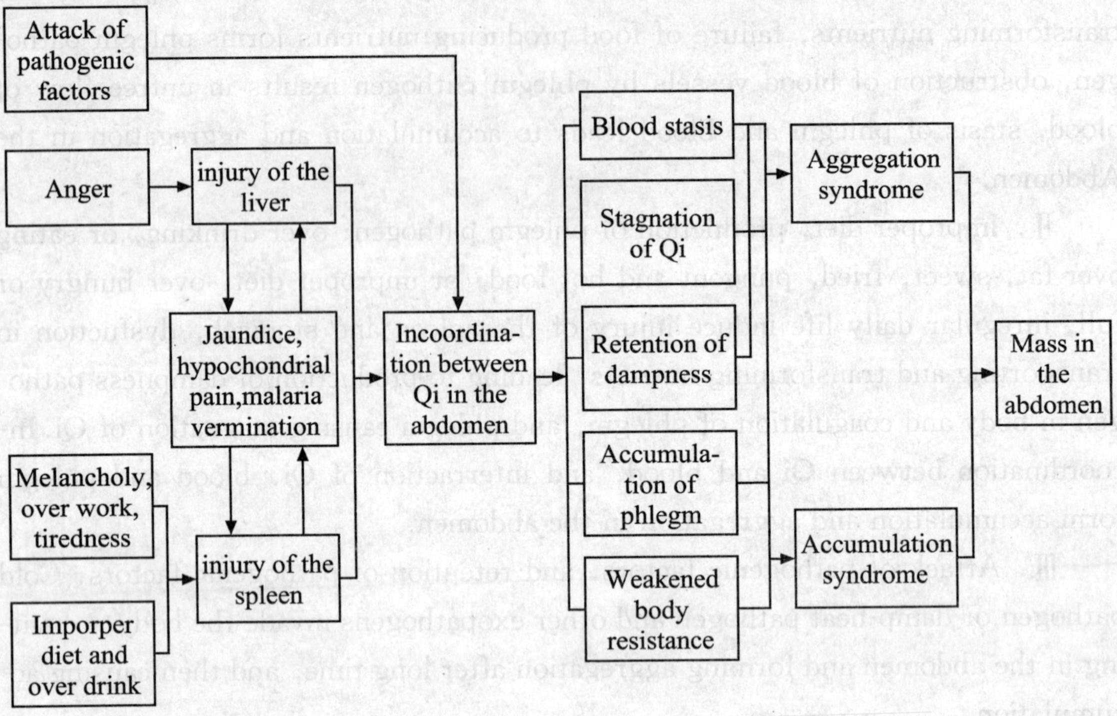

〔Treatment Based on Differentiation of Symptoms and Signs〕

Accumulation and aggregation attack and develop often slowly, and they are related and transformed with jaundice, hypochondrial pain, malaria, vermination, tympanites, and other syndromes each other. Accumulation and aggregation are difficult to be absolutely differentiated at initial stage. So, they should be divided into three stages, initial, middle and late stages according to duration of disease, characteristics of syndrome, pathological changes, and then give treatment based on differentiation of symptoms and signs. In differentiation of symptoms and signs, should differentiate over stagnation of Qi, over blood stasis, over accumulation of phlegm, retention of food, over coagulation of phlegm, or over vital deficiency, and should combine with parts of accumulation and aggregation, in the abdomen or in hypochondrium.

Ⅰ. Main Points of Differentiation of Symptoms and Signs

(1) Differentiation of initial, middle and late stages: At initial stage occurrence of accumulation and aggregation, and diseases of the liver and spleen are

caused by stagnation of Qi, blood stasis and retention of dampness. Retention in abdomen belongs to injury of the spleen and stomach and it is caused by stagnation of Qi, food retention, retention of dampness as main; retention in hypochondrium belongs to injury of the liver and spleen and it is caused mainly by stagnation of Qi and blood stasis. At the middle stage, stagnation of Qi and blood stasis, accumulation of dampness into phlegm, coagulation of Qi, blood and phlegm into mass in the abdomen or in the hypochondrium. At the latter stage, pathogenic factors do not decline and vital Qi has had impaired, deficiency of vital Qi, and excessive pathogens, so it belongs deficiency in origin and excess in superficiality.

(2) Differentiation of in Qi or in blood, and belonging to dampness, phlegm or deficiency; at the initial stage, often seen stagnation of Qi, marked by distending pain as main, with no fixed part. At chronic stage, it attackes collaterals, marked by blood stasis, with a fixed pain part and touchable mass, often being hard in property. Disease of the spleen easily produces dampness pathogen, marked by fullness in the stomach, disgestion, loose stool, dull complexion, lassitude of limbs. Protracted retention of dampness coagulates into phlegm, marked by expectoration, or swelling distention with a shape, thicker in size, movable as touching it. Protracted retention of pathogenic factors exhausts vital Qi, manifesting Yin-deficiency of Qi, deficiency of Qi and blood, or deficiency of Yang-Qi.

Ⅱ. Differentiation of Mass in the Abdomen, Mass at the Right Hypochondrium and Tympanites

Accumulation and aggregation are marked by mass in the abdomen with distention or pain. Aggregation can form or resolve, and accumulation has a shape with no resolution for long time.

Mass at the right hypochondrium is marked by feeling of fullness in the chest and upper abdomen, with no shape. It has differences of deficiency and excess syndromes, being deficiency before meal, hunger, and being excess after meal, fullness.

Tympanites is marked by enlargement of abdominal distention, pale-yellow skin, exposition of blood vessels in the abdominal skin. Tympantes has differences of Qi tympanites, blood tympanites, water tympanites, tympanites due to parasitic infestation, but it is characterised by unique water-vibrated sound, or like abdomen-pressed capsel filling water, and it is developed from accumulation and aggregation due to lack of treatment and delayed treatment.

Ⅲ. Main Points of Therapeutic Principle

(1) According to the law of clinical changes for mass in the abdomen, at initial stage, it is caused often by stagnation of Qi, food retention, blood stasis and retention of dampness, promoting the flow of Qi, promoting digestion and relaxing the bowels, activating circulation of blood, removing dampness should be uesd as main methods; at middle stage, it is caused often by stagnation of Qi, blood stasis, accumulation of phlegm, promoting the flow of Qi, removing blood stasis and clearing away phlegm should be used as main methods; at late stage, excess of pathogen and deficiency of vital Qi are often seen, so strengthening the body resistance to eliminate pathogenic factors, reinforcement and elimination in combination should be adopted.

(2) Protracted mass in the abdomen impairs Qi and blood, so in treatment should protect vital Qi, and should not use over amount of drugs resolving mass, for avoiding injury of vital Qi.

(3) Because aggregation is milder that accumulation, aggregation syndrome is in the Qi system, regulating Qi is main method for its treatment, and accumulation syndrome is in the blood system, activating circulation of blood should be main method. Therapeutic effects is more easily attained for aggregation syndrome and accumulation syndrome is difficult to be cured.

Ⅳ. Classification of Syndromes and Treatment

(1) Initial stage

Main symptoms: Distenting pain in the abdomen, Qi aggregates or disperses with emotional change.

Accompanying symptoms: Anorexia, nausea, even vomiting of phlegm and saliva, constipation, distention and fullness sensation in the hypochondrium.

Tongue and pulse: Dark tongue with white and greasy fur, taut and slippery pulse.

Analysis: incoordination between Qi and blood, infree circulation of Qi and blood, stagnation of Qi and blood in the abdomen induce distention and pain in the abdomen, and aggregation of Qi; emotional change induces disorder of Qi, so state of syndrome exacerbates. Ease of mind causes free flow of Qi. Injury of both the liver and spleen, dysfunction in transporting and transforming nutrients, production of pathogenic dampnes in interior, checking ascending and descending function of Qi, so occur anorexia and nausea, even vomiting of phlegm and saliva, constipation, or distention and fullness sensation in the hypochondrium. Infree circulation of Qi and blood results in dark tongue, retention of pathogenic dampness in the interior induces greasy fur. Taut and slippery pulse are sings of incoordination between the liver and spleen.

Therapeutic principle: regulating Qi and activating circulation of blood, eliminating dampness and resolving aggregation.

Prescription: Modified Mu Xiang Shun Qi Powder. In the prescription, more drugs of regulaing Qi are used for regulating functional activity of Qi in the three Jiao. Fruit of citron or trifoliate orange for the upper-Jiao; aucklandia root, tangerine peel and green tangerine orange peel for the middle-Jiao; sichuan chinaberry and lindera root for the lower-Jiao. Functional activity of Qi is strengthened, so distention and pain disappear and aggregation of Qi is dispersed. Chuanxiong rhizome is a herb for regulating Qi in blood and nutgrass flatsedge is a herb for promoting circulation of blood. The both are used in combination for regulating Qi and blood. Amomun fruit and atractylodes rhizome can remove dampness and promote function of the spleen. A small amount of bark of Chinese cassia tree can resolve aggregation and relieve pain. For the patient with serious stagnation of the liver-Qi, marked by more severe distention and fullness sansation in the hypochondium, upleurum root, red peony root, curcumaa root or turmeria rhizoma can be added for strengthening action of soothing the liver and regulating Qi, or it is treated with Chai Hu Shu Gan Powder. For the patient with vomiting more phlegm and saliva, Xiao Ban Xia plus Fu Ling Decoction are used in combination, or Ling Gui Zhu Gan Decoction is used in combination; for production of heat induced by retention of fluid, Gan Sui Ban Xia Decoction can be used in combination; for the patient with dry mouth and bitter taste, redish margin and tip of tongue with thin, yellowish and greasy fur, Zuo Jin Pill can be added for clearing away heat in the liver; for food retention, stagnation of dampness, and unfree flow of Qi of Fu-organs, Liu Mo Yin can be selected. In the prescription, rhubarb, fruit of immature citron or trifoliate orange, betel nut are used for removing stagnation and relaxing the bowels; eagle wood, aucklandia root and lindera root for promoting flow of Qi; for the patient complicated with stagnation of phlegm, Ban Xia Hou Po Decoction can be used in combination. In the prescription, magnolia bark, purple perilla can promote circulation of Qi and alleviate stagnation in the middle-Jiao; pinellia tuber and poria can eliminate phlegm and resolve mass; for protracted disease with obvious blood stasis and dark tongue with ecchymosis, Shi Xiao Powder can be used in combination; for long duration of disease, excess of the liver and deficiency of the spleen, mental tiredness and loose stool, dangshen and white peony root can be added for supplementing Qi and strengthening the spleen.

Example of prescription: 10g fried fruit of citron or trifoliate orange, 10g aucklandia root, 6g green tangerine orange peel, 6g tangerine peel, 10g lindera root, 10g Chuanxiong rhizome, 10g prepared nutgrass flatsedge rhizome, 10g pinellia tuber, 10g atractylodes rhizome, 3g amomum fruit, 10g magnolia bark, 12g fried red peony root.

(2) Middle stage

Main symptoms: Mass in the abdomen with immobilization and fixation part of distending pain.

Accompanied symptoms: Darkish complexion and emaciation, anorexia, viscous phlegm, cold and heat now and then, squamous and dry skin and amenorrhea for women.

Tongue and pulse: blue-purple tongue proper, or ecchymosis on the tongue, with greasy fur, taut pulse, slippery or fine and uneven pulse.

Analysis: Protracted aggregation of Qi forms gradually accumulation syndrome, stagnacy of Qi, blood stasis and coagulation of phlegm in the abdomen, hence mass in the abdomen with immobilization, and fixation part of distending pain. Incoordination between the liver and spleen, infree circulation of Qi and blood, dysfunction in transport and transformation, insuficiency of nutrients, induce drakish complexion and general thin, anorexia and viscous phlegm, squamous and dry skin. Stagnacy of Qi, blood stasis and incoordination between the Ying and Wei, result in cold and heat now and then. Stagnation of the liver-Qi and blood stasis leads to amenorrhea for women. Blue-purple tongue proper with ecchymosis, fine and uneven pulse all are signs of blood stasis and stagnacy of Qi. Greasy fur on the tongue markes retention of phelgm turbit in the interior; taut and slippery pulse are signs of incoordination between the liver and the spleen.

Therapeutic principle: Promoting circulation of Qi and blood, resolving phlegm and removing stagnation of Qi.

Prescription: Modified Ge Xia Zhu Yu Decoction. In the prescription, dried rehmannia root is deducted from Tao Hong Si Wu Decoction and moutan bark is added for strengthening power of nourishing blood and actvating blood circulation, resolving masses and removing stagnation of Qi. Trogopterus dung for removing blood stasis to relieve pain, fruit of citron or trifoliate orange, lindera root for regulating functional activity of Qi; nutgrass flatsedge rhizome and corydalis tuber for promoting flow of Qi to relieve pain, flow of Qi promotes blood circulation, strengthening power of removing blood stasis; pinellia tuber, fritillary bulb, red tangerine peel, poria, burreed tuber, zedoary can be added for strengthening function of resolving phlegm and removing masses.

For the patients of accumulation and aggregation syndromes with cold and heat, pantalgia, white fur on the tongue, floating pulse and so on, who are affected by exopathogenic wind and cold, the therapeutic principles of dispelling the superficial syndrome and regulating Qi, and removing stagnation and accumulation should be adopted, and Wu Ji Powder can be used. The prescription joints the drugs for relieving exterior syndrome, dispelling cold, removing dampnees, resolving phlegm, promoting flow of Qi, diuresis, promoting blood circulation, dredging colletaral, warming the middle-Jiao and relieving pain, which can treat simunitaneously disease involving both exterior and interior, which is induced by dysfunction of Qi activity with affection by exopathogenic factors at early stage of accumulation and aggregation with affection by exopathogenic factors, and syndromes due to retention of many pathogenic factors in the abdomen.

For the patients of more severe stagnation of Qi and blood stasis, accompanied by cold sign, Da Qi Qi Decoction can be used, in which green tangerine orange peel, tangerine peel, root of balloon flower, nutgrass flatsedge rhizome, wrinkled giant-hyssop can promote flow of Qi to resolve masses; bark of Chinese cassia tree, burreed tuber, zedoary can remove obstruction of small boold vessels by warmness, and soften and resolving hard masses.

The patient with hard mass and tendeness can take Bie Jia Pill for removing blood stasis and shorftening hard mass and relieving pain; The patient of amenorrhea, and squamous and dry skin can take Da Huang Zhe Chong Pill for removing blood stasis and removing accumulation and dredging channels. The above two prescriptions and Liu Jun Zi Decoction can take alternately for invigorating Qi of the spleen and stomach, which is a method of reinforcement and elimination in combination. At the stage, there are more severe stagnation of Qi, blood stasis and coagulation of phlegm, gradual enlargement of mass, with hardness and pain, such insect drugs for removing blood stasis and accumulation as ground beetle, pillb driedug, fresh-water turtle shell, oyster shell, sargassum, etc. can be used for elevating therapeutic effects.

For enlargment of masses, with burnibing heat and pain, reddish tongue with yellowish fur, heat-clearing and detoxifying drugs such as forsythia fruit, dandelion herb, barbat skullcap, lyrate nightshade, oldenlandia, etc. can be added. For more severe phlegm turbit, dried coix seed, trichosanthes fruit, fritillary bulb, pinellia tuber, airpotato yam, etc. drugs for removing phlegm and resolving masses can be added.

Example of prescription: 10g whole Chinese angelica root, 10g red peony root, 10g white peony root, 10g chuanxiong rhizome, 10g peach kernel, 6g safflower, 6g burred tuber, 6g zedoary, 10g green tangerine orange peel, 10g tangerine peel, 10g moutan bark, 10g fritillary bulb, 10g pinellia tuber, and 15g poria.

Main symptoms: Hard, enlarged and firm mass gradually, lingering retention of mass in the abdomen, increasingly violent pain.

Accompanying symptoms: Sallow or dark complexion, a greatly reduced appetite, emaciation, lassitude and weakness, dry mouth and tongue, feverish sensation in the five centers, palpitation, dream-disturbed sleep or insomnia, or aversion to cold, cold limbs, clear urine and loose stool.

Tongue and pulse: Thin red tongue with less tongue coating or glossy red tongue without coating, or with ecchymosis on the tongue; or light purple and enlarged tongue with thin greasy coating, and taut thready pulse or deep thready pulse.

Analysis: At this stage, anti-pathogenic qi deficiency and accumulation of blood stasis. Lingering retention of mass and protracted stagnation of phlegm and blood stasis in the body cause hard, enlarged and firm mass gradually, and pain increasingly violent.

Retention of blood stasis prevents the production of new blood leading to insufficient nutrient qi; its symptom is sallow or dark complexion. This also damages the spleen qi in transportation and transformation, then appetite is reduced, emaciation, lassitude and weakness result. Dry mouth and tongue, feverish sensation in five centers are resulted from deficiency of yin. Palpitation, dream-disturbed sleep can be seen in patient with insufficiency of both qi and blood. Aversion to cold, cold limbs, loose stool and clear urine are the signs of decline of yang qi. The picture of deficiency of both qi and yin with accumulation of blood stasis shows thin red tongue with less tongue coating or glossy red tongue without coating, or with ecchymosis on the tongue, and a taut thready pulse. The indication of depletion of both qi and blood or great decline of yang qi with retention of blood coagulation is light purple and enlarged tongue with thin greasy coating, and deep thready pulse.

Therapeutic principle: Strengthening the body resistance to eliminate pathogenic factors.

Prescription: Ba Zhen Decoction combined with Hua Ji Pill. In the former, Si Jun Zi Decoction and Si Wu Decoction are used for invigorating Qi and blood, and in the later, nutgrass flatsedge rhizome, sappan wood, trogopterus dung are used for regulating Qi and removing stasis; and burreed tuber, zedoary, asafetida, pumice, etc., for sorftening and resolving hard mass. The two prescriptions are used in combination for strengthening the body resistance to eliminate pathogenic factors, and treating both the principal and the secondary aspects of a disease at the same time.

For the patient with deficiency of both Qi and Yin, manifesting as obvious deficiency-fire, Ba Zhen Decoction could be replaced by Yi Wei Decoction and pseudostellaria root, siberian solomonseal rhizome and other drugs for invigorating Qi and nourishing Yin are added. For decline of Yang-Qi and production of Yin-cold in the interior, it is used in combination with Fu Zi Li Zhong Decoction, for increasing the power of warming the middle-Jiao and strengthening the spleen, For weak spleen and strong stomach, and cold-spleen and heat stomach, and biter mouth and yellowish fur on the tongue, loose stool and weak pulse, Ban Xia Xie Xin Decoction or Wen Pi Decoction could be used for treatment. For protracted disease involving the kidney, deficiency of both Yin and Yang, lassitude in loin and knee, dizziness, aversion to cold, tonifying both Yin and Yang should be adopted with Bu Tian Da Zhao Pill and Hua Ji Pill are used alternately.

For Accumulation syndrome, no matter short or long duration of disease, external treatment can be used in combination. At present, clinically, A Wei Gao or Shui Hong Hua Gao are generally applied for promoting resolving accumulation and removing stasis.

Example of prescription: 3g ginseng powder, 10g poria, 10g fried bighead atractylodes rhizome, 10g whole Chinese angelica root, 10g red peony root, 10g white peony root, 10g chuanxiong rhizome, 6g burreed tuber, 6g zedoary, 10g prepared nutgrass flatsedge rhizome, 10g fried trogopterus dung, 10g fresh cattail pollen, 3g notoginseng powder.

〔Measures of Prevention and Nursing Care〕

1. Stable mention, avoid restlessness, deppress and anger.

2. Regular diet, abstain from peppery, greasy and sweet, fried food, do not drink wine.

3. Pay attention to personal hygiene and enviromental hygiene, for prevention from invasion of exopathogenic factors.

4. Actively treat jaundice, hypocondrial pain, mass in the abdomen, and schistosomiasis, etc.

〔Analysis of Typical Case〕

Case 1, Lu XX, female, aged 40 years, presented herself first visit on 7 July, 1976.

She found suddenly a small mass on the left lower abdomen several months ago, which gradually enlarged, and it had a size like an egg. Examination found that general weekness, shortness of breath when motion, distending pain on the hypochondium and lower abdomen on both sides, anorexia, loose stool 2～3 times each day, frequent belching, spontaneous perspiration, aversion to cold, pale tongue with less fur, taut and fine pulse.

Diagnosis of traditional Chinese medicine: Mass in the abdomen (stagnation of the liver-Qi and deficiency of the spleen).

Therapeutic principle: Soothing the liver and regulating the circulaton of Qi, warming Yang and strengthening the spleen.

Prescription: 9g bupleurum root, 12g white peony root, 9g fruit of immature citron or trifoliate orange, 9g nutgrass flatsedge rhizome, 9g dangshen, 9g bighead atractylodes rhizome, 9g poria, 6g common fennel fruit, 9g magnolia bark, 6g aucklandia root, 12g charcoal of sichuan chinaberry, 3g liquorice.

The second visit: After the above prescription was took four doses, belching alleviated, appetite increased, and then litchi seed and tangerine seed were added.

The third visit: After took 8 doses, the mass in the left lower abdomen was resolved completely and following taking several doses, appetite recoveried gradually to normal, without symptoms of shortness of breath, spontaneous persipiration, and aversion to cold, etc., and following-up did not find relapse.

Note: Mass in the abdomen in differentiation of syndrome belongs hyperactive liver-Qi attacking the spleen, stagnation of the liver-Qi and deficiency of the spleen, treatment should adopt therapeutic princples of soothing the liver and regulating the circulation of Qi, warming Yang and strengthening the spleen, with bupleurum root, white peony root, fruit of immature citron ot trifoliate orange, nutgrass flatsedge rhizome, charcoal of sichaun chinaberry are used for soothing the liver and regulating the circulation of Qi, and dangshen, bighead stractylodes rhizome, poria, liquorice for tonifying the spleen, and common fennel fruit, magnolia bark, aucklandia root for dredging the lower abdomen with warming, and ictchi seed and tangerine seed were added for strengthening the power of resolving masses in the lower abdomen. The above drugs carried commonly out the functions, so that stagnation of the liver-Qi was removed, and the spleen was strengthened. (LI Si CHi' Medical Records)

Accumulation and aggregation are referred to mass in the abdomen, or distension or pain. There is a form with fixed position and fixed pain part for accumulation; and there is no form and wandering pain for aggregation. The causitive factors are for accumulation and aggregation are mainly mental upsets, improper diet, pathogenic attacking and jaundice, hypochondail pain, malaria, and schistosomiasis can turn to accumulation and aggregation syndromes. Its pathological pathogenic factors are stagnation of Qi, blood stasis, and coagulation of phlegm, and deficiency of vital-Qi is internal factors of attacking.

Clinically, should pay attention to differentiation of mass and tympanites. Mass is characterized by spontaneous discomfort due to fullness in the stomach with no shape, and tympanites are characterized by abdominal distension and fullness, pale and explosion of small blood vessel on the abdomen.

In treatment, the method of regulating Qi should mainly be used for aggregation syndrome and the method of regulating blood for accumulation syndrome, which can be divided into three stages, early, middle and later stages for treatment. The drugs for removing stasis and resolving mass are often used to enimilate excess, but for accumulation and aggregation, the vital-Qi is certainly deficiency and often are deficiency accomanied with excess, or excess with deficiency, so, in the treatment, should correctly treat relationship among the "vital-Qi", "eliminate"and "tonifying".

Questions for Review

1. What is the conception of accumulation and aggregation? What relationship is

there between the accumulation and mass?

2. What is the pathogenic key of accumulation and aggregation? Which Zang- and Fu-organs are closely related to accumulation and aggregation syndromes?
3. Try to discuss laws of differentiation of syndrome and treatment for the accumulation and aggregation syndromes.
4. Try to discuss relationship of accumulation and aggregation syndromes with jaundice, hypochondrial pain, tympanites?

Tympanites

〔General Description〕

Tympanites means abdominal distention. Hollow inside and tense outside, the abdomen is beaten like a drum. Tympanites is clinically characterized by abdominal distention, sallow skin, blood vessels seen, mass in the hypochondria or abdomen, and thin limbs. In ancient literature, there are a lot of names for the disease. According to its etiology, pathology and clinical manifestations, ancient people divided the disease into tympanites due to stagnation of qi, tympanites due to blood stasis, ascites, and tympanites due to parasitic infestation. The disease lingers for a long time, and is difficult to be cured. Hematemesis, hemafecia and coma will appear at its late stage.

The disease is mainly ascites due to cirrhosis in western medicine. In addition, ascites due to tubercular peritonitis or tumor in the abdomen, similar to symptoms of tympanites, can be diagnosed and treated in reference to this article.

〔Etiology and Pathology〕

Tympanites occurs slowly. Although related to improper diet, emotional depression and schistosomiasis, the disease is directly caused by dysfunction of the liver, spleen and kidney and by stagnation of qi, blood and water in the abdomen due to no treatment or mistreatment of jaundice, hypochondriac pain and abdominal mass for a long time.

A. Direct Cause

Lingering jaundice, hypochondriac pain and abdominal mass cause tympanites.

Pathological changes of jaundice mainly are yang jaundice and yin jaundice. Yang jaundice is always caused by disorder of qi and by incoordination between the liver and spleen due to stagnation of damp-heat in the middle jiao. Yin jaundice is caused by obstruction of cold-dampness, or by stagnation of blood stasis, or by deficiency of the spleen and blood. Obstruction of cold-dampness or stagnation of blood stasis can cause disorder of qi in the middle jiao and accumulation of dampness, leading to impairment of the liver and spleen. Deficiency of the spleen and blood and failure to transport and transform nutrients cause stagnation of dampness and disorder of qi, giving rise to impairment of the liver and spleen. Treated improperly for a long time, impairment of liver and spleen causes dysfunction of the kidney and retention of water, leading to stagnation of qi, blood and water.

Pathology of hypochondriac pain can be summarized as stagnation of blood stasis, stagnation of the liver-qi, damp-heat in the liver and gallbladder, and deficiency of the liver-yin. The first three can cause dysfunction of the liver, disorder of qi, invasion of the spleen by hyperactive liver-qi, failure of the spleen to transport and transform nutrients, and retention of dampness. Untreated promptly, the disease will affect the kidney, eventually causing impairment of the liver, spleen and kidney, and stagnation of qi, blood and water. Deficiency of the liver-yin can cause malnutrition of the liver, incoordination between channels, disorder of qi, and incoordination between the liver and spleen. Lingering deficiency of the liver-yin can also cause deficiency of the kidney-yin. Yin deficiency of the liver and kidney, if treated improperly, will eventually lead to impairment of the liver, spleen and kidney, and stagnation of qi, blood and water.

Main pathological manifestations of abdominal mass are impairment of the liver and spleen, incoordination between visceral organs, stagnation of qi, stagnation of blood stasis, stagnation of phlegm-dampness, and indigestion. If treated improperly for a long time, the disease will cause dysfunction of the kidney and retention of water, eventually leading to stagnation of qi, blood and water.

B. Predisposing Cause

(A) Emotional Depression: Anxiety, anger, dysfunction of the liver and stagnation of qi cause hypochondriac pain and blood stasis. Stagnation of qi and blood cause abdominal mass. Lingering hypochondriac pain and abdominal mass cause tympanites.

(B) Improper Diet: Over-drinking and over-eating fatty and sweet food cause impairment of the spleen and stomach, failure to transport and transform nutrients, stagnation of dampness in the middle jiao, and invasion of the skin by bile to form jaundice. In addition, accumulation of dampness into phlegm, stagnation of phlegm in qi system, incoordination between qi and blood, and stagnation of qi, blood and phlegm in the abdomen form mass. Lingering jaundice and hypochondriac pain cause tympanites.

(C) Schistosomiasis: Obstruction of channels by schistosome, incoordination between the liver and spleen and between qi and blood, failure of the spleen to transport and transform nutrients cause phlegm. Stagnation of qi, blood stasis, and accumulation of phlegm form abdominal mass, leading to tympanites.

If emotion is not regulated and diet is not restricted or the patient is infected with schistosome, tympanites will be further aggravated.

In the process of forming tympanites, qi stagnation, blood stasis, and water retention are cause and result to one another, forming the main contents of excessive pathogen. Weakened body resistance is an inevitable trend for the development of qi stagnation, blood stasis and water retention, mainly involving the liver, spleen and kidney. Tympanites is a complicated syndrome with deficiency in origin and excess in superficiality.

〔Diagnosis and Treatment〕

A. Key Points for Differentiating Symptoms

Tympanites is a complicated syndrome with deficiency in origin and excess in superficiality. Excess in superficiality has its stress on qi stagnation, blood stasis or water retention. Deficiency in origin has its stress on deficiency of the spleen-qi, deficiency of qi and yin, deficiency of the spleen-yang, deficiency of the spleen and kidney or yin deficiency of the liver and kidney. Therefore, although the main symptom is abdominal distention, there are differences in clinical manifestations. Qi stagnation is often accompanied with hypochondriac distention, sigh, eructation, bitter taste in the mouth, and taut pulse. Abdominal distention can be slightly alleviated after passing flatus. Blood stasis is often accompanied with thin limbs, vessels seen in the abdomen, mass in the hypochondria or abdomen, darkish complexion, vascular nevus in cheeks, chest and arms, squamous and dry skin, liver palm, darkish lips and nails, and ecchymosis on tongue edge. Water retention is often accompanied with abdominal distension, water-vibrating sound in the abdomen, lassitude all over the body, scanty urine and loose stool. Deficiency of the spleen-qi is often accompanied with sallow complexion, lassitude, anorexia, pale tongue and slow pulse. Deficiency of qi and yin is often accompanied with deficiency of the spleen-qi, thirst with no desire to drink, hunger with no desire to eat, thinness, dysphoria with feverish sensation in chest, palms and soles, dry and hot skin, and red thin tongue with scanty saliva. Deficiency of the spleen-yang is often accompanied with sallow complexion, aversion to cold, cold limbs, loose stool, pale enlarged tongue, and deep, thready and powerless pulse. Yang deficiency of the spleen and kidney is often accompanied with cold pain in the waist and knees, damp-cold scrotum, impotence, premature ejaculation, and delayed and scanty menstruation. Yin deficiency of the liver and kidney is often accompanied with dizziness, tinnitus, lassitude in loin and knees, insomnia due to vexation, red cheeks, epistaxis, red tongue with scanty fur, and taut and thready pulse.

B. Distinguishing Tympanites from Edema

It is very difficult to distinguish tympanites from edema at their late stage. However, tympanites and edema at their early stage can be clearly distinguished as follows:

name of disease / distinguish	tympanites	edema
distension	stiffness and fullness sensation in the enlarged abdomen, normal or thin limbs	swelling face and limbs, flat and soft abdomen
accompanying symptoms	vessels seen in the abdomen, vascular nevus in the neck and chest, hematemesis, hemafecia, jaundice, fever, dysphoria, coma	oppressed feeling in the chest, palpitation, dyspnea, nausea, vomiting, dysphoria, lethargy
location of disease	liver, spleen, kidney	lung, spleen, kidney
pathology	qi stagnation, blood stasis and water retention in the abdomen, weakened body resistance	retained water in the skin

name of disease / distinguish	tympanites	edema
therapeutic principle	regulating the flow of qi to yeliminate distention, promoting blood circulation to remove blood stasis, promoting diuresis to dispel retained water, strengthening the body resistance and restoring normal function of the body to consolidate the constitution	inducing diaphoresis, inducing diuresis, purgation, strengthening the spleen, warming the kidney, removing blood stasis
commonly used recipes	Mu Xiang Shun Qi Pill, Zhong Man Fen Xiao Pill, Tiao Ying Decoction	Yue Bi Jia Zhu Decoction, Shu Zao Decoction, Wu Ling Powder, Shen Ling Bai Zhu Powder

C. Key Points for Therapeutic Principle

Tympanites due to qi stagnation should be treated with drugs of regulating the flow of qi to eliminate distension. Tympanites due to blood stasis should be treated with drugs of promoting blood circulation to remove blood stasis. Tympanites due to water retention should be treated with drugs of promoting diuresis to dispel retained water. Tympanites due to weakened body resistance should be treated with drugs of strengthening the body resistance and restoring normal function of the body to consolidate the constitution. It is appropriate to eliminate pathogen at the early stage, and to purge and nourish simultaneously at middle and late stages. The key point is to induce diuresis and eliminate distension at middle stage and to prevent and treat serious accompanying symptoms at late stage.

D. Diagnosis and Treatment at Different Stages

According to course of illness and relation between vital energy and pathogenic factor, tympanites is divided into early, middle and late stages. Symptoms at early stage mainly are incoordination between the liver and spleen, qi stagnation, blood stasis and dampness obstruction in the abdomen. No treatment or mistreatment at early stage will make vital qi to be gradually impaired and the disease enter middle stage with symptoms of weakened body resistance and excessive pathogen. At late stage, vital qi gradually depletes, serious accompanying symptoms appear one after another, and pathological changes are interwoven and complicated.

Schematic Diagram for Etiology and Pathogenesis of Tympanites

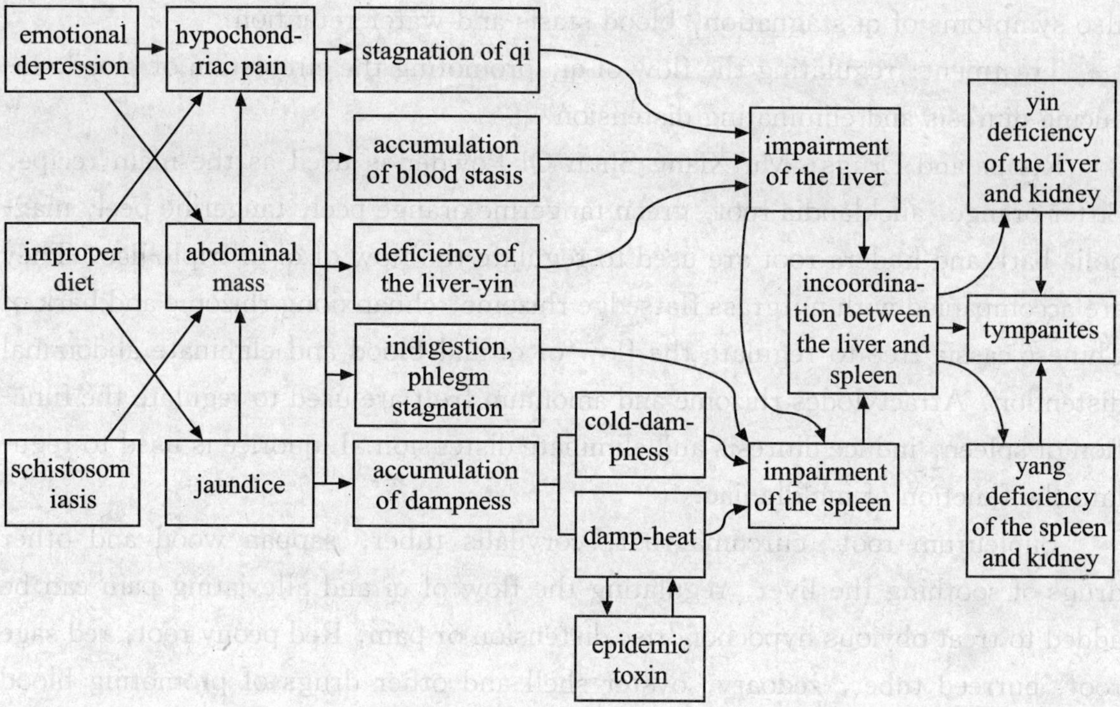

(A) Diagnosis and Treatment at Early Stage

Main Symptom: distended abdomen is beaten like a drum. The main symptom is not alleviated for a long time.

Accompanying Symptoms: hypochondriac distending pain, anorexia, lassitude and scanty urine. Abdominal distension is aggravated after meal and alleviated after eructation and passing flatus.

Tongue and Pulse: darkish tongue or with ecchymosis, white and greasy fur, and taut and slippery pulse.

Analysis: Jaundice, hypochondriac pain and abdominal mass, if untreated or mistreated, will cause incoordination between the liver and spleen, stagnation of the liver-qi, failure of the spleen to transport nutrients, qi stagnation, blood stasis and water retention, hence abdominal distention. Serious qi stagnation and blood stasis and slight water retention make the distended abdomen beaten like a drum. Deep-rooted and serious disease lasts a long time without alleviation. Dysfunction of the liver and stagnation of qi cause hypochondriac distention or pain. Indigestion due to unhealthy spleen and stomach causes anorexia. Abdominal distension is aggravated after meal and alleviated after eructation and passing flatus. Qi stagnation and water retention cause lassitude and scanty urine. Darkish tongue or with ecchymosis, white and greasy fur, and taut and slippery pulse are also symptoms of qi stagnation, blood stasis and water retention.

Treatment: regulating the flow of qi, promoting the circulation of blood, inducing diuresis and eliminating distension.

Recipe and Drugs: Mu Xiang Shun Qi Powder is used as the main recipe. Bitter orange, aucklandia root, green tangerine orange peel, tangerine peel, magnolia bark and lindera root are used to regulate the flow of qi in triple-jiao. They are accompanied with nutgrass flatsedge rhizome, chuanxiong rhizome and bark of Chinese cassia tree to regulate the flow of qi and blood and eliminate abdominal distention. Atractylodes rhizome and amomum fruit are used to regulate the function of spleen, induce diuresis and eliminate distension. Liquorice is used to regulate the function of middle-jiao.

Bupleurum root, curcuma root, corydalis tuber, sappan wood and other drugs of soothing the liver, regulating the flow of qi and alleviating pain can be added to treat obvious hypochondriac distension or pain. Red peony root, red sage root, burreed tuber, zedoary, oyster shell and other drugs of promoting blood circulation, removing blood stasis and softening and resolving hard masses can be added to treat hypochondriac mass with prickling pain. Bao He Pill or Yue Ju Bao He Pill (decocted in wrapped form) of promoting digestion can be added to treat anorexia and distension in the stomach and abdomen after meal. Plantain seed, oriental water plantain rhizome, umbellate pore-fungus, fuling and other drugs of eliminating dampness and inducing diuresis can be added to treat lassitude and scanty urine. Morning glory seed, shell of areca nut, radish seed, macrostem onion and other drugs of sending down adverse qi, eliminating distension and resolving mass can be added to treat obvious abdominal distention.

Example of Recipe:

Fried bitter orange 10g, aucklandia root 10g, green tangerine orange peel 6g, tangerine peel 10g, magnolia bark 10g, lindera root 10g, prepared nutgrass flatsedge rhizome 10g, chuanxiong rhizome 6g, atractylodes rhizome 10g, amomum fruit 3g, shell of areca nut 10g, seed of areca nut 10g.

(B) Diagnosis and Treatment at Middle Stage

Main Symptom: serious distension, stiffness and fullness of abdomen; water-vibrating sound in motion; sunken area appearing after pressing.

Accompanying Symptoms: sallow and dim complexion, lassitude, abdominal distension, no desire to eat, thirst with no desire to drink, vascular nevus and spider nevus scatted on neck, cheeks, chest and back, vessels seen in abdomen, liver palms, constipation or loose stool, and scanty urine.

Tongue and Pulse: pale enlarged tongue with teeth-prints, or dark purple tongue with ecchymosis, thick and greasy fur, and thready and slippery pulse.

Analysis: Lingering tympanites makes more and more Qi, blood and water accumulated in the abdomen, so the abdomen becomes seriously enlarged, stiff and full, bringing unbearable sufferings to the patient. The abdomen with water retained in it produces water-vibrating sound in motion, or has a sunken area on it after pressed. Impairment of the liver, spleen and kidney by pathogen causes sallow and dim complexion and lassitude. Dysfunction of the spleen and stomach and disorder of qi cause distension of the stomach and abdomen. The patient does not dare to eat because the distension will become aggravated after eating. Water retention and indigestion cause thirst with no desire to drink, constipation or loose stool, and scanty urine. Blood stasis causes vascular nevus and spider nevus scatted on neck, cheeks, chest and back, vessels seen in abdomen, and liver palms. Pale enlarged tongue with teeth-prints, or dark purple tongue with ecchymosis, thick and greasy fur, and thready and slippery pulse are signs of dysfunction of the liver, spleen and kidney, weakened body resistance, and excessive qi, blood and water.

Treatment: strengthening the body resistance, promoting the flow of qi, removing blood stasis, inducing diuresis, and treating symptoms and causes simultaneously.

Recipe and Drugs: In a self-prescribed recipe of strengthening the body resistance and eliminating tympanites, large doses of astragalus root and Siberian solomonseal rhizome are used to reinforcing the spleen, replenish qi and strengthen the body resistance. Although the liver, spleen and kidney are impaired, the spleen and stomach should be first treated. Auchlandia root, shell of areca nut, seed of areca nut and bottle gourd peel are used to promote the flow of qi, eliminate distension and induce diuresis. Motherwort, Herba Lycopi, and princeplume ladysthumb fruit are used to promote blood circulation, remove blood stasis and eliminate dampness. Bighead atractylodes rhizome, umbellate pore-fungus, fuling, plantain seed or plantain herb are used to especially induce diuresis and eliminate dampness. All these drugs are used together to strengthen the body resistance, eliminate pathogenic factors, treat symptoms and causes simultaneously, and eliminate distension.

Dried ginger and cinnamom twig, or cinnamom bark and prepared aconite root of inspiring the spleen-yang can be added to treat obvious ascites and white and greasy fur. Oriental water plantain rhizome, red bean and tetrandra root can be also added to strengthen the effects of eliminating dampness and inducing diuresis. Oriental wormwood, smilax glabra rhizome, lysimachia and other drugs of removing damp-heat should be added to treat damp-heat and jaundice. Talc, rice-paper pith, cricket powder of inducing diuresis can be added to treat difficulty in micturition with dark urine. Straight ladybell root, fragrant solomonseal rhizome and ophiopogon root of nourishing yin and reinforcing the stomach can be added to treat deficiency of both qi and yin and pink tongue. Chinese angelica root, fleece-flower root, donkey hide gelatin and other drugs of nourishing the blood and tranquilizing the mind can be added to treat deficiency of both qi and blood, pale tongue, palpitation and insomnia. Pinellia tuber, tangerine peel, fresh ginger, bamboo shavings and other drugs of regulating the stomach and sending down the adverse flow of qi can be added to treat retention of dampness in the middle-jiao, failure of the stomach-qi to descend, nausea and vomiting. Scutellaria root and coptis root can be added to remove damp-heat in the middle-jiao. Phellodndron bark and pittosporm root can be added to remove damp-heat in the lower-jiao. For severe ascites with dyspnea, ephedra, apricot kernel and platycodon root can be added to promote the dispersing function of the lung and induce diuresis. Or mulberry bark and lepidium seed can be added to remove heat from the lung and induce diuresis. Or loquat leaf and trichosanthes peel can be added to moisten the lung and induce diuresis.

Severe ascites with no response to conventional treatment can be treated with a method of purgation and diuresis according to the following principles. (1) Severe ascites is accompanied with unbearable abdominal distension. (2) Unimpaired spleen and kidney can bear purgation. (3) The method is used until ascites decreases by 70%～80%. (4) After purgation, the spleen and stomach should be regulated to consolidate the curative effect. Commonly used recipes are Zhou Che Pill and Shi Zao Decoction.

Example of Recipe:

Stir-fried astragalus root 30g, Siberian solomonseal rhizome 30g, aucklandia root 10g, shell of areca nut 10g, bottle gourd peel 20g, motherwort 12g, princesplume ladysthumb fruit 20g, umbellate pore-fungus 20g, fuling 20g, plantain herb 30g, Folium Herba Lycopi 10g.

(C) Diagnosis and Treatment at Late Stage: Pathogen has not eliminated completely, weakened body resistance is the main cause of illness, and accompanying symptoms are coma, hematemesis and hemafecia.

1. Weakened Body Resistance and Excessive Pathogenic Factors

Main Symptoms: abdominal distension with more uncomfortable feeling in the evening than in the morning, lassitude, inclination to move, short breath, low voice, and a mere skeleton.

Accompanying Symptoms: sallow or pale complexion, cold pain in the waist and knees, aversion to cold, cold limbs, impotence, menolipsis, dysphoria with feverish sensation in chest, palms and soles, squamous and dry skin, dizziness, tinnitus, insomnia and night sweat.

Tongue and Pulse: pale tongue, white fur, deep and thready or feeble or taut pulse.

Analysis: Lingering retention of qi, blood and water impairs the spleen and kidney. Dysfunction of qi further aggravates retention of water. Uncomfortable feeling caused by abdominal distension is severer in the evening than in the morning with the vital qi weakened and strengthened. Deficiency of vital qi leads to lassitude, inclination to move, short breath and low voice. Difficulty in generation of essence and blood gives rise to a mere skeleton and sallow or pale complexion. Yin excess due to yang deficiency of the spleen and kidney causes cold pain in the waist and knees, aversion to cold, cold limbs, impotence, menolipsis, pale enlarged tongue, and deep, thready and feeble pulse. Hyperactivity of fire due to yin deficiency of the liver and kidney causes dysphoria with feverish sensation in chest, palms and soles, squamous and dry skin, dizziness, tinnitus, insomnia, night sweat, pink enlarged tongue, and deep, thready and taut pulse.

Treatment: mainly warming and recuperating the spleen and kidney, or nourishing the liver and kidney.

Recipe and Drugs: Fu Zi Li Zhong Pill and Ji Sheng Shen Qi Pill are used to warm and recuperate the spleen and kidney. Mai Wei Di Huang Pill is mainly used to nourish the liver and kidney. Fu Zi Li Zhong Pill is mainly used to warm the middle-jiao, strengthen the spleen and inspire yang in the middle-jiao. Ji Sheng Shen Qi Pill is mainly used to warm the kidney, invigorate yang, promote the flow of qi and induce diuresis. The two recipes can be used alternatively to treat yang deficiency of the spleen and kidney. Mai Wei Di Huang Pill can nourish yin in the liver, spleen and kidney simultaneously.

Weakened body resistance should not be treated quickly but slowly. Superficiality-treating method should not be used in order to avoid further impairing vital qi. Due to predisposing cause, weakened body resistance can become syndrome of deficiency in origin and excess in superficiality, which should be treated moderately.

Example of Recipe:

Stir-fried aconite root 6g, baked ginger 5g, dangshen 10g, dried rehmannia root 10g, prepared rehmannia root 10g, dogwood fruit 10g, fuling 15g, oriental water plantain rhizome 10g, red sage root 10g, parched bighead atractylodes rhizome 10g, Chinese yam 10g.

2. Hematemesis and Hemafecia

Main Symptom: in mild case, vomiting with fresh blood or blood clot, or darkish feces; in severe case, serious hematemesis or dark red loose stool.

Accompanying Symptoms: bitter taste in dry mouth, burning heat in the stomach, bowel sound, abdominal distension, palpitation, short breath, perspiration, and cold limbs.

Tongue an Pulse: reddish yellow or pale tongue, taut, slippery and rapid or deep, thready and rapid pulse.

Analysis: incoordination between the liver and spleen, heat due to lingering stagnation of qi in the middle-jiao, and oppression of blood vessels by heat cause hematemesis, hemafecia, bitter taste in dry mouth, burning heat in the stomach, bowel sound and abdominal distention.

Deficiency of qi and blood causes palpitation, short breath, perspiration and cold limbs. Red tongue, yellow fur, and taut and slippery pulse are signs of excessive heat in the middle-jiao. Pale tongue and deep, thready and rapid pulse are signs of depletion of qi and blood.

Treatment: Patients with depletion of qi and blood should be treated with drugs of supplementing qi and inducing astringency to purge heat, calm vessels, remove heat from blood and stop bleeding.

Recipe and Drugs: Paste made from rhubarb powder 2g and hyacinth bletilla powder 6～9g with cool boiled water is taken 2～3 times a day. Fierce hematemesis and hemafecia with focus around the cardia can be treated in this way: A tri-cavity tube is inserted into the stomach, the stomach-balloon is inflated, half dosage of powder of rhubarb and hyacinth bletilla is swallowed, and esophagus-balloon is inflated to strengthen the styptic effect.

For depletion of qi and blood, respiration and cold limbs, ginseng powder 3g can be added to the above-mentioned recipe to supplement qi and induce astringency, or Huang Tu Decoction can be taken.

Example of Recipe:

Thin paste made from rhubarb powder 2g, hyacinth bletilla powder 6g, and notoginseng powder 3g with cool boiled water is slowly taken 2～3 times a day.

3. Coma

Main Symptoms: dysphoria, gradual lethargy and coma; or divagation, gradual lethargy and coma.

Accompanying Symptoms: oppressed feeling in the stomach, anorexia, nausea, vomiting, and disorder of visceral function.

Tongue and Pulse: red tongue with yellow and greasy fur, or normal tongue with greasy fur, and slippery pulse.

Analysis: Invasion of the pericardium by accumulated damp-heat causes dysphoria, gradual lethargy and coma. Red tongue, yellow and greasy fur and slippery pulse are signs of damp-heat. Invasion of the pericardium by accumulated phlegm-dampness causes divagation, gradual lethargy and coma. Normal tongue with greasy fur is a sign of phlegm. Disorder of qi in the middle-jiao, and failure of the stomach-qi to descend cause oppressed feeling in the stomach, anorexia, nausea, vomiting, and disorder of visceral function.

Treatment: refreshing the mind and inducing resuscitation.

Recipe and Drugs: Powder of Ju Fang Zhi Bao Pill is taken by mouth or nose to remove heat and induce resuscitation with cool drugs in the treatment of invasion of pericardium by damp-heat. Powder of Su He Xiang Pill is taken by mouth or nose to induce resuscitation with warm drugs in the treatment of invasion of pericardium by phlegm-dampness.

Qing Kai Ling 20ml and 5% glucose saline 200ml can be used for intravenous drip 1～2 times a day. Qing Kai Ling is used to treat invasion of pericardium by damp-heat with the best curative effect.

Example of Recipe:

Powder of a Ju Fang Zhi Bao Pill is taken by nose 2 times a day.

〔Prevention and Nursing Measures〕

1. Attention should be paid to recuperation. Serious patients should mainly stay in bed.

2. The patient should take proper low-salt diet, should not eat seafood, uncooked, cold, fatty, pungent, oil-fried, rough and solid food, should not drink wine, and should reduce smoking cigarettes.

3. The patient should keep emotion stable, eliminate fearful psychology and strengthen confidence in treatment of abdominal mass, jaundice and hypochondriac pain.

4. The patient should pay attention to climatic changes to prevent body resistance from weakened.

〔Analysis of A Typical Case〕

Mr. Ren, 44.

Chief Complaint: repeated fits of abdominal distension, and scanty urine for nearly 2 years.

History of Illness: Having suffered from "icterohepatitis" from October 1973. The patient was treated in a contagious hospital with unremarkable curative effect. After leaving the hospital, he gradually had abdominal distension and scanty urine. Mr. Ren paid his first visit here in July 1977.

Present Symptoms: abdominal distension with vessels seen, thinness, darkish complexion, thirst, vexation, epistaxis, gum bleeding, scanty dark urine, spider nevus on neck and chest, red tongue, scanty saliva, no fur, and thready and rapid pulse.

Medical Check-up: heart and lung(—), spider nevus on neck and chest, hepatic lower boundary at 2.5cm below xiphoid process, spleen at 3.5cm under hypochondria, circumference of abdomen 84cm, shifting dullness(+), and liver palms.

Physiochemical Examination: (1) liver function: icteric index 21 units, and glutamic-pyruvic transaminase 120 units; (2) serum total protein: 7.8g%, albumin: 3.79g%, and globulin: 4.01g%.

TCM Diagnosis: tympanites (yin deficiency of the liver and kidney, and water retention in the middle-jiao).

Western Medical Diagnosis: cirrhosis.

Therapeutic Principle: nourishing the liver and kidney, softening mass, removing blood stasis, and inducing diuresis.

Recipe: self-prescribed recipe.

Chinese angelica root 24g, chuanxiong rhizome 12g, red peony root 15g, glossy privet fruit 24g, fragrant solomonseal rhizome 18g, dried rehmannia root 12g, zedoary 12g, oyster shell 30g, bupleurum root 15g, isatis root 30g, scrophularia root 15g, moutan bark 15g, umbellate pore-fungus 15g, oriental water plantain rhizome 18g, oriental wormwood 30g, and liquorice 10g.

Second Visit: After more than 40 doses of the above-mentioned recipe had been taken, symptoms were alleviated drastically, with liver function: icteric index 3 units; serum total protein: 8.1g%, albumin: 4.63g%, globulin: 3.47g%; and circumference of abdomen 74cm. The patient was given drugs to nourish the liver and kidney and strengthen the spleen-qi:

Chinese angelica root 24g, red peony root 24g, prepared rehmannia root 24g, Chinese yam 30g, glossy privet fruit 30g, fragrant solomonseal rhizome 24g, Siberian solomonseal rhizome 18g, dangshen 24g, straight ladybell root 15g, ophiopogon root 15g, scrophularia root 15g, and fuling 12g.

Third visit: After nearly 60 doses of the above-mentioned recipe Jia Jian had been taken, symptoms were alleviated drastically with yellowish complexion, no spider nevus, better appetite, normal urination and defecation, slightly red tongue, thin and white fur, thready and forceful pulse, no touch of liver, and still enlarged spleen. No relapse was found in later follow-up survey.

Note: This is a serious case of tympanites with yin deficiency and dampness, and with deficiency of origin and excess of superficiality. Its therapeutic principle is to strengthen the body resistance and eliminate pathogenic factors, to nourish yin and enrich blood without impairing the stomach, and to remove heat and eliminate pathogenic factors without weakening the body resistance. Chinese angelica root, red peony root and bupleurum root regulate the liver, nourish the blood and promote blood circulation. Glossy privet fruit, fragrant solomonseal rhizome, moutan bark, dried rehmannia root and scrophularia root can nourish yin and remove heat from the blood. Isatis root and oriental wormwood remove heat and eliminate dampness. Zedoary, oyster shell and red peony root soften and resolve mass and remove blood stasis. After more than 40 doses had been taken, symptoms were alleviated drastically, but the patient was still in low spirit. Dangshen, fuling and Chinese yam replenish qi and strengthen the spleen. Chinese angelica root, red peony root, fragrant solomonseal rhizome, glossy privet fruit, prepared rehmannia root, ophiopogon root, Siberian solomonseal rhizome and scrophularia root enrich the blood, promote blood circulation and nourish the liver. Having taken nearly 60 doses, the patient was almost cured and left the hospital ("Collection of Experiences Achieved by Famous Veteran TCM Practitioners in Henan Province" issued by Health Bureau of Henan Province).

Lingering tympanites with its focus at the liver and spleen will impair the kidney. Its main pathological mechanism is stagnation of qi, blood and water, and impairment of the liver, spleen and kidney. At early stage, no treatment or mistreatment of jaundice, hypochondriac pain and abdominal mass causes incoordination between the liver and spleen, stangnation of qi, obstruction of dampness, and stagnation of cold-dampness or damp-heat in the spleen. At middle stage, impairment of the liver and spleen affects the kidney, causing syndrome of deficiency in origin and excess in superficiality with qi stagnation, blood stasis, water retention, yin deficiency of the liver and kidney, or yang deficiency of the spleen and kidney. At late stage, lingering retention of qi, blood and water aggravates deficiency of the liver, spleen and kidney, with accompanying symptoms of coma, hematemesis and hemafecia.

Tympanites should be treated according to its superficiality, origin, deficiency and excess. At early stage, excessive pathogen is the main factor, but the vital qi has not declined. Stress should be put on expelling pathogen, or promoting the flow of qi to remove dampness, or warming the middle-jiao to disperse dampness, or removing heat to induce diuresis, in order to coordinate the liver and spleen, eliminate water retention and relieve distension. At middle stage, pathogen impairs the vital qi. Elimination of qi stagnation, blood stasis and water retention should be accompanied with protecting the vital qi, and warming and nourishing the spleen and kidney or nourishing the liver and kidney. At late stage, weakened body resistance is the main factor, and pathogen is still lingering with accompanying symptoms. It is rather difficult for tympanites at late stage to be treated with unfavorable prognosis. At that time, weakened body resistance should mainly be treated, but only with slow-acting drugs. Excess in superficiality should also be treated simultaneously. Emergency treatment should be actively given to accompanying symptoms of coma, hematemesis and hemafecia with drugs to refresh the mind, induce resuscitation, remove heat from the blood and stop bleeding.

Questions for Review

1. How to recognize the pathological changes of tympanites?
2. Try to describe the law governing the diagnosis and treatment of commonly encountered types of tympanites.
3. How to grasp the key points of using hydragogue method to treat tympanites?
4. How to nurse the patient with tympanites in normal times?

Headache

〔General Description〕

Headache is a disease with pain in the head as the main symptom caused by exopathy or by internal injury. Headache is divided into acute and chronic pain in the whole head or in its part. Headache can be seen in many acute and chronic diseases. Headache to be discussed here is an internal disease with pain in the head as its main symptom. Headache as an accompanying symptom of a disease will not be included in this article.

Headache can be caused by exopathy or by internal injury. Headache due to exopathy is mainly treated with drugs to dispel wind and eliminate pathogen. Headache due to internal injury is mainly treated with drugs to calm the liver, remove heat, resolve phlegm, eliminate blood stasis, nourish yin, enrich the blood, and replenish qi.

Headache can be seen in various diseases at departments of internal medicine, surgery, neurology, psychosis as well as eye, ear, nose and throat in Western medicine. Infective fever, hypertension, intracarnial disease and neurosis with headache as the main symptom can be diagnosed and treated in reference to this article.

〔Etiology and Pathology〕

Head is "confluence of all yang channels", "home of lucid yang" and place of sea of marrow. Blood from five zang-organs and lucid yang-qi from six fu-organs flow upward to the head. Rich qi and blood, orderly ascension and descension of yin and yang and no worry make people clearheaded and wise-minded. Headache can be caused by six exopathic factors invading seven orifices directly or flowing through channels upward to invade head, or by phlegm and blood stasis obstructing channels and lucid yang. Failure of lucid yang to ascend due to heavy qi, malnutrition of seven orifices due to blood deficiency, flaring-up of fire due to yin deficiency of the liver and kidney, and hyperactivity of the liver-yang due to lingering depression can also cause headache. In spite of many causes, headache can be summarized as due to exopathy and internal injury.

A. Headache due to exopathy is mainly caused by careless daily life. Exopathic factors of wind, cold, summer heat, dampness and fire enter the skin, mouth and nose and move through channels upward to invade the vertex. Obstruction of lucid yang-qi and stagnation of qi and blood cause headache. Wind is the chief of six exopathic factors. "The head is first attacked by wind." "Only wind can invade the vertex." Headache is often caused by wind accompanied with seasonal pathogens, such as difficulty in blood circulation due to wind-cold, invasion of seven orifices by wind-heat or by wind-dampness, and failure of lucid yang to rise.

B. Headache due to Internal Injury: "The brain is sea of marrow." It is nourished by blood from the liver and kidney and by food essence transported by the spleen and stomach. Therefore, headache due to internal injury is closely related to the liver, spleen and kidney. Headache is caused by deficiency of the liver-yin and hyperactivity of yang in deficiency condition or by invasion of seven orifices by fire due to lingering stagnation of the liver-qi. Headache is caused by deficiency of the spleen in transforming nutrients, failure of lucid yang to ascend due to qi deficiency, and malnutrition of seven orifices due to blood deficiency. Headache is caused by failure of the spleen to transport nutrients, stagnation of phlegm, disorder of qi, and invasion of seven orifices by turbid yin. Headache is caused by depletion of sea of marrow due to loss of blood and essence, or by deficiency of the kidney-yin, failure of water to nourish wood, and upward invasion by wind-yang. Headache is caused by deficiency of the kidney-yang and malnutrition of seven orifices, or by generation of endopathic cold due to deficiency of yang and obstruction of lucid yang. Lingering headache with stabbing pain is caused by obstruction of vessels by blood stasis.

In addition, headache is also caused by obstruction of vessels by blood stasis due to external injury.

〔Diagnosis and Treatment〕

A. Key Points for Differentiating Symptoms

(A) Differentiating Headache due to Exopathy from Internal Injury: Headache due to exopathy occurs acutely and seriously, often with continuous drawing pain, jumping pain, burning pain, distending pain and choking pain. Headache due to expathy is mainly an excess syndrome. Exopathic factors of wind, cold, dampness, summer heat and fire should be clinically differentiated. Summer heat is similar to fire in nature.

Headache due to internal injury occurs chronically and mildly, often with vague pain, hollow pain and dizzy pain. The pain fits intermittently and is aggravated at work and alleviated at rest. The pain has its nature of deficiency, excess or deficiency complicated with excess. Qi deficiency, blood deficiency, essence deficiency, liver-yang, yang in deficiency condition, phlegm and blood stasis should be clinically differentiated. Headache due to qi deficiency fits at work, mainly with vague pain. Headache due to blood deficiency is aggravated after bleeding, mainly with hollow pain. Hollow pain in the head due to essence deficiency is severer than headache due to blood deficiency and accompanied with xenophthlmia, photophobia and lassitude in loin and knees. Headache due to liver-yang often has distending pain, conjunctival congestion and bitter taste in the mouth. Headache due to yang in deficiency condition often has dizzy pain and tinnitus. Headache due to phlegm often has dizzy pain, nausea and anorexia. Headache due to blood stasis often has continuous stabbing pain in a fixed area, or history of external injury and lingering pain.

(B) Differentiating Channels of Headache: Head is confluence of all yang channels. The Three Yang Channels of the Hand and the Foot run through the head and face. The Jueyin Channel reaches the vertex. The location of headache varies depending on visceral channel attacked by pathogen. Taiyang headache is often in the rear part of the head and neck. Yangming headache is often in the forehead and supra-orbital bone. Shaoyang headache is often in the two sides of the head and ears. Jueyin headache is often in the vertex and eye system.

B. Key Points for Treatment

Headache due to exopathy should be mainly treated with drugs to expel wind pathogen. Headache due to internal injury should be treated according to superficiality, origin, deficiency and excess. Deficiency should be nourished, excess purged, and deficiency complicated with excess nourished and purged simultaneously.

In addition, guiding drugs can be selectively added according to the location of headache in reference to the channel-running line in order to strengthen curative effect. Notopterygium root, chastetree fruit and chuanxiong rhizome are selected for Taiyang headache. Pueraria root and dahurian angelica root can be used for Yangming headache. Bupleurum root, chuanxiong rhizome and scutellaria root are selected for Shaoyang headache. Evodia fruit and ligusticum root are selected for Jueyin headache. Notopterygium root and ledebouriella root can be used for pain in the whole head. These experiences accumulated by our ancestors can be used for reference during clinical practice.

C. Treatment of Various Types of Headache

(A) Headache due to Exopathy

1. Headache due to Wind-cold

Main Symptoms: pain in the head, neck and back; preference for warm in the head; and severe headache in wind-cold.

Accompanying Symptoms: aversion to wind-cold, pain in the body without sweat, and no thirst.

Tongue and Pulse: normal tongue, thin and white fur, and floating and tense pulse.

Analysis: Wind-cold runs through Taiyang Channel upward to invade the vertex and obstruct lucid yang-qi, causing headache to fit suddenly and continuously. Taiyang Channel governs the skin of the whole body, and runs upward to the vertex and downward to the neck and back, so headache affects the neck and back. Invasion of the skin by wind-cold causes dysfunction of wei-yang, leading to aversion to wind-cold, pain in the body and no sweat. Cold is a yin pathogen and dispersed by warm, so the patient with headache prefers warm. Headache is aggravated in wind-cold. Cold with no heat causes no thirst. Thin and white fur and floating and tense pulse are signs of invasion of the skin by wind-cold.

Schematic Diagram for Etiology and Pathology of Headache

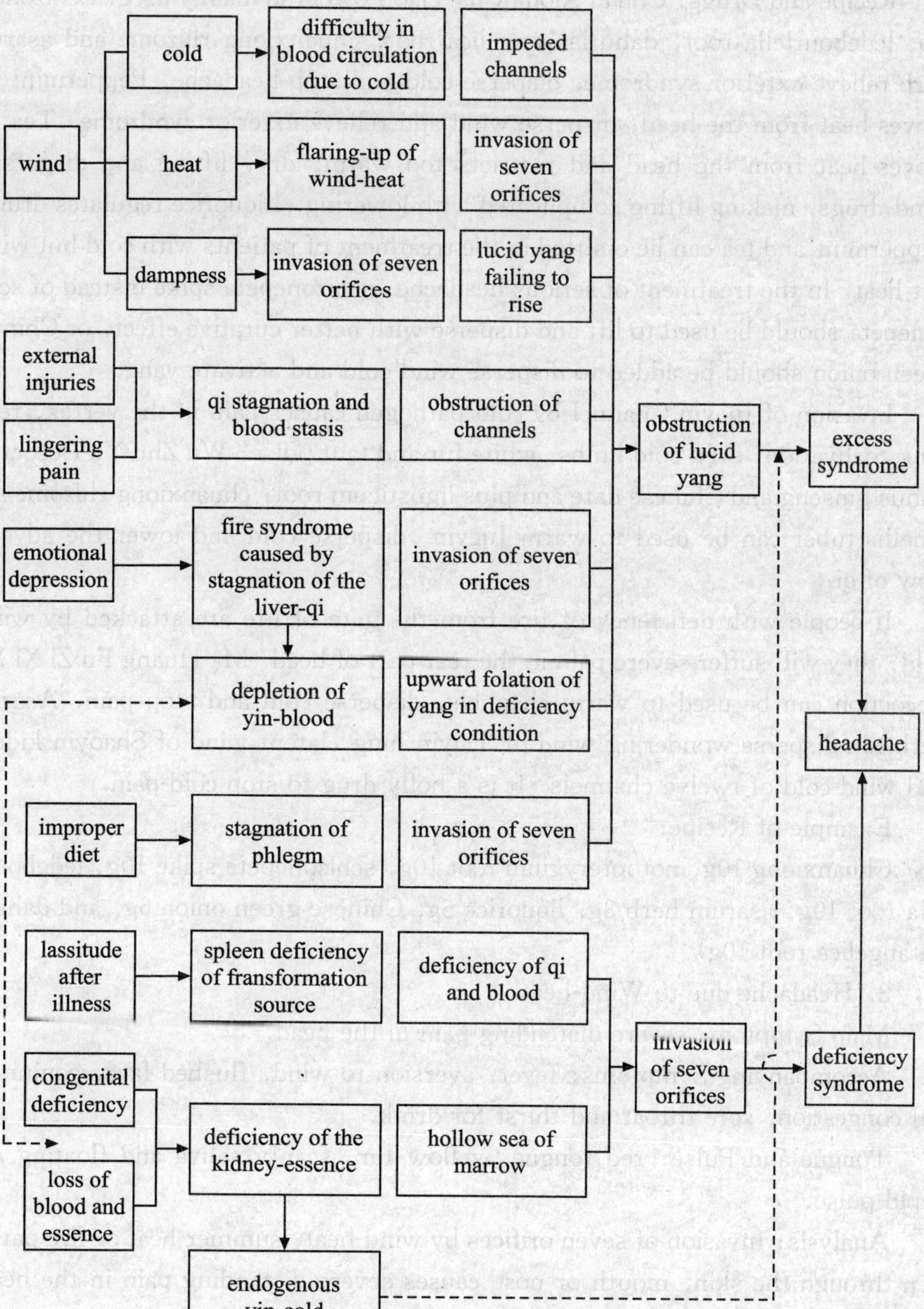

Treatment: expelling wind, dispersing cold and stopping pain.

Recipe and Drugs: Chuan Xiong Cha Tiao Powder is mainly used. Schizonepeta, ledebouriella root, dahurian angelica root, chuanxiong rhizome and asarum herb relieve exterior syndrome, disperse cold and stop headache. Peppermint removes heat from the head, disperse wind and relieve exterior syndrome. Tea removes heat from the head and restricts too warm, dry, lifting and dispersing wind-drugs, making lifting complicated with lowering. Liquorice regulates drugs. Peppermint and tea can be omitted in the treatment of patients with cold but without heat. In the treatment of serious headache, schizonepeta spike instead of schizonepeta should be used to lift and disperse with better curative effect, or Chinese green onion should be added to disperse wind-cold and activate yang.

Invasion of Jueyin Channel by cold pathogen causes pain in the vertex, retching, salivation, even cold limbs, white fur and taut pulse. Wu Zhu Yu Decoction minus ginseng and Chinese date and plus ligusticum root, chuanxiong rhizome and pinellia tuber can be used to warm Jueyin, disperse cold and lower the adverse flow of qi.

If people with deficiency of fire from the gate of life are attacked by wind-cold, they will suffer severe pain in the rear part of head. Ma Huang Fu Zi Xi Xin Decoction can be used to warm channels, disperse cold and stop pain. Asarum herb can disperse wondering wind of Taiyin lung, latent wind of Shaoyin kidney and wind-cold of twelve channels. It is a holly drug to stop cold-pain.

Example of Recipe:

Chuanxiong 10g, notopterygium root 10g, schizonepeta spike 10g, ledebouriella root 10g, asarum herb 3g, liquorice 6g, Chinese green onion 6g, and dahurian angelica root 10g.

2. Headache due to Wind-heat

Main Symptom: severe distending pain in the head.

Accompanying Symptoms: fever, aversion to wind, flushed face, conjunctival congestion, sore throat and thirst for drink.

Tongue and Pulse: red tongue, yellow fur, scanty saliva and floating and rapid pulse.

Analysis: Invasion of seven orifices by wind-heat, summer-heat or fire pathogen through the skin, mouth or nose causes severe distending pain in the head, flushed face and conjunctival congestion. The throat is the gate of lung. Attack on the throat by heat causes swelling pain. Depletion of saliva due to excessive heat causes thirst for drink. Red tongue, yellow fur, scanty saliva and floating and rapid pulse are signs of impairment of the lung by wind-heat.

Treatment: dispelling wind and removing heat.

Recipe and Drugs: Xiong Zhi Shi Gao Decoction is mainly used. Chuanxiong rhizome, dahurian angelica root, chrysanthemum flower and gypsum disperse wind-heat to stop headache. Ligusticum root and notopterygium root, pungent in taste and warm in nature, can be omitted for excessive heat. Mulberry leaf and peppermint, pungent in taste and cool in nature, are added to remove heat. Fresh eupatorium and fresh lotus leaf should be added to remove summer-heat. Scutellaria root, pittorsporm root and forsythia fruit should be added to remove fire-heat and toxin.

Fresh reed rhizome, scrophularia root and trichosanthes root can be added to produce saliva to quench thirst for depletion of body fluid by excessive heat. Gentian root and shave grass can be added to remove heat from the liver for flushed face and conjunctival congestion. Isatis root, honeysuckle flower and danlelion herb can be added to remove heat and toxin for obvious sore throat.

Pittosporm root, rhubarb and dried glauber's salt can be added to purge heat and clear the visceral passage for accumulated heat in the viscera, severe headache and constipation. The recipe can be used together with Huang Lian Shang Qing Pill. The recipe, bitter in taste, cold in nature and removing fire in function, can stop headache.

Example of Recipe:

Chuanxiong rhizome 10g, dahurian angelica root 10g, gypsum 30g (decocted first), chrysanthemum flower 10g, mulberry leaf 10g, peppermint 6g (decocted later), parched scutellaria root 10g, honeysuckle flower 10g, forsythia fruit 10g, platycodon root 6g, and liquorice 6g.

3. Headache due to Wind-dampness

Main Symptom: pain and heaviness sensation in the head, aggravated when it is cloudy or rainy.

Accompanying Symptoms: lassitude, oppressed feeling in the chest, anorexia, sticky feeling in the mouth, difficulty in micturition, and loose stool.

Tongue and Pulse: white and greasy fur and soft pulse.

Analysis: Obstruction of wei-yang and invasion of seven orifices by wind-dampness cause pain and heaviness sensation in the head. The symptom is aggravated when it is cloudy or rainy. Obstruction of wei-yang causes lassitude.

Stagnation of dampness and indigestion cause oppressed feeling in the chest, anorexia and sticky feeling in the mouth. Water retention causes difficulty in micturition and loose stool. White and greasy fur and soft pulse are signs of excessive dampness.

Treatment: dispelling wind and eliminating dampness.

Recipe and Drugs: Qiang Huo Sheng Shi Decoction is mainly used. In the recipe, Xin Wen Powder of notopterygium root, pubescent angelica root, chuanxiong rhizome, ledebouriella root, chastetree fruit and ligusticum root dispels wind and eliminates dampness. Agastache, eupatorium and Liu Yi Powder remove summer-dampness. Huo Po Xia Ling Decoction can be used together with the above-mentioned recipe to treat stagnation of dampness.

Example of Recipe:

Notopterygium root 10g, chuanxiong rhizome 10g, chastetree fruit 10g, atractylodes rhizome 10g, Agastache 10g, eupatorium 10g, ledebouriella root 10g, ligusticum root 6g, and lotus leaf 10g.

(B) Headache due to Internal Injury

1. The Liver-yang Headache

Main Symptom: distending pain in the head, aggravated after the patient is angry, and mainly seen as migraine.

Accompanying Symptoms: flushed face and ears, bitter taste in the mouth, dry throat, distending pain in the hypochondria, vexation, liability to anger, insomnia and nightmare.

Tongue and Pulse: red edge and tip of tongue, thin and yellow fur, and taut, slippery and forceful pulse.

Analysis: impairment of the liver by anger, fire syndrome caused by stagnation of the liver-qi, and invasion of seven orifices by hyperactive liver-yang cause distending pain in the head, that is aggravated after the patient gets angry. Jueyin Channel runs through one side of the head, so migraine is often seen. Flaring-up of qi-fire causes flushed face, conjunctival congestion, bitter taste in the mouth, and dry throat. Jueyin Channel runs through hypochondria, so disorder of the liver-qi cause distending pain in the hypochondria. Hyperactive fire in the heart and liver disturbs mental activity, causing vexation, liability to anger, insomnia and nightmare. Red edge and tip of tongue, thin and yellow fur, and taut, slippery and forceful pulse are signs of excessive fire and hyperactive yang.

Treatment: calming the liver and suppressing yang.

Recipe and Drugs: Tian Ma Gou Teng Decoction is mainly used. Gastrodia tuber, hooked uncaria and abalone shell calm the liver and suppress yang. Scutellaria root and pittosporm root can remove heat from the liver. Achyranthes root, loranthus mulberry mistletoe and eucommia bark nourish the liver and kidney, strengthen the waist and back, and guide drugs and pathogenic heat to go down. Fleece-flower stem and fushen nourish the heart and calm the mind. Motherwort fruit should replace motherwort to promote blood circulation, clear channel and stop headache. Chrysanthemum flower and tribulus fruit calm the liver and stop the wind for headache and dizziness due to upward invasion by wind-yang. Gentian root, prunella spike and antelope's horn powder should be added to treat excessive liver-fire, flushed face, conjunctival congestion, vexation and liability to anger. Dried rehmannia root, white peony root, glossy privet fruit and eclipta can be added to nourish the liver and kidney for yin deficiency of the liver and kidney due to impairment of yin by excessive fire.

Example of Recipe:

Gastrodia tuber 10g, hooked uncaria 10g, abalone shell 30g (decocted first), scutellaria root 10g, pittosporm root 10g, cyathula root 10g, motherwort fruit 10g, red peony root 10g, white peony root 10g, chrysanthemum flower 10g, and gentian root 6g.

2. Headache due to Deficiency of the Kidney

Main Symptom: hollow pain in the head, aggravated at excessive work and alleviated after sleep.

Accompanying Symptoms: fatigue, dizziness, tinnitus, lassitude in loin and knees, seminal emission, leukorrhea, palpitation and insomnia.

Tongue and Pulse: pink tongue, scanty fur and thready and powerless pulse.

Analysis: The kidney stores essence and produces marrow. The brain is sea of marrow. Depletion of sea of marrow due to deficiency of kidney-essence causes hollow pain in the head. The hollow pain is aggravated by impairment of the kidney due to excessive work and alleviated by restoration of essence after sleep. Deficiency of essence and blood due to deficiency of the kidney can not nourish the brain, causing dizziness, tinnitus and lassitude. The waist is the home of kidneys, so deficiency of the kidney causes lassitude in loin and knees. Deficiency of the kidney causes seminal emission and leukorrhea. Mental hypoactivity due to deficiency of essence and blood causes palpitation and insomnia. Pink tongue, scanty fur and thready and powerless pulse are signs of deficiency of the kidney-essence.

Treatment: reinforcing the kidney and producing essence.

Recipe and Drugs: Da Bu Yuan Decoction is mainly used. Prepared rehmannia root, dogwood fruit, Chinese yam and wolfberry fruit nourish the liver and kidney. Ginseng vigorously reinforces the primordial qi. Chinese angelica root enriches the blood. Eucommia bark nourishes the kidney and strengthen the waist. Chuanxiong rhizome and asarum herb can be added to activate collaterals and relieve severe headache. Deficiency of the kidney-yang, hollow pain in the head, aversion to cold, pale complexion, cold limbs, pale tongue, and deep, thready and slow pulse can be treated with You Gui Pill to warm the kidney, reinforce yang, and replenish essence and blood.

Fits of hollow pain in the head can often be treated with Ji Ju Di Huang Pill to reinforce the liver and kidney and suppress floating yang.

Dragon's bone and oyster shell can also be added to suppress floating yang for headache and dizziness.

Example of Recipe:

Prepared Rehmannia Root 12g, dogwood fruit 10g, wolfberry fruit 10g, antler glue 10g (melted by heat), tortoise-plastron glue 10g (melted by heat), dodder seed 10g, chuanxiong rhizome 6g, asarum herb 3g, loranthus mulberry mistletoe 30g, and parched eucommia bark 12g.

3. Headache due to Deficiency of Qi

Main Symptom: lingering headache, aggravated with fatigue.

Accompanying Symptoms: sallow complexion, thinness, lassitude, tasteless in the mouth, anorexia, and loose stool.

Tongue and Pulse: pale enlarged tongue, thin and white fur and thready, feeble and powerless pulse.

Analysis: The spleen is in charge of lifting lucid yang. Deficiency of the spleen causes failure of lucid yang to ascend, failure of turbid yin to descend, and failure of seven orifices to be nourished, leading to lingering headache. Headache will be aggravated with fatigue and alleviated after rest. Failure to transport nutrients due to deficiency of the spleen and failure of the yang-qi to reach limbs and bones cause sallow complexion, thinness and lassitude, Indigestion due to weak spleen and stomach causes tasteless in the mouth, anorexia and loose stool. Pale enlarged tongue, thin and white fur, and thready, feeble and powerless pulse are signs of weakness of the spleen and deficiency of qi.

Treatment: strengthening the spleen, reinforcing qi and lifting lucid yang.

Recipe and Drugs: Shun Qi He Zhong Decoction is mainly used, with Bu Zhong Yi Qi Decoction as the basic recipe to strengthen the spleen, reinforce qi and lift lucid yang. Chastetree fruit, chuanxiong rhizome and asarum herb can be added to dispel wind and stop pain. Curative effect can often be achieved by reinforcing complicated with dispelling, and treating both superficiality and origin. If the disease is accompanied with syndrome of blood deficiency, the recipe should be used together with Si Wu Decoction to reinforce both qi and blood. If excessive phlegm is caused by failure to transport nutrients due to deficiency of the spleen, phlegm-resolving drugs should be added to the recipe to purge and nourish simultaneously.

Example of Recipe:

Dangshen 10g, stir-fried astragalus root 15g, parched bighead atractylodes rhizome 10g, bupleurum root 10g, cimicifuga rhizome 6g, chuanxiong rhizome 10g, chastetree fruit 10g, asarum herb 3g, fuling 15g, and stir-fried liquorice 6g.

4. Headache due to Deficiency of Blood

Main Symptom: hollow pain in the head, mainly in supra-orbital bone, aggravated after bleeding.

Accompanying Symptoms: dim complexion, lassitude, palpitation and scanty menstruation.

Tongue and Pulse: pale tongue, thin and white fur and thready and feeble pulse.

Analysis: Malnutrition of seven orifices due to deficiency of blood causes hollow pain in the head, mainly in supra-orbital bone. Bleeding will aggravate deficiency of blood, causing severer headache. Failure of the blood to nourish the face causes dim complexion. Failure of the blood to nourish the muscle causes lassitude. The heart governs the blood, so deficiency of blood causes malnutrition of the heart, leading to palpitation. Debility of Chong and Ren Channels due to deficiency of blood causes scanty menstruation. Pale tongue, thin and white fur and thready and feeble pulse are signs of deficiency of blood.

Treatment: nourishing and enriching the blood.

Recipe and Drugs: Jia Wei Si Wu Decoction is mainly used. The recipe consists of Si Wu Decoction plus chrysanthemum flower, chastetree fruit, scutellaria root and liquorice. Chinese angelica root, rehmannia root and white peony root replenish yin and enrich blood. Chuanxiong rhizome, chastetree fruit and chrysanthemum flower refresh the head and stop pain. Liquorice regulates the stomach and coordinates the actions of all drugs. Scutellaria root can be omitted for patients without heat signs. If deficiency of blood is accompanied with deficiency of qi, for example, slightly hard work will aggravate lassitude, then the recipe can be used together with Ju Yuan Decoction. For deficiency of blood with dizziness, tinnitus and lassitude in loin and knees, the dose of chuanxiong rhizome can be reduced, and fleece-flower root, wolfberry fruit, donkey-hide glue, glossy privet fruit and other drug to nourish yin and enrich blood can be added. Blood deficiency and blood stasis with lingering pain and ecchymosis can be treated with motherwort fruit, chuanxiong rhizome and other drugs to promote blood circulation and remove blood stasis.

Example of Recipe:

Fleece-flower root 12g, wolfberry fruit 10g, Chinese angelica root 10g, red peony root 10g, white peony root 10g, chuanxiong rhizome 6g, prepared rehmannia root 10g, amomum fruit 3g, chastetree fruit 10g, chrysanthemum flower 10g, and hooked uncaria 10g.

5. Headache due to Phlegm

Main Symptom: dizzy pain in the head.

Accompanying Symptoms: fullness and oppressed feeling in the chest, anorexia, nausea, vomiting and phlegm.

Tongue and Pulse: white and greasy fur and slippery or soft and slippery pulse.

Analysis: Improper diet, dysfunction of the spleen to transport nutrients, stagnation of phlegm, disorder of qi, failure of turbid yin to descend, and obstruction of seven orifices cause dizzy pain in the head. Stagnation of phlegm causes fullness and oppressed feeling in the chest and stomach. Failure of the stomach-qi to descend causes anorexia and nausea, even vomiting and phlegm. White and greasy fur and slippery or soft and slippery pulse are signs of stagnation of phlegm.

Treatment: regulating the spleen, resolving phlegm and lowering the adverse flow of qi.

Recipe and Drugs: Ban Xia Bai Zhu Tian Ma Decoction is mainly used. In the recipe, Er Chen Decoction eliminates dampness, resolves phlegm and normalizes function of qi. Bighead atractylodes rhizome regulates the spleen and eliminates dampness. Gastrodia tuber resolves phlegm, calm the endopathic wind and stop dizzy pain in the head. Fresh ginger and Chinese date regulate the stomach. All these drugs make turbid yin descend to stop headache. If dampness is complicated with summer-heat, xing tou cao, agastache and lotus leaf can be added to eliminate summer-heat and dampness. Tribulus, chastetree fruit, notopterygium root and other wind-dispelling drugs can be added to treat severe headache. For obvious stagnation of dampness in the middle-jiao, atractylodes rhizome, magnolia bark and round cardamon seed can be added to regulate the stomach, eliminate dampness and normalize the function of qi.

For phlegm-heat with distending pain in the head, vexation, insomnia, yellow and greasy fur, and slippery and rapid pulse, bighead atractylodes rhizome can be omitted, and bamboo shavings, immature bitter orange and scutellaria root, or coptis root and pittosporm root can be added to remove phlegm-heat.

If stagnation of both phlegm and blood stasis affects seven orifices to cause severe headache and dizziness incurable for a long time, only by treating phlegm and blood stasis simultaneously, can curative effect be achieved.

Example of Recipe:

Pinellia tuber 10g, parched tangerine peel 10g, gastrodia tuber 10g, bighead atractylodes rhizome 10g, lotus leaf 10g, Xing Tou Cao 10g, tribulus fruit 10g, chastetree fruit 16g, fuling 10g, and fresh ginger 3 pieces.

6. Headache due to Blood Stasis

Main Symptom: lingering prickling or dull pain in a fixed area of the head, or the patient has a history of external injury at the head.

Accompanying Symptoms: darkish and dim complexion, staring blankly, insomnia, or scar of external injury.

Tongue and Pulse: dark purple tongue or with ecchymosis, and thready and uneven pulse.

Analysis: Stagnation of blood stasis due to external injury at the head causes lingering prickling or dull pain in a fixed area of the head. Failure of blood to nourish the face causes darkish and dim complexion. Failure of blood to nourish the brain causes staring blankly and insomnia. Dark purple tongue or with ecchymosis, and thready and uneven pulse are signs of blood stasis.

Treatment: promoting the circulation of blood to remove blood stasis, and promoting the flow of qi to induce resuscitation.

Recipe and Drugs: Tong Qiao Huo Xue Decoction is mainly used. Peach kernel, safflower, chuanxiong rhizome and red peony root promote the circulation of blood to remove blood stasis. Musk, Chinese green onion and fresh ginger warm the channel to promote the flow of qi. Musk has the best pain-stopping effect. However, musk is rare, so it can be substituted with proprietary Chinese medicine containing musk if necessary. Motherwort fruit, curcuma root, calamus, asarum herb and dahuria angelica root can also be added to regulate the flow of qi, promote the circulation of blood, induce resuscitation and stop pain.

For lingering pain due to blood stasis and deficiency of qi and blood, Chinese angelica root, fleece-flower root, astragalus root and dangshen should be added to reinforce qi, enrich blood and promote the circulation of qi and blood. For severe headache, scorpion, centipede, ground beetle, long-noded pit viper and earthworm and other drugs of removing obstruction in the channels can be added. However, these drugs should not taken in large doses or for a long time. For severe headache and stagnation of blood stasis, leech, winged euony twigs and other drugs of promoting blood circulation to remove blood stasis can be added.

Heat syndrome due to lingering blood stasis and qi stagnation has symptoms of vexation, insomnia and red dry tongue. Schizonepeta spike, prunella spike and sweet warmwood can be added to remove stagnated heat from qi system. Or moutan bark, red sage root and pulsatilla root can be added to remove latent heat from the blood system. If headache due to blood stasis is caused by cold, cinnamom twig and asarum herb can be added to warm channels, dispel cold and remove obstruction in the channels.

Headache due to stagnation of blood stasis and phlegm in seven orifices should be treated with drugs of promoting blood circulation to remove blood stasis and eliminating dampness to resolve phlegm. The above-mentioned recipe can be used in combination with Dao Tan Decoction or Qian Zheng Powder.

Example of Recipe:

Motherwort fruit 12g, chuanxiong rhizome 10g, red peony root 10g, earthwrom 10g, peach kernel 10g, safflower 10g, hooked uncaria 10g, calamus 6g, asarum herb 3g, curcuma root 10g, and Chinese green onion 6g.

In addition, laws governing the diagnosis and treatment of some clinically special types of headache should be grasped. For example.

(1) "Thunder-headache" is characterized by headache like thunder with nodules or swelling pain in the head, and is mainly caused by damp-heat, alcohol toxin and phlegm. The recipe of Qing Zhen Decoction plus ingredients can be used to remove heat and toxin and resolve dampness and phlegm. Obvious heat-toxin can be treated with the recipe and Pu Ji Xiao Du Decoction.

(2) Migraine is characterized by pain on one side or two sides of the head. It fits suddenly and acutely with pain affecting eye and teeth. Migraine is mainly caused by invasion of the head by wind-fire in the liver-channel. Chrysanthemum flower, gastrodia tuber, chuanxiong rhizome, dahurian angelica root, chastetree fruit, hooked uncaria, scorpion and earthworm are often used to calm the liver, dispel wind, remove obstruction in channels and stop pain. Pittosporm root, scutellaria root, gentian root and moutan bark can be added to treat hyperactivity of the liver-fire. Pinellia tuber, arisaema tuber, bamboo juice, fresh ginger juice or white mustard seed can be added to treat stagnation of phlegm in channels. Red peony root, peach kernel, safflower, pangolin scales, chuanxiong rhizome and other drugs of resolving phlegm and removing obstruction in channels can be added to treat lingering illness affecting channels.

〔Prevention and Nursing Measures〕

1. Headache due to exopathy should be prevented with leading a regular life, wearing clothes according to weather, doing physical exercise, and strengthening the body resistance.

2. Headache due to internal injury should be prevented with calming emotions, ensuring adequate sleep, eating light food, and reducing work and sex for patients who fall ill for a long time, are old or feeble.

3. Patients with severe headache should take rest in bed, live in a quiet environment with soft light, give up wine and smoking, avoid emotional stimulation, not eat pungent and fatty food.

4. If condition permits, massage, acupuncture and other auxiliary treatments can be used.

〔Analysis of A Typical Case〕

Mr. Liu, 38.

He had headache, dizziness and vexation for several years. He was impetuous and had obviously reduced memory. His symptoms were yellowish urine, normal defecation, normal appetite, slightly floating, taut, thready and forceful pulse, red tongue with uneven edge, and yellow and slightly greasy fur. His illness was caused by excessive fire in the liver and gallbladder and by exopathic wind, and should be treated with drugs to remove heat, replenish yin and dispel wind. The recipe consisted of mulberry leaf 6g, chrysanthemum flower 6g, batryticated silkworm 6g, tribulus fruit 10g, chuanxiong rhizome 5g, ligusticum root 6g, moutan bark 5g, parched capejasmine fruit 6g, gentian root 5g, scrophularia root 6g, liquorice 3g, lotus leaf 10g, abalone shell (calcined) 15g, and five-leaf akebia stem 5g. The patient should take 3 doses of the decoction.

Return Visit: Headache disappeared. The patient had dizziness sometimes, taut, thready and slow pulse, reduced fur, and other symptoms as before. Pills were used to slowly nourish yin, enrich blood and regulate the intestine and stomach.

The recipe consisted of Chinese angelica root 10g, chuanxiong rhizome 10g, white peony root 12g, dried rehmannia root 18g, red sage root 10g, parched capejasmine fruit 10g, acrophularia root 12g, chrysanthemum flower 15g, wolfberry bark 15g, tribulus fruit 15g, cassia seed (parched) 15g, dondrobium stem 15g, desertliving cistanche 15g, linseed (parched and pulverized) 15g, sesame seed (parched and pulverized) 15g, Jian Qu 30g, and prepared nutgrass flatsedge rhizome 30g. These drugs were pulverized into fine powder and mixed with honey evenly to make pills. A pill weighing 9g was taken every morning and evening. The patient chewed it carefully and then swallowed it with boiled water. With two doses taken, all the symptoms disappeared. The patient was advised to calm emotions in order to avoid flaring up again of ministerial fire in the liver and gallbladder.

Note: "Fire syndrome due to hyperactivity of five emotions" put forward by Zhu Danxi is clinically often seen. The patient was impetuous, had excessive fire in the liver and gallbladder, and was attacked by exopathic wind. Headache, dizziness, vexation, yellow urine and taut, thready and forceful pulse were signs of deficiency syndrome complicated with excess symptoms. Drugs of removing heat, replenishing yin and dispelling wind were used to treat deficiency syndrome and excess symptoms simultaneously. Decoction was first used to suppress the flaring fire, and pill was then used to slowly distinguish the suppressed fire, so the patient is cured (quoted from "Pu Fuzhou's Medical Records").

Headache is a clinically common disease caused by exopathy and internal injury. The key point of its diagnosis is to differentiate exopathy from internal injury, and deficiency from excess. Headache due to exopathy is mainly caused by wind-cold, wind-heat (or summer-heat and fire) or wind-dampness. Headache due to internal injury is mainly caused by dysfunction of the viscera, qi and blood, and closely related to the liver, spleen and kidney. Headache due to exopathy is mainly excess syndrome. Headache due to internal injury is mainly deficiency syndrome, but there is also excess syndrome or deficiency syndrome complicated with excess symptoms. Headache due to exopathy is mainly treated with drugs to dispel exopathic wind, and ingredients are added or omitted depending on accompanying symptoms. Headache due to internal injury is mainly treated with drugs to regulate visceral function. Deficiency syndrome is treated with nourishing drugs, while excess syndrome is treated with purging drugs. For example, the liver-yang is treated with drugs to calm the liver and suppress hyperactivity of the liver-yang, phlegm is treated with drugs to resolve phlegm, and blood stasis is treated with drugs to promote blood circulation and remove blood stasis. Deficiency syndrome complicated with excess symptoms is treated with drugs to purge and nourish simultaneously. The illness condition of headache is complicated and changeable, so it is necessary to distinguish the principal cause from secondary cause, and to diagnose and treat according to its etiological and pathological changes and characteristics of symptoms. The physician should pay attention to the location of headache, and use guiding drugs to enhance curative effect. The physician should not merely attach importance to analgesics, while neglecting overall differentiation of symptoms. In addition to medicinal treatment, acupuncture, massage and other external therapies can also be used to achieve better curative effect according to illness conditions.

Questions for Review

1. Try to describe the etiology and pathology of headache.
2. Try to describe the symptoms of headache due to exopathy and the law governing its diagnosis and treatment.
3. Try to describe the symptoms of headache due to internal injury and the law governing its diagnosis and treatment.
4. What guiding drugs are often used to treat headache?

Dizziness

〔General Description〕

Dizziness is the general name for giddiness and vertigo. Giddiness is referred to as dim eyesight or blackened and blurred vision. Vertigo means that patients feel themselves or surrounding scenery revolving and can not stand firm. Giddiness and vertigo can often be seen simultaneously, hence the name dizziness. Mild dizziness can disappear immediately after sufferers close their eyes. Serious patients feel as if riding a car or boat and even can not stand firm, or with nausea, vomiting, sweating, coma and other symptoms.

Dizziness can be caused by exopathy or by internal injury. Its pathology is closely related to wind, fire, phlegm, deficiency syndrome and blood stasis.

Many diseases in Western medicine, such as aural dizziness, cerebral dizziness, hypertension, hypotension, anemia and neurosis, with dizziness as their main symptom, can be diagnosed and treated in reference to the disease.

〔Etiology and Pathology〕

The disease is mainly caused by hyperactivity of the liver-yang, by deficiency of the kidney-essence, qi and blood, and by stagnation of phlegm and blood stasis. It is generally a deficiency syndrome and described separately as follows:

A. Hyperactivity of the Liver-yang: The liver is an organ of wind and wood. Excessive yang and hyperactive fire in the heart and liver easily cause upward invasion by wind-yang, leading to dizziness of pure excess syndrome. Deficiency of yin, failure of water to nourish wood, stirring-up of endopathic wind of deficiency type, and upward invasion of seven orifices also cause dizziness of deficiency syndrome complicated with excess symptoms.

B. Deficiency of the Kidney-essence: The kidney is the origin of congenital constitution, stores the kidney-yin, kidney-yang and essence, and generates marrow. Congenital deficiency, old age, lingering illness, and loss of blood and essence cause deficiency of the kidney-essence, depletion of sea of marrow, and malnutrition of the brain, leading to dizziness.

C. Deficiency of Qi and Blood: The spleen and stomach are the material basis of acquired constitution, and the source of qi and blood. Improper diet, anxiety and fatigue impair the spleen and stomach. Weakened spleen and stomach or lingering illness and indigestion cause deficiency of qi and blood. Qi deficiency causes failure of lucid yang to ascend and turbid qi to descend, and malnutrition of seven orifices, leading to dizziness. Blood deficiency causes failure to produce essence and marrow to nourish seven orifices, malnutrition of the liver, stirring-up of endopathic wind of deficiency type and upward invasion of seven orifices, leading to dizziness.

D. Stagnation of Phlegm: Obesity and addiction to wine and meat impair the spleen and stomach and cause stagnation of phlegm due to accumulation of dampness, disorder of qi and invasion of seven orifices by phlegm, leading to dizziness. Transformation of stagnant phlegm into heat, and upward invasion by phlegm-heat cause severe dizziness.

E. Stagnation of Blood Stasis: Cerebral damage due to fall or drop with blood stasis obstructing channels causes malnutrition of seven orifices, hence dizziness. With blood stasis staying there, it is difficult for fresh blood to generate, further aggravating malnutrition of seven orifices and dizziness. Obstruction of seven orifices by blood stasis causes headache and dizziness. Obstruction of seven orifices by blood stasis and phlegm makes dizziness difficult to be cured.

F. Affection of Exopathy: The head is the confluence of all yang-channels, and related to twelve regular channels and eight extra-channels. Six exopathic factors enter the skin, mouth and nose through channels upward to invade the vertex and seven orifices, causing dizziness. Wind, summer-heat, dampness and fire are most harmful among six exopathic factors. If entering half exterior and half interior or entering the interior to transform into heat, exopathic factors can move upward through channels to interfere with seven orifices to cause dizziness.

Dizziness can be caused by more than one pathogenic factor. Its etiology and pathology can be transformed into each other. For example, deficiency of both qi and blood can cause dizziness. However, deficiency of both qi and blood is caused by deficiency of the spleen, deficiency of the spleen can produce phlegm, and phlegm often aggravates dizziness. Deficiency of the kidney-essence can cause dizziness. However, the liver and the kidney have a common source, so deficiency of the kidney-essence causes malnutrition and stirring-up of the liver, and upward invasion by wind-yang to make dizziness severer.

〔Diagnosis and Treatment〕

A. Key Points for Differentiating Symptoms

1. Differentiation of Internal Injury from Exopathy: Dizziness can be caused by internal injury or by exopathy. Dizziness due to exopathy often has obvious exterior syndrome, occurs acutely and transforms rapidly. Exopathic factors can be wind, cold, summer heat, dampness and fire. Exopathic factors entering the interior can invade Shaoyang or Yangming. Dizziness due to internal injury is mainly caused by impairment of the liver, kidney, spleen and stomach. Impairment of the liver causes deficiency of yin-blood, failure of yin to suppress yang, and

upward floating of yang in deficiency condition, or causes fire syndrome due to stagnation of the liver-qi, fire and wind stirring up each other, and hyperactivity of the liver-yang. Impairment of the kidney causes deficiency of essence and depletion of sea of marrow. Impairment of the spleen and stomach causes failure to transport and transform nutrients, deficiency of both qi and blood, and malnutrition of seven orifices. Although dizziness due to internal injury is mainly deficiency syndrome, it is also caused by endogenous wind, fire, phlegm and blood stasis.

2. Differentiation of Deficiency from Excess: Dizziness is mainly a deficiency syndrome. Deficiency and excess should be differentiated according to main symptom, accompanying symptom, tongue picture and pulse condition. The main symptom for dizziness of deficiency syndrome is hollow and heaviness sensation in the head. Its accompanying symptom is weakened liver, kidney, spleen and stomach. The tongue is thin or enlarged, and pink and smooth or pale. The pulse is deep and thready or feeble and taut. The main symptom for dizziness of excess syndrome is dizzy and distending pain in the head. Its accompanying symptom is exterior syndrome, phlegm, blood stasis, or liver-fire. The tongue is red or darkish with ecchymosis, thick, greasy and yellow fur, and scanty saliva. Deficiency syndrome complicated with excess symptoms should be carefully differentiated.

3. Differentiation of Superficiality from Origin and Slow from Quick Treatment: Dizziness is mainly caused by internal injury and characterized by deficiency syndrome complicated with excess symptoms. Therefore, it is appropriate to differentiate superficiality from origin and slow from quick treatment. In general, weakened body resistance is origin, while superficiality is pathogenic factors of wind, phlegm, blood stasis and fire. It is urgent to eliminate pathogenic factors if they are obviously hyperactive. Weakened body resistance leads to deficiency of blood, essence and qi. Obviously weakened body resistance and unnoticeable pathogenic factors should be treated slowly. If none of them is excessive or deficient, they should be treated at the same time.

B. Key Points for Treatment

Dizziness due to exopathy should be mainly treated with drugs to eliminate exopathic factors. Dizziness of exterior syndrome should be treated with drugs to dispel wind, cold, summer-heat, dampness and fire. Dizziness of half-exterior and half-interior syndrome should be treated with regulating drugs. Dizziness of interior syndrome should be treated with purging drugs. Dizziness due to internal injury should be treated after differentiation deficiency from excess. Dizziness of deficiency syndrome should be treated with nourishing, replenishing or warming drugs according to conditions. Dizziness of excess syndrome should be treated with drugs to purge excessive fire, suppress hyperactive yang, resolve stagnant phlegm, eliminate retained dampness, and remove blood stasis. Dizziness of deficiency and excess syndromes should be treated with drugs to purge and nourish simultaneously, or first purge and then nourish, or first nourish and then purge.

Schematic Diagram for Etiology and Pathology of Dizziness

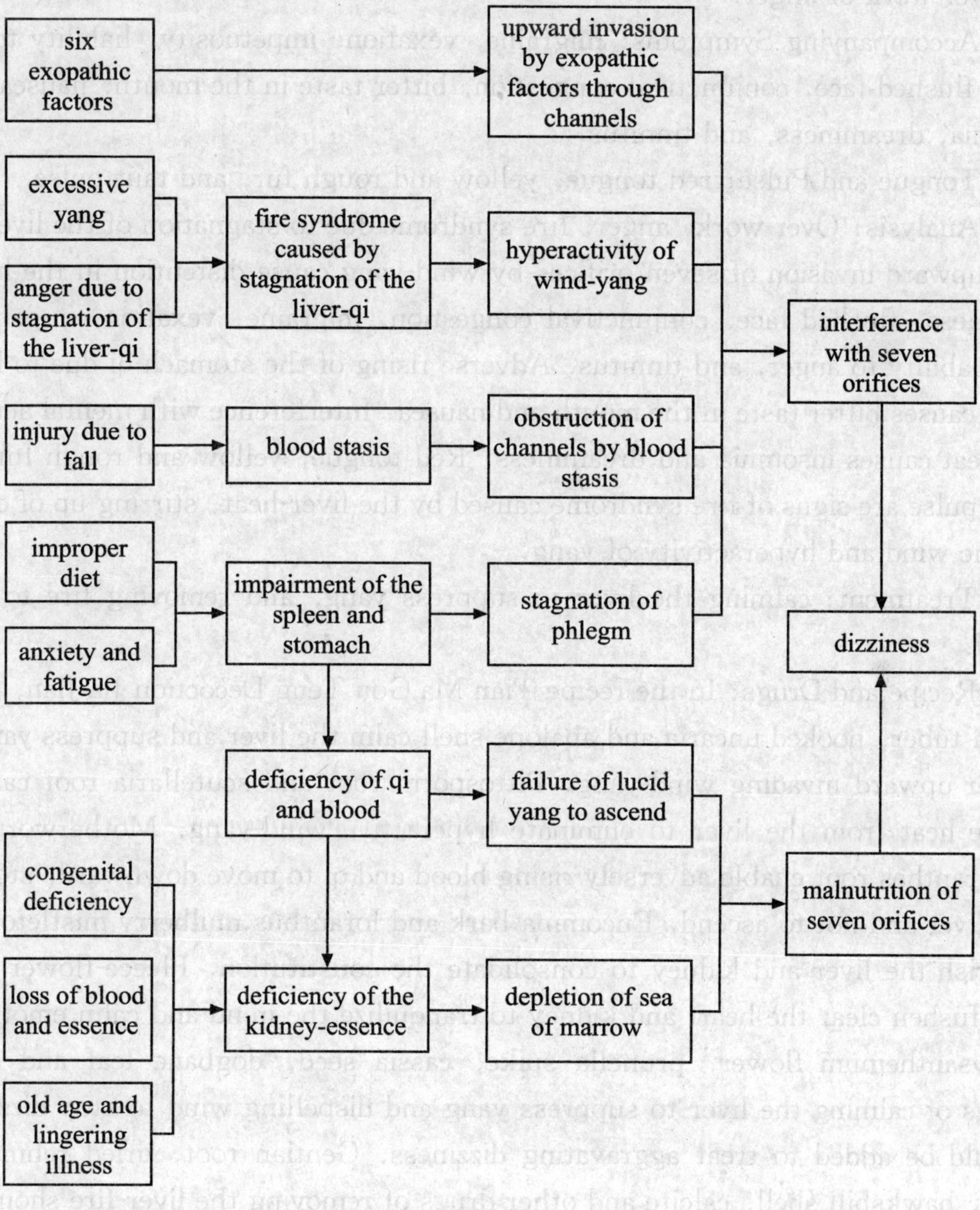

C. Diagnosis and Treatment of Dizziness of Various Types

The diagnosis and treatment of dizziness due to exopathy can be seen in Treatise on Febrile Diseases and Doctrine of Epidemic Febrile Diseases, and is similar to that of "Common Cold" and "Headache due to Exopathy" in this book. Therefore, only dizziness due to internal injury is summarized as follows:

(A) Hyperactivity of the Liver-yang

Main Symptom: distention in the head and dizziness, which are aggravated by over-work or anger.

Accompanying Symptoms: migraine, vexation, impetuosity, liability to anger, flushed face, conjunctival congestion, bitter taste in the mouth, nausea, insomnia, dreaminess, and tinnitus.

Tongue and Pulse: red tongue, yellow and rough fur, and taut pulse.

Analysis: Over-work, anger, fire syndrome due to stagnation of the liver-qi, and upward invasion of seven orifices by wind-yang cause distention in the head, dizziness, flushed face, conjunctival congestion, migraine, vexation, impetuosity, liability to anger, and tinnitus. Adverse rising of the stomach-qi due to liver-heat causes bitter taste in the mouth and nausea. Interference with mental activity by heat causes insomnia and dreaminess. Red tongue, yellow and rough fur and taut pulse are signs of fire syndrome caused by the liver-heat, stirring-up of endopathic wind and hyperactivity of yang.

Treatment: calming the liver to suppress yang, and removing fire to stop wind.

Recipe and Drugs: In the recipe Tian Ma Gou Teng Decoction Jia Jian, gastrodia tuber, hooked uncaria and abalone shell calm the liver and suppress yang to lower upward invading wind-yang. Pittosporm root and scutellaria root can remove heat from the liver to eliminate hyperactive wind-yang. Motherwort and achyranthes root enable adversely rising blood and qi to move downward, store in the liver and not to ascend. Eucomma bark and loranthus mulberry mistletoe can nourish the liver and kidney to consolidate the constitution. Fleece-flower stem and fushen clear the heart and kidney to tranquilize the mind and calm emotions. Chrysanthemum flower, prunella spike, cassia seed, dogbane leaf and other drugs of calming the liver to suppress yang and dispelling wind to stop dizziness should be added to treat aggravating dizziness. Gentian root, dried rehmannia root, hawksbill shell, calcite and other drugs of removing the liver-fire should be added to treat hyperactive liver-fire and dysphoria. Antelope's horn can be used, if necessary, to strengthen the effect of removing the liver-fire and dispelling wind. If drug source is tense, a large dose of buffalo horn can be used to replace antelope's horn. If yin deficiency of the liver and kidney is obvious, Er Zhi Pill should be added to strengthen nourishing effect. Dragon's bone, oyster shell, tortoise plastron, fresh water turtle shell and other drugs of tranquilizing the liver-wind can be added to treat stirring-up of endogenous wind of deficiency type with tremor of limbs and muscular twitching and cramp. Dang Gui Long Hui Pill or Shou Feng Shun Qi Pill and other drugs of removing the liver-fire and clearing the viscera should be added to treat dry intestine due to fire and constipation. The patient with constipation should not sit on a closet for a long time or defecate too forcefully.

Dizziness as if in a boat, lassitude in loin and knees, xenophthalmia, photophobia, nocturnal emission, irregular menstruation, taut, thready and slippery pulse, pink and smooth tongue, and scanty or no fur belong to deficiency of the liver and kidney, and upward floating of yang in deficiency condition. Da Ding Feng Pill can be used to nourish yin and suppress yang. With symptoms alleviated after taking the drugs, the patient should often take Ji Ju Di Huang Pill to nourish the liver and kidney and consolidate the curative effect.

Example of Recipe:

Gastrodia tuber 10g, hooked uncaria 12g, abalone shell 30g (decocted first), chrysanthemum flower 10g, prunella spike 10g, scutellaria root 10g, pittosporm root 10g, achyranthes root 15g, magnetite 30g (decocted first), red ochre 30g (decocted first), and loranthus mulberry mistletoe 20g.

(B) Deficiency of Both Qi and Blood

Main Symptom: dizziness, easily occurring or aggravated when the patient is tired.

Accompanying Symptoms: pale and dim complexion, pale lips and nails, lassitude, anorexia, palpitation, short breath, insomnia and dreaminess.

Tongue and Pulse: pale tongue, thin fur, and thready and feeble pulse.

Analysis: Qi deficiency causes failure of lucid yang to rise. Blood deficiency causes malnutrition of the brain. Fatigue causes impairment of the heart and spleen. Deficiency of qi and blood and malnutrition of seven orifices causes or aggravates dizziness. Blood deficiency causes malnutrition of the heart, leading to palpitation, dreaminess, pale and dim complexion, and pale lips and nails. Qi deficiency causes failure of the spleen to transport and transform nutrients, leading to lassitude, short breath and anorexia. Pale tongue, thin fur, and thready and feeble pulse are signs of deficiency of both qi and blood.

Treatment: strengthening the spleen, replenishing qi, nourishing the heart and enriching the blood.

Recipe and Drugs: The recipe Gui Pi Decoction Jia Jian is mainly used to strengthen the spleen and replenish qi. The spleen is the source of qi and blood. A healthy spleen can normally transport and transform nutrients, making qi and blood fully supplied. Ginseng, astragalus root, atractylodes rhizome, liquorice, fresh ginger and Chinese date, sweet in taste and warm in nature, are used to strengthen the spleen and replenish qi. Chinese angelica root, sweet and pungent in taste and warm in nature, is used to nourish and generate the blood. These drugs are used together to reach the goal of nourishing qi and blood. Fuling, Chinese date, longan aril and polygala root nourish the heart and tranquilize the mind. Aucklandia root regulates the flow of qi and enlivens the spleen to prevent drugs of replenishing qi and nourishing the blood from stagnation of qi, to smoothly transport and transform nutrients and to facilitate generating qi and blood. For anorexia, loose stool and obviously weakened spleen and stomach, amomum fruit, calamus, lotus seed, hyacinth bean and Chinese yam should be added, aucklandia root roasted in ashes, and Chinese angelica root stir-fried with wine, to reinforce the effect of strengthening the spleen and stomach. For normal appetite but severe deficiency of blood, white peony root, donkey-hide gelatin, fleece-flower root and other drugs of nourishing and generating the blood should be added. For deficiency of the spleen-yang, aversion to cold, and cold limbs, baked ginger, stir-fried cinnamom twig and other drugs of warming the middle-jiao and strengthening the spleen should be added. For sinking of qi in the middle-jiao, hollow sensation in the head, dizziness, short breath, lassitude, and proctoptosis aggravated when the patient is standing and slightly alleviated when the patient is lying down, Bu Zhong Yi Qi Pill (decoction of a wrapped drug) can be added.

Example of Recipe:

Dangshen 10g, stir-fried astragalus root 20g, wine-fried Chinese angelica root 10g, parched white peony root 10g, donkey-hide gelatin10g (melted by heat), parched bighead atractylodes rhizome 10g, roasted aucklandia root 6g, fuling 15g, polygala root 10g, longan aril 10g, and roasted pueraria root 10g.

(C) Deficiency of the Kidney-essence

Main Symptom: dizziness, lassitude and amnesia.

Accompanying Symptoms: listlessness, xenophthalmia, photophobia, and lassitude in loin and knees. The patient with yin deficiency has dysphoria with feverish sensation in the chest, palms and soles, night sweat, nocturnal emission, irregular menstruation.

Tongue and Pulse: For kidney yin deficiency: pink tongue with scanty fur, and taut thready pulse. For kidney yang deficiency: pale tongue, and deep, thready and powerless pulse.

Analysis: deficiency of the kidney-essence, depletion of sea of marrow and malnutrition of seven orifices can cause dizziness, lassitude, amnesia and listlessness. The liver is in charge of eyes. The liver and kidney have a common source. Deficiency of essence and blood causes xenophthalmia, photophobia, and lassitude in loin and knees. Hyperactivity of the ministerial fire of deficiency type causes dysphoria with feverish sensation in the chest, palms and soles, night sweat, nocturnal emission and irregular menstruation. Pink tongue, scanty fur, and taut and thready pulse are signs of hyperactivity of fire due to yin deficiency. Deficiency of the kidney-yang causes decline of the fire from the gate of life, with yang-qi failing to warm the viscera and skin, leading to aversion to cold, lassitude in loin and knees, impotence and coldness of the genitals. Pale tongue and deep, thready and powerless pulse are signs of decline of the fire from the gate of life.

Treatment: nourishing yin and reinforcing the kidney for yin deficiency, warming the kidney and restoring yang for yang deficiency.

Recipes and Drugs: Zuo Gui Pill is mainly used to nourish yin and reinforce the kidney. You Gui Pill is mainly used to warm the kidney and restore yang. In the two recipes, prepared rehmannia root, dogwood fruit, Chinese yam, wolfberry fruit and dodder seed reinforce the kidney and replenish essence. Antler glue nourishes essence and blood. In Zuo Gui Pill, tortoise-plastron glue nourishes yin-blood to astringe floating yang, and achyranthes root reinforces the kidney, strengthens the muscle and guides drugs downward to return to the kidney. In You Gui Pill, eucommia bark can nourish the liver and kidney and strengthen the muscle and bone, and Chinese angelica root can nourish and enrich the blood. The essence and blood have a common source, so generation of blood causes exuberant essence. Cinnamom bark and prepared aconite root warm the kidney, restore yang and strengthen the effect of drugs of replenishing essence and nourishing marrow.

For obvious hyperactivity of fire due to yin deficiency, anemarrhena rhizome and phellodendron bark can be added to purge ministerial fire, or dragon's bone and oyster shell can be added to suppress floating yang. If the patient feels uncomfortable in the stomach after taking the decoction, amomum fruit and tangerine peel can be added to regulate the spleen and stomach and eliminate greasy food. For deficiency of both yin and yang, morinda root, curculiga rhizome and aerial part of Epimedium Brevicornum can be added to normally nourish. For obvious dizziness, magnetite and red ochre can be added to heavily suppress hyperactive yang.

Examples of Recipes:

For deficiency of the kidney-yin: dried rehmannia root 10g, prepared rehmannia root 10g, dogwood fruit 10g, wolfberry fruit 10g, white peony root 12g, glossy privet fruit 10g, eclipta 10g, loranthus mulberry mistletoe 20g, achyranthes root 10g, dragon's bone 20g (decocted first), oyster shell 20g (decocted first), tortoise-plastron glue 10g (melted by heat), and chrysanthemum flower 10g.

For deficiency of the kidney-yang: prepared rehmannia root 12g (mixed with amomum fruit 2g), dogwood fruit 10g, wolfberry fruit 10g, dodder seed 10g, parched eucommia bark 12g, morinda root 12g, curculigo rhizome 10g, prepared aconite root 6g, antler glue 10g (melted by heat), magnetite 20g (decocted first), and gastrodia tuber 10g.

(D) Stagnation of Phlegm

Main Symptoms: dizziness with a heavy sensation

Accompanying Symptoms: obesity, addiction to fatty and sweet food, feeling of stuffiness and tightness in the chest, anorexia, nausea and lassitude.

Tongue and Pulse: white and greasy fur, and soft and slippery pulse.

Analysis: Fat people have abundant phlegm, and addiction to fatty and sweet food promotes dampness to produce phlegm. Stagnation of phlegm causes disorder of qi. Turbid qi failing to descend invades seven orifices, and clear qi failing to ascend causes malnutrition of seven orifices, leading to dizziness. Stagnation even adverse ascension of qi in the middle-jiao causes feeling of stuffiness and tightness in the chest, anorexia, and nausea. Stagnation of phlegm-dampness in the spleen causes yang-qi not to function, leading to lassitude. White and greasy fur and soft and slippery pulse are signs of stagnation of phlegm-dampness.

Treatment: eliminating dampness, resolving phlegm, regulating the spleen and stopping dizziness.

Recipe and drugs: In the recipe Ban Xia Tian Ma Bai Zhu Decoction Jia Jian, Er Chen Decoction is used as a basis to eliminate dampness, resolve phlegm, regulate the stomach and lower the adverse flow of qi. Bighead atractylodes rhizome regulates the spleen and eliminates dampness. Gastrodia tuber dispels wind and stops dizziness. All these drugs are used together to resolve phlegm, normalize the flow of qi and stop dizziness. For severer dizziness due to wind-phlegm, batryticated silkworm and arisaema with bile can be added to stop wind and resolve phlegm. For abundant phlegm, parched perilla fruit, bamboo shavings and immature bitter orange can be added to resolve phlegm, or inula flower and loquat leaf can be added to lower qi and resolve phlegm. For dizziness with nausea and vomiting, hooked uncaria, ochre and oriental water plantain rhizome can be added to strengthen the effect of stopping wind, lowering the adverse flow of qi, eliminating dampness and resolving phlegm. For dizziness with tinnitus, calamus and curcuma root can be added to resolve phlegm and induce resuscitation. For tightness sensation in the stomach and anorexia, radish seed, nutmeg and amomum fruit can be added to induce appetite and regulate the spleen.

Fire syndrome due to stagnation of phlegm causes distending pain in the head, vexation, liability to anger, dizziness changeable with emotion, bitter taste in the mouth, vomiting, insomnia, nightmare, yellow and greasy fur, and taut and slippery pulse. Wen Dan Decoction, coptis root, scutellaria root, hooked uncaria and gastrodia tuber should be used to resolve phlegm, remove heat, dispel wind and stop dizziness.

Example of Recipe:

Pinellia tuber 10g, parched tangerine peel 10g, fuling 15g, bamboo shavings 10g, parched immature bitter orange 10g, parched bighead atractylodes rhizome 10g, hooked uncaria 12g, gastrodia tuber 10g, polygala root 10g, amomum fruit 5g, and red ochre 20g (decocted first).

(E) Obstruction of Channels by Blood Stasis

Main Symptom: dizziness due to external injury in the head or dizziness with no cure after treatment for a long time.

Accompanying Symptoms: relapses of headache in a fixed area or prickling pain with no response to conventional treatment, darkish complexion and lips, insomnia, amnesia, lassitude and palpitation.

Tongue and Pulse: dark purple tongue, or with ecchymosis, and taut and slippery or thready and uneven pulse.

Analysis: External injury in the head causes blood stasis to obstruct channels, or lingering dizziness with no response to conventional treatment causes illness to enter channels. Obstruction of channels by blood stasis causes malnutrition of seven orifices, leading to prickling pain in a fixed area, insomnia and amnesia. No generation of blood due to blood stasis causes malnutrition of the heart, leading to palpitation and lassitude. Darkish tongue, or with ecchymosis, and taut and slippery or thready and uneven pulse are signs of obstruction of channels by blood stasis.

Treatment: removing blood stasis, clearing channels, promoting blood circulation, and inducing resuscitation.

Recipe and Drugs: In the recipe Tong Qiao Huo Xue Decoction Jia Jian, red peony root, chuanxiong rhizome, peach kernel and safflower promote blood circulation to remove blood stasis. Chinese green onion and musk activate yang and induce resuscitation. Fresh ginger and Chinese date regulate the spleen and stomach and make the above-mentioned drugs not to impair the stomach. For obvious blood stasis in the head, motherwort fruit pangolin scales, scorpion and centipede can be added to promote blood circulation and clear channels. For emotional depression and stagnation of the liver-qi with pain in the chest and hypochondria and sigh, bupleurum root, bitter orange and curcum root can be added to sooth the liver and regulate qi circulation. For qi deficiency with lassitude, abundant sweat and aversion to wind, astragalus root and dangshen can be added to strengthen the spleen and replenish qi. For yang deficiency and excessive cold with aversion to cold and cold limbs, prepared aconite root and cinnamom twig can be added to warm yang and promote blood circulation. For yin deficiency with hectic fever, consumptive fever, and squamous and dry skin, moutan bark, anemarrhena rhizome, phellodendron bark and dried rehmannia root can be added to nourish yin and remove heat.

Example of Recipe:

Chuanxiong rhizome 10g, motherwort fruit 10g, parched red peony root 12g, scorpion powder 3g, (infused separately), 2 centipedes, Chinese angelica root 10g, peach kernel 10g, safflower 10g, Chinese green onion 2cun, hooked uncaria 10g and gastrodia tuber 10g.

〔Preventive and Nursing Measures〕

1. The environment should be quiet and comfortable without noise and with soft light. When dizziness fits, the patient should lie down calmly and reduce movement, and particularly should not turn round.

2. The patient should be happy, avoid harmful stimulation to its mind, and relieve or reduce its anxiety and fear.

3. Diet should be light. It is particularly important for patients with abundant phlegm to take light diet. The patient with deficiency syndrome should be gradually nourished with taking frequent small meals, and should not indulge in crapulence.

4. The patient with serious dizziness, drastic vomit, vibration of eyes, numb limbs, vague mind and unstable blood pressure should be promptly treated to avoid delaying illness condition.

〔Analysis of A Typical Case〕

Mr. Xue, 59.

He suffered from dizziness for more than 10 years. When dizziness fitted, he felt as if riding a boat or car with nausea and vomiting. His dizziness mainly fitted in the spring with insomnia, dreaminess, anorexia, abdominal distention, eructation, thirst for hot drinks, sometimes vibration of fingers, constipation, sometimes diarrhea, normal urine, slightly enlarged liver, and normal function of the liver. His pulse was taut and thready at cun and chi, but taut, forceful and hollow at guan. His tongue was normal without fur and with teeth prints on its edge. The patient was diagnosed as suffering from Meniere's syndrome belonging to yin deficiency and yang floating. The disease should be treated with the following recipe to reinforce yin, suppress yang and regulate the spleen and stomach.

red ginseng 30g, fushen 30g, dogwood fruit 60g, wolfberry fruit 30g, desertliving cistanche 60g, Chinese yam 90g, Siberian solomonseal rhizome 60g, stir-fried tortoise plastron (smashed) 120g, sesame seed (parched) 90g, magnetite (smashed) 60g, pearl shell (smashed) 60g, flatstem 60g, amomum fruit (smashed) 15g, bighead atractylodes rhizome 30g, tangerine peel 15g, lotus seed (smashed) 60g, and longan aril 30g.

Three doses of the drugs were decocted, concentrated after residue removed, and mixed with honey into a paste. Every morning and evening, the patient took

10g of the paste infused with warm boiled water. He stopped taking the paste when catching cold.

The patient took the paste for about 3 months with dizziness disappearing and appetite improved. After he had stopped taking the paste, distending pain in the abdomen, reduced appetite and other symptoms of yin deficiency, weakened spleen, dysfunction of the intestine and stomach relapsed. Another dose of the above-mentioned recipe plus and minus ingredients was taken to consolidate the curative effect.

Note: The case belonged to yin deficiency, weakened spleen, upward floating of yang in deficiency condition, and dysfunction of the spleen and stomach. Drugs were used to nourish the liver and kidney, replenish yin, suppress yang, and regulate the spleen and stomach with curative effect achieved. Lingering illness and repeated fits should be slowly treated with paste. (quoted from "Medical Experiences of Pu Fuzhou")

Dizziness is a clinically common disease. Mild dizziness fits momentarily and disappears after a while. Serious patients feel everything around revolving and have symptoms of vomiting, no appetite, dysphoria and insomnia. Although the pathogenesis of dizziness is complicated, its causes can be summarized as factors of wind, fire, phlegm, deficiency syndrome and blood stasis. Dizziness can be caused by one factor or jointly by several factors. For example, yin deficiency of the liver and kidney, hyperactivity of the liver-yang, phlegm and blood stasis can jointly cause dizziness. Clinically, there is a trend of increase in dizziness of deficiency syndrome and deficiency syndrome complicated with excess symptoms. Its pure excess syndrome is rarely seen. In its treatment, purging drugs should be used for excess syndrome, nourishing drugs for deficiency syndrome, and purging and nourishing drugs altogether for deficiency in origin and excess in superficiality. Acute dizziness is mainly excess syndrome, which can be treated with measures to calm the liver, stop wind, suppress yang, clear away heat, resolve phlegm and remove blood stasis. Chronic dizziness is mainly deficiency syndrome, which should be treated with measures to invigorate qi, enrich the blood, strengthen the spleen, nourish the liver and reinforce the kidney. One measure or several measures can be used to treat dizziness according to its illness condition of deficiency or excess syndromes.

Frequent fits of dizziness in middle-aged and old people are mainly caused by deficiency of the liver and kidney, which is liable to trigger stirring-up of the liver.

Serious patients can suddenly fall in a faint and possibly develop into a stroke, so they should be treated actively. Dizziness sufferers should refrain from eating fatty, sweet and pungent food, drinking wine, getting angry and having sex. They should pay attention to proper balance between work and rest, and carry out appropriate physical activities. Serious patients can practise qigong and should follow medical order to take drugs for recuperation.

Question for Review

1. Try to describe the pathology of dizziness.
2. How to understand the significance of the liver, spleen, stomach and kidney in the invasion of dizziness.
3. Try to describe characteristics of symptoms for common types of dizziness and their interrelations.
4. Try to describe treatments, recipes and drugs for common types of dizziness.
5. How to recognize the relations between dizziness and stroke.

Apoplexy

〔Introduction〕

Apoplexy, or stroke, is a group of signs of disease characterized by its main clinical manifestations as falling down abruptly, unconsciousness, hemiplegia, numbness all over the body, speech disorder or aphasia. It also may occur without falling but with hemiplegia, convulsion, distortion of mouth and tongue as its essential features. Since its acute onset, swiftness in coming up, multiplicity in symptom complex, rapid change and its clinical appearance of falling and convulsion are similar to the characters of 'wind' in easiness in moving and having a series of changes. Therefore, in ancient medicine, this kind of diseases was recognized and studied in a more broad sense, the commonly used method as grouping the similarities and comparison the dissimilarities was adopted. Those groups of diseases with above mentioned characters were named as apoplexy. The disease entity was followed afterward, and understanding on it had been improved continuously. An unique theory of pathogenic factors and pathogenesis of apoplexy was established and rich experiences on its prevention and treatment has been accumulated.

Above described distinguished clinical feature of apoplexy is fundamentally different from so called exterior syndrome of Tai Yang Zhong Feng (apoplexy) as stated in the chapter of《Shang Han Lun • Bian Tai Yang Bing》. Where it was stated "Tai Yang disease those with fever, sweating, wind-phobia, bradycardia are called apoplexy". So called Tai Yang apoplexy(Zhong Feng) in《Shang Han Lun》belongs to exterior syndrome originated from external invasion, similar to such kind of diseases as we called"catch cold""common cold" today. It is similar only in nomination but different substantially from apoplexy that will be discussed in this chapter. They should not be mixed up with each other, especially in studying ancient literature.

Diseases with essential manifestation as described above such as cerebral hemorrhage, obliterative cerebral vascular disease, and stroke due to tumor, different kind of intracranial arterities in modern medicine may fall into this category and may be referred to in the treatment by differential symptoms.

〔Pathogenic Factors and Pathology〕

Occurrence of apoplexy lies mainly on imbalance in Yin and Yang in daily life, deficiency in Qi and blood, lack of adjustment, with worrisome mental status and angry, or uncontrolled in dietary intake, injury by too much sexual activities, destruction of resistance by fatigue, invasion by external seasonal pathogens. As a consequence, the circulation of Qi and blood become stagnant, muscle, skin, tendon and vessels are less nutrient. Result in descend of Yin, liver Yang extend and enlarge suddenly which transformed into current of wind, reversed and distorted circulation of Qi and blood, carrying phlegm and fire, attack and disturb channels and collateral vessels, obscure and obstruct heart foramen. Thus, induce sudden onset of coma and hemiplegia. with the appearance of critical syndrome of a status in which excess in the upper part and deficiency in the lower part exists and disconnection between Yin and Yang. The pathogenesis changing rapidly and frequently will be stated separately as following.

1. Insufficiency in vital-Qi, emptiness in collateral branch of the large channel, invasion by external pathogenic factors. External wind is one of six pathogenic factors. Wind invades into the body through skin and hair, either retaining in between muscle masses and tendons or wandering along with channels and collateral vessels. Wind comes into mostly under the condition as deficiency in

vital-Qi, untightness of spaces, low defensive function to exterior pathogenic factors. By taking this advantage wind brings harm to the channels and collateral vessels and causes loss of nourishment in muscle and skin. On the other hand, due to excess in phlegm in ordinary life, external wind induces phlegm disperse over channels and collateral vessels. The attack of wind is rather superficial, mostly Yang channels and cephalic or facial region are essentially to be diseased. Therefore, the main clinical features are distortion of mouth and eye, parenthesis of muscle and skin, hemiplegia.

2. In case of under stress either mentally or physically, weakness after illness, debility in elderly, imbalance in Yin and Yang, endogenous wind send forth. Overloading may move up Yang Qi, which run upward and transformed into wind. Additionally overloading may exhaust and destroy essence of life and blood. After a long course of illness or in frail old ones, hyperactivity of liver Yang occur due to similar reason of deficiency in essence of life and blood; deficiency in liver and kidney Yin, deprivation of liver from its nourishment. Under condition of severe disturbance in Ying and Yang, additional induction factors, such as emotional upset, alcoholism, fatigue, climate change, may cause Yin deficiency in lower part and excess Yang in upper part and Yang transformed into current of wind. Qi and blood ascend, mentality become confused and develop to apoplexy. This is endogenous wind. While endogenous wind blows up, it should have floating upward of Qi and fire, forcing the blood spring upward, otherwise wind bringing phlegm and stagnant blood together disturbing channels and collateral vessels, crowding in mind. In more severe condition, Qi accompanied with blood run upward, forcing blood separated from channel, lead to coma lastly. Most of this disease are progressed by incite of internal wind, and the situation is more serious.

3. Uncontrol in diet, internal injury by strain and fatigue, spleen deprived of normal transportation, accumulation of dampness producing phlegm, stagnation of phlegm transform into fire, obstruction in channels and collateral, lead to loss of consciousness. Otherwise frequent hyperfunction of liver Yang, wood restrict spleen earth, which causes dysfunction of spleen transportation and phlegm turbid rises up endogenously. Otherwise internal fire burns vigorously, dried up the secretion into phlegm. Liver wind carrying phlegm and fire runs upward and disturbs channels and collateral of vessels, obscures the mind, then, sudden falling down with coma, paralysis occur. Overall, this is dysfunction in spleen

transportation producing phlegm turbid endogenously. Phlegm can be classified into damp phlegm, heat phlegm and wind phlegm which may be interchangeable with each other.

4. Exaggeration of five kinds of emotion, extreme excess in heart fire, wind and fire interact with each other, or liver suppres with stagnation of liver Qi, stagnancy of Qi with blood stasis. Great angry injury liver, hyperactivity in liver Yang, all these easily elicit Qi and blood retrogressed flow disorder and lead to confusion and falling down with loss of sensation, developing to apoplexy lastly. Apoplexy caused by injury to liver under condition of bursting into extreme angry is most commonly seen in clinics. Under extreme angry, liver Yang extends significantly within a moment, both Qi and blood float upward, forcing blood rushes to the brain. Both Qi and blood run side by side in the upper part, then symptoms of coma develop suddenly. The disease is more prevalent in one under emotional stress commonly, enduring worry or with an irritable temperament.

Above all, although the pathogenesis and mechanism of apoplexy is rather complicate, but its pathogenic changes is not beyond six groups: wind, fire, phlegm, Qi, blood, deficiency. Wind may be differentiated into internal or external wind; fire may be separated into heart fire and liver fire; in the phlegm there is difference in wind phlegm, damp phlegm, and fire phlegm, in addition there are Qi deficiency, Qi stagnancy, reversed flow of Qi, blood deficiency, stagnancy of blood, Yin deficiency, et al. But overall stagnancy of blood is most commonly seen. Among Qi deficiency, spleen deficiency, kidney deficiency, liver and kidney Yin deficiency is the base. Endogenous wind, phlegm turbid, and stagnancy of blood often in accompany and intermingled with each other in disease developing process.

If the disease comes from invasion by external pathogenic factors it is called external apoplexy also named as true apoplexy. While it developes without external invasion is called internal apoplexy, or apoplexy-like. Although in the early stage of disease, according to deepness in localization of disease, severity of disease it may be classified into apoplexy involving the channels and collateral and apoplexy involving internal organs but the fundamental pathogenic changes are indifferent.

〔Diagnosis and Treatment〕

Although apoplexy is caused by many factors, but the fundamental pathogenic changes are relative excess of Yin Yang, retrogressed flow of Qi and blood. Superficially it appears as wind and fire stirring up each other, stagnancy of turbid phlegm, obstruction by blood stasis, leading to the formation of complex syndromes of both excess in origin but deficiency in superficiality and excess in upper part but deficiency in lower part. Since the strength of vital energy and pathogenic factors is quite different and individuality in body constitution of relative excess of Yin and Yang, so there are differences either in severity of disease, deepness of pathologic localization, or syndromes belonging to cold, heat, deficiency, excess, progress of disease is improveing or worsening. Under so intermingled complicate circumstances, that to master the critical points for differentiation is the essence for correct differentiation of syndroms in clinics.

Skematic Diagram for Pathogenic Factors and Pathogenesis of Apoplexy

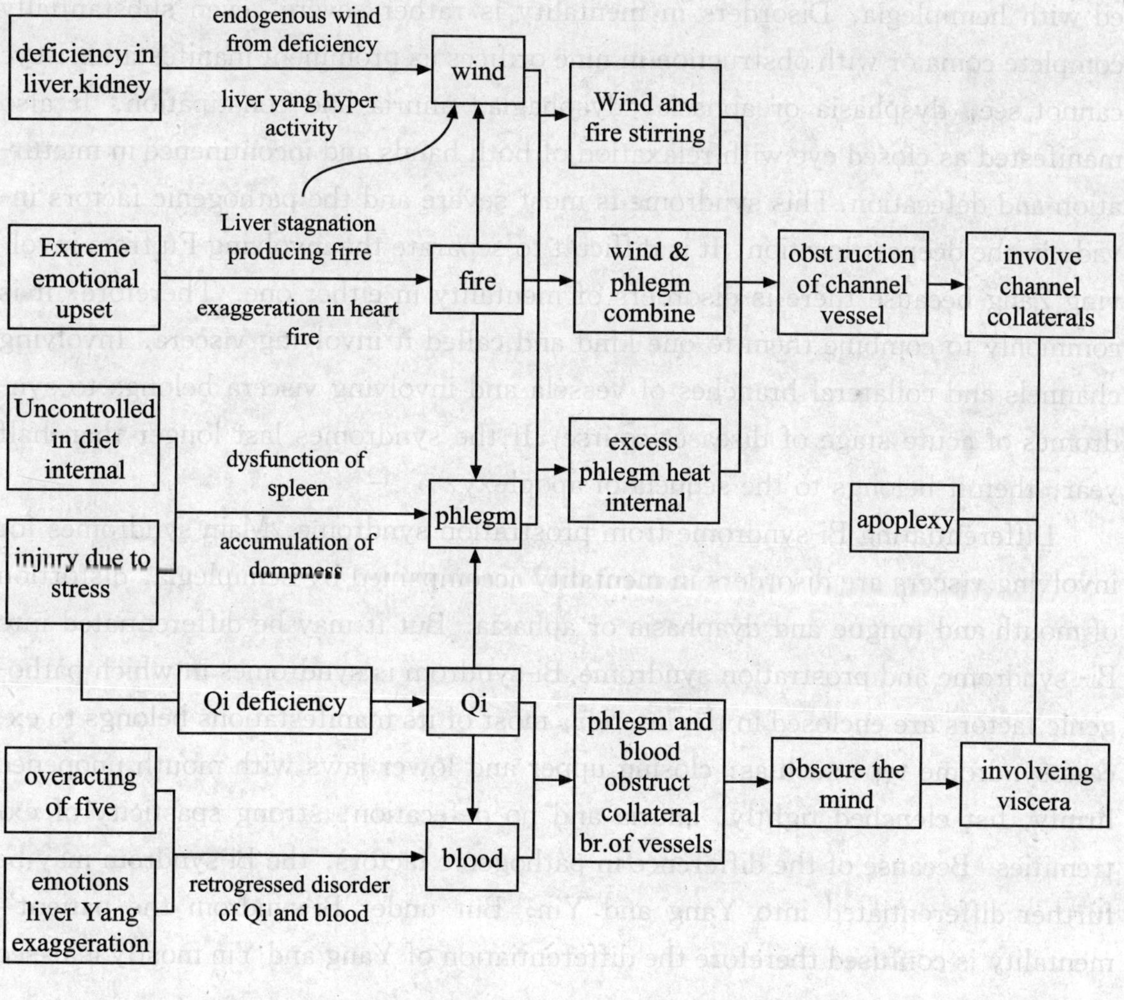

Differentiation of deepness of pathologic location and severity of disease: The syndromes in acute stage of apoplexy may be classified into two kinds; involving channel and collateral and involving visera. The main symptoms for involving collateral branch of vessels are distortion of mouth and tongue and numbness in muscle and skin which usually occur in one side of the body or extremities of one side. In this condition the pathogenic factors localized superficially and disease is rather mild. The main syndromes of involving channels are hemiplegia, distortion of mouth and tongue, numbness in one side and dysphasia, no coma. This condition is more severe than involving collaterals. In the clinics this two conditions are belonged to one group and named it involving channel and collateral.

The main syndromes in involving Fu are: hemiplegia, distortion of mouth and tongue, paresthesia of one side of body, dysphasia and unconsciousness. But the character of loss of consciousness in this condition is rather mild only some confusion or sleepiness present. Involving Zang is sudden onset of coma associated with hemiplegia. Disorders in mentality is rather severe, even substantially complete coma or with obstruction in nine orifices as prominent manifestation: eye cannot see, dysphasia or aphasia, dysphagia, anuria and constipation. It also manifested as closed eye with relaxation of both hands and incontinence in micturation and defecation. This syndrome is most severe and the pathogenic factors invade in the deepest location. It is difficult to separate the involving Fu from involving Zang because there is disorders of mentality in either one. Therefore, it is commonly to combine them to one kind and called it involving viscera. Involving channels and collateral branches of vessela and involving viscera belongs to syndromes of acute stage of diseases'course. If the syndromes last longer than half year, then it belongs to the sequela of apoplexy.

Differentiating Bi-syndrome from prostration syndrome: Main syndromes for involving viscera are disorders in mentality accompanied by hemiplegia, distortion of mouth and tongue and dyaphasia or aphasia. But it may be differentiated into Bi- syndrome and prostration syndrome. Bi-syndrom is syndromes in which pathogenic factors are enclosed in the interior, most of its manifestations belongs to excess syndrome type such as: closing upper and lower jaws with mouth unopened firmly, fist clenched tightly, anuria and no defecation, strong spasticity of extremities. Because of the difference in pathogenic factors, the Bi-syndrom may be further differentiated into Yang and Yin. But under Bi-syndrom the patient's mentality is confused therefore the differentiation of Yang and Yin mostly is based essentially on inspection of the tongue or pulse-taking. Prostration-syndrome is the syndrome in which the Yang-Qi dispersed externally, its manifestation mostly belongs to deficiency syndrome, such as closed eyes with opened mouth, superficial and weak breathing, hands relaxed with incontinence in urination, All this is the indication for decaying and exhaustion of vital energy of five hollow organs leading to unfavorable prognosis. Its treatment is stregthening the body resistance and restore the normal function of the body to against prostration.

Differentiating degree of seriousness of disease is improving or worsening: In acute stage of apoplexy, the syndrome changes rapidly, which may be differed in improving or worsening. It will be helpful in prognosis if the degree of seriousness may be differentiated as worsening or improving and the trend of development of the disease kept in mind. Generally speaking, the changes in mentality is an important criteria in differentiating the degree of seriousness of disease. Under condition of involving viscera at first, if the mentality become wake up gradually and symptoms like hemiplegia et, al. either not aggravated or with some recovery, the disease is transformed from involving viscera to involving channewls and collateral branches of vessels, the degree of seriousness of disease is improving. Symptoms like unconsciousness, hemiplegia et al. may be aggravated or fluctuated by internal excess in phlegm heat or deficiency in vitality, which is most commonly seen in acute stage of apoplexy. This degree of seriousness still belongs to improving. If hiccup occurs frequently, either with sudden onset of coma, continuous convulsion of four extremities, or extreme high temperature in abdomen and back region in contrast with low temperature in extremities, or hemoptysis, hematochezia occurs, all these indicate disease is developing and degree of seriousness is worsening.

Apoplexy should be differentiated from epilepsy, flaccidity syndrome, and syncope.

Although in epilepsy there is sudden onset of loss of sensation with convulsion but mostly it is transient and wake up shortly with normal appearance. No hemiplegia, no distortion of mouth and tongue, no dysphasia in epilepsy. The history of recurrent onset of similar attacks in epilepsy is very useful in differentiation.

In flaccidity syndrome there is paralysis of extremities and disability in movement but its slow onset and usually occurs only in two lower extremities accompanied by muscular weakness is different.

In syncope, although coma and sudden onset of loss of sensation associated with cold in extremities may also occur, but usually wake up shortly, after that without hemiplegia, distortion of mouth and tongue, dysphasia.

Apoplexy is a syndrome of deficiency in origin and excess in superficiality. In the origin there is liver and kidney deficiency, blood and Qi deficiency; while in the superficiality there is wind and fire stirring up each other, excess of phlegm pathogenic factors, functional disorder of Qi, obstruction of stagnant blood. Because of the difference in deepness of pathogenic location, the degree of seriousness, sequence and acuteness of origin and superficiality, and sequence and acuteness of deficiency and excess, therefore in clinics usually divide apoplexy into involving channels and colateral branches of vessels, involving viscera and residuals for differentiation syndromes and treatment.

1. Involving channels and collateral vessels

(1) Emptiness in collateral branches of vessels and invasion by wind pathogenic factors

Main symptoms: wind invades from outside, distortion of mouth and tongue occurs suddenly. Else, there is dizziness in ordinary time, numbness of one side of body and loss of perception in muscle and skin occur abruptly. Otherwise, dysphasia, salivation overflow from corner of mouth, and even hemiplegia occur.

Accompanying symptoms: either headache, nasal obstruction, or aversion to cold with fever, soreness and pain in joints, et, al.

Tongue and pulse: tongue fur is thin and white or thin and yellow, type of pulse is floating and tense or taut and thready.

Analysis: Because of insufficient vital energy and low defensive function, or in the situation of sweating after exertion resulting in skin and sebaceous gland open up or lying facing a swift of wind, wind as pathogenic factor invades into channels and collateral vessels. As a result, Qi and blood become stagnant with unsmooth circulation, which brings in loss of nutrients in muscles and vessels. Wind as a pathogenic factor attacks the upper portion firstly, the head as the converge of a lot of Yang and locates at the upper most region, therefore, distortion of mouth and eye are commonly seen. If the body with phlegm and dampness excess internally or those already diseased by endogenous wind are invaded by external wind, the external wind enters interior, activates phlegm pathogen or motivate endogenous wind, endogenous and external pathogens combine up, wind and phlegm combining with each other, disturb channels resulting to hemiplegia and dysphasia. Otherwise wind phlegm disturbs collateral branches of vessels, Qi and blood circulate unevenly, resulting in dysfunction of nutrition and defense and leading to numbness of muscles and skin. Wind invades externally cause disharmony between Yin (nutrition) and Wei (defense) and induce the symptoms of aversion of cold with fever and pain and soreness in joints. Tongue fur is thin and white. Floating and tense pulse is sign of invasion internally by superficial pathogen. Taut and thready pulse is the sign of deficiency in Qi and blood.

Method of treatment: dispelling wind and removing obstruction in the channels. nourishing blood and enforcing nutrition.

Prescription: Modified Da Qin Jiao Decoction. This prescription is composed of drugs inducing diaphoresis to dispel wind mainly, combined with drugs nourishing blood, promoting blood flow and clearing heat. Gentian as the main drug induces dispel wind and remove the pathogen. Rhizoma seu Radix Notopterygii, Ledebouriella root dissipate the wind pathogen in Tai Yang channel. Radix Angelicae Dahuricae dissipate the wind pathogen in Yang Ming channel. Herba Asari and Radix Angelicae Pubescentis search the wind pathogen in Shao Yang channel. Due to the characteristics of drugs inducing diaphoresis and dispelling wind is rather dryness so adjusted with Radix Paeoniae Alba astringing Yin and nourishing blood, Radix Rehmannia, Rhizoma Ligustici Chuangxiong, Radix Angelicae Sinensis nourishing blood and regulating the nutrient. In addition Rhizoma Atractylodis Macrocephalae, Poria, and Radix Glycyrrhizae, et al., reinforcing the spleen and replenishing Qi, altogether make up a prescription of nourishing blood, enforcing Qi, dispelling wind, for strengthening the body resistance and eliminating pathogenic factors. Wind belongs to Yang pathogenic factor, invasion internally by which easily transformed into heat. Therefore Radix Scutelariae and Gypsum Fibrosum are added. If after treatment the symptoms such as distortion of mouth and eyes, numbness in limbs are not relieved, the cause of which is usually due to obstruction in collateral vessels by stagnant blood of damp phlegm. Then drugs promoting blood as Radix Salviae Miltiorrhizae, Caulis Spatholobi may be added for strengthening the effect of eliminate stasis and promoting circulation; Semen Sinapis Albae, Rhizoma Typhonii, and Scorpio are added to remove wind phlegm, promote circulation, dispel the resistant pathogen in channels and collateral vessels. When wind-heat syndromes are accompanied, remove Rhizoma seu Radix Notopterygii, Ledebouriella root, Radix Angelicae Sinensis and drugs dispelling wind and clearing heat like Folium Mori, Flos Chrysanthemi, Herba Menthae are added. If there are syndromes of rigidity of neck, spasticity in nape and numbness Radix Puerariae, Rsmulud Cinnamomi may be added for dispel wind and relaxing muscles. If hiccup occur with excessive phlegm, tongue covered with white greasy fur, Radix Rehmannia, Radix Paeoniae Alba, and Radix Angelicae Sinensis may be removed and Rhizoma Pinelliae, Rhizoma Arisaematis, Exocarpium Citri for drying dampness and reducing phlegm are added.

If only distortion of mouth and hemiplegia are seen, Modified Qian Zheng Powder may be used with the addition of Herba Schizonepetae, Radix Angelicae Dahuricae, Ledebouriella root for dispel wind eliminate pathogenic factors and Flos Carthami for promoting blood and eliminating stasis.

For example:

Gentian 6g, Ledebouriella root 10g, Radix Paeoniae Alba 10g, Radix Scutelariae 6g, Lumbricus 10g, Rhizoma Ligustici Chuangxiong 9g, Poria 15g, Atractylodis Macrocephalae 6g, Radix Angelicae Sinensis 10g, Cortex Moutan Radicis 10g, Scorpio 3g, Radix Glycyrrhizae 6g.

(2) Liver and kidney Yin deficiency, Wind Yang invades upper portion

Main Symptoms: Dizziness and giddiness in usual time, headache, tinnitus, less sleep with frequent dream, lumbar soreness with weak legs, sudden onset of heaviness and numbness in limbs, hemiplegia, distortion in mouth and tongue, dysphasia or rigidity in tongue with aphasia.

Accompanying Symptoms: little salivation in mouth, constipation or hard stool in usual time, deep color urine.

Tongue and pulse: red tongue proper, yellow fur, pulse taut, thready and rapid or taut and slippery.

Analysis: Due to liver kidney Yin deficiency in ordinary live, excessive liver Yang, disharmony in Yin and Yang, deficiency of essence of live in the lower part, Yang float in the upper part, stagnancy in blood(?) and retrogression of Qi, excess in upper part and deficiency in lower part are resulted and syndromes of dizziness, headache, tinnitus, giddiness occur. It comes from the theory that kidney storing of essence of live, being in charge of bone, and liver being the window of eye, therefore deficiency in liver and kidney results in insufficient filling of sea of marrow, less nourishing in ears and eyes. Diminished sleep with frequent dream, lumbar soreness and weak legs are caused by breakdown of the normal physiological coordination between the heart and the kidney, deficiency in kidney.

Sometimes syndromes of deficiency in Yin and excess in Yang may occur, such as face dried with heat, worrying, agitating, easily to become angry, feeling of heaviness in head and lightness in legs while walking. Deficiency in liver Yin and liver Yang being lost of control become hyperactive, which brings to activation of liver wind. Wind is pathogenic factor of Yang. If liver wind carrying phlegm runs upward or carrying with stagnant blood disturbs channel, syndromes like distortion of mouth and tongue, dysphasia, hemiplegia would occur abruptly. Analyzing from type of pulse, taut pulse being in charge of liver wind, slippery is phlegm dampness, taut thready and rapid pulse comes from endogenous heat raised from deficiency in liver and kidney Yin, heat pathogen disturbs internally and even burned up Yin liquid, resulting wind Yang floating. Red tongue proper is endogenous heat injured by Yin. Greasery fur is accompanied by phlegm dampness. Yellow fur is the manifestation of transmission of heat.

In this syndrome hemiplegia is the main feature but without mental disorder. It belongs to involving channel, many changes may occur within the first week after onset. If treatment is on-time and good adjustment being carried out, endogenous wind would be calmed down and degree of severity of disease would gradually become stable. Prognosis is better under condition of phlegm turbidity being transmitted, endogenous heat cleared up, stagnant blood eliminated and symptoms like hemiplegia and dysphasia diminished, recovery gradually occurs. In severe cases or the disease not under good adjustment or drugs of promoting Yang with producing heat being taken, bringing to motivation of unstopping endogenous wind, within one week after onset, the disease is worsened gradually and hemiplegia aggravated, furthermore mental status become confused, disease transformed into involving internal organs. Particular attention should be paid to those with liver and kidney Yin deficiency, and those endogenous wind blow up commonly in usual time, intensive carcful adjustment is needed, preventing from worrisome, anger is important. Great angry will cause exaggeration of liver Yang, sudden onset of wind Yang brings to phlegm turbid pathogen, forcing blood runs retrogressed upward, and resulting to critical signs of syncope.

Method of treatment: cultivating yin with suppresing yang, tranquilizing liver with calming down wind.

Prescription: Modified Zhen Gan Xi Feng Decoction. Radix Paeoniae Alba, Radix Scrophulariae, Radix Asparagi, Plastrum Testudinis in the prescription nourish liver and kidney Yin, softening liver calming wind. Os Dragonis Fossilia

Ossis Mastodi, Concha Ostreae, Orchra Haematium check hyperfunction of liver to suppressing Yang, descend retrogression with tranquilizing excitation. Combination with Rhizoma Gastrodiae, Ramulus Uncarine cum Uncis, Flos Crysanthemi, intensify the effect of tranquilizing liver and calming wind. Put emphasiz on Radix Achyranthis Bidentatae and helped by Fructus Meliae Toosendan may conduct blood downward. Combination with Herba Artemisiae Capillaris, Fructus Hordei Germinatus is used to clear liver removing stagnancy, restore stomach balancing the middle. In those excess in phlegm-heat, remove nourishing and greasy ones as, Plastrum Testudinis and Radix Asparagi Arisaema cum Bile, Succus Bambosae are added to clear phlegm-heat. in those irritable, Radix Scutellariae, Capejasmine, Gypsum Fibrosumare added to clear heat and sedation. While in severe headache Concha Haliotidis, Spica Prunellaeare added to dispel and calm wind Yang. In insomnia with frequent dream, pearl, Fossilia Dentis Mastodiare, Caulis Polygoni Multiflori, Poria cum Ligno Hospite added as tranquilizer to ease mental stress. According to the individual condition other drugs of rescucitating and promoting collateral circulation may be added such as Calamus, Radix Polygalae, Lumbricus, Flos Carthami, Caulis Spatholobi, et al.

Example for prescription: Rhizoma Gastrodiae 10g, Ramulus Uncarine cum Uncis 30g, Flos Crysanthemi 6g, Radix Paeoniae Alba 12g, Radix Scrophulariae 12g, Lumbricus 6g, Radix Achyranthis Bidentatae 10g, Concha Ostreae 30g (ahead), Radix Rehmanniae 20g, Capejasmine 6g, Orchra Haematium 30g (ahead), Radix Asparagi 10g.

(3) Wind-phlegm disturb upward, phlegm-heat with excess Fu-organ

Main Symptoms: sudden onset of distortion in mouth and tongue, hemiplegia, numbness over one side of body, excessive salivation and phlegm, constipation.

Accompanying Symptoms: either dizziness, tongue rigidity with dysphasia, or abdominal fullness and distention, or fever.

Tongue and pulse: red tongue proper, yellow fur or with thick greasy fur, pulse taut and slippery or with rapidity.

Analysis: Without control in ordinary diet, over intake of fatty, sweaty, heavy taste food injure spleen. Large amount in drinking produce damp-heat endogenously. Otherwise internal injury like overloading and fatigue cause dysfunction of spleen transportation, accumulation of dampness producing phlegm. Long time accumulation of pathogenic factor as phlegm-dampness transformed to heat.

In case of worrying or anger, endogenous wind blow up abruptly, which carrying phlegm-heat obstructs channels and collaterals, then hemiplegia and distortion of mouth and tongue suddenly come. Obstruction in middle burner by pathogenic factor as phlegm-heat, dysfunction in transportation, abnormality in ascending of clearness and descending of turbidity cause stagnancy of Qi of hollow Fu-organ and constipation resulted. Clear Yang Qi not ascends, turbid Qi ascends into brain resulting dizziness. Wind-phlegm pathogenic factor obstruct the origin of tongue, disorder in Qi and blood circulation cause tongue spasticity and dysphagia. This syndrome may also be raised from obstruction by stagnant blood, obstruction in channels, causing dysfunction of solid and hollow internal organs, phlegm-heat produced endogenously and inducing manifestation of endogenous wind carrying phlegm-heat and stagnant blood. Yellow tongue fur, or yellow and greasy; pulse taut and slippery demonstrate excess phlegm-heat internally.

This syndrome is commonly seen in clinics. Though it belongs to involving channels and collateral, but excess interior or stagnant in Fu-organ Qi, in case of phlegm-heat enclosed internally for long time confusion in mental status such as blurring, sleepiness may also present. If it is treated not on-time, phlegm-heat aggravated day by day, heart forum obstructed, it will develop into Bi-syndrom of involving internal organs. Therefore, it is suitable to consider this syndrome is a syndrome placed in between involving channels and collateral and involving internal organs. For treatment, removing obstruction in internal hollow organs and eliminating phlegm may be put on the first step. As obstruction in Fu-Qi being relieved, drugs for clearing away heat with resolving phlegm and promoting collateral branches of vessels may be prescribed secondary. As phlegm-heat cleared up, then the main direction is to promoting blood circulation and removing the stagnancy, recovery from hemiplegia and related syndromes would be expected.

Method of treatment: resolving phlegm with release obstruction in hollow organs.

Prescription: Modified Xing Lou Cheng Qi Decoction. Fructus Trichosanthis, Arisaema cum Bile, Radix et Rhizoma Rhei, Natrii Suphas are consisted in. Arisaema cum Bile and Fructus Trichosanthis are used for clearing phlegm-heat, while Radix et Rhizoma Rhei and Natrii Suphas for removing stagnancy and conducting hollow organs. This prescription is modified from Set prescription Cheng Qi Decoction. If had been constipated for long time with marked abdominal fullness and distension, drugs for regulating the flow of Qi such as immature bitter orange, Cortex Magnoliae Officinalis may be added. In case of relieving of constipation after taking the prescription, Fu-Qi flows smoothly with phlegm-heat reduced, then disorders in mental status and hemiplegia will be recovered gradually. If no improvement after first dose, next dose may be followed. Dosage for Radix et Rhizoma Rhei and Natrii Suphas should not over 10g. Hyperactivation of bowel and diarrhea should be avoided in order not bring in injury to vital-Qi. For treatment in those being injured in both Yin and Qi accompanied by accumulation of phlegm-heat, it is suitable to combine reinforcement and elimination aimed at increasing liquid and continuing Qi. Drugs nourishing vital essence and remove dryness such as Radix Rehmanniae, Radix Scrophulariae, and Radix Ophiopogonis are added to above prescription. If unstopping diarrhea occurs after purgative therapy, it means vital-Qi being injured greatly, purgatives should not be used anymore. After release of stagnancy in hollow organs, prescription with clearing heat and resolving phlegm, activating blood circulation and promoting collateral vessels are used Such as: Arisaema cum Bile, Fructus Trichosanthis, Radix Salviae Miltiorhizae, Radix Paeoniae Rubra, Caulis Spatholobi, et al. In dizziness Ramulus Uncarine cum Uncis, Flos Crysanthemi, Concha Haliotidis are added.

Examples for prescription: Fructus Trichosanthis 30g, Arisaema cum Bile 10g, Radix et Rhizoma Rhei 10g (after), Natrii Suphas 10g (take as infusion and in divided dosage) Calamus 10g, Bambosae textilis Meclure 10g, Radix Salviae Miltiorhizae 20g.

2. Involving internal organs

Involving internal organs is the acute dangerous critical type of apoplexy. One of them manifested as sudden onset of coma, unconsciouness, paralysis of extremities; the another one is transmitted from involving channels and collatrals. According to its clinical manifestation it may be differentiated into Bi-syndrome and prostration syndrome. Treatment for these two syndromes are substantially different, it should be investigated carefully in clinics. Discussed separately as following:

(1)Bi-syndrom: Main symptoms for Bi-syndrome are sudden onset of coma, unconsciousness, trismus, mouth unopened, both hands clenched fist firmly, spasticity in extremities, constipation and dysuria.

Although it is similar in pathogenic factors enclosed in heart forum, the clinic manifestation varies due to the difference in causes of diseases, the body constitution being strong or weak. Therefor Bi-syndrome is further divided into two types: Yang-Bi and Yin-Bi.

1) Yang-Bi

Main Symptoms: In additional to main syndromes commonly seen in Bi-syndrome such as; sudden onset of coma, unconsciousness, trismus, mouth unopened, both hands clenched fist firmly, spasticity in extremities, constipation and dysuria; also other syndromes are accompanied as: face red and moistened or flushed face with hot body, excessive salivation and phlegm, coarse breathing, agitation.

Accompanied Symptoms: contraction of extremities, hiccup.

tongue and pulse: red tongue proper, yellow greasy fur, pulse taut, slippery and strong.

Analysis: Because of liver Yang in usual time is hyperactive, liver Yang exaggerates significantly under emotional upset, Yang ascending stirring up wind, blood following Qi retrogresses upward and carrying phlegm and fire, covering and blurring the mind, unclear in heart and mind then coma with unconsciousness occurs promptly. Yang-Bi syndrome is produced by wind and fire enclosed interior, phlegm and heat combining with each other, obstruction in heart forum, obstruction in channels and vessels. Thus symptoms causing by fire and heat pathogenic factors may also present such as red face, flushed face, hot body, agitation. Red tongue proper, yellow greasy fur, taut, slippery and strong pulse, all are signs for endogenous wind, phlegm and fire.

Yang-Bi is an acute critical disease of apoplexy, in which pathogenic factors are in excess while the vital energy have not been defeated. If it is treated ontime, pathogenic factors be eliminated and heart forum opened, then consciousness gradually restored and prognosis may be better. After mental status recovers completely some hemiplaegia or dysphasia et al. may remain, and involving internal organs transmit to involving channels and collateral. Gradual recovery may be expected. In case of long term coma or pathogenic factors having not been defeated by vital energy, or incomplete and making mistake in treatment, Bi-syndrome transmits to prostration syndrome. This is due to consumption of vital energy through burning up Yin liquid by injury of wind fire and phlegm heat. It is the manifestation of degree of severity of disease being more serious. In condition of pathogenic heat enclosed internally in Qi and blood, dissociation of Yin and Yang, various syndromes may present such as hemoptysis, hematemesis, hematochezia, continuous convulsion, or fever in the ventral and dorsal surface of the body but with cold extremities. All these indicate bad prognosis.

Method of treatment: opening forums with drugs pungent in flavor and cool in property, clearing liver with wind calmed up.

Prescription: At first, nasal feeding or forced feeding with Zhi Bao Pill for open forum with drugs of pungent in flavor and cool in property. Then followed by Ling Yang Jiao Decoction for clear liver with calming wind, nourishing Yin and suppressing Yang. In the prescription Cornus Saigae Tataricae, Flos Crysanthemi Spica Prunellaeare clear liver and calm wind, Radix Paeoniae Alba, Plastrum Testudinis, Concha Haliotidis cultivate Yin and suppressing Yang, Radix Rehmanniae and Cortex Moutan Radicis clear heat and cold blood, Radix Achyranthis Bidentatae and Herba Leonuri conduct blood downward. In case of large amount of phlegm with coma, drugs resolving phlegm open forum such as Succus Bambosae, Arisaema cum Bile, Bambusa textilis Meclureare added. In convulsion of extremities Scorpio, Centipede, dead and stiffened Bombyx Batryticatus are used as spasmolytics and calming wind. In those with foul breath, abdominal distention and constipation, Radix et Rhizoma Rhei, immature bitter orange, Natrii Suphas are added for dysphoria and relieve obstruction in hollow organs. In those with hematemesis and hematochezia, Inner Cortex of Bamboo, Radix Scutellariae, Radix Sanguissorbae, powder of Rhizoma Bletillae may be added. Those with fever Gypsum Fibrosum and Rhizoma Anemarrhena asphodeloides are added.

Example for prescription: Flos Crysanthemi 6g, Spica Prunellaeare 10g, Radix Paeoniae Alba 10g, Radix Sanguissorbae 30g, Cortex Moutan Radicis 12g, Concha Haliotidis 30g(ahead). Calamus 10g, Radix et Rhizoma Rhei 6g. (after), Cornus Saigae Tataricae powder 1g(divided dose and mix up with decoction).

2) Yin-Bi

Main Symptoms: In additional to main syndromes commonly seen in Bi-syndrome such as; sudden onset of coma, loss of sensation, trismus, mouth unopened, there are pale face with dark lips, lying quietly without agitation, extremities rather less warmed, excessive salivation and phlegm.

Accompanying Symptoms: abdominal distention and fulness, spontaneous perspiration.

Tongue and pulse: tongue proper dark or pale with white greasy fur, pulse deep and slippery or slow.

Analysis: This syndrome susceptible to those with Yang deficiency. Because of Yang deficiency and Yin excess in ordinary time, spleen and kidney hypofunction, heart Yang deficient and weak, dysfunction in transportation and transformation result in turbid dampness stagnancy internally. Under the condition of emotional upset, endogenous wind stirring up and carrying turbid dampness, phlegm pathogenic factor upward obstructs mind. Damp turbidity and phlegm pathogen belongs to Yin, thus transmission of pathogenic factors from Yin leads to Yin-Bi syndrome. Damp turbidity and phlegm pathogen obstruct Yang-Qi, body organ cannot to be warmed up by Yang-Qi, so syndromes like pale face with dark lips, less warmed extremities and lying quietly without agitation were seen. White greasy fur and deep, slippery, slow pulse are indication for obstruction by phlegm turbidity.

Yin-Bi is also an acute critical condition of apoplexy. If effective treatment is carried out on-time, mental status gradually awakened it is also possible to transmit into involving channels and collateral and prognosis will be better. However if Yin pathogen is excessive, Yang-Qi exhausted, vital energy cannot be restored at last, it will easily transmit to prostration syndrome, difficult to be treated. Enclosed Yin for long period, functional activities of Qi in transformation cannot continue, stagnation of pathogenic factor of damp phlegm also can be transmitted into heat and resulting into Yang-Bi syndrome of phlegm-heat enclosed internally.

Method of treatment: opening orifice with drugs pungent in flavor and warm in property, resolv and dispelling phlegm and calme wind.

Prescription: Enema or nasal feeding with Su He Xiang Pilll instantly. Open orifice with drugs pungent in flavor and warm in property. Modified Di Tan Decoction is followed, which is composed of modified Er Chen Decoction acting as drying damp, resolving phlegm, regulating flow of Qi and function of middle-Jiao. Among the decoction Pericarpium Citri Reticulatus, Rhizoma Pinelliae used to remove dampness and resolve phlegm; Inner cortex of Bamboo, Poria to remove dampness and resolving phlegm, immature bitter orange to descend Qi and regulate middle-Jiao; Calamus, Arisaema cum Bile to resolve phlegm open forum, Rhizoma Gastrodiae, Ramulus Uncarine cum Uncis and dead and stiffened Bombyx Batryticatus are added to tranquilize liver and calm wind. Radix Salviae Miltiorhizae, Rhizoma Ligustici Chuangxiong and Lumbricusare used to reinforce the effect of promoting blood circulation and relieve stasis.

Example of prescription: Rhizoma Pinelliae 10g, Pericarpium Citri Reticulatus 10g, Poria 20g, Inner Cortex of Bamboo 6g, immature bitter orange 9g,

Calamus 10g, Radix Polygalae 10g, Arisaema cum Bile 6g, dead and stiffened Bombyx Batryticatus 9g.;

take Su He Xiang Pill with this decoction.

(2)Prostration syndrome

Main Symptoms: prompt coma, loss of consciousness, closed eyes, faint breath, paralysis of four limbs, incessant sweating over the extremities.

Accompanying Symptoms: curled-up tongue and ascend testes, faint pulse going to stop.

Analysis: Yang Qi is the motivation origin for functional activities of internal organs, being the fundamental elements of life. Prostration syndrome of apoplexy is weakening of Yang Qi to critical point wherever tendency of dissociation of Yin and Yang happens. Thus all manifestation of exhaustion of function of five organs going to the end are demonstrated such as closed eyes, opened mouth, curled and retracted tongue. Failing of heart function cause faint pulse going to stop. Failing lung function cause weak breath. Curling and retraction of tongue, incessant sweating also are important indications for failing heart. Spontaneous urination and defecation are manifestation for failing kidney function. The syndrome due to Yin exhausted internally with isolated Yang going separately is dangerous condition of apoplexy.

Prostration syndrome usually transmit from Bi syndrome. The essential contradiction lies on excess in pathogenic factors and deficiency in vital energy. In the treatment restoring normal function of the body is the fundamental requirement. If after first aid, Bi syndrome manifestoes or both bi and prostration syndrome are seen, the treatment of strengthening the body resistance to eliminate pathogenic factors should be administered.

Method of treatment: Supplementing Qi and restoring Yang, restoring normal function of the body to protect from further collapse.

Prescription: Modified Shen Fu Decoction. Ginseng in the prescription supplements primodial-Qi greatly, and Radix Aconiti preparata restoring Yang and rescuing the patient from collapse. In those with incessant sweating drugs for arresting sweating and preventing from collapse such as Radix Astragali seu Hedysari, Orchra Haematium, Fructus Schisandrae are added.

If Yang restores after treatment and syndromes like red face with cold extremities, vexation due to deficiency, faint pulse or floating large pulse without root are seen, which is caused by deficiency in genuine Yin, floating of Yang in deficiency condition. Genuine Yin deficient internally with upward floating of defecient Yang. During this situation, Yang in deficiency condition floats upward tend to collapse, it is suitable to use Di Huang Yin Zi for tonifying Yin, invigorate kidney Yang by warmth, aimed at tonifying both Yin and Yang. In the prescription Radix Rehmanniae preparata, Radix Ophiopogonis, Herba Dendrobi, Radix Morindae Officinalis, Herba Cistanchis, Fructus Corni, Fructus Schisandrae are used for arrest sweating and protecting from collapse.

Example of prescription: prepared Asonite 10g, Ginseng 10g, Fructus Schisandrae 12g. Radix Astragali seu Hedysari 20g, Radix Ophiopogonis 10g.

However, in Bi and prostration syndromes the clinical manifestation varies with the variations in relative strength of vital energy and pathogenic factors, speciality in Yin and Yang of pathogenic factors. Generally speaking, Bi- syndrome are more commonly seen in the beginning of apoplexy and in acute stage. Prostration syndromes are less seen and rather difficult to treat. These two syndromes are inter-changeable with each other, but sometimes they may be associated. In treatment, for Bi-syndrome the essential is treating the superficiality as emission of pathogenic factors and open orifice. While in prostration syndrome the first important is tonifying vital energy and rescuing collapse. If both of them are seen, it is necessary to differentiate the primary and secondary, treat either the originality or the superficiality, supplemenying vital-Qi and eliminating pathogenic factors.

3. Sequelae

Apoplexy comes on promptly with tremendous variations in the acute stage. After vigorous effective treatment disease may become stable gradually, symptoms like hemiplegia, dysphasia may recover gradually. But in some cases, because of excess in pathogenic factors and failure in vital energy, in spite of treatment from various aspects in acute and convalescent stage, some symptoms cannot be eliminated easily and remain as sequelaes afterward; such as hemiplegia, dysphagia or aphasia, abnormality in emotion or mind, some syndrome and dementia. For treatment of sequelaes, in addition to following the principle of treatment according to differentiating of syndrome some modification along with syndromes, combining with different principles of treatment such as promoting blood, resolve stagnancy, promoting collateral, supplement Qi, et al. to select drugs intelligently is necessary. Additionally, combination with acupunctue and moxibustion, massage, and functional training may increase the effectiveness of treatment. For treatment of residuals, on one hand promoting functional rehabilitation, on the other hand is to prevent recurrence within short period. For syndromes like disorder in mental activity, dementia, convulsive attack, treat them according to treatment through differentiating syndromes in madness, dementia, and epilepsy. Discuss separately the treatment for hemiplegia and dysphasia by treatment according to differentiating syndromes as following:

(1) Hemiplegia

1) Qi deficiency and blood stagnancy, obstruction in channels and collaterals

Main Symptoms: flaccid and weak limbs, disused muscular atrophy, fatigue and weakness, or numbness of limbs, distortion of mouth and tongue.

Accompanying Symptoms: less amount of food intake with soft stool, dysphasia.

Tongue and pulse: dark purple tongue or with ecchymosis, white fur, pulse thready and uneven or weakened under pressing.

Analysis: Under long course of apoplexy, primodial energy is extremely injured. Qi deficiency cannot transport blood, Qi cannot move, blood cannot nourish. Stagnancy in Qi and blood, channels and vessels obstruction result in flaccidity and weakness in extremities and muscular atrophy by disuse. Numbness of limbs is caused by Qi deficiency and blood stagnancy, dysfunction in channels and vessel. Purple tongue with ecchymosis is the evidence for blood stasis.

Method of treatment: supplementing Qi, activating blood flow, promoting circulation in collaterals

Prescription: Modified Bu Yang Huan Wu Decoction. In the prescription put great emphasis on Radix Astragali seu Hedysari for supplementing Qi; Radix Angelicae Sinensis, Radix Paeoniae Rubra, Rhizoma Ligustici Chuangxiong Semen Persicae, Flos Carthami are used for activating blood flow and resolving stasis, Lumbricusare promoting channels and circulation in collaterals. All together make up the effect of supplement Qi and activating blood circulation. If dysphasia is accompanied Rhizoma Pinelliae, Calamus, Radix Polygalae are added for dispel phlegm and benefiting orifice. In case with distortion of mouth and tongue Rhizoma Typhonii, Scorpio, dead and stiffened Bombyx Batryticatus are added for dispel wind and resolve phlegm. In case of palpitation of heart with deficiency in heart Yang, Ramulus Cinnamomi, Radix Glycerrrhizae prepara are used to supplement Qi and warm Yang. If accompanied by numbness of limbs, Fructus Chaenomelis, Radix Lycopodium clavatum L., Radix Stephaniae Tetrendrae are added to relax muscles and activate collaterals. Rhizoma Pinelliae, Arisaema cum Bile, Pericarpium Citri Reticulatus, Poria for replenish Qi, dry up dampness and remove wind phlegm pathogen. In incontinence in micturation Ootheca Mantidis, Fructus Alpiniae Oxyphyllae are added for warm up Yang and supplementing kidney. In weakness of limbs Radix Dipsaci, Ramulus Loranthi, Cortex Eucommiae, Radix Achyranthis Bidentatae, et al. Are used for tonifying kidney and strengthening muscle and bone. In condition of disease of long time with severe blood stasis, Hirudo, Squama Manitis drastic drug with removing blood stasis and promoting circulation are selected.

Examples for prescription: Radix Astragali seu Hedysari 30g, Semen Persicae 6g, Flos Carthami 6g, Radix Salviae Miltiorhizae 20g, Lumbricusare 10g, Paeoniae Rubra 12g, Radix Angelicae Sinensis 10g, Rhizoma Pinelliae 10g; Poria 30g.

2) Yin deficiency with Yang excess, Stasis in collateral vessels

Main Symptoms: apoplexy for long course, hemiplegia, spasm, rigidity or contrcture in affected limbs, stiff joint, dizziness, headache, flushed face, tinnitus as cicada singing.

Accompanying Symptoms: irritability, dysphasia, numbness in limbs.

Tongue and pulse: red tongue with yellow fur, pulse taut and forceful.

Analysis: Due to liver and kidney deficiency, Yin fails to keep Yang well, liver Yang hyperactive, fire flare upward wind motivated, Qi and blood run retrogressed upward, so red face, headache, dizziness, tinnitus follow up. Loss of nourishment in tendon and vessels, collateral are obstructed by stagnant blood resulting to hemiplegia, spaasticity and contracture of affected limbs, immobility of joints. red tongue with yellow fur, pulse taut and strong are signs of hyperactivity of Yang.

Method of treatment: calming liver and suppressing Yang hyperactivity, calming wind and promoting circulation

Prescription: Modified Zhen Gan Xi Feng Decoction or Tian Ma Gou Teng Decoction. In Decoction of Gastrodia and Uncaria, Rhizoma Gastrodiae, Ramulus Uncarine cum Uncis adix, Concha Haliotidis, for calm liver and descend retrogression, Ramulus Loranthi, Cortex Eucommiae for reinforce kidney; Herba Leonuri, Poria cum Ligno Hospite, and Caulis Polygoni Multiflori for nourishing blood and tranquilizing mind; Radix Achyranthis Bidentatae conduct Qi and blood downward flow; Radix Pittospori, Radix Scutellariae for clear heat; In addition,

Radix Sanguissorbae, Radix Paeoniae Alba, Radix Ophiopogonis supplementing Yin and suppressing Yang; Fructus Chaenomelis, Herba Lycopodii for relieve rigidity of muscles and joints, Radix Salviae Miltiorhizae, Cortex Moutan Radicis, Flos Carthami et al. for activating blood and circulation removing stasis.

Example for prescription: Rhizoma Gastrodiae 10g, Ramulus Uncarine cum Uncis 30g, Concha Haliotidis 30g. (ahead), Ramulus Loranthi 12g, Cortex Eucommiae 10g, Herba Leonuri 15g, Radix Sanguissorbae 20g, Radix Paeoniae Alba 10g, Orchra Haematium 30g(ahead), Radix Pittospori 6g, Radix Salviae Miltiorhizae 15g, Radix Achyranthis Bidentatae 10g.

(2) Dysphasia

1)Obstruction of collateral by wind-phlegm

Main Symptoms: stiff tongue and dysphasia, even curled tongue with difficulty in protruding, difficulty in speak or dysphasia, or large amount thick phlegm, difficulty in expectoration, difficulty in free movement of extremities, numbness of extremities.

Accompanying Symptoms: dizziness and headache, tremor of extremities.

Tongue and pulse: red or dark tongue with white or yellow and greasy fur, pulse taut and slippery.

Analysis: Tongue as the sprout of the heart. Expression of language is intimately related to mind and movement of tongue proper. When the mind is clouded no words can be expressed. Disabled to speak freely also associated with stiff tongue, curled-up tongue, or without free movement of tongue. Heart, liver, spleen and kidney channels contact with each other in tongue. Heart channel connects with root of tongue. Liver channel goes upward along the back of throat into the nasopharynx, Spleen channel connected to tongue proper and dispersed underneath. Kidney channel goes along throat interspersed in tongue proper. Therefore, unclearity in speech, flaccid tongue with aphasia are caused by obstruction of channels in tongue proper by wind-phlegm and stagnant blood.

Method of treatment: calming wind and removing phlegm, opening orifice and promoting circulation in collateral.

Prescription: Modified Jie Yu Pill. Rhizoma Gastrodiae, Scorpio, Arisaema cum Bile, et al. used in the prescription for tranquilizing liver, calming wind and remove phlegm; Bambusa textilis Meclure, Radix Polygalae, Calamus, Radix Curcumae, Radix Aucklandia et al. For opening orifice and normalize Qi and promote circulation. It is suitable to take drugs as pill or powder.

Examples for prescription: Rhizoma Gastrodiae 10g, Scorpio 6g, Arisaema cum Bile 10g, Calamus 10g, Radix Polygalae 10g, Bambusa textilis Meclure 10g, Radix Aucklandia 6g, Radix Curcumae 9g, Rhizoma Pinelliae 10g, Lumbricusare 10g, Radix Salviae Miltiorhizae 30g, Paeoniae Rubra 10g.

2) Kidney deficiency and diminished essence of life

Main Symptoms: flaccid tongue and aphasia, weakness and soreness of lumbar region and knee joint, palpitation and shortness of breath.

Accompanying Symptoms: incontinence in defecation and micturation, dizziness and giddiness.

Tongue and pulse: slender tongue proper or curled-up with white fur, deep and thready pulse.

Analysis: having apoplexy for long period, stagnancy in channel and vessels, dysfunction in transportation of both Qi and blood, affect on kidney and result to kidney deficiency and loss of essence of life. Qi of essence of life cannot go upward.

Method of treatment: supplementing Yin and replenishing kidney and opening orifice.

prescription: Modified Di Huang Yin Zi. Almond and radix platycodi are added for promoting opening orifice and relieve aphasia.

In case of kidney deficiency with excess liver, hyperactivity of liver Yang, associated with obstruction by wind-phlegm, calm up liver and reduce Yang is suitable. Modified Zhen Gan Xi Feng Decoction or Tian Ma Gou Teng Decoction can be selected and drugs for removing phlegm and opening foramen such as Calamus, Radix Polygalae, Arisaema cum Bile and Bambusa textilis Meclure, et al. may be added. In case associated with vexation and asomnia drugs for sedation as pearl oyster, succinum may be added.

Examples for prescription: Radix Rehmanniae preparata 30g, Herba Cistanchis 20g, Fructus Corni 12g, Herba dendrobii 15g, Fructus Schisandrae 10g, Calamus 10g, Radix Polygalae 10g, pearl oyster 30g (ahead), Cortex Moutan Radicis 12g, Radix Salviae Miltiorhizae 20g, Rhizoma Gastrodiae 10g, poria 20g.

(3) Deviation of the eye and mouth: If it is the only sequale mostly is caused by obstruction of collaterals by wind-phlegm. Obstruction in channels and collaterals by wind-phlegm and stagnant blood, circulation of Qi and blood is disturbed. Being lasted for long time unnourishing of muscle and tendon brings to contracture. For treatment remove wind and eliminate phlegm to promote circulation

is selected. Usually modification of Qian Zheng powder are used. In the prescription Radix Aconiti preparata remove wind eliminate phlegm, release spasticity, promote circulation; Scorpio clear phlegm, calm wind, release spasm. If accompanied with twitch of eye and mouth, Gastrodia, Uncaria, Concha Haliotidis, et al. are added for calming liver and stop wind, Radix Paeoniae Alba, Fructus Chaenomelis are added to nourishing the tendon and promote circulation Examples for prescription: Radix Aconiti preparata 6g, Scorpio 6g, Bombyx Batryticatus 6g, Gastrodia 10g, Rhizoma Ligustici Chuangxiong 10g, Fructus Chaenomelis 30g, Paeoniae Rubra 10g.

〔Prevention and nursing〕

1. Prevention

1) Pay attention to observation on premonitory aura. Although onset of apoplexy is acute, but the pathological changes develops slowly really. Before onset of the disease, there are premonitory symptoms commonly. Wang Qing Ren in Qi Dynasty recorded 34 premonitory symptoms for apoplexy: occasional a short period of headache, hearing of a swift of wind sound with no reason, stiffness of eye of no reason for a short period, salivation out of mouth during sleep, sudden loss of memory in a intelligent man, continuous hand tremor for long time, unreasonable arm numbness, unexplained muscle contraction, unexplained eye twitch. Prevention of apoplexy carried out from three aspects: carefulness of daily activities, adjustment in psychology, dietary control. In careful daily activities it means not only keep regularity in daily living, suitable work and refreshment arrangement, but also pay attention to physical exercise particularly in aged people, in order to maintain good functional activity, smooth blood circulation, free joint mobility for prevention of apoplexy. In Psychologically adjustment means keep a happy mind, stable emotion not to be harmed by seven emotions. Over emotional excitation usually is the induced factor for apoplexy. Therefore adjustment in emotion, preventing from depression and angry is quite important. Dietary control means food mainly composed of light tasted with less fat and sweet. Free from cigar and alcoholism. Not to be satiated.

2) Enhancing early treatment on prodromal symptoms. If dizziness, tinnitus, muscle twitch or contraction et al. are seen, it is sign for hyperactivity of liver Yang, tendency of moving of liver wind. Drugs for calm liver and stop wind such

as Uncaria, Flos Crysanthemi, Fructus Tribuli, Concha Ostreae, Radix Paeoniae Alba, et al are used. In case of numbness and heaviness of extremities, causes of which is stagnancy of circulation of Qi and blood in vessels and collaterals, drugs for promoting circulation and removing stagnancy may be used such as Radix Salviae Miltiorhizae, Paeoniae Rubra, Semen Persicae, Flos Carthami, Caulis Spatholobi, et al.

3) For relapse: Apoplexy may be recovered after energetic treatment, but it relapses easily. It is called as second attack, which must be more severe even fatal. Therefore particular attention must be paid on prevention.

2. Nursing care

In acute stage usually patients are disabled in five activities: turning over, coughing, speech, eating, incontinence in defecation and micturation. In order to promote self recovery, diminish complications and sequale, Close observation, intense nursing, energetic treatment are required:

1) Close observation on changes of disease is important for judging the progress of the disease. In case of mental status change from coma to consciousness it means becoming better, otherwise retrogressed to worsen. Frequency of convulsive episode, its manifestation and lasting period, occurrence of symptoms like floating Yang, hemoptysis, hematochezia should be observed and recorded down carefully. The changes in pulse is also very important for judging the progress of disease. In case of Yang-Bi, occurence of deep slow pulse or intermittent pulse indicates the possibility of sudden death. Hemiplegia as a sequale of apoplexy belongs to Qi deficiency with slow pulse, if pulse changes to taut, forceful and rapid second attack may come. All these should be discovered by intense observation.

2) Dietary forbidden: Principle for food of apoplexy patients should be light less salty. Especially in acute stage, in patient with dysphagia nasal feeding with mixed milk and vegetable juice. Fatty, sweet, heavy tasted, hot and stimulating substances should be avoided. Fatty sweet food is harmful for stomach producing damp transforming to phlegm. Hot substance would move up fire which is unbenefit to disease. In addition alcoholism will aggravate or induce apoplexy, wine should be avoided.

3) Prevention of bedsore: Bedsore most easily prevail in acute stage of apoplexy while bed rest without movement. Frequent turning over is needed. In unconscious patient regular observation on the skin is necessary. Clothes and

bedsheet should be dry, smooth and soft. If the skin under pressure become red, should be massaged by palm of the hand or local application of tincture of Flos Carthami, for promoting channels and collaterals and blood circulation.

4) Functional training: encourage and help patient to do exercise training is the essential nursing work in recovery stage and with residuals. Massage on limbs disabled to move voluntary and passive movement be carried out to promote blood circulation, enhance recovery, and prevent from contracture of joints. In patients with voluntary activity, direction to training according to his capability in mobility. In dysphasia patients teach them in pronunciation patiently to be able to speak gradually.

〔Typical case study〕

Case 1: Yu-male 64 yr. Worker admitted in on July 9, 1984

The patient is rather fatty, had history of hypertension for more than 10 years with frequent headache. Two days before fell down in work place suddenly. Develop left hemiplegia, fatigue and somewhat less alert. Admitted in under emergency. During admission the patient is confused mentally, wake up occasionally during deep cough, stiff tongue and dysphasia, left sided hemiplegia, distortion of tongue and mouth, having constipated for 3 days, dark red tongue less moistened with yellow greasy fur, slippery taut pulse, left hand pulse larger than right. Modified decoction of Arisaema and Trichosanthis for supplementing Qi was prescribed:

Fructus Trichosanthis 30g, Arisaema cum Bile 6g, Bambusa textilis Meclure 6g, Cortex Moutan Radicis 10g, Radix Salviae Miltiorhizae 30g, Natrii Sulphas 6g. (taking this by infusion), Radix et Rhizoma Rhei 10g. (after), Calamus 6g.

Having had 6～7 times of defecation with slimy foul stool after taking two doses, mental status become alert. Pulse was still slippery and taut. Other symptoms remained as before. Prescription was changed to drugs for clearing heat, removing phlegm, promoting circulation.

Fructus Trichosanthis 15g, Arisaema cum Bile 6g, Bambusa textilis Meclure 6g, Radix Salviae Miltiorhizae 30g, Cortex Moutan Radicis 10g, Caulis Spatholobi 30g, Preparata Radix et Rhizoma Rhei 6g.

After 12 doses, thick yellow fur was dissolved, speech become clear than before, the diseased limb begin to rise up slightly. Prescription for promoting blood and relieve stagnation, removing phlegm free collaterals was given more.

Emphasizing on drugs with promoting circulation in above prescription, and change its content according to the symptoms. Having taken more than 20 doses, the patient can walk under help, speak fluently. He was treated by acupuncture further for recovery.

Note: In this case, the disease belongs to syndrome of phlegm heat Fu excess with up-stirring of wind phlegm at the onset. Wind fire carrying phlegm turbid go upward covering brain and obstructing vessels and collaterals, result into mental confusion, dysphasia and hemiplegia. After treatment by removing phlegm and conduct free movement of internal organs, Qi in internal organs relaxed, phlegm heat reduced, mental status become clear up and syndrome transmitted from involving internal organs to involving channels. Then prescription for clear heat and resolve phlegm, activate blood and collateral circulation was used. Gradually phlegm heat and stagnant blood eliminated, and recovery took place. Thus grasping the main points of differentiating syndromes, treatment according to the syndrome is critical for successful treatment in this case. Apoplexy is a common and highly prevalent dissuasion clinics. Due to its rapid change, variation in changes and its high mortality in the acute stage, although recovered from acute stage through energetic treatment some residuals as hemiplegia, disabled to speech normally may still remain, even for life span. In spite of variations in causes the fundamental basis lies on dysfunction of internal organs, imbalance in Yin and Yang. In condition of empty in channels and collaterals exogenous pathogen invades into involving channels and collaterals it is known as real apoplexy. While so called apoplexy-like is caused by stirring of wind Yang, upward retrogression of Qi and blood carrying phlegm and fire, flow over channels and vessels covering and obstructing brain. In clinics, depending on whether there is mental disturbance or not it is differentiated into involving internal organs and involving channels and collaterals. In involving channels and collaterals it is further divided into invasion by exogenous wind and harmed by endogenous wind. Usually there is no aura in exogenous invasion but accompanied with exopathic symptoms and the treatment for which should be supplementing vital essence to remove pathogen, clear wind release the superficiality, increase the resistance and activate circulation. In case of involving internal organs, there is mental confusion and further divided into Bi- and prostration syndrome. Bi-syndrome is classified into Yang-Bi and Yin-Bi according to the difference in phlegm fire and phlegm damp with their own peculiarities. For the treatment of Yin-Bi, principles of pungent cool open orifice, clear liver and calm wind should be taken. For Yang-Bi pungent and warm drugs to open orifice, remove phlegm and calm wind. As for prostration syndrome, weakening of vital energy, Yin and Yang is going to its end, first aid is necessary, the first requirement is replenishing Qi and stop prostration.

Gradual recovery usually take place after acute stage of apoplexy through adequate adjustment. But a lot of them remains with sequale. Treatment for hemiplegia should be Energetic, such as if it belongs to Qi deficiency and stagnancy of blood, main method is supplementing Qi, activating circulation; if it belongs to hyperactivity of liver Yang leading to obstruction in vessels and collaterals, treated by calm liver and reduce Yang, stop wind free colaterals. Syndrome of dysphasia is differentiated to wind phlegm obstructing collaterals and kidney deficiency with less vital energy, accordingly the treatment should be either eliminate wind removing phlegm or replenish kidney fulfilling vital energy. Otherwise if it is due to obstruction by phlegm heat, the treatment should be clearing heat resolve phlegm facilitate opening of orifice, eliminating stagnancy and free colaterals. Since apoplexy is liable to relapse, preventive measures are essential. Once aura presented energetic treatment should be taken in order to protect from recurrence.

Questions for Review

1. What are main characteristics of apoplexy?
2. What is the basic pathogenic factors of apoplexy and the concrete pathologic changes?
3. What is the main difference between involving internal organs and involving channels and collateral?
4. What is the emergency treatment for Bi- and prostration syndrom?
5. How to nursing and adjusting the apoplexy patient?

Edema

〔Introduction〕

Edema is a morbid state in which there is water retention within the body, as water overflowing in the muscle and skin resulting to edema of face and head, extremities, abdominal and back region, scrotum, even whole body. In severe cases, water may remain in the thoracic and abdominal cavity and transmitted to other diseases, critical to survival.

In《Nei Jing》it is named as "edema"and classified into "Wind edema" "Stony edema" "Yong edema", et al. according to variation in symptoms. Details in the pathogenic factors, pathogenesis and classification were described in it. For the treatment three kinds of method was suggested as: purgation, inducing diaphoresis, and diuresis. In《Jin Gui Yao Lue》, it was called as "Edema" and was discussed in a special chapter, in which according to the pathogenic factors and pulse, edema was classified into"Wind edema" "Severe edema due to hypofunction of spleen" "Anasarca with shortness of breath""Stony edema" "Tawnysweat". According to the characteristics of syndromes related to five viscera, edema was further classified into heart edema, liver edema, lung edema, spleen edema and kidney edema. It is suggested that treatment for edema should be varies with variation in location of edema, i.e. "In edema localized below lumbar region diuresis should be used, in above lumbar region should induce diaphoresis."

In《Dan Xi Xin Fa》, edema was classified into Yin and Yang edema two large groups, which was suitable for practical use. After Song and Yuan Dynasty great progress made in knowledge on pathogenesis and in the pathogenesis of edema emphasizing on the important role of dysfunction of lung, spleen, kidney played in Qi-transmission. For the treatment, instead of eliminate pathogen alone, method of reinforce spleen, tonify kidney, warm up Yang and reinforcement and elimination in combination was adopted. Thus a complete theoretical system was established.

It may be referred on in treatment of edema found in acute and chronic nephritis, congestive heart failure, endocrine gland dysfunction and nutritional disorders in western medicine.

〔Pathogenic factors and pathogenesis〕

Normal transportation of the water in the human body depends on regulatory and ventilation function of lung, transportation and transmission function of spleen, discharge and retention function of the kidney, thus three Jiao is effective in charge of water circulation, urinary bladder in normal Qi-transmission and normal excretion of urine. On the contrary, if regulatory function of three organs on water metabolism are affected on anyway and failure of three Jiao in charge of water circulation, dysfunction of urinary bladder in Qi-transmission, disturbance in water and fluid circulation, retention, accumulation and overflowing of water resulting to edema.

There are two groups of causes of edema: exopathic and internal injury. Among exopathic factors wind cold and dampness is frequent. While in internal injury, diet, over strain, sexual strain and deficiency in whole body may be the common causes.

1. Wind pathogen invades from outside, impairment of regulatory and ventilatory function of the lung: Lung is in charge of ventilation and dispersion, being the upper origin of water. It relates to the skin and hair and in charge of the exterior of the whole body. Wind cold or wind heat invades muscle and exterior, dysfunction of lung in ventilation and descending, disability in regulate water passage to flow downward to urinary bladder, result to wind block free movement of water, struggle between wind and water, overflow of water into muscle and skin and edema formed.

2. Water damp infiltrate and immerse, impairment in normal transportation function of spleen: Spleen is in charge of transformation and transportation, like dry averse damp. Under condition of living in low and damp room, free from sunlight and cold, or immersing in water in rainy days, cold pathogen and water damp invade interior. Otherwise uncontrolled in wine and diet in usual time, too much raw and cold substances in the food, dampness accumulates in the middle. Due to suppression of spleen by dampness, impaired in transportation function resulting to failure of lucid Yang ascending and turbid Yin descending, water damp stops interior, overflows in muscle and skin, edema occurs. If water damp remaining on, long time stagnancy transmitted to heat, evaporation alternately by damp and heat, abnormal function of Qi-transmission of urinary bladder, edema also occurs.

3. Damp heat and sore toxins invade interior to spleen and lung: In case of long staying uncured sore, abscess and ecchymosis, wind-toxins damp-heat stagnant and obstruct body exterior, injured interior to lung and spleen. Result to disturbances in water metabolism and edema formed from overflow.

4. Diet, over strain harm to spleen and stomach: Spleen is in charge of transformation and transportation, while stomach is in charge of reception. Inadequate regulation in food, irregularity in hungry and fullness must be harmful to spleen and stomach. Over working and fatigue will induce spleen deficiency and Qi consumption, dysfunction of spleen transportation. Earth fails to control water, dampness stay and water cumulate lead to edema. In addition, spleen deficiency bring to loss of originality in transformation, weakness in Qi and blood, failure in transmission of water by Qi then deficiency edema formed.

5. Indulging in sexual activity and multiple birthing, injure interior to kidney Qi: Essence of life are stored in kidney, being the origin of congenital constitution. Kidney governs the water, being the root of Qi. Congenital insufficiency in body constitution, or indulge in sexual activity with multiple birth consume kidney Qi. Kidney deficiency impairs Qi-transmission and circulation of water. Retention and cumulating of water and fluid lead to overflow to muscle and skin and edema formation.

Overall, the causes of onset of edema are: Invasion by external wind pathogen, loss of lung function interior, failure in lung regulatory and ventilatiory function, and uneliminated sore, carbuncle, ecchymosis of the muscle and skin, inflammatory toxic substance return to spleen and lung; Residing in damp area, immerse in water in rainy days, water damp pathogen invades interior, or uncontrolled in diet, satiating in cold raw substance bring in suppress and impairment in normal transportation function of spleen. Long staying damp heat or transmission to heat by stagnant damp results in interior excess of damp heat, failure of three Jiao to ascend and descend causing stagnancy and obstruction in three Jiao. Uncontrolled in diet, fatigue and overstrain harm to spleen and stomach in loss the function of transformation and transportation. Indulging in sexuality, uncontrolled birth injure kidney Qi interior cause failure in Qi-transmission. Among these causes, some are exopathic and the others are internal injury. Raised by exopathic factors mostly are Yang edema, while Yin edema commonly are induced by internal injury. The pathogenic factors may be either single or complex. However, Yin or Yang edema are not remained unchanged always, but interchangeable with each other. If Yang edema not recover for long time, water damp infiltrate, immerse and stayed everlasting result to weakening of vital-Qi day by day, spleen and kidney Yang deficiency, made the disease more lingering and transformed into Yin edema. On the contrary, under condition of external pathogen invades additionally on Yin edema, dysfunction of lung in dispersing made edema severe abruptly, then it would be treated as Yang edema. Treat the exterior at first. If Yang syndromes appear in Yin edema attacked by exopathic pathogen, instead of considering the degree of disease become better rather the case is more complicated by deficiency in vital-Qi and excess in pathogen. The main pathologic changes in edema lie on lung, spleen and kidney. Failure of lung in regulation and ventilation, impairment of transformation and transportation function of the spleen, failure of kidney in discharge and retention function, result to functional disorder of Qi-transmission in the whole body, retention and overflow of water and fluid then edema formed. They are interconnected and influenced on each other. Such as in kidney water overflow upward, it would attack heart and injure lung, lead to dysfunction of lung in descending, without free movement in water passage. Then make more deficiency in kidney Qi, more excess of water pathogen. On the contrary, the similar result seen when lung channel is invaded by pathogen and transmitted to kidney channel. Kidney deficiency fails to warm up the spleen earth causing dysfunction of spleen in normal transportation, retention and cumulating of water damp would aggravate distress to spleen by damp. Spleen Qi deficiency become more severe, loss of originality of blood and Qi, failure of blood in transforming to essence of life. Exhaustion of kidney in essence of life disabled to govern water, more severe edema resulted. Among the three viscera, kidney is the originality, lung is the superficiality, spleen being the viscera for control water is really the critical one in treatment of edema. In addition, obstruction by stagnant blood injures water passage in three Jiao, make edema more resistant to treatment. Long standing edema exhaust the kidney essence. Upward invasion of turbid pathogen or liver wind move up endogenously would produce prostration, the prognosis would be not good.

〔Treatment according to differentiation of syndromes〕

In the beginning, edema usually starts from the eyelid, then extends to head, face, extremities, lumbar, abdomen and whole body, but may also start from the lower extremity and then to the whole body. In mild cases only regional edema on face or lower extremities are seen. In severe cases the whole body is edematous, even fullness in abdomen and sensation of oppression in chest, palpitation of heart and shortness of breath, cannot lie down in supine position. For the method of treatment as said in… "Su Wen. Tang Ye Lao Li Lun". It is still impotent as a guide for clinics up to now.

1. Important points in differentiating syndrome

1)Differentiating between Yin and Yang edema: Yin and Yang is the outline for differentiating syndromes of edema. Syndromes of exterior, heat and excess are more commonly seen in situation caused by external invasion of wind pathogen, water damp immersion and infiltration, extreme excess in damp heat, inflammatory toxins invasion interior. It should be treated as Yang edema. On the other hand interior, deficiency, cool syndromes are more commonly seen in the situation caused by diet, fatigue, overstrain, deficiency of body constitution, indulging in sexuality and multiple birth. It should be treated as Yin edema.

2) Pay attention to the transmission of diseases: Generally Yang edema belongs to excess syndrome and Yin edema belongs to deficiency syndrome or deficiency in origin and excess in exterior. But these two may be intermingled or interchanged. Long lasting Yang edema lead to weakening of vital-Qi day by day, excess in water pathogen and transmission to Yin edema. External pathogen invasion adding on Yin edema would induce edema much severe and exterior syndrome of excess may be seen, then treat the exteriort. Treat it as Yang edema. But it is different form yang edema beginning from the start and in the treatment deficiency in origin and excess in superficiality should be considered on.

3) Differentiating associated syndrome in pathologic region: In sever edema, internal organ are affected on. Syndromes like retention of water and fluid, palpitation of heart, shortness of breath, swelling of abdomen, obstruction and rejection, dysuria and vomiting, et al. may be associated with. Should differentiate between origin and superficiality, acute and chronic. Edema may be classified into five viscera, that is heart edema usually associated with palpitation of heart; liver edema usually associated with fullness and distention of abdomen and hypochondrium; large abdomen, disabling in turn to one side voluntarily; spleen edema usually associated with fullness and sensation of oppression in epigastrium and poor appetite, heaviness in four extremities; lung edema is commonly associated with cough, panting; kidney edema is commonly associated with swelling in

umbilicus and lumbago, damp and cool in pudendal region. Knowledge on the pathological localization and its associated syndromes is important in guiding choice of drugs.

Diagrammatic sketch for Pathogenic Factors and Pathogenesis of Edema

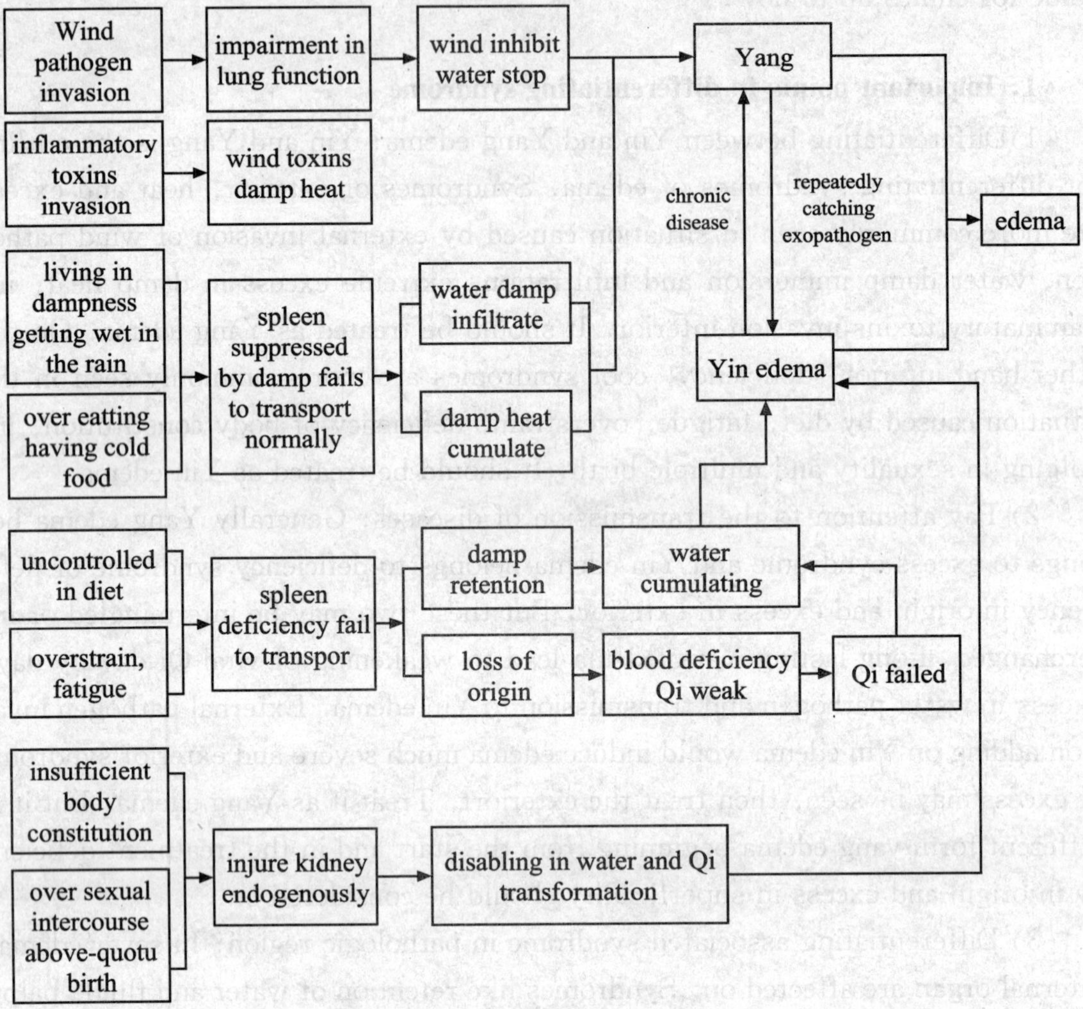

2. Principles for treatment

Methods for treatment of edema consists of: inducing diaphoresis, diuresis elimination of water, et al., to remove pathogen and render water circulate; supplementing Qi, tonifying spleen, warm up kidney to help vital-Qi in Qi-transmission and water flow. Additionally other methods may be used in combination such as regulating Qi, activating blood, detoxication, descending turbidity, et al. Main treatment for Yang edema is elimination of pathogen, while help to the vital-Qi is the first for Yin edema. When either transmission from excess to deficiency in Yang edema or external pathogen invades on the base of Yin edema, then elimination of pathogen and help to vital-Qi should be carried out simultaneously. Treatment goes on orderly according to differentiation in degree of severity, which one is more severe and which one is mild. Edema located in upper part with exterior syndrome should be treated by inducing diaphoresis, if it locates in the lower part then diuresis is the choice. In condition of excess in body constitution with moderate edema purgative method is suitable. The basis of edema lie on lung, spleen and kidney. Regulating and supplementing internal organs may increase Qi and render water circulate, tonifying spleen to transport water, warm up kidney to transmitte water. Especially in case of deficiency in origin after relieve of edema, should supplement according to deficiency in Zang-Fu, visera(hollow organs), Qi, blood, Yin and Yang. In clinical practice different methods are selected according to various condition such as: one method only, several methods in combination, remove pathogen at first followed by helping vital-Qi, or help to vital-Qi at first followed by remove pathogen, or consider vital-Qi and pathogen simultaneously.

3. Treatment according to different types

1) Yang edema

1.1 overflow of wind water

Main symptoms: Edema starts from eyelid and spreads to extremities, thorax, back, abdomen and the whole body. It develops rapidly, and marked in head and face. Skin become fresh, bright and thin, the concave formed under pressure easily disappear, oliguria.

Accompanying symptom: mostly with averse to cold and fever, soreness of joints and extremities, or cough and panting, or sore throat, red and swelling of tonsils.

Tongue and pulse: In inclination to wind cool type, white thin slippery fur, floating slippery or tight pulse. In inclination to wind heat type, tongue proper red with thin yellow fur, floating rapid slippery pulse. In overflowing of water pathogen and moderate edema, deep pulse may be seen.

Analysis: lung is in charge of dispersing and dispelling, related to skin and hair exterior. It governs descending and purification, regulates and makes water passage free. Wind pathogen invasion, dysfunction of lung in dispersing, disabled in regulating water passages downward to urinary bladder result to less urination.

Overflowing of cumulated water to muscle and skin develops to edema. Wind pathogen being Yang pathogen is light and raising, liable to move with multiple changes. Wind and water catch each other, make a stormy sea stormier. Thus edema starts from face, involving the extremities rapidly. The disease being caused by wind, lodges exterior. Vital-Qi just in excess, Yang Qi circulates freely, so the skin is fresh, bright and thin. The concave formed under pressure easily recovers. Pathogen lodges in muscle exterior, body resistance is suppressed, disharmony between Ying and Wei, result into fever and averse cold, heaviness and soreness in joints and extremities. External pathogen invades lung, dysfunction of lung in dispersing; or attack lung by retained water, impairment in dispersing and descending function of lung, result to cough and panting. Wind heat stirring upward bring to sore, swelling throat. Thin white fur and slippery, floating slippery or tight pulse is wind water inclined to cool. Red tongue proper with thin, yellow fur, floating rapid pulse is wind water inclined to heat. In severe edema, Yang Qi being suppressed, deep pulse seen.

Method of treatment: dispelling wind and clearing heat, promoting diuresis by activating dispersing function of lung

Prescription: Modification of Yue Bi Jia Zhu Decoction. Herba Ephedrae in the prescription removes wind and promotes dispersing function of the lung, removes edema by promoting movement of water. Gypsum Fibrosumclear clears lung and purges heat; Rhizoma Atractylodis Macrocephalae tonyfing spleen and diuresis; Rhizoma Zingiberis Recens, Radix Glycyrrhizae, Fructus Ziziphi Jujubae used for regulating Ying and Wei; Combination of these drugs in order to eliminate obstruction of lung Qi, clear and dispelling lung heat, downward movement of water damp, wind edema would disappear automatically. In case with moderate heat and oliguria, put emphasize on Gypsum Fibrosumclear and Rhizoma Imperatae, semen Phasoli Calcarati added for clear heat and diuresis. In case of moderate superficial pathogen with inclination to cold, reduce or remove Gypsum Fibrosum, and Rhizoma seu Radix Notopterygii and Radix Sileris are added for dispelling wind, expelling cold and release exterior. In case of red and swelling sore throat, Radix Isatidis, Radix Platycodi, Rhizoma Belamcandae, Fructus Arctii are added for clear heat toxin, benefit to the throat and reduce edema. In case of injury to Yin by excess heat with dysphoria with sensation of smothering and thirsty, less moistened red tongue, Radix Scrophulariae, Rhizoma Phragmitis, Rhizoma Anemarrhenae are added for supplementing Yin and clearing heat. In case of cough, panting with large amount of sputum, Semen Armeniacae Amarum, Radix Platycodi, Radix Peucedani, are added for releasing lung and antitussives. In sever cases Cortex Mori Radicis, Semen Lepidii seu Descurainiae, Fructus Perillaee are used for purging heat from lung and relieving asthma.

If exterior syndrome is relieved gradually but heaviness in body and edema not eliminated, the disease may be treated with method as in water damp infiltration and immersing syndrome. Combination of Wu Ling Powder and Wu Pi Powder, et al. are used in order to activating Yang and promoting diuresis, tonyfing spleen and resolving damp. If sweating and averse to wind, heaviness of the body with edema indicates deficiency in body resistance Yang, modification of Fang Ji Huang Qi Decoction would be used for increasing body resistance and promoting movement of water damp.

Example for prescription: Herba Ephedrae 6g, Gypsum Fibrosum 15g, Rhizoma Atractylodis Macrocephalae 12g, Semen Phaseoli 30g, Radix Platycodi 9g, Semen Plantaginis 30g, Rhizoma Zingiberis Recens 4g, Preparata Radix Glycyrrhizae 4g.

1. 2 Infiltrate and immerse of water damp

main symptoms: edema over the whole body especially in lower extremities, concave under pressure, oliguria, gradual onset and course of disease extend long time.

Accompanying symptom: drowsiness and fatigue, sensation of oppression in chest and distention in abdomen, poor appetite with nausea.

Tongue and pulse: white greasy or white slippery fur, deep slow pulse.

Analysis: Housing in a low damp place or immerse in water in a rainy day; wearing wet and cold clothes or over intake of raw and cold substance, water damp invades interior, suppress middle earth, result to dysfunction of spleen transportation; retention and accumulation of water damp. Water damp cumulates internally, three Jiao fails to govern water circulation, dysfunction of urinary bladder in Qi-transmission bring to oliguria. Pathogen of water damp increases day by day, infiltrate and immerse muscle and skin, remaining and cause obstruction, thus edema formed in whole body and extremities. The severity of edema aggravates gradually, tip of the finger drops into the concave formed under pressure. Damp being Yin pathogen is characterized by slimy and greasy, unlikely to change suddenly, therefore the disease would be long lasting not easily to recover. Retention of damp in middle Jiao, failure of stomach in descending bring to poor appetite and nausea. Spleen distressed by damp, Yang Qi cannot extend, bring to sensation of oppression in chest and distention of abdomen, heaviness of body and drowsiness. White greasy fur or white slippery fur and deep slow pulse are signs for distress by damp.

Method of treatment: Invigorating yang and promoting diuresis, invigorating the spleen and drying dampness.

Prescription: Modified Wu Ling Powder and Wu Pi Powder. Modification of combination of Powder of five Drugs with Poria and Decoction of Peel of five Drugs. In the prescription Rhizoma Atractylodis Macrocephalae, Cortex Poria, Umdellate Pore, Rhizoma Alismatis are light and sweet in taste infiltrating into damp and diuretic; Ramulus Cinnamomi pungent in flavor and warm activating Yang, promote function of Qi in moving water. Pericarpium Zingiberis Recens pungent in flavor to disseminate water; Pericarpium Citri Reticulatae, Pericarpium Arecae activate Qi removing damp; Cortex Mori Radicis descends lung Qi and regulating water passage; Rhizoma Atractylodis Macrocephalae, Poria, Cortex Pericarpium Citri Reticulatae tonify spleen resolving damp; Combination of these drugs has the effect of release Yang, activating Qi to circulate water, tonyfing spleen, resolving damp and reduce edema. In case of marked edema in upper half of the body with cough, asthma and reversing flow of Qi, Herba Ephedrae, Semen Armeniacae Amarae are added for dispersing lung relieving asthma. ; in severe case even semen Lepidii seu Descurainiae is used to expelling heat from lung and relieving asthma. In case of tasteless and mental depression, sensation of oppression in hypochondrium and distention in abdomen, poor appetite and nausea, with thick white fur, it indicates obstruction in middle Jiao by damp, dysfunction of stomach in descending, Cortex Magnoliae Officinalis and Rhizoma Atractylodis may be added just similar to Wei Ling Decoction to tonyfing spleen resolving damp. Qi circulate rendering water move up. In case of marked edema in lower extremities Semen Plantaginis and Pericarpium Laenariae used for diuresis and eliminate edema.

Examples for prescription: Cortex Poria 30g, Cortex Mori Radicis 10g, Umdellate Pore 15g, Rhizoma Alismatis 15g, Preparata Rhizoma Atractylodis Macrocephalae 10g, Ramulus Cinnamomi 6g, Pericarpium Zingiberis Recens 6g, Cortex Magnoliae Officinalis 6g, Fructus Amomi 3 g.

1.3 Toxins from infectious disease invades interior

Main symptoms: having had skin or other external infection or swelling, pain, ulceration of pharynx or throat, edema of eyelids spread to whole body, disorders in urination.

Accompanying symptoms: averse to cold, fever, or itching over the body.

Tongue and pulse: red tongue proper with yellow thin fur, floating rapid or slippery rapid pulse.

Analysis: Skin and muscle is the region governed by spleen and lung, inadequate treatment in external infection make damp toxins not cleared and eliminated on-time, invades interior to viscera, resulting dysfunction of spleen in transporting water damp, dysfunction of lung in regulating water passage thus disorders in urination. Wind pathogen lodged in exterior, disorders in lung Qi, disharmony in Ying and Wei, result to averse to cold and fever. Damp pathogen accumulates interior, wind and water catch each other, cause edema starting from eyelid then spreading over the whole body. Red tongue proper with thin yellow fur, rapid floating pulse or slippery rapid pulse are caused by wind pathogen carrying damp toxins.

Method of treatment: promoting dispersion function of lung and detoxication, inducing diuresis and alleviate edema.

Prescription: Modification of Ma Huang Lian Qiao Chi Xiao Dou Decoction. Herba Ephedrae and Fructus Forsythiae used for promoting dispersion function of the lung and facilitate flow of water, Preparata cortex Mori Radicis, Semen Phaseoli clear heat relieve damp and dispell edema. Fructus Forsythiae clears heat, detoxication and alleviating carbuncle. Rhizoma Zingiberis Recens, Radix Glycyrrhizae, Fructus Ziziphi Jujubae promote regulating Ying and Wei. In marked septic condition, Wu Wei Xiao Du Powder is added for intensifying the effect of detoxication and alleviate carbuncle. In case of marked excess in damp with sloughing, Radix Sophorae Flavescentis, Poria are added to clear heat and dried up damp In case of marked excess in wind with pruritus Cortex Dictamni Radicis and Fructus Kochiae added for eliminate wind and antipruriginous. In case with constipation Radix et Rhizoma Rhei and Natrii Sulphas are added for promote movement of hollow organs to dispel turbid.

Examples for prescription: Preparata Herba Ephedrae 5g, Fructus Forsythiae 15g, Semen Phaseoli 30g, Poria 30g, Flos Chrysanthemi 10g, Herba Violae 10g, Flos Lonicerae 10g, Herba Plantaginis 15g, Tetrapanacis 6g, Radix Angelicae Dahuricae 10g.

1.4 Stagnancy of excess damp-heat

Main symptoms: edema over the whole body, skin stretched and extended tightly and brightened. Degree of edema is rather significant, oliguria and dark colored urine. hard aggromulated stool.

Accompanying symptoms: dysphoria with smothery sensation and thirsty, stuffiness and distention of epigatrium.

Tongue and pulse: yellow greasy fur, rapid deep or slippery rapid pulse.

Analysis: invaded by damp heat or water-damp pathogen, retention of damp and transmitted to heat, overflowing to muscle, skin and in-between channels and cannels, result to edema over whole body with moistened, stretched tensely, brightened appearance. Due to excessive heat-damp, severity of edema is significant. Owing to evaporation of damp-heat, disorders in Qi-transmission of three Jiao, dysfunction of Qi in descending and ascending, result to oliguria with dark colored urine, distention in chest and epigastrium. Excessive heat burned up fluid leads to dysphoria with sensation of smothery and thirsty, oliguria with dark colored urine. Abnormal conduction brings to dried aggromulated stool. Yellow greasy fur and rapid deep or slippery rapid pulse are signs for excessive damp-heat.

Methods of treatment: dispersing heat and eliminating dampness both inside and outside the body.

Prescription: Modified Shu Zao Yin Zi. This prescription is effective in get rid off water-damp through dividing to different path such as upper, lower, exterior and interior. Pass out retend water by urine and stool, heat cleared and water withdrawn, edema would disappear spontaneously. In the prescription Rhizoma et Radix Notopterygii, Radix Gentianae Macrophyllae expelling wind and promoting exterior, remove water in the exterior through perspiration. Radix Phytolaccae, Zanthoxylum schinifolium Sieb. et Zucc. seed, Semen Phaseoli, Rhizoma Alismatis, Caulis Aristolochiae Manshuriensis promote delivery of stool and urine, remove out water located interior through downward passage; Percarpium Arecae, Semen arecae promote circulation of Qi to induce diuresis, Qi in motion rendering blood circulate normally. These are purgatives usually administered generally in whole body edema originated from excess in both superficiality and originality, stagnancy of damp-heat in excess. In condition of distended abdomen with stuffiness, scanty stool and urine, Ji Jiao Li Huang Pill are used in combination in helping the effect of purgation, leading water pass out in stool. In severe edema accompanied by stuffiness in chest and coarse breath, marked cough and asthma to unable to lie down in supine position, rapid taut forceful pulse, it indicates water located in chest, pressed upward on lung, lung Qi failed to descend, purgation of lung to remove water is necessary. Wu Ling Powder, Wu Pi Powder, et al in combination with Ting Li Da Zao Xie Fen Decoction for removing Phlegm from lung are used in order to get rid of water Qi in the chest.

Example for prescription: Radix Phytolaccae 6g, Cortex Poria 30g, Pericarpium Arecae 15g, Rhizoma Alismatis 10g, Semen Plantaginis 30g (separated), Radix Ledebouriellae 6g, Semen arecae 30g, Zanthoxylum schinifolium Sieb. et Zucc. seed 6g, Radix Stephaniae Tetrandrae 10g, Semen arecae 10g.

2) Yin edema

2.1 Hypofunction of spleen Yang

Main symptoms: edema more prominent below lumbar region, concave appeared under pressure not easily disappear.

Accompanying symptoms: sallow complexion, sensation of oppression in epigastrium and distention of abdomen, poor appetite with soft stool, fatigue with cold limb, oliguria.

Tongue and pulse: pale and enlarged tongue coated with white greasy or slippery fur. Deep slow or deep thready weak pulse.

Analysis: Starving and eaten fully, overwork, frail elderly, deficiency due to chronic disease bring to deficiency in middle Yang, dysfunction of spleen in transportation, failure of Qi in water transmission, retention of water damp causing oliguria. Owing to Water-damp descends downward, overflowing in lower Jiao, edema more prominent below lumbar region and concave formed under pressure not recover. Hypofunction of spleen Yang disabled in transportation leads to sense of oppression in epigastrium and abdominal distention, poor appetite and soft stool. Insufficiency in spleen Qi, also deficiency in Wei Yang, pale face, mental depression and cold extremities with dim complexion, pale and enlarged tongue with white greasy or slippery fur. Deep slow or deep thready weak pulse are signs for hypofunction of spleen Yang, disorders in fluid and liquid transmission, retention and accumulation of water-damp.

Method of treatment: warming Yang and tonyfying spleen, rendering qi circulation to diuresis.

Prescription: Modification of Shi Pi Powder. In the prescription Poria, Rhizoma Atractylodis Macrocephalae tonify spleen and diuresis; Radix Aconiti praeparata, Rhizoma Zingiberis warm and move Middle Yang to remove water damp; accompanied by Pericarpium Arecae, Radix Aucklandiae, Fructus Chaenomelis for activate Qi in induce diuresis; Cortex Magnoliae Officinalis, Fructus Tsaoko dry up damp and motivate Qi; Radix Glycyrrhizae, Fructus Ziziphi Jujubae. supplement spleen regulate middle Jiao. Combination of these drugs is effective in warm Yang tonyfying spleen, activate Qi induce diuresis. If water-damp is too excess, Ramulus Cinnamomi, Rhizoma Alismatis, Umdellate Pore are added for helping urinary bladder function and diuresis. In Qi deficiency with shortness of breath Radix Codonopsis Pilosulae, Radix Astragali seu Hedysari are added for supplementing spleen and stomach Qi; In case with sensation of oppression in chest and nausea, white thick greasy fur Rhizoma Atractylodis, Herba Eupatorii, Herba Agastachis are added for tonifying spleen and drying up damp, while fragrant in flavor removing turbid.

Example of prescription: Poria 30g, Rhizoma Atractylodis 10g, Rhizoma Atractylodis alba 10g, Rhizoma Zingiberis 6g, Preparata Aconiti 6g, Radix Aucklandiae 10g, Cortex Magnoliae Officinalis 10g, Fructus Tsaoko 10g, Pericarpium Arecae 12g, Fructus Chaenomelis 10g, Rhizoma Alismatis 10g.

2. 2 Weakness of Kidney Yang

Main symptoms: having edema for long time, recurrent and lasting, not recovered from pressed concave, quantity of urine reduced or increased.

Accompanying symptoms: darkish-grey or pale complexion, lumbago and heaviness in loins, cold four extremities, afraid of cold and listlessness. Palpitation and shortness of breath in severe cases.

Tongue and pulse: Pale and corpulent tongue with white thin fur, deep and thready pulse or deep and slow pulse.

Analysis: Kidney is in charge of water metabolism, Qi-transmission- in three Jiao depends on normal function of kidney in warming and vaporization. In case of congenital insufficiency or failed to keeping it in a long period of disease, or not recovered from long lasting edema, exhaustion of kidney Qi occur and lead to insufficiency in kidney Yang, dysfunction in Qi-transmission bringing in retention of water and fluid, which overflow in muscle and skin and edema induced. Kidney Qi governs region below loin and knee, thus weakness in kidney Yang, excess of Yin in lower part, edema would be more prominent in region below loin, pressed concave not disappear. Kidney is in charge of excretion, related exterior-interior with urinary bladder. Insufficiency in kidney Yang, dysfunction of bladder in Qi-transmission lead to oliguria. Unconsolidation in the kidney gate, more discharge with less retention bring to polyuria. Loin is the residence of kidney, kidney deficiency cause excess of water interior with lumbago and soreness and heaviness in loin. Kidney deficiency and weakness in fire, disabled to warm and nutrient extremities resulting to cold extremities, aversion to cold and listlessness. Yang Qi disabled to warm up upper portion result to pale complexion. Yin cold excess interior, Qi and blood become stagnant and coagulate result to darkish-grey complexion. Water pathogen retrode upward, cold up heart and hurt lung, result to palpitation and shortness of breath. Pale and corpulent tongue with white thin fur, deep and thready pulse or deep and slow pulse are signs for weakness of kidney Yang with excess of water damp interior.

Method for treatment: warming kidney and helping Yang, transforming qi and rendering water circulation.

Prescription: Modified Ji Sheng Shen Qi Pill or Zhen Wu Decoction. Kidney is an organ of water and fire, storing kidney Yin and kidney Yang. Owing to interdependence of Yin and Yang, one who skilled to supplement Yang, would get Yang from Yin. In the former prescription Liu Wei Di Huang Pill is used for supplementing kidney Yin; Radix Aconiti praeparata, Cortex Cinnamomi warm kidney and help Yang, render Qi move to circulate water; Accompanying Bolus of Six Drugs Including Rehmannia would supplementing fire within the water, warm Yang in the kidney; Semen Plantaginis diuresis and eliminate edema. While in the latter one Radix Aconiti praeparata warm kidney help Yang to remove Yin covering; Rhizoma Atractylodis Macrocephalae, Poria tonifying spleen and diuresis; Rhizoma Zinghiberis Recens warm and dispel water-cold, Radix Paeeoniae Alba harmonize regulate Ying Yin beneficial for water circulation. The former prescription is indicated for deficiency in both Yin and Yang, but mainly deficiency in Yang, retention of water pathogen interior; while the latter one is indicated for weakness in spleen and kidney Yang, excess in Yin cold interior with retention of water pathogen. In case with extreme excess of Yin cold, Semen Trigonellae, Radix Morindae Officinalis, et al added to warm and supplement kidney Yang, for helping Qi-transmission; In case of weakness of kidney and unconsolidation, with large amount of light urine take away Rhizoma Alismatis, Semen Plantaginis and add in Fructus Psoraleae, Fructus Alpiniae Oxyphyllae, Semen Trigonellae, Radix Morindae Officinalis to warm and consolidate kidney Yang. In case of asthma and shortness of breath, more expiration with less inspiration, exaggerated after movement, perspiration with cold extremities, it suggests water pathogen affect on lung, dysfunction of kidney in receipt air. Radix Ginseng, Fructus Schisandrae,

Gecko, Calcining Concha Ostreae or Hei Xi Pill are used for help Yang in receipt air, preventing from changing to prostration due to asthma. In case of palpitation and feeling of oppression in chest, cyanosis in lips and tongue, rapid weak pulse or arrhythmic pulse, it means water pathogen retrogressed upward, inhibit heart Yang, heart and blood stagnancy and obstruction, Radix Aconiti Praeparata should be emphasized on and accompanied by Ramulus Cinnamomi, Radix Glycyrrhizae, Radix Salviae Miltiorrhizae, Flos Carthami for warm Yang and resolve stagnancy. In case of heaviness in head with nausea, sleepy and lassitude, even confusion of mind, with urinary smell in mouth, it indicates critical condition caused by damp pathogen runs upward and covering mind. Wen Pi Decoction combined with Ping Wei Powder and Herba Agastachis, with addition of Herba Pogostemi, Herba Eupatorii are added for warming Yang and purging turbidity, regulate stomach descending retrogression; otherwise Radix Aconiti praeparata combined with Radix and Rhizoma Rhei, Rhizoma Coptidis, Rhixoma Pinelliae for detoxication and descending turbidity. In case of long lasting unrelieved edema attacked additionally by exterior pathogen, edema is aggravated significantly, fever with aversion to cold but without sweating, it should be treated as wind-edema. But drugs for dispelling superficity should not be over-used, it is necessary to protect and considering vital-Qi, strengthening the body resistance to eliminate pathogenic factors. In the last stage of the disease, deficiency and weakness of kidney Yang, disorder of Yang affecting Yin, lead to deficiency and weakness of kidney Yin. Syndromes like lingering edema, dizziness and lassitude, soreness of loin and emission, dryness in mouth and throat, dysphoria with smothery sensation and night sweat, red tongue with less fur, thready rapid pulse, it should be treated by supplementing kidney Yang, nourishing kidney Yin, accompanied with diuresis to eliminate water pathogen. Large dose on Da Bu Yuan Jian may be put on, but drugs for nourishing Yin with too cool and greasy character to block water pathogen should not be used, diuresis should not be too strong to avoid damage to Yin fluid.

Examples of prescription: Radix Rehmanniae Praeparata 10g, Poria 30g, Radix Aconiti Praeparata 9g, Rhizoma Dioscoreae 10g, Rhizoma Atractylodis alba 10g, Radix Paeoniae Alba 10g, preparata Radix Glycyrrhizae 6g, Cortex Cinnamomi 6g, Herba Leonuri 30g, Rhizoma Alismatis 12g.

In addition, for treatment of edema method of motivating blood and resolve stagnancy are usually used in combination. As said in《Xue Zhang Lun》: "stagnant blood transformed into water, also lead to edema, which is blood disease accompanied by edema."Blood in motion renders water circulating normally. Therefore in treatment for edema, especially whenever ineffective by ordinary treatment but with signs of blood stagnancy, addition of Herba Leonuri, Rhizoma Lycopus Lucidus Turez, Semen Persicae, Flos Carthami may increase the effect of diuresis and eliminating edema.

〔Prevention and nursing care〕

1. Salt is forbidden《Shi Ji De Xiao Fang》: "Salt should forbidden in all kinds of edema." Therefore in early stage of edema, non-salted food must be taken; then transfer to low salted food gradually after dissemination of edema and at last ordinary food.

2. Raw and cold, oily and greasy, spicy, alcohol and other stimulating food should not be taken. Prefer easily absorbable, richly nutrient food.

3. Regulate to and take care of environmental cold and warm, avoid invasion by exterior pathogen; escape from great angry, take emotional adjustment, establish confidence on fight against disease, do not indulge in sexual activity and overworking to protect from damage to premodial Qi and aggravate severity of disease.

4. Treat the skin infection, ecchymosis, sore throat on-time to prevent from invading interior by toxins of infection.

5. In severe cases pay close attention to changes in disease, preventing from occurrence of transformation of syndromes such as prostration due to asthma, motivation of wind, mental disturbances and confused mind.

〔Analysis on typical case〕

Case 1: Chang, male, 15 years of age, case no. 1382.

Admitted on 26th Nov. 1983. Had influenza and headache ten days before with fever aversion to cold, swelling and sore throat, edema of face, eyes and edema over whole body for 4 days. In examination the followings are found: edema of face and eyes, eyes cannot open, swelling of abdomen, slight edema in lower extremities, less quantity dark urine, averse to cold, neck rigidity, fatigue and listlessness, cough with thin sputum, poor appetite, white thin fur, float slow pulse.

This case was attacked by exterior wind pathogen, heat-transmission in retention and staying of pathogen. Interconnection of water and heat, struggle between wind and water, stagnancy and obstruction of lung Qi, dysfunction in dispelling and descending, failure in governing and regulation, result to disorder in Qi-transmission in three Jiao, water pathogen failed to transport downward to urinary bladder, overflow of water damp transversely and retroversely induce edema over whole body. The method of treatment should be promote the dispersing function of the lung and expelling exterior pathogen, diuresis and eliminating edema. Prescription:

Herba Ephedrae 12g, Gypsum Fibrosum 50g, Rhizoma Atractylodis 12g, Fructus Ziziphi Jujubae 25g, Herba Brassiae Oleiferae 15g, Rhizoma Alismatis 15g, Umdellate Pore 15g, Semen Plantaginis 25g, Rhizoma Imperatae 25g, Spica prunellae 15g, Herba Leonuri 15g, Radix Stephaniae Tetrandrae 25g, Radix Glycyrrhizae 6g.

Taking above prescription for six doses, amount of urine increased, edema eliminated. Recovery after another 10 doses with slight changes in the prescription. Urine examination normal. Followed up for 5 months no relapse occured. 《Si Chuan ZhoYi》, 1985 (6):24)

Note: Pathogenic factor in this case is exterior pathogen, diseased location is lung, wind water overflow, degree of edema is more severe in the face and eyes than lower extremities. Course of disease is 4 days, signs found in four diagnostic methods demonstrate disease belongs to wind edema. Pathogenesis of disease is dysfunction of lung in dispelling and descending. Therefore for promoting the dispelling function of the lung, rendering circulation of water, modification of Decoction for relieving edema was selected and recovery was expected.

Edema is a morbid state in which the main manifestation is retention of water fluid within the body, overflowing in the muscle and skin even remaining in chest and abdomen. Either exterior invasion or interior injury may be the pathogenic factor. Usually attack by exterior pathogen, water damp invades harmfully, excess interior in damp heat and infection toxins, and indulge in sexual activity and multiple birth result to dysfunction of lung in regulation and ventilation, dysfunction of spleen in transforming and transporting, dysfunction of kidney in discharge and retention, retention of water damp and overflowing in muscle and skin leading to edema.. The disease is intimately related to lung, spleen, and kidney; especially kidney is the most important one among these three organs.

The guide line for differentiating edema is Yin and Yang. Disease caused by overflow of wind water, water damp invasion and immerse, excessive damp heat and infected toxins mostly belong to Yang edema, excess syndrome. Diseased location is lung and spleen. Edema raised from hypofunction in spleen Yang or weakness in kidney Yang mostly belongs to Yin edema, deficiency syndrome, diseased location is spleen and kidney. Nevertheless, in the clinics, usually Yin and Yang is intermingled, deficiency and excess may be seen simultaneously, particular attention should pay to their transmission. Methods for treatment of edema various as: inducing diaphoresis, diuresis, purging water, tonyfying spleen, warm kidney, descending turbidity, resolving stagnancy, et al. In treatment for Yang edema syndrome, main method administered is inducing diaphoresis and diuresis. If there is obstruction of damp turbid with constipation, purging water downward may be used temporary and stop purging immediately after the effect seen to prevent from harm to the vital-Qi. In Yin edema warm transmission is the main choice. Among them in those with spleen deficiency warm spleen consolidate earth and warm kidney helping Yang in those with kidney deficiency. In deficiency and excess mixed up cases reinforcement and elimination in combination, or superficiality at first then originality. Generally after elimination of edema, signs of deficiency commonly seen, regulation and supplementation according to deficiency in Zang-Fu, Qi-blood, Yin Yang are required.

As prognosis for edema, if therapy carried out on-time, the prognosis would be good in disease lasting not long or edema raised from disorders in nutrition. But in those of long lasting cases with multiple recurrence, deficiency in vital Qi and retention of pathogen, the disease would be lingering and hard to recover. In moderate edema with symptoms like: palpitation, cyanotic lips, shortness of breath with difficulty to lie on supine position, or black lip, no concave in supraclavicular fossa, protrusion of umbilicus, foot not straight but back straight, or with nausea and vomiting, urine smell in mouth, confused mind, or dizziness and headache, tremor of limbs even contracture or anuria, nose-bleeding, hematuria, hematochezia, all of them are critical case with poor prognosis.

Additionally, salt should be forbidden in edema and food with spice and heavy taste should be avoided. Protect from common cold and over strain in order to free from relapse.

Questions for Review

1. Describe briefly the important role of lung, spleen, kidney functional disorders

play in the pathogenesis of edema.

2. What is the main point in differentiation of syndroms in edema and their principles of treatment ? How to use them?

3. What is the characteristics for Yin and Yang edema? How to treat according to differentiation of syndroms?

4. Prognosis of edema.

5. How to regulate and take care of the edematous patient?

Stranguria

(Appendix: turbid urine)

〔Introduction〕

Stranguria is the disease which character is frequent and urgent or dribbling in micturition with prickling pain, desiring but difficulty in urination, with spastic distension in the lower abdomen or pain expanding to waist and abdomen.

Stranguria is first recorded in "Nei Jing". "Jin Gui Yao Lue" named this disease "Lin" or "Lin Bi", and pointed out stranguria had the character of dripping and difficuly in micturition with prickling pain in the urethra. The "urine like millet" means there is millet like things obstructed in urethra and cause pungent and unbearable pain, on the other hand the character of the stones that move out of urine are like millets. It is vivid description of TCM stranguria. "Zhang Zhong Jing" had recognized stranguria belonged to whole body disease. For example, five zang-organ unclear, six fu-organ disharmony, mass in triple-jiao and deficiency of Ying-wei etc. all can cause stranguria. According to the difference of pathogeny and clinical manifestation stranguria can be divided into 8 types, they are cold stranguria, heat stranguria, Qi-Stranguria, overstrain stranguria, chyluria stranguria, sand stranguira, deficiency stranguria and excess stranguria. It makes the clinical embryonic types of stranguria. "Wai Tai Mi Yao" pointed out concrete contents of five stranguria: "The 5 stranguria are: stone stranguria, Qi stranguria, chyluria stranguria, overstrain stranguria and heat stranguria." Today clinical physicians still use them but the content has a little difference. Five stranguria of today are Qi stranguria, blood stranguria, stone stranguria, overstrain stranguria and chyluria stranguria. About the pathogenesis, Dan Xi held it belonged to heat, He Jian pointed out it had relation with stagnation of Qi and blood; "Jing Yue Quan Shu" regarded it "come from cold, heat and deficiency", which is complete description of the pathogenesis of stranguria. About the therapeutic principle, the treatment methods from "Dan Xi Xin Fa Lin" and "Jin Gui Yi" have important instructive significance to clinical practice.

If the west medicine diseases i. e. urinary infection, urinary calculus, tumor, prostatosis and chyluria etc. have the symptom of stranguria all can be treated referring to the TCM treatment of stranguria.

〔Etiopathology〕

The main etiology of stranguria is accumulation of damp-heat in lower-jiao. "Jin Gui Yao Lue · Wu Zang Feng Han Ji Ju Bing Mai Zheng Bing Zhi" regarded the etiology of this disease is "heat in lower-jiao". "Dan Xi Xin Fa Lin" said: "There are five types of stranguria, they all belong to heat." "Zhu Bing Yuan Hou Lun · Lin Bing Zhu Hou" pointed out "All stranguria come from deficiency of kidney and heat in bladder." Which suggested the initial state of stranguria belonged to a cumulation of heat-damp in bladder then it changed from excess to deficiency or excess mixing with deficiency.

According to the description of past physicians we can conclude the etiology of stranguria in three aspects:

1. Damp-heat in the bladder: damp-heat comes from external or gives rise to internal production. Damp-heat from external is caused by contaminated lower orifice then the filthy evil invading into bladder, or heat pathogen of other zang-fu organs moving to bladder i. e. excessive heart-fire moves into small intestine and invade into the bladder. Damp-heat from internal is caused by overeating pungent, heat, fat and sweat food or overdrinking alcohol which generate damp-heat and it moving into bladder, causing disturbance in Qi transformation, inducing abnormality of water passageway and caused stranguria. If the stranguria patient has scorching hot urine with prickling pain is heat stranguria; If the stranguria with excess heat of bladder hurting the vessel, causing blood to circulate rashly and wildly and resulting in difficult urination with pain and blood is blood stranguria. If the stranguria with damp-heat invading into lower body causing disturbance in bladder-Qi transformation, unseparating of lucid and turbid and urine like oil or fat is chyluria stranguria. If the stranguria with accumulation of damp-heat burning urine the impurity of urine solidifying sand and stone is stone stranguria.

In brief, heat, blood, chyluria and stone stranguria all can be caused by damp-heat in bladder.

2. Deficiency of kidney and spleen: Deficiency of kidney and spleen is resulted from prolonged stranguria, the damp-heat consuming vital-Qi, old body, prolonged disease, overstrain and indulging in sexual intercourse. Deficiency of spleen will cause collapse of middle-jiao energy and deficiency of kidney falling to hold form which will result in continue urination. Kidney is the origin of congenital constitution, spleen is the origin of acquired constitution. The two organs help and promote each other. So deficiency of spleen can cause deficiency of kidney, conversely, deficiency of kidney also can cause deficiency of spleen. With deficiency of spleen and kidney external evil can easily invade into bladder to cause stranguria. After suffered from stranguria damp-heat injure spleen, kidney, and make the patient's condition difficult to recover. It is obviously that deficiency of spleen and kidney and damp-heat in bladder are all important etiology of stranguria. If rest make stranguria condition better, overworking make the condition worse the stranguria is overstrain stranguria. If deficiency of Qi in middle-jiao causing sinking of Qi is Qi stranguria. If deficiency of Qi in kidney causing unconsolidation of lower-jiao, oil can not be restrained, the oil sinking and the turbid urine like oil and fat is chyluria stranguria. If Yin deficiency causing hyperactivity of fire, deficiency type of fire burning vessel, causing urination with blood is blood stranguria.

3. Stagnation of the liver-Qi: It is caused by anger hurting liver leading to the stagnation and undispersion of Qi. Stagnation of Qi will generate pathogenic fire in lower-jiao and disturbance of bladder-Qi transformation can cause distending pain in the lower abdomen, urination with uneven pain and result in excess type Qi stranguria. The Qi stranguria caused by sinking of Qi in middle-jiao is deficiency type.

In brief the etiology of stranguria is mainly caused by damp-heat in bladder, its location is at bladder and kidney and have relation with liver and spleen. Its pathogenesis is accumulation of damp-heat in lower-jiao causing the disturbance of bladder-Qi transformation. At the initial state of the disease is excessiveness of pathogen, then the syndrome turns from excess to deficiency. If pathogenic factor has not fallen into decline and the vital-Qi hurted is complex of excess and deficiency.

〔Differentiation and treatment of common syndromes〕

Ⅰ. Main point of differentiating syndrome

1. Differentiating the classification of stranguria: All strangurias have the symptom of frequent and urgent or dribbling micturition with prickling pain, desiring but difficulty in urination, with spastic distention in the lower abdomen or pain expand to waist and abdomen. But each type of stranguria has its own characters. The main symptom of stone stranguria is micturition with sand and stone. The main symptom of chyluria is turbid urination with cloudy rice-water like or oily urine. The main symptom of blood stranguria is hematuria with pungent pain. The Qi stranguria is distension and pain lower abdomen and with uneven dripping urination. The main symptom of heat stranguria is scorching hot urination with stabbing pain. The main symptom of overstrain stranguria is dripping and continue mictruation which is caused or exacerbated by overworking.

Diagrammatic Sketch of Stranguria Etiopathology

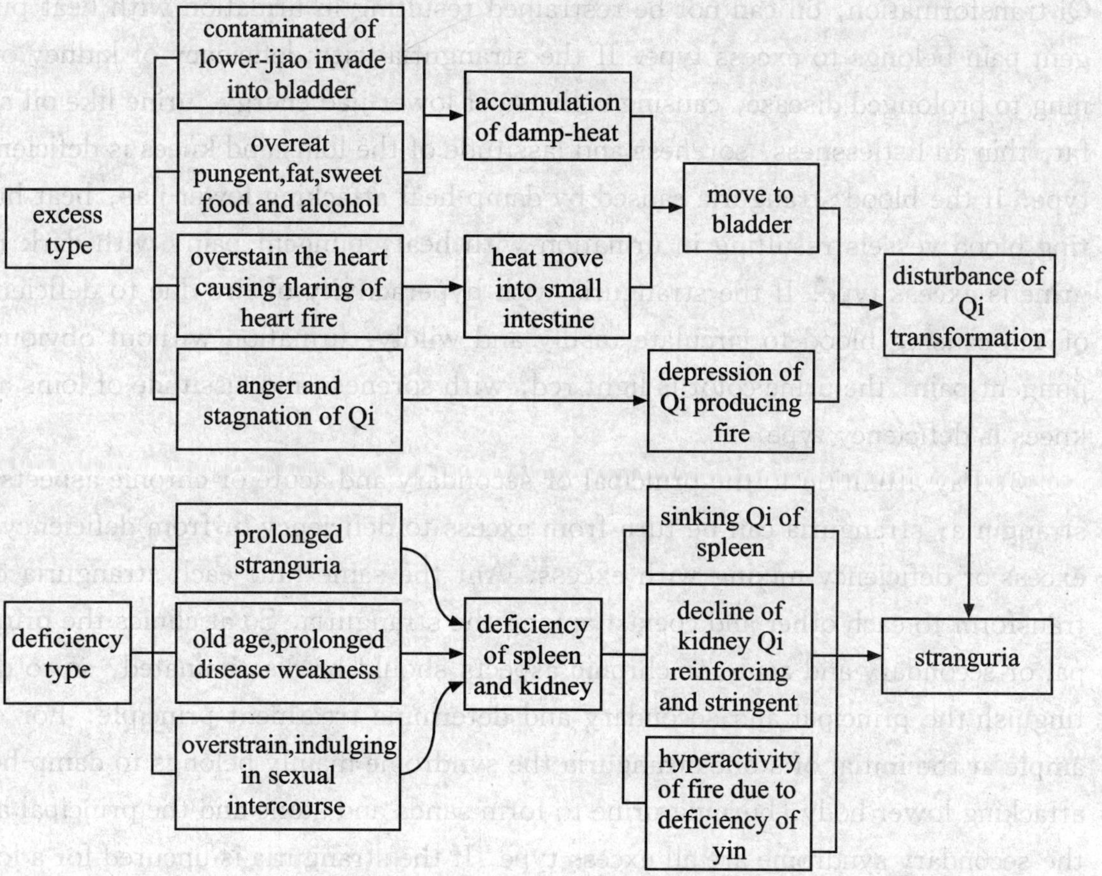

2. Observing excess and deficiency of syndrome: On the base of differentiation types of stranguria physician should observe the excess and deficiency of syndrome. Differentiation is according to etiology, course of disease, part and whole symptom and the color properties of urine. Generally, at the initial or acute stage of the disease the syndrome belongs to excess type, which main property is damp-heat in bladder, stone forming and stagnation of Qi. Prolonged disease belongs to deficiency and the disease location is in spleen and kidney, at most time is mainly deficiency of spleen, kidney and deficiency of Qi and Yin. If the urine is heat with obviously stabbing pain, urinate turbid and red without deficiency of zang-fu and Yin-Yang belongs to excess type; If the urine with no obviously heat and stabbing pain, urinate clear and light and with deficiency of zang-fu and Yin-Yang belongs to deficiency type. One type of stranguria can be excess or deficiency according to etiopathology. If stone stranguria caused by sinking damp burning urine to forming stone is excess type; If the stranguria is with consumption of Yin caused by prolonged stranguria or deficiency of spleen and kidney is deficiency type. If the chyluria heat stranguria caused by damp-heat attacking the lower-jiao, disturbing Qi transformation, oil can not be restrained resulting in urination with heat pungent pain belongs to excess type. If the stranguria with deficiency of kidney owning to prolonged disease, causing collapse of lower-jiao energy, urine like oil and fat, thin an listlessness, soreness and lassitude of the loins and knees is deficiency type. If the blood stranguria caused by damp-heat attacking lower-jiao, heat hurting blood vessels resulting in urination with heat, pungent pain, with dark red urine is excess type. If the stranguria with hyperactivity of fire due to deficiency of Yin causing blood to circulate rashly and wildly, urination without obviously pungent pain, the urine color is light red, with soreness and lassitude of loins and knees is deficiency type.

3. Pay attention to the principal or secondary and acute or chronic aspects of stranguria: stranguria can be turn from excess to deficiency or from deficiency to excess or deficiency mixing with excess. Ant the same time each stranguria can transform to each other and coexist among the stranguria. So at clinics the principal or secondary and acute or chronic aspects should be discriminated, so to distinguish the principal and secondary and determine treatment principle. For example at the initial of stone stranguria the syndrome mainly belongs to damp-heat attacking lower body, burning urine to form sands and stone and the principal and the secondary syndrome are all excess type. If the stranguria is uncured for a long

time it will hurt Qi and Yin, the manifestation of deficiency of Qi or Yin can be seen. The syndrome gradually transformed from excess to deficiency type and display excess of principal syndrome and deficiency of secondary syndrome. Overstrain stranguria mainly is deficiency of spleen and kidney if it attacked by exopathogen, damp-heat evil invading bladder will cause heat stranguria and it will display deficiency of principal syndrome and excess of secondary syndrome. According to the principle of symptomatic treatment in acute condition and radical treatment in chronic condition firstly damp-heat should be eliminated to treat the secondary syndrome — heat stranguria; then the body resistance restoring Qi should be strengthened to treat principal syndrome—overstrain stranguria.

4. Classified differentiation:

1) Dysuria: Dysuria is the disease which character is difficulty in urination, scanty urine in amount even dribbling or nothing. Its urine scanty in amount and difficulty in urination is same as stranguria. But the character of stranguria is frequent micturition with pain and the total amount urine is normal and the character of dysuria is urination without pain, the total amount urine is less than normal amount, at severe situation the urination is blocked up and without urine.

2) Hematuria: Blood stranguria and hematuria are all urination with blood or blood lumps, even urinating pure blood; The difference is urination with pain or not, hematuria is always urination without pain but blood stranguria is urination with unbearable pain.

3) Turbid urine: Chyluria stranguria and turbid urine are all turbid in urine like rice-water; but turbid urine is without pain and pungent feeling and chyluria stranguria is with pain and pungent feeling.

Ⅱ. Treatment principles and contraindication

The basic treatment principle of stranguria are eliminating excess evil to excess type, restoring Qi to deficiency type, tonifying Qi and purging pathogenic evil to excess mixing with deficiency type. If the excess type is taken damp-heat in bladder as main factor the treatment should be clearing away heat and promoting diuresis. If the excess type is taken heat hurting blood vessel as main factor the treatment should be cooling the blood to stop bleeding. If the excess type is taken stone forming as main factor the treatment should be purging stranguria and eliminating stone. If the excess type is taken difficulty in urination as main factor the treatment should be promoting and regulating Qi. If deficiency type is taken deficiency of spleen as main factor the treatment should be invigorating the spleen and restoring Qi. If deficiency type is taken deficiency of kidney as main factor the treatment should be restoring Qi and invigorating kidney.

About the therapy method of stranguria there were ancient wordings of avoiding diaphoresis and invigoration. If stranguria is really induced by external pathogenic factor or infected by new evil, the symptom is averting to cold, fever, nasal obstruction, running nose and itching throat, it should be treated both superficies and interior, cooperating compatible durgs of dispelling wind. As for avoiding invigoration is pointed to excess type, if stranguria with deficiency of spleen and collapse of middle-Qi or deficiency of kidney and collapsing of lower energy the therapy method of invigorating spleen Qi and kidney Qi and stop nocturnal emission should be used. The ancient saying must not be sticked to.

Ⅲ. Treatment according to type differentiation

1. Heat stranguria

Main symptoms: frequent and scant urination with scorching hot and stabbing pain, yellowish and red urine.

Accompanied symptoms: spastic distending pain in the lower abdomen or pain in loins and tenderness, or fever and chills, bitter mouth, nausea, vomiting or constipation.

Tongue and pulse: yellow and greasy fur, soft and rapid pulse.

Analysis: Damp-heat in lower-jiao, disturbing the Qi transformation is the main pathogenesis of heat stranguria so frequent and scant urination with hot and stabbing pain, yellow and red urine is seen. Damp-heat obstruction and dysfunction of Qi transformation will cause spastic distending pain in the lower abdomen; If the damp-heat evil attacks kidney so the pain in loins with tenderness is seen. Internal damp-heat steaming, the evil attacking Shao Yang causing fever chill exchanged, bitter mouth, nausea and vomiting can be seen; If evil spread to large intestine the constipation is seen. Yellow and greasy fur, soft and rapid pulse are all phenomena of damp-heat.

Treatment: clearing away pathogenic heat and dampness, relieving stranguria.

Prescription: modified "Ba Zheng Powder". The function of the recipe is clearing away heat and purging fire, inducing diuresis for treat stranguria. It is the general recipe for treating heat stranguria. Chinese pink herb (herba dianthi), prostrate knotweed (herba polygoni avicularis), fiveleaf akebia stem (caulis akebiae) plantain seed (semen plantaginis) and talc (talcum) in the recipe can treat stranguria by inducing diuresis, clearing away pathogenic heat to dredge orifice. Rhubab (radix et rhizoma rhei), capejasmine fruit (fructus gardeniae) and liquorice (radix glycyrrhizae) can clear away heat and purges fire, promotes heat downaway by inducing diuresis. If there are the sensation of consitipation and spastic distending pain in the abdomen unprepared rhubarb (radix et rhizoma rhei) can be used in larger dosage and used with fruit of immature citon or trifolate orange (fructus aurantii immaturus) to purge heat and loosen the bowels. If the disease manifested fever-chill, bitter mouth, nausea and vomitting, "Xiao Chai Hu Decoction" can be used to treat Shao-Yang disease by mediation. If loin with severe pain, achyranthes and cythula root (radix achyranthis bidentatae et radix cyathulae) is used to reinforce kidney and promote blood circulation, cure stranguria by inducing diuresis to relieve pain. If damp-heat hurt Yin or deficienc of Yin suffered by heat stranguria, manifested by red tongue with little fur, thready and rapid pulse use "Zhu Ling Decoction" with cogongrass rhizome (imperata rhizome) to tonify Yin, induce diuresis and treat stranguria.

Prescription case:

Chinese pink herb (herba dianthi) 10g, Prostrate knotweed (herba polygoni avicularis) 10g, Plantain herb (herba plantaginis) 30g, Fiveleaf akebia (caulis akebiae) 6g, Capejasmine fruit (fructus gardeniae) 10g, Unprepared rhubarb (Radix et rhizoma rhei) (decocted later than other drugs) 6g, "Liu Yi Powder" 10g (decocted with wrappings), Giant knotweed rhizome (rhizoma polygoni caspidati) 15g.

2. Stone stranguria

Main symptom: Difficulty in urination sometimes with sand and stone, or suddenly interruption in micturition, urgent pain in urethra, yellow red urine even with blood.

Accompanied symptoms: Spastic distension in lower abdomen or colicky pain in loins and abdomen expanding lower abdomen and perineum. If the disease uncured for a long time, continuing hematuria or unexpelled sand and stone will cause listlessness and fatigue, aching dull pain in loin, feverish sensation in palms and soles.

Tongue and pulse: At the beginning of the disease is with thin yellowish fur, taut or taut and rapid pulse; Prolonged disease will marked red tongue with little fur or pale tongue whose edges are covered with teeth prints; the pulse is thready and rapid or thready and weak pulse.

Analysis: Damp-heat moves downward to the lower jiao, and causes the urine to solidify into stones, leading to stone stranguria. Stones block the urethra, resulting in difficulty in urination, or suddenly interruption in micturition, and painful urination. Damage to the blood vessels by sands and stones causes the yellow red urine, even with blood. If sands and stones hinder the function of bladder-qi transformation and the smooth flow of qi in the lower jiao, the disease is marked as the symptoms of spastic distension in lower abdomen or colicky pain in loins and abdomen expending lower abdomen and perineum. Due to the excessive damp-heat as main at the initial stage, there are thin yellow fur and taut rapid pulse. Listlessness and fatigue, weakness in the lumbar and legs, feverish sensation in palm and soles, red tongue with little fur, and thready rapid pulse are the results of insufficiency of both qi and yin at the prolonged stage.

Treatment: Dispersing heat, eliminating dampness, relieving stranguria and dispeling stones.

Prescription: Modified Shi Wei Powder. The function of this prescription is eliminating the heat and dampness, inducing diuresis to treat stone stranguria. The recipe contains pyrrosia leaf, semen malvae, herba dianthi, semen plantaginis, and tale plantain seed. Its eliminating heat function is weaker than "Ba Zheng Powder", but the inducing diuresis and treating stranguria function is better than "Ba Zheng powder". In order to inforce eliminating excess evil removing stone and dissloving hard masses function, Lysimachis (herba lysimachiae), Climbing field (spora lygoddii), Chicken's gizzard membrane (endothelium cormeum gigeriae galli) and asteriscus pseudociaenae can be used. If the patient is with colicky pain in loins and abdomen, red peony root (radix paeoniae rubra), white peony root (radix paeoniae alba), liquorice (radix glycyrrhizae), frankincense (resina olibani) myrrh (myrrha) and eagle wood (lignum aquilariae resinatum) can be used to relive spasm and pain, promot the flow of Qi and blood. If the patient is with fever, dandelion herb (herga taraxaci), forsythia fruit (fructus forsythiae) and phellodendron bark (cotex phellodendri) can be added in this recipe to clear heat and detoxicate. Unprepared phubarb (radix et rhizoma rhei) can be used to purge heat and loosing the bowels to treat constipation. Prolonged stone stranguria can cause deficiency of vital Qi. This is mixture type of excess and deficiency, the treatment should done to both the principle and the secondary aspects of the stranguria. If there is deficiency of Qi and blood "Ba Zhen Decoction" should be added; If there is deficiency of kidney Yin "Liu Wei Di Huang Pill" should be added; If there is deficiency of kidney Qi "Ji Sheng Shen Qi Pill" should be added.

Prescription case:

Pyrrosia leaf (folium pyrroslae) 30g, cluster mallow fruit (fructus malvae veticillatae) 12g, Chinese pink herb (herba dianthi) 10g, talc (talcum) 12g, plantain seed (semen plantaginis) 15g (to be wrapped before it is decocted with other drugs), Chicken's gizzard-skin (Endothelium corneum gigeriae galli) 30g, climbing fern spore (spora lygodii) 12g, lysimachia (herba lysimachiae) 30g.

3. Qi stranguria

1) Excess type (stagnation type of Qi stranguria)

Main symptoms: difficulty in urination and distension in lower abdomen.

Accompanied symptoms: fullness and discomfort in the chest and hypochondrium.

Tongue and pulse: thin and white fur of the tongue, deep stringy pulse.

Analysis: Liver governs the flow of Qi, its channel passes lower abdomen, distribute chest and hypochondrium, relating external genitalia. If emotional depression cause liver falling to sooth will cause fullness in lower abdomen, chest and hypochondrium. Stagnation of Qi can cause disturbance of Qi transformation and result in the difficulty in urination. Stagnation of the liver Qi can not be soothed, in most case will cause deep stringy pulse and thin white fur. Stagnation of Qi and blood stasis will show dark tongue.

Treatment: Regulating the flow of qi and blood, inducing diuresis and treating stranguria.

Prescription: "Chen Xiang Powder" with additional ingredients. In the recipe eagle wood (lignum aquilaras) and tangerine peel (pericrpium citri reticulatae) can promote the circulation of Qi. Chinese angelica root (radix angelicae sinesnsis) and white peony root (radix paeoniae alba) can nourish the liver and regulate blood flow. Prossia leaf (folium pyrrosiae), talc (talum), cluster mallow fruit (fructus malvae vertillatae) and vaccaria seed (semen vaccariae) are used as adjuvant drugs to induce diuresis and treat stranguria. Liquorice (radix glycyrrhizae) can moderate the properties of other drugs and eliminate heat. These drugs cooperate with each other and have the function of regulating the flow of Qi and blood, inducing diuresis and treating stranguria. If there is distending pain in chest and hypochondrium, Corydalis tuber (rhizoma corydalis), sichuan chinaberry (fructus meliae toosendan) and green tangerine orange peel (pericarpium citri reticulatae viride) can be used to sooth the liver and regulate the circulation of Qi. If there is distending pain in lower body, lindera root (radix linderae), mutgrass flatsedge rhizome (rhizoma cyperi) and aucklandia root (radix aucklandiae) can be used to regulate the folw of Qi to alleviate pain. If there is obviously stabbing pain in chest, hypochondrium and lower abdomen with dark tongue and ecchymosis, Red peony root (paeoniae rubra) safflower (flos carthamia) shiny bugleweed herb (herba lycopi) cyathula root (radix cyathulae) and motherwort (herba leonuri) can be added to activate blood flow, remove blood stasis and induce diuresis.

Prescription case:

White peony root (radix paeoniae alba) 15g, Chinese angelica root (radix angelicae sinensis) 12g, green tangerine orange peel (pericarpium citri reticulatae viride) and tangerine peel (pericarpium citri reticulatae) 10g, respectively, pyrrosia leaf (folium pyrrosiae) 30g, eagle wood powder (lignum aquilarae resinatum) (to be taken after infused in finished decoction) 1g, talc (talcum) 10g, achyranthes root (radix achyranthis bidentatae) 12g, chuster mallow fruit (fructus malvae vertillatae) 10g.

2) Deficiency type

Main symptoms: distending pain in lower abdomen, void pain which is relieved by pressing, frequent urination, clear and dripping urine without stopping.

Accompanied symptoms: pale complexion, listlessness and fatigue, loose stool.

Tongue and pulse: pale tongue, weak and thready pulse.

Analysis: Spleen is in charge of sending up essential substance and transporting nutrients, its channel passes abdomen, prolonged stranguria or overusing bitter in taste, cold in nature and soothing drugs will consume middle-jiao energy. Insufficency of middle-jiao energy and collapse of spleen-Qi will cause distending pain in lower abdomen, with void pain which is relieved by pressing; the deficiency of Qi will fall to absorb and digest, which will cause frequent urination, clear and dripping urine without stop. Deficiency of spleen-Qi will cause dysfunction in transport, little source of growth and development, which will cause pale complexion, listlessness and fatigue, loose stool with pale tongue, weak and thready pulse.

Treatment: Invigorating the spleen and replenishing Qi.

Prescription: Modified "Bu Zhong Yi Qi Decoction". In the recipe, astragalus root (radix astragali aeu hedysai) acts as a principal drug with the effects of replenishing Qi and elevating Yang; dangshen (radix codlonopis pilosulae), bighead atractylodes rhizome (rhizoma atractylodis macrocephalae) and liquorice (radix glycyrrhizae) as assistant drugs share the efforts of invigorating the spleen and replenishing Qi. Functioning as an adjuvant drug, Chinese angelica root (radix angelicae sinesis) can nourish blood and regulate the nutrient system. While tangerine peel (pericarpium citri reticulatae) promote the flow of Qi to remove stagnation. Cimicifuga rhizome (rhizoma cimicifugae) and bupleurum root (radix bupleuri) use as guiding drugs for sending up lulcid Yang to assistant Astragalus root (radix astragali seu hedysai) and dangshen (radix codonopsis pilosulae). If there is with sallow complexion, dizziness, palpitation use white peony root (radix paeoniae alba) and prepared rehannia root (radix rehmanniae praeparata) to tonify blood. If there is weakness and soreness of waist and knees with dull pain achyranthes root (radix achyranthis bidentatae), eucommia bark (cortex eucommiae) and wolfberry fruit (fructus lycii) can be used to tonify kidney.

Prescription case:

Astragalus root (radix astagali seu hedysari) 15g, dangshen (radix codonopsis pilosulae) 10g, bighead atractylodes rhizome (rhizoma atractylodis macrocephalae)10g, prepared liquorice (radix glycyrrhizae praepartae) 6g, Chinese angelica root (radix angelicae sinensis) 10g, tangerine peel (pericarpium citri reticulatae) 10g, cimicifuga rhizome (rhizoma cimicifugae) 6g, bupleurum root (radix bupleuri) 4g, lindera root (radix linderae) 6g, eagle wood powder (lignum aquilariae resinatum) (to be taken after being infused in finished decoction) 1g.

4. Blood stranguria

1) Excess type

Main symptoms: frequent and urgent urination with hot, pungent stabbing pain, red urine or with blood lump or blood streak.

Accompanied symptoms: fullness and pain in lower abdomen or showing vexation.

Tongue and pulse: yellow fur, slippery and rapid pulse.

Analysis: Damp-heat moving to bladder and heat suffering the superficial venules will result in the excess type of blood stranguria. Flaring of heart-fire move to the small intestine, heat pressing up to the bladder and heat hurting vessel will cause dark-red urination with blood lump or blood streak. Damp-heat accumulating in lower-jiao, blood lump obstructing urethra will cause frequent and urgent urination with hot, pungent and stabbing pain. Damp-heat moving to lower-jiao, dysfunction of Qi transformation and stagnation of Qi will cause fullness and pain in lower abdomen. Flaring of heart-fire disturbing spirit will cause vexation. Yellow fur and slippery and rapid pulse are all phenomena of excess type.

Treatment: purging heat and treat stranguria, cooling blood to stop bleeding.

Prescription: "Xiao Ji Yin Zi" with "Dao Chi Powder". In the recipe, field thistle (herba cephalanoploris) and dried rehmannia root (radix rehmanniae) remove heat from the blood to stop bleeding and eliminate pathogenic heat. Cat-tail pollen (pollen typhae) and node of lotus rhizome (nodus nelumbinis rhizomatis) can cool blood and remove blood stasis. Talc (talcum), fiveleaf akebia (caulis akebiae), lophatherum (herba lophatheri) and capejasmine fruit (fructus gardeniae) can remove heat, induce diuresis, clear away the heart fire and relieve dysphoria. Chinese angelica root (radix angelicae sinensis) and liquorice (radix glycyrrhizae) nourish the blood, relieve spasm and pain. Cooperation of these drugs have the function of removing heat, treating stranguria and cooling blood to stop bleeding. If there are overbleeding and severe pain, powder of amber (succinum) and notoginseng (radix notoginseng) can be infused in prepared decoction to remove blood satsis and treat stranguria to stop bleeding.

Prescription case:

Field thistle (herba cephalanoploris) 30g, dried rehmannia root (radix rehmammiae) 30g, capejasmine fruit (fructus gardeniae) 10g, node of lotus rhizome (nodus nelumbinis rhizomatis) 15g, talc (talcum) 12g, cat-tail pollen (pollen typhae) (parched) 10g, fiveleaf akebia (caulis akebiae) 6g, lophatherum (herba lophatheri) 6g, cogongrass rhizome (rhizoma imperatae) 30g, amber powder (succinum) (infused in prepared decoction) 3g.

2) Deficiency type

Main symptoms: light red urine without severe difficult pain

Accompanied symptoms: weakness and soreness in waist and knees, listlessness and fatigue.

Tongue and pulse: red tongue with little fur, thready and rapid pulse.

Analysis: Prolonged disease, damp-heat hurting Yin, deficiency of kidney Yin, deficiency fire hurting vessel, and vessel injury causing bleeding will result in light red urine without severe difficult pain. Deficiency of kidney Yin will cause soreness of waist and fatigue. red tongue with little fur and thready and rapid pulse are phenomena of heat due to deficiency of Yin.

Treatment: Nourishing and enriching the kidney Yin, clearing away heat to stop bleeding.

Prescription: "Zhi Bai Di Huang Pill" with additional ingredients. In the recipe "Liu Wei Di Huang Pill" can nurish and enrich kidney Yin. Anemarrhena rhizome (rhizoma anemarrhenae) and phellodendron bark (cortex phellodendri) can clear away heat to stop bleeding. Eclipta (Heaba ecliptae), glossy privent fruit (fructus ligustri lucidi) and donkey-hide gelatin (colla corii asini) are added to remove heat from the blood to stop bleeding. If the bleeding can not stop, biota tops (cacumen biotae), cogongrass rhizome (rhizoma imperatae) and hairy vein agrimony (herba agrimoniae) can be added to stop bleeding.

Prescription case:

Dried rehmannia root (radix rehmanniae) (stir-baking) 30g, poria (poria) 12g, Chinese yam (rhizoma dioscoreae) 12g, dogwood fruit (fructus corni) 10g, moutan bark (cortex moutan radicis) 10g, phellodendron bark (cortex phellodendri) 6g, anemarrhena rhizome (rhizoma anemarrhemae) 10g, eclipta (herba ecliptae) 30g, biota tops (cacumen biotae) 10g, donkey-hide gelatin (colla corii asini) (melting by heating) 10g.

5. Chyluria stranguria

1) Excess type

Main symptoms: Urination with cloudy rice-water like, after laid the urine precipitation like folccule, with floating oil like fat, or mixed with solidifying blood lump or blood, with hot, pungent pain in urethra.

Accompanied symptoms: dry mouth and throat or thirst without fondness of drink.

Tongue and pulse: red tongue with greasy fur, soft and rapid pulse.

Analysis: Damp-heat accumulating in lower-jiao cause dysfunction of Qi transformation of bladder, unclearing of lucid and turbid, fat not be restrained, so will cause urine like cloud rice-water with pungent, hot pain in urethra. If heat hurt the blood vessel will cause urination with blood lump or blood. Excess of heat will cause dry mouth and throat. Obstruction of damp will cause thirst without fondness of drink. Red tongue with yellow greasy fur and soft and rapid pulse are all phenomena of damp-heat.

Treatment: clearing away heat and promoting diuresis, eliminating turbid from lucid.

Prescription: Modified "Chen Shi Bi Xie Fen Qing Yin". In the recipe hypoglauca yam (rhizoma dioscoreae hypoglaucae) and grassleaved sweetflag rhizome (rhizoma acori graminei) can eliminate turbid from lucid. Phellodendron bark (cortex phellodendri) and plantain seed (semen plantaginis) can clear away heat and promote diuresis. Smilax glabra rhizome (rhizoma smilacis glabrae) and white atractylode rhizome (rhizoma atractylodis macrocephalae) can renforce the spleen and induce diuresis. Lotus seeds (semen melumbinis) and red sage root (radix salviae miltiorrhizae) can remove heat from heart and as tranquilizer, promote blood circulation to remove obstrution in the channels. All the drugs cooperated can clear turbid and lucid, eliminate damp and heat, dredge blood vessel, make oil and fat coming back to its channel. If there is yellow-red urination with severe pungent and hot pain talc (talcum) and manshurian aristolochia stem (caulis aristolochiae manshuriensis) can be used to eliminate heat and induce diuresis. If there is fullness and distension in lower abdomen, difficulty in urination lindera root (radix linderae) and green tangerine orange peel (pericarpium citri peticulate viride) can be used to promote the flow of Qi and relieve distension. While urination with blood field thistle (herba cephalanoploris), node of lotus rhizome (nodus nelumbinis rhizomatis) and cogongrass rhizome (rhizoma imperatae) can be used to remove heat from blood to stop bleeding. If damp-heat gradually become weaker or heat leaving and damp remaining during a long course will cause deficiency of spleen and kidney. The treatment should be warming and tonifying kidney to promote diuresis, eliminating turbid from lucid, the "Bi Xie Fen Qing Yin" of "Dan Xi Xin Fa" should be selected to treat the disease.

Prescription case:

Hypoglauca yam (rhizoma dioscoreae hypoglaucae) 24g, grassleaved sweetflag rhizome (rhizoma acori graminei) 10g, plantain seed (semen plantaginis) (to be wrapped) 10g, smilax glabra rhizome (rhizoma smilacis glabrae) 15g, phellodendron bark (cortex phellodendri) 10g, lotus seed (semen nelumbinis) 12g, red sage root (radix salviae miltiorrhizae) 12g, white atractylode rhizome (rhizoma atractylodis macrocephalae) 10g, bugleweed 10g, liquorice (radix glycyrrhizae) 4g.

2) Deficiency type

Main symptoms: prolonged disease can not be cured or repeat attack, stranguria urine like fat without obviously pungent pain.

Accompanied symptoms: thin in appearance, weakness and soreness in loins and knees, dizziness and fatigue.

Tongue and pulse: pale tongue with white greasy fur, deep and weak pulse.

Analysis: Prolonged disease, repeating attack and can not be cured, causing damp-heat become weaker, so vital-Qi turns to deficiency. Deficiency of kidney cause primordial Qi unconsolidiation, fat overflowing, so manifest the stranguria urination like fat, weak in appearance, weakness and soreness in loins and knees, dizziness and fatigue. Pale tongue with white greasy fur and deep and weak pulse are phenomena of obstruction of damp and deficiency of kidney.

Treatment: Tonifying kidney and inducing astringency.

Prescription: Modified "Gao Lin Decoction". In the recipe prepared rehmannia root (radix rehmanniae praeparate) and gorden euryale seed (semen euryales) can tonify kidney. Dangshen (radix codonopsis pilosulae) and Chinese yam (rhizoma dioscoreae) can reinforce spleen. Dragon's bone (os craconis fossilia), oyster shell (concha ostreae) and white peony root (radix paeoniae alba) can induce astringency. If the disease with deficiency of spleen and sinking Qi of middle-jiao "Bu Zhong Yi Qi decoction"should added in the recipe. If the disease with the deficiency of kidney and spleen,"Jin Gui Shen Qi Pill" can added in the recipe.

Prescription case:

Prepared rehmanniam root (radix rehmanniae praeparate) 10g, Chinese yam (rhizoma dioscoreae) 15g, gorden euryale seed (semen euryales) 12g, dangshen (radix codonopsis pilosulae) 12g, calcined dragon's bone (os craconis fossilia), oyster shell (concha ostreae) 30g, respectively, (decocted earlier than other drugs), poria (poria) 12g, dodder seed (semen cuscutae) 10g, mantis egg-cass (Oŏtheca mantidis) 12g.

6. Overstrain stranguria

Main symptoms: dripping urination without obvious red, difficulty and pain, repeat attacking, work will induce it and make it more severe.

Accompanied symptoms: listlessness and fatigue, weakness and soreness in loins and knees.

Tongue and pulse: pale tongue, thready and weak pulse.

Analysis: prolonged stranguria or overtaking cold and cool drugs, or prolonged disease causing weakness, or overworking result in deficiency of spleen and kidney. Damp-evil retaining and dysfunction of Qi transformation can cause the urination without obvious difficult and pain, but dripping without stop, work will induce it. Qi deficiency of spleen and kidney cause listlessness and fatigue, weakness and soreness in lions and knees, pale tongue, thready and weak pulse.

Treatment: strengthening the spleen and tonifying the kidney.

Prescription: Modified "Wu Bi Shan Yao Pill". This recipe can tonify spleen and kidney and induce diuresis. Chinese yam (rhizoma diosoreae) is the main drug which not only tonify spleen and kidney but also replenish Qi and Yin. Poria (poria) can strengthen the spleen, while prepared rehmannia root (radix rehmanniae praeparata). dogwood fruit (fructus corni), morinda root (radix morindae officinalis), desertliving cistanche (herba cistachis), dogger seed (semen cuscutae), eucommia bark (cortex eucommiae), achyranthes and cyathula root (radix achyranthis bidentatae et radix cyanthulae) and schisandra fruit (fructus schisandrae) can tonify the kidney and induce astringency. Oriental water plantain rhizome (rhizoma alismatis) is as adjuvant drug to promote diuresis. If there is deficiency of the spleen and collapsing of Qi, distension and fullness in lower abdomen, urination with difficulty, "Bu Zhong Yi Qi Decoction" can be used with to replenish Qi and elevating the Qi. If there is deficiency of kidney Yin manifesting low fever, flushing of zygomatic region, dysphoria with feverish sensation in chest, palms and soles, red tongue with little fur and weak and rapid pulse, morinda root (radix morindae officinalis)should be removed and desertliving cistanche (herba cistachis) and add glossy priventfruit (fructus ligustri lucidi), eclipta (herba ecliptae) should be added to nourish Yin and tonify the kidney. If the patient manifests obvious fever of deficiency type, "Zhi Bai Di Huang Pill" can be used with to nourish Yin to eliminate fire. If there is weakness of kidney Yang, cold of extremities and frequent urination in night, bitter cardamon (fructus alpiniae oxyphyllae), raspberry (Fructus Rubi) and antler (Cornucervi) powder should be used to warm kidney and induce astringency.

Prescription case:

Chinese yam (rhizoma diosoreae) 30g, prepared rehmannia root (radix rehmanniae praeparata) 12g, schisandra fruit (fructus schisandrae) 10g, dogwood fruit (fructus corni) 12g, poria (poria) 12g, desertliving cistanche (herba cistachis) 10g, dodder seed (semen cuscutae) 12g, eucommia bark (cortex eucommiae) 10g, achyranthes and cyathula root (Radix achyranthis bidentatae et radix cyathulae) 12g, oriental water plantain rhizome (rhizoma alismatis) 10g.

Though every type of stranguria mentioned above has it own characters but they have certain relation with each other. The clinical manifestation may take one type of stranguria as main symptoms, or express symptoms of two or three types of stranguria symptoms, i. e. heat stranguria mixed with blood stranguria or stone stranguria complicated with heat stranguria and blood stranguria. About the transformation, there are transformation between deficiency and excess and transformation among stranguria types, i. e. on one hand the excess type of Qi stranguria, blood stranguria and chyluria stranguria can turn to deficiency type; the deficiency type can manifest excess type due to repeat attack or exacerbation. On the other hand excess type of heat stranguria and blood stranguria can turn to deficiency type or deficiency type of heat stranguria, Qi stranguria and blood stranguria. When damp-heat has not fallen into decline and vital-Qi has been suffered, the disease is at the transition state between excess and deficiency type or deficiency type express excess symptom due to domination of pathogen all can manifest mixture type of deficiency and excess. So the physician should master it flexiblely in clinical operation.

At most time the prognosis of stranguria has relation with its type, slight or severe state and whether being treated in time and thoroughly or not. Generally at the initial state of stranguria it can cured. i. e. the initial state of blood stranguria, Qi stranguria and chyluria stranguria are all can be cured and will not turn to chronical types if they have be treated positively, suitably at initial state and be taken care of. If stranguria are not being systemic treated or error treated it will become delaying type or repeat attacking, and turn into overstrain stranguria which can not be easily cured. Because of long course, slowly developing, slight symptoms and sometime attacking sometime stopping the stranguria is neglected for long course of treatment and become deficiency of Qi, blood, Yin and Yang and turn into consumptive disease. Or due to dysfunction of Qi transformation, retention of water in the body turns to edema. If reverse of upward flow noxious water and damp-evil confuse mental can cause the deteriorations: cough with dyspnea, palpitation, vomiting, nausea, drowsiness and coma etc.

〔Measure of prevention and nursing〕

1. Strengthen vital-Qi, prevent emotional discord, eliminate the relating factors of all kinds of invasion of exthogen and internal damp-heat, i. e. bearing urination, overeating fat and sweet food, indulgeing in sexual intercourse and overstrain, unclean of vulva, etc.

2. It has important significance for preventing child stranguria and postpartum stranguria that pay attention to health of pregnancy and postpartum;

positively treat the diseases of deficiency of the kidney such as diabetes and tuberculosis can decrease the occurrence of stranguria.

3. Drink more water, eat light food, avoid fat, sweet, aromatic, dry, pungent and hot food, take note of suitable rest and keep emotional happy.

4. Avoid sexual intercourse.

〔Appendix: turbid urine〕

The main symptoms of turbid urine were cloudy urination white like rice-water with no pain.

The occurrence of this disease are eating fat and sweet food causing the spleen falling to transport and convert and generating phlegm, or damp-heat evil remaining after disease, moving to bladder and causing disclear of turbid and lucid. Or prolonged disease causing spleen and kidney damage, deficiency of spleen causing collapse of Qi, unconsolidication of kidney Qi, causing refined nutritious substance and fat flowing to lower-jiao, so turbid urine is caused. If damp-heat hurt vessel and vessel damage result in bleeding will cause turbid urine with blood. If deficiency of spleen fall to absorb or deficiency of kidney Yin cause fire of deficiency type hurting vessel also can cause turbid urine with blood. If greedy and indulge in fat and sweet food or overstrain and indulging in sexual intercourse will cause turbid urine more severe or make it repeat attacking. The location of the disease is mainly in spleen, kidney and bladder. At initial state it belongs to damp-heat and excess type, the treatment should be removing heat to induce diuresis. Prolonged of the disease will cause deficiency of spleen and kidney, the treatment should be strengthening the spleen and kidney, solidifying the vital-Qi of lower-jiao; If the disease belongs to deficiency mixing with excess type should treat both vital-Qi and evil. Now the treatment of turbid urine are respectively described as follows:

1. Damp-heat attacking lower-jiao

Main symptoms: turbid urination like cream color with stasis lump and float oil, or with blood color, or with blood stick and lump, overeating fat and sweet food will make it more severe.

Accompanied symptoms: fullness in chest, thirsty but without fondness for drinking or with hot and pungent sensation in urethra.

Tongue and pulse: yellow and greasy fur, soft and rapid pulse.

Analysis: Because of overeating fat and sweet food cause internal damp-heat attacking bladder and disclearing of turbid and lucid.

Treatment: removing heat to induce diuresis.

Prescription: Modified "Cheng Shi Bi Xie Fen Qing Yin".

2. Collapse of Qi due to deficiency of spleen

Main symptoms: Repeat attacking of turbid urine can not be cured for a long time, turbid urination like white rice-water; overstrain or overeating fat and sweet food will induce its attack or make it more severe.

Accompanied symptoms: Weight and fullness in lower abdomen, frequently wanting to urinate, listlessness and fatigue, with no lusture on the face.

Tongue and pulse: pale tongue, feeble and weak pulse.

Analysis: Prolonged disease cause collapsing of Qi due to deficiency of spleen result in refined nutritious substance flowing to lower-jiao.

Treatment: Tonifying spleen and nourishing Qi, elevating lucid Yang and inducing astringence.

Prescription: Modified "Bu Zhong Yi Qi decoction". Chinese yam (rhizoma dioscoreae), gordon euryale seed (semen euryales) and gingko nut (semen gingko) can be added in the recipe to tonify kidney and strengthen kidney to induce astrigency. If deficiency of Qi can not display vigour and turbid urine with blood, notoginseng (radix notoginseng) and node of lotus rhizome (nodus nelumbinis rhizomatis) should be added in the recipe to induce astringence to stop bleeding. If there is cold extremities and loose stool baked ginger carbon and psoralea fruit (fructus psoraleae) can be added in the recipe to warm spleen and tonify kidney to stop diarrhea.

3. Deficiency of kidney falling to hold firm

Main symptoms: Delaying turbid urine can not be cured, turbid urination like condensed fat or jellied glue, soreness and weakness in lions and knees.

Accompanied symptoms: If the disease is stressed on deficiency of kidney Yin is with dizziness, tinnitus, fever accompanied with restlessness and dry mouth; if the disease is stressed on deficiency of kidney Yang is with pale complexion, cold body and extremities.

Tongue and pulse: If the disease is stressed on deficiency of kidney Yin is with red tongue, thready and rapid pulse; if the disease is disease is stressed on deficiency of kidney Yang is with pale tongue, deep and week pulse.

Analysis: Prolonged disease cause deficiency of the kidney falling to store essence, cause essence and fat flowing to lower-jiao.

Treatment: If the disease is stressed on deficiency of kidney Yin should nurishing Yin and tonify the kidney; if the disease is stressed on deficiency of kidney Yang should warm the kidney to induce astringence.

Prscription: If the disease is stressed on deficiency of kidney Yin should use "Zhi Bai Di Huang Pill"; if the disease is stressed on deficiency of kidney Yang should use "You Gui Pill" with additional ingredients.

〔Typical case analysis〕

Case 1: Song, female, 35 year old, cadre.

Short and red urination with blood about half year, having a cold will make it more severe, frequent urination with pain, having the sensation of scorching hot, soreness in waist and fatigue in back, fullness in lower abdomen with straining sensation, the pulse is feeble and rapid. She has been treated many times, but sometime stop and sometime attacking, so ask for treatment. Differentiation: blood stranguria of damp-heat in lower-jiao. Treatment: removing heat to induce diuresis, cooling the blood to stop bleeding.

Honeysuckle flower (flos lonicerae) 25g, dried rehmannia root (radix rehmanniae) 12g, chinese pink herb (herba dianthi) 12g, manshurian aristolochia stem (caulis aristolochiae manshuriensis) 10g, plantain seed (semen plantaginis) (wrapped) 12g, phellodendron bark (cortex phellodendri) 6g, prostrate knotweed (herba polygoni avicularis) 12g, oriental water plantain rhizome (rhizoma alismatis) 10g, chimbing fern spore (spora lygodii) 10g, liquorice tip (radix glycyrrhizae) 9g, lophatherum (herba lophatheri) 10g.

Second visit: the patient had taken 6 doses of the medicine, short and red urinatin with blood and scorching hot pain had taken a favourable turn, but waist pain turned no better, so tonifying kidney and strengthening waist drugs should be added in the recipe.

Red poria (poria rubra) 12g, oriental water plantain rhizome (rhizoma alismatis) 10g, prostrate knotweed (herba polygoni avicularis) 12g, capejasmine fruit carbon (fructus gardeniae) 6g, donkey-hide gelatin (colla corii asini) (melting by heating) 12g, dipsacus root (radix dipsaci) 12g, dried rehmannia root carbon (radix rehmanniae) 10g, eucommia bark barbon (cortex eucommiae) 8g, lophatherum (herba lophatheri) 9g, liquorice tip (radix glycyrrhizae) 9g.

The patient recuperates with the recipe mentioned above for one month, the disease is recovered, survey followed up two years the situation is good. ("Xu Yu

Shan Yi An")

Note: The blood stranguria patient of this case is with deficiency of kidney with damp-heat in the lower-jiao, damp-heat steaming and burning bladder, pressing the blood to circulate rashly and wildly so cause the hematuria. Vessel damage causing bleeding, stasis and heat entangled, obstructed in urethra, dysfunction of Qi transformation will cause frequent urination with pain, scorching and hot, fullness and urgency in lower abdomen with straining sensation. Prolonged disease causing consuming of kidney so will result in soreness in waist and fatigue in back. The treatment should be symptomatic treatment in acute condition—removing heat to induce diuresis, cooling blood to stop bleeding. Waiting for the damp-heat condition quitting, then should treat both principal and secondary symptoms, support the healthy energy and eliminate the evil factors, use the drugs of cooling blood and stopping bleeding are used, so the patient was cured about 1 month.

Stranguria is the disease which character is frequent urination, dribbling in micturition with stabbing pain, desiring but difficulty in urination, spasmatic distension in the lower abdomen or pain expanding to waist and abdomen. Its pathogency is taken damp-heat in bladder as main factor, the location of the disease is at kidney and bladder. At most time the initial state belongs to excess type, prolonged disease cause it from excess to deficiency type or manifesting excess mixed with deficiency. There are two types of clinical symptoms: one is symptoms causing by dysfunction of bladder-Qi transformation; the other is special symptoms of stranguria causing by different pathogency. The former is foundation for diagnosis of the stranguria, the latter is the characters for distinguishing different stranguria. At the same time they should be discriminated with dysuria, hematuria and turbid urine.

Stranguria is divided into 6 types: heat stranguria, stone stranguria, Qi stranguria, blood stranguria, chyluria stranguria and overstrain stranguria. At differentiation the physician should pay attention to the classification of stranguria, observe the excess and deficiency of syndrome, the principal or secondary and acute or chronical aspects, treat and prescribe combining with the course of disease and constitution and carry out direct treatment. The initial excess type is taken damp-heat accumulating lower-jiao and dysfunction of bladder-Qi transformation as main factors, the treatment should be removing and inducing diuresis to treat stranguria, assisting promoting the flow of Qi. Deficiency type is taken deficiency of spleen and kidney, dysfunction of bladder-Qi transformation as main factors, the treatment should be tonifying spleen and nourishing kidney. The excess with deficiency type should treat both principal and secondary aspects. And according to the characters of different stranguria consult the methods of stopping bleeding, eliminating stone and eliminating turbid from lucid. About the ancient physicians' wordings of avoiding diaphoresis and invigoration in treating stranguria should make a concrete analysis, not to be lumped together.

Among the strangurias they have certain relations. i. e. the transformation: one is the change between excess and deficiency, there exist this condition among stranguria and one type stranguria itself; the other is the change among all types of stranguria or manifesting two stranguria, excess and deficiency symptoms at the same time. It has important instructive significance to clinical operation knowing the relationship.

Besides, the stranguria patient should avoid overworking, avoiding eating fat, sweet, pungent and hot food, pay attention to his own health.

Questions for Review

1. Try to describe the characters and classification of stranguria.
2. Simply describe the clinical characters of every kind of stranguria.
3. How to distinguish stranguria from dysuria, hematuria and turbid urine?
4. Simply describe the etiopathology of stranguria.
5. Try to describe the relationship of every kind of stranguria.
6. How to differentiate and treat to stranguria?
7. How to prevent stranguria?

Retention of Urine

〔Introduction〕

Retention of urine, long-bi in Chinese, is defined as: the urine, the amounts of which is small, passes as drops, or even be completely retained. Long, a mild situation, refers to difficult urination, urine passes as drops, with small amount; Bi, is a severe one, that the patient is unable to pass any urine at all. The two symptoms, though between which has difference to some extent, both refer to dysuria; it is naturally called them long-bi as a whole.

The term long-bi, first appeared in《Nei Jing》. According to this book, the etiology pathogenesis and location of the disease were demonstrated in details. The pathology of the disease, as the book concluded, is that the urinary bladder and triple-jiao fail to control the urine and body fluid.《 Zhu Bing Yuan Hou Lun Xiao Bian Zhu Hou 》pointed out that the heat of the kidney and bladder is the etiology of retention of urine and difficulty in urination. The treatment of the disease with urethral catheterization was first recorded in《Bei Ji Qian Jin Yao Fang》, the serious consequence to death of this disease is also realized in the same book.

Zhu Dan Xi, a famous doctor of Yuan Dynasty, considers the disease as a result of several pathologic factors such as qi deficiency, blood deficiency, phlegm, wind blocking, excess heat. He, who treats this disease with emetic therapy that opens the upper switch to induce the diuersis.

Zhang Jing Yue, a skillful therapist of Ming Dynasty, reduced the etiology of the disease to four factors, especially the qi deficiency, of which he discussed in details.

Li Nian Cui, who lived in Qing Dynasty, summarized the documents before his age. In his book《Zheng Zhi Hui Bu long-bi》, he divided the etiology of the disease into seven types and put forward the concrete therapeutic method, which set the seal on the study and treatment of the disease.

In western medicine, the retention of urine and anuria caused by various kinds of factors can be treated by symptom complex differentiation referring to this chapter.

〔Etiology and Pathology〕

The normal urine of a person depends on the normal functional activity of qi of the triple-jiao. the activity can't be completed unless it depends on the dispersing and descending of lung qi, the transportation and transformation of the spleen qi, and the function of open and close of the kidney. Otherwise, the stasis of liver qi and obstruction of the urinary tract can also lead to long-bi by affecting the functional activity of qi of triple-jiao, the etiology and pathology are explained in detail as follows:

1. Accumulation of dampness heat

Constitutional excess dampness heat inside the body, preference for pungent and ratty food and wine produce dampness heat. The pathogenic dampness heat move downward from the middle-jiao to the urinary bladder, or the heat of other zang organs transmit to the urinary bladder, the accumulated dampness heat restrain the functional activity of the urinary bladder, the control of urination is impaired, retention of urine is occur.

2. Lung heat and stagnant of lung qi

The lung is the upper source of water, and regulates the body's water passages. If persistent lung heat in the body or evil heat attack the lung, it may restrain the descending function of lung qi, and impair the transportation and arrangement of liquid; the water passage is blocked, the water can't be transport downward to the urinary bladder; otherwise, the downward movement of excess lung heat to the urinary bladder block qi in both the upper and lower jiao, the passage of urine is blocked, retention of urine take place.

3. Failure of the spleen qi to ascend

Spleen controls of transportation and transformation; it also controls the ascending of clear qi. Too much anxiety, overstrain, improper diet or bad health after a prolonged illness or poor health in old age may cause the deficiency of spleen, the clear qi can't ascend while the turbid qi can't descend, the urine is blocked.

4. Kidney deficiency

The kidney dominates the water. Pathogenesis as congenital defeat, postnatal overstrain, weak resistance due to old age or following prolonged illness may cause kidney yang deficiency and the declining of the fire of the life gate. Here the control of urination is impaired, then retention of urine occurs. On the other hand, accumulation of dampness heat in the lower-jiao over a long period of time consumes fluid, and causes deficient kidney yin, yang qi fails to be produced because of yin deficiency, and it can also lead to retained urine.

5. Stagnant liver qi

Liver regulates the flow of qi that guarantees the orderly functioning of triple-jiao, the socalled water pathway. Emotional trauma blocks the free flow of liver qi, the functional activity of triple-jiao is affected, the water pathway is blocked, and the retention of urine occurs. On the other hand, the liver channel curves around the external genitalia and passes through the lower abdomen, this is why illness of the liver channel can lead to retained urine.

6. Blockage of the urinary tract

Blockage by stagnant blood, stale essence, lumps or stones make it difficult to urinate.

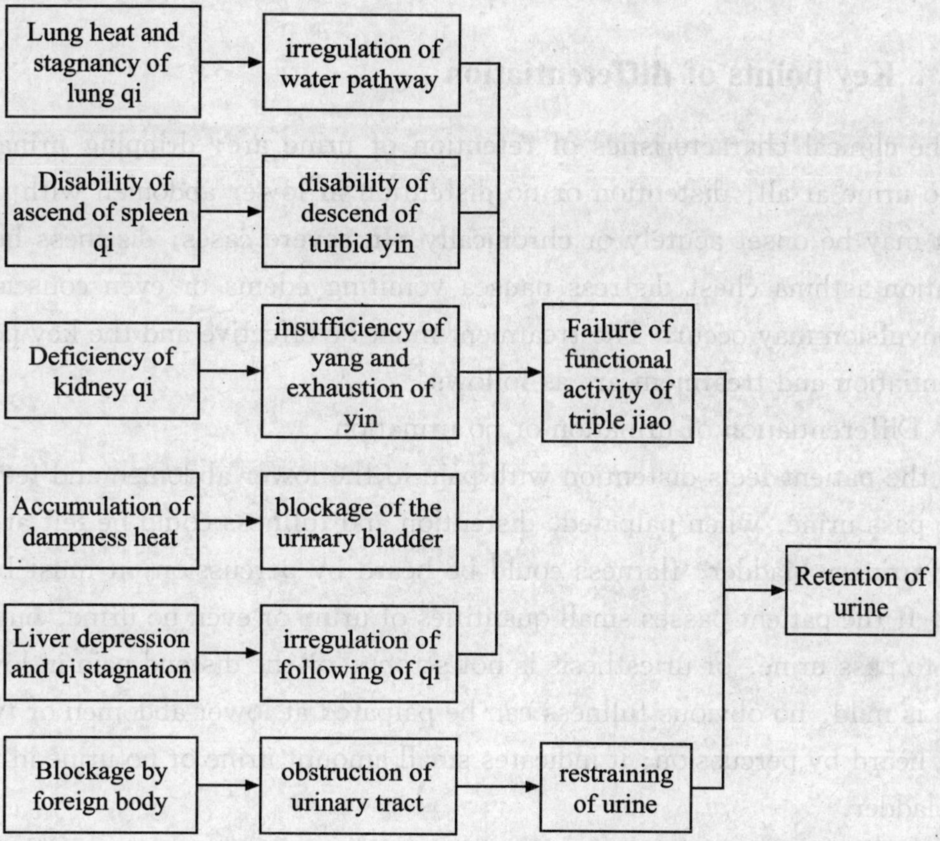

To sum up, the formation of retention of urine closely related with triple-jiao, lung, spleen and kidney, though it is a disease of urinary bladder. The dysfunction of qi of upper-jiao, as a result of lung heat and stagnation of lung qi, leads to the impairment of regulating and dispersing the water pathway. The dysfunction of middle-jiao is caused by the failure of ascending of clear yang and descending of turbid yin as a result of the accumulation of dampness heat or spleen deficiency. The failure of transportation and transformation of lower-jiao which relate closely with the kidney, is caused by downward movement of dampness heat or deficiency of kidney yang that can't transform water, all these can lead to the dysfunction of urinary bladder, retention urine forms. Stagnation of liver qi or blockage of urinary bladder caused by various reasons can also give rise to retention of urine.

〔Differentiation and treatment〕

Ⅰ. Key points of differentiation

The clinical characteristics of retention of urine are: dripping urination or even no urine at all; distention or no distention in lower abdomen with painless felt. It may be onset acutely or chronically. In severe cases, dizziness headache palpitation asthma chest distress nausea vomiting edema or even consciousness and convulsion may occur. The treatment must be effective and the key points of differentiation and treatment are as follows.

1. Differentiation of urination or no urination

If the patient feels distention with pain in the lower abdomen and feels difficult to pass urine, when palpated, distention and fullness could be felt at the region of urinary bladder, flatness could be heard by percussion, it must be uroschesis. If the patient passes small quantities of urine or even no urine, but has no desire to pass urine, or uriesthesis is not strong, or the distend pain in lower abdomen is mild, no obvious fullness can be palpated at lower abdomen or tympany can be heard by percussion; it indicates small amount urine or no urine in the urinary bladder.

2. Differentiation of deficiency and excess

Relative large amount of urine means excess syndrome. Little quantities of urine or no urine indicates deficiency syndrome. The retention of urine, which caused by accumulation of dampness heat, lung heat and stagnation of lung qi, stagnation of liver qi or blockage of urinary tract, belongs to excess syndrome, however, the syndrome of deficiency type can be caused by failure to ascend of spleen qi or deficiency of kidney, primordial qi. For the excess syndrome, the onset is usually acute, the manifestation is: distention or pain in the lower abdomen, scanty dark urine with burning sensation, a yellow and greasy tongue coating or a thin yellow coating, a taut smooth or rapid pulse. The deficient syndrome often onset chronically and give rise to vitality fatigue, shortness of breath, low and faint voice, white color of complexion without luster, no strength to urinate with drops of urine or even no urine, a pale tongue, a deep tready and faint pulse.

3. Differentiation of mildness and severity

Generally, the situation of long is chronic, while bi is severe. If long changes into bi it indicates the situation becomes worse, contrarily, it is better. If the distention and painfulness in the lower abdomen, chest distress, asthma nausea and vomiting appears, it means the situation is more serious, if coma, restlessness, convulsion take place, that means the situation is severe.

Ⅱ. Treating principle

The principle of treating retention of urine focuses on removing any obstructions, while superficiality and origin, mildness and severity of the disease should be concern about. Based on the principle of fu organs function better when unobstructed, emphasis should be laid on clearing. For the excess syndrome, clearing refers to dispersing dampness heat and stagnant blood and promoting the smooth circulation of qi, for the deficient cases, it means replenishing the spleen and kidney and assisting the regulation of body fluid. In addition, according to the theory of opening the upper gate to clear the lower orifice of the ancestor, the treatment of retention of urine is often effective by ascending the lung qi.

In the mean time, differentiation and treatment must be based on the causes and on which organs are diseased. Herbs that promote diuresis should not be abused. If the retention of urine is caused by little drink, hyperhidrosis, or consumption of yin by the heat diseases, the principle of treatment should be nourishing yin but not inducing diuresis.

Ⅲ. Treating according to type differentiation

1. Urinary bladder dampness heat

Main symptoms: Retention of urine or discharge of small quantities of hot dark yellow urine, distention and fullness in the lower abdomen.

Accompanied symptoms: A bitter taste and stickiness in the mouth, or thirsy with no desire to drink, constipation.

Tongue and pulse: A red tongue with sticky yellow coating, a rapid pulse.

Analysis: The accumulation of damp-heat in the lower jiao and the disturbance of the function activity of urinary bladder impair the control over urination, thus causing dysuria with hot dark yellow urine or retention of urine in severe cases. Stagnant qi of lower jiao due to retained dampness heat leads to distention and fullness in lower abdomen and constipation. Excess dampness heat inside the body gives rise to a bitter taste and stickiness in the mouth. The inability to distribute fluid causes a dry mouth with no desire to drink, a red tongue with yellow sticky coating and a rapid pulse are signs of dampness heat in the lower jiao.

Treatment: To disperse heat, eliminate dampness and promote diuresis.

Prescription: Modified Ba Zheng Powder. In the formula, Fiveleaf akebia, plantain seed, prostrate knotweed, chinesepink herb act together to disperse heat and eliminate dampness and promote the diuresis. Capejasmine fruit clear away of the triple -jiao, Talc and licorice root clear dampness-heat in the lower jiao, rhubarb reduces fire and relieves constipation. If the tongue coating is yellow sticky and thick, atractylodes rhizome and phellodendron should be added to dispersing heat and eliminating dampness. If the dampness heat turns the urine into stone that block the urinary tract, the treatment should take the treating method of stranguria as reference. If it is accompanied with dysphoria, oral ulceration, the treatment should be clearing heart fire and removing dampness heat combined with Daochisan. The dampness heat accumulates in the lower jiao for a long period, the kidney yin is injured, thirst, dry throat, hectic fever, night sweating, a hot sensation in the palms and soles, and a glossy red tongue or yellow sticky coating at the bottom will be onset. The treatment should be nourishing kidney yin and removing dampness heat and promoting the functional activity of qi. The prescription is Zi Shen Tong Guan pill while rhizome of rehmannia, plantain seed, achyranthes root are added. If dampness heat stagnation obstruct the functional activity of the triple jiao, which give rise to little amount of urine or even no urine, dirty complexion, lassitude, poor appetite, chest stressness, restlessness, nausea and vomiting, smell of urine in the mouth or even coma delirium. These indicates the attacking of toxin of urine, Huang Lian Wen Dan Decoction should be used as plantain seed congongrass rhizome, fiveleaf akebia are added to regulate stomach and purge turbid and to clear heat and eliminate dampness. For the severe case, An Gong Niu Huang Pill should be used to clear away heat and toxic material, to eliminate phlegm and induce resuscitation. If constipation is accompanied, rhubarb is added to relax bowels and expel toxin.

Formula for example:

Fiveleaf akebia 6g, plantain seed 15g(to be wrapped alone), prostrat knotweed 12g, Chinese pink herb 10g raw rhubarb 5g(to be decocted later), talc 10g raw tail of licorice root 6g, capejasmine fruit 10g, phellodendron bark 10g.

2. Stagnation of excess lung heat

Main symptoms: Difficulty of urination or retention of urine, scanty dark urine, with little quantities, shortness of breath

Accompanied symptoms: Coughing with dry throat, thirsty.

Tongue and pulse: A thin yellow tongue coating, a rapid pulse.

Analysis: Excess heat in the lungs prevents them from sending fluid down to the urinary bladder, resulting in difficulty of urination with scanty dark urine in small amount or retention of urine. Excess heat in the lungs also causes the upward movement of lung qi couples with a shortness of breath and coughing. The stagnation of the lung heat obstructs the distribution of fluid, that give rise to dry throat and thirst. A thin yellow tongue coating and a rapid pulse are symptoms of evil heat inside the body.

Treatment: To disperse heat in the lungs and regulate the water passage

Prescription: Modified Qing Fei decoction. Of the ingredients in the recipe, scutellaria root and wolfberry bark act as the principle drugs to disperse heat in lungs; capejasmine fruit, poria, fiveleaf akebia stem, plantain seed are served as assistant drugs for clearing heat and remove dampness. Lilyturf root, take the part as adjacent drug for nourishing yin and clearing heat. All the drugs combine to clear the upper jiao and disperse the lower jiao, to pass the urine. If irritable heart and red tongue lip has shown which refer to excess of heart firé, coptis root and lophatherum should be added to removing heart fire. If the lung yin is insufficient, which give rise to red tongue with less fluid on it, glehnia root, tricho sabthes root and fragrant solomonseal rhizome are needed for tonifying yin and clearing heat. If the fecal is obstructed, rhubarb, platycodon root should be used to promote the dispersing function of the lung to remove the feces. If headache, stuffy nose and superficial pulse are accompanied, peppermint and platycodon root should be combined to disperse the lung qi and relieve exterior syndrome.

Prescription for example:

Wolfberry bark 15g, scutellaria root 10g, capejasmine fruit 10g, fiveleaf akebia stem 6g, plantain seed 12g (to be wrapped alone), poria 12g, platycodon root 6g, lilyturf root 10g, cicada slough 6g, licorice root 6g.

3. Stagnation of liver qi

Main symptoms: Depression or irritability, retention of urine or difficulty in passing urine.

Accompanied symptoms: Distention and fullness or pain of the hypochondrium and chest.

Tongue and pulse: A red tongue with a thin or yellow thin coating, a taut pulse.

Analysis: Emotional injury affects the flowing of liver qi, the stagnation of liver qi impairs the ability of triple jiao to promote qi and regulate fluid, the passing of liquid is blocked, depression irritability, retention of urine or difficulty in passing urine will occurs. The liver channel passes through the lower abdomen and diaphragm and branch out in the coastal and hypochondriac region, thus the stagnation of qi of liver channel lead to distention and fullness or pain of the hypochondrium and abdomen. The taut pulse indicates the excess liver qi, red tongue with thin yellow coating refers to the tendency of stagnant liver qi turning into fire.

Treatment: To regulate qi circulation and promote diuresis.

Prescription: Modified Chen Xiang Powder. In the prescription, eagle wood and tangerine peek promote the smooth circulation of liver qi. White peony root, licorice root nourish the liver and relieve spasm; Chinese angelica root and vaccaria seed activate the blood circulation and promote the flow of qi, pyrcosia leaf, talc and cluster mallow fruit are combined to regulate the water passages. If the distention and fullness or pain of hypochondrium and abdomen is severe, nutgrass, flatsedge, spicebush root should be added to strengthen the function of the formula, sooth the liver and regulate the circulation of qi. For irritability accompanied with red tongue and thin yellow coating, it indicates the fire transmission of the stagnant qi; moutan bark, capejasmine fruit and gentian root should be added to clear away liver fire. If eructation, nausea and vomiting are accompanied, it indicates the hyperactive liver qi attacking the stomach, perilla stem and pinellia tuber should be used to regulate the stomach and check upward adverse flow of qi.

Prescription for example:

Eagle wood powder 2g(taking by infusion of the decoction), tangerine peel 10g, white peony root 15g, nutgrass flatsedge10g, talc 10g, cluster mallowfruit 10gvaccria seed 10g, Chinese angelica root 10g, licotice root 6g.

4. Blockage of the Urinary tract

Main symptoms: Dripping urine, urinating with a stream as fine as a thread, or retention of urine in severe cases.

Accompanied symptoms: Distention fullness and pain in the lower abdomen

Tongue and pulse: A dark purplish tongue or a tongue with purple spots, an unsmooth pulse.

Analysis: Blockage of the urethra by stagnant blood, stale essence and stone leads to distention, fullness and pain in the lower abdomen. A dark purplish tongue or a tongue with purple spots and an unsmooth pulse are signs of stagnant qi and blood

Treatment: To remove stagnant blood, disperse stagnation and regulate water passages.

Prescription: Modified Da Di Dang Pill. In the prescription, Chinese angelica root, pangolin scales, peach kernel, rhubarb, mirabilite are used to disperse blood stagnation and remove obstruction. Achyranthes, safflower, herba lycopi can be added to strengthen the function of activating blood circulation and dissipating blood stasis. If stone blocks the urinary tract, lysimachia, climbing ferspore, talc should be used to remove urinary calculus and induce diuresis. If the disease last for a long period and the patient is in the situation of both deficiency of qi and blood with dim complexion, dstragalus root、Chinese angelica root、red sage root should be combined to replenish qi, nourish blood and promote blood circulation. If the blockage of urinary tract caused the retention of urine, which results in unendurable distention and pain in the lower abdomen, little amount of musk powder should be taken to promote flow of qi and blood circulation to alleviate pain. If blood urine is accompanied, some amber and notoginseng powder should be used to activate the blood circulation to stop bleeding.

Prescription for example:

Chinese angelica root 15g, peach kernel 10g, prepared pangolin scales 6g, raw rhubarb 5g(to be decocted later), achyranthes 12g, lysimachia 15g, pyrcosia leaf 12g, herba lycopi 10g, musk 0.13g(take by infusion).

5. Sinking of qi of middle jiao

Main symptoms: A weighted sensation in the lower abdomen, retention of urine, or dysuria with only small quantities of urine.

Accompanied symptoms: Lassitude, shortness of breath, a feeble voice, poor appetite, slow digestion, constant desire to defecate, a long time diarrhea and prolapse of rectum.

Tongue and pulse: A pale tongue with a thin coating, a weak pulse.

Analysis: The spleen qi fails to ascend while the turbid yin is unable to descend, the result is dysuria. The spleen qi is weak, the resource of qi and blood is absent, thus give rise to lassitude, shortness of breath, feeble voice; if the deficiency of middle qi fails to transport and transform, the result is poor appetite and slow digestion. If Qi of middle jiao sinks, a constant desire to defecate, persistent diarrhea and prolapse of rectum will develop. A pale tongue with a thin coating and a weak pulse are symptoms of qi deficiency.

Treatment: To send the clear qi upward and the turbid yin downward, produce qi and circulate water

Prescription: Modified Bu Zhong Yi Qi Decoction with Wu Ling Powder. Bu Zhong Yi Qi Decoction can nourish qi of middle jiao, send the clear yang upward. Wu Ling Powder can strengthen the spleen and eliminate dampness, produce qi, and circulate water. The cooperation of the two formulae completes the function of ascending clear yang and circulating the spleen qi, descending the turbid yin. As a result, the qi can circulate smoothly and the water pathway is unobstructed. For the patient presents poor appetite and the slow digestion, amomum fruit, medicated leaven, germinated barkey should be added to regulate the stomach and induce appetite and digestion. If constant desire to defecate, or long term diarrhea and prolapse of rectum appear, fruit of citron orange should be used to ascend qi of middle jiao.

Prescriptions for example: Astragalus root 30g, bighead atractylodes 10g, pilose asiabell root 10g, poria 10g, umbellate pore fungus 12g, oriental water plantain rhizome 12g, Chinese angelica root 10g, cimicifuga rhizome 9g, bupleurum root 3g, licorice root 6g.

6. Deficiency of kidney yang

Main symptoms: Retention of urine or experience of dripping urination, no strength to pass urine.

Accompanied symptoms; Lassitude in loin and knees, aversion to cold, a cold sensation, a pale complexion, weakness of vitality qi

Tongue and pulse: A pale tongue with a white coating, a deep, thready and weak pulse

Analysis: The deficiency of fire of the life gate can't circulate the qi of urinary, as a result, retention of urine or dripping urination occur. Insufficiency of the primordial qi of the kidney result in weakness of urination, pale complexion, weakness if vitality and qi. The deficient kidney yang fails to warm the body, symptoms of soreness and weakness of lumbar region and knees, averse to cold, cold sensation of the limbs may present. A pale tongue with a white coating, a deep thready pulse that weak at chi position indicate the insufficiency of kidney qi.

Treatment: To warm yang and replenish qi, nourish the kidney and promote diuresis.

Prescription: Modified Ji Sheng Shen Qi Pill. Cinnamon bark and aconite root in this prescription warm and nourish the kidney yang, promote the kidney qi. Liu Wei Di Huang Pill tonify the kidney yin, achyranthes plantain seed are used to promote diuresis. If the patient is old and weak with failure of spirit and body, soreness and pain of the waist and spine, that means exhaustion of primordial qi, and the du channel is affected, red ginseng, antler glue, epimedium, curculigo rhizome should be combined to tonify essence and blood, activate yang and disperse diuresis. If the weakness of kidney yang affect the activity of triple jiao, small amount urine or no urine in severe case, nausea and vomiting, restlessness, unconsciousness will develop, 《Qian Jin》 Wen Pi Decoction and Wu Zhu Yu Decoction should be combined to warm and replenish the spleen and kidney, regulate the stomach and lower and the adverse flow of qi.

Prescription for example:

Prepared rhizome of rehmannia 12g, Chinese yam 15g, dog wood fruits 10g, poria 15g, oriental water plantain rhizome 12g, cinnamon bark 5g, prepared aconite root 10g, achyranthes 10g, plantain seed 12g(to be wrapped alone), morinda root 12g.

If the retention of urine can be treated effectively and immediately, the amount of urine increase, that indicates the situation becomes better or even be cured completely. If the disease doesn't be treated or treated incorrectly, manifested with dizziness, palpitation, chest stressness, asthma, nausea, vomiting, edema, or even coma, convulsion. It means the situation gets worse, and transform to obstruction and rejection. if the patient does not be rescued, death will not be avoidable.

〔Precaution and nursing method〕

1. Do physical exercise to improve the body resistance.

2. Keep happiness and prevent depress and anger.

3. Keep out of relative factors that can lead to exopathogen attacking and dampness heat producing such as enduring of urination, taking too much fatty food, over strain of sexual activity and physical work.

4. It's important to treat stranguria and edema actively for the precaution of retention of urine

〔Typical case analysis〕

First visit: Zhang ××, male, 70years old, worker. The patient came to the outpatient at autumn, the season is dominated by dry-gold, chief complains: he had suffered from constant urgency of urination every other period of time since last year. Some day this summer, he suddenly developed the retention of urine, manifested with unendurable distention and pain in the lower abdomen, dry mouth but no desire to drink, restlessness, he had been treated with catheterization for three days. Diagnosis showed deep thready and rapid pulse, white coating constipation. Differentiation: stagnation of dampness disperses diuresis.

Dried rehmannia root 10g, phellodendron bark 6g, Chinese pink herb 10g, lophatherum 9g, plantain seed 12g, talc 12g licorice root 6g.

Second visit: After took the prescription above for three bags, the patient is still suffered from the retention of urine, constipation for three days. The tongue coating changed to dry yellow, the pulse is deep and rapid, and these are the symptoms of accumulation of dampness heat in the colon. The evil heat goes upward and consumes the lung fluid, which result in the dryer of the colon. For the treatment, the two aspects should be considered, the method of timely purgation to preserve yin accompanied with clearing away heat and moistening the lung should be taken.

Prepared rhubarb 9g, mirabilite 9g (to be wrapped alone and taken for twice), Chinese pink herb 12g, prostrate knotweed 12g, phellodendron bark 6g, lilyturf root 15g, fire leaf akebia stem 10g, capejasmine fruit 6g.

Third visit: After taken one bag, the feces was removed, the urine was dispersed, the dry mouth was getting better the lower abdomen feels comfortable, when another two bags was taken, the symptoms was disappeared.

Analysis: Constitutional dampness heat accumulated inside body, which lead to intermittent anuria. As the evil heat of summer attack the internal organs, the stagnant dampness heat may occur, which result in the accumulation of water and heat, stagnant dryness in the bowel organ. The constipation caused by the dryness of the colon leads to the impairment of descending of the lung, which blocked the function of regulating the water pathway of the lung. For the location of the disease is not in the urinary bladder, the treatment of clearing way dampness heat and dispersing diuresis was not effective. The correct method of treatment is to remove the stagnant dryness in the colon and clear away lung heat, so as to promote the descending of the lung, while accompanied with disperse diuresis. The stool is removed, the stagnant dampness heat is expelled, and the disease is cured.

Retention of urine is a disease of small amount urine and dripping urination or even auria as its main symptoms. It should be differentiated from stranguria while if the patient has or has no urine should be made clear.

Retention of urine develops as a result of dysfunction of activity of the triple jiao. The disease is located in urinary bladder, and its occurrence relates closely with the triple jiao, liver, spleen and kidney. The etiology and pathology of the disease include accumulation of dampness heat, heat of the lung and lung qi stagnant, the liver qi stagnation blockage of the urinary tract, descending of qi of the middle jiao and deficiency of kidney yang. The disturbance in qi transformation of the urinary bladder caused by the former four factors will develop a excess syndrome, the later two factors which obstruct the functional activity of bladder will present as a deficient syndrome.

The differentiation of retention of urine: Firstly, the deficiency and excess of the syndrome should be made clearly. Secondly, the disease should be treated according to the mild and severe, chronic and acute situation of the disease

The key point of the treatment is to regulate the transformation of the urinary bladder. For the excess syndrome, the method should be clearing away dampness heat, eliminating the blood stagnation, smoothing the flowing of qi to disperse the water pathway; for the deficient type, the method of tonifying the spleen and the kidney assisting the transformation of qi to disperse diuresis should be adopted. For the severe situation, if the dysuria presents and the intake of decoction could not help, some external treating methods such as acupuncture and massage should be used to disperse diuresis. If dysuria lasting for a period of time, the bladder is fullness with unendurable distend pain, the urethral catheterization should be used. If the distention of urine is caused by the renal failure, the treatment is difficult for the complex state of illness.

Questions for Review

1. Try to explain the meaning of the concept of long-bi (retention of urine).
2. How to realize the importance of the lung, spleen, kidney and liver in the occurrence of the retention of urine?
3. Try to integrate the principle of treating diseases in the lower part by managing the upper and ascending first when descending needed.
4. What is the key point of differentiation of the retention of urine? How to treat

the disease by differentiation of the syndrome?

5. How is the prognosis of the retention of urine? How many external therapies are commonly used to treat the disease?

Diabetes (Xiao Ke)

〔Summary〕

Xiao is interpreted as polyrexia, water of consumption or waste; Ke refers to thirst with taking of fluids and not getting rid of thirst after drinking. Xiao Ke is a pathocondition characterized by polydipsia, polyphagia, polyuria, and emaciation or sweet urine. Ancient healer divided it into diabetes involving with upper-jiao, middle-jiao, lower-jiao according to inclination of different symptoms.

The clinic features of diabetes in Western Medicine are consistent with them in the pathcondition. Diabetes insipidus has the symptoms of polydipsia and polyuria. So these two diseases are all selected treatment based on the differential diagnosis in light of the content of this chapter.

〔Etiological factors and morbid mechanism〕

The disease is primarily caused by dietary irregularity, disorder of emotion, overstrain or overindulgent for a person of yin-deficiency constitution.

1. Accumulated heat hurting liquid due to dietary irregularity:

Long-term overtake of greasy highly-flavored pungent food or indulgence in alcohol drinking leads to dysfunction of the spleen and stomach transporting and transforming, accumulation of heat and fluid-deficiency caused by dryness turned from accumulated, which causes diabetes.

2. Accumulated fire hurting yin due to disorder of emotion:

Long-term mental stimulus results in inhibition of vital energy which further turns into fire. Intense fire consumes yin-fluid of the lung and stomach which causes diabetes.

3. Deficiency of the kidney essence due to overindulgent:

Overstrain and excessive sexual activities lead to consumption of yin-essence, deficiency of the kidney yin and asthenic fire produced in the interior. Namely, Fire becomes even intenser because of exhaustion of water; water becomes even shorter because of flaming of fire. Finally it causes diabetes that deficiency of the kidney、dryness of the lung and heat of the stomach due to hyperactivity of fire caused by deficiency of yin flaming up the lung and stomach occur simultaneously.

The constitution of yin-deficiency, as an elementary factor in etiology of diabetes, arises from innate deficiency and is also formulated by lackness of proper care in postnatal life for a long period of time.

To sum up, several characteristics of pathogenesis of diabetes are as follows:

Yin-deficiency serving as a primary factor and dryness-heat serving as a secondary factor: The pathogenesis of diabetes includes deficiency of yin-fluid and excessive of dryness-heat which are often reciprocal causation. Namely, much more dryness-heat can lead to severe yin-deficiency and severe yin-deficiency can also lead to much more dryness-heat. Although the pathologic change involves with five Zang-organs, especially with the lung, the stomach and the kidney. The kidney is the key visceral. The lung is responsible for the coordination of visceral activities and is the upper source of water. Dysfunction of regulating coordination of visceral activities caused by dryness-heat hurting the lung results in body-fluid flowing straightly downward, which is marked as frequent micturition and polyuria. The lung fails to distribute body fluid to all parts of the body, which marked as thirst and liking drink. The stomach is a reservior of food-stuff. Intense stomach fire caused by dryness-heat hurting the stomach brings about polyorexia, constipation. The kidney controls water metabolism, stores essence and hides primordial yang and yin. It leads to disturbance in functioning of qi, failure of opening and closing, dysfunction of the kidney in storing essence that deficiency of the kidney-yin, asthenic fire produced in the interior and dryness-heat hurting the kidney. On this condition, polyuria with frequent micturition will occur. Refined nutritious substances flowing down comes about urine with sweet smell. Three viscera are injured in a different extent which still affect each other in the course of pathological changes. For example, failure of seminal fluid nourishing and dispersing to all parts of the body caused by the lung-yin deficiency due to lung-dryness leads to the stomach failing to be moistened and the kidney failing to be nourished. The excessive stomach-heat may consume the lung-fluid and impair the kidney-yin, while the hyperactive fire caused by deficiency of the kidney may also flame up the lung and stomach. In the end, for the lung-dryness, the stomach-heat and the kidney-deficiency exists together, polydipsia, polyphagia and polyuria will occur simultaneously.

Deficiency of both yin and yang due to impairment of qi and yin: With the prolongation of the course of the disease, deficiency of yin affecting yang and qi deficiency due to loss of body fluid leads to impairment of both qi and yin or deficiency of both yin and yang, even marked by syndrome of declination of the kidney-yang. On the other hand, the onset of the disease is complicated with deficiency of qi or yang, which is generally related to the constitution of yang deficiency, the unfavorable factors in diet, emotion and defatigation. Yang or qi are easy to be affected by impairment of yin. But the latter rarely occurs in clinic.

Dryness-heat due to deficiency of yin causing various deteriorated cases: Because of dryness-heat and yin-deficiency, diabetes may bring about many deteriorated cases. For example, long-term impairment of nourishing and moistening function of the lung will be complicated with tuberculosis of lung. Diabetes will be also complicated with cataracta, nyctalopia, deafness on account of essence and blood of the kidney and liver being unable to nourish eyes upward which is caused by the kidney-yin deficiency and the liver failing to be nourished. It causes carbuncle, furuncle, ulcer that dryness-heat stagnating in the interior, nutrient yin being burned, blood stasis in collaterals and accumulated poisonous pathogen turning into pus. Intense dryness-heat in the interior due to yin-deficiency refines body fluid into phlegm stagnating in the meridian, marked by numbness or pain of the limbs and the pain in the chest due to stagnation of phlegm and blood stasis, etc. Phlegm blocking the clear orifices can bring about apoplexy or hemiplegia. Exhaustion of the spleen and kidney due to deficiency of yin affecting yang may carry about accumulation of the body fluid which runs rampant to the skin and muscles, marked as edema. If extreme consumption of body-fluid can cause phlegm-fire attacking upwards and upwards floating of yang in deficiency condition, it is characterized by flushed face, headache, dysphoria, nausea and vomiting, sunken eyes, dryness of the lips, red tongue, deep and long breathing, even coma. The crsis of coma, extreme cold of the limbs, faint pulse being about to disappear, etc. will occur because of extinction of yin and yang.

Furthermore, in etiology, diabetes connects with blood-stasis. Blood-stasis with blood deficiency is caused by interior heat due to deficiency of yin consuming body fluid. Deficiency of both yin and yang due to yin deficiency affecting yang with cold congelation due to yang deficiency can also result in blood stasis which may not get body fluid to be transforted again, so that the symptoms of diabetes will be more serious.

schematic diagram of etiological factors and morbid mechanism of diabetes

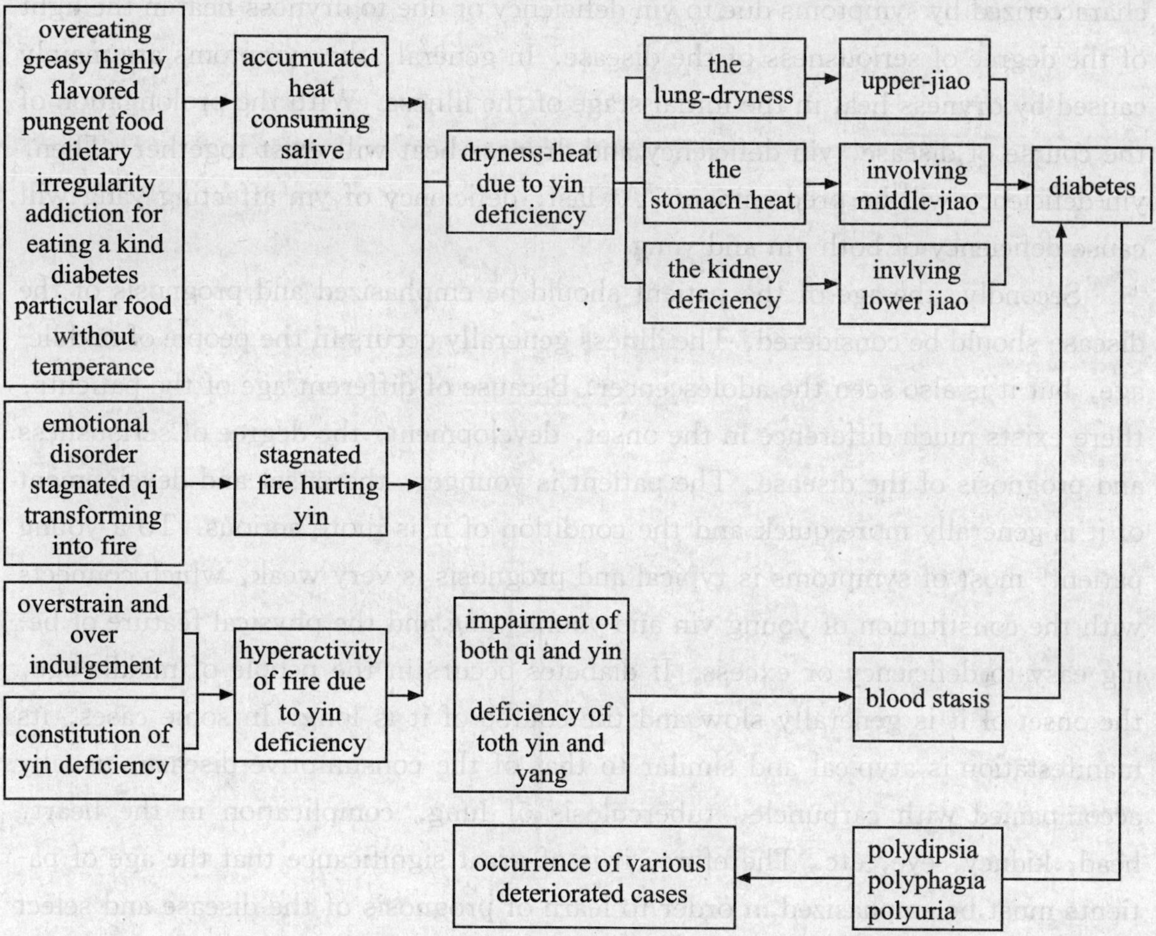

〔Diagnosis and treatment according to differentiation〕

1. Main points of differentiation of symptoms and signs

At first, the type of diabetes should be determined. Although it can be divided into diabetes involving upper-jiao due to the lung-dryness, diabetes involving middle-jiao due to the stomach-heat, diabetes involving lower-jiao due to kidney deficiency. Actually, as seen in clinic, the symptoms of polydipsia, polyphagia and polyurian often occur simultaneously. Diabetes involving upper-jiao is characterized by polydipsia with slight polyphagia, polyuria. Diabetes involving middle-jiao is characterized by polyphagia with slight polydipsia and polyuria, Diabetes involving lower-jiao is characterized by polyuria with slight polydipsia and polyphagia. Yin-deficiency is known as a principal factor in etiology of the diseses and dryness-heat as secondary factor, both of which are reciprocal causation. It is characterized by symptoms due to yin deficiency or due to dryness-heat in the light of the degree of seriousness of the disease. In general, the symptoms are mainly caused by dryness-heat in the initial stage of the illness. With the prolongation of the course of disease, yin deficiency and dryness-heat will exist together. Then, yin-deficiency will be predominant. At last, deficiency of yin affecting yang will cause deficiency of both yin and yang.

Secondly, the age of the patient should be emphasized and prognosis of the disease should be considered. The illness generally occurs in the people of middle-age, but it is also seen the adolescencer. Because of different age of the patients, there exists much difference in the onset, development, the degree of seriousness and prognosis of the disease. The patient is younger, the onset and development of it is generally more quick and the condition of it is more serious. To a young patient, most of symptoms is typical and prognosis is very weak, which connects with the constitution of young yin and young yang and the physical feature of being easy to deficiency or excess. If diabetes occurs in the people of middle-age, the onset of it is generally slow and the course of it is long. In some cases, its manifestation is atypical and similar to that of the consumptive disease, usually accompanied with carbuncle, tuberculosis of lung, complication in the heart, head, kidney, eye, etc. Therefore, it is of great significance that the age of patients must be emphasized in order to learn of prognosis of the disease and select the remedy.

Thirdly, pay attention to identify the risk syndromes of diabetes. With the prolongation of course of the disease, the factors such as affectation of other diseases, pregnancy, delivery and improper treatment can make symptoms serious. The serious syndrome, marked by flushed face, headache, restless, nausea and vomiting, anorexy, deep and quickly breathing with smell of rotten apples, dry cherry lips and tongue, even lethorgy or unconsciousness, is caused by phlegm-fire blocking the orifice of the heart due to extreme consumption of body fluid, yin failing to keep yang well and upward floating of yang in deficiency. The crisis such as coma, extreme cold of the limbs, faint pulse being about to disappear, etc. is caused by extinction of yin and yang. It will easily occur if diabetes is accompanied with severe carbuncle, tubercosis of lung, diarrhea.

Finally, because the onset of diabetes is similar to that of goiter, the clinical doctors should pay attention to distinguish them. Hyperthyroidism in modern medicine belongs to the category of "yin bing"in TCM. It is characterized by impatience, polyorexia, gradual emaciation, palpitation, exophthalmus swelling in one side or both of anterior cervical region. When its clinical manifestation is polyorexia, emaciation, no exophthalmus and neck swelling, it is very similar to diabetes involving middle-jiao, but both of them differs slightly in morbid mechanism. Concretely speaking, goister is caused by hyperactivity of heart-fire and liver-fire, yin-deficiency of both the heart and stomach due to stagnation of phlegm and qi converting into fire. The infectious Zang Fu-organs involve with the liver, the heart and the stomach. If it is difficult to distinguish them in symptoms and medical history, routine laboratary examination of blood and urine should be made if necessary.

Typical diabetes is marked as polydipsia, polyuria, polyorexia, gradual emaciation and can be easily diagnosed in general. However, to the people of middle-age or more, if there appears fat, listlessness, sometimes palpitation, a feeling of hungry with or without polydipsia, carbuncle or urcer of skin which will occur repeatedly or rise one after another, complication such as apoplexy, catarct, obstruction of qi in the chest, stranguria with turbid urine. It is considered that they might suffer from diabetes. Necessarily, they should make laboratory, examination of blood or urine.

2. Therapeutic principle

According to pathogenetic features of dryness-heat and yin-deficiency, the foundational therapeutic principle of diabetes. is determined as nourishing yin to promote the production of body fluid, moistening for dryness and clearing away heat. No matter that diabetes involves with upper-jiao, middle-jiao, or lower-jiao, the treatments of them are all based on benefiting the kidney and nourishing yin. Clearing away heat-fire or heat-torxin should be also employed in terms of different degree of dryness-heat. Those of the two others should be considered in selecting the therapeutic method of one of the three types of diabetes. As"Yi Xue Xin Wu · San Xiao" said, treatment of diabetes involving upper -jiao should be moistening the lung besides clearing away the stomach heat; treatment of diabetes involving middle-jiao should be clearing away the stomach heat, besides nourishing the kidney; treatment of diabetes involving lower-jiao should be nourishing the kidney besides tonifying the lung. As the pathogenesis changes, for the case of deficiency of both qi and yin, treatment should be tonifying qi and yin to promote the production of body fluid. For the case of deficiency of both yin and yang treatment should be nourishing the kidney-yin and warming the kidney-yang, i.e. tonifying both yin and yang. For the case of stagnated blood, treatment should be added for activating blood circulation to dissipate blood stasis.

3. Treatment according to type differentiation

3.1 Diabetes involving upper-jiao (Consumption of body fluid due to the lung-heat)

Main symptoms: thirst, polydipsia, dry mouth and tongue.

Accompanying symptoms: frequent and profuse urine, gradual emaciation.

Tongue and pulse: red color on the lip and edge of tongue, thin and yellow coating, full and rapid pulse.

Analysis: Dry mouth and tongue are caused by excessiveness of the lung-heat consuming body fluid under normal conditions, the lung has the function of regulating the whole body. If it is destroyed because of dryness-heat hurting the lung, water will fail to be transformed into body fluid and flow straight downward, which will be marked as frequent and profuse urine. Outflowing of body fluid leads to gradual emaciation. Red color on the tip and edge of tongue with thin and yellow coating, full and rapid pulse are manifestations of excessiveness of the interior heat.

Treatment: Clearing away heat and moistening the lung, promoting the production of body fluid to quench thirst.

Prescription: Modified Xiao Ke Decoction. In the recipe, trichosanthes root is used in large dosage to promoting the production of body fluid. It assists coptis root to clear away heat and keep the adverse fire downwards, Dried rehmannia root and juice of hindu lotus large rhizome are used to increase yin-fluid.

Modification: In order to strengthen the force of promoting the production of body fluid to quench thirst and nourishing yin to relieve dryness, ophiopogon root, scrophularia root, pueraria root should be added to the recipe in accordance with practical conditions.

In case of full and rapid pulse without strength, continous excessive thirst, frequent micturition caused by deficiency of both qi and yin of the liver and kidney. Modified Er Dong Decoction can be selected. In the recipe, ginseng is often used to tonify qi to promote the production of body fluid. Ophiopogon root, plolygala root, trichosanthes root, scutellaria root and anemarrhena rhizome are used to clear away heat to quench thirst.

In case of yellow and dry tongue, thirst and polydipsia, full and large pulse caused by excessive heat of the lung and stomach consuming qi and yin, Bai Hu Jiao Ren Shen Decoction should be used to clear away remove heat from the lung and stomach and to quench thirst.

Prescription for example:

Trichosanthes root 20g, glehnia root 15g, pueraria root 10g, scrophularia root 12g, plolygala root 10g, ophiopogen root 10g, anenarrheria rhizome 10g, unprepared gypsum 30g (decocted first).

3.2 Diabetes involving middle-jiao (Excessiveness of the stomach-heat)

Main symptoms: polyorexia, constipation.

Accompanying symptoms: emaciation

Tongue and pulse: dry and yellow coating, slippery and forceful pulse

Analysis: Hyperactivity of stomach-fire promotes digestion of food, marked by polyorexia. Impairment of body fluid and blood due to intense heat of Yang Ming leads to failure of nourishing muscles, which is marked by emaciation. Due to deficiency of stomach-fluid, intestines can not be nourished, which is marked by constipation or even stasis of excrement. Excessiveness of the stomach-heat shows as dry and yellow coating, slippery and forceful pulse.

Treatment: clearing away the stomach fire, tonifying yin-fluid.

Prescription: Yu Nu Decoction with coptis root and capesjasmine fruit. In the recipe, gypsum and anemarrhena rhizome are used to clear away heat of the stomach and lung. Rehmannia root and ophiopogen root have the effect of nourishing the stomach-yin and the kidney-yin. Coptis root and capejasmine fruit are used to clear away heat-fire. Achyranthes and cyathula root are used to guide the heat to go downwards.

Modification: If the patients suffer from constipation or stasis of execrement, Use Zeng Yie Cheng Qi Decoction for supplementing fluid to relax the bowels, moistening for dryness and purging the bowels. The above recipe should be used again after the bowels are relaxed.

Prescription for example:

Rehmannia root 15g, unprepared gypsum 30g (decoctated first), anemarhena rhizome 10g, achyranthes root 10g, ophiopogon root 10g, scrophularia root 10g, stir-barked capejasmine fruit 10g, coptis root 4g.

3. 3 Diabetes involving lower-jiao

3. 3. 1 Deficiency of the kidney-yin

Main symptoms: frequent micturition with profuse urine, feverish sensation in the palms and soles.

Accompanying symptoms: turbid or sweet urine, dry mouth and lips, or even feverish sensation in the chest, palms and soles.

Tongue and pulse: red tongue, deep, rapid and thready pulse.

Analysis: Water fluid can not be controlled inside due to deficiency of the kidney, which is marked as frequent micturition with profuse urine. Refined materials in food-stuff flowing down due to dysfunction of the kidney consolidating and governing may lead to turbid urine with sweet smell just like greasy paste. Asthenic fire stirring up due to deficiency of the kidney-yin shows as dysphoria with feverish sensation in the chest, palms and thready pulse.

Treatment: nourishing yin and reinforcing the kidney

Prescription: Modified Liu Wei Di Huang Decoction. In the recipe, dogwood fruit and chinese yam in large dosage should be used, because Chinese yam has the effect of nourishing the spleen-yin to pretect the food essence and dogwood fruit has the effect of reinforcing the kidney, tonifying essence and keeping the refined materials in foodstuff from flowing down. Prepared rehmannia root is used to nourish the kidney for replenishing the essence of life. The three drugs are used in common to nourish the apleen-yin, the kidney-yin and liver-yin. Poria cooperates with them to excrete dampness from the spleen. Oriental water plantain is used to clear away the ministerial fire in the kidney and to pretect prepared rehmannia root from showing retention in nature. Moutan bark is used to clear away the liver-fire and to protect dagwood fruit from showing warm in property. They both are acted as adjuvant drugs. It is proved in clinical practice that the recipe has the effect of treating diabetes and solidfy the curative. It is fit for the patient suffering from diabetes to admistrate the recipe for a long period of time.

Modification: If the patient suffers from hectic fever, dysphoria, insomnia emission, red tongue, rapid and thready pulse caused by hyperactivity of fire due to yin deficiency, anemarrhena rhizome, phellodendron bark, schisandra fruit, tortoise plastron, dragons bone and oyster shell should be added to the above recipe for nourishing yin, clearing away heat, controlling nocturnal emission and checking exuberance of yang.

In case of profuse and turbid urine as greasy, bitter cardamon, mantis egg-case, schisandra fruit, silkworm cocoon, Chinese gall should be added for tonifying the kidney and reducing urination.

For those of deficiency of both qi and yin accompanied with tiredness, lassitude, shortness of breath, unwillingness to speak, pale tongue, the ingredients tonifying qi such as dangshen, astragalus root and so on should be added in accordance with practical conditions

Prescription for example:

Rehmannia root 12g, prepared rehmannia root 12g, dogwood fruit 12g, chinese yam 12g, moutan bark 10g, ophiopogon root 10g, schisandra fruit 10g, oriental water plantain 10g, scrophularia root, 12g.

3. 3. 2 Deficiency of both yin and yang

Main symptoms: frequent micturition, drinking one cup of water and running two cups of urine, aversion to cold.

Accompanying symptoms: Turbid urine like greasy paste, darkish complexion, extremely dry helix, lassitude in loin and knees, impotence.

Tongue and pulse: pale tongue with white coating, deep and thready pulse without strength.

Analysis: Dysfunction of the kidney in storing and controlling the essence of life leads to frequent micturition and turbid urine as grease paste. Deficiency of the kidney-qi leads to dysfunction in controlling the water-fluid, which is marked by drinking one cup of water and running two cups of urine. Refined materials in foodstuff together with urine flowing down can not nourish the skin and muscles, which is marked by darkish complexion. The kidney is in charge of the bones and has its specific orifice in the ear. The lumbar region is the house of the kidney. Therefore, deficiency of the kidney will result in extremely dry helix, lassitude in loin and knees. Decline of fire from the gate of life results in coldness of the body with chills and impotence. Deficiency of both yin and yang shows as pale tomgue with white coating, deep and thready pulse without strength.

Treatment: warming yang and nourishing the kidney to recover the function of controlling

Prescription: Modified Jin Gui Shen Qi Pill. In the recipe, prepared lateral root of asonite and chinnamon bark are used for warming are recuperating the kidney-yang; the ingredients of Liu Wei Di Huan Pill for regulating and nourishing the kidney-yin.

Modification: In case of deficiency of yin, yang, qi and blood, Lu Rong Pill should be used. In the recipe, prepared rehmannia root, ophiopogon root, scrophularia root, dogwood fruit, wolfberry bark, schisandra fruit are used for nourishing the kidney-yin, replenishing vital essence and promoting the production of blood; pilose antler, psoralea fruit and desertliving cistanche for invigorating the kidney-yang; ginseng, astragalus root for invigorating qi; poria tasteless in flavour for excreting dampness; membrance of chicken's gizzard for reinforing digestion; achyranthes root for guiding other drugs to the kidney. So the recipe has the effect of invigorating qi, enriching blood and supplementing yin- yang without retention.

In case of drinking one cup of water and running two cups of urine, chinese raspberry, mantis egg-case, cherokee rose-hip should be added to the above mentioned recipe in accordance with practical conditions for tonifying the kidney to recover the controlling function

Prescription for example:

Prepares rehmannia 15g, dogwood fruit 10g, scrophula root 12g, psoralea fruit 10g, atractylodes rhizome 6g, astragalus root 15g, Chinese yam 12, schisandra fruit 10g, chinnamon bark 3g, red sage root 12g.

If the syndrome of blood stasis occurs in the above types of diabetes, the ingredients which have the function of promoting blood circulation to remove blood stasis, such as red sage root, hawthorn fruit, safflower, peach kernel and so on should be added to the recipe for requiring the good curative effect.

4. Accompanying syndrome

Cataracta, nyctalopia, deafness are caused by of deficiency of the liver-blood and kidney-essence failing to nourish ears and eyes upward. Qi Ju Di Huang Pill or Yang Gan Pill may be used to deal with the syndromes for nourishing the liver and kidney.

Carbuncle, ulcer: In the onset of the syndromes, noxious heat hurts ying. Detoxicating and removing heat from the blood should be applied to treatment. The prescription is modified Wu Wei Xiao Du Decoction. It the syndromes has delayed for a long time, deficiency of both qi and yin, blood stasis in collaterals, accumulated poisonous pathogen turning into pus will occur. Tonifying qi and detoxicating should be applied to treatment. Use Huang Qi Liu Yi Decoction and Xi Jiao Pill with honeysuckle stem, forsythia fruit in accordance with practical conditions.

If diabetes is complicated with tuberculosis of lung, edema, apoplexy, stranguria, syncope, etc., it is necessary that referring to the mentioned chapters determine diagnosis and treatment based on pathogenesis obtained through differentiation of symptoms and signs.

5. Critical syndrome

5.1 Upward floating of yang in deficiency condition: marked by dysphoria and thirst getting heavier, headache, nausea, vomiting, red lips with dry tongue deep and quick breathing, rapid and thready pulse without strength. The therapeutic principle is nourishing yin and suppressing the excesseve yang. Shen Mai Powder with dogwood fruit, plolygala root, oystershell, tortoise plastron should be decoctated quickly and administrated instananeously. The therapeutic method of the western medicine is also used to treat it in combination with that of TCM.

5.2 Yin being intent to exhaustion and yang being intent to deleption: marked by coma, extreme cold of limbs, faint pulse being about to disappear. The therapeutic principle is supplementing qi and astringing yin fluit, recupering depleted yang and rescuing the patient from collapse. Prescription: modified Sheng Mai Powder with Shen Fu Decoction. The therapeutic methods of the western and Chinese medicine are used for rescuing the risk patients positively.

Some simple recipe may be also used in combination according to diagnosis and treatment based on pathogenesis obtained through differentiation of symptoms and signs. Besides drug treatment, keep the patient from mental intensation and suppress hypersexuality. In diet, the patients should not eat too much, but eat tasteless food such as proper rice, vegetable, egg, bean, thin mice and so on. Pungent and irritating food is prohibited.

〔Prevention and nursing measurement〕

1. Pay attention to have a rest and do not overstrain. The patient suffering from serious illness should have a rest in bed.

2. Keep a mental state of peace and suppress hypersexality. The patient should prevent himself from dysphoria and depression.

3. The patients should have regular diet. Every day they may not eat more than 500g of rice or powder, but eat much vegetable.

4. Pay attention to personal hygiene. Prevent the occurance of complication. Pungent and greasy food with containing lots of starch should be prohibited.

Drinking and smoking can't be admitted.

〔**Typical case analysis**〕

Case one: Zhang××, male, fifty -two years old, candre.

The patient suffered from thirst and polydipsia (about 1000ml everyday), polyorexia with a feeling of hunger after eating two hours, dry and fissural lips, constipation, red tongue with thin and yellow coating, rapid pulse about two months.

Laboratory examination: fasting blood-glucose: 220mg %

glucose in urine: (+++)

Diagnosis in TCM: Xiao Ke (syndome of hyperactivity of stomach-fire)

Diagnosis in western medicine: diabetes

Therapeutic principle: clearing away the stomach fire, supplementing qi and nourishing yin.

Prescription: modified Yu Nv Decoction.

Gypsum 20g, anemarrhena rhizome 20g, scutellaria root 10g, coptis root 10g, capejasmine fruit 5g, rehmannia root 15g, scrophularia root 15g, dangshen 20g, astraglaus root 100g; ophiopogon root, 20g; schisandra fruit 10g.

After his taking twenty-five dose of it, the laboratory examination showed: fasting blood-glucose: 120mg%; glucose in urine: (—). The symptoms disappeared. (Pang Mei hong treat 15 cases of diabetes based on pathogenesis obtained through differentiation of symptoms and signs; Chinese medicine of Hei Long Jiang. 1988, (1): 21)

The case belongs to diabetes involving middle-jiao, differentiated as syndrome of hyperactivity of the stomach fire. Doctors should selected clearing away the stomach fire, supplementing qi and nourishing yin as the therapeutic method. In the recipe, gypsum and anemarrhena rhizome are used to clear away the heat of the lung and stomach; rehmannia root, ophiopogon root, scrophularia root, schisandra fruit are used to nourish the lung-yin and stomach-yin; coptis root, scutellaria root and capejasmine fruit are used to clear away heat - fire; dangshen and astragalus root are used to supplement qi. The above drugs are used together so as to keep the adverse stomach fire downwards, persevere the yin fluid and eliment all the symptoms and signs.

Diabetes is a disease characterized by polydipsia, polyphagia, polyuria and emaciation. The etiologic factor includes constitution of deficiency of yin, dietary irregularity, disordr of emotion, over fatigue or over indulgement. Main pathogenesis includes dryness-heat due to deficiency of yin besides impairment of both qi and yin, deficiency of both yin and yang. Dryness-heat due to deficiency of yin can lead to many pathogenetic changes, so that a lot of complications will occur.

The location of the disease is in the lung, the stomach and the kidney, above all, the kidney. In clinical differentiation of symptoms, at first, determine the type of diabetes and infer which is main factor between deficiency of yin and dryness-heat; secondly, emphasize the pathogenic age of the patient so as to learn about the prognosis of the disease; finally, pay attention to identify critical syndromes and differ in the onset of diabetes and goister, moreover, to people of middle - age or more, pay attention to find patients of diabetes by their tending to complicate with carbuncle, boil rising one after another and cartarct.

The foundmental therapeutic principle is nourishing yin to promote the production of body fluid, moistening for dryness and clearing away heat. In spite of the type of diabetes, nourishing the kidney-yin should be rooted as a theraputic method, assisted with clearing away heat. Others should be considered in accordance with practical conditions. In order to get well curative result a simple recipe consisting of a herb should be employed in combination with nourishing the patient's health. In addition, pay attention to rescue the patients suffering from critical symptoms caused by upward floating of yang in dificiency condition, ying being intent to exhaustion and yang being intent to deleption.

Questions for Review

1. Try to explain that main points of pathogenesis in diabetes are deficiency of yin due to dryness-heat through clinical manifestations and explain the relationship between deficiency of yin and dryness-heat.
2. Why say that the location of diabetes is in the lung, the stomach and the kidney?
3. Try to explain respectively diagnosis and treatment based on pathogenesis obtained through differentiation of symptoms and signs of diabetes involving upper-jiao, middle-jiao and lower-jiao.
4. How many complications of diabetes will occur? what are they ? What do critical syndromes show?

Arthralgia syndrome

〔**Summary**〕

Arthralgia syndrome is caused by blockage of channels and qi and blood flowing unsmoothly due to invasion of exogenous pathogenic wind, cold, dampness and heat, marked by pain, numbness, a heavy feeling, swelling, incapability of flexing and extending or even a feeling of burning heat in muscles, bones and joints. Zhang Zhong Jing argued with wind-dampness syndrome, damp arthralgia, severe and migratory arthralgia; there are also illness names such as li jie feng, bai hu feng, bai hu li jie feng, tong feng, (severe and migratory arthralgia), he xi feng, gu chun feng, (arthroncus of knee) in later generation. They all belong to the category of arthralgia syhdrome.

Huang Di Nei Jing divides arthralgia syndrome into wind arthralgia, arthralgia aggravated by cold, damp arthralgia according to the invasive degree of wind, cold, dempness pathogen. Arthritis of heat type is also added to it in later generation. In addition, it is called arthralgia of five body constituents (bone, vessel, tendon, muscle, and skin) on account of the location of the illness and the season when exogenous pathogen invades the body. If arthralgia of five body constituents has delayed for a long time and can not be get rid of, it will involve with five viscera and turn into syndromes caused by obstructed qi flow in the five Zang-organs. For example, obstruction of heart-qi, often seen in clinic, is marked by blocked pulse, restlessness and severe palpitation dyspnea due to "suddenly rising of abnormal qi, dry sensation in pharynx and frequent eructation, a feeling of fear due to upward adverse flow of qi"; obstruction of the kidney channel is manifestated as inability to stand up straightly as if the function of heels is replaced by the sacral bone, and humped thoracic vertebrae seeming higher than head, etc. It is of great significance that we identify the clinic characteristics of arthralgia syndrome and know of progression of it.

In western medicine, the diseases such as rheumatic arthritis, rheumatoid arthritis, bony arthritis. sciatica, periarthritis humeroscapularis, gout, and so on can also refer to this syndrome for diagnosis and treatment based on pathogenesis obtained through differentiation of symptoms and signs.

〔**Etiological factors and morbid mechanism**〕

Arthralgia syndrome is mainly caused by invasion of wind, cold, dampness, heat pathogen on the condition of deficiency of vital-qi. The brief explanation is as follows:

1. Deficiency of vital-qi causing failure of superficial-qi protecting the body against diseases, striae of skin, muscles and viscera being loose will lead to exogenous pathogen invading the body and retaining in the interspaces of muscles, tendons and channels due to dificiency of vital-qi, so that normal flow of qi and blood is obstructed. Deficiency of vital-qi is related inmitately to innate weakness of the body, imbalance between work and test, shortness of physical exercises, menstruation and postpartum for female.

2. Pathogenic wind, cold and dampness invading the body, or infecting pathogenic heat, or wind, cold and dampness pathogen retained for a long time turning into heat. If it is warm, a person who falls asleep in the wind after sweating will easily infect wind pathogen; if it is cold and the earth is frozen, a person will easily infect wind and cold pathogen; if a person has lived in damp place for a long time or a person catches in the rain, he will easily infect dampness pathogen; wind and heat pathogen, in combination with dampness pathogen can invade the body; if arthritis of heat type delays for a long time and stagnation of pathogen converts into heat, wind, cold, dampness and heat pathogen can invade the body.

Deficiency of vital-qi and invasion of exogenous pathogen are the etiological factors of arthralgia syndrome. Concretly speaking, invasion of exogenous pathogen is a external factor and deficiency of vital-qi is a basic internal factor during the occurrence of the disease. Only when the former combines with the latter, will the disease occur. In the case of preponderance of yang-qi, hyperactivity of fire due to yin deficiency or infectation of wind, dampness and heat pathogen, arthritis of heat type will easily occur. In the case of deficiency of yang-qi or infectation of wind-cold-dampness pathogen, arthritis of heat type will easily occur. The former can interchange with the latter under the specific condition. Besides, wheather arthritis of heat type or arthralgia due to wind-cold-dampness lasts for a long time, blood and qi will stagnate in channels and collaterals which causes the syndrome of phlegm accumulating with stagnant blood, marked by ecchymosis, subcutaneous nodule and peri-articular nodule or joint deformity, etc. Moreover, because of retention of pathogenic qi in the channels, stagnated blood can't be get rid of so that fresh blood can't be produced, which leads to impairment of qi and blood, even the syndrome of deficiency of the liver and kidney due to the joints being lack of movement. At last, because arthralgia syndrome has delayed for a long time, together with invasion of exogenous pathogen, the arthralgia of five body constituents will convert into syndromes caused by obstructed qi flow in the five Zang-organs, among which obstruction of the heart-qi and obstruction of the kidney channel often occur.

Schematic diagram of etiological factors and pathogenesis of arthralgia syndrome

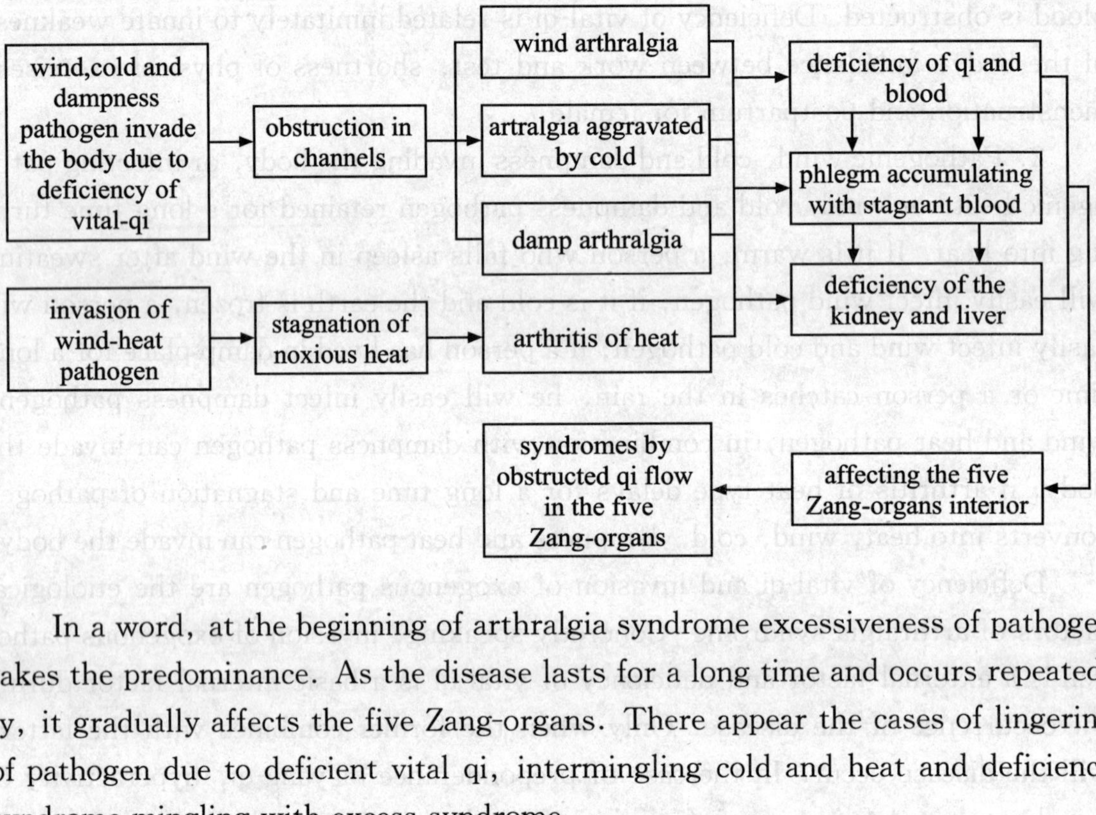

In a word, at the beginning of arthralgia syndrome excessiveness of pathogen takes the predominance. As the disease lasts for a long time and occurs repeatedly, it gradually affects the five Zang-organs. There appear the cases of lingering of pathogen due to deficient vital qi, intermingling cold and heat and deficiency syndrome mingling with excess syndrome.

Diagnosis and treatment according to differentiation

1. Identification of similiar syndromes

The disease and flaccidity syndrome are all marked by symptoms of limbs or joints, both of them may interchange. So it is necessary to distinguish these two disease. But arthralgia syndrome is mainly characterized by aching pain, a heavy feeling, swelling in tendons, bones, muscles and joints, incapability of flexing and extending. Sometimes, it is accompanied with numbness, but no paralysis. While flaccidity syndrome is characterized by atrophy and debility of the limbs, wasting and atrophy of muscle, no pain in the limbs or joints.

If arthralgia syndrome lasts for a long time, the patient can hardly motion due to pain of limbs, which leads to wasting and atrophy of muscles, joint deformity, ankylosis. But it is accompanied with flaccidity and weakness of the lower limbs. So it is seen in clinic that arthralgia syndrome coverts into flaccidity syndrome. For a patient of arthralgia syndrome, due to deficiency of vital-qi he infects exogenous pathogen that obstructs the channels causing stagnation of qi and blood, then, arthralgia syndrome will occur. So it is seen in clinic that flaccidity syndrome accompanies with arthralgia syndrome.

2. Main points of differentiation of symptoms and signs

2.1 Identifying arthralgia due to wind -cold-dampness pathogen with arthritis of heat of type: The former is marked as wandering pain and swelling of limbs or joints, no heat symptoms. The latter is marked by redness,. swelling, burning sensation, pain of joints with irritability.

2.2 Identifying excess of wind, cold, dampness pathogen: Excess of wind pathogen leads to wandering aching pain in the limbs and joints; excess of cold pathogen leads to steady pain in the limbs and joints; excess of dampness pathogen leads to swelling, a heavy feeling, aching pain in the joints.

2.3 Identifying blockage of phlegm and blood stasis in channels: With the prolongation of the course of the disease, it is marked as swelling of joints, even joint deformity, incapability of flexing and extending, purplish tongue with greasy coating, uneven thready pulse.

2.4 Differentiation of excess and deficiency of syndromes: At the beginning of arthralgia syndrome, if marked by continuous pain in the limbs and joints, even fever, it mostly belongs to the category of excess syndrome. When arthralgia syndrome is not cured through long-term treatment and occurs reapeatedly, marked by obscure pain in the limbs and joints, symptoms of deficiency of the liver and kidney such as listlessness, lassitude in loin and knees, dysphoia with feverish sensation in the chest, palms and soles, etc. it belongs to deficiency syndrome or deficiency syndrome miggling with excess syndrome.

3. Therapeutic principle

Arthralgia syndrome is caused by invasion of pathogenic wind, cold, dampness, heat, so its basic therapeutic principle is expelling the wind, dispersing cold, eliminating dampness, clearing away heat and dredging the channels. In the late stage of it, the method of tonification should be used in combination for the consumptive case. "Yi Xue Xin Wu · Bi" generalized the treatment of arthralgia syndrome. Namely, expelling the wind is the basic principle in treatment of wind arthralgia assisted with dispersing cold and eliminating dampness. The ingredients enriching the blood are generally used in combination. It is so called that drugs connecting with blood system can be used to treat the syndrome caused by invasion of pathogenic wind. Blood flowing smoothly in the vessels can get wind pathogen to be dispelled by itself. Dispersing cold is the basic principle in treatment of arthralgia aggravated by cold, assisted with eliminating wind-dampness. The ingredients warming yang are generally used in combination. It is so called that drugs of warm nature can make qi and blood flow smoothly which will not lead to pain, yet cold make blood coagulate which will lead to pain. Eliminating dampness is the basic principle in treatment of damp arthralgia, assisted with expelling wind and clearing away cold. The ingredients reinforcing the spleen are generally used in combination. It is so called that sufficient spleen-qi can remove dampness and numbness will not occur on account of sufficiency of qi and blood. The above content may be referred to in differentation.

4. Classific syndrome and treatment

4.1 arthralgia due to wind -cold-dampness

4.1.1 Wind arthralgia

Main symptoms: wandering aching pain in the limbs or joints.

Accompanying symptoms: aversion to wind, fever, a feeling of wind in the joints, incapability of flexing and extending.

Tongue and pulse: light red tongue with thin and white coating.

Analysis: Pathogenic wind-cold retaining in channels can obstruct qi and blood flowing in vessels, which is marked as aching pain in the limbs or joints, incapability of flexing and extending. Wind arthralgia is characterized by pain wandering in right, left, upper, lower joints. Qi and blood flowing unsmoothly in the channels of limbs, disharmony of nurient qi with defensive qi can lead to a feeling of wind in the joints, aversion to wind, fever. Pathogenic wind-cold-dampness invading the skin, muscles and channels shows thin and white coating, floating pulse.

Treatment: expelling wind and dredging channel, dispelling cold and removing dampness, assisted with enriching blood and promoting blood circulation.

Prescription: modified Fang Feng Decoction. In the recipe, ledebouriella root, ephedra are used to expel wind and disperse cold; chinese angelica root, large-leaf, chinnamon bark, pueraria root, gentian root are used for promoting blood circulation to remove obstruction in the channels and expelling pathogenic factors from muscles and skin to relieve pain. Drugs connecting with blood system can be used to treat the syndrome caused by invasion of pathogenic wind and blood flowing smoothly in vessels can get wind pathogen to be dispelled by itself, which was considered as a therapeutic article by the ancient healer. Chinese angelica root combined with chinnamon bard are used for nourishing blood to stop wind. Poria is used for eliminating dampness and removing obstruction in the channels. Prepared licorice root, fresh ginger, Chinese dates are used for regulating middle-jiao and mutrient qi and coordinating the actions of various ingredients. Scutellaria root will be expunged in the case of no fever.

In case of aching pain mainly in the joints of the upper limb such as the shoulder and eldow joint, notopterygium root, dahurian angelica root, turmaria, chuanxiong rhizome, clematis root, mulberry twigs should be added to the above recipe for expelling wind and removing obstruction in the channels to relieve pain. In the case of aching pain mainly in the joints of lower limb such as the knee and ankle joint, pubescent angelica root, achyranthes and cyathula root, chaenomeles fruit, dipsacus root, pyrola may be added for strengthening the tendons and removing obstruction in the channels to relieve pain. In the case of aching pain along spinal column, eucommia bark, loranthus mulberry mistletoe, epimedium, drynaria rhizome may be added for tonifying the kidney and removing obstruction in the channels to relieve pain. Modified Du Huo Ji Sheng Decoction may be used.

In the case of swelling in the joints, thin and yellow coating caused by stagnation of wind, cold, dampness pathogen converting into heat, modified Gui Zhi Shao Yao Zhi Mu Decoction may be used for dredging the blocked meridians to relieve pain.

Prescription for example:

Red peony root 12g, ledebouriella root 10g, gentian root 10g, notopterygium root 10g, pubescent angelica root 10g, Chinese angelica root 10g, clematis root 15g, cinnamon twig 6g.

4. 1. 2 Arthralgia aggravated by cold

Main symptoms: steady pain in the limbs and joints, which becomes severe when accompanied with the affection of coldness, and gets alleviated when warmed.

Accompanying symptons: ankylosis, incapablity of flexing and extending, no red color and swelling of the skin, and no heat sensation in the joints.

Tongue and pulse: normal tongue, thin and white coating or white and moist coating, floating and tense pulse.

Analysis of symptoms: Pathogenic wind, cold, dampness obstructing the meridians and excess of cold pathogen lead to severe pain with fixed spots, because pathogenic cold is a kind of yin pathogen and has the property of coagulation and constriction. Qi and blood in meridians flow smoothly when warmed, so that pain may get alleviated. Qi and blood coagulates in meridians when accompanied with the affection of coldness, so that pain will get more severe. Stagnation of yang -qi due to cold coagulation leads to qi and blood flowing unsmoothly, which is marked as ankylosis, incapability of flexing and extending, no redness, swelling, heat sensation in the local skin. Severe pain caused by cold coagulation shows thin and white coating or white and moist coating, tense and tout pulse.

Treatment: expelling pathogenic cold from channel, expelling wind and removing dampness.

Prescription: modified WuTou Decoction. In the recipe, sichuan aconite root and ephedra are used to expell pathogenic cold from channel, eliminate dampness to relieve pain; unprepared astragalus root is used for tonifying qi to strengthen the superficies, promoting blood circulation to dredge the blocked meridians; peony root and licorice root are used to nourish yin, dredge the collaterals, relieve spasm and pain. In the case of severe pain caused by excess of pathogenic cold, cinnamon twig or bark, wild ginger may be added to the recipe. Sichuan aconite root with wild aconite root is used to reinforce the effect of expelling pathogenic cold from channel. If arthralgia aggravated by cold lasts for a long time without recovery, the ingredients warming the kidney and reinforcing yang such as drynaria rhizome, psoralea fruit, morinda root, deglued antler powder, etc. may be added in accordance with practical conditions.

Modified Yang He Deciction may be used for the patients having the constitution of yang-deficiency whose illness is cured difficulty.

Prescription for example: prepared aconite root 5g, prepared wild aconite root 5g, red peony root 10g, white peony root 10g, cinnamon twig 10g, ephedra 5g, unprepared licorice root 10g, unprepared astragalus root 30g, fresh ginger 3 pieces, Chinese dates 7 pieces.

4.1.3 Damp arthralgia

Main symptoms: swelling, a heavy feeling, fixed pain in the limbs and joints, numbness.

Accompanying symptoms: aching of the whole body, listless, heavy sensation in hands and feet, limited movement.

Tongue and pulse: normal tongue with white and greasy coating, soft and moderate pulse.

Analysis: Because damp pathogen is heavy, turbid, viscous and stagnant in nature, invasion of pathogenic wind, cold, dampness and excess of damp pathogen leads to swelling, a heavy feeling, pain in the limbs and joints. Damp pathogen obstructs the meridians, so that qi and blood flow roughly in vessels, which is marked by numbness. Dampness is a kind of yin pathogen and causes stagnation of yang -qi, which is marked as aching in the whole body, listlessness, heavy sensation in hands and feet, incapability of flexing and extending. Pathogenic dampness not being eliminated shows white and greasy coating, soft and moderate pulse.

Treatment: removing dampness and dredging channel, expelling wind and clearing away cold.

Prescription: modified Yi Yi Ren Decoction. In the recipe, atractylodes rhizome, coix seed are used to remove dampness and dredge channel. Because wind can disperse dampness, as the drugs expelling wind, motopterygium root, pubescent angelica root, ledebouriella root are also used to eliminate dampness. Sichuan acnoite root, ephedra, cinnamon twig are used to expel pathogenic cold from channel, eliminate dampness and dredge channel. Chinese angelica root and chuanxiong rhizome with a pungent flavor and warm nature are used to dredge vessels, enrich blood and promote blood circulation. Fresh ginger, licorice root are used to regulate middle-jiao and resolve dampness. In the case of severe swelling caused by dampness, wolly or mealy yam, manshurian aristolochia stem, tetrandra root, chaenomels fruit may be added to the recipe for removing dampness by diuresis and dredging channel. In the case of numbness, ledebouriella root, white atractylode rhizome, peony root or erythrina bark, siegesbeckiae herb may be added for eliminating wind-dampness of skin. Then, qi and blood flow smoothly in vessels due to harmony between ying and wei.

At the beginning of arthralgia syndrome, if retainment of pathogenic wind-cold -dampness in the superfices causes of exterior syndrome of excess type marked as no perspiration, Ma Huang Jia Zhu Decoction may be used to induce lightly dysphoria. Also use modified Wu Ji Powder. For those of exterior syndrome of deficient type marked by perspiration, Gui Zhi Fu Zi Decoction may be used.

Prescription for example:

Coix seed 30g, wolly or mealy yam 10g, atractylodes rhizome 10g, motopterygium root 10g, pubcescent angelica root 10g, ledebouriella root 10g, tetrandra root 10g, ephedra 5g, cinnamon twig 10g, Chinese angelica root 10g, chuanxiong rhizome 10g.

4.2 Arthritis of heat type:

Main symptoms: Swelling pain and a feeling of burning heat in joints with red color of the skin. The pain is either single or multiple, which becomes severe when pressed, gets alleviated when cooled.

Accompanying symptoms: fever, aversion to wind sweating, thirst, dysphoria.

Tongue and pulse: red tongue with yellow and dry coating slippery and rapid pulse.

Analysis: Pathogenic heat stagnating in meridians and joints results in accumulation of qi and blood, which is marked by pain and a feeling of burning heat in joints with red color of the skin, severe pain in one or many joints. Accumulation of heat leads to stagnation qi and blood, which is marked by pain becoming severe when pressed and getting allievated when cooled. Pathogenic heat lingering and disharmony between ying and wei lead to fever, aversion to cold. Inward invasion of pathogenic heat causes excess of internal heat, which is marked as high fever, sweating, thirst and liking drink, dysphorsia. Accumulation of heat and blockage of dampness show as red tongue with yellow and dry coating, rapid and slippery pulse.

To the patients of arthralgia syndrome, due to wind-heat -dampness and excess of pathogenic qi or hyperactivity of yang-qi the local and general symptoms will be severe. The onset of the disease is sudden and it easily affects five Zang-organs, which make the pathogenic changes various.

Treatment: clearing away heat and dredging channel, expelling wind and eliminating dampness.

Prescription: modified Bai Hu Gui Zhi Decoction. In the recipe, Bai Hu Decoction are used for clearing away heat and relieving restlessness, nourishing the stomach to regulate the middle-jiao. Cinnmon twig is used to expel wind and dredge channel. In the case of swelling sore throat, platycodon root, scrophularia root, chinese white olive are used to relieve swelling sore throat. Also perlingual Liu Shen Pill. If excess of pathogenic heat causes fever and aversion to wind, honey-suckle stem, forsythia fruit, capejasmine fruit, giant knotweed rhizome are used to clear away heat and toxic material. For treatment of high fever and thirst, besides unprepared gypsum used in large dosage, fresh reed rhizome, trichosanthes root, scrophularia root, rehmannia root may be added for clearing away heat to promote the production of body fluid. For treatment of conspitation, capejasmine fruit, rhubard, irabillte are used to clear away heat and purge the bowels. For treatment of pain in the joints with dysphoria, mulberry twigs, siegesbeckia herb, clematis root, gentian root, frankincense, myrrh, lumbricus are used for dredging channel to relieve the pain. For treatment of ankylosis with red color of the skin and a feeling of burning heat, moutan bark, rehmannia root, red peony root, arnebia or lithosperm root are used for removing pathogenic heat from the blood and toxic material from the body.

Modified Xuan Bi Decoction is used for the case accompanied with red color of the skin, swelling, heat sensation, pain in the joints, yellow and greasy coating. In the recipe, tetrandra root, excrementa bombycum, coix seed and red phaseolus bean are used for expelling wind, eliminating dampness, clearing and activating the channels and collaterals; forsythia fruit, capesjasmine fruit, talcum are used to clear away heat and promote diuresis. The ingredients of the recipe have the effect of eliminating mildly pathogenic dampness and heat from the channels and collaterals, so that qi and blood can flow smoothly and pain can be relieved. For treating the manifestations of the lower limbs, San Miao Pill may also be used in combination to strengthen the force of eliminating pathogenic dampness and heat from the lower-jiao.

Toxic heat converting into fire invades inward the bones and muscles. Then, body fluid is impaired, which is marked as redness and swelling joints, extreme pain, spasm of muscles and vessels light at day and severe at night, high fever, thirst, red and dry tongue, tout and rapid pulse. In order to treat them, modified Xi Jiao Powder with Bai Hu Decoction is used for removing pathogenic heat from the blood and toxic material from the body to relieve the pain. Also add scrophularia root, rehmannia root, moutan bark, ophiopon root for nourishing yin and removing heat from the blood in accordance with pratical conditions. Caulis aristolochiae manshuriensis, coix seed, excrementa bombycum, chaenomeles fruit is added for clearing away heat and eliminating dampness, dredging channel to relieve pain. If the source of rhinoceros horn is scarce, it is replaced by buffalo horn in large dosage.

Prescription for example:

Unprepared gypsum (decocted first) 30g, anemarrhena rhizome 10g, purple gromwell root, 10g; forsythia fruit 10g, honey-suckle stem 30g, cinnamon twig 10g, red peony root 10g, white peony root 10g, caulis aristolochiae manshuriensis 6g, unprepared licorice root 10g, unprepared coix seed 30g, polished round-grained nonglutinous rice 10g.

4.3 Wang Bi

Wang Bi is a syndrome characterized by arthrocele, ankylosis, joint deformity, wasting of limbs. If arthralgia syndrome lasts for a long time, it will occur. The illness name has been accepted in civil lecture discussion and clinic. Wang Bi is similar to obstruction of the kidney channel. As Huang Di Nei Jing said obstruction of the kidney channel is manifestated as inability to stand up straightly as if the function of heels is replaced by the sacral bone and humped thoracic vertebrae is higher than head. We discuss it in the chapter. It is favorable to clinic study and treatment of it.

Main symptoms: arthrocele, joint deformity, ankylosis, incapability of flexing and ankyloses of the whole body.

Accompanying symptoms: aching pain in the limbs and joints getting severe obviously, a feeling of pain arising from the bones. The pain is light in the daytime and becomes serious at night or in cloudy and rainy day. On the initial stage of the illness, will ankylosis occur in the morning, further in all day, often accompanied by lassitude in loin and knees, fatigue and weakness, liking warm and aversion to cold, irregular menstruation for female, emission and impotence for male.

Tongue and pulse: red, pale of dark tongue with ecchymoses; white or yellowing coating; deep thready or tout pulse with weakness in chi.

Analysis: The kidney, as congential foundation, houses the primordial yin and yang; stores essence; forms marrow and dominates the bones. The liver stores blood and is in charge of tendons. The liver and the kidney have a common source. Blood and vital essence produce each other. Due to inherent defect, malnutrion after birth, deficiency of the kidney and liver and faint muscles and bones, exogenous pathogen easily affects the body. Therefore, to a person of constitution of yin- deficiency, wind-cold pathogen invades the body and easily retains in the tendons and bones. With the prolongation of arthralgia syndrome, the kidney-yin is impaired so as to make exogenous pathogen enter the tendons and bones. Deficiency of blood and vital essence failing to nourish the tendons and bones leads to spasm with loose bones, then, joint deformity, ankylosis and incapblity of flexing and extending, finally, debility of limbs. Invasion of cold pathogen which is coagulative and constrictive in nature causes extreme pain getting severe in rainy and day as if it arises from the bones, liking warm and aversion to cold. Daytime belongs to yang dominating stability; night belongs to yin dominating movement. Movement makes blood and qi flow smoothly; stability makes blood and qi flow roughly. So the pain is light in the daytime and severe at night. Ankylosis will occur in the morning and get allievated after movement. The loin is the residence of the kidney. The liver dominates tendons. Deficiency of the liver and kidney causes lassitude in loin and knees, fatigue and weakness. Malnutrion of Chong and Ren channels leads to menstruation for female. The kidney-essence fails to control for male who is marked by emission and impotence. The case of deficiency of yin is marked by red tongue; the case of yang-deficiency is marked by pale tongue. Stagnation of collaterals due to deficiency of blood and vital essence leads to dark tongue, or even with ecchymoses and petechiae. Excess of pathogenic cold-dampness leads to white coating or greasy coating. Accumulation of pathogen converting into heat leads to yellow or greasy coating. Deep pulse indicates interior syndrome; thready pulse indicates deficiency syndrome; tout pulse indicates pain; faint pulse in chi indicates deficiency of the kidney.

Treatment: tonifying the kidney and dispersing cold, assisted with expelling wind and eliminating dampness, nourishing the liver and the tendons, clearing and activating the channels and collaterals.

Prescription: proved recipe of modified Zhi Wang Decoction consisting of modified Gui Zhi Shao Yao Zhi Mu Decoction with Hu Gu Powder (selected from Jian Yi Fang). In the recipe, psoralea fruit, dipsacus root, prepared aconite root and prepared rehmannia root are used to tonify the kidney and disperse cold. Cinnamon twig, red peony root and white peony root are used to regulate ying wei. Drynaria rhizome and prepared tiger bone are used to expel wind from bones and to strengthen muscles and bones. Epimedium, clematis root and pubescent angelica root are used to warm kidney-yang and to expel wind-dampness. Ledebouriella root and ephedra are used to expel wind and disperse cold. Atracylodes rhizome is used to eliminate dampness and recuperate the spleen. Prepared pangolin scales, buck grass and nodular branch of pine are used to clear and activate the channels and collaterals in order to relax tendons to ease joint movement. Anemarrhena rhizome is used to clear away asthenic heat and to inhabit prepared aconite root and cinnmon bark with hot in property and pungent in flavour. Achyranthes root is used to tonify the liver and kidney, dredge channel and guide other drugs into the kidney channel. For those of obvious aching pain in loin and knees, atractylodes rhizome should be expunged; loranthus mulberry mistletoe, cibot rhizome, pyrola should be added; otherwise, dipsacus root, achyranthes root, posoralea fruit and eucommia bark should be used in large dosage. For those of spasm of muscles, unprepared coix seed, chaenomeles fruit, unprepared licorice root should be added to the recipe or white peony root should be used in large dosage. For those of wasting and atrophy of muscles, fatigue and weakness, astragalus root, dangshen and white atractylodes rhizome should be added. For those of arthrocele, obvious arthroncus, severe pain in the joints and edema of lower extremity, wolly or mealy yam, tetrandra root, unprepared coix seed and round cardamon seed should be added, otherwise, clematis root should be used in large dosage. If arthralgia syndrome lasts for a long time, pathogen will infect the blood collaterals which causes symptoms of blood stasis. To treat it, safflower, earthworm, frankincense and myrrh should be added. In case of intermingling cold and heat, tonifying the kidney and dispersing cold should be used, assisted with clearing away heat, eliminating dampness and dredging collaterals. The dosage of drugs warm or got in nature in the above recipe should be reduced; rehmannia root, phellodendron bark, honeysuckle stem, Chinese starjasmine should be added to it so that warming and heat-clearing are used simultaneously. In case of cold converting into heat, the drugs tonifying the liver and kidney such as rehmannia root, spatholobus stem, fleece-flower stem and hornet nest are used in large dosage for treatment of it which should refer to arthritis of heat type. If the illness lasts for a long time, long-noded pit viper, black-tail snake and scorpoin should be added.

Prescription for example: prepared rehmannia root 12g, posoralae fruit 10g, drynaria rhizome 10g, dipsacus root 15g, cinnamon twig 10g, prepared aconite root 6g, red peony root 5g, white peony root 5g, ephedra 5g, prepared pangolin scales 10g, clematis root 12g, pabcescent angelica root 10g, ledebouriella root 10g, unprepared coix seed 15g, achyranthes root 15g, prepared licorice root 6g.

If arthralgia syndrome lasts for a long time, deficiency of vital -qi leads to lingering of pathogen; pathogen attacks the blood collaterals which causes blood stasis; coagulated body fluid turns to phelgm. Finally blockage of phlegm and blood stasis will occur simultaneously. It is marked by spasmodic pain, arthrocele, lusterless skin or ever joint deformity, ankylosis, incapblity of flexing and extending, dark purplish tongue with ecchymoses and petechiae, thready and uneven pulse, etc. Eliminating phelgm, expelling wind and dredging channel should be used to treat it. Prescribe Tao Hong Decoction with pangolin scales, earthworm, ground beetle for nourishing the blood, promoting blood circulation and removing blood stasis to dredge channel. White mustard seed, bamboo juice, fresh ginger juice and arisaema tuber may be added to it for eliminating phlegm, removing the obstruction of channels and resolving mass; scorpoin and black-tail snake may be added to it for expelling wind and dredging channel to relieve pain.

If arthralgia syndrome lasts for a long time, besides the symptoms caused by obstruction of pathogenic cold -dampness in the meridian and joints, yet there appears symptoms caused by deficiency of qi and blood or deficiency of the liver and kidney due to impairment of vital-qi. To treat them, doctors should give consideration to both the incidental and fundamental. Reinforcement and elimination are used in combination, i. e, expelling wind, dispersing cold and eliminating dampness assisted with either tonifying qi and blood or nourishing the kidney and liver. In order to tonify qi and blood, doctors use modified Si Jun Zi Decoction, Si Wu Decoction, Yang Rong Decoction or Gui Pi Decoction; in order to nourish the liver and kidney, docters use modified You Gui Pill, Zuo Gui Pill, Du Huo Ji Sheng Decoction or Jian Bu Hu Qian Pill. Arthralgia syndrome affects inward the heart with the prolongation of the course of the disease, which is marked by palpitation and shortness of breath which become aggravated after movement, lusterless complexion, pale tongue, rapid and feeble or knotted and intermittent pulse. Tonifying qi and nourishing the heart are used to treat them. Prescibe modified Zhi Gan Cao Decoction. It is of benefit for patients to use acupuncture and moxibustion, massage, fumigation and washing in combination besides oral drugs.

〔Prevention and nursing measure〕

1. If there occurs extreme pain in the joints, arthroncus, limited movement and high fever at the initial stage of the disease, the patient should have a rest in bed and will make himself comfortable by regulating his posture so that the pain can be eased.

2. When the condition of the disease is steady and pain in limbs and joints is alleviated, the patient should increase movement in order to strengthen his health, above all, recover the joint function.

3. The residence of the patient should have proper temperature and fresh air. Especially, keep the affected limb warm so as to relieve the pain, promote recovery and prevent reoccurence of the disease.

4. Pay attention to eat nutrient food so as to strengthen the resistance force. Eat little pungent and irritant food. The patient of arthralgia aggravated by cold shouldn't eat uncooked and cold food, but eat food warm in nature, such as mutton, beaf and so on. They should also eat much vegetable or fruit.

5. Also apply a heat bag of herbs or plaster to the affected part. Steam or wash the whole body by decoction. Necessarily, therapy of acupuncture, moxibustion and massage may be used in combination.

6. If its complication occurs, the illness should be diagnosed and treated in time.

〔Typical case analysis〕

Case one: Su ××, female, 31 year old.

She went shopping and caught in the heavy rain in the third month after delivery. She was right at night, but she couldn't get up the next day and had a feeling of paralysis under the waist. She couldn't turn over; only lie on the back due to pain in the two legs. By checking, redness, swelling, compression pain were not seen in the lumbosacral joint. The pulse was faint and tout in Guan, no strength in the cun and chi. The arthralgia syndrome is obviously caused by invasion of pathogenic wind-cold which combines with interior dampness due to deficiency of qi and blood. Expelling pathogenic cold from channel and regulating ying and wei are used to treat it.

Prescription: modified Huang Qi Gui Zhi Decoction.

Ingredients: loranthus mulberry misteletoe 15g, astragalus root 15g, cinnamon twig 9g, white atractylodes rhizome 9g, fresh ginger 9g, prepared aconite root 6g, prepared licorice root 6g, parched coix seed powder 30g, Chinessdate 4 picieces.

After taking it, she had a heat sensation in the abdomen. The next day the pain was allievated. Menstrual onset after delivery with slight pain in the lower abdomen occured in two days. She could go to a clinic by herself after taking three doses of it. The pulse was tout and rapid. Then, the following recipe is used to regulate qi and blood and to eliminate wind-dampness. Ingredients of it: chinese angelica root 6g, chuanxiong rhizome 6g, gentian root 6g, white atractylodes rhizome 6g, cyathula root 6g, white peony root 9g, cinnamon twig 9g, rehmannia root 9g, loranthus mulberry mistletoe 9g, astragalus root 15g, eucommia bark 12g, ledebouriella root 5g, wild ginger 3g, prepared licorice root 3g. After her taking three doses of it, the pain was again eased and the pulse was moderate. Wholly speaking, it was cured. Tian Ma Pill, Hu Gu Mu Gua Pill or Da Huo Luo Dan were taken continously for those of constitution of deficiency of the liver and kidney marked by dizzness and tinnitus.

The patient caught in heavy rain at the time of no less than one hundred days after delivery. Pathogenic wind-cold-dampness attacked the body. So expelling cold from the channel and regulating ying and wei were used to treat her. The obvious effect that menstrual pain was allievated was required after her taking three doses of it. The arthralgia pain was cured after she administrated three doses again.

Arthalgia syndrome is often seen in clinic. Deficiency of vital-qi, as a interior factor, combining with invasion of pathogenic wind, cold, dampness, heat which is considered as a exterior factor, leads to the disease. It is characterized by pain, aching or heavy sensation and numbness in the muscles 、bones, joints, arthrocele, incapability of flexing and extending. The condition of the disease is closely related to the changes of climate. The pathogenesis of arthralgia syndrome is that qi and blood can't flow smoothly due to blockage of collaterals and channels. Clinically, it is divided into two types: arthalgia due to wind-cold-dampness and arthritis of heat type. In recent years, with the deep study of Wang Bi, the range of it isenlarged. In arthralgia due to wind-cold-dampness, wind arthralgia is mainly caused by invasion of pathogenic wind, marked by wandering pain; arthralgia aggravated by cold is mainly caused by invasion of pathogenic cold, marked by extreme pain in fixed position; damp arthralgia is mainly caused by pathogenic dampness, marked by pain in fixed position with a heavy sensation, arthroncus and numbness. Arthritis of heat type is marked by redness, swelling, burning heat and pain in the joints. Wang Bi is a obstinate disease, marked by pain slight in the daytime and severe at night as if it arises from the bones, arthrocele, joint deformity.

Before doctors treat arthralgia syndrome, they should figure out the relationship between vital-qi and pathogen. According to the course, the onset, the condition of the disease and characteristics of syndrome, it is necessary to define the nature of it, the urgency and severity of the fundamental and the incidental. In general, on the initial stage of the disease, it is manifested as excess syndrome and it should be treated by eliminating the pathogenic factor, clearing and activating the channels and collaterals. The protracted disease that is marked by deficiency syndrome miggling with excess syndrome should be treated by strengthening the body resistance to eliminate pathogenic factors, clearing and activating the channels and collaterals or by eliminating the pathogenic factor, promoting blood circulation and resolving masses accompanied with strengthening the body resistance. It is so called that doctors should treat the incidental under urgent situation; when the condition of the disease permits, both the incidental and the fundamental are taken in consideration. Expelling wind, dispersing cold, eliminating dampness and clearing away heat, as basic therapeutic methods of arthralgia syndrome, are assisted with eliminating phlegm, resolving masses, promoting blood circulation to remove blood stasis, strengthening the spleen, replenishing qi, warming yang, nourishing the kidney, enriching the blood and nourishing the liver according to the practical conditions. Moreover, in treatment of pain in the various parts, the medicinal guide should be added to the recipe for promoting the curative effect. For those of pain in the upper limbs, notopterygium root, chuanxiong rhizome, turmaria and cinnamon twig are used; for those of pain in the lower limbs, achyranthes root, pubescent angelica root, chaenomeles fruit and manshurian aristolochia root are used; for those of pain in the neck or nape, pueraria root are used; for those of pain in the lumbar vertbrae, loranthus mulberry mistletoe, eucommia bark, cibot rhizome and pyrola are used. Pay attention to regulate the function of the spleen and stomach during treatment of arthralgia syndrome, which is favorable to treatment and recovery. Besides, when arthralgia due to wind-cold-dampness is marked by extreme pain, prepared aconite root and sichuan aconite root are used for expelling wind, eliminating dampness and warming the channels to relieve pain. Because poisonous prepared aconite root and sichuan aconite root are pungent in flavor and hot in nature, it is unfit to take them for a long time or in large dosage. They should be administrated in small dosages at the beginning and increased gradually. After taking them, if the patient is marked by intoxication symptoms such as tingling sensation in lips and tongue, numbness in hands and feet, nausea, palpitation, slow pulse and so on, the dosage of them should be reduced in accordance with practical conditions or discontinued. If necessarily, the measures should be made to rescue him in time. For those of dragging pain and spasm of limbs which can't be cured by ordinary drugs due to long-term course of the disease, the animal drugs expelling wind from collaterals and channels such as agkistrodon acutus, black-tail snake, prepared pangolin scales, earthworm, hornet nest and scorpoin are used for dredging channel to relieve pain. The drugs are mostly pungent in flavour, hot in nature and drastic in function. Some of them are poisonous and some are irritant. So it is unfit to take them in large dosage or for a long time. They are used in pills or powders. As soon as the patients' condition improves, they can't be taken.

During the treatment of arthralgia syndrome, the patients should increase physical exercises, prevent the invasion of pathogenic wind-cold-dampness and change the clothes according to the weather, which plays an important role in prevention of reoccurence and treatment. Generally, if arthralgia syndrome is treated in time, its prognosis will be favorable. But it occurs repeatedly and it is lingering. As a protracted disease, it can lead to obstruction of phlegm and blood-stasis which is marked by joint deformity; it can also affect interior Zang-organs which leads to deficiency of qi and blood or deficiency of liver-yin and kidney-yin. On this condition, it is so deep and serious that it can be difficulty cured and its prognosis is poor. Doctors should deal it with positively referring to this chapter.

Questions for Review

1. Try to give the etiological factor and pathogenesis of arthralgia syndrome.
2. What about diagnosis and treatment of arthralgia syndrome due to pathogenic wind-cold-dampness based on differentiation of symptoms and signs?
3. What about diagnosis and treatment of arthritis of heat type based on differentiation of symptoms and signs?
4. How should doctors diagnose and treat arthralgia syndrome when it is

accompanied with obstruction of phlegm and blood stasis, deficiency of qi and blood or deficiency of kidney-yin and liver-yin?

5. How many syndromes will occur when arthralgia syndrome affects the interior Zang-organs? What are they?
6. How is the complex therapy applied to the treatment of arthralgia syndrome?
7. What should doctors pay attention to when they use prepare aconite root, sichuan aconite root and animal drugs to treat arthralgia syndrome?

Wei-syndrome

〔Introduction〕

Wei-syndrome refers to a condition when the muscles and tendons are week and flaccid or when muscles have atrophied. Clinical manifestations are muscular atrophy and debility of the whole body or parts of the body. Atrophy and debility of lower limbs with atrophic and impaired mobility are commonly present, therefore, wei-syndrome are named "wei bi". "wei" suggests atropby and debility of limbs, persistent errection of tendons; "bi" suggests muscles are weak and flaccid in lower limbs with impaired mobility.

Myelitis, acute infections polyradiculitis, progressive myotrophy, myasthenia gravis, periodic paralysis, progressive spinal paralysis, amyotrophic paralysis, hysterical paralysis and multiple sclerosis, syrinyomyelia and following abstruction of sensation manifesting flaccid and atrophic muscles. belong to modern medical science may be diagnosed and treated according to Wei-syndrome.

〔Etiology and pathogenesis〕

1. Consumption of Fluid due to Heat in the Lungs: A disability in fighting against external pathogenic factor due to deficiency of the lung qi allows the dampness-heat or wind-cold to invade the body, which may turn into heat, when a high fever produces or residual pathogenic factor after an illness produces a low fever or heat in five zang organs removed to the lung leads to consumption of fluid and malnutrition of the muscles and tendons due to pulmonary heat, thus atrophy and debility of limbs results in wei-syndrome. As the lung is huagai and delicate organ, lying in the upper-warmer, it is normal for it to inhale fresh air and

clarifying and sending down the qi. As a result, it is open to attack from every kind of external pathogenic factor, then, the diseases occur.

The lung has the function of disseminating food essence and body fluid due to all the blood vessels meet in the lungs. If the qi and yin fluid of the lung are damaged by pathogenic heat, the lung can't disseminating food essence and body fluid, therefore, malnutrition of the muscles and tendons due to weakness and flaccidity of muscles leads to wei-syndrome.

2. Invasion by Dampness-Heat: If the patient lives in a damp place or is caught in the rain, this allows dampness to remain inside the body. Over a long period of time, the dampness turns into heat. If dampness-heat invade the spleen and stomach and reaches the lower-warmer, or the spleen and stomach are damage as a result of improper diet, such as excess greasy or spicy food or excess alcohol, then dampness is produced, which may also turn into heat over a long period of time. Once produced, dampness-heat will invade the muscles and tendons, and impair qi and blood circulation thus, malnutrition of the muscles and tendons will lead to wei-syndrome.

3. Splenic and Gastric Deficiency: Because the spleen and stomach are the foundation of life and the sources of qi, blood and body fluid, the five zang and six fu and the muscles and tendons rely on them. If the patient suffers from constitutional deficiencies or has suffered from a prolonged illness, the stomach is too weak to absorb food essence and body fluid and the spleen can't transmit and transport the nutrient fluid, for the stomach, this means that the sources are insufficient. Malnutrition of the muscles and tendons leads to wei-syndrome.

〔Differention and Treatment〕

Clinically, wei-syndrome is one of common disease and is characterized by flaccid and weak muscles; The pathogenesis can be both external and internal. It should be diagnosed weather the syndrome is caused by deficiencies or by excesses. Wei-syndrome caused by external pathogenic warmth and heat or by the invasion of dampness-heat, has an acute onset and develops rapidly, weakness and flaccidity of the limbs often occur during or after an illness, it is usually caused by excesses. Wei-syndrome caused by a weak spleen and stomach or hepatic and renal deficiency develops gradually over a long time; atrophy and debility of both lower limbs are commonly present; this usually caused by deficiencies or by deficiencies complicated by excesses. If wei-syndrome caused by external pathogenic factors is treated in time, the dampness-heat will go away, the qi and blood will move in harmonious way, the tendons will drege, the symptoms of atrophy and debility of limbs will be gradually recovered, the disease will be improved and the patient will be in general health after a treatment. If the case is caused by consumption of qi and yin by pulmonary heat, the stagnant dampness-heat and debility of tendons may cause deteriorated case, manifested as dyspnea and short breath, stagnation of qi and blood, purple lips and nails dripping sweat, cold extremities and faint pulse, then yang-depletion. Wei-syndrome caused by internal injury, weakness of the liver and kidney due to injuried spleen and stomach affecting the sources and deprives the muscles and tendons of nourishment with the result that flaccidity is hard to cure.

Wei-syndrome should be discerned from apoplexy. Patients suffering from apoplexy may also produce paralysis of limbs, the accompanying symptoms include numbness of muscles and limbs, facial paralysis, this is not accompanied by any of the symptom exogenous. If weakness and flaccid of limbs accompanied with tremor, swaying step, slurred speech, this is wei-syndrome accompanied by Fei-syndrome, which should be diagnosed and treated according to them.

Some patients with bi-syndrome may lose the use of their muscles and when bi-syndrome is in its later stages, they may suffer from muscular atrophy; this is wei-syndrome. If the case accompanied by rigidity in the joint, muscular contracture, this is wei-syndrome accompanying with jing-syndrome, which should be diagnosed treated combining with bi and jing-syndrome.

The principal of getting rid of wei-syndrome is treating the Yangming meridians. It should be said that eliminating the evil qi of Yangming meridians and replenishing deficient Yangming merdians are two ways to treat the case. The disease caused by external pathgenic facter is of the excess type, treatment aims to eliminate evil qi or disperse heat or eliminate dampness; the disease caused by internal injury, efforrs should be made to replenish deficient stomach and spleen-qi, and to restore organic function of spleen and stomach, to invigorate qi and blood and to nourish the tendons and muscles. However, the principal of treating the Yangming meridians cannot be use for all kinds of wei-syndrome. In order to treat the wei-syndrome correctly, we must make prescription in accordance with the syndromes and conditions to replenish the liver and kidney or to nourish blood and dredge the meridians.

1. Consumption of Fluid due to Pulmonary Heat

Main symptoms: fever then high fever, weakness and flaccidity of the limbs, atrophic muscles.

Accompanying symptoms: restlessness, thirst, coughing, dry throat, scandy dark or anuria, constipation, pain in the joint and limbs or numbness.

Tongue and pulse: red tongue with a yellow coating, thready and rapid pulse.

Analysis: The lungs control and defend external pathogenic factor. If the lung is invaded by pathogenic dampness-heat and warmth-heat due to weakness of defending qi. Consumption of fluid by pulmonary heat prevent it from being distributed the body to warm and benefit muscles and skin. Malnutrition of the muscles and tendons leads to weak and flaccid muscles and flaccid limbs and atrophic muscles. Restlessness, thirst and dry throat are signs of fluid consumption by internal heat. If the lung qi does not descend due to pulmonary heat, a cough will occur. The qi that transforms between the lung and bladder is the source of water and plays a significant effect in metabolism. If consumption of fluid due to pulmonary heat can't be distributed, fluid passage is abstructed and qi transformation of bladder is in dysfunction, a scandy dark urine or unuria will occur. The exterior and interior relationship between the lung and the large intestine moves pulmonary heat into the large intestine and result in consumption of fluid, the function of transporting can't work. The stoppage of the qi of the bowels, constipation, red tongue with yellow coating and thready and rapid pulse are signs of fluid consumption by internal heat.

Treatment: To disperse heat, moisten dryness, nourish the lungs and produce body fluid.

Prescription: Modified Qing Zao Jiu Fei Decoction. Radix Ginseng and Radix Ophiopogonis tonify lung and produce fluid; Gypsum Fibrosum, Folium Mori and Fructus Cannabis dispel heat and moisten dryness; Semen Armeniacae Amarurn promotes the smooth circulation of lung qi. In cases of high fever, thirst and sweating, add Rhizoma Anemarrhenae. Flos Lonicerae and Flucture Forsythiae to disperse heat and other pathogenic factors. Use large doses of Gypsum Fibrosum, Folium Eriohotryae, Colla Corii Asim moisten the lung and produce body fluid. Cortex Mori Radicis, Radix scrophularilariae and Radix Rehmanniae may also be added. In cases of cough and a small amount of sputum, add Bulbus Fritillariae

Cirrhosae and Fructrs Trichosanthis. If the patient is suffering from dry mouth and throat, poor appetite and red tongue with scanty coating after fever has subsided, this suggests that pulmonary and gastric yin have been damaged. Decoction for benefiting stomach should be prescribed with Semen Coicis, Rhizoma Atractylodis Macrocephalae, Rhizoma Dioscreae and Fructus Oryzae Germinatus to benefit the stomach and produce body fluid.

If the patient is treated in time, his pulmonary heat will be eliminated, qi and yin will be restored, nutrition of the muscles and tendons will lead to atrophic limbs alleviating, urination and defecation may be ease. If excessive pathogenic heat is difficult to eliminate, qi and yin are seriously damaged and configuration and constitution of the body is in a bad condition, this may result in deteriorating case. The magnifestations include dyspnea with rapid and short breath, purple lips and nails, a difficulty in swallowing, splurred speech, drippling sweat, extreme cold of the limbs, even yin and yang exhaust. Deteriorated case occurs because deficiency of qi and yin from the lung to the kidney. The kidney is in charge of water and the lung is the source of water. If the lung yin is too deficient to reach the kidney and fluid of the kidney can not go upward to the lung, the lung is serious dry, it is said that the source is in failure. The lung is in charge of qi, the kidney is the root of qi and has the function of controlling and promoting inspiration. If the lung qi is seriously damaged, a dyspnea with rapid and short breath will occur. The vessels converge in the lung which are in charge of coordination of visceral activities. As the same time, the vessels rely on the heart and lung to make their circulation regulated. If the lung qi is flaccid, blood vessels are stagnated, purple lips and nails will occur. The stoppage of the root of tongue result in difficulty in swallowing, splurred speech. The lung channel of Hand-Taiyin lies in both side of the root of tongue charging throat, the kidney channel of Foot-Shaoyin lies in both side of the base of tongue; the heart channel of Hand-Shaoyin connects with the root of tongue. Consumption of fluid and flaccid qi, channels stagnation, weakness and flaccidity of the heart and lung and kidney will lead to the base of tongue disorder.

If fluid has been seriously damaged due to qi deficiency and excessive sweating and yin exhaustion, this will lead to yang lose and turn into coldness-syndrome. In order to treat the case, prescription for recuperating the depleted yang to cure collapse-zheng should be prescribed, Shen Fu Decoction, Sheng Mai power may be selected.

Prescription for example:

Gypsum Fibrosum 30g, Radix Ophiopogonis 10g, Folium Mori 6g, Cortex Mori Radicis 10g, Semen Coicis 30g, Forsythiae 10g, Semen Armeniacae Amarum 10g, Radix glycyrrhizae 10g.

2. Invasion by Dampness-Heat

Main symptoms: Heaviness or swelling, flaccidity, weakness, numbness of the limbs, particularly the lower limbs.

Accompanying symptons: feveror dyspnea, a burning sensation on passing urine sweating, constipation and anuresis, difficulty in swallowing.

Tongue and pulse: red tongue with yellow coating, soft and rapid pulse.

Analysis: Retention of dampness-heat in the interior leads to consumption of fluid and excessive dampness retaining in the spleen. Dampness is yin and heavy and turbid in nature. If downward flow of turbid dampness invades the skin, havness will produce. Invasion of the meridians by dampness-heat blocks qi and blood circulation causing the limbs to become swell and numb. Invasion of the tendons by dampness causes the muscles and tendons to become flaccid, weak and atropy. Dampness-heat retained in the chest and diaphragm leads to distress and stuffiness there. Its downward movement gives rise to difficult and painful urination with dark yellow urine. A stick yellow tongue coating and a soft and rapid pulse are signs of retained dampness-heat.

Treatment: To disperse heat and eliminate dampness-heat.

Prescription: Modified Er Miao Powder. Cortex phellodendri disperses heat, Rhizoma Atractylodis dispels dampness, and Rhizoma Dcoscoreae Septemlobae and Radix Stephaniae Tetrandrae dissipate heat and eliminate dampness. Radix Angelicae Sinensis and Radix Achyranthis Bidentate tonish blood and remove obstruction from the meridians. In case of excess dampness when the limbs are heavy and swell and the tongue coating is sticky and thick, add Poria and Talcum to eliminate dampness. To eliminate dampness and remove obstructions from the meridians, add caulis Akebiae. Semen Coicis and Fructus Chaenomelis. In case of choking sensation over the chest, add Cortex Magnoliae officinalis and Herba Agstachis to regulate qi and eliminate dampness. Aromatics such as Herba Agastachis and Herba Eupatorii can be added to resolve dampness in the summer and fall. If Yin is damaged by dampness-heat with signs including emaciation, restless, a thready and rapid pulse and a tongue with a red tip and border or a tongue with extoliated coating in the center, remove Rhizoma Atractylodis and add Radix Rehmanniae; Radix Ophipogonis to disperse heat and produce fluid. In cases where the limbs are numb and there is only limited flexibility of the joints complicated by signs of stagnant blood such as a purple tongue and an unsmooth pulse, add Flos Carthami, Radix Paeoniae Rubra, Radix Salviae Miltiorrhizae, Fructus Chaenomelis and Lumbricus to activate blood circulation and remove obstructions from the meridians. In case where lumbar and lower extremity are cold, suggests that dampness-heat stagnates the meridians and Yang qi is warmless, removes Cortex phellodendri, add Ramulus Cinnamomi to warm and remove obstructions from the meridians.

If the patient is treated in time, dampness-heat is eliminated, qi and blood flows smoothly. Nutrition of muscles and tendons makes the patient better. If dampness flows downward to tendons, it is not easy to eliminate rapidly because of its turbid and sticky nature. A dysfunction of the spleen in transporting, distributing and transforming nutrients will cause the limbs heaviness and flaccidity and incapability to raise. Consumption of fluid by heat and damaged qi lead to the function of taking charge of qi abnormal, dyspnea, stagnation of blood circulation and Yang exhaustion will occur, this suggests heat has changed. The principle of treatment should benefit qi and save Yang, Shen fu decoction may be selected.

Prescription for example: Cortex Phellodendri 10g, Radix Achyranthis Bidentatae 12g, Rhizoma Atractylodis 9g, Semen Coicis 30g, Poria 20g, Rhizoma Pinelliae6g Fructus Chaenomelis 20g, Lumbricus 9g, Talcum 15g, Radix Glycyrrihizae 10g.

3. Splenic and Gastric Deficiency

Main symptoms: Weakness and flaccidity of the limbs or muscular atrophy develops gradually.

Accompanying symptoms: poor appetite, loose stools, pale complexion and puffy face or accumulation and obstruction of sputum and celostomia.

Tongue and pulse: thin white tongue coating and thready pulse.

Analysis: The spleen and stomach provide the material basis of the acquired constitution, deficiency of these organs means that the source of qi and blood are insufficient, thus, the limbs are deprived of nourishment and become flaccid and weak, with pronounced muscular atrophy. The sinking of clear qi due to impaired transport causes to poor appetite and loose stools. Lassitude a puffy, a pale complexion and a thready pulse are caused by deficiencies of the qi and blood flowing weakness of the spleen and stomach. Spleen is the source of producing phlegm, deficiency of the spleen prouduces sputum. The root of tongue is obstructed by sputum, celostomia occurs.

Treatment: To invigorate the spleen and benefit qi.

Prescription: Modified Shen Ling Bai Zhu powder. Radix Codonopsis Pilosulae, Rhizoma Atractylodis Macrocephalae, Rhizoma Dioscoreae, Semen Dolichoris and Semen Nelumbinis invigorate the spleen and benefit qi; and Poria, Semen Coicis invigorate the spleen, eliminate dampness; Fructus Amomi, Pericarpium Citri regulate qi and harmonize the stomach. In case of poor appetite, add Endothelium Corneum Gigeriae Galli; In cases where the patient has an aversion to cold and cold limbs, add Radix Aconiti Lateralis preparata and Rhizoma Zingiberis to warm spleen yang. In cases where both qi and blood are deficient, add Radix Astragali, Radix Angelicae sinensis and Kadix paeoniae Alba to help replenish qi and blood.

If spleen yang of the patient is restored gradually and both qi blood are invigorated by treatment, nutrition of muscles helps the body of patient is in good condition. If the spleen and stomach deficient as a result of improper diet and temperature, happiness, angry and anxiety and overwork, or qi is damaged by infecting pathogenic factor, developing atrophy and debility may damage the lung and kidney along with dyspnea, aphasia, this is said "shortness of breath, qi duo after stomach diseases by Li Dong Yuan, which leads to hoarseness and dyspnea with rapid respiration and damaged spleen and stomach." Finally, five zang must also be damaged, it is difficult to heal.

Prescription for example: Radix Codonopsis Pilosulae l0g, Rhizoma Atractylodis Macrocephalae 12g, Poria 20g, Rhizoma Dioscoreae 10g, Pericarpium Citri 10g, Semen Coicis 30g, Fructus Amomi 6g, Radix Angelicae Sinensis 10g, Radix Astragali 15g, Radix Aconiti Lateralis Preparata 6g, Radix Zingiberis 3g, Radix Glycyrrhizae 10g;

4. Hepatic and Renal Deficiency

Main symptoms: The disease develops gradually, weakness, flaccidity occur in the lower, soreness and weakness of the lumbar region.

Accompanying symptoms: anigestations, dizziness, tinnitus, spermatorrhea or incontinence of urination and defecation, or muscular twitching and cramp, splurred speech or irregular menstruation or atrophy of limbs and muscles and trembling tongue.

Tongue and pulse: red tongue with a little coating, or thin tongue body with a small amount of fluid, thready and rapid pulse.

Analysis: Congenital defect or malnutrition after birth or excess of sexual intercourse lead to deficiency of the liver and kidney. Malnutrition of tendons due to deficiency of blood of the liver leads to atrophy of tendons; Deficiency of the essence of life in the kidney fails to take charge of bone leads to debility of bone.

Malnutrition of the muscles and tendons due to deficiencies of liver and kidney lead to atrophy of limbs. The lumbar region is the house of the kidney of nourishment, causing soreness and weakness. Urination and defecation and urinary bladder are out of control due to renal deficiency causes incontinence of urination and defecation. Internal pathogenic wind produces due to deficiency of the liver and kidney results in muscular twitching and cramp. Malnutrition of chongren pulse leads to irregular menstruation; a cough during swallowing and splurred speech is caused by tongue disease following deficiency of the liver and kidney. A red tongue with only small amounts of tongue coating and a thready and rapid pulse are signs of deficient yin and hyperactive fire.

Treatment: To replenish the liver and kidney, nourish yin and disperse heat

Prescription: Modified Hu qian Bolus. Os Tigris and Radix Achyranthis Bidentatae strengthen the tendons and bones; Herba Cynomorii warms kidny and benefits essense. Radix Angelicae Sinesis, Radix Paeoniae Alba soothe the liver and nourish blood; Cortex phellodendri, Rhizoma Anemarrhenae, Radix Rehimanniae Preparata and Carapax et Plastrum Testudinis nourish yin and disperse heat. In case where the patient suffers from yellow complexion, palpitations, and thready and weak pulse, add Radix Astragali, Radix Codonopsis and caulis Spatholobi to replenish qi and blood. If the treatment of wei-syndrome caused by yin deficiency by heat, remove Herba Cynomorii and Rhizoma Zingiberis. In cases of yin deficiency affecting yang with symptoms of aversion to cold, atrophic muscles, large quantities of clear urine, pale tongue and deep thready pulse, this is caused by decline of Ming-Men Yang without warmness and obstruction of the meridians by accumulated blood. The principle of treatment should warm kidney assist yang, strengthen the tendons and bones and active the meridians. Modified Jin-gang Bolus should be prescribed. Radix morindae. Cortex Eucommiae, Herba Cistanchis, Herba Epimedii and Semen Cuscutae replenish the kidneys and assist yang, Semen Strychni preparata, Fructus chaenomelis, Radix Achyranthis Bidentatae benefit the liver kidney and comfort the tendons; Rhizoma Gastrodiae, Scolopendra, Bombyx Batryticatus and zaocys eliminate wind and dredge the collateral; Rhizoma Dioscoreae and regulate stomach and eliminate dampness. A proper amount of herbs such as Radix Angelicae Sinensis, Radix Paeoniae Alba soothe the liver and benifit blood; Lumbricus, and Flos Carthami promote blood circulation to dredge the collateral. It is appropriate to use Flos Dolus because this disease has a long course.

Prescription for example: Radix Astragali 15g, Herba Cynomorii 10g, Fructus Psoraleae 12g, Herba Epimedii 10g, Radix Aconiti Lateralis Preparata 6g, Radix Morindae 10g, Radix Angelicae Sinensis 12g, Radix Paeoniae Alba 12g, Radix Rehmanniae Preparata 9g, Radix Achy ranthis Bidentatae 12g, Cortex Phellodendri 3g, Rhizoma Atractylodis Macrocephalae 10g.

It is help to prevent atrophy and deform of the limbs and restore normal function of the body when medication is used along with acupuncture, massage physical therapy and proper exercise.

〔Preventive and nursing treatment〕

It is difficult to recover his health after the patient suffers from wei-syndrome which often develops gradually or keep in a certain extent. Therefore, it is of important not to treat disease but to prevent it, this is accord with the idea of traditional Chinese medicine which main to prevent the diseases and not to treat it. In order to prevent the patient from wei-syndrome, he should keep regular habit of life, keep away from damp places over a long times and has a proper and nutritious diet, keep clean and hygiene, pay attention not to damage the spleen and stomach, take care not to get tired, refrain from sexual activity, avoid damaging the liver and kidney and treat some diseases such as internal injury and affection of exogenious heat in time. Pay attention to exercise to help to keep the normal function of muscles. It was said in ancient-proverb that running water is never stale and a door-hinge never gets worm-eaten.

The patient should have proper understanding and keep optimistic manner and full of confidence to struggle against this disease after he suffers from wei-syndrome. He should insist on treating and exercising for a long time.

Noursing work should be done to help patient setting up proper manner toward this disease. The patient should exercise his atrophic muscles and limbs on his initiative and passivity massage may be use twice a day to exercise patient's muscles and pay attention to have a nutritious diet.

Sometimes, an infection of exogenic wind-cold and dampness-heat may lead patient to a serious condition and a difficult treatment due to deficient body of patient.

The patients who lie in bed should prevent bed-injury and often turn the body over and pad their back and massage projecting part of bone which is having pressed; Take care of urination and defecation not to soak pressed muscles; The patient who suffers from incontinence of urination or difficult in urination may set catheterzation, patients who can move parts of body should pay attention not be damaged suddenly impact injury and other unexpected accident.

〔Typical Case analysis〕

A five years old child suffered from fever for four days after a caught which attain a highest temperature at 40 degree. Atrophy and flaccidity of muscles of left leg following walking lamely after the heat had subsided for ten days. West doctor diagnosises his disease as poliomyelitis, and injects Lan Ta Min 1 mg a time, there are taken twice dailyinto his muscles, Vitamin B are taken orally, the patients are told to please Chinese doctor to treat. When the child first visited, his signs included a pale complexion, a poor appetite, a dry mouth and lips a red tongue with a small amount of coating, a thready pulse and soft debility of muscles in left leg without atrophy and lame. It was diagnosised as wei-syndrome following consumption of his fluid of the lung and stomach. Treatment aimed at dispersing heat and nourishing the lung and stomach. The main ingredients of the prescription included Cortex Mori Radicis, Colla Cotii Asini, Radix Ophiopogonis, Folium Mori, Semen Coicis, Rhizoma Atractylodis macrocephalae, Fructus Oryzae Germinatus and Fructus Hordei; Germinatus, Endothelium Corneum Gigeriae Galli, etc. The child's appetite was better and a lame remained undanged, accompanying manifestation included light a red tongue with a white and thin coating and a lame after l0-odd doses of the decoction. Now, the main pathogenesis are deficiencies and weak of the spleen and stomach due to consumption of fluid having recovered. Treatment invigorated the stomach, nourished the spleen, and liver kidney. The ingredients of the prescription included Radix Codonopsis, Rhizoma Atractylodis Macrocephalae, Poria, Semen Coicis, Simen Dolichos Album, Pericarpium Citri Reyiculatae viride, Pericarpium Citri Reticulatae, Cortex

Phellodendri, Racix Dipsaci, Radix Achyranthis Bidentatae. His symptoms were stable after he was taken 10-odd doses continuously, but the muscle of left leg slack obviously.

It was suggested that pills should be taken for several months which only had a slightly changing of the prescription.

Discuss: This case was caused by the weakness and flaccidity of limbs due to consumption of their fluid by pulmonary heat following a febrile disease. Fluid fails to distribute leads to malnutrition of the muscles and skin. The method of treatment adopted should be dispersing heat and produced fluid, but when the patient visited, the high fever had subsided, only red tongue with a small amount of coating and poor appetite were observed, this was diagnosed as a surplus pulmonary heat resulting in consumption of fluid of the lung and stomach. The symptoms were stable after nouring the lung and stomach and changed the prescription to regulate the spleen and stomach according to the principle of treating flaccidity by treating Yang-ming meridian first; so the kidney is in charge of lower limb added these herbal medicine and the liver is in charge of the tendons to benefit kidney and regulate the liver.

It was suggested that pills should be take over a long time after a stable symptoms, and the patient was advised to do proper exercises to strength ill limb.

Weakness and flaccidity of tendons and limbs or atrophy of muscles are main manifestations of wei-syndrome, particularly, atrophy and debility of or impaired mobility of lower limb are commonly present. The pathogenesis included consumption of fluid due to pulmonary heat, stagnation of qi and blood due to invasion of dampness-heat, exhausted source due to deficiency of the spleen and stomach and alnutrition of muscles and tendons due to deficiency of the liver and kidney. The basic principle of treating wei-syndrome is to treat Yang-ming meridian first, the emphasis should be placed on regulating the function of the spleen and stomach. The syndrome which caused by invasion of external pathogenic heat is of excess type, treatment is to eliminate external pathogenic factor, or to disperse the heat in the Yang-ming meridians, or to dispel heat and eliminate dampness. The syndrome which caused by internal ones is of the deficiency type, the stress should be laid on replenishing and recovering the function of transports and transmition of spleen and stomach. Qing Zao Jiu Fei Decoction, Shen Ling Bai Zhu powder, Modified Er Miao powder, HuQian Bulous were often used. Many diseases in nervous system manifesting flaccidity and atrophy of muscles and limbs may be treated accorin to wei-syndrome.

Diagrammatic sketch of etiology and pathogenesis of Wei-Syndrome examination

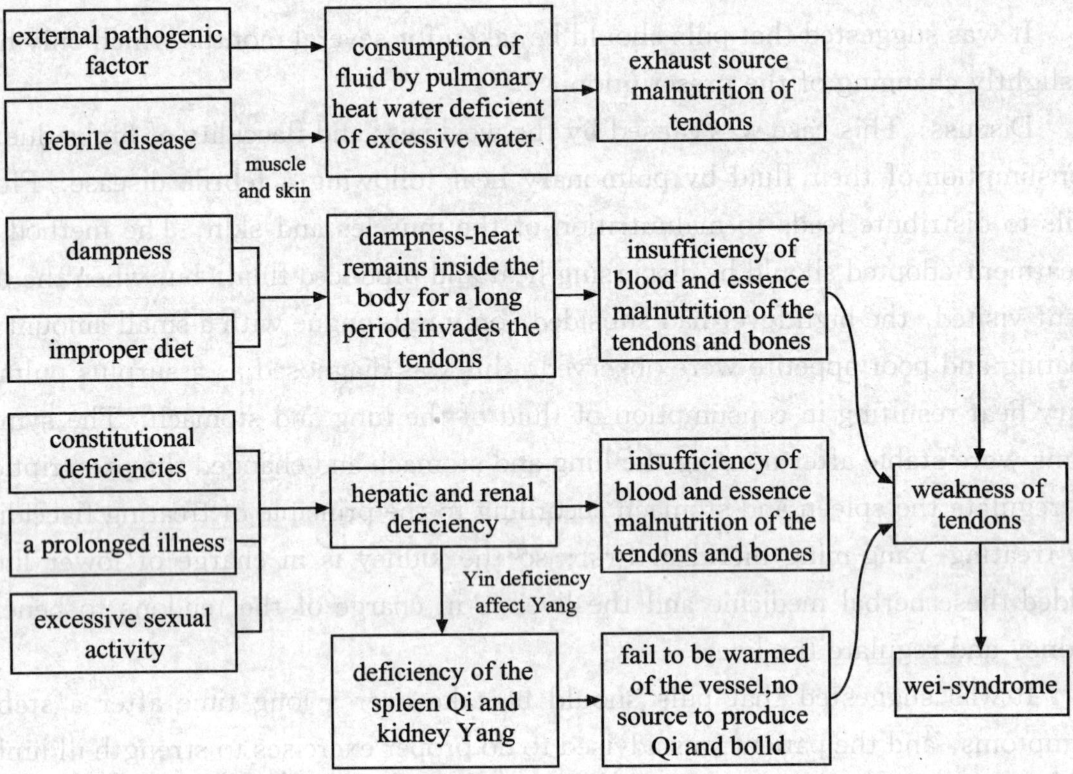

Questions for Review

1. Which is the etiology of Wei-syndrome?
2. How many symptoms and signs are common in Wei-syndrome?
3. How to understand correctly the principle that treating Wei-syndrome is to treat Yangming meridians first?

Fever Due to Internal Disorders

〔Introduction〕

Fever due to internal disorders refers to fever caused by maladjustment of the zang-fu organs and deficiency of qi, blood, yin and yang. Clinical characteristics of the disease can be described as follows: a long period of low fever in most cases, sometimes high fever, subjective fever, or restlessness and hot sensations in the palms, soles and chest, but in most circumstances the patient's temperature will not rise. Symptoms as a result of internal injury or liver depression, blood stasis, dampness accumulation may appear at the same time.

Internal fever is an independent syndrome, which can also be presented as a symptom of some chronic diseases, is discussed in these chapters. The disease with fever as its main symptom and internal injury as its etiology.

In western medicine, functional fever, fever caused by tumor, blood disease, disease of connective tissue, endocrinpathy, tuberculosis and chronic infective diseases, some idiopathic fever may manifest the syndrome of fever due to internal disorders. The treatment can refer to the contents of this chapter.

〔Etiology and pathology〕

Fever due to internal disorder is mainly caused by the disorder of emotion injury, improper diet and overstrains. For some cases, the disease is also the result of imbalance of zang-fu organs and yin, yang, qi and blood caused by exopathy. If the fever is caused by deficiency of zang-fu organs and qi, blood, yin and yang, we call it fever of deficiency type or fire of deficiency type and it belongs to deficiency syndrome. If the fever is the production of qi stagnation, blood stasis, retention of food, dampness heat retardation, it is considered as excess syndrome or deficiency-excess complex. The different diseased zang-fu organs are the bases of the different type of the fever. The detail contents are illustrated as follows:

1. Deficiency of yin

Essence constitutional yin deficiency or consumption of yin by persistent febrile disease or chronic diarrhea, erroneous or excessive use of warm and drying drugs with pungent flavor, all these can cause the deficiency of yin essence. The water can't inhibit the fire, thus the yang qi is relatively excessive and fever occurs, this is called fever caused by yin deficiency

2. Deficiency of qi of middle jiao

Overstrain, improper diet or failure of recuperation after illness, all these can lead to qi deficiency of spleen and stomach, thus fever develops. For this type of fever, we call it fever caused by qi deficiency. The pathology: the upward floating of deficient yang, attacking up of the yin fire, failure of resistance of wei-qi and disharmony between ying and wei. Yin fire is a relative concept to yang fire, another name for primordial qi. Yin fire usually refers to fire of deficient type or evil fire, insufficient qi of middle jiao and collapsed qi cause the up attacking of the fire of deficiency or evil fire

3. Ying and blood deficiency

Prolonged illness may result in blood deficiency of heart and liver; spleen deficiency means inability to produce blood, loss of blood due to hemorrhage and child birth, or surgery may cause blood deficiency. Blood is related to yin, deficient yin and blood can't check yang and thus give rise to floating yang accompanied by fever. This type is named as fever caused by blood deficiency.

Illustration of etiology and pathology of fever due to internal disorder

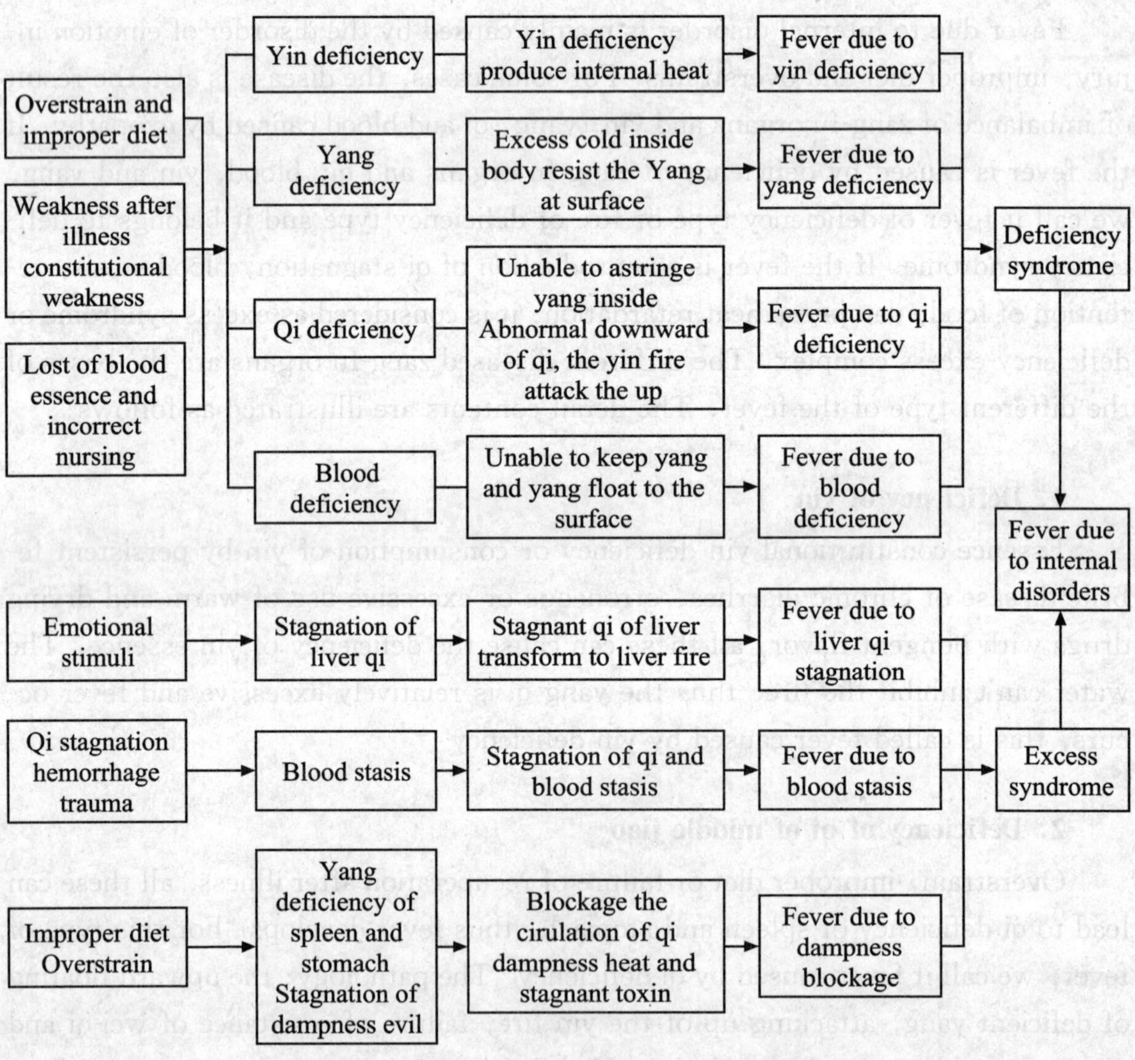

4. Deficiency of kidney yang

Yang is kept externally by the excessive cold-qi, and floating superficially, thus fever appears. Prolonged qi deficiency of the spleen and stomach may also result in yang deficiency of kidney and spleen, which can also lead to fever. These kind of fever, is called fever caused by yang deficiency.

5. Stagnant heat of liver channel

Depression impairs the liver's ability to regulate the free flow of qi and the stagnant qi turns into fire and produce fever. Excess anger leads to hyperactive liver fire with fever. This kind of fever relates to emotional changes, so it is called the fire of five emotions.

6. Blood stasis

The blood stasis produced by emotional injury, overstrain trauma, hemorrhage accumulates inside the body, therefore block the channel and collaterals along with unsmooth circulation of qi and blood. The stagnation of qi and blood lead to fever. It's usually named as fever caused by blood stasis

7. Blockage and streaming of the dampness evil

Fever caused by dampness stagnancy or dampness heat streaming can be identified as exopathy or internal disorder. For the cases of internal disorder, the deficient spleen and stomach qi affect the function of the spleen, as a result, the dampness accumulates, and dampness heat will be produced if the condition persists, fever will onset by the streaming of the stagnant dampness heat.

To sum up, fever due to internal disorder can be classified as excess and deficiency type. For the deficiency type, qi, blood, yin, yang deficiency should be the reason, and for the excess type, the pathology is the emotional injury, blood stasis and the streaming of the stagnant dampness heat. The pathology of the fever of the two types some times can also combined together to cause the syndrome, such as qi and blood deficiency and dampness obstructer, for a prolonged fever, the condition is always belongs to deficiency and the condition is serious. Since the fever lasts a long period of time, the situation will change. Usually to be more serious; and the syndrome will turn from excess type to deficiency type. For example, the fever due to blood stasis, if it persists a long time, thus the qi, blood, yin and yang will be consumed, syndromes of deficiency of qi, blood, yin and yang will present. A long period of qi stagnation accompanied with qi deficiency can also lead to fever. If the heat consumes yin fluid, the type of the fever syndrome will turn into qi stagnation and yin deficiency, except these, long term dampness evil accumulation, spleen qi deficiency or stagnant dampness evil with yin deficiency can also cause fever, which is usually seen in clinical practice.

〔Treatment according to differentiation of syndrome〕

Ⅰ. Differentiation of similar syndrome

Fever due to internal disorder should be identified from fever caused by excess pathogens. It's not difficult to distinguish the two syndromes if we consider the difference between them such as the onset, etiology, duration of the disease, the characteristic of the fever, accompanied symptoms, properties of aversion to cold, the tongue and pulse. The main points of the difference between the two syndromes are listed in the table below:

type	Fever due to internal disorder	Fever due to excess pathogens
Onset	Chronic	Acute
Etiology	Internal injury improper diet, emotion, trauma, overstrain	Exopathic six evil qi
Duration	Long	Short
Character of fever	Low fever or subjective fever or heat sensation in palms and toes Intermittent fever that onset regular or irregular	High fever Persistent fever unless the exopathy is eliminated High fever easy to transform heat will be reduced by perspiration
Character of aversion to cold	Mostly without aversion to cold when fever occur, or feel cold and the sensation of cold will relieved by wearing more clothes	Aversion to cold is always accompanied with fever at primary, and unable to be relieved by wearing more clothes

type	Fever due to internal disorder	Fever due to excess pathogens
Accompanied symptoms	Accompanied with symptoms of internal injury and deficiency such as dizziness lassitude shortness of breath no desire to speak spontaneous sweating light sweating fever can't be relieved with perspiration	Accompanied with nasal obstruction runny nose headache
Tongue and pules	Red or pale tongue with purple spots thin or no coating or thick and greasy coating	White or yellow thin coating with floating rapid slippery tense pulse

To differentiate the syndrome of fever, deficiency and excess of the syndrome should be noticed first. For the deficiency type, we should identify the mildness and severity of the deficiency of qi, blood, yin and yang, and which zang-fu organ is injured seriously. For the cases of excess, which is the main complains of qi stagnation, blood stasis or dampness blockage should also be identified. Some notes should be also taken if the syndrome belongs to the pure deficiency type or pure excess type or type of a mixture of deficiency and excess. The changing of the pathology should be paid attention to that if the syndrome transforms from excess to deficiency or as the opposite. All the mentioned above are not difficult to determine by manifestation and medical history. For the second step, the slightness and severity of the situation of the disease should be identified. Generally speaking, if the course of the fever is long, and the treatment is difficult, or the fever is extremely high, or the fever persists, accompanied with symptoms caused by the failure of stomach qi, severe deficiency of vital qi, exhaustion of yang and yin, and these indicated that the situation is severe. It is the basic principle that the treatment is focused on the etiology and pathology of the different type. The treating method such as tonifying yin and clearing away heat, nourishing qi and strengthening the spleen, reinforcing qi and blood, warming yang and tonifying kidney, soothing the liver and regulating the circulation of qi and blood dispersing dampness and clearing away heat are commonly used. Prescriptions with the property of dispersing or formula to purge the pathogenic fire with property of cold and bitter in nature should not be abused when treating the syndrome. For herbs with the property of dispersing is liable to exhaust qi and fluid, herbs with cold flavor and bitter nature will injury yang-qi the middle jiao, or will injury yin if it transform to dryness though they can remove heat and tonify yin when properly used, and the situation will get worse. For the treating of the chronic disease, stomach qi should be paid more attention to. If the fever last a long period and cause the spleen and stomach deficiency, formula of reinforcing is used excessively, and the deficient qi can't transform and transport the nourishing herbs; if herbs of tonifying yin is overused, the transportation of the spleen is obstructed, the dosage, therefore, would rather be small, the treatment should be carried out gradually instead of anxiously, or the situation will get worse.

Ⅱ. Treatment by differentiation of the type of the syndrome

1. Fever due to yin deficiency

Main symptoms: Persistent hectic fever in the afternoon, or fever at night or heat sensation in palms and toes, or hectic fever due to yin deficiency with flushing of zygomatic region.

Accompanied symptoms: Dry mouth, restlessness, insomnia with dreamful sleep, vexation and night sweating, dry feces, yellow small amount of urine

Tongue and pulse: A red dry tongue with cracks with little or without coating, a thready and rapid pulse.

Analysis: Yin deficiency produce internal heat that located in yin system, the water is unable to control the fire, the yin deficiency and yang excess is the pathology. The syndrome characterized by fever accompanied with symptoms of yin deficiency and excess fire. The deficient yin essence leads to excess fire of deficient type, thus hectic fever in the afternoon or fever at night heat sensation in palms and toes, flushing of zygomatic region will present. If the deficient fire burns the upper part of the body and disturb the spirit of the heart, vexation, insomnia with dreamful sleep will occur. The internal heat forces the fluid outward, and night sweating appears. Yin deficiency with fire burning leads to consumption of fluid, then dry mouth and throat, dry feces and small amount of urine will be onset, a red dry tongue with little coating or without coating, a thready and rapid pulse are symptoms of hyperactivity of fire due to yin deficiency.

Treatment: To nourish yin and disperse heat.

Prescription: Modified Qing Gu Powder. This formula can clear away fever of deficiency type and remove hectic fever due to yin-deficiency. Stellaria root, wolfberry bark, picrorhiza rhizome, wind-weed rhizome, sweet wormwood and large-leaf gentian root disperse heat caused by deficiencies and relieve hectic fever. Fresh-water turtle shell provides the effect of replenishing yin, checking exuberance of yang, and moistening dryness. Licorice root acts as the coordination of various effects of the herbs in the recipes. For the patient with night sweating, sweet wormwood should be removed, prepared oyster shell, light wheat should be added to constrict the body surface and check sweating. In case of insomnia, wild jujube seed, arborvitae seed and fleece-flowe stem are used to nourish the heart and calm the mind. If there is obvious yin deficiency, add scrophularia root, dried rehmannia, prepared fleece-flowe root to nourish the yin essence. If signs of qi deficiency also appear, such as lassitude, dizziness and shortness of breath, glehnia root, ophiopogon root and schisandra fruit can be used to tonify qi and yin. If signs of yin deficiency are pronounced, this can be done by prescribing Da Bu Yin Pill, or Zhi Bai Di Huang Pill.

2. Fever due to qi deficiency

Main symptoms: Fever, which could be lower or high, is induced or aggravated by overwork.

Accompanied symptoms: Dizziness, lassitude, spontaneous sweating, shortness of breath, unwilling to speak, susceptibility to common cold, poor appetite, loose stools.

Tongue and pulse: Pale tongue with thin and white coating, and thready weak pulse.

Analysis: Pathology: deficiency of spleen and stomach qi, and upward attacking of yin fire inside. Characteristic of syndrome: fever comes from deficiency of spleen and stomach qi following stress as the result of overwork. Spleen is "the foundation of postnatal life" and "the source for the produce of qi and blood". When the function of spleen and stomach is impaired, giving rise to the malnutrition and malnourishment of Zang-Fu organs, dizziness, lassitude, and shortness of breath can be induced. Deficiency qi can't govern the body surface, there are spontaneous sweat and susceptibility to common cold. The failure of spleen in transportation and transformation is manifested as poor appetite and loose stool. Pale tongue with thin white coating, thready weak pulse are signs of insufficiency of qi.

Treatment: to replenish qi, tonify the spleen to eliminate heat with sweet and warm herbs.

Prescription: Modified Bu Zhong Yi Qi Decoction. The prescription is a representative formula for reinforcing qi and elevating the spleen yang and relieving fever with drugs of sweet flavor and warm nature. In the prescription, astragalus root, pilose asiabell root, bighead atractylodes, licorice root are combined together to replenish qi and reinforce the spleen. Chinese angelica root nourishes yin and promotes blood circulation. Langerine peel regulates qi and the stomach, cimicifuga rhizome and bupleurum root can not only elevates clear yang but also remove heat from interior. For the cases with much spontaneous perspiration, prepared oyster shell, prepared Dragon's bone or light wheat, glutinous rice root should be combined to consolidate exterior and to astringe to suppress sweating. If the patient feels cold and hot by turn with aversion to wind and perspiration, cinnamon twig and white peony root should be used to regulate ying and wei. When fullness in chest and abdomen with a white greasy coating appears, it means the sign of dampness, atractylodes rhizome magnolia bark should be added to invigorate the spleen and eliminate dampness or herbs with aroma in nature like agastache eupatorium should be used to remove dampness. If the dampness intend to turn into dampness heat with the presents of a dry mouth with a thin yellow coating, herbs removing dampness without dry nature such as coix seed, bamboo shavings can be combined

Prescription for example: Pilose asiabell root 10g astragalus root 15g bighead atractvlodes rhizome 10g Chinese angelica root 10g poria 10g bupleurum root 10g cimicifuga rhizome 6g tangerine peel 10g prepared licorice root 5g

3. Fever due to blood deficiency

Main symptoms: Low fever, pale lip and nail, dim and sallow complexion

Accompanied symptoms: Dizziness and dim eye sight, lassitude, palpitation

Tongue and pulse: A pale tongue, a thready and weak pulse.

Analysis: The pathology is that the deficient blood can't inhibit yang. The character is fever with symptoms of blood deficiency. Blood belongs to yin, deficient blood yin is unable to astringe yang thus fever is produced. Deficient blood can't tonify head and eye and limbs, so caused dizziness and lassitude. Blood doesn't nourish the heart, palpitation occurs. If the deficient blood can't replenish the face and the blood vessel isn't filling, as a result, dim and shallow complexion, pale lip and nail, a pale tongue a thready and weak pulse will be onset.

Treatment: to reinforce qi and blood.

Prescription: Modified Gui Pi Decoction. The prescription can nourish the heart and spleen, restore qi and blood, it fit for the syndrome of deficiency of qi and blood of the heart and spleen. In the formula, astragalus root, polose asiabell root, bighead atractylodes rhizome are combined together to tonify qi and the spleen. Chinese angelica root, longan aril are used to nourish blood; wild orspiny jujuba seed, plolygala root can nourish the heart and tranquilize the spirit; costus root can strengthen the spleen and regulate qi. As the resource of qi and blood are the same, in severe cases of blood deficiency, if fever occurs as a result of exhaustion of qi due to hemorrhage, the treatment should comply to the principle that the invisible qi must be arrested immediately as for visible blood is unable to be produced at once. Dang Gui Bu Xue Decoction can severed as basic prescription. Because essence and blood can transform mutually, symptoms of yin and blood deficiency can both present, the treatment should be tonifying yin and blood cooperated with replenishing qi and blood. Modified Ba Zhen Decoction can be used.

Prescription as an example: Astragalus root 20g, pilose asiabell root 10g, poria 10g, bighead atractylodes rhizome 10g, chinese angelica root 10g, plolygala root 10g, white peony root 10g, fleece-flower stem 20g, siberian solomonseal rhizome 20g.

4. Fever due to yang deficiency

Main symptoms: Fever with preference for clothes, cold body with cold limbs.

Accompanied symptoms: Pale complexion, lassitude, aching pain in waist and knees, diarrhea before dawn, retention of urine or micturition.

Tongue and pulses: A pale swollen tongue with teeth markings, a white and greasy coating, a deep thready and weak pulse or a big floating pulse of weakness or big pulse floating in cun gun region but weak in chi region.

Analysis: Pathology: Kidney yang deficiency, and floating outward of the deficiency yang. Characteristic of syndrome: Fever accompanied with symptoms of kidney yang deficiency. The deficient kidney fails to warm the body, thus leads to low fever with preference for clothes, cold body and cold limbs. The head is the location of all yang channel, the waist is the home of kidney. If the kidney yang is deficient, and fails to warm and nourish, symptoms such as dizziness, lassitude, pale complexion will appears. If the kidney yang is insufficient, the yin coldness will be excess before dawn, therefore diarrhea before dawn occurs. The deficient yang fails to warm and transform the fluid and control the function of open and close, retention of urine or frequency of urine will be onset. A pale swollen tongue with tooth markings, a white greasy coating, a deep thready and weak pulse or big floating weak pulse are signs of yang deficiency.

Treatment: To warm yang and tonify the kidney.

Prescription Modified Jin Gui Shen Qi Pill or You Gui Decoction. In the former prescription, Liu Wei Di Huang Pill is used to tonify the kidney yin essence, prepared aconite root cinnamon bark is combined to replenish the fire in the water, warm and nourish kidney yang, promote the kidney qi. Ancient physician considers the prescription as the right formula treating the cold kidney and life gate of deficient type, the excellent method taking the dragon back to the sea. In the later prescription, prepared rhizome of rehmannia, Chinese yam, dogwood fruit, wolfberry fruit cooperate to tonify kidney yin, cinnamon bark, and aconite root work together to warm and nourish kidney yang. To reinforce the middle jiao, prepared licorice root is used. Bark of eucommoa here to strengthen and tonify essence. If deficiency of yang and qi cause the serious shortness of breath and weakness, ginseng and bighead atractylodes rhizome should be added to reinforce the prominary qi. If the fire is unable to produce earth and give rise to the symptom of diarrhea, dried ginger, bighead atractylodes rhizome are needed to warm the middle jiao and nourish the spleen. For the cases with diarrhea before dawn, schisandra fruit and nutmeg should be used to tonify the kidney and astringe the bowel. For the cases who presents frequency of urine or seminal emission, spermatorrhoea, soreness of waist, psoralea fruit, gordon euryale and cherokee rose hip should be added to arrest seminal emission

Prescription for example: Prepared aconite root 10g, cinnamon bark 6g, prepared rhizome of rehmannia 12g, dogwood fruit 10g, poria 10g, oriental water plantain rhizome 10g, Chinese yam 10g, prepared bighead atractylodes rhizome 10g, dodder seed 10g, eucommoa bark 10g.

5. Fever due to liver depression

Main symptoms: a hot sensation in the body with restlessness, fever fluctuates along with the emotions

Accompanied symptoms: Depression, irritability, stuffiness in the chest, distention of the hypochondriac region, sighing, a bitter and dry mouth, irregular menstruation, dysmenorrhea or distending sensation in the breasts.

Tongue and pulse: A thin yellow tongue coating, a taut and rapid pulse.

Analysis: Pathology: stagnant of liver qi, and fire produced by liver qi stagnation. Character of syndrome: fever fluctuates along with the emotions accompanied with the symptoms caused by liver depression and liver qi stagnation. Most patients are females. Liver stores the blood and controls the regulation of qi, prefer for smooth, while its channel dispatch through hypochondriac region and passthrough the diaphragm. If the live qi is stagnant and fail to regulate the circulation of qi that lead to the qi stagnation, therefore depression restlessness irritability, distention and fullness of chest and hypochondriac or irregular menstruation, distention in the breasts will present. As sighing can promote the circulation of qi, so it occurs. The stagnant qi turns into fire and produces fever, which fluctuate along with emotion, accompanied symptoms such as hot sensation inside body, restlessness, a dry and bitter mouth will appear. A thin yellow tongue coating and a taut rapid pulse are signs of attacking of the stagnant liver fire.

Treatment: To soothe the liver, regulate the circulation of qi, clear away heat.

Prescription: Modified Dan Zhi Xiao Yao Powder. The prescription has the function of soothing the liver and regulating the circulation of qi restoring blood and clearing away heat, it's fit for the treatment of syndromes of fever and irregular menstruation caused by liver depression and blood deficiency. In the formula, moutan bark and capejasmine act together to clear away liver heat, bupleurum root peppermint are cooperated to soothe the liver and remove heat; Chinese angelica root, white peony root are combined to nourish blood and liver. Bighead atractylodes rhizome, poria, licorice root are used to replenish the spleen. The excess stagnant fire will to red facial complexion with red eyes, restlessness, irritability, dark urine and constipation, red tongue and rapid pulses. Gentian root, scutellaria root pranella spike, dried rehmannia root should be added to strengthen the function of clearing heat. The modified prescription Long Dan Xie Gan Decoction should also be used to clear away stagnant fire and dampness heat. If the symptoms caused by qi stagnation such as hypochondriac pain and distensible sensation in the breasts, curcuma root, nutgrass flatsedge, Sichuan china berry, green tangerine, orange peel, cory dalis tuber should be added to regulate the circulation of qi and alleviate pain. For the cases accompanied with irregular menstruation, herba lycopi and motherwort should be used to regulate the menstruation and promote blood circulation. In some cases, if the qi stagnation last a long period of time, and the stagnant heat injuries blood or constitutional yin deficiency with liver depression, the modified prescription Zi Shui Qing Gan Decoction should be used to tonify the liver and kidney, soothe the liver and clear away heat. In this formula, Liu Wei Di Huang Pill acts to tonify yin. Dan Zhi Xiao Yao Powder completes the function of soothing the liver, tonifying the blood and clearing away heat. Licorice root and bighead atractylodes rhizome are selected to reduce the dryness of the prescription. The combination of the two formulas is functioning better than either of them. If the stagnant wood restrict the earth, the spleen fails to transport and transform, and the dampness accumulates, manifested as thick and greasy tongue coating, stuffiness in the chest and fullness in the abdomen. Symptoms caused by qi stagnation complicated with dampness heat and phlegm evil may also be onset. For the treatment, Yue Ju Pill or Yue Ju Bao He Pill combined by bupleurum root should be used.

Prescription for example

Moutan bark 10g, capejasmine root 10g, Chinese angelica root 10g, white peony root 10g, poria 12g, bupleurum root 10g peppermint 3g(to be decocted later), curcuma root 10g, scutellaria root 10g.

6. Fever due to blood stasis

Main symptoms: Fever in the afternoon or at night, or hot sensation in part of the body.

Accompanied symptoms: Dry mouth and throat with no desire to drink, pain in the limbs at a fixed location, palpable mass, squarose and dry skin, a dark and sallow complexion, ecchymosis and purple spots in the body.

Tongue and pulse: Bluish purple tongues or tongue with ecchymosis and purple spots, an unsmooth pulse.

Analysis: pathology: Blood stasis and blockage of qi and blood. Characteristic of the syndrome: Fever accompanied with symptoms caused by blood stasis. Blood accumulates inside the body, the flow of qi and blood is restrained, and fever occurs. Since the xue system is diseased and blood is related to yin, fever usually occurs in the afternoon or at night. Stagnant blood blocks qi and blood circulation, thus produce a fixed pain or palpable masses. Heat restrains the ying and blood, a dry mouth and throat, no desire to drink will occur. Stagnant blood prevents the production of new blood, and the head, face and skin are failed to be nourished. Dark complexion and squarose and dry skin. Bluish-purple lips and tongues or tongue with purple spots, unsmooth pulse are further signs of blood stagnation.

Treatment: To activate blood circulation, remove blood stasis and clear away heat.

Prescription: Modified Xue Fu Zhu Yu Decoction. In the formula, Tao Hong Si Wu Decoction can promote blood circulation and remove blood stasis. Si Ni Powder can promote the smooth circulation of qi. Platycodon root which moves upward in qi system, and fruit of citron orange, which moves downward in qi system, are act together to regulate the circulation of blood. Therefore, the prescription can regulate both qi and blood circulation. In the case of severe fever, swallowwort root, moutan bark rhubarb, ground beetle should be added to cool the blood and activate the circulation of blood. In cases of aversion to cold and cold limbs, cinnamon twig should be added to replenish qi and circulate blood. If there are palpable masses in the hypochondrium, Bie Jia Jian Pill should be added to soften hard masses.

If the patient has an identified history of trauma, modified Fu Yuan Ho Xue Decoction should be used.

Prescription for example:

Mirabilite 10g, safflower 10g, Chinese angelica root 10g, prepared rhubarb 6g, bupleurum root 10g, fruit of citron orange 10g, chuan xiong rhizome 10g, red peony root 10g, swallowwort root 10g.

7. Fever due to dampness stagnation

Main symptoms: Low fever, the fever become serious in the afternoon, stuffiness in the chest and fullness in the stomach, a chronic onset.

Accompanied symptoms: No thirst, vomiting after drinking nausea, poor appetite heaviness sensation of the limbs, loose stool or viscid stool.

Tongue and pulse: A white greasy tongue coating or a yellow greasy tongue coating, a soft rapid pulse or deep smooth pulse.

Analysis: pathology: the spleen fails to transport and transform, therefore, dampness evil is produced, and stagnant dampness turns into heat. Character of the symptoms: fever accompanied with symptoms caused by dampness or dampness heat stagnation. The dampness is a yin evil, and it of cause is active in yin time; therefore the fever is serious in the afternoon. For dampness evil has the character of viscosity, the onset, is of course a chronic process. Dampness blocks the circulation of qi, and give rise to stuffiness in chest and fullness in epigastria and abdomen, heaviness sensation the limbs. Accumulation of dampness at the middle jiao leads to poor appetite, or even nausea and vomiting, no thirsty or vomiting after drinking. The failure of transportation and transformation of the spleen result in the downward moving of dampness evil to large bowel, loose stool appears. The accumulated dampness turns into heat and blocks the bowel that leads to viscid stool and difficult feeling to defecate. A white greasy tongue coating and a deep smooth pulse are signs of dampness stagnation. A yellow greasy tongue coating and a soft rapid pulse are symptoms of stagnation dampness turning into dampness heat.

Treatment: To promote the dispersing function of upper jiao and the transforming function of middle jiao, to eliminate dampness and clear away heat.

Prescription: Modified San Ren Decoction. In this formula, bitter apricot kernel promote the dispersing function of the lung and open the upper jiao. katsumadai seed, fragrance in nature, removes dampness evil, regulate the function of middle jiao. Coix seed replenish the spleen and excrete dampness, it can also regulate the function of the lower jiao. Pinellia tuber, magnolia barks are added to eliminate dampness by warming. Ricepaper pith, talc bamboo leaf act together to clear away heat and eliminate dampness. All the drugs combined together to clear away heat. The stagnant dampness turns into fire and obstructs the regulation of Shao yang channel, which give rise to chills and fever like malaria, the cold is mild and the fever is severe, bitter mouth and nausea. Sweet wormwood and scutellaria root should be added to clear away the heat from Shao yang channel, or use Hao Qin Qing Dan Decoction to clear away the dampness heat from the liver and gallbladder. As the stagnation of dampness heat persists, the essence of food stuff can't be transformed regularly, yin deficiency complicated with dampness heat symptoms as dry mouth, red tongue with yellow thick coating will present. Lilyturf root and trichosanthes root, which can tonify yin without producing dampness, should be added in the prescription for eliminating dampness, the modified Huang Qin Hua Shi Decoction combined with sweet wormwood, adenophora root, moutan bark should be used to tonify yin and eliminate dampness.

Prescription for example:

Reed rhizome 30g, talc 12g, scutellaria root 10g, coix seed 20g, bamboo leaf 10g, magnolia bark 6g, katsumadai seed 6g, sweet wormwood 12g, ricepaper pith 3g.

〔Methods for precaution and nursing〕

1. Take precaution to deal with the factors that can cause the fever due to internal disorder, in cases of constitutional weakness, the degree of deficiency of qi, blood, yin and yang should be measured and treated timely to prevent the disease. A proper balance between work and rest should be made ordinarily. Excessive fatigue must be avoided. for the patient who suffer from emotion trauma or blood stasis caused by injury or excessive dampness, the treatment should be aimed at the cause on time.

2. Strengthen the patient's conviction and free his mind of misgivings while serious examination and treatment should be taken. Because the situation of the fever due to internal disorder is usually complex and the duration often last for years. If the patient lack of the confidence or has a heavy burden on his mind, the disease will become serious.

3. Protect the spleen and stomach the patients should take light and nutrious food. The drugs used should protect the function of transformation of the spleen and stomach.

4. Preventing from affection by exopathogen: preventing wind and keep warm, especially for the patients with spontaneous perspiration and night sweating, of which, the wei system will be attacked more easily.

5. Make careful observation and pay more attention to the transformation of the pathology, so as to differentiate and treat the disease more effectively.

〔Typical cases analysis〕

Fever due to yin deficiency. Lu××, female, 20 years old, intellectual,

First visit: august 31, 1976.

The patient suffered a low fever for over one month, which occurs every other day or persists several days. The main symptoms are malar flush, hot sensation in palms and toes, dry mouth and throat. The treatment is ineffective. The diagnosis is lung tuberculosis made by a tuberculosis hospital. In the past few days, the patient presents dry cough with no phlegm, chest pain, night sweating, sourness in the joint, lassitude, insomnia with dreamful sleep, a red tongue with little liquid, a thready pulse. For the differentiation, the lung was burning by heat, and the function of dispersing is impacted, the lung yin is deficient, thus the disease occur, the treating method is tonifying yin and clearing way heat.

Stellaria root 15g, white peony root 20g, wind-weed rhizome 15g, scrophu 15g, fresh water turtle shell 15g, oyster shell 50g.

6 bags decocted with water.

Second visit: September 9, 1976.

The low fever was lured and other symptoms were relieved obviously. Prescriptions should be modified to tonify yin and qi. Rehmannia rhizome 15g, gelhnia root 20g, lilyturf root 15g, pilose asiabell root 20g, schisandra fruit 10g, scrophu 20g, lucid asparagus root 15g, Chinese yam 25g, oyster shell 30g.

6 bags, decocted by water.

The symptoms were disappeared one by one after the patient took the decoction for half a month. The X-ray examination was normal and the patient recovered.

Analysis: this case is a syndrome as《Su Wen Tiao Jing Lun》indicates: deficient yin leads to internal heat. The first step is to treat the superficiality with Qing Gu Powder. The second step is to treat the origin with the complex of Sheng Mai Powder and Zeng Ye Decoction.

Fever due to internal disorder may results of emotion injury, improper diet overstrain, trauma and usually, the manifestation is low fever, the deficiency of qi, blood, yin and yang and dysfunction of the zang-fu organs are the pathology. For clinical differentiation, the fever can be put into two categories, the deficient fever and the excessive fever. The deficient fever can be caused by deficiency of qi, blood, yin and yang. The fever always accompanied with symptoms caused by both qi, blood, yin and yang, or symptoms caused by both deficient qi and blood, yin and blood, qi and yin or yin and yang, the excessive fever includes fever caused by qi stagnancy, blood stasis and dampness stagnation. The fever always accompanied with the symptoms caused by liver depression and liver qi stagnancy, blockage of blood stasis, accumulation of dampness evil. The principle for treatment is that the treating method must be focused on the etiology and pathology of the disease, because human body is a whole unit, fever caused by various kinds of pathogenesis often related to each other, or transform mutually or coexist at the same time. Different kinds of fever must be recognized and treated according to the view of developing and integrating. It's incorrect to consider a prolonged fever as a fever caused by internal disorder. For the treatment, it is also unsuitable to use drugs of pungent flavor or bitter flavor with cold nature, which will make many malpractice.

Because the situation of the fever due to internal disorder is complicated, and causes of the disease is unclear, and frequently the disease lasts few more years or attacks repeatedly. It is more important to make a careful observation, pay attention to the transformation of the pathogenesis, and to adjust the treating plan in time. If the patient strike a proper balance between work and rest, take an optimistic attitude, take a light and easily digested food with rich nutrition, prevent from exopathic diseases, all these will make the treating more effective.

Questions for Review

1. What is the definition of fever due to internal disorder?
2. Try to expound the etiology and pathology of the disease?
3. How to differentiate the fever due to internal disorder from fever due to exopathic attack?
4. How many types do the fever due to internal disorder include? What is the key point of differentiation, treating method and commonly used prescription?
5. What should be pay attention to when treating the disease by differentiation?

Prescriptions in the Book

No	NAME	SOURCE BOOK	COMPOSITION OF THE PRESCRIPTION
1	A Wei Extract	Jing Yue Quan Shu	notopterygium root, pubescent angelica root, scophularia root, red peony root, pangolin scales, storax oil, fresh rehmannia gastrodia tuber, safflower, musk, mirabilite, asafetida, frankincense, myrrh, etc.
2	An Gong Niu Huang Pill	Wen Bing Tiao Bian	cow-bezoare, curcuma root, rhinoceros horn, coptis root, cinnabar, borneol, Concha Margaritiferajusta, Gardenia Jasminoides, realgar, suctellaria root, musk, etc.
3	An Shen Ding Zhi Pill	Yi Xue Xin Wu	poria, poria with host wood, polygala root, ginseng, glassleaved sweetflag, dragon's teeth
4	Ba Zhen Decoction	Zheng Ti Lei Yao	ginseng, bighead atractylodes rhizome, poria, liquorice, Chinese angelica root, white peony root, chuanxiong rhizome, prepared rehmannia root, fresh ginger, Chiness-date
5	Ba Zheng Powder	Tai Ping Hui Min He Ji Ju Fang	Caulis Aristolochiae Manshuriensis, Plantain seed, Prostrate Rnotweed, Chinese pink herb, tale, liquorice tip, Rhubarb, Gardenia Jasminoides, rush pith
6	Bai Bu Jian Ji Decoction	Yan Fang	stemona root
7	Bai He Gu Jin Pill	Yi Fang Ji Jie Yin Zhao Ji An Fang	dried rehmannia root, prepared rehmannia root, ophiopogon root, sichuan fritillary bulb, lily bulb, Chinese angelica root, baked peony root, liquorice, scrophularia root, platycodon root

No	NAME	SOURCE BOOK	COMPOSITION OF THE PRESCRIPTION
8	Bai Hu Decoction	Bai Hu Tang	Anemarrhena asphodeloides, gypsum, prepared liquorice, stalk rice
9	Bai Hu Jia Gui Zhi Decoction	Jin Gui Yao Lue	Anemarrhena asphodeloides, gypsum, liquorice, stalk rice, cinnamom twig
10	Bai Hu Jia Ren Shen Decoction	Shang Han Lun	Anemarrhena asphodeloides, gypsum, liquorice, stalk rice, ginseng
11	Bai Jin Pill	Yan Fang	alum, curcuma root
12	Bai Tou Weng Decoction	Shang Han Lun	pulsatilla root, ash bark, coptis root, phellodendron bark
13	Bai Ye Decoction	Jin Gui Yao Lue	biota tops, dried ginger, argyi leaf, etc.
14	Ban Liu Pill	Tai Ping Hui Min He Ji Ju Fang	pinellia tuber, Sulphur
15	Ban Xia Bai Zhu Tian Ma Decoction	Yi Xue Xin Wu	pinellia tuber, bighead atractylodes rhizome, gastrodia tuber, tangerine peel, poria, liquorice, fresh ginger, Chinese-date
16	Ban Xia Hou Po Decoction	Jin Gui Yao Lue	pinellia tuber, magnolia bark, perilla frutescens, poria, fresh ginger
17	Ban Xia Xie Xin Decoction	Shang Han Lun	pinellia tuber, scutellaria root, dried ginger, ginseng, prepared liquorice, coptis root, Chiness-date
18	Ban Xia Zhu Mi Decoction	Nei Jing	pinellia tuber, etc.
19	Bao He Pill	Dan Xi Xin Fa	medicated leaven, hawthorn fruit, poria, pinellia tuber, tangerine peel, forsythia fruit, radish seed

No	NAME	SOURCE BOOK	COMPOSITION OF THE PRESCRIPTION
20	Bao Yuan Decoction	Qing Ai Xin Jian	ginseng astragalus root, bark of Chinese cassia tree, liquorice, fresh ginger
21	Bie Jia Jian Pill	Jin Gui Yao Lue	fresh-water turtle shell, scutellaria root, buplearum root, pillb driedug, dried ginger, Rhubarb, peony root, cinnamom twig, cimicifuga rhizome, Pyrrosia Leaf, magnolia bark, moutan bark, Chinese pink herb, Campsis Grandiflora, pinellia tuber, ginseng, ground beetle, donkey-hide gelatin, hornet, nestpeach kernel etc.
22	Bu Fei Decoction	Yong Lei Qian Fang	ginseng, astragalus root, prepared rehmannia root, schisandra fruit, Aster Tataricus, mulberry bark
23	Bu Gan Decoction	Yi Zong Jin Jian	Chinese angelica root, white peony root, Chuanxiong rhizome, prepared rehmannia root, jujuba seed, chaenoleles fruit, prepared liquorice
24	Bu Qi Yun Pi Decoction	Tong Zhi Fang	ginseng, bighead atrctylodes rhizome, poria, liquorice, astragalus root, tangerine peel, amomum fruit, pinellia tuber, fresh ginger, Chinese-date
25	Bu Tian Da Zao Pill	Yi Xue Xin Wu	ginseng, bighead atractylodes rhizome, Chinese angelica root, jujuba seed, prepared astragalus root, polygala root, white peony root, Chinese yam, poria wolfberry fruit, Placenta Hominis, tortoise plastron, anter, prepared rehmannia root
26	Bu Yang Huan Wu Decoction	Yi Lin Gai Cuo	Chinese angelica root, Chuanxiong rhizome, astragalus root, peach kernel, earthworm, red peony root, safflower

No	NAME	SOURCE BOOK	COMPOSITION OF THE PRESCRIPTION
27	Bu Zhong Yi Qi Decoction	Pi Wei Lun	ginseng, astragalus root, bighead atractylodes rhizome, liquorice, Chinese angelica root, tangerine peel, cimiciguga rhizome, bupleurum root
28	Cang Zhu Er Chen Decoction	Za Bing Yuan Liu Xi Zhu	atractylodes rhizome, bighead atractylodes rhizome, poria, tangerine peel, liquorice, pinellia tuber
29	Chai Hu Bai Hu Decoction	Chong Ding Tong Cu Shang Han Lun	bupleurum root, gypsum, trichosanthes root, stalk rice, scutellaria root, Anemarrhena Asphodeloides, liquorice, fresh lotus leaf
30	Chai Hu Gui Zhi Gan Jiang Decoction	Shang Han Lun	bupleurum root, cinnamom twig, dried ginger, scutellaria root, trichosanthes root, oyster shell, prepared liquorice
31	Chai Hu Qing Gu Powder	Yi Zong Jin Jian	large-leaf gentian root, fresh-water turtle shell, bupleurum root, wolfberry bark, sweet wormwood, Anemarrhena Asphodeloides, picrorhiza rhizome, macrostem onion, liquorice, trildren's urine, pig's spinal cord, pig's bile
32	Chai Hu Shu Gan Powder	Jing Yue Quan Shu	bupleurum root, nutgrass flatsedge rhizome, chuanxiong rhizome, Liquorice, white peony root, and fructus citri auratil.
33	Chai Hu Si Wu Decoction	Su Wen Bing Ji Qi Yi Bao Ming Ji	chuanxiong rhizome, prepared rehmannia root, Chinese angelica root, peony, bupleurum root, ginseng, scutellaria root, liquorice, pinellia tuber, yeast
34	Chai Zhi Ban Xia Decoction	Yi Xue Ru Men	bupleurum root, scutellaria root, pinellia tuber, trichosanthes seed, Fructus Aurantii, platycodon root, bitter apricot kernel, green tangerine orange peel, liquorice

No	NAME	SOURCE BOOK	COMPOSITION OF THE PRESCRIPTION
35	Chen Xiang Jiang Qi Powder	Zhang Shi Yi Tong	eagle wood, amomum fruit, liquorice, nutgrass flatsedge rhizome, Sichuan chinaberry, corydalis tuber
36	Chen Xiang Powder	Jin Gui Yi	eagle wood, Pyrrosia Leaf, tale, Chinese angelica root, tangerine peel, white peony root, Semen Malvae, liquorice, Vaccaria Segetales
37	Cheng Shi Bi Xie Fen Qing Drink	Yi Xue Xin Wu	seven-lobed yam, plantain seed, poria, lotus plumule, gastrodia tuber, phellodendron bark, red sage root, bighead atractylodes rhizome
38	Chu Bi Powder	Yi Xue Xin Wu	asarum herb, Gladitsia Sinensis, pinellia tuber
39	Chuan Xiong Cha Tiao Powder	Tai Ping Hui Min He Ji Ju Fang	chuanxiong rhizome, schizonepeta, peppermint, notopterygium root, asarum herb, (or nutgrass flatsedge rhizome), dahurian angelica root, liquorice, ledebouriella root
40	Chen Yang Zheng Qi Pill	Cheng Yao	tangerine peel, cloves, poria, lance atractylodes rhizome, bighead atractylodes rhizome, agastache, prepared pinellia tuber, bark of Chinese cassia tree, dutchmanspipe root, pepertree leaf, Hongling pellet
41	Chun Ze Decoction	Yi Fang Ji Jie	bighead atractylodes rhizome, cinnamom twig, Umbellate Pore, Alisma Orientale, poria, ginseng
42	Cong Bai Qi Wei Drink	Wai Tai Mi Yao	Chinese green onion, pueraria root, ophiopogon root, dried rehmannia root, fermented soya beans, fresh ginger, etc.

No	NAME	SOURCE BOOK	COMPOSITION OF THE PRESCRIPTION
43	Cong Chi Decoction	Zhou Hou Bei Ji Fang	Chinese greenonion, fermented soya beans, (or) pueraria root, cimicifuga rhizome, (or) ephedra
44	Cong Chi Jie Geng Decoction	Tong Su Shang Han Lun	Chineses green oniom, fermented soya beans, notopterygium root, forsythia fruit, Ganminoides, Tamarisk Tops, platycodon root, liquorice
45	Da Ban Xia Decoction	Jin Gui Yao Lue	pinellia tuber, ginseng, white honey
46	Da Bu Yin Pill	Dan Xi Xin Fa	Anemarrhena asphodeloides, phellodendron bark, prepared rehmannia root, tortoise plastron, pig spinal cord
47	Da Bu Yuan Jian	Jing Yue Quan Shu	ginseng, baked Chinese yam, prepared rehmannia root, eucommia bark, wolfberry fruit, Chinese angelica root, dogwood fruit, prepared liquorice
48	Da Chai Hu Decoction	Shang Han Lun	bupleurum root, scutellaria root, pinellia tuber, Immature Bitter Orange, white peony root, rhubarb root, fresh ginger, and Chinese dates
49	Da Cheng Qi Decoction	Shang Han Lun	Rhubarb, magnolia bark, Immature Bitter Orange, mirabilite
50	Da Ding Feng Zhu	Wen Bing Tiao Bian	white peony root, donkey-hide gelatin, fresh tortoise plastron, dried rehmannia root, hemp seed, schisandra fruit, fresh oyster shell, ophiopogon root, prepared liquorice, egg ylok, fresh-water turtle shell
51	Da Huang Fu Zi Decoction	Jin Gui Yao Lue	Rhubarb, prepared aconite root, asarum herb

No	NAME	SOURCE BOOK	COMPOSITION OF THE PRESCRIPTION
52	Da Huang Gan Cao Decoction	Jin Gui Yao Lue	Rhubarb, liquorice
53	Da Huang Xiao Shi Decoction	Jin Gui Yao Lue	Rhubarb, phellodendron bark, cape-jasmine, etc.
54	Da Huang Zhe Chong Decoction	Jin Gui Yao Lue	Resina Toxicodendrin, dried rehmannia root, liquorice, leech, white peony root, bitter apricot kernel, scutellaria root, peach kernel, gradfly, Rhubarb, etc.
55	Da Jian Zhong Decoction	Jin Gui Yao Lue	pepertree, dried ginger, ginseng, maltose
56	Da Qi Qi Decoction	Yi Xue Ru Men	green tangerine orange peel, tangerine peel, platycodon root, agastache, liquorice, burreed tuber, zedoary, nutgrass flatsedge rhizome, bitter cardamon, fresh ginger, Chinese-date, etc.
57	Da Qin Jiao Decoction	Su Wen Bing Ji Qi Yi Bao Ming Ji	large-leaf gentian root, Chinese angelica root, liquorice, notoptery gium root, ledebouriella, dahurian angelica root, prepared rehmannia root, poria, gypsam, Chuanxiong rhizome, white peony root, pubescent angleica root, scutellaria root, dried rehmanni a root bighead atractylodes rhizome asarum herb
58	Da Qing Long Decoction	Shang Han Lun	ephedra, bitter apricot kernel, cinnamom twig, liquorice, gypsum, fresh ginger, Chiness-date
59	Dai Di Dang Pill	Zheng Zhi Zhun Sheng	Rhubarb, Chinese angdica root, dried rehmannia root, peach kernel, bark of Chinese cassia tree
60	Dai Ha Powder	Yan Fang	natural indigo, clam shell
61	Dan Shen Drink	Yi Zong Jin Jian	red sage root, sandalwood, amomum fruit

No	NAME	SOURCE BOOK	COMPOSITION OF THE PRESCRIPTION
62	Dan Zhi Xiao Yao Powder	Yi Tong	Chinese angelica root, white peony root, bighead atractylodes rhizome, bupleurum root, poria, liquorice, ginger, peppermint, moutan bark, pittosporm root
63	Dang Gui Bu Xue Decoction	Nei Wai Shang Bian Huo Lun	astragalus root, Chinese angelica root
64	Dang Gui Liu Huang Decoction	Lan Shi Mi Cang	Chinese angelica root, dried rehmannia root, prepared rehmannia root, coptis root, scutellaria root, phellodendron bark, astragalus root
65	Dang Gui Long Hui Pill	Xuan Ming Lun Fang	Chinese angelica root, gentian root, Gardenia Jasminoides, coptis root, scutellaria root, phellodendron bark, Rhubarb, natural indigo, aloes, auchlandia root, musk
66	Dang Gui Shao Yao Powder	Jin Gui Yao Lue	Chinese angelica root, peony root, poria, bighead atractylodes rhizome, Alisma Orientale, chuanxiong rhizome
67	Dao Chi Powder	Xiao Er Yao Zheng Zhi Jue	dried rehmannia root, Akebia Trifoliata, Lophatherum, liquorice
68	Dao Tan Decoction	Ji Sheng Fang	pinellia tuber, tangerine peel, Immature Bitter Orange, poria, liquorice, prepared arisaema tuber
69	Di Huang Yin Zi	Xuan Ming Lun	dried rehmannia root, morinda root, dogwood fruit, dendrobium, desertliving cistanche, schisandra fruit, bark of Chinese cassia tree, poria, ophiopogon root, prepared aconite root, grassleaved sweetflag rhizome, polygala root, fresh ginger, Chiness-date peppermint

No	NAME	SOURCE BOOK	COMPOSITION OF THE PRESCRIPTION
70	Di Tan Decoction	Ji Sheng Fang	prepared pinellia tuber, prepared arisaema tuber, tangerine peel, Immature Bitter Orange, poria, ginseng, grassleaved sweetflag rhizome, Caulis Bambasae in Taeniam, liquorice, fresh ginger
71	Di Yu Powder	Yan Fang	sanguisorba root, rubia root, scutellaria root, Gardenia Jasminoides, poria
72	Dian Kuang Meng Xing Decoction	Yi Lin Gai Cuo	peach kernel, pupleurum root, nutgrass flatsedge, Caulis Aristolochiae Manshuriensis, red peony root, pinellia tuber, shell of areca nut, green tangerine orange peel, tangerine peel, mulberry bark, liquorice, etc.
73	Ding Chen Tou Ge Powder	Tai Ping Hui Min He Ji Ju Fang	bighead atractylodes rhizome, nutgrass flatsedge rhizome, ginseng, amomum fruit, cloves, germinated barley, aucklandia root, nutmeg, medicated leaven, prepared liquorice, eagle wood, green tangerine orange peel, magnolia bark, agastache, tangerine peel, pinellia tuber tsaoko
74	Ding Chuan Decoction	She Sheng Zhong Miao Fang	gingko nut, ephedra, mulberry bark, coltsfoot flower, pinellia tuber, bitter apricot kernel, perilla fruit, scutellaria root, liquorice
75	Ding Xian Pill	Yi Xue Xin Wu	gastrodia tuber, Sichuan fritillary bulb, arisaema with bile, prepared pinellia tuber

No	NAME	SOURCE BOOK	COMPOSITION OF THE PRESCRIPTION
76	Ding Xiang Powder	Gu Jin Yi Tong	cloves, kaki calyx, galangal rhizome, prepared liquorice
77	Ding Zhi Pill	Bei Ji Qian Qin Yao Fang	dangshen, poria with hostwood, grassleaved sweetflag rhizome, polygala root, liquorice, poria, bighead atractylodes rhizome, ophiopogon root
78	Du Huo Ji Sheng Decoction	Bei Ji Qian Jin Yao Fang	pubescent angelica root, loranthus mulberry mistletoe, large-leaf gentian root, ledebouriella root, asarum herb, Chinese angelica root, peony, chuanxiong rhizome, dried rehmannia root, eucommia bark, achyranthes root, ginseng, poria, liquorice, bark of Chinese cassia tree
79	Du Shen Decoction	Jing Yue Quan Shu	ginseng
80	Er Chen Decoction	Tai Ping Hui Min He Ji Ju Fang	pinellia tuber, tangerine peel, poria, prepared liquorice
81	Er Dong Decoction	Yi Xue Xin Wu	lucid asparagus (root), ophiopogon root, trichosanthes root, scutellaria root, Anemarrhena Asphodeloides, liquorice, ginseng, lotus leaf
82	Er Miao Pill	Dan Xi Xin Fa Xi Zhuo	phellodendron bark, atractylodes rhizome
83	Er Shen Powder	Za Bing Yuan Liu Xi Zhu	climbing fern spore, talc
84	Er Xian Decoction	Zhong Yi Fang Ji Lin Chuang Shou Ce	curculigo rhizome, epinedium, morinda root, phellodendron bark, Anemarrhena Asphodeloides, Chinese angelica root

No	NAME	SOURCE BOOK	COMPOSITION OF THE PRESCRIPTION
85	Er Yin Jian Decoction	Jing Yue Quan Shu	dried rehmannia root, ophiopogon root, date seed, fresh liquorice, scrophularia root, poria, Caulis Aristolochiae Manshuriensis, rush pith, Tamarisk Tops, coptis root, Lophatherum
86	Er Zhi Wan	Yi Fang Ji Jie	glossy privet fruit, eclipta
87	Fang Feng Decoction	Xuan Ming Lun Fang	ledebouriella root, Chinese angelica root, red poria, bitter apricot kernel, scutellaria root, large-leafgentian root, pueraria root, ephedra, bark of Chinese cassia tree, fresh ginger, liquorice, Chinese-date
88	Fang Feng Tong Sheng Powder	Xuan Ming Lun Fang	ledebouriella root, chuanxiong rhizome, Chinese angelica root, peony, Rhubarb, mirabilite, forsythia fruit, pepper mint, ephedra, gypsum, platycodon root, scutellaria root, atractylodes rhizome, capejasmine, schizonepeta spike, tale, liquorice, fresh ginger
89	Fang Ji Huang Qi Decoction	Jin Gui Yao Lue	tetrandra root, bighead atractylodes rhizome, astragalus root, liquorice, ginger, Chinese-date
90	Fu Yuan Huo Xue Decoction	Yi Xue Fa Ming	bupleurum root, trichosanthes root, Chinese angelica root, safflower, liquorice, pangolin scales, Rhubarb, peach kernel
91	Fu Zi Geng Mi Decoction	Jin Gui Yao Lue	prepared aconite root, stalk rice, pinellia tuber, liquorice, Chinese-date

No	NAME	SOURCE BOOK	COMPOSITION OF THE PRESCRIPTION
92	Fu Zi Li Zhong Pill	Tai Ping Hui Min He Ji Ju Fang	prepared aconite root, ginseng, bighead atractylodes rhizome, prepared ginger, prepared liquorice
93	Fu Zi Xie Xin Decoction	Shang Han Lun	Rhubarb, coptis root, scutellaria root, prepared aconite root
94	Gan Cao Gan Jiang Decoction	Jin Gui Yao Lue	liquorice, dried ginger
95	Gan Cao Xie Xin Decoction	Shang Han Lun	prepared liquorice, scutellaria root, Chinese-date, dried ginger, pinellia tuber, coptis root, ginseng
96	Gan Lu Xiao Du Pellet	Wen Re Jing Wei	tale, oriental wormwood, scutellaria root, grassleaved sweetflag, Sichuan fritillary bulb, Caulis Aristolochiae Manshuriensis, agastache, belamcanda rhizome, forsythia fruit, peppermint, etc.
97	Gan Mai Da Zao Decoction	Jin Gui Yao Lue	liquorice, Triticum Aestivum, Chinese-date
98	Gan Sui Ban Xia Decoction	Jin Gui Yao Lue	kansui root, pinellia tuber, peony, liquorice
99	Gao Lin Decoction	Yi Xue Zhong Zhong Can Xi Lu	Chinese yam, gordom euryale seed, dragon's bone, oystershell, dried rehmannia root, dangshen, white peony root
100	Ge Gen Decoction	Shang Han Lun	pueraria root, ephedra, cinnamom twig, fresh ginger, liquorice, peony root, Chiness-date
101	Ge Gen Qin Lian Decoction	Shang Han Lun	pueraria root, scutellaria root, coptis root, prepared liquorice

No	NAME	SOURCE BOOK	COMPOSITION OF THE PRESCRIPTION
102	Ge Xia Zhu Yu Decoction	Yi Lin Gai Cuo	trogopterus dung, Chinese angelica root, chuanxiong rhizome, peach kernel, moutan bark, red peony root, lindera root, corydalis tuber, liquorice, nutgrass flatsedge rhizome, safflower, Immature Bitter Orange
103	Geng Yi Pill	Xian Xing Zhai Yi Xue Guang Bi Ji	aloes, cinnabar
104	Gua Lou Gui Zhi Decoction	Jin Gui Yao Lue	trichosanthes root, cinnamom twig, peony, liquorice, fresh ginger, Chinese-date
105	Gua Lou Xie Bai Bai Jiu Decoction	Jin Gui Yao Lue	trichosanthes fruit, macrostem onion, alcohol
106	Gua Lou Xie Bai Ban Xia Decoction	Jin Gui Yao Lue	trichosanthes fruit, macrostem onion, alcohol, pinellia tuber
107	Gui Pi Decoction	Ji Sheng Fang	pilose asiabell root, astragalus root, bighead atractylodes rhizome, poria with hostwood, wild or sping jujuba seed, longan aril, aucklandia root, prepared liquorice, Chinese angelica root, polygala root, fresh ginger, Chiness-date
108	Gui Zhi Decoction	Shang Han Lun	cinnamom twig, peony, fresh ginger, prepared liquorice, Chinese-date
109	Gui Zhi Fu Ling Pill	Jin Gui Yao Lue	cinnamom twig, poria, moutan bark, baked peach kernel, peony
110	Gui Zhi Gan Cao Long Gu Mu Li Decoction	Shang Han Lun	cinnamom twig, prepared liquorice, dragon's bone, oyster shell

No	NAME	SOURCE BOOK	COMPOSITION OF THE PRESCRIPTION
111	Gui Zhi Jia Hou Pu Xing Ren Decoction	Shang Han Lun	cinnamom twig, peony, prepared liquorice, fresh ginger, Chinese-date, magnolia bark, bitter apricot kernel
112	Gui Zhi Shao Yao Zhi Mu Decoction	Jin Gui Yao Lue	cinnamom twig, peony, prepared liquorice, ephedra, bighead atractylodes rhizome, Anemarrhena Asphodeloides, ledebouriella root, prepared aconite root, fresh ginger
113	Guo Min Jian Decoction	Yan Fang	bupleurum root, white peony root, ledebouriella, black plum
114	Hua Gan Jian	Jing Yue Quan Shu	green tangerine orange peel, tangerine peel, peony root, moutan bark, capejasmine, Alisma Orientale, fritillary bulb
115	He Che Da Zao Pill	Fu Shou Jing Fang	Placenta Hominis, prepared rehmannia root, eucommia bark, lucid asparagus, ophiopogon root, tortoise plastron, phellodendron bark, achyranthes root
116	Hei Xi Pellet	Tai Ping Hui Min He Ji Ju Fang	Heixi Pellet, sulphur, sichuan chinaberry, fenugreek seed, auchlandia root, prepared aconite root, untmeg, actinolite, eagle wood, Fructus Foeniculi, bark of Chinese cassia tree, psoralea fruit
117	Hu Qian Pill	Dan Xi Xin Fa	tortoise plastron, phellodendron bark, Anemarrhena Asphodeloides, prepared rehmannia, white peony root, cynomorium, tangerine peel, tiger bone, dried ginger

No	NAME	SOURCE BOOK	COMPOSITION OF THE PRESCRIPTION
118	Hua Ji Pill	Lei Zheng Zhi Cai	burreed tuber, zedoary, asafetida oscostaziae, nutgrass flatsedge rhizome, realgar, areca seed, sappan wood, ark shell, trogopterus dung
119	Huai Jiao Pill	Dan Xi Xin Fa	sophora fruit, sanguisorba root, scutellaria root, Chinese angelica root, Immature Bitter Orange, ledebouriella root
120	Huang Bing Jiang Fan Pill	Yan Fang	magnolia bark, lance atractylodes, tangerine peel, liquorice, Chinese-date
121	Huang Lian E Jiao Decoction	Shang Han Lun	coptis root, donkey-hide gelatin, scutellaria root, yolk, peony
122	Huang Lian Jie Du Decoction	Zhong Yao Zhi Ji Shou Ce	scutellaria root, coptis root, phellodendron bark, capejasmine, cimicifuga rhizome, honeysuckle flower, ledebouriella root, baked arctium fruit, rhubarb, Chinese angelica root, red peony root, liquorice
123	Huang Lian Qin xin Drink	Shen Shi Zun Sheng Shu	coptis root, fresh rehmannia root, Chinese angelica root, liquorice, jujuba seed, poria with hostwood, polygala root, ginseng, lotus seed
124	Huang Lian Shang Qing Pill	Gu Jin Yi Fang Ji Cheng	sculellaria root, coptis root, phellodendron bark, capejasmine, chrysanthemum flower, platycodon root, peppermint, chuanxiong rhizome, rhubard, forsythia fruit, Chinese angelica root, pueraria root, scrophularia root, pollen, turmeria

No	NAME	SOURCE BOOK	COMPOSITION OF THE PRESCRIPTION
125	Huang Lian Wen Dan Decoction	Qian Qin Fang	pinellia tuber, tangerine peel, poria, liquorice, Immature Bitter Orange, Caulis Bambusae in Taeniam, coptis root, Chinese-date
126	Huang Lian Xiang Ru Drink	Lei Zheng Huo Ren Shu	coptis root, elscholtzia, magnolia bark
127	Huang Qi Bie Jia Powder	Wei Sheng Bao Jian	astragalus root, fresh-water turtle shell, lucid asparagus, wolfberry bark, large-leaf gentian root, bupleurum root, Aster Tataricus, pinellia tuber, poria, Anemarrhena Asphodeloides, fresh rehmannia root, white peony root, mulberry bark, ginseng, bark of Chinese cassia tree, platycodon root, liquorice
128	Huang Qi Decoction	Ji Gui Yi	astragalus root, tangerine peel, hemp seed, white honey
129	Huang Qi Jian Zhong Decoction	Jin Gui Yao Lue	astragalus root, white peony root, cinnamom twig, prepared liquorice, fresh ginger, Chinese-date, maltose
130	Huang Qi Liu Yi Decoction	Tai Ping Hui Min He Ji Ju Fang	astragalus root, liquorice
131	Huang Qin Hua Shi Decoction	Wen Bing Tiao Bian	scutellaria root, tale, Umbellate Pore, poria peel, shell of areca nut, round cardamon seed, rice paper pith
132	Huang Tu Decoction	Jin Gui Yao Lue	loess in stor, liquorice, dried rehmannia root, bighead atractylodes rhizome, prepared aconite root, donkey-hide gelatin, scutellaria root

No	NAME	SOURCE BOOK	COMPOSITION OF THE PRESCRIPTION
133	Huo Ren Bai Du Powder	Nan Yang Huo Ren Shu	ginseng, notopterygium root, pubescent angelica root, root of purple-flowered peucedanum, bupleurum root, chuanxiong rhizome, Fructus Aurantii, platycodon root, poria, prepared liquorice, fresh ginger
134	Huo Xiang Zheng Qi Powder	Tai Ping Hui Min He Ji Ju Fang	agastache, Perilla Frutescens, dahurian angelica root, plagycodon root, bighead atractylodes rhizome, magnolia bark, pinellia tuber, shellof areca nut, poria, tangerine peel, liquorice, Chiness-date
135	Ji Chuan Jian	Jing Yue Quan Shu	Chinese angelica root, achyranthes root, desertliving cinstanche, Alisma Orientale, cimicifuga rhizome, Fructus Aurantii
136	Ji Jiao Li Huang Pill	Jin Gui Yao Lue	tetrandra root, lepidium seed, Rhubarb, etc.
137	Ji Sheng Shen Qi Pill	Ji Sheng Fang	rehmannia root, Chinese yam, dogwood fruit, moutan bark, poria, Alisma Orientale, prepared aconite root, cinnamom twig, achyranthes root, plantain seed
138	Jia Jian Cheng Qi Decoction	Yan Fang	Rhubarb, Immature Bitter Orange, phlogopite, Gleditsia Sinensis, Pig's bile enema, vinegar, etc.
139	Jia Jian Wei Rui Decoction	Tong Su Shang Han Lun	fragrant solomonseal rhizome, Chinese green onion, platycodon root, swallowwort root, peppermint, prepared liquorice, Chiness-date, prepared sogbean
140	Jia Jian Xie Bai Powder	Yi Xue Fa Ming	mulberry bark, wolfberry bark, stalk rice, liquorice, green tangerine orange peel, tangerine peel, schisandra fruit, ginseng, white poria

No	NAME	SOURCE BOOK	COMPOSITION OF THE PRESCRIPTION
141	Jia Wei Er Miao Powder	Dan Xi Xin Fa	scutellaria root, atractylodes rhizome, Chinese angelica root, achyranthes root, tetrandra root, seven-lobed yam, tortoise plastron
142	Jia Wei Gan Mai Da Zao Decoction	Fu Ke Ji Yao	liquorice, Triticum, Chiness-date, peony root, Fluoritum
143	Jia Wei Jie Geng Decoction	Yi Xue Xin Wu	platycodon root, liquorice, sichuan fritillary bulb, red tangerine peel, honeysuckle flower, coix seed, lepidium seed, hyacintybletilla
144	Jia Wei Jin Gang Pill	Yan Fang	morinda root, eucommia bark desertliving cistanche, epimedium, dodderseed, chaenomeles fruit, phellodendron bark, gastrodia tuber, centipedefern, batryticated silkworm, black snake, seven-lobed yam, cuttle-bone, etc.
145	Jia Wei Qing Wei Powder	Zhang Shi Yi Tong	dried rehmannia root, moutan bark, Chinese angelica root, coptis root, forsythia fruit, rhinoceros horn, cimicifuga rhizome, fresh liquorice
146	Jia Wei Si Jin Decoction	San Yin Ji Yi Bing Zheng Fang Lun	desertliving cistanche, achyranthes root, dodder seed, chaenomdes fruit, pilose antler, prepared rehmannia root, gastrodia tuber, schisandra fruit
147	Jia Wei Si Jun Zi Decoction	San Yin Fang	ginseng, poria, bighead atractylodes rhizome, prepared liquorice, astragalus root, white hyaciath bean
148	Jia Wei Si Wu Decoction	Jin Gui Yi	white peony root, Chinese angelica root, dried rehmannia root, chuanxiong rhizome, chastetree fruit, chrysanthemum flower, scutellaria root, liquorice

No	NAME	SOURCE BOOK	COMPOSITION OF THE PRESCRIPTION
149	Jia Wei Ze Xie Decoction	Yan Fang	Alisma Orientale, bighead atractylodes rhizome, uncaria, stem with hooks, Conchamargaritlfera wsta, achyranthes root, etc.
150	Jiao Mu Gua Lou Decoction	Yi Chun Sheng Yi	Fructus Trichosanthis Seed, cimicifuga rhizome, mulberry bark, perilla fruit, pinellia tuber, poria, red tangerine peel, tribulus fruit, fresh ginger
151	Jiao Tai Pill	Han Shi Yi Tong	coptis root, bark of Chinese cassia tree
152	Jie Geng Bai Powder	Wai Tai Mi Yao	platycodon root, fritillary bulb, croton seed
153	Jie Geng Xing Ren Jian Decoction	Jing Yue Quan Shu	platycodon root, bitter apricot kernel, liquorice, honeysuckle flower, fritillary bulb, Fructus Aurantii, sargentgloryvine, forsythia fruit, prunella spike, lily bulb, ophiopogon root, donkey-hide gelatin
154	Jie Yu Pellet	Yi Xue Xin Wu	ginant typhenium tuber, glassleaved sweetlag, polygala root, gastrodia tuber, scorpion, notopterygium root, arisaema tuber, aucklandia root, liquorice
155	Jin Bo Zhen Xin Pill	Tai Ping Hui Min He Ji Ju Fang	Placenta Hominis Chinese yam, prepared liquorice, ginseng, poria, cinnabar, borneol musk, etc
156	Jin Fo Cao Powder	Tai Ping Hui Min He Ji Ju Fang	inula flower, ephedra, root of purpleflowerd peucedanum, schizonepeta spike, prepared liquorice, prepared pinellia tuber, red peony root, fresh ginger, Chinese-date

No	NAME	SOURCE BOOK	COMPOSITION OF THE PRESCRIPTION
157	Jin Gui Shen Qi Pill	Jin Gui Yao Lue	cinnamom twig, prepared aconite root, prepared rehmannia root, dogwood fruit, Chinese yam, poria, moutan bark, Alisma Orientale
158	Jin Ling Zi Powder	Su Wen Bing Ji Qi Yi Bao Ming Ji	Sichuan chin berry, corydalis tuber
159	Jin Shui Liu Jun Jian	Jing Yue Quan Shu	Chinese angelica root, poria, pinellia tuber, prepared rehmannia, tangerine peel, prepared liquorice, fresh ginger
160	Jin Suo Gu Jing Pill	Yi Fang Ji Jie	tribulus fruit, gordon euryale seed, lotus stamen, dragon's bone, oyster shell, lotus plumule
161	Jing Fang Bai Du Powder	Wai Ke Li Li	schizonepeta, ledebouriella root, root of purple-flowered peucedanum, Chuanxiong rhizome, Fructus Aurantii, poria, platycodon root, liquorice, bupleurum root, notopterygium root, and pubescent angelica root
162	Ju Pi Zhu Ru Decoction	Jin Gui Yao Lue	gingseng, tangerine peel, liquorice, fresh ginger, Chiness-date, bamboo shavings etc.
163	Ju Yuan Jian Decoction	Jing Yue Quan Shu	ginseng, prepared astragalus root, prepared liquorice, baked cimicifuga rhizome, baked bighead atractylodes rhizome
164	Juan Bi Decoction	Yi Xue Xin Wu	notoptery gium root, pubescent, angelica root, bark of Chinese cassia tree, large-leaf gentian root, Chinese angelica root, chuanxiong rhizome, prepared liquorice, futokadsura stem, mulberry twigs, aucklandia root, etc.

No	NAME	SOURCE BOOK	COMPOSITION OF THE PRESCRIPTION
165	Kai Jin Powder	Yi Xue Xin Wu	ginseng, coptis root grassleaved sweetflag, red sage root, lotus fruit, poria, tangerine peel, waxgourd seed, long-stored rice, stalk of Folium Nelumbinis
166	Kong Xian Pellet	San Yin Ji Yi Bing Zheng Fang Lun	kansui root, knoxia root, white mustard seed
167	Li Zhong Pill	Shang Han Lun	ginseng, bighead atractylodes rhizome, dried ginger, prepared liquorice
168	Lian Li Decoction	Zhang Shi Yi Fang	ginger, bighead atractylodes rhizome, dried ginger, prepared liquorice, coptis root, poria
169	Lian Po Drink	Sui Xi Ju Chong Ding Huo Luan Fang	prepared magnolia bark, coptis root, grassleaved sweetflag rhizome, prepared pinellia tuber, parched fermented soya beans, burnt capejasmine, reed rhizome
170	Liang Fu Pill	Liang Fang Ji Ye	galangal rhizome, nutgrass flatsedge rhizome
171	Liang Ge Powder	Tai Ping Hui Min He Ji Ju Fang	Rhubarb, liquorice, lapejasmine seed, peppermint leaf, scutellaria, forsythia fruit, Lophatherum, honey
172	Ling Gan Wu Wei Jiang Xin Dection	Jin Gui Yao Lue	poria, liquorice, shisandra fruit, dried ginger, asarum herb
173	Ling Gui Zhu Gan Decoction	Gin Gui Yao Lue	poria, cinnamom twig, bighead atractylodes rhizome, liquorice

No	NAME	SOURCE BOOK	COMPOSITION OF THE PRESCRIPTION
174	Ling Yang Gou Teng Decoction	Tong Su Shang Han Lun	antelope's horn, mulberry leaf, sichuan fritillary bulb, fresh dried rehmannia root, uncaria stem with hoods, chrysanthemum flower, white peony root, fresh liquorice, poria with hostwood, etc.
175	Ling Yang Jiao Decoction	Yi Chun Sheng Yi	antelope's horn, tortoise plastron, fresh rehmannia root, moutan bark, white peony root, bupleurum root, peppermint, cicada slough, chrysanthemum flower, prunella spike, abalone shell
176	Liu Jun Zi Decoction	Yi Xue Zheng Zhuan	ginger, prepared liquorice, poria, bighead atractylodes, tangerine peel, prepared pinellia
177	Liu Jun Zi Decoction	Yi Fang Ji Jie	ginseng, bighead atractylodes rhizome, poria, liquorice, astragalus root, Chinese yam
178	Liu Mo Decoction	Zheng Zhi Zhun Sheng	eagle wood, aucklandia root, areca seed, lindera root, Immature Bitter Orange, Rhubarb
179	Liu Wei Di Huang Pill	Xiao Er Yao Zheng Zhi Jue	prepared rehmannia root, Chinese yam, poria, moutan bark, Alisma Orientale, dogwood fruit
180	Liu Yi Powder	Shang Han Biao Ben Xin Fa Lei Cui	Talc, liquorice
181	Long Dan Xie Gan Decoction	Lan Shi Mi Cang	gentian root, Alisma Orientale, Akebia Trifoliata, plantain seed, Chinese angelica root, buplearum root, dried rehmannia root, (scutellaria root, capejasmine)

No	NAME	SOURCE BOOK	COMPOSITION OF THE PRESCRIPTION
182	Long Hu Pill	Yan Fang	cow-bezoare, defatted powder of croton seed, cinnabar, arsenolite
183	Lu Jiao Jiao Pill	Yi Xue Zheng Zhuan	antler glue, deglued antler powder, prepared rehmannia root, cyathula root, white poria, dodder seed, ginseng, Chinese angelica root, bighead atractylodes rhizome, eucommia bark, tigger bone, tortoise plastron
184	Lu Rong Pill	Shen Shi Zun Sheng Shu	pilose antler, ophiopogon root, prepared rehmannia root, astraga; is rppt. scjosamdra fruit, desertliving, chicken's gizzard-skin, dogwood fruit, psoralea fruit, ginseng, achyranthes root, scrophularia root, poria, wolfberry bark
185	Ma Huang Decoction	Shang Han Lun	ephedra, cinnamom twig, bitter apricot kernel, prepared liquorice
186	Ma Huang Fu Zi Xi Xin Decoction	Shang Han Lun	ephedra, prepared aconite root, asarum herb
187	Ma Huang Jia Zhu Decoction	Jin Gui Yao Lue	ephedra, cinnamom twig, prepared liquorice, bitter apricot kernel, bighead atractylodes rhizome
188	Ma Huang Lian Qiao Chi Xiao Dou Decoction	Shang Han Lun	ephedra, bitter apricot kernel, forsythia fruit, red bean, liquorice, fresh ginger, Chinese-date
189	Ma Xing Shi Gan Decoction	Shang Han Lun	ephedra, bitter apricot kernel, gypsum, prepared liquorice
190	Ma Xing Yi Gan Decoction	Jin Gui Yao Lue	ephedra, prepared liquorice, coix seed, bitter apricot kernel

No	NAME	SOURCE BOOK	COMPOSITION OF THE PRESCRIPTION
191	Ma Zi Ren Pill	Shang Han Lun	Hemp Seed, peony, prepared Immature Bitter Orange, Rhubarb, prepared magnolia bark, bitter apricot kernel
192	Mai Men Dong Decoction	Jin Gui Yao Lue	ophiopogon root, ginseng, pinellia tuber, liquorice, stalk rice, Chinese date
193	Mai Wei Di Huang Pill	Yi Ji	prepared rehmannia root, dogwood fruit, Chinese yam, moutan bark, Alisma Orientale, poria, ophiopogon root, schisandra fruit
194	Meng Shi Gun Tan Pill	Yang Sheng Zhu Lun	Lapis chloriti, eagle wood, Rhubarb, scutellaria root, etc.
195	Miao Xiang Powder	Shen Shi Zun Sheng Shu	Chinese yam, poria, poria with hostwood, polygala root, liquorice, aucklandia root, cinnabar, musk
196	Mu Fang Ji Decoction	Jin Gui Yao Lue	tetrandra root, gypsum, cinnamom twig, ginseng
197	Mu Li Powder	Tai Ping Hui Min He Ji Ju Fang	calcining oyster shell, astragalus root, ephedra root, light wheat
198	Mu Li Ze Xie Powder	Shang Han Lun	calcining oyster shell, Alisma Orientale, baked lepidium seed, baked pokeberry root, sargassum, trichosanthes root
199	Mu Xiang Shun Qi Powder	Shen Shi Zun Sheng Shu	aucklandia root, green tangerine, tangerine peel, liquorice, aurantii immaturus peel, magnolia bark, lindera root, nutgrass flatsedge rhizome, atractylodes rhizome, amomum fruit, bark of Chinese cassia tree, chuanxiong rhizome
200	Niu Huang Qing Xin Pill	Dou Zhen Shi Yi Xin Fa	cow-bezoare, cinnabar, coptis root, scutellaria root, capejasmine curcuma root

No	NAME	SOURCE BOOK	COMPOSITION OF THE PRESCRIPTION
201	Nuan Gan Jian	Jing Yue Quan Shu	bark of Chinese cassia tree, Fructus Foeniculi, poria, lindera root, wolfberry fruit, Chinese angelica root, eagle wood, fresh ginger
202	Ping Chuan Gu Ben Decoction	Nan Jing Zhong Yi Xue Yuan Fu Yuan Yan Fang	dangshen, schisandra fruit, cordyceps, walnut, eagle wood, perilla fruit coltsfoot flower, Rhizoma Pinelliae Praeparata, red tangerine peel, etc.
203	Ping Wei Powder	Tai Ping Hui Min He Ji Ju Fang	atractylodes rhizome, magnolia bark, tangerine peel, liquorice, ginger, Chinese-date
204	Pu Ji Xiao Du Drink	Dong Huan Shi Shu	scutellaria root, coptis root, forsythia fruit, scrophularia root, isatis root, puff-ball, arctium fruit, batry ticated silkworm, cimicifuga rhizome, bupleurum root, tangerine peel, platycodon root, liquorice, notopterygium root
205	Qi Ge Powder	Yi Xue Xin Wu	adenophora root, poria, red sage root, Sichuan fritillary bulb, curcuma root, amomum fruit shell, lotus leaf stalk, chaff
206	Qi Ju Di Huang Pill	Yi Ji	wolfberry fruit, chrysanthemum flower, prepared rehmannia root, dogwood fruit, Chinese yam, Alisma Orientale, moutan bark, poria
207	Qi Wei Du Qi Pill	Yi Zong Ji Ren Pian	rehmannia root, dogwood fruit, Chinese yam, poria, moutan bark, Alisma Orientale, schisandra fruit
208	Qian Gen Powder	Jing Yue Quan Shu	rubia root, scutellaria toot, donkey-hide gelatin, biota tops

No	NAME	SOURCE BOOK	COMPOSITION OF THE PRESCRIPTION
209	Qian Jin Wei Jing Decoction	Bei Ji Qian Jin Yao Fang	fresh reed rhizome, coix seed, wax-gourd seed, peach kernel
210	Qian Zheng Powder	Yang Shi Jia Cang Fang	giant typhonium tuber, batryticated silk worm, scorpion
211	Qiang Huo Sheng Shi Decoction	Nei Wai Shang Bian Huo Lun	notopterygium root, pubescent angelica root, chuanxiong rhizome, chastetree fruit, liquorice, ledebouriella root, sweet wormwood
212	Qin Jiao Bie Jia Powder	Wei Sheng Bao Jian	wolfberry bark, bupleurum root, large-leaf gentian root, Anemarrhena Asphodeloides, Chinese angelica root, fresh-water turtle shell, sweet wormwood, black plum
213	Qing E Pill	Tai Ping Hui Min He Ji Ju Fang	psoralea fruit, eucommia bark, walnut kernel, garlic
214	Qing Fei Drink	Zheng Zhi Hui Bu	poria, scutellaria root, mulberry bark, ophiopogon root, plantain seed, Gardenia Jasminoides, Caulis Aristolochiae Manshuriensis
215	Qing Gu Powder	Zheng Zhi Zhun Sheng	stellaria root, picrorhiza rhizome, large-leaf, gentian root, fresh-water turtle shell, wolf berry bark, sweet wormwood, Anemarrhena Asphodeloides, liquorice
216	Qing Jin Hua Tan Decoction	Tong Zhi Fang	scutellaria root, Gardenia Jasminoides, platycodon root, ophiopogon root, malberry bark, sichuan fritillary bulb, Anenarrhena Asphodeloides, trichosanthes seed, red tangerine peel, poria, liquorice

No	NAME	SOURCE BOOK	COMPOSITION OF THE PRESCRIPTION
217	Qing Re Zhen Jing Decoction	Yi Zong Jin Jian	abalone shell, Fluortum, gentian root, Gardenia Jasminoides, Caulis Aristolochiae Manshuriensis, fresh Rhubarb, dried ginger, root of purple-flowered peucedanum, ophiopogon root, Comeretio Silicea Bambusae, arisaema with bile, polygala root, glassleaved sweetflag gastrodia tuber uncarid stem with hoods
218	Qing Shu Yi Qi Decoction	Wen Re Jing Wei	root of American ginseng, dendrobium, ophiopogon root, copits root, lophatherum, lotus petiole, Anemarrhena Asphodeloides, liquorice, stalk rice, watermelon peel
219	Qing Wei Powder	Lan Shi Mi Cang	Chinese angelica root, dried rehmannia root, moutan bark, cimicifuga rhizome, coptis root
220	Qing Zao Jiu Fei Decoction	Yi Men Fa Lu	mulberry leaf, gypsum, bitter apricot kennel, liquorice, ophiopogon root, ginseng, donkey-hide gelatin, baked pedaliaceae seed, prepared lopuat leaf
221	Qing Zhen Decoction	Su Wen Bing Ji Qi Yi Bao Ming Ji	cimicifuga rhizome, atractylodes rhizome, lotus leaf
222	Ren Shen Yang Ying Decoction	Tai Ping Hui Min He Ji Ju Fang	ginseng, liquorice, Chinese angelica root, white peony root, prepared rehmannia root, bark of Chinese cassia tree, Chiness-date, astragalusroot, bighead atractylodes rhizome, poria, schisandra fruit, polygala root, tangerine peel, fresh ginger
223	Ru Jin Jie Du Powder	Jing Yue Quan Shu	platycodon root, liquorice, scutellaria root, coptis root, phellodendron bark, Garderia Jasminoides

No	NAME	SOURCE BOOK	COMPOSITION OF THE PRESCRIPTION
224	Run Chang Pill	Shen Shi Zun Sheng Shu	Chinese angelica root, fresh rehmannia root, Hemp Seed, peach kernel, Fructus Aurantii
225	San Ao Decoction	Tai Ping Hui Min He Ji Ju Fang	ephedra, bitter apricot kernel, fresh liquorice
226	San Cai Feng Sui Pellet	Wei Sheng Bao Jian	lucid asparagus root, prepared rehmannia root, ginseng, phellodendrom bark, amomum fruit, liquorice
227	San Ren Decoction	Wen Bing Tiao Bian	bitter apricot kernel, coix seed, magnolia bark, pinellia tuber, rice-paper pith, tale, tamarisk tops, etc.
228	San Sheng Powder	Ru Min Shi Qin	Muskmelon Pedicel, ledebouriella root, Veratrum Nigrum
229	San Zi Yang Qin Decoction	Han Shi Yi Tong	perilla fruit, white mustard seed, radish seed
230	Sang Bai Pi Decoction	Jing Yue Quan Shu	mulberry bark, pinellia tuber, perilla fruit, bitter apricot kernel, fritillary bulb, scutellaria root, coptis root, capejasmine
231	Sang Ju Drink	Wen Bing Tiao Bian	mulberry leaf, chrysanthemum flower, forsythia fruit, peppermint, platycodon root, bitter apricot kernel, reed rhizome, liquorice
232	Sang Piao Xiao Powder	Ben Cao Yan Yi	mantis egg-case, polygala root, grassleaved sweetflag rhizome, dragon's bone, poria with hostwood, Chinese angelica root, tortoise-plastron

No	NAME	SOURCE BOOK	COMPOSITION OF THE PRESCRIPTION
233	Sang Xing Decoction	Wen Bing Tiao Bian	mulberry leaf, bitter apricot kernel, adenophora root, fritillary bulb, fermented soya beans, capejasmine, pear peel
234	Sha Shen Mai Dong Decoction	Wen Bing Tiao Bian	adenophora root, ophiopogon root, fragrant solomonseal rhizome, mulberry leaf, liquorice, trichosanthes root, fresh hyacinth bean
235	Sha Shen Qing Fei Decoction	Yan Fang	glehnia root, fresh astragalus root, pseudostellaria root, albizia bark, hyacinth bletilla, fresh liquorice, platycodon root, coix seed, wax-gourd seed
236	Shao Fu Zhu Yu Decoction	Yi Lin Gai Cuo	common fennel fruit, dried ginger, corydalis tuber, myrrh, Chinese angelica root, chuanxiong rhizome, bark of Chinese cassia tree, red peony root, cat-tail pollen, trogopterus dung
237	Shao Yao Decoction	Su Wen Bing Ji Qi Yi Bao Ming Ji	scutellaria root, peony root, prepared liquorice, coptis root, Rhubarb, areca seed, Chinese angelica root, aucklandia root, bark of Chinese cassia tree
238	Shao Yao Gan Cao Decoction	Shang Han Lun	white peony root, prepared liquorice
239	She Gan Ma Huang Decoction	Jin Gui Yao Lue	belamcanda rhizome, ephedra, asarum herb, Aster Tataricus, coltsfoot flower, pinellia tuber, schisandra fruit, fresh ginger, Chinese-date
240	Shen Fu Decoction	Fu Ren Liang Fang	ginseng, aconite root ginger, Chinese-date

No	NAME	SOURCE BOOK	COMPOSITION OF THE PRESCRIPTION
241	Shen Jie Powder	Ji Sheng Fang	ginseng, gecko
242	Shen Ling Bai Zhu Powder	Tai Ping Hui Min He Ji Ju Fang	ginseng, poria, bighead atractylodes rhizome, platycodon root, Chinese yam, liquorice, white hyaciath bean, lotus seed, amomum fruit, coix seed
243	Shen Su Drink	Tai Ping Hui Min He Ji Ju Fang	ginger, perilla leaf, pueraria root, root of purple-flowered peucedanum, Rhizoma Pinellinae Praeparata, poria, red tangerine peel, liquorice, Fructus Aurantii, aucklandia root, tangerine peel, ginger, Chinese-date
244	Shen Tong Zhu Yu Decoction	Yi Lin Gai Cuo	large-leaf gentian root, chuanxiong rhizome, peach kernel, safflower, liquorice, notoptery gium root, myrrh, nutgrass flatsedge, trogopterum dung, achyranthes root, earthworm, Chinese angelica root
245	Shen Xi Pellet	Wen Re Jing Wei	rhinoceros horn, grassleaved sweetflag rhixome, scutellaria root, fresh rehmannia root, honeysuckle flower, forsythia fruit, isatis root, fermented soya beans, scrophularia root, trichosanthes root, purple gromwell root
246	Shen Zhu Powder	Yi Xue Xin Wu	atractylodes rhizome, tangerine peel, magnolia bark, liquorice, agastache, amomum fruit
247	Sheng Jiang Powder	Sai Wen Tiao Bian	parched batryticated silkworm, cicada slough, turmeria, Rhubarb
248	Sheng Mai Drink	Bei Ji Qian Jin Yao Fang	ginseng, ophiopogon root, schisandra fruit

No	NAME	SOURCE BOOK	COMPOSITION OF THE PRESCRIPTION
249	Sheng Tie Luo Drink	Yin Xue Xin Wu	lucid asparagus root, ophiopogon root, fritillary bulb, arisaema with bile, red tangerine peel, polygala root, grassleaved sweetflag rhizome, forsythia fruit, poria, poria with hostwood, scrophularia root, uncaria stem with hooks, red sager root, cinnabar Pig Iron Cinder
250	Shi Hui Powder	Shi Yao Shen Shu	Japanese thistle, field thistle, biota tops, lotus leaf, rubia root, Gardenia Jasminoides, Cogongrass rhizome, Rhubarb, moutan bark, palmae bark
251	Shi Pi Drink	Ji Sheng Fa	prepared aconite root, dried ginger, bighead atractylodes rhizome, liquorice, magnolia bark, aucklandia root, tsaoko, areca seed, chaenomeles fruit, fresh ginger, Chinese-date, poria
252	Shi Quan Da Bu Decoction	Tai Ping Hui Min He Ji Ju Fang	prepared rehmannia root, white peony root, Chinese angelica root, chuanxiong rhizome, ginseng, bighead atractylodes rhizome, poria, prepared liquorice, astragalus root, bark of Chinese cassia tree
253	Shi Wei Powder	Zheng Zhi Hui Bu	Pyrrosia Leaf, Semen Malvae, Chinese pink herb, tale plantain seed
254	Shi Xiao Powder	Tai Ping Hui Min He Ji Ju Fang	trogopterus dung, cat-tail pollen
255	Shi Zao Decoction	Shang Han Lun	knoxia root, genkwa, kansui root, Chiness-date

No	NAME	SOURCE BOOK	COMPOSITION OF THE PRESCRIPTION
256	Shu Yu Pill	Jin Gui Yao Lue	Chinese Yam, ginseng, bighead atracty lodes rhizome, poria, liquorice, Chinese angelica root, peony root, chuanxiong rhizome, dried rehmannia root, donkey-hide gelatin, ophiopogon root, bitter apricot kernel, platycodon root, ledebourella root, bupleurum root cinnamom twig medicated leaven dried ginger ampelopsis root Chiness-date etc.
257	Shu Zao Yin Zi	Shi Yi De Xiao Fang	pokeberry root, Alisma Orientale, red bean, Caulis Aristolochiae Manshuriensis, poria peel, shell of arecanut, areca seed, fresh ginger, notoptery gium root, large-leaf gentian root
258	Shui Hong Hua Extract	Jing Yue Quan Shu	Polygonum Orientale, Rhubarb, lime, alcohol yeast
259	Shui Lu Er Xian Pellet	Zheng Zhi Zhun Sheng	cherokee rose-hip, gordoneuryale seed
260	Shun Qi He Zhong Decoction	Zheng Zhi Zhun Sheng	astragalus root, ginseng, bighead atractylodes rhizome, tangerine peel, Chinese angelica root, peony, prepared liquorice, cimiciguga rhizome, bupleurum root, chastetree fruit, Sichuan aconite root, asarum herb
261	Si Jun Zi Decoction	Tai Ping Hui Min He Ji Ju Fang	dangshen, bighead atractylodes rhizome, poria, liquorice
262	Si Miao Pill	Cheng Fang Bian Du	atractylodes rhizome, phellodendron bark, achyranthes root, coix seed
263	Si Ni Decoction	Shang Han Lun	prepared liquorice, dried ginger, prepared aconite root

No	NAME	SOURCE BOOK	COMPOSITION OF THE PRESCRIPTION
264	Si Ni Powder	Shang Han Lun	prepared liquorice, Immature Bitter Orange, bupleurum root, peony root
265	Si Qi Decoction	Tai Ping Hui Min He Ji Ju Fang	prepared pinelliae tuber, magnolia bark, poria, fresh ginger, Chinessdate, etc.
266	Si Shen Pill	Zheng Zhi Zhun Sheng	psoralea fruit, nutmeg, dogwood fruit, schisandra fruit, fresh ginger, Chinese-date
267	Si Wei Hui Yang Drink	Jing Yue Quan Shu	ginseng, prepared aconite root, prepared ginger, prepared liquorice
268	Si Wu Decoction	Tai Ping Hui Min He Ji Ju Fang	Chinese angelica root, white peony root, chuanxiong rhizome, prepared rehmannia root
269	Su He Xiang Pill	Tai Ping Hui Min He Ji Ju Fang	bighead atractylodes rhizome, dutchmanspipe root, rhinoceros hore, nutgrass flatsedge rhizome, cinnabar, chebula fruit, sandalwood, benzoin, eagle wood, musk, cloves, long pepper, storax oil, borneol, etc.
270	Su Zi Jiang Qi Decoction	Tai Ping Hui Min He Ji Ju Fang	perilla fruit, tangerine peel, pinellia tuber, Chinese angelica root, root of purple -flowered peucedanum, magnolia bark, bark of Chinese cassia tree, liquorice, fresh ginger
271	Suan Zao Ren Decoction	Jin Gui Yao Lue	wild or sping jujuba seed, Anemarrhena Asphodeloides, chuanxiong rhizome, poria, liquorice
272	Tao Hua Decoction	Jin Gui Yao Lue	red halloysite, dried ginger, stalk rice

No	NAME	SOURCE BOOK	COMPOSITION OF THE PRESCRIPTION
273	Tao Ren Hong Hua Jian	Su An Yi An	red sage root, red peony, peach kernel, safflower, prepared nutgrass flat sedge rhizome, corydalis tuber, green tangerine peel, Chinese angelica root, chuanxiong rhizome, fresh rehmannia root
274	Tian Ma Gou Teng Drink	Za Bing Zhen Zhi Xin Yi	gastrodia tuber, uncaria stem with hooks, abalone shell, cyathula root, roranthus mulberry, scutellaria root, motherwort, poria, fleece flower stem, capejasmine fruit and bark of eucommia
275	Tian Wang Bu Xin Dan	She Sheng Mi Ji	ginseng, scrophularia root, red sage root, poria, schisandra fruit, polygala root, Chinese angelica root, lucid asparagus, ophiopogon root, arborvitae seed, wild or sping jujuba seed, dried rehmannia root, cinnabar
276	Tiao Wei Cheng Qi Decoction	Shang Han Lun	Rhubarb, prepared liquorice, mirabilite
277	Tiao Ying Drink	Zheng Zhi Zhun Sheng	zedoary, chuanxiong rhizome, Chinese angelica root, corydalis tuber, red peony root, Chinese pink herb, rhubarb, areca seed, tangerine peel, shell of areca nut, lipidium seed, red poria, mulberry bark, asarum herb, prepared liquorice, ginger, Chinese-date, dahurian angelica root
278	Tiao Ying Lian Gan Drink	Yi Chun Teng Yi	Chinese angelica root, white peony root, baked gecko powder, donkey-hide gelatin, wolfberry fruit, schisandra fruit, chuanxiong rhizome, jujuba seed, tangerine peel, aucklandia root, fresh ginger, Chinese-date
279	Ting Li Da Zao Xie Fei Decoction	Jin Gui Yao Lue	lepidium seed, Chiness-date

No	NAME	SOURCE BOOK	COMPOSITION OF THE PRESCRIPTION
280	Tong Qiao Huo Xue Decoction	Yi Lin Gai Cuo	red peony root, chuan xiong rhizome, peach kernel, safflower, musk, old onion, fresh ginger, Chinese-date, alcohol
281	Tong Xie Yao Fang	Jing Yue Quan Shu Yin Liu Cao Chuang Fang	bighead atractylodes rhizome, white peony root, ledebouriella root, baked tangerine peel
282	Tong You Decoction	Lan Shi Mi Cang	fresh rehmannia root, prepared rehmannia root, peach kernel powder, safflower, Chinese angelica root, prepared liquorice, cimicifuga rhizome
283	Tong Yu Jian	Jing Yue Quan Shu	Chinese angelica root, hawthorn fruit, nutgrass flatsedge rhizome, safflower, lindera root, green tangerine orange peel, aucklandia root, Alisma Orientale
284	Wei Ling Decoction	Dan Xi Xin Fa	atractylodes rhizome, magnolia bark, tangerine peel, liquorice, fresh ginger, Chinese-date, cinnamom twig, bighead atractylodes rhizome, Alisma Orientale, poria, Umbellate Pore
285	Wen Dan Decoction	Bei Ji Qian Jin Yao Fang	pinellia tuber, tangerine peel, liquorice, Immature Bitter Orange, fresh ginger, poria, bamboo shavings
286	Wen Pi Decoction	Bei Ji Qian Jin Yao Fang	prepared aconite root, ginseng, Rhubarb, liquorice, dried ginger
287	Wu Bi Shan Yao Pill	Tai Ping Hui Min He Ji Ju Fang	Chinese yam, desertliving astanche, prepared rehmannia root, dogwood fruit, poria, dodder seed, schisandra fruit, red halloysite rhizome, eucommia bark, achyranthes root, etc.

No	NAME	SOURCE BOOK	COMPOSITION OF THE PRESCRIPTION
288	Wu Fu Ma Xin Gui Jiang Decoction	Cheng Du Zhong Yi Xue Yuan Dai Yun Bo Fang	Sichuan aconite root, prepared aconite root, ephedra, asarum herb, cinnamom twig, dried ginger, liquorice, honey
289	Wu Ji Powder	Tai Ping Hui Min He Ji Ju Fang	dahurian angelica root, tangerine peel, magnolia bark angelica root, chuanxiong rhizome, white peony root, poria, platycodon root, atractylodes rhizome, Fructus Aurantii, pinellia tuber, ephedra, dried ginger, bark of Chinese cassia tree, liquorice, ginger
290	Wu Ling Powder	Shang Han Lun	cinnamom twig, bighead atractylodes rhizome, poria, dysuria, Alisma Orientale
291	Wu Mei Pill	Shang Han Lun	black plum, coptis root, phellodendron bark, ginseng, Chinese angelica root, prepared aconite root, cinnamom twig, peppertree, dried ginger, asarum herb
292	Wu Mo Yin Zi	Yi Fang Ji Jie	lindera root, eagle wood, areca seed, Immature Bitter Orange, aucklandia root
293	Wu Pi Powder	Zhong Cang Jing	mulberry bark, tangerine peel, gin ger peel, shell of areca nut, fuling peel
294	Wu Ren Pill	Shi Yi De Xiao Fang	peach kernel, bitter apricot kernel, arborvitae seed, pine nut, bush-cherry seed, tangerine peel
295	Wu Sheng Drink	Shi Yi De Xiao Fang	arisaema with bile, dried pinellia tuber, dried giant typhonium tuber, Sichuan aconite root, black soybean

No	NAME	SOURCE BOOK	COMPOSITION OF THE PRESCRIPTION
296	Wu Tou Chi Shi Zhi Pill	Jin Gui Yao Lue	peppertree, Sichuan aconite root, prepared aconite root, dried ginger, red halloysite
297	Wu Tou Decoction	Jin Gui Yao Lue	Sichuan aconite root, ephedra, peony, astragalus root, liquorice
298	Wu Tou Gui Zhi Decoction	Jin Gui Yao Lue	cinnamom twig, peony, liquorice, ginger, Chinese-date, Sichuan aconite root
299	Wu Wei Xiao Du Drink	Yi Zong Jin Jian	honeysuckle flower, wild chrysanthemum flower, dandelion herb, Viola Yedoensis, etc.
300	Wu Zhi An Zhong Drink	Yan Fang	Chinese chies juice, milk, ginger juice, pear juice, lotus rhizome juice
301	Wu Zhu Yu Decoction	Shang Han Lun	dogwood fruit, ginseng, fresh ginger, Chinese-date
302	Wu Zi Yan Zong Pill	Dan Xi Xin Fa	wolfberry fruit, raspberry, dodder seed, schisandra fruit, plantain seed
303	Xi Huang Pill	Wai Ke Zheng Zhi Quan Sheng Ji	Xihuang, musk, myrrh, etc.
304	Xi Jiao Di Huang Decoction	Bei Ji Qian Jin Yao Fang	rhinoceros horn, dried rehmannia root, moutan bark, peony root
305	Xi Jiao Powder	Bei Ji Qian Jin Yao Fang	rhinoceros horn, coptis root, cinicifuga rhizome, Gardenia Jasminoides, oriental wormwood
306	Xiang Fu Xuan Fu Hua Decoction	Wen Bing Tiao Bian	fresh nutgrass flatsedge rhizome, inula flower, perilla fruit, coix seed, pinellia tuber, poria, tangerine peel

No	NAME	SOURCE BOOK	COMPOSITION OF THE PRESCRIPTION
307	Xiang Lian Pill	Tai Ping Hui Min He Ji Ju Fang	coptis root, aucklandia root
308	Xiang Ru Drink	Tai Ping Hui Min He Ji Ju Fang	baked hyacinth bean, manolia bark, elsoholtzia
309	Xiang Sha Liu Jun Zi Decoction	Shi Fang Ge Kuo	aucklandia root, amomum fruit, tangerine peel, penellia tuber, dangshen, bighead atractylodes rhizome, poria, liquorice
310	Xiang Su Powder	Tai Ping Hui Min He Ji Ju Fang	nutgrass flatsedge rhizome, Folium Perillae, Caulis Perillae, tangerine peel liquorice
311	Xiao Ban Xia Decoction	Jin Gui Yao Lue	pinellia tuber, fresh ginger
312	Xiao Ban Xia Jia Fu Ling Decoction	Jin Gui Yao Lue	pinellia tuber, fresh ginger, poria
313	Xiao Chai Hu Decoction	Shang Han Lun	bupleurum root, scutellaria root, pinellia tuber, ginseng, liquorice, fresh ginger, Chinese-date
314	Xiao Cheng Qi Decoction	Shang Han Lun	Rhubarb, magnolia bark, Immature Bitter Orange
315	Xiao Ji Yin Zi	Ji Sheng Fang	dried rehmannia root, field thistle, tale, ricepaper pith, parched cat-tail pollen, lophatherum, node of lotus rhizome, Chinese angelica root, pittosporm root, liquorice
316	Xiao Jian Zhong Decoction	Shang Han Lun	cinnamom twig, white peony root, liquorice, fresh ginger, Chinessdate, malt extract

No	NAME	SOURCE BOOK	COMPOSITION OF THE PRESCRIPTION
317	Xiao Ke Fang	Dan Xi Xin Fa	coptis root powder, trichosanthes root powder, fresh rehmannia root juice, lotus rhizome juice, breast milk, ginger juice, honey
318	Xiao Qing Long Decoction	Shang Han Lun	ephedra, cinnamom twig, peony root, liquorice, dried ginger, asarum herb, pinellia tuber, schisandra fruit
319	Xiao Qing Long Jia Shi Gao Decoction	Jin Gui Yao Lue	ephedra, cinnamom twig, peony root, liquorice, dried ginger, asarum herb, pinellia tuber, schisandra fruit, gypsum
320	Xiao Shi Fan Shi Powder	Jin Gui Yao Lue	alum, etc.
321	Xiao Xian Xiong Decoction	Shang Han Lun	coptis root, pinellia tuber, trichosanthes fruit
322	Xiao Yao Powder	Tai Ping Hui Min He Ji Ju Fang	bupleurum root, bighead atractylodes rhizome, white peony root, Chinese angelica root, poria, prepared liquorice, peppermint, sewed ginger
323	Xie Bai Powder	Xiao Er Yao Zheng Zhi Jue	mulberry bark, wolfberry bark, fresh liquorice, stalk rice
324	Xie Xin Decoction	Jin Gui Yao Lue	Rhubarb, scutellaria root, coptis root
325	Xin Jia Xiang Ru Drink	Wen Bing Tiao Bian	elscholtzia, fresh hyacinth-bean flower, magnolia bark, honeysuckle flower, coptis root
326	Xing Su Er Chen Pill	Yan Fang	bitter apricot kernel, pinellia tuber, tangerine peel, poria, perilla fruit, liquorice

No	NAME	SOURCE BOOK	COMPOSITION OF THE PRESCRIPTION
327	Xing Su Powder	Wen Bing Tiao Bian	bitter apricot kernel, Folium Perillae, tangerine peel, pinellia tuber, fresh ginger, Fructus Aurantii, platycodon root, root of purple-flowered peucedanum, poria, liquorice, Chinese-date
328	Xiong Zhi Shi Gao Decoction	Yi Zong Jin Jian	chuanxiong rhizome, dahurian angelica root, gypsum, chrysantyemum flower, ligusticum root, notopterygium root
329	Xuan Bai Cheng Qi Decoction	Wen Bing Tiao Bian	gypsum, fresh rhubarb, bitter apricot kernel powder, trichosanthes peel
330	Xuan Bi Decoction	Wen Bing Tiao Bian	tetrandra root, bitter apricot kernel, forsythia fruit, tale, coix seed, pinellia tuber, silkworm excrement, red bean, Gardenia Jasminoides
331	Xuan Fu Dai Zhe Decoction	Shang Han Lun	inula flower, red ochre, ginseng, pinellia tuber, prepared oqiproce. fresh ginger, Chinese-date
332	Xuan Fu Hua Decoction	Jin Gui Yao Lue	inula flower, onion, etc
333	Xue Fu Zhu Yu Decoction	Yi Lin Gai Cuo	Chinese angelica root, prepared liquorice, peach kernel, safflower, Fructus Aurantii, peony root, bupleurum root, liquorice, platy condon root, chuan xiong rhizome, achyranthes root
334	Yang Gan Pill	Lei Yuan Fang	bat's faces, cicada slough, shave grass herb, Chinese angelica, Yanggan

No	NAME	SOURCE BOOK	COMPOSITION OF THE PRESCRIPTION
335	Yang He Decoction	Wai Ke Quan Sheng Ji	Prepared nehmannia root, bark of chinese cassis free, ephedra, autler glue, white mustard seed, baked ginger, ang licorice root
336	Yang Wei Decoction	Zheng Zhi Zhun Sheng	adenophora root, ophiogogon root, fragrant solomonseal rhizome, fresh dolicholis mulberry leaf, liquorice
337	Yang Xin Decoction	Zheng Zhi Zhun Sheng	astragalus root, poria, poria with hostwood, Chinese angelica root, chuanxiong rhizome, prepared liquorice, pinellia tuber, arborvitae seed, jujuba seed, polygala root, schisandra fruit, ginseng, bark of Chinese cassiatree
338	Yi Guan Jian	Liu Zhou Yi Hua	adenophora root, ophiopogon root, Chinese angelica root, dried rehmannia root, wolfberry fruit, Sichuan chinaberry
339	Yi Qi Cong Ming Decoction	Zheng Zhi Zhun Sheng	astragalus root, ginseng, cimicifuga rhizome, pueraria root, chastetree fruit, peony, phellodendron bark, prepared liquorice
340	Yi Wei Decoction	Wen Bing Tiao Bian	adenophora root, ophiopogon root, fresh rehmannia root, fragrant solomonseal rhizome, crystal sugar
341	Yi Yi Ren Decoction	Lei Zheng Zhi Cai	coix seed, chuanxiong rhizome, Chinese angelica root, ephedra, cinnamomtwig, notopterygium root, pubescent angelica root, ledebouriella root, atractylodes rhizome, liquorice, fresh ginger, etc.

No	NAME	SOURCE BOOK	COMPOSITION OF THE PRESCRIPTION
342	Yin Chen Hao Decoction	Shang Han Lun	orintal wormwood, Gardenia Jasminoides, Rhubarb
343	Yin Chen Wu Ling Powder	Jin Gui Yao Lue	Oriental wormwood, cinnamom twig, poria, bighead atractylodes rhizome, Alisma Orientale, Umbellate Pore
344	Yin Chen Zhu Fu Decoction	Yi Xue Xin Wu	Oriental Wormwood, bighead atractylodes rhizome, prepared aconite root, dried ginger, prepared liquorice, bark of Chinese cassia tree
345	Yin Qiao Powder	Wen Bing Tiao Bian	honey suckle flower, forsythia fruit, fermented soya beans, arctium fruit, natopterygium root, schizonepeta spike, platycodon root, liquorice, Tamarisk Tops, fresh reed rhizome
346	You Gui Drink	Jing Yue Quan Shu	prepared rehmannia root, dogwood fruit, wolfberry fruit, Chinese yam, poria, liquorice
347	You Gui Pill	Jing Yue Quan Shu	prepared rehmannia root, Chinese yam, dogwood fruit, wolfberry fruit, eucommia bark, dodder seed, prepared aconite root, bark of Chinese cassia tree, Chinese angelica root, antler glue
348	Yu Nu Jian	Jing Yue Quan Shu	gypsum, prepared rehmannia root, ophiopogon root, Anemarrhena Asphodeloides, achyranthes root

No	NAME	SOURCE BOOK	COMPOSITION OF THE PRESCRIPTION
349	Yu Ping Feng Powder	Shi Yi De Xiao Fang	astragalus root, bighead atractylodes rhizome, ledebouriella root
350	Yu Shu Dan	Bai Yi Xuan Fang	pleione rhizome, moleplant seed, knoxia root, musk, cinnabar, Chinese gall
351	Yue Bi Jia Ban Xia Decoction	Jin Gui Yao Lue	ephedra, gypsum, fresh giner, Chiness-date, liquorice, pinellia tuber
352	Yue Bi Jia Zhu Decoction	Jin Gui Yao Lue	ephedra, gypsum, liquorice, Chiness-date, bighead atractylodes rhizome, fresh ginger
353	Yue Ju Pill	Dan Xi Xin Fa	Chuanxiong rhizome, atractylodes rhizome, nutgrass flatsedge rhizome, baked Gardenia Jasminoides, medicated leaved
354	Zao Jia Pill	Jin Gui Yao Lue	Gleditsia Sinensis, Chinese-date
355	Ze Xie Decoction	Jin Gui Yao Lue	Alisma Orientale, bighead atractylodes rhizome
356	Zeng Ye Cheng Qi Decoction	Wen Bing Tiao Bian	Rhubarb, mirabilite, scrophalaria root, ophiopogon root, dried rehmannia root
357	Zeng Ye Decoction	Wen Bing Tiao Bian	scrophalaria root, ophiopogon root, dried rehmannia root
358	Zhen Gan Xi Feng Decoction	Yi Xue Zhong Zhong Can Xi Lu	dragon's bone, fresh white peony root, lucid asparagus root, germinated barley, redochre, oyster shell, scrophularia root, sichuan chinaberry, oriental wormwood, liquorice, tortoise plastron, etc.

No	NAME	SOURCE BOOK	COMPOSITION OF THE PRESCRIPTION
359	Zhen Ren Yang Zang Decoction	Zheng Zhi Zhun Sheng	chebula fruit, poppy peel, nut meg, bighead atractylodes rhizome, ginseng, aucklandia root, prepared liquorice, fresh ginger, Chinese-date
360	Zhen Wu Decoction	Shang Han Lun	prepared aconite root, bighead atractylodes rhizome, poria, peony, fresh ginger
361	Zhen Zhong Pellet	Bei Ji Qian Jin Yao Fang	tortoise plastron, dragon's bone, polygala root, grassleaved sweetflag rhizome
362	Zhi Bai Di Huang Pill	Yi Zong Jin Jian	Anemarrhena Asphodeloides, Phellodendron Bark, prepared rehmannia root, dogwood fruit, Chinese yam, poria moutan bark, A lisma Orientale
363	Zhi Bao Pellet	Tai Ping Hui Min He Ji Ju Fang	cinnabar, musk, benzoin, rhinoceros horn, cow-bezoare, amber, realgar, hawksbill shell, porneol, etc.
364	Zhi Gan Cao Decoction	Shang Han Lun	prepared liquorice, ginseng, cinnamom twig, fresh ginger, donkey-hide gelatin, fresh rehmannia root, ophiopogon root, hemp seed, Chinese-date
365	Zhi Shi Dao Zhi Pill	Nei Wai Shang Bian Huo Lun	Rhubarb, Immature Bitter Orange, scutellaria root, coptis root, medicated leaven, bighead atractylodes rhizome, poria, Alisma Orientale
366	Zhi Sou Powder	Yi Xue Xin Wu	schizone peta, platycodon root, liquorice, swallowwort rhizome, tangerine peel, stemona root, etc.

No	NAME	SOURCE BOOK	COMPOSITION OF THE PRESCRIPTION
367	Zhi Zhu Pill	Nei Wai Shang Bian Huo Lun	bighead atractylodes rhizome, baked Immature Bitter Orange
368	Zhi Zi Bai Pi Decoction	Shang Han Lun	capejasmine, liquorice, phellodendron bark
369	Zhi Zi Qing Gan Decoction	Lei Zeng Zhi Cai	capejasmine, moutan bark, bupleurum root, Chinese angelica root, peony, poria, chuanxiong rhizome, arctium fruit, liquorice
370	Zhong Man Fen Xiao Pill	Lan Shi Mi Cang	magnolia bark, Immature Bitter Orange, coptis root, pinellia tuber, tangerine peel, poria, Umbellate Pore, Alisma Orientale, amomum fruit, dried ginger, turmeria, ginseng, bighead atractylodes rhizome, prepared liquorice
371	Zhong Qi Tian Xiang Powder	Zheng Zhi Zhun Sheng, from Liu He Jian's Prescription	lindera root, nutgrass flatsedge rhizome, dried ginger, Perilla Frutescens, tangerine peel
372	Zhou Che Pill	Jing Yue Quan Shu Yin Liu He Jian Fang	kansui root, genkwa, knoxia root, Rhubarb, morning glory seed, aucklandia root, greentangerine orange peel, tangerine peel, calome, areca seed.
373	Zhou Fei Pill	Bai Yi Xuan Fang	schisandra fruit, ginseng, cinnamom twig, coltsfoot flower, Aster Tataricus, bitter apricot kernel, etc.
374	Zhou Shi Hui Sheng Pellet	Quan Guo Zhong Cheng Yao Chu Fang Ji	Chinese gall, sandalwood, aucklandia root, eagle wood, musk, realgar powed, cloves, liquorice, moleplant seed, knoxia root, pleione rhizome, borneol, cinnabar powder, medicated leaven powder

No	NAME	SOURCE BOOK	COMPOSITION OF THE PRESCRIPTION
375	Zhu Che Pill	Bei Ji Qian Jin Yao Fang	coptis root, donkey-hide gelatin, Chinese angelica root, dried ginger
376	Zhu Li Da Tan Pill	Gu Jin Yin Jian	Lapis Chloriti eagle wood, Rhubarb, scutellaria root, bamboo juice, pinellia tuber, red tangerine peel, liquorice, ginger guice, poria, ginseng
377	Zhu Ling Decoction	Shang Han Lun	umbellate pore, poria, Alisma orientale, donkey-hide gelatin, tale
378	Zhu Ru Decoction	Ben Shi Fang	pinellia tuber, dried ginger, liquorice, fresh ginger, Chiness-date, etc.
379	Zhu Sha An Shen Pill	Yi Xue Fa Ming	coptis root, cinnabar, dried rehmannia root, prepared liquorice, etc.
380	Zhu Ye Shi Gao Decoction	Shang Han Lun	Lophatherum, gypsum, ophiopogon root, ginseng, pinellia tuber, stalk rice, prepared liquorice
381	Zi Jin Pellet	Pu Ji Ben Shi Fang	white arsenic, fermented soya beans
382	Zi Shen Tong Guan Pill	Lan Shi Mi Cang	Anemarrhena asphodeloides, phellodendron bark, bark of Chinese cassia tree
383	Zi Shui Qing Gan Drink	Yi Zong Ji Ren Pian	dried rehmannia root, dogwood fruit, poria, Chinese angelica root, Chinese yam, moutan bark, Allsma orientale, white peony root, bupleurum root, Gardenia Jasminoides, wild or sping jujuba seed
384	Zi Xue Pellet	Tai Ping Hui Min He Ji Ju Fang	tale, gypsum, calcite, magnetite, antelope's horn, dutchmanspipe root, rhinoceros horn, eagle wood, cloves, cinnicifuga rhizome, scrophularia root, liquorice, cinnabar benzoin, etc.

No	NAME	SOURCE BOOK	COMPOSITION OF THE PRESCRIPTION
385	Zuo Gui Pill	Jing Yue Quan Shu	prepared rehmannia root, Chinese yam, dogwood fruit, cyathula root, antler glue, tortoise-plastron glue
386	Zuo Gui Yin	Jing Yue Quan Shu	prepared rehmannia root, dogwood fruit, wolfberry fruit, Chinese yam, eucommia bark, liquorice, prepared aconite root, bark of Chinese cassia tree
387	Zuo Jin Pill	Dan Xi Xin Fa	coptis root, dogwood fruit

中 医 内 科 学

总 论

第一章 中医内科学发展简况

中医内科学是祖国医学宝库中的重要组成部分，古称“大方脉”，这是人类在长期的医疗实践中不断积累、逐渐形成的。

由于中医内科学在祖国医学中的特殊地位，因此，它的起源亦可以像祖国医学一样追溯到原始社会。如《山海经》一书中，就可以看到“风”、“症”、“疫疾”、“腹痛”等内科病证的名称和症状。进入封建社会，生产力发展到一定的水平，医学理论开始产生。奴隶社会，奴隶们创造越来越丰富的财富，给科学文化的发展创造了条件，阶级的出现与社会分工的进一步扩大，使各行各业日趋专业化，内科学就逐渐从医疗实践中突出和独立出来。据《周礼·天官》记载，当时的宫廷医生已分为疾医、食医、疡医、兽医四种，其中疾医相当于内科医生，而扁鹊被人们视为分科的先师。由于内科疾病的普遍存在和医疗实践的深入发展，使内科学的理论知识和临床经验得到迅猛的发展，尤其是《黄帝内经》的问世，被视为战国以前医学知识的总结。

殷周之际出现的阴阳五行学说是朴素的唯物主义学说，至春秋战国时代，则被广泛用以阐述和解释一切自然现象，与此同时也被祖国医学所采纳，用以探讨和认识人体生理病理现象，从而促进了医学的发展，为祖国医学奠定了比较坚实可靠的理论基础。因此，自战国迄秦汉这一时期，为祖国医学理论体系的奠基时期。

《黄帝内经》包括《素问》、《灵枢》两部分，共 18 卷，各 81 篇。其基本理论可以概括为：①强调整体观念：人体是一个有机的整体；人的健康和病态与自然环境有一定的关系。② 将阴阳五行学说贯穿于生理、病理、诊断及治疗等各个方面，摸索出人体疾病变化与治疗的粗略规律。③重视脏腑、经络，论述人身五脏六腑、十二经脉、奇经八脉等的生理功能、病理变化及其相互关系。④在以上理论指导下叙述六淫、七情、饮食、劳伤等病因，以及脏腑六气经络的病理变化。⑤论述望、闻、问、切四诊的诊断方法和具体内容。⑥确定治未病，因时、因地、因人制宜，标本、正治反治，制方、饮食宜忌、精神治疗及针刺大法等治疗法则。形成了比较系统的理论体系，已见理法方药的雏型，成为内科学理论的渊源。

另外，《黄帝内经》还记叙了 200 多种内科病证，从病因、病理、病性转化及预后等方面作了简要的论述，有些病证还专篇加以讨论，如“热论”、“咳论”、“痿论”、“疟论”、“痹论”等，从而为内科学的发展打下了基础。

张仲景继承了《内经》等古典医籍的基本理论，以六经论伤寒，以脏腑言杂病，提出了包括理、法、方、药在内的比较系统的辨证施治原则，使祖国医学的基础理论与临床实践密切结合起来，走上了科学发展的轨道。

《伤寒论》以六经论伤寒，分别讨论各经病证的特点和相应的治法，此外，还阐述了各经病证的传变关系，以及合病、并病或失治、误治引起的变证、坏证的辨证与治疗方法。通过六经辨证，又可以认识证候变化方面的表里之分、寒热之异、虚实之别，再以阴阳加以总概括，从而为后世的八纲辨证打下了基础。

《金匮要略》以脏腑论杂病，以病证设专题、专篇并加以论述，如肺痈、肺痿、痰饮、黄疸、痢疾、水肿等病证的辨证与治疗。

张仲景开创辨证论治的先河，临证时因证立法、以法系方、按方遣药，而且注意剂型对治疗效果的影响。书中共制375首方剂，有不少功效卓著的名方，一直沿用至今。因此，《伤寒杂病论》在中医学术上及内科学的发展上占有重要的位置。

经隋至唐，由于祖国医学理论与临床的发展，医学教育也达到比较完善的程度。宫廷医学校的课程规定，必须先学《素问》、《神农本草经》、《脉经》等基础课，然后再学习包括内科在内的临床各科，加强了理论与实践之间的有机联系，亦可以看出内科在当时所处的位置和所具的规模。隋唐时代，对内科中的多种疾病已有详细的论述，如对伤寒、中风、天行、温病、脚气病、地方性甲状腺肿等都积累了一定的治疗经验，对绦虫病、麻风、恙虫病、狂犬病的预防和治疗亦具有较高的水平。《外台秘要》已记载消渴病患者的尿是甜的，以及通过对黄疸病患者治疗效果的观察，提出"每夜小便中浸白帛片，取色退可验"。孙思邈进一步总结了消渴病的发病过程及其药物、食治等疗法，并规定了饮食、起居的某些禁忌。《诸病源候论》是我国现存最早的病因病机学及证候学专著，其中记载内科病27卷，内科症状784条，对每一个病证的病因、病理、证候分类进行了深入的探讨和总结。如对泄泻与痢疾、痰证与饮证，一反过去而分别立论；对寸白虫的病因、疟疾的分类、麻风病的临床表现都具有极其深刻的认识。

宋代对于医学人才的选拔与培养比较重视，规定各科人员之间的比例关系。《元丰备对》记载宋神宗时"太医局九科学生额三百人"分科中属内科的大方脉120人，风科80人，可见当时对内科之器重。从宋代起，金、元、明三代均设有大方脉科，为治疗成人各种内科疾病的专科，促进了内科的进步。特别值得提出的是金元时代四大医家的出现，他们各自结合当时的社会形势、人体状况及发病特点，总结了具有特色的理论和治疗方法。如刘完素对《内经》中五运六气学说有深刻的研究，他根据临床实践经验，参照《内经》病机十九条精神，认为"火热"是引起疾病的重要原因，故力倡火热致病的机理，创立"火热论"，在治疗上，他极善于使用寒凉药物，故后世称之为"寒凉派"。张子和受刘完素的学术影响并加以发挥，认为疾病发生的根本原因全在于病邪之侵害，不论外因、内因致病，一经损害人体，即应设法驱邪外出，不能让其滞留体内为患。他把汗、吐、下三法广泛运用于临床，并有独到的见解。由于他治病以攻邪为主，后人称他为"攻下派"。李杲生活于金元混战、社会动荡之年，人们饥寒交迫，民不聊生，体质虚弱，从而使脾胃在人体中的地位更加突出。所以，他指出"内伤脾胃，百病由生"，治病时则多用补气升阳的药物。由于他擅长温补脾胃，后世称他为"补土派"。朱丹溪研究了先世医家的学术思想和著作，熔各家学说于一炉，独树"相火论"、"阳有余，阴不足"两论。在治疗上，竭力主张滋阴降火之法，故后世称他为"滋阴派"。此四者形成了对后世影响极大的四大学派。

金元四大家及其弟子创建的四大学派，除了其本身的学术价值外，则是他们结合实践中出现的疾病，敢于和善于从临床到理论进行探索、总结，乃至提出自己的见解，证明了祖国医学发展过程中的内在联系——即继承性，同时在继承过程中可以得到发展，这一点对后世具有极大的启迪。

自金元四大家起掀起学术争鸣之风，遂至后世历代诸家纷纷而起，各抒己见，使中医的理论与实践日趋深入、成熟、系统和完整。如历代对中风之争，或言真中，或言类中，或言"非风"，越辨越明。又如补脾、补肾及脾肾双补的推敲，使脾肾的生理、病理、在人体中的重要性以及二者之间的联系也更加明确。再如对臌胀的病机认识，从东垣与丹溪的“湿热论”到赵养葵、孙一奎的“火衰论”，再至喻昌的“水裹气结血瘀论”，也是越分析越透彻，从而能更好地指导临床实践，提高了治疗效果。

金元时代的成就不仅限于金元四大家。与此同时，《圣济总录》有 18 卷专论诸风，反映当时对“风证”的专题研究已有一定的水平。张锐著《鸡峰普济方》，把水肿分为多种类型，根据起始部位的特征区别不同性质的水肿，施以不同治法。另外，还有一些内科病的专著问世，如宋代董汲著《脚气治法总要》，对脚气病的病因、发病情况、治疗方法均有详细论述，并订出 64 方，是一部现存较全面的脚气病专书。元代葛可久著《十药神书》是一部治疗肺痨病的专著，书中所拟 10 首名药方，分别具有止血、止嗽、祛痰、补养等作用，对肺痨全过程的分型和治疗总结了一套可以遵循的经验。

病因学在此时也有重要发展，陈无择的《三因极一病证方论》一书在《伤寒论》病因分类的基础上，结合《内经》理论，创立外因、内因、不内外因的三因学说，此说概括性强，适于临证应用，沿用至今。

金元以后，在中医学术界掀起了发展、创新的风气，如对人体某一脏腑生理、病理的新的探讨，或某脏腑代谢产物被重视，以及某个内科病证证治的见解不断有新的突破，使祖国医学及其内科学在广度与深度上都得到迅速发展。

明代继承了金元的学术成就并有新的发展，如薛己的《内科摘要》在学术上受李杲善于温补的影响，而有所发展，是我国最早用内科命名的医书。虞抟的《医学正传》则发展了朱丹溪的学说。王纶明确指出：“外感法仲景，内伤法东垣，热病用河间，杂病用丹溪”，是对当时内科学术思想的总结。另外，龚廷贤所著《寿世保元》先基础，后临床，先论述，后列方，并附医案，取材丰富，立论精详，选方切用，适于内科临床参考。《景岳全书》为纠正金元刘、张嗜用寒凉攻伐之偏，倡导人之生气阳为主，指出人体“阳非有余，阴常不足”，而主温补之法。该书论内科杂病部分计 28 卷，记述 70 余种病证的证治，每病证均引录古说，参以己见。张氏对内科许多病证病理之分析与归纳极为精辟，治则方药也多有心得，张氏结合病证对温补学说进行了充分的阐述。

明清时代，温病学说的形成和发展，使内科学之外感病的实践与理论进入更高、更完善的境地。吴又可的《温疫论》，是我国传染病学中较早的专门论著。他认为，瘟疫有别于其他热性病，它不因感受“六气”所致，而以感染“戾气”和机体机能状况不良为发病主因，并指出“戾气”的传染途径是其与人体接触，自口鼻而入，无论老少强弱，触之皆病。这一认识，在我国医学发展史上也是一个突破性的见解。叶天士的《温热论》为温病学的发展提供了理论与辨证的基础，其贡献在于：首先提出了“温邪上受，首先犯肺，逆传心包”之说，概括了温病的发病途径和传变规律，成为外感温病的纲领；其次，根据温病的发病过程，分为卫、气、营、血 4 个阶段，表示病变由浅入深的 4 个层次，作为辨证施治的纲领；再者，在温病诊断上，总结前人经验，创造地发展了察舌、验齿、辨别斑疹与白痦的方法。这就为温病学说奠定了理论与实践基础。吴鞠通在叶氏学说基础上著成《温病条辨》，以三焦为纲，病名为目，论述风温、温热、瘟疫等 9 种温病的证治，并提出清络、清营、育阴等各种治法，使温病学说更趋系统和完整，建立了温病辨证论治体系。其后薛生白著《湿热病篇》，对湿温病进行了深入研讨；王孟英著《温热经纬》将温病分为新感与伏气两大类进行辨证施治。也都对温病学说作了发挥和补充，促进了温病学说的发展。

在内科杂证方面，明清也有一定发展。喻昌《寓意草》中提出疾病发生与时代背景密切相联的观点，加深了对疾病发生的本质的认识，故而提高了疾病诊疗和理论水平。另外，如林佩琴的《类证治裁》极为实用。再者熊笏著的《中风论》及尤在泾著的《金匮翼》对中风病的叙述，胡慎柔著的《慎柔五书》、绮石著的《理虚元鉴》对虚痨病的分析，卢之颐著的《痎疟论疏》对疟疾的认识，都可称之为内科专篇专著，有一定学术水平。此时，对血证的认识有新的突破，如王清任著的《医林改错》，对瘀血证的论述和所创立的活血化瘀诸方，特别是为气虚血瘀所制益气活血之补阳还五汤更属创举，直到今日，仍有很高的实用价值。唐容川的《血证论》是论述血证的专著，对血证的认识更深入一步，并提出治血证四大要法，对后世影响较大。

鸦片战争以后，中国逐渐沦为半殖民地半封建社会，西医学传入我国，不可避免地影响了祖国传统医学的发展，所谓中西汇通派就是在这种条件下产生的。由于旧中国反动统治阶级的昏庸与无能，不可能正确引导中西两种医学取长补短，相互为用，反而企图扼杀中医，这是非常错误的。

新中国成立以后，在毛主席的“古为今用，洋为中用”思想指引下，继承发扬祖国医学的工作不断取得新进展。中医院校和中医医院的建立，使内科学同其他各学科一样，取得日新月异的发展。《中医内科学》统编教材的几次修订和使用，一些中医名家整理了自己的心得体会，著书立说，如秦伯未的《谦斋医学讲稿》，蒲辅周的《医案》、《医话》，任应秋的《论医集》都有一定的见解和发挥。这类书在党的“振兴中医”精神鼓舞下，必将越来越多，越来越好。1983 年的《衡阳会议》和 1985 年的《合肥会议》对振兴中医起了巨大推动作用，特别是中共中央书记处关于卫生工作的决定中，明确指出：“要把中医和西医摆在同等重要的地位。一方面，中医药学是我国医疗卫生事业所独具的特点和优势，中医不能丢，必须保存和发展；另一方面，中医必须积极利用先进的科学技术和现代化手段，促进中医药事业的发展。”这一决定得到全国的响应，各类中医院校和中医医院像雨后春笋般地出现，中医药队伍不断成长，造就出一大批内科专业人才，创造更高更新的内科理论，更好地指导临床实践，促进内科学的迅速发展。

复习思考题

1.《黄帝内经》、《伤寒杂病论》和《诸病源候论》对中医内科学的形成有何贡献？

2. 金元四大家对中医内科学的发展起到哪些推动作用？

3. 1985 年《合肥会议》上宣布的中共中央书记处关于卫生工作的决定的内容是什么？

第二章 中医内科学基础

第一节 病因学

祖国医学的病因学说是在古代医与巫斗争中逐渐发展起来的。春秋时期，秦国著名的医生医和提出六气病因学说，指出晦淫过度可以使人发生内热蛊惑之疾，可谓是比较原始的病因学说。《内经》已经清楚认识到疾病与自然环境的关系，并且提供防病的知识，这种预防思想的提出证实了当时对病因的认识已经相当深刻。《伤寒杂病论》把复杂的病因粗略地概括为三大类，已见病因学之端倪。该书指出："千般疢难，不越三条，一者，经络受邪入脏腑，为内所因也；二者，四肢九窍，血脉相传，壅塞不通，为外皮肤所中也；三者，房室、金刃、虫兽所伤。此以详之，病由都尽。"至隋巢氏《诸病源候论》被视为我国最早的病因病机学专著，书中对一些疾病病因、病理的描述比较详尽而科学，如某些寄生虫病的感染，已明确指出与饮食有关，如寸白虫病即认为是吃了不熟的肉类所致；还指出一些传染病是因感受外界的有害物质（乖戾之气）所致；某些病证的发生与人体的过敏体质有关，如接触生漆而生漆疮则与素质有关等等。以后的医学著作对病证的论述中，常先论病因，然后再论脉证方药等，如《太平圣惠方》、《圣济总录》，说明病因已为人们重视。

至宋代，陈言在仲景病因学的基础上，结合《内经》理论，对病因进行了深入研究，遂著成我国第一部病因学专著《三因极一病证方论》，系统地阐述了"三因学说"，指出：内因为七情，即喜、怒、忧、思、悲、恐、惊，所谓"七情动之，内伤脏腑，外形于肢体"；外因为六淫，即风、寒、暑、湿、燥、火，起于经络，发于脏腑，如伤寒、中暑、温疫等；不内外因为饮食饥饱，叫呼伤气，虫兽所伤，中毒金疮，跌损压溺等。这种分类方法更符合临床实际，而且明确、具体。后世医家虽结合当时社会背景对发病的影响，对具体的病因不断有新的发挥，如李杲的"饮食劳倦"，朱丹溪的"郁"及"房劳"，吴又可的"戾气"，王孟英的"新感"与"伏气"等，但都未出三因之约，至今，三因学说仍被沿用。

（一） 六淫

即风、寒、暑、湿、燥、火六种外感病邪的统称。六淫是外感病的主要致病因素，当人体内外环境失调时，感受六淫之气即能发病。

1. 风：风性多动善变，流行最广，常因季节不同，随其气候变化，而有风温、风寒、风暑、风燥之异，又常与其他邪气结合为风湿、风火等，故古人称"风为百病之长"。

感受风邪发病，轻者在上焦气分为"伤风"，重者在经络脏腑为"中风"。

2. 寒：寒为阴邪，性主收引。伤于体表者为"伤寒"，直接伤于里者为"中寒"。

3. 暑：暑是夏令的主气。暑热挟风伤表，邪在上焦。若在烈日下长途奔走或劳作等，感受暑热而发病，称之为"中暑"，也叫"中暍"。中暑是热症，多因动而得之，阳主动，故也称阳暑；相反，暑令因静而得病，就称为阴暑。暑热多挟湿气，这是由于天热地湿郁蒸的结合，故古人治暑多兼治湿。

4. 湿：湿为重浊之邪，黏滞难化。若气候潮湿、涉水淋雨、居处潮湿、汗出沾衣等均可使湿邪侵袭人体。湿属阴性，与风邪结合为风湿，与寒邪结合为寒湿，与热邪结合为湿热。

5. 燥：燥为秋季主气，亦为火之余气。燥邪为病又有温燥、凉燥之分，初秋有夏热之余气，燥与温热结合侵犯人体，则多见温燥病证，深秋又有近冬之寒气，燥与寒邪结合侵犯人体，则多见凉燥病证。

6. 火：火（热）为阳盛所生，火与热只是程度不同，多由外感温热邪气所化，古人有“五气化火”之说，凡风、寒、暑、湿、燥五气均可转化为火。

另外，疫疠之邪亦为外来致病因素之一。疫是互相染易，不问老少，病状相似，即传染之意；疠是指自然界一种毒戾之气，危害人体大而不同于普通的六淫之邪。

感染六淫之邪立即发病，称为“新感”；感染六淫之邪不立即发病，经过一个时期方才出现病证，称为“伏邪”。新感与伏邪相对，主要是从症状的表里、轻重和传变的迟速加以区别。

（二） 七情

七情即喜、怒、忧、思、悲、恐、惊七种情态变化。七情过激，可使人体气机紊乱，脏腑阴阳气血失调，导致疾病的发生。《内经》指出：“怒则气上，喜则气缓，悲则气消，恐则气下，思则气结。”又指出：“喜伤心，怒伤肝，思伤脾，忧伤肺、恐伤肾。”但这只说明七情致病的一般规律，并非绝对如此。七情引起的病变，最初是气的变化，而气血相关，病情进一步发展则影响到血。

七情致病，与刺激的强弱以及病人的体质和敏感性有一定的关系。另外，已病之人的情志异常波动，常可使病情加重或急剧恶化。

（三） 饮食

饮食是人体营养的主要来源，若饮食不节或不洁、偏嗜等常能使脾胃纳化失调而致病，即伤食。可造成肠胃病，即《内经》所说“饮食自倍，肠胃乃伤”。伤食还可聚湿、凝痰、化热、生虫或变生他证。

（四） 内生五邪

内生五邪即内风、内寒、内湿、内燥、内火（内热）的统称，是脏腑功能失调所产生的病理产物，同时又是致病因素。

1. 内风：多由肝阳、阴虚、痰火过甚所变生而成，常导致眩晕、抽搐、昏厥、麻木、角弓反张等。

2. 内寒：多由气虚、阳虚而产生，如心阳虚、肺气虚、脾阳虚、肾阳虚等均可变生相应的病证，称其为虚寒，常导致脘腹隐痛、腹泻、肢冷、脉微等。

3. 内湿：嗜食膏粱厚味，或过食生冷瓜果、甜腻食物，或外湿入里，均可使脾气不运，湿浊内生，常导致胸闷脘痞、纳呆泛呕、尿少便溏、面浮肢肿等。

4. 内燥：热病之后，津血耗伤，或过服温热之品，或汗、吐、下法克伐太过，也能伤津亡液，燥症易起。常导致皮肤干燥、口唇燥裂、目中干涩、鼻孔燥热、渴饮善饥、咽干噎隔、大便不畅，甚则酿成痿躄、劳嗽、痉病等。

5. 内火：可分为实火与虚火两类。实火多由五脏功能亢进所生，称为“五志之火”，常导致口疮、心烦、不寐目赤、口苦、头昏胀痛、咽痛、咳血、吐血、痰黄、腹痛、便秘、溲赤、遗精、淋证等。虚火多由阴血亏损所生，常导致潮热盗汗、颧红耳鸣、虚烦不眠等。

（五） 痰饮

痰饮主要是肺、脾、肾功能失调，水液代谢障碍所变生。古人有“水泛为痰”、“水沸为痰”之说。痰黏稠而饮清稀，痰无处不到，症状多端，而饮易停留于空腔或组织疏松之处。

(六)瘀血

凡血脉中血液流行不畅、停滞，或离经之血停积体内，称之瘀血。多由气滞、气虚、血寒、血热、阴血不足、阳气不振、以及外伤等产生。常导致疼痛如刺、固定不移、肿块、肌肤甲错、唇舌青紫、瘀斑、瘀点等。

(七)劳逸太过

劳指劳累，逸指安逸。过度劳累或过度安逸均可致病。劳包括劳力过度，劳神过度，房劳过度。逸包括长期既不劳动，也不运动，致使人体气血不畅，脾胃功能减弱，《内经》所说“久卧伤气”就是此意。

(八)外伤

包括枪弹伤、金刃伤、跌打损伤、持重努伤、烧烫伤、冻伤、虫兽伤、食物中毒或药物中毒等，这些因素不仅引起外科病证，而且能使脏腑功能失调，导致内科病证。

六淫之邪属于外因，七情、饮食、内生五邪、痰饮、瘀血属于内因，劳逸太过、外伤属于不内外因。

第二节　病理学

《黄帝内经》奠定了祖国医学理论的基础，对人体的生理、病理已有相当深刻的论述，为后世病理学的发展创造了条件。《伤寒杂病论》对病理学作出了创造性的发挥，提出“六经辨伤寒，脏腑辨杂病”的方法，开创了六经辨证和脏腑辨证的先导。以后医家又将六经辨证运用于杂病，脏腑辨证也日渐发展并深化，特别是金元四大家从不同的方面作了深入的阐述。由于历代医家的不断努力，脏腑辨证逐渐完善，而且对脏腑变化的病理产物如气、血、风、火、痰、湿、瘀血等的认识，也日益深刻，经过不断整理与充实而日趋系统和完整。明清温病学说的发展，提出和完善了卫气营血辨证和三焦辨证的具体内容，亦形成完整的病理学说。从实践中人们认识到，祖国医学丰富的病理学说，在不同类型的疾病中应用，如六经、卫气营血、三焦多用于外感病，而脏腑、气血、风火痰湿等多用于内伤病，但两者也是可以互相影响、互相渗透的。后世逐步认识到，诸多辨证方法都可以统一到脏腑生理、病理上来。诚然，这项工作还有待进一步去探索，它必将促进病理学的不断发展。

一、脏腑病机、病证的基本概念

脏腑病机，是探讨疾病发生演变过程中脏腑功能活动病理变化的机制。脏腑病证，是脏腑病理变化反映于临床的不同证候。

从脏腑病理生理学理解，心主血脉，血脉充足则面色红润光泽；又主神明，主宰情志思维活动；舌为心之苗，又为心窍，心与小肠互为表里，故心热常反映出舌尖色红，而移热于小肠，则见舌疮心烦、小溲短赤。心包为心之外卫，保护心主，故外邪内侵，则心包代心受邪为病。肺主气，司呼吸，外合皮毛，开窍于鼻，主一身之治节，且肺为娇脏，不耐寒热，故外感诸病，常先犯肺卫为患。肺与大肠互为表里，大肠职司传导，有赖肺气之肃降而排泄通调；反之，大肠积滞不通，也能影响肺气肃降。脾胃为后天之本，气血生化之源，主受纳、腐熟、运化水谷。脾有统血功能，四肢肌肉亦为脾所主。脾性升清，胃宜通降。二者功能一旦失健，必将影响水谷之纳化，出现一系列胃肠病变。肝性刚强，喜疏泄条达，藏血，濡养筋与爪甲，开窍于目，其经脉络胆，会巅，绕阴器。胆附于肝，互为表里。若肝阳亢盛，则胆火亦旺，可见面红、目赤、头痛诸症；肝血不足，则胆气亦衰，而现头晕、目涩、视力减退及雀盲等症。肾为水火之脏，命门附于两肾，内寄真阴真阳，主藏精，有温润五脏的功能，为人体精髓之源泉，故称先天之本。脑健、骨坚、发荣、耳聪、齿固，是为肾气充实；生育、发育、月事为肾所司，亦反映肾气之盈亏。肾与膀胱互为表里，膀胱为州都之官，主藏津液，其气化赖肾气之开阖。所以肾脏有病，就会出现骨不坚、脑不健、发不荣、耳不聪、齿不固，甚至发育迟缓、月事中断、胎产障碍、气化失职。并可为喘逆、肿满、癃闭、遗尿诸证。

因为脏腑是构成人体的一个密切联系的整体，五脏之间有生克乘侮，脏与腑又互为表里，所以在疾病演变过程中，反映出来的病理变化和证候就极为错综复杂；尤其是病机的演变发展，虚实寒热的参合更迭，都是辨证施治的关键。若能明确脏腑病机的基本概念，就能由浅入深，分辨各种内科杂病的不同证候，分清病情主次、病性虚实、病理转化，从而运用理、法、方、药，一线贯通，为临床实践和深入钻研打下良好基础。

兹分别就心与小肠、肺与大肠、脾与胃、肝与胆、肾与膀胱等脏腑的生理、病理、病证范围、证候分类以及辨证论治要点，分述如下。至于心包为心之外卫，三焦是脏腑的外腑，前者附入于心，后者基本上包括了脏腑的病机病证，故不列专题讨论。

（一）心（附小肠）

1. 生理：心居胸中，心包围护其外，与小肠互为表里，在体为脉，其经脉下络小肠，舌为心之窍。心主血脉，故为人体生命活动的中心；又主神明，故为情志思维活动之中枢。

2. 病理：因为心之生理功能主要为主血脉和神明，因此在病理条件下，反映在临床上的证候就离不开血脉运行的障碍和情志思维活动的异常。又心包为心之外卫，故温邪逆传，多为心包所受，而心本脏之病多起于内伤，如禀赋不足，脏气虚弱，或病后失调，以及思虑过度，伤及心脾，都是导致心阴虚或心阳虚的病因。心阴虚的主要病机为心血亏耗，心阳虚的主要病机是心气不足，两者皆能表现为心神不宁。若思虑太过，气机郁结，津液凝聚，生痰化火，痰火上扰，或气滞脉中，瘀血阻络，或饮邪阻遏心阳，均可出现心之热证和实证。

心之病理机制示意图

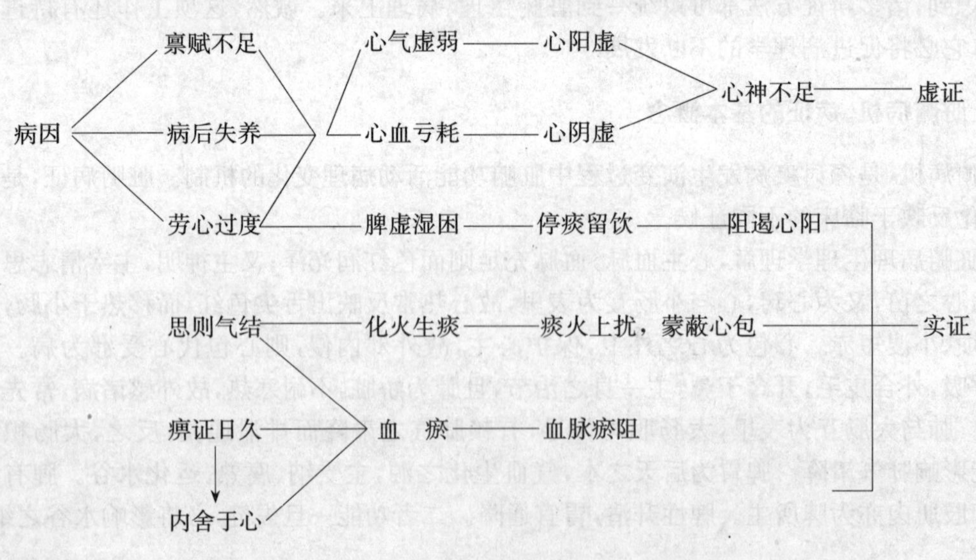

3. 病证范围：主要有心悸、心痛、健忘、失眠、癫狂、昏迷、气喘、吐血、衄血、舌疮、尿血、遗精等。

4. 证候分类

(1)虚证

①心阳虚

病机概要：为思虑伤神，劳心过度，心气不足所致。

主要脉症：心悸，气喘，心痛，舌苔淡白，脉细弱或虚大无力等，为心阳虚之主症。心悸的特点为心中空虚，惕惕而动，动则尤甚。气喘的表现为阵阵发作，气短而息促，行动尤甚。心痛系暴作，并现肢冷，脉疾数而散乱，甚则手足唇鼻青紫晦暗，或面色皖白，自汗，形寒等症参见。

②心阴虚

病机概要：思虑劳心过度，以致营血亏虚，阴精暗耗，阴不敛阳，心阳浮越。

主要脉症：心悸，心痛，少寐，心嘈，舌质淡红，苔少或舌尖干赤等为心阴虚之主症。其心悸心痛的特点为心悸而烦，隐隐作痛，惊惕不安。少寐多伴梦扰不宁，心嘈乃心中灼热似饥。此外，或见健忘，梦遗，盗汗，多疑善虑等证。

治疗：滋阴养心安神。用天王补心丹或朱砂安神丸之类。

(2)实证

①痰火内扰

病机概要：思则气结，津液凝聚为痰，或脾不健运，湿痰内蕴，蕴久化火，痰热内扰，甚则上蒙心包，心神不宁。

主要脉症：心悸，癫狂，不寐，舌质红赤或干裂，苔黄，脉滑数为其主症。其心悸为时时动悸，胸中烦热躁动；癫狂的特点为神志痴呆，或急躁易怒，甚则哭笑无常，如癫如狂。不寐多见恶梦纷纭，躁扰难寝，或面赤，口渴喜冷饮，吐血，衄血，小便热赤，溲血淋痛等症。

治疗：清心豁痰。用黄连温胆汤或礞石滚痰丸。

②饮邪阻遏心阳

病机概要：水湿内停，积久成饮，停于胸中，阻遏心阳。

主要脉症：心悸，眩晕，呕吐，舌苔白腻，脉象滑或沉紧为主证。本证之心悸为悸而胸闷，气机不畅。眩晕多伴泛恶欲吐。呕吐皆为痰涎。有时兼见畏寒，痞满，肠鸣。

治疗：温阳化饮。用小半夏加茯苓汤或苓桂术甘汤之类。

③心血瘀阻

病机概要：劳倦伤心，心气不振，气滞脉中，或痹证日久，内舍于心，血脉痹阻，络道不和。

主要脉症：心悸不宁，胸部刺痛或牵及两胁肩背，舌质暗红，并见紫色瘀点，苔少，或见面青，唇甲青紫，脉涩等。

治疗：活血化瘀通络。用失笑散或血府逐瘀汤之类。

(3)兼证

①心脾两虚：面色萎黄，食少倦怠，气短神怯，健忘，怔忡，少寐，妇女月经不调，脉细软无力，苔白舌淡。治宜补益心脾，用归脾汤之类。

②心肾不交：虚烦不眠，夜寐梦遗，潮热盗汗，咽干，目眩耳鸣，腰酸腿软，夜间尿多，舌红无苔，脉虚数。治宜交通心肾，用黄连阿胶汤或交泰丸之类。

③痰瘀互结：心烦不寐，多梦善惊，纳呆泛呕，头晕目眩，胸脘痞闷，胸中刺痛，胸痛彻背，舌

质紫暗或有瘀斑，苔腻，脉滑。治宜化痰祛瘀，用温胆汤合丹参饮之类。

④热移小肠，详见小肠实热。

5. 证治要点

(1)心气不足和心血亏耗，为鉴别心阳虚和心阴虚的主要病机。

(2)临证时如遇有阴阳两虚、气血俱亏者，应两者兼治，如炙甘草汤之阴阳并调，十全大补汤之气血双补。

(3)心阳虚与饮邪阻遏心阳两证，与脾阳不运也有关系，治疗还应温运脾阳，健脾养心。

(4)心阴虚与痰火内扰两证，与肝经的虚实也有关系，前者是血亏木失荣，后者是火旺木被焚，治疗时应联系整体处理。

(5)痰瘀同源于心火，也可同源于心脾两虚，故痰瘀互阻之证可以同现。治疗时则宜消痰与祛瘀兼施，或补益心脾以化痰祛瘀。

(6)虚证一般均可佐用安神宁心之品，如枣仁、柏子仁、茯神、龙眼肉等。实证均可使用镇静开窍之品，如龙齿、牡蛎、郁金、菖蒲、琥珀等。

(7)小肠病由于心移热者，均为实证，治宜清心火，导热下行。小肠本经之病，多与脾、胃、大肠相关，临证时应联系互参。

心病辨证施治见简表。

心病辨证施治简表

证别	虚证		实证		
	心阳虚	心阴虚	痰火	饮邪	瘀血
病机	心气不足	心血亏耗	痰火内扰 蒙蔽心窍	饮邪上逆阻遏心阳	瘀血阻络
神志	喜静怕动 气惫形寒 面白虚浮	神情多疑 面色少华	神志痴呆 或躁扰不 宁语无伦次	畏寒背冷 身体瞤动 呕吐痰涎	痛楚不安 指甲青紫
心悸	空虚而悸	虚烦而悸	烦而悸躁 胸中烦热	悸而胸闷 或见喘息	悸惕心痛 时作时止
心痛	隐痛	隐痛或烦痛	闷痛或灼痛	闷痛或悸痛	刺痛
睡眠	嗜睡	少睡多梦	不寐躁扰 梦扰纷纭	喘息悸而 难以安卧	痛时难寐
出汗	易见自汗	易见盗汗	易见自汗	易见自汗	痛剧见汗出
舌苔	舌质淡白	舌质嫩红 或尖红少苔	舌红苔黄厚	舌苔白腻	舌质紫黯 或有瘀斑瘀点
脉象	虚弱或大 而中空	细数	滑数	沉紧或小滑	涩
治法	益心气温心阳	滋养 心阴	清火豁痰	化饮除痰	活血行瘀通络
方剂	养心汤 四逆汤	天王补心丹 朱砂安神丸	小陷胸汤 礞石滚痰丸	小半夏加茯苓汤 苓桂术甘汤	失笑散 血府逐瘀汤

附:小肠

1. 生理:小肠上接幽门,与胃相通,下连大肠,两者相合处为阑门,其经脉络心。小肠受盛胃中水谷,主转输清浊,清者输于各部;浊者渗入膀胱,下注大肠。

2. 病理:小肠之病,多因饮食失节,损伤脾胃下传而引起。小肠与心互为表里,故心亦移热于小肠。一旦小肠为病,其病理表现主要为浊清不分,转输障碍,症见小便不利、大便泄泻,临床上可分为虚寒、实热、气痛三证。

3. 证候分类

(1)小肠虚寒:小腹隐痛喜按,肠鸣溏泻,小便频数不爽,舌淡苔薄白,脉细而缓。治以温通小肠,用吴茱萸汤之类。

(2)小肠实热:心烦口疮,咽痛耳聋,小便赤涩,或茎中痛,脐腹作胀,矢气后稍快,舌红苔黄,脉滑数。治以清利实热,用导赤散或凉膈散之类。

(3)小肠气痛:小腹急痛,连及腰背,下控睾丸,苔白,脉沉弦或弦滑。治以行气散结,用天台乌药散之类。

(二)肝(附胆)

1. 生理:肝在胁下,胆附其中。肝在体为筋,开窍于目,其经脉连目系,交于巅。肝主血液之贮藏调节,目得其养而视明。肝又司全身筋骨关节之屈伸,其性刚强,喜条达而恶抑郁,凡精神情志功能之调节,均与肝气有密切关系。

2. 病理:肝病的病理表现,也可概括为虚实两证,而以实证为多见。因肝为刚脏,主藏血,体阴而用阳,由于情志所伤,致肝气不得疏泄,郁而化火,火动则阳失潜藏,阳亢则风自内生,风火相煽,上升巅顶,或横窜经络,以致血不归藏,随气火而并走于上。根据其病情轻重之不同,又可分为肝气郁结、肝火内炽、肝阳上亢等实热证候。若肾阴亏虚,精不化血,肝失濡养,则成肝阴不足、虚阳上扰的虚证。外寒入侵,滞留于肝脉,亦属肝之实证。

肝病的病机示意图

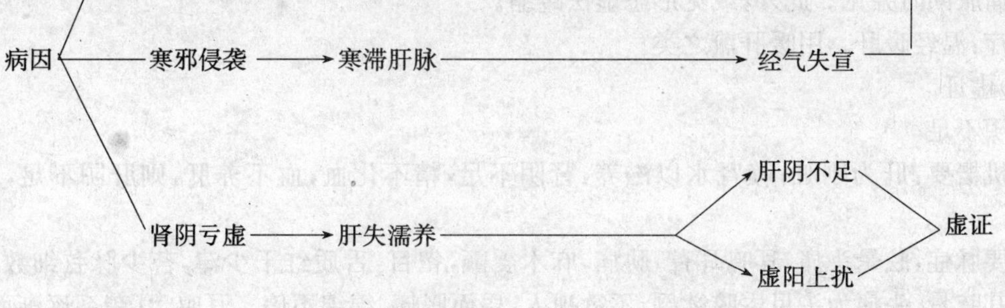

3. 病证范围:肝与胆的病理变化,反映于临床上,主要有眩晕、头痛、惊恐、不寐、耳聋、耳鸣、吐血、衄血、痉、痫、麻木、震颤、昏厥、中风、积聚、疝、等病证。

4. 证候分类

(1)实证

①肝气郁结

病机概要:郁怒伤肝,木失条达,肝气横逆,疏泄无权,气机阻滞不畅,为痛为聚;血行瘀阻,经脉痹塞,为痞为积。

主要脉症:胁痛,呕逆,腹痛便泄,便后不爽,积聚,苔薄,脉弦等为其主要症候。其胁痛为气闷不舒,流窜作痛,不得转侧。呕逆为气逆吐酸或呕出黄绿苦水。腹痛便泄,便后不爽之特点,系时有少腹作痛不适、泻后不减,每因情志不遂而发。积聚之部位在胁下,癖积或左或右,或聚散无常,时觉胀痛或刺痛。此外,尚可出现易怒、食欲不振等。

治疗:疏肝理气,破积散聚。用柴胡疏肝散或血瘀丸之类。

②肝火内炽

病机概要:肝胆疏泄无权,气郁化火,火随气窜,或火性炎上,上扰巅顶。

主要脉症:胁痛,呕吐,眩晕,头痛,狂怒,耳聋,耳鸣,目赤,吐衄,舌边光红,苔黄或干腻,脉象弦数等为其主症。其胁痛为灼痛而烦。呕吐苦水或黄水。眩晕、头痛为头晕不支,自觉筋脉跳动,额热而痛,痛若刀劈,或为胀痛。耳鸣、耳聋均为暴作,鸣声如潮,阵作阵平,按之不减。目赤为眼结膜发红,暴痛或肿。吐衄亦为骤然暴作,血涌量多,冲口而出。此外,尚可见小便热涩黄赤,面赤而热,口苦而干等。

治疗:清泄肝胆。用龙胆泻肝汤之类。

③肝阳上亢

病机概要:肝气化火,阳气暴张,火随气窜,横逆络道,血随气升,上冲巅顶。

主要脉症:昏厥,痉挛,麻木,眩晕,头痛,脉弦,舌体歪斜颤动,舌质红,苔薄黄等为其主症。其昏厥为卒然晕仆,不省人事,或抽搐,或吐涎。痉挛表现为项强,四肢挛急,不能屈伸,角弓反张。麻木为手足面唇等部有如蚁行。眩晕、头痛为头眩眼花,行走飘浮,头部抽掣作痛。此外,还可在昏厥之后,出现口眼㖞斜,语言謇涩,半身不遂等症。

治疗:平肝熄风。用天麻钩藤饮之类。

④寒滞肝脉

病机概要:外感寒邪入侵厥阴肝经,肝气失宣,络气痹阻。

主要脉症:少腹胀痛,睾丸坠胀,或阴囊收缩,舌润滑,苔白,脉象沉弦或迟为其主证。少腹胀痛常牵及睾丸偏坠剧痛,受寒则甚,得热而缓。阴囊收缩为寒滞厥阴,致少腹之脉收引,故多与少腹痛胀同时并见。此外,或见形态虚怯踡缩。

治疗:温经暖肝。用暖肝煎之类。

(2)虚证

肝阴不足

病机概要:肝为刚脏,赖肾水以滋养,肾阴不足,精不化血,血不养肝,则肝阴不足,肝阳上亢。

主要脉症:眩晕头痛,耳鸣耳聋,胁痛,麻木震颤,雀目,舌质红干少津,苔少脉弦细数等为主症。其眩晕、头痛为头目昏眩欲倒,不欲视人,昏而胀痛,绵绵不停。耳鸣、耳聋系逐渐而起,鸣声低微,经常不已,按之可减。麻木为肢体不仁之感,抚之觉快。胁痛多为隐痛,拂之则减。震颤为肢体筋肉瞤动,或自觉或他觉发抖动摇,甚者四肢筋挛拘急。雀目为两目干涩,入夜视力大减，或成夜盲。此外，尚可见面部烘热，午后颧红，口燥咽干，少寐多梦等。

治疗：柔肝滋肾，育阴潜阳。用一贯煎或大补阴丸之类。

(3)兼证

①肝气犯胃：胸脘痞闷时痛，两胁走窜，食入不化，嗳气吐酸，舌苔薄黄，脉弦。治以泄肝和胃，用四逆散合左金丸之类。

②肝脾不和：不思饮食，腹胀肠鸣，便溏，舌苔白腻，脉弦缓。治以调和肝脾，用逍遥散之类。

③肝胆不宁：虚烦不眠，或恶梦惊恐，触事易惊或善恐，短气乏力，目视不明，口苦，苔薄白，脉弦细。治以养肝清胆宁神，用酸枣仁汤之类。若属痰热扰动，苔腻而黄，脉弦滑者，用黄连温胆汤。

④肝肾阴虚：面色憔悴，两颧嫩红，头眩目干，腰膝酸软，咽喉干痛，盗汗，五心烦热或大便艰涩，男子遗精，女子经水不调或带下，舌红无苔，脉细。治以滋阴降火，用杞菊地黄丸之类。

⑤肝火犯肺：胸胁刺痛，咳嗽阵作，咳吐鲜血，性急善怒，烦热，口苦，头眩目赤，苔薄舌红，脉弦数。治以清肝泻肺，用黛蛤散或泻白散之类。

5. 证治要点

(1)肝为刚脏，属春木而主风，性喜升发，故肝病多见肝阳的证候。肝之寒证，仅见寒凝少腹厥阴肝经。

(2)在肝病的实证中，肝气郁结、肝火内炽、肝阳上亢三者同出一源，多由情志郁结，肝气有余，化火上冲，致阴血不足而阳妄动。三者关系极为密切，不能截然分割，临床应掌握主次，随证论治。

(3)肝阳上亢为危重之证，有上冲巅顶和横窜经络之别。上冲者宜熄风潜阳，横窜者当和络熄风，挟痰则兼以涤痰。

(4)实证久延，易耗伤肝阴，形成本虚标实证。临床颇常见，辨证时须予注意。

(5)肝病虚证多因肾阴不足，精不化血，以致肝阴不足，阳亢上扰，应与实证对照，详细鉴别。其病机与肾阴亏乏有极为密切的关系，故临床多取肝肾并治之法。

肝病辨证施治见简表。

肝病辨证施治简表

证别	虚证	实证			
病机	肝阴不足 肾阴亏损 肝失濡养	肝气郁结 气机不畅 疏泄无权	肝火内炽 气郁化火 肝火内炽	肝阳上亢 血随气升横逆络道	寒客肝脉 寒客厥阴凝滞经络
眩晕	头目眩晕 不欲睁眼	眩晕偶作	头晕而胀烘 热阵阵上冲	头目眩晕 头重脚轻 行走飘浮	头晕欲倒
头痛	绵绵不休	两侧微胀痛	额热而痛如刀割	头顶抽搐而痛	偶作偏头痛
耳鸣	渐起如蝉鸣 按之可减	偶作耳鸣	耳鸣如潮按之不减	耳鸣轰响	偶作耳鸣

续表

证别	虚证	实证			
神态	抑郁	抑郁或易怒	躁怒或狂妄不避亲疏	口眼㖞斜语言不利甚则不省人事	恶寒踡缩
心胁腹痛	胁肋作痛隐然不快	胁肋胀痛走窜不定	心烦灼痛		腹痛引胁得热为快
眼征	两目干涩入夜失明	间有视物不清	目赤暴痛或肿	斜视不正	间有视物不清
二便	大便干涩	便秘或泄泻	大便干结小便赤热	可见遗尿	睾丸坠胀或囊缩便清
舌苔	舌质红少苔或光中裂	苔薄白或薄黄	舌质红苔黄少津	舌歪斜颤动舌红苔微黄	舌润滑苔白
脉象	弦细而数	弦	弦数	弦滑有力	沉弦
治法	养阴柔肝	疏肝理气	清泄肝胆	平肝熄风	温经暖肝
方剂	杞菊地黄丸	柴胡疏肝散	龙胆泻肝汤	天麻钩藤饮	暖肝煎

附:胆

1. 生理:胆附于肝,内藏清汁,其经脉络肝。胆中所藏为清净之汁,与其他传化之腑所盛之浊质不同,故《千金要方》又称之为"中清之腑"。所以,胆既属六腑,又属奇恒之腑。胆性刚直,豪壮果断,所以《素问》说:"胆者,中正之官,决断出焉。"

2. 病理:胆因寄附于肝,禀春生之气,其性刚直,故在病理情况下,多现阳亢火旺之证。火热可灼津为痰,故胆病又多兼痰证。痰火郁遏,常扰心神,故辨证施治之时,既要泻胆化痰,又要清心安神。

3. 证候分类

(1)胆虚证:头晕欲呕,易惊少寐,视物模糊,舌苔薄滑,脉弦细。治以养心神,和胆胃,用酸枣仁汤之类。

(2)胆实证:目眩耳聋,头晕,胸满胁痛,口苦,呕吐苦水,心烦易怒,寐少梦多,或往来寒热,或面目俱黄,脉弦数实,苔黄舌红。治以清胆泻热,用龙胆泻肝汤之类。伴黄疸者合用茵陈蒿汤。若心烦易怒,躁扰不宁,少寐多梦,痰黏纳少,苔腻而黄,脉弦滑者,治以清化痰热,用黄连温胆汤之类。

(三)脾(附胃)

1. 生理:脾与胃以膜相连,位于腹内,互为表里。脾胃为仓廪之官,在体为肉,开窍于口。胃主受纳,腐熟水谷,脾主运化,输布水谷精微,升清降浊,共为生化之源,五脏六腑,四肢百骸皆赖以养。脾又有益气、统血、主肌肉四肢等重要生理功能,故古人合称脾胃为"后天之本"。

2. 病理:脾胃的功能主要为受纳和运化,其致病因素多系饥饱劳倦所伤,影响水谷的消化吸收,使脾胃之受纳、腐熟、转输、传导等功能失调。脾经之病,不外虚实寒热等方面。如脾阳虚衰,中气不足属虚证;寒湿困脾,湿热内蕴属实证。脾虚不运则水湿不化,故脾病多与湿有关,而见本虚标实证候。而且脾虚也常影响他脏,出现兼证。

脾脏本经发病机制示意图

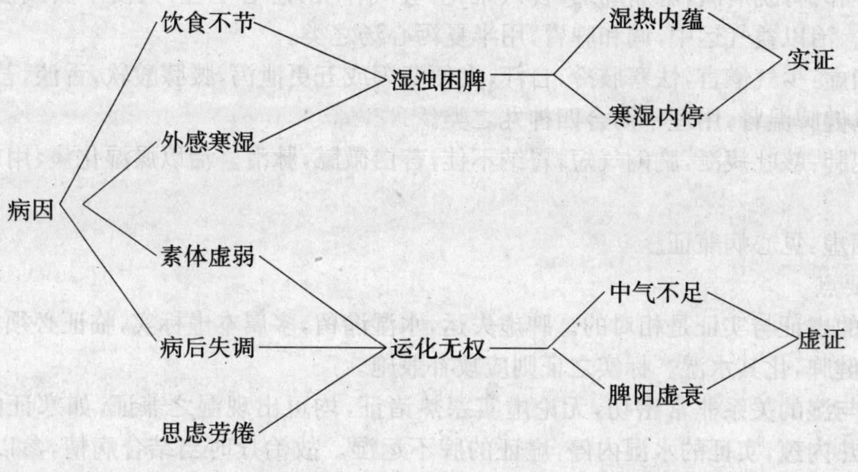

3. 病证范围：临床常见的脾胃病有泄泻、霍乱、黄疸、胃脘痛、呕吐、呃逆、水肿、臌胀、痰饮、吐血、便血、妇科崩漏等。

4. 证候分类

(1)虚证

①脾阳虚衰

病机概要：胃病日久，饮食生冷肥甘，或过用寒凉药物，及年高体弱或病后失养，脾阳不足，运化无权。

主要脉症：面黄少华，脘冷喜暖，喜热饮，便溏，溲清，或见肌肉消瘦，畏寒肢冷，少气懒言等，舌淡，苔白，脉濡弱为其主症。

治疗：温运中阳。用理中汤之类。

②中气不足

病机概要：素体气虚，或因病久耗伤脾胃之气，升清降浊无权。

主要脉症：声低气短，四肢乏力，肠鸣腹胀，大便溏薄而便意频，舌淡，苔薄白，脉缓或濡细等为其主症。或见肌肉消瘦，动则气坠于腰腹，脱肛等。

治疗：健脾益气。用四君子汤之类；中气下陷者，治以益气升阳。用补中益气汤。

(2)实证

①寒湿困脾

病机概要：涉水淋雨，坐卧湿地，或内湿素盛，中阳被遏，脾失运化。

主要脉症：饮食不香，中脘饱闷，口甜而黏，头身重困，便不实或泄泻，舌苔白腻，脉象濡细。

治疗：运脾化湿。用胃苓汤之类。

②湿热内蕴

病机概要：因感外邪，或素嗜酒酪，伤脾胃，脾失健运，湿停化热，湿热交阻，气机升降失司。

主要脉症：胸脘痞胀，不思饮食，口中黏腻，恶心呕吐，身重体困，小便色赤不利，苔黄而腻，脉濡数等为主症。或见口渴，口苦等症。

治疗：清热利湿。用小陷胸汤、连朴饮之类。

(3)兼证

①脾胃不和：胃脘痞满，隐痛绵绵，食入难化，嗳气作呃，恶心呕吐，大便不实或便次增多，脉细，苔薄白。治以益气运中，调和脾胃，用半夏泻心汤之类。

②脾肾阳虚：少气懒言，怯寒肢冷，自汗，大便溏泻或五更泄泻，腰膝酸软，舌淡，苔薄白，脉象沉细。治以健脾温肾，用理中汤合四神丸之类。

③脾湿犯肺：咳吐痰涎，胸闷气短，胃纳不佳，苔白微腻，脉滑。治以燥湿化痰，用二陈汤或平胃散之类。

④心脾两虚：见心病兼证。

5. 证治要点

(1)脾病的虚证与实证是相对的。脾虚失运，水湿潴留，多属本虚标实，临证必须注意。一般轻证，当先健脾，化其水湿。标实之证则应攻补兼施。

(2)脾病与湿的关系非常密切，无论虚实寒热诸证，均可出现湿之兼证，如寒证的寒湿困脾，热证的湿热内蕴，实证的水湿内停，虚证的脾不运湿。故治疗时当结合病情，参以燥湿、利湿、逐水、化湿之品，湿去则脾运自复。

(3)脾与胃的病理可相对地来看，古人认为“实则阳明，虚则太阴”，所以脾病多虚多寒，胃病多实多热。

(4)从脏腑整体观念分析，不但脾与胃肠有关，其病理演变与其他脏腑也有关，如脾病日久不愈，常影响及它脏；同样，他脏有病，也常传及于脾。所以，治脾能使其他脏腑疾病转归良好，而治疗其他脏腑也有助于脾病的恢复。

脾病辨证施治见简表。

脾病辨证施治简表

鉴别	虚证		实证	
	脾阳虚衰	中气不足	寒湿困脾	湿热内蕴
病机	中气亏耗 脾阳不振	脾胃不健 中气虚弱 甚则下陷	寒湿困遏 脾失运化	湿热交阻 升降失司
主症	脘冷腹胀 其痛隐隐 畏寒肢冷 渴喜热饮 少气懒言 溲清便溏	气短声怯 纳少不食 肢倦神疲 大便不实 便意频作 腰腹坠胀 甚则脱肛	中脘饱闷 纳食不香 恶心作呕 头身困重 口甜而黏 大便不实 或泄泻	胸脘痞胀 恶心呕吐 口中黏腻 大便溏薄 小便赤涩不利 身重体困
舌苔	舌淡体肥苔薄白	舌淡苔白	苔白腻	苔黄腻
脉象	沉细缓而迟	细缓无力	濡细	濡数
治法	温中健脾	益气健脾升阳	运脾化湿	清利湿热
方剂	理中汤	四君子汤或补中益气汤	胃苓汤	小陷胸汤

附：胃

1．生理：胃在膈下，上连食道，下通小肠，其经脉络脾。胃之上口为贲门，下口为幽门；贲门部又名上脘，幽门部又为下脘，其间为中脘，三部共称胃脘。胃主受纳、腐熟水谷，脾代胃输水谷之精微，故脾胃表里相合，共司升降清浊。《灵枢》称"胃者，太仓也"。

2．病理：胃为水谷之海。凡饮食不节，饥饱失常，或冷热不适，都能影响胃的功能，使之发生病变。胃为燥土，故性喜润恶燥，所以一般易致食结郁热，以和降为顺，所以胃病易于气逆作嗳泛吐。

3．证候分类

(1)胃寒：胃脘胀满疼痛，绵绵不止，喜热喜按，泛吐清水，呕吐呃逆，苔白滑，脉迟。治以温胃散寒，用良附丸之类。

(2)胃热：口渴思冷饮，消谷善饥，呕吐嘈杂，或食入即吐，口臭，牙龈肿痛，腐烂或出血，舌赤苔黄少津，脉滑数。治以清胃泄火，用清胃散之类。

(3)胃虚：胃脘痞满，食不化，时作嗳气，大便不实，脉软弱，苔少。治以益气健脾，用建中汤之类。

(4)胃实：食滞胃脘，脘腹胀满，大便不爽，口臭嗳腐，或呕吐，舌苔薄黄，脉滑。治以消导化滞、和胃通降，用香苏饮、保和丸之类。

(四)肺(附大肠)

1．生理：肺位于胸中，上连气道，开窍于鼻，合称肺系。肺在体为皮毛，其经脉下络大肠，互为表里。肺主气属卫，为宗气出入之所，司呼吸，为气机出入升降之枢，助心主治节，故《素问》说："肺者，相傅之官，治节出焉。"

2．病理：肺主气，所以肺之病理表现，主要为气机出入升降的失常。因肺为娇脏，不耐寒热，又为呼吸之孔道，所以外感及肺痨之病，常先犯肺。又肺气贯百脉而通它脏，故它脏有病，也常累及于肺。

肺的病证，可分为虚实两大类。虚证又有阴虚、气虚之分；阴虚多系津液消耗，肺失濡养所致；气虚多为久病亏耗，或被它脏之病所累。实证则多由痰浊水湿内聚，寒邪外束或邪热乘肺所致。

肺病病机示意图

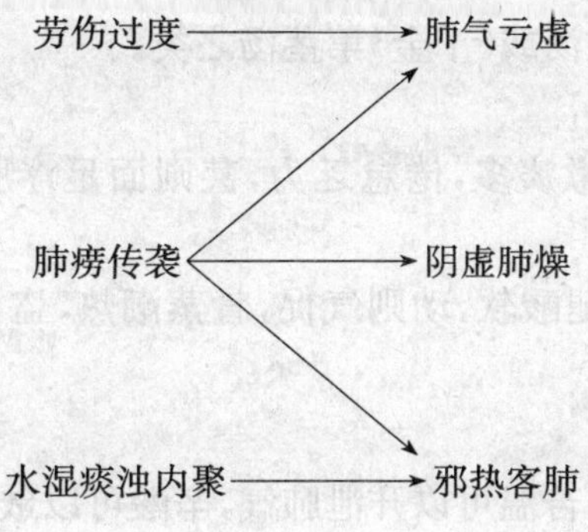

3. 病证范围：肺系的疾病，临床上常见者有感冒，咳嗽，哮喘，肺痈，肺痨，肺痿，咳血，失音，衄血，胸痛等。

4. 证候分类

(1)虚证

①阴虚肺燥

病机概要：外感燥邪或肺痨邪毒，或久咳伤肺，以致肺阴不足，虚热内生，耗灼肺金。

主要脉症：咳呛气逆，痰少质黏，咳吐不利；痰中带血，或为血丝，或见血块；潮热盗汗，午后颧红，少寐失眠；口干咽燥，或声音嘶哑；舌红少苔，脉象细数。

治疗：滋阴润肺。用百合固金汤之类。

②肺气亏虚

病机概要：劳伤过度，病后元气未复，或久咳伤肺，致肺气亏虚，失其温煦。

主要脉症：咳而短气，痰液清稀；倦怠懒言，声音低怯；面色㿠白，畏风形寒，或有自汗；舌淡苔薄白，脉虚弱。

治疗：补益肺气。用补肺汤之类。

(2)实证

①痰浊阻肺

病机概要：形寒饮冷，水饮痰浊内聚，阻塞肺气，气机不得宣降。

主要脉症：咳嗽气喘，喉中痰鸣，痰黏稠；胸胁支满疼痛，倚息不得卧；苔腻色黄，脉滑。

治疗：化痰降气去壅，用三子养亲汤或葶苈大枣泻肺汤。

②风寒束肺

病机概要：风寒外束，肺气不宣，或寒饮内阻，肺失肃降。

主要脉症：风寒在表，则恶寒发热，头痛身楚，无汗，鼻塞流涕，咳嗽痰稀薄，苔薄白，脉浮紧。寒饮内阻，则咳嗽频剧，气急身重，痰黏色白量多，发热恶寒，苔白滑，脉浮紧。

治疗：发散风寒，用三拗汤；或温化寒饮，用小青龙汤之类。

③邪热客肺

病机概要：风热上受，或寒郁化热，或痰热内阻，邪热壅肺，肺失清肃。

主要脉症：咳声洪亮，气喘息促，痰稠色黄，或咯吐腥臭脓血，咳则胸痛引背；鼻干或鼻衄鼻煽；或流脓涕，气息觉热；身热，烦渴欲饮，咽喉肿痛；大便干结，小便赤涩不利，舌干质红，苔黄燥，脉数。

治疗：清肺泄热。用桑白皮汤或《千金》苇茎汤之类。

(3)兼证

①脾虚及肺：纳呆便溏，咳嗽痰多，倦怠乏力，甚则面足浮肿，苔白，脉濡弱。治以培土生金，用四君子汤之类。

②肺肾两亏：咳嗽夜剧，腰腿酸软，动则气促，骨蒸潮热，盗汗遗精，舌红苔少，脉细数。治以滋阴养肺，用生脉散之类。

5. 证治要点

(1)肺主气，味宜辛，用药辛苦温可以开泄肺气，辛酸可以敛肺益气，除非必要，一般不用血分药。

(2)肺为娇脏，清虚而处高位，选方宜轻清，不宜重浊，正所谓“治上焦如羽，非轻不举”。

又，治疗肺气之病，大法当用肃降；且肺为娇脏不耐寒热，辛平甘润最为适宜。

(3)肺主气为娇脏，故治疗肺之虚证，补肺不宜温燥，润肺切忌滋腻。

(4)肺之病证，可以通过脏腑关系作间接治疗，如虚证可用补脾（补母），滋肾（补子）的治法，而实证可用泻肝的治法。

(5)肺与大肠互为表里，所以肺经实证、热证可泻大肠，使肺热从大肠下泄而气得清肃。因肺气虚致大肠津液不布而便秘者，则用滋养肺气之法，以通润大肠。

(6)肺经病证，从病因上分析，可分外感内伤，辨证则不外虚实两类，其中又有寒、热、痰之别，医者应掌握这些要领，灵活辨治。肺病辨证施治见简表。

肺病辨证施治简表

证别	实	证		虚	证
	痰浊阻肺	风寒束肺	邪热乘肺	阴虚肺燥	肺气亏虚
病机	水饮痰浊阻塞肺气	风寒或寒饮伤肺气失肃降	寒郁化热，或痰火、风热内炽	肺痨。燥邪伤肺，阴津亏损	劳伤过度久咳伤气
咳嗽	咳声不扬痰稠量多	咳频而剧咳声重浊痰多稀薄	咳声洪亮痰黏色黄	咳呛气逆，痰少而黏，咯吐不利	咳而乏力气怯痰稀而量不多
气息	气喘不利。甚则不得平卧	气急	气粗鼻煽气息发热	烦扰气微促	气短形怯动则喘甚
胸痛	胸痛而闷两胁支满	胸闷或疼痛	咳则牵引胸背作痛	时有胸胁隐痛	时有胸胁隐痛
咳血			痰中带血，色红或黯。亦可咯血量多色鲜红	痰中带血丝或血块，有时量多色红	偶见淡红血痰，其量不多
寒热	寒热不明显	寒重热轻，无汗	发热面赤，烦热引饮，有汗	潮热盗汗	形寒怕冷，四肢欠温，自汗
咽喉	喉中痰鸣	或见音哑	咽喉干燥红肿作痛	咽干痒或痛	
舌苔	苔腻或黄	苔薄白而滑	质红苔黄燥	舌红少苔	质淡苔白
脉象	滑	浮　紧	数	细　数	虚　弱
治法	涤浊化痰以开肺	发散风寒化痰止咳	清热泄肺	养阴润肺	补益肺气
方剂	三子养亲汤或葶苈大枣泻肺汤	三拗汤小青龙汤	桑白皮汤《千金》苇茎汤	百合固金汤	补肺汤

附：大肠

1. 生理：大肠包括回肠和广肠（直肠）。回肠上接阑门，下接广肠，广肠下端为魄门（肛门),其经脉络肺。大肠司传送糟粕以排出。《素问》说:“大肠者,传导之官,变化出焉。”

2. 病理:因大肠为“传导之官”,所以大肠的病理主要反映在大便方面,特别是大便秘结。一切热证,均可灼伤津液而产生便秘;肺脏清肃之气不能下降,也能发生便秘;肾水不足,肠中津液缺乏,亦能造成大便秘结。此外,因大肠属于脾胃系统,故凡脾胃虚弱,运化失健,也可直接影响大肠,而致传导功能失常。

3. 证候分类

(1)寒证:腹痛肠鸣,大便溏泄,溲清,脉缓,舌苔白滑。治以散寒止痛,用胃苓汤合良附丸之类。

(2)热证:口燥唇焦,大便秘结,或便腐臭、肛门灼热肿痛,小便短赤,苔黄燥,脉数。治以通便泻热,用凉膈散之类。若症见下利赤白或脓血,里急后重,发热身重,脉滑数,舌苔黄腻,为湿热痢疾。治以清热利湿,用芍药汤或白头翁汤之类。

(3)虚证:久痢泄泻,肛门下脱,四肢欠温,舌淡苔薄,脉细数。治以厚肠固摄,用真人养脏汤之类。

(4)实证:腹痛拒按,或发热呕逆便秘,或便而不爽,苔黄,脉沉实。治以清热导滞,用承气汤之类。

(五)肾(附膀胱)

1. 生理:肾左右各一,命门附焉,内藏元阴元阳,为水火之脏,其经脉络膀胱,互为表里。肾在体为骨,开窍于耳。肾的生理功能:主藏精,为生殖发育之源;主五液以维持水液代谢平衡;主骨生髓;听力乃肾气所充。肾的生理功能极为重要,故古人称“肾为先天之本”,实为生命之根。

2. 病理:肾为先天之本,藏真阴而寓元阳,为水火之脏,只宜固藏,不宜泄露,所以肾多虚证,其病因多为劳倦淫欲过度,久病失养,致肾气耗伤。临床表现为阴虚、阳虚两大类型;阳虚包括肾气不固,肾不纳气,肾阳不足和肾虚水泛;阴虚包括肾阴亏虚和阴虚火旺。又肾与膀胱互为表里,肾气不足直接影响膀胱气化,故膀胱虚证,也是肾虚的病理表现。

肾病病机示意图

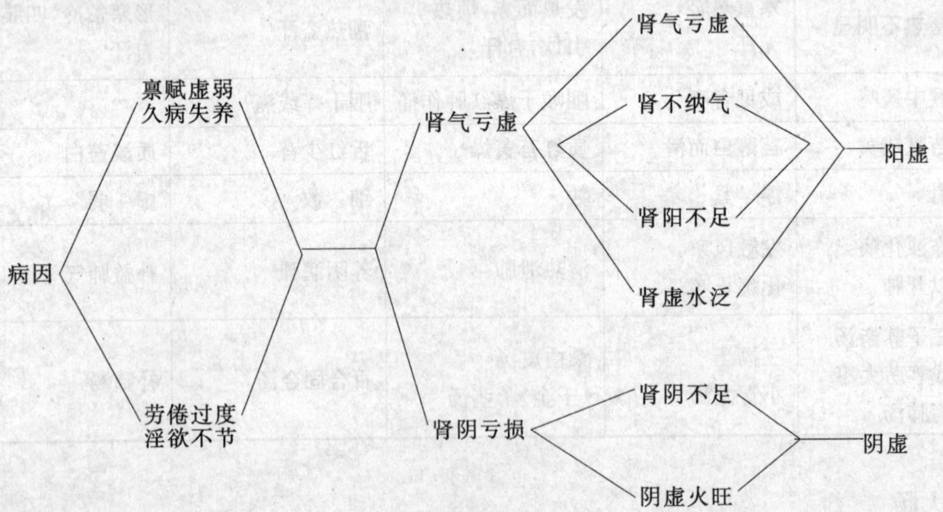

4. 证候分类

(1)阳虚

①肾气不固

病机概要：肾阳素亏，劳损过度，久病失养，肾气亏耗，失其封藏固摄之权。

主要脉症：面色淡白，腰脊酸软，听力减退，小便频数色清，甚则失禁，滑精早泄，尿后余沥，舌淡苔薄白，脉细弱。

治疗：固摄肾气。用大补元煎之类。

②肾不纳气

病机概要：劳伤肾气，或久病气虚，气不归元，肾失摄纳之权。

主要脉症：短气喘逆，动则尤甚，咳逆汗出，小便常随咳嗽而出，甚则痰鸣，面浮色白，舌淡苔薄，脉虚弱。

治疗：纳气归肾。用人参胡桃汤或参蛤散之类。

③肾阳不足

病机概要：禀赋薄弱，久病不愈，或房劳伤肾，下元亏损，命门火衰。

主要脉症：面色淡白，腰酸腿软，阳痿，头昏耳鸣，形寒尿频，舌淡白，脉沉弱。

治疗：温补肾阳。用右归丸或金匮肾气丸之类。

④肾虚水泛

病机概要：禀赋素虚，久病失调，肾阳亏耗，不能温化水液，致水邪泛滥而上逆，或外溢肌肤。

主要脉症：水溢肌肤，则为周身浮肿，下肢尤甚，按之如泥，腰腹胀满，尿少；水泛为痰，则咳逆上气，痰多稀薄，动则喘息，舌淡白，脉沉迟。

治疗：温阳化水。用真武汤或济生肾气丸之类。

(2)阴虚

①肾阴亏虚

病机概要：酒色思虑过度，或久病之后，真阴耗伤。

主要脉症：形体虚弱，头昏耳鸣，少寐健忘，腰酸腿软，或有遗精，口干，舌红少苔，脉细。

治疗：滋养肾阴。用六味地黄汤之类。

②阴虚火旺

病机概要：欲念妄动，或热病后耗伤肾阴，阴虚生内热，水亏则火浮。

主要脉症：颧红唇赤，潮热盗汗，腰脊酸痛，虚烦不寐，阳强梦遗，口咽干痛，或呛咳，小便黄，大便秘，舌红苔少，脉细数。

治疗：滋阴降火。用知柏地黄汤之类。

(3)兼证

①肾虚土衰：大便溏泄，完谷不化，滑泻难禁，腹胀少食，神疲形寒，肢软无力，舌淡苔薄，脉沉迟。治以补火生土，用四神丸之类。

②肾水凌心：心悸不宁，水肿，胸腹胀满，咳嗽短气，不能平卧，指唇青紫，四肢厥冷，舌淡苔薄，脉虚数。治以温化水气，用真武汤之类。

5. 证治要点

(1)一般而论，肾无表证和实证。肾之热，属于阴虚之变；肾之寒，为阳虚之化。临床必须掌握。

(2)肾虚之证，一般分为阴虚、阳虚两类。总的治则是“培其不足，不可伐其有余”。阴虚证治忌辛燥、苦寒，宜甘润壮水以补阴配阳，使虚火降而阳归于阴，所谓“壮水之主，以制阳光”。阳虚证治忌凉润、辛散，宜甘温益气以补阳配阴，使阴霾散而阴从于阳，所谓“益火之源，以消阴翳”。至于阴阳俱虚、精气两亏证，治当阴阳双补。

(3)肾阴虚者，往往导致相火偏旺，此为阴虚生内热之变，治则滋阴为主，参以清泻相火。肾阳虚者，在温肾补火的原则下，必须佐以填精益髓，当用血肉有情之品，资其化生之源。

(4)肾与膀胱互为表里，膀胱病变属虚寒者，多由肾阳虚衰，气化失职所致，当以温肾化气为主。而实热癃闭之证，可由他脏移热所致，也可因膀胱本脏湿热壅结而成，治当清利通窍为主。

(5)肾与其他脏腑的关系非常密切，如肾阴不足，可致水不涵木，肝阳上亢；或子盗母气，耗伤肺阴；或水不上承，心肾不交。而肾阳亏虚，又易形成火不生土，脾阳衰弱。上述病证，通过治肾参治他脏，可加快病情恢复。

肾病辨证施治见简表。

肾病辨证施治简表

证别	阳	虚		阴	虚	
病机	肾气不固	肾不纳气	肾阳不足	肾虚水泛	肾阴亏虚	阴虚火旺
	肾气亏耗，封藏固摄无权	肾失纳气之能气不归元	下元亏损命门火衰	命火虚衰温化无力水湿泛滥	劳伤久病真阴耗伤	真阴亏损虚火浮越
形态	面色淡白	面色沉白	面色淡白	肢体浮肿下肢尤甚	形体虚弱	颧红唇赤
精神	神倦乏力听力减退	咳喘不宁	形寒怕冷耳鸣	少气懒言	头晕耳鸣健忘少寐	虚火不寐潮热盗汗
腰腿	腰脊酸软	腰脊酸软	腰腿酸软	腰腹胀满	腰腿酸软	腰脊酸楚
咳喘		短气喘息，呼多吸少动则尤甚咳而汗出	咳逆气喘痰稀薄起沫	喘促痰多稀白多沫		咽干咳呛
遗精	滑精早泄		阳痿		遗精	阳强梦遗
二便	尿后余沥	小便常阻随咳而出	尿频	尿少	尿黄	小便黄大便秘
舌苔	淡白	淡薄	淡白	淡白	舌红少苔	舌红体瘦苔少
脉象	细弱	虚弱	沉弱	滑迟	细	细数
治法	固摄肾气	纳气归肾	温补肾阳	温阳化水	滋养肾阴	滋阴降火
方剂	大补元煎	人参胡桃汤	右归丸	真武汤	六味地黄丸	知柏地黄丸

附：膀胱

1. 生理：膀胱位于少腹，其经脉络肾；生理功能主要为贮存津液，化气行水，故《素问》说：“膀胱者，州都之官，津液藏焉，气化则能出矣。”小便之源为津液，津液之余入膀胱，气化则为小便。

2. 病理：膀胱既有化气行水功能，故病理变化主要表现为气化无权，癃闭，小便不利，频数，失禁等。肾主水液，与膀胱互为表里，肾气不足必影响膀胱气化，此为膀胱虚证的主要病机。至于膀胱实热证，系由他脏移热或本腑湿热壅结而成。

3. 证候分类

(1)虚寒：小便频数，淋漓不禁，或遗尿，舌淡苔润，脉沉细。治以固摄肾气，用桑螵蛸散之类。

(2)实热：小便短赤不利，尿色黄赤，或浑浊不清，尿时茎中热痛，甚则淋沥不畅，或见脓血砂石，舌红苔黄，脉数。治以清利湿热，用八正散之类。

二、气血病机、病证的基本概念

气和血，是人体生命活动的动力和源泉，它既是脏腑功能的反映，又是脏腑活动的产物，人体病理变化无不涉及气血，所以认识和分析气血的病机、病证，就能更深入地探讨脏腑病理变化，对指导临床实践有重要意义。

(一)气

1. 生理：气的来源，一为禀受先天父母所赐，称为元气，入藏于肾；其二源于后天水谷之气，此气承脾胃之输布，充泽于五脏，就成为各脏之气。两气相合，即成为人体生命活动的动力，正如《灵枢》所谓："真气者，所受于天，与谷气并而充身者也。"

人体之气，包括元气、宗气、营气、卫气及五脏之气。元气乃先天精气所化，发源于肾，借三焦之道通达全身，以推动五脏六腑的功能活动。宗气为水谷之气与自然界之清气相合而成，积于胸中，出喉咙而司呼吸，贯心脉以行气血。营气亦由水谷所化，源于脾胃，为营运于脉中之精气，内注五脏六腑，外营四肢百骸。卫气同营气，生于水谷，源于脾胃，所不同者，乃运行于脉外，循皮肤之中，分肉之间，以温养肌肉皮肤，其主要功能为保卫体表，抵御外邪入侵。五脏之气，则指五脏功能的具体表现，有关内容已如前述，不再重复。

2. 病理：由上所述，气的活动范围较为广泛，因此，疾病之发生演变与气的关系极为密切，即《素问》所谓："百病皆生于气。"

气病的病因，不外外感内伤。外感疾病中，风寒外束，则致肺气失宣，而为咳嗽；寒与气结，则为疝为痞；风热上乘内炽，肺气失于肃降，而见咳吐黄痰，鼻翼煽动；邪热内扰心包，心气逆乱，故有神昏惊厥之证，湿浊阻遏气机，在肺则气机壅塞而喘逆吐涎，在脾则清气不升而见泄泻。至于内伤之病，劳损过度，则气耗血虚；饮食失节，则胃失和降；七情无制，怒则气上，喜则气缓，悲则气消，恐则气下，劳则气耗，思则气结。说明劳倦、饮食和情志所伤，亦与气病的发生有一定。综上所述，外感内伤，均可引起气病，由于病因、病机的不同，其病理变化所反映出来的证候亦有区别。

气病与脏腑的关系非常密切，气来源于脾肾，升降出入治节于肺，升发疏泄于肝，统血贯脉而周行于心，故脏腑一旦受病，就会直接或间接地反映出气的病理变化，出现不同的气病证候。如肺气不宣，则为喘咳；肺气不足，则神倦气短。心气逆乱，则心神被扰而昏迷癫狂；气血亏耗，则心气不足而心悸怔忡。脾胃不和，则胃气上逆而泛恶呕吐；脾失运化，则胃气虚衰而纳呆泄泻，生湿生痰。肝气郁结，则化火上炎；肝阳暴张而上扰神明；肝气虚则胆亦虚，而头晕心悸，胆怯肢麻。肾气虚弱，固摄失权则遗泄；肾气不纳，故动则喘息；气不化水，而水泛为痰为肿。

气病虽有虚实之分,然多见于升降出入之变。升降出入为气机运动的基本形式,亦是脏腑功能活动的基本表现,如心火下降,肾水上济;肝性升发,肺主肃降;脾主升清,胃主降浊;肺主呼气,肾主纳气。其中,脾胃为气机升降之枢纽,肝肺为气机升降之道路,心肾为气机升降之动力。心肺胃之气以降为顺,肝脾肾之气以升为健。脏腑协调,维持气机升降出入。病理情况下,脏腑功能失调,进而影响气机之升降出入,因此为病。

3. 气病证候:上面已经提到,气病的病理与脏腑直接相关,因此,气病的证候也包括在脏腑的不同证候之中,具体内容也如前述。现反将气病概括为虚实两证,分述如下:

(1)气虚:凡因劳伤过度,久病失养而耗伤元气者,皆属气虚。其主要表现为:少气懒言,语声低微,自汗,心悸,怔忡,头晕耳鸣,倦怠乏力,食少,小便清或频,脉虚弱或虚大等。此外,气虚易下陷,久病阳亦虚,故脱肛及子宫脱出等,亦属气虚范畴。

(2)气实:气实证多由痰火、食滞、湿热、郁结等所致,也可因外感治疗不当而引起。其主要表现有:胸闷,脘痞,痰多喘满,气粗,腹胀,大便秘结,脉弦滑或数实等。此外,气实易上逆,逆则可见恶心,呕吐,呃逆,嗳气,噎嗝等。气实易化火,故有“气有余便是火”之说。

4. 气病的治疗:治疗气病的基本原则是:气虚宜补气,气实宜理气、行气、降气。气虚者,其补气主要是补肺肾脾之气,因脾胃为元气生化之源,脾胃虚衰则元气不足,其他脏腑亦因元气不足而虚弱,如李东垣说:“脾胃之气既伤,元气亦不能充,而诸病之所由生也。”肺为脾之子,脾气不足,最易导致肺气出入升降失常,加重病情的发展。肾为先天之本,主藏精气,又为气化之司,故肾气不足,则可引起一系列水液气化失调的病证,因此,气病的治疗,一般是根据气虚的不同病机,以补肺脾肾之气为主。补脾胃气虚,常用四君子汤、补中益气汤;补肺气常用补肺汤;补肾气常用大补元煎、金匮肾气丸等。如果出现兼有痰火等虚中挟实证候,则须根据具体情况,分清主次,视其轻重缓急进行处理。

至于气实证,主要因气郁、气滞、气逆以及外邪侵犯所致,与肝肺脾三脏关系较为密切,故多采用泄肝、理脾、宣肺、降逆、散寒、化结等法。一般气实之证多较复杂,故当分别其与脏腑的关系,针对治疗。如肺气郁阻者宜开,胃气积滞者宜导,肝火上逆者宜降,肝气郁结者宜疏,胆气壅滞者宜和,肝胆火盛者宜泄,气滞而痛者宜调。如湿、食、痰、火夹杂为患,则当分清轻重缓急进行调治。

(二)血

1. 生理:血来源于水谷之精气,通过脾胃的生化输布,注之于脉,化而为血。另外,血与肾的关系也极为密切,精血互生,故有“肾为水脏,主藏精而化血”之说。血的功能主要是充润营养全身。目之视,足之步,掌之握,指之摄,以及皮肤的感觉,五脏六腑功能之协调,无不赖血之营养。

血液之所以能循行脉中,周流不息,除了与“心主血脉”的功能有直接联系外,与气的功能亦密切相关。因血属阴,赖阳气以运行,气行则血行,气滞则血瘀,气脱则血失,故有“血随气行,气为血帅”之说。

2. 病理:血病的表现一般分为出血、血瘀、血虚,三者的病因病机既有区别,又有联系。如出血既是血虚的病因,又可能是瘀血的病机,当出血蓄积于内而为瘀者,就是这种联系的反映。现将三者的病理分述如下:

(1)出血:正常情况下血液循行于脉中,若脉络受伤,血溢脉外,即为出血。从上而出,称为上溢,如咳血、吐血、衄血等;从下而出,称为下溢,如便血、尿血、崩漏等。

出血之病机，大多由火引起，亦有因气之不足、血无所依而导致者。因此，归纳出血的病机，不外风火燥热损伤脉络；过食酒酪辛辣动火之品，或肥厚甘甜蓄积为患；七情因素之激扰，五志之火内燔；素有血病，复因恣情纵欲，耗伤肾阴，虚火伤络；以及跌打损伤，用力超重等。

(2)瘀血：凡离经之血未出体外，停滞于内，或脉中之血为邪气或痰火或湿热所阻，均能成瘀。其病机可归纳为：邪毒入营，或外阻脉道；出血后处理不当，余血内留；产后恶露不下；挫伤脉络，以及其他气病、血病等。

(3)血虚：主要由于失血过多或生血不足两个方面。如吐血、衄血、产后以及外伤性出血等，血失过多，新血未生；或因脾胃素弱，水谷之精微不能化生营血；以及久病不愈，肠中虫积，营血消耗等，均能使脏腑百脉失养，而出现一系列血虚的病理反应。

3. 血病证候

(1)出血：多以出血之部位或器官而分证。如咳嗽咯痰而出者，为肺系之出血；随食物呕吐而出者，为胃之出血；随大小便而出者，为便血、尿血；由鼻窍而出者，是为衄血；女子月事过多或经血频频者，是为崩漏。此外，尚有从龈、耳、目、肌肤等处出血者。其临床症状，则根据其病因、病机及出血部位各有不同。有关内容，均分述于各论血证诸篇中。

(2)瘀血：主要表现为疼痛，部位随瘀血所在而定，痛处不移，状若针刺，得寒温不移，常兼痞闷、胀满，自觉烦热，眼睑乌黑，唇色枯萎，皮肤紫斑，或有血丝红缕，甚则甲错，舌质暗，或见瘀斑，脉细涩。

(3)血虚：面色苍白，唇舌爪甲色淡无华；头眩晕，心悸怔忡，气微而短，疲倦乏力，或手足发麻，脉细。

4. 血病的治疗

血病的治疗，主要根据上述证候，血虚者补血，出血则止血，血瘀者宜活血化瘀。

(1)出血：凡由火热引起出血者，以泻热止血为主法，如肝胆火热内炽出血，用龙胆泻肝汤之类；血热妄行出血用犀角地黄汤之类；胃火内炽出血，用《金匮》泻心汤之类；阴虚火旺咯血用沙参麦门冬汤之类；肠风下血用槐花散之类；热在下焦尿血，用小蓟饮子之类；如因脾不统血或气不摄血致出血者，法当益气摄血，可用归脾汤或补中益气汤之类。

(2)瘀血：瘀血的治疗，视病情而定，如瘀血内结，可行血破瘀，用桃仁承气汤或抵当汤之类；如瘀血阻滞，可行气活血，或活血化瘀，用血府逐瘀汤之类；因寒滞经脉而血瘀者，可温经活血，用温经汤之类。因正虚无力推动血行而瘀者，又当扶正祛瘀同用，用补阳还五汤之类。

(3)血虚：主要是补气养血，用人参养荣汤或十全大补汤。妇人血虚，多用四物汤或当归补血汤之类。若精血双亏，则应佐以益肾填精之品。

三、风火湿痰病机、病证的基本概念

风、火、湿(痰)，既是六淫之气，也是脏腑病理变化产物，还是脏腑疾病的临床表现。因此，又是直接或间接致病的内外因素。

(一)风

风有内外之分。外风为六淫病毒之一；内风系人体阳气所化，多呈火热炽盛、肝阳偏亢或阴血亏虚所引起的一系列气血逆乱的证候。

1. 风证特点

(1)外风：病起急骤，身热而渴，或兼咳嗽，肢体酸痛，或骨节红肿，游走不定，或皮肤出现风疹作痒，或口歪舌强等。

(2)内风：多系肝阳肝风、阴血亏虚所产生，或因情志、起居、饮食失节而诱发，根据病情轻重不同，多有头目眩晕，抽搐震颤，癫狂，或卒中，口眼㖞斜，语言蹇涩，半身不遂等。

2. 风证病机

(1)外风：风为六淫之首，四季皆能伤人，经口鼻或肌表而入。经口鼻而入者，多先犯肺系；经肌表而入者，多始自经络，正虚邪盛则内传脏腑。此两者感受途径又可同时兼有。

风邪为病，很少单独袭人，往往兼邪同犯或随时气而发病，如冬多兼寒；天气由寒转暖，则多与温邪病毒入侵而为温病；时令多湿，或居处潮湿，则兼湿为患；也有风、寒、湿同时感受而致病者。风为阳邪，其性善行数变，故若侵犯经络骨节，其痛多游走流窜而无定处。挟热者为风热，风热上受多犯头面咽喉；若兼湿，湿性下流，故多犯下肢。风气刚劲，常卒然伤人，留滞经络，而出现口歪舌强，肢体拘急挛痛等症。

(2)内风：内风系自内而生，产生内风的病机如下：

①热极生风：凡热极之证，必灼伤津液，消灼营血；营血既伤，心肝受病，邪热上扰，可出现惊厥神昏证候，此即所谓“热极生风”的病机。

②肝风内动：肝为刚脏，性喜条达，每因情志不遂，致肝气不得疏泄，郁而化火。则肝火偏亢而上炎；火升阳亢，血随气逆，风动于内，横窜络道，上冲巅顶，直扰神明，可出现眩晕、抽搐，或卒中不省人事等证候，此即“肝风内动”和“诸风掉眩，皆属于肝”的病机。

③血虚生风：肝脏体阴用阳，肝为藏血之脏，其性刚强，赖血以濡养。血虚则肝阴不足，肝阳偏亢，风自内生，也会出现瘈疭、眩晕、痉厥等症。

由前述可知，内风为病，多与心肝肾三脏有关，病本在肝肾，病标则在心。此外，内风与痰也有一定关系，如内有痰火郁结，则更易生风；反之，肝风内动，痰浊随之上逆，易出现卒中。有关痰的病机见后节述。

3. 风证的辨证论治

(1)外风

①风寒：风寒外袭，肺卫郁闭，症见头项强痛，恶寒或发热无汗，鼻塞，苔薄白，脉浮紧等。治以疏风散寒，用葱豉汤或荆防败毒散之类。

②风热：风热外感，多犯上焦，症见头胀，咽喉肿痛，发热不恶寒，或少汗恶风，目赤胀痛羞明，咳吐黄痰，也可见头面焮红肿痛，乳蛾，鼻渊；如风热伤络，则为咯血，小便色黄，脉洪数等；治以疏风清热，用桑菊饮或银翘散之类。

③风湿：风湿为患，表现为体表经络的症候可为头痛而重，骨节疼痛，走窜不定，湿疹，水疱等；表现为肠胃的症候则为肠鸣腹痛，泄泻清稀如水等。治以散风化湿，在体表经络者用羌活胜湿汤之类，在肠胃可用藿香正气散之类。

(2)内风

病情轻者，主要表现为头目眩晕，心绪不宁，手足颤动；重者可突然出现昏迷，口眼㖞斜，角弓反张，半身不遂等症。热极生风，必兼热盛症状；虚风内动，必兼肝肾阴虚、肝阳上亢的症状；血虚生风，必兼血虚内燥症状。

内风的治疗，凡热极生风者，宜平肝熄风，用天麻钩藤饮之类，酌情可加用安宫牛黄丸、至宝丹、紫雪丹；如虚阳妄动者，宜滋阴潜阳，用大定风珠之类；血虚生风者，宜养阴熄风，用加减复脉汤之类。

(二)火

火为热之甚。火既是六淫病邪之一,亦可在疾病过程中产生。火有虚实之分,实火多因直接感受火热,或它邪化火而成;虚火则是脏腑病理变化的产物,多由阴液耗伤,精血亏损而生。

1. 火证特点:火系热之甚,其性上炎,故火证与热证相似,但比热更重,其主要特点如下:

实火:多由外感所致,病势急速,病程短,多有壮热,面红耳赤,口渴心烦,喜冷饮,甚者狂躁,谵语,昏迷,小便短赤,大便秘结,唇焦,苔黄燥或起刺,脉洪数等。

虚火:多因内伤而起,病势缓慢,病程长,症见潮热盗汗,午后颧红,虚烦失眠,口干咽燥,干咳无痰,或痰中带血,耳鸣健忘,腰酸遗精,舌质红绛少津或光剥无苔,脉细数等。

2. 火证病机:在生理状态下,人体脏腑活动,赖水谷之气以营养,从而生火生热以为用;反过来,人体又赖此火热之能,以腐熟水谷,化生精气,而维持生命,这种火称之为"少火"。病理状态下,精血耗伤,脏腑功能失常,阴阳失其相对平衡,因脏腑阳偏亢所生之火称为"壮火",是反常之邪火,能伤人正气而致病,即《内经》所谓"壮火食气,少火生气"。言少火为正常之火,物赖以生;壮火为反常之火,物因以耗。

火的病机,不外内伤外感两个方面。凡感受六淫之邪而为火证者,可因直接感受火热所起,亦可由它邪衍化而生。因感受火热之邪而出现火热证者,乃由火热灼伤津液营血,内损脏腑所致。因感它邪而为火证者,则须渐趋化热,再由热化火。如寒之化火,必须由寒化热,热极而后生火;湿之化火,必须与热相结,或湿蕴化热,湿热极盛而成痰火。一般认为,这种由外感引起的火,多属实火,反映于临床就是实火证候。

内伤亦可生火,如劳伤过度,情志抑郁,淫欲妄动,均可影响脏腑正常生理功能,使阴液耗伤,或久病失养,精血亏损,均可导致内火的发生,而出现火证。这种因内伤所致之火,多属虚火,反映于临床多是虚火证候。

3. 火证的辨证论治

辨火之证,首别虚实,虚者宜养宜滋,浮者宜引宜敛,实者宜清宜泻。由于受病的脏腑不同,虚实有别,必须详细辨证。

(1)实火

①心火炽盛:主症为面红耳赤,五心烦热,口燥唇裂,舌碎糜破,甚则喜笑无常,谵语,神昏,吐衄等。治以清泻心火,用泻心汤之类。

②肝胆火盛:主症为胁痛耳聋,少寐多梦,头昏目赤,口苦,筋痿,或淋浊溺血等。治以清泄肝胆,用龙胆泻肝汤之类。

③肺火壅盛:主症为气粗鼻煽,咳吐稠痰,烦渴欲饮,大便燥结,或鼻衄咳血等。治以清肃肺热,用《千金》苇茎汤或桑白皮汤之类。

④胃火炽盛:主症为烦渴引饮,牙龈腐烂而痛或出血,呕吐嘈杂,消谷善饥等。治以清泻胃热,用清胃散之类。

⑤大肠火热:大便秘结不通,或暴泻黄赤,肛门灼热等。治以泻下积热,用大承气汤之类。

⑥小肠火热:主症为少腹坠痛,血淋热浊等。治以清心降火,用导赤散之类。

⑦脾火内炽:主要为口唇干燥,烦渴易饥等。治以清脾泻火,用泻黄散之类。

⑧膀胱有火:主症为癃闭淋沥,遗溺混浊,尿血腹痛等。治以清利火热,用八正散之类。

⑨火热入心,蒙蔽清窍:主症为神昏谵语,抽搐等。治以清心开窍,用安宫牛黄丸、至宝丹之类。

(2)虚火

①肾虚火动：肾阴不足，相火妄动，主症为虚热骨蒸及其他阴虚证候。治以滋阴降火，用知柏地黄丸之类；骨蒸者用清骨散之类。

②脾胃虚火：主症为嘈杂，口干不欲饮，知饥而不纳，便干等。治以养阴清胃，用益胃汤之类。

(三)湿

湿有内外之分。外湿为六淫之一，常先伤于下，湿留体内，或从热化，结为湿热，或从寒化，聚为寒湿，或致泄泻，或为水肿。内湿为病理产物，与脾的病理变化有密切关系。

1. 湿证特点

湿为阴邪，得温则化，得阳则宣。但湿邪性黏腻而滞，故不易速去，常反复经久不已。

外湿：外湿起病，与气候环境有关，如阴雨连绵，或久处雾露潮湿，均易发生湿病；又脾胃素弱，也容易感受外湿。其临床表现多有身重体酸，关节疼痛，甚者屈伸不利，难以转侧，其痛常限于一处不移，苔白微腻，脉濡缓等。

内湿：内湿之证，皆与脾胃有关，故以脾胃症状为主，如口淡乏味而腻，食欲不振，或食而不多，胸脘痞闷，嗳气泄泻，肢软无力，头痛身重，苔白厚而腻，脉濡弱等。

2. 湿证病机

湿的形成及其病机，有外来与内生之别。外湿乃外来之邪，多由肌肤体表侵入，浅则伤人皮肉筋脉，或流注关节，甚则可入脏腑。湿邪伤人，常兼寒、热与风。湿邪侵入人体，可从阴化寒，亦可从阳化热，视人体脏腑功能的不同，禀赋之强弱，以及治疗失当而转化。如肾阳素虚者易从寒化，胃热之人易从热化；过用寒凉易寒化，妄加温燥易于热化。

内湿的形成，多因饮食不节所致。如恣食生冷酒醴肥甘，或饥饱失时，损伤脾胃；脾伤则运化功能失常，致津液不得运化敷布，故湿从内生，聚而为患，或为泄泻，或为肿满，或为痰饮。此即《内经》“诸湿肿满，皆属于脾”的病机。在内湿基础上，更易感受外湿，两者互相影响，可出现各种不同的湿证。

3. 湿证的辨证论治

(1)外湿

①寒湿：全身疼痛，以关节痛为重，行动不便，无汗，便溏，或见四肢浮肿，苔白腻，脉濡缓。治以蠲痹通络，用蠲痹汤之类。

②风湿：见风证辨证论治。

③湿热：发热心烦，口渴自汗，四肢关节肿痛，胸满黄疸，小便黄赤，舌苔黄腻，脉濡数。治以清热化湿，如苍术白虎汤之类；以关节肿痛为主者用桂枝白虎汤之类；以黄疸为主者，用茵陈五苓散之类。

④暑湿：呕吐泄泻，发热汗出，胸闷腹满，不思饮食，苔白滑，脉虚濡。治以芳香化湿，用藿香正气散之类。

(2)内湿

①脾为湿困：肢体沉重，困倦疲惫，脘闷饱胀，大便溏稀，或见呕逆，脉虚濡，苔白滑而腻。治以理脾除湿，用胃苓汤之类。

②湿从热化：湿热蕴于心经，则口舌生疮糜烂；湿热注于下焦，或为痢疾，或为淋浊血尿、癃闭，或为带下；湿热浸淫肌肤，则为疮疥；流注关节，则红肿疼痛。治疗可参照火证，酌加除湿之

品。皮肤湿热所致的疥癣疹疮，可用解毒化湿法，如苦参汤或蛇床子散之类。

(四)痰

痰和饮，都是病理变化的产物，是水液停集于体内空腔等部位的两种不同证候。古人谓“积水成饮，饮凝成痰”，水、饮、痰三者的区别即稠浊者为痰，清稀者为饮，更清者为水。痰饮之产生，与脾肺肾三脏关系最为密切。

1. 痰和饮的特点：从发病部位而言，饮多见于胸腹四肢，故与脾胃关系较为密切。痰之为病，全身各处均可出现，与五脏之病均有关系。张景岳说：“饮惟停积肠胃，而痰则无处不到。水谷不化，而停为饮者，其病全由脾胃；无处不到而化为痰者，凡五脏之伤，皆能致之。”现将痰与饮的临床表现分述如下：

(1)痰之主症：胸部痞闷，胁胀痛，咳嗽痰多，恶心呕吐，腹泻，心悸，眩晕，癫狂，皮肤麻木，关节痛或肿胀，皮下结节或结肿，溃破流脓，久不收口，苔白滑或厚，脉滑。

(2)饮之主症：临床部位多随饮停部位而异，如见心下痞硬，泛吐清涎，肠鸣漉漉，是为痰饮，饮在肠胃；如咳吐引胁下作痛，不利转侧，则为悬饮，饮停胸胁；如体重肢肿，为溢饮，饮在四肢；如喘咳吐涎沫，不能平卧，为支饮，饮在膈上。

2. 痰和饮的病机：人体在生理状态下，水谷之精气得脾之健运，肺之调节，肾之煦蒸，三焦之气化，或化为血，或化为津液，以营养全身；或变为汗，或变为气，或变为溺，而排出体外。而在病理状态下，脏腑失去正常生化输布功能，使游溢之水谷精气，遇阴寒聚而为水为饮，得火气之煎熬变津成痰。脾虚，中阳不振，运化失职，水谷精气敷布失常，则可聚而成饮成痰；阴虚生热，或肝郁化火，火热上炎，灼熬津液，因而生痰；风寒犯肺，气机郁阻，或化热化燥，蒸灼肺津而成痰。痰迷心窍，则神昏癫痫；犯肺则咳嗽痰多；留滞中焦而肠鸣腹泄；流窜肌肉筋骨而为瘰疬痰核。饮在肌肉，溢而为肿：留胁则咳吐引胁而痛，心下痞硬；居膈上则咳喘不能平卧，下注肠中则漉漉有声。

3. 痰和饮的辨证论治

(1)痰证

①风痰咳嗽：即一般伤风所出现的表证咳嗽，咯痰。治以宣肺化痰，用杏苏散之类。

②痰湿犯肺：咳嗽痰多，色白质稀。治以燥湿化痰，用三子养亲汤之类。

③痰热伏肺：肺有伏热，痰黏而黄。治以清热化痰，用清金化痰汤之类。

④痰蒙心窍：卒然昏仆，痰涎壅塞。治以化痰开窍，用稀涎散之类。

⑤痰核瘰疬，项下痰核瘰疬。治以清痰散结，用消核散之类。

⑥痰气相搏：气为痰滞，痰因气结，痰涎壅塞，喘咳气急，胸膈噎塞。治以降气化痰，用苏子降气汤之类。

(2)饮证

①痰饮：症见思水不欲饮，肠中水声漉漉，呕吐清水，胸腹胀满，苔白，脉弦滑。治以温化痰饮，用苓桂术甘汤之类。

②悬饮：咳吐引胁肋痛，转侧不利，发热汗出，苔白或腻，脉弦。治以攻逐水饮，用十枣汤之类。

③溢饮：干呕发热而渴，面目四肢浮肿，身体痛重，苔白或微黄，脉浮而散。治以发汗逐饮，用小青龙汤之类。

④支饮：咳逆倚息，短气不能平卧，身体微肿，脉弦细，苔白。治以泻肺逐饮，用葶苈大枣泻

肺汤之类。

四、六经病机、病证的基本概念

张仲景在继承《内经》、《难经》等古代医学知识的基础上，创立了六经辨证论治的体系，运用于外感病。六经辨证，是把各种外感病的临床表现，综合划分为太阳、阳明、少阳、太阴、少阴、厥阴六种不同的类型。外感病的临床表现，是各脏腑经络受到以风寒为主邪气侵袭后所引起的病理反映，掌握和运用这种规律，是非常必要的。因一则由于邪气性质的差异，二则由于脏腑、经络属性有阴阳，部位有浅深，加之人体禀赋有强弱，年龄有老幼，故病情演变就会出现寒、热、虚、实的不同，辨证时，就需要在原有基础上灵活运用。

六经辨证，临床意义有二：一是对风寒外感病发展不同阶段、六经不同证候的概括，即太阳病、阳明病、少阳病、太阴病、少阴病、厥阴病；二是表明了风寒邪气所在部位与转化及其发展变化的一般规律，即太阳病→阳明病→少阳病→太阴病→少阴病→厥阴病。显示病情由表及里，由浅入深的六个阶段。

六经辨证的基本内容概括如下：

(一)太阳病

太阳病主表，为外感病初起，风寒侵袭肌表之证。

1. 提纲：太阳之为病，脉浮，头顶强痛而恶寒。

2. 病理：风寒袭表，营卫失和，则为经证；经证不解，内传膀胱，则为腑证；邪入气分为蓄水证，邪入血分为蓄血证。

3. 证治

(1)经证：分中风、伤寒两证。

中风证：恶风发热，汗出，头顶强痛，脉浮缓。又称表虚证。治宜调和营卫，以桂枝汤为主方。

伤寒证：恶寒发热，无汗，头痛身痛，项背强，脉浮紧。又称表实证，治宜辛温解表，以麻黄汤为主方。

(2)腑证：分蓄水证、蓄血证。

蓄水证：恶风发热，小便不利，烦渴喜饮，饮入则吐，脉浮。治宜解表利水，以五苓散为主方。

蓄血证：恶风发热，少腹硬满，小便自利，神志错乱，甚则发狂，脉沉细。治宜破血逐瘀，以桃核承气汤为主方。

(二)阳明病

阳明病主里，为风寒之邪由表入里，由寒化热而致邪热炽盛之证。

1. 提纲：阳明之为病，胃家实是也。

2. 病理：寒邪由表入里化热，热蕴胃肠，倘若未见肠中有燥屎则称为经证，若已见肠中有燥屎停积则称为腑证。

3. 证治

(1)经证：高热，汗自出，不恶寒，反恶热，烦渴引饮，脉洪大而数，舌苔黄燥。治宜清热泄火，以白虎汤为主方。

(2)腑证：腹满而痛，大便秘结，潮热谵语，脉沉实。治宜泻热通腑，以诸承气汤为主方。

(三)少阳病

少阳病，主半表半里，为病邪已脱离太阳之表，而尚未进入阳明之里。

1. 提纲:少阳之为病,口苦咽干目眩。

2. 病理:病邪由表内传,或由里外传,或起于本经而停留于表里之间,正邪相争,枢机不运,升降不利。

3. 证治:少阳证为往来寒热,胸胁苦满,默默不欲饮食,心烦喜呕,口苦,咽干,目眩等。治宜和解少阳,以小柴胡汤为主方。若太阳少阳合病,则兼见头痛身痛,汗出等,治宜和解疏表,以柴胡桂枝汤为主方。若少阳阳明合病,则兼见脘腹胀满,痞硬,大便或秘结或下利,治宜和解通里,以大柴胡汤为主方。

(四)太阴病

太阴病主脾阳虚衰。病邪可由三阳病转变而来,也可直接侵入,损伤脾胃,导致脾阳不振。本病为邪入于阴的早期阶段。

1. 提纲:太阴之为病,腹满而吐,食不下,自利益甚,时腹自痛,若下之,必胸下结硬。

2. 病理:寒邪由表入里,损伤脾胃,脾阳不振,运化无权。

3. 证治:太阴病为腹满而痛,下利,食不下而吐。治宜温中健脾,以理中汤为主方。若太阴病兼有表证,则宜根据证情缓急,相应采用先解表,后温里,或表里兼顾之法。

(五)少阴病

少阴病主心肾虚衰,为病邪传入少阴,损伤心肾,导致心肾之阴阳虚衰。本病可由他经传变而来,或直中而病,为病情危重的后期阶段。

1. 提纲:少阴之为病,脉微细,但欲寐。

2. 病理:病邪深入伤及心肾,或致阳气耗伤则内生虚寒,或致阴血亏损则内生虚热,少阴病属虚寒者多而属虚热者少。

3. 证治

(1)少阴虚寒证为恶寒身蜷,四肢厥逆,精神萎靡而欲睡,脉微细,或下利清谷,小便清长。治宜回阳救逆,以四逆汤为主方。

(2)少阴虚热证为心烦,不得眠,口燥咽干,舌红少苔,脉细数等。治宜育阴清热,以黄连阿胶汤为主方。

(3)少阴水泛证为心下悸,头眩,筋肉跳动,全身颤抖,有欲倒于地之势,甚则浮肿,小便不利,或四肢沉重疼痛,或下利,或腹痛等。治宜温阳行水,以真武汤为主方。

(4)少阴病兼证为或兼见太阳证,或兼见阳明证。治宜两者兼顾,分别用助阳解表的麻黄附子细辛汤,或急下存阴的大承气汤。

(六)厥阴病

厥阴病主寒热错杂。为伤寒后期,病邪入里,使人体气血津液和脏腑功能遭到严重损伤,病情复杂,常表现为寒热互见,阴阳错杂。

1. 提纲:厥阴之为病,消渴,气上撞心,心中疼热,饥而不欲食,食则吐蛔,下之利不止。

2. 病理:病邪损伤气血津液,脏腑功能发生障碍,而致阴阳失调,导致内外或上下寒热错杂之证。

3. 证治:

(1)寒热错杂证为时心烦,得食而呕,甚则吐蛔,或见吐利。治宜寒温并用,以乌梅丸为主方。

(2)厥阴寒证为干呕,吐涎沫,头痛,手足厥冷,脉细欲绝等。治宜养血通脉,温经散寒,以当归四逆加吴茱萸生姜汤为主方。

(3)厥阴热证为热利，下重，口干欲饮水，脉数。治宜清热利湿解毒，以白头翁汤为主方。

五、卫气营血病机、病证的基本概念

卫气营血病机，是探讨温热病发生演变过程中，按病变的浅深轻重而分成卫、气、营、血四个阶段的变化机制。叶天士在《温热篇》指出："大凡看法，卫之后方言气，营之后方言血。"概括了温热病邪气传变规律。卫气营血病证，是温邪传至卫、气、营、血各阶段反映于临床的不同证候，即包括卫分证候、气分证候、营分证候、血分证候。它们的一般变化规律是卫分→气分→营分→血分，病变由浅入深，由轻转重，反之，由营、血传至卫、气，是病变由深出浅，由重转轻。

(一)卫分证

卫分证主要见于温热病初起。温邪从口鼻或皮毛而入，侵犯肺卫。

1. 主症：发热，微恶风寒，头痛，无汗或少汗，咳嗽，口渴，舌边尖红，苔薄白，脉浮数等。

2. 病理：温邪上受或侵袭肌表，肺卫失于宣肃。

3. 证治：

(1)风温卫分证：症同主症。治宜辛凉解表，以银翅散为主方。

(2)秋燥卫分证：症见恶寒发热，头痛无汗，咽干唇燥，鼻干，干咳，舌苔薄白而干，脉浮细。秋燥有凉燥与温燥之分。凉燥治宜散寒解表，宣肺润燥，以杏苏散为主方。温燥治宜辛凉解表，宣肺润燥，以桑杏汤为主方。

(3)暑温，湿温之卫分证可参考三焦病机之上焦证。

(二)气分证

气分证主要见于温邪由卫分入里化热，病变部位有胃、脾、肠、胆、胸膈等，其中以热盛阳明较为常见。

1. 主症：壮热，不恶寒但恶热，汗多，渴欲冷饮，舌苔黄燥，脉洪大。

2. 病理：邪入阳明气分，正邪剧烈抗争，津液耗伤。

3. 证治：

(1)热积肺胃：症见如主症。治宜清热生津，以白虎汤为主方。若兼见汗出过多而伤津耗气，可用人参白虎汤为治。若兼见痰黄而稠，胸痛气喘，可用麻杏石甘汤加清化痰热药治疗。若兼见大便秘结或泻下黄臭稀水，腹痛拒按，可用调胃承气汤为治；再有伤阴之症，可用增液承气汤为治。

(2)里热夹湿证可参考三焦病机之中焦证。

(三)营分证

营分证多由卫分、气分传来，也有起病即为营分证者。是温热病的严重阶段。

1. 主症：

(1)身热夜甚或身灼热，渴不欲饮或反不渴，心烦不寐，时有谵语，舌质红绛，脉细数。

2. 病理：温热之邪入里，热势内盛，损伤营阴，或热扰心神，或热极生风。

3. 证治：

(1)热灼营阴，症见如主症，或斑疹隐隐，舌绛无苔。治宜清营泄热，以清营汤为主方。

(2)热入心包，症见高热神昏谵语，或四肢厥冷，抽搐。治宜清心开窍，以清营汤送服安宫牛黄丸或局方至宝丹。

(3)热极生风:症见高热,躁扰不宁,抽搐,或四肢拘急,项强,角弓反张,舌颤,舌红或绛,脉弦数。治宜清热熄风,以白虎汤加羚羊角、钩藤之类。

(四)血分证

血分证多从营分发展而来,也有由卫分、气分直入血分的,个别情况也有起病即现血分证者,是温热病的危重阶段。

1. 主症:吐血,衄血,便血,溺血,斑疹密布,身热,或低热,手足心热,口干舌燥,齿枯唇焦,躁扰不宁,或神昏谵语,舌质红绛或光红如镜,或手足抽搐,痉厥。

2. 病理:热盛迫血,热瘀交结,阴液被灼,虚风内动。

3. 证治:

(1)热在血分:症见如主症。治宜清热凉血解毒,以犀角地黄汤为主方。

(2)气血两燔:症见壮热口渴,心烦躁扰,甚或昏狂谵妄,吐血,衄血,肌肤发斑,舌绛,苔黄燥,脉数。治宜清气凉血化斑,以化斑汤。若热毒充斥表里上下,内侵脏腑,外窜经络,症见寒战高热,大渴饮冷,头痛如劈,烦躁谵妄,神昏,出血等。治宜清气凉血,泻火解毒,以清瘟败毒饮为主方。

(3)血热动风:症见壮热神昏,头晕胀痛,手足抽搐,颈项强直,角弓反张,舌干绛,脉弦数。治宜凉肝熄风,以羚羊钩藤汤为主方。

(4)血热伤阴:因邪气的强弱和阴液耗伤程度不同,表现有异,治疗总离不开清热凉血和滋阴增液两法,具体运用时酌情取舍。

第三节 分 类 学

中医内科学所包含的疾病,随着医疗实践的不断深入和历代医家的积累和整理而与日俱增。为了方便学习研究与临床应用,探讨内科疾病分类的必要性早就引起人们的普遍重视。《金匮要略》一书中,已经作了简单的疾病分类,易于辨证施治。尽管粗糙,但在疾病分类方面的探索却是有益的。《诸病源候论》是我国现存第一部证候学专著,其以“候”类述,共1739则,可见书中证候分类之细。《千金方》则由博返约,进行初步归纳。《太平惠民和剂局方》虽是宋代的一种成药处方配本,但此书按病分类,在疾病分类方面也作了一些尝试。宋代陈言《三因极一病证方论》,试图按三因将疾病分类,但某些病症之中,又包含了内因、外因、不内外因等不同证治,所以也说明此法分类尚未达到尽善之地。《明医杂著》将当时常见内科病证分题讨论,重点突出。

张从正《三法六门》把疾病按病因而分为风、寒、暑、湿、燥、火、内伤、外伤、内积、外积共十门,这对后世《医门法律》影响颇大,是书将前六者及诸杂证,分门别类,著成一书。《医学纲目》则按脏腑分部加以分类,可以看出著者在分类学上所下的苦心,价值较大。《证因脉治》将所论病证的每一“症”又以外感、内伤分类,可以说是以外感、内伤对疾病进行分类的雏形。《证治汇补》将内科杂病分为八门,探讨了按部分类的方法。《医学实在易》以表证、里证、寒证、热证、实证、虚证分类讨论疾病的证治。

纵观历代医家对内科疾病的分类,尚未统一看法。为了便于指导临床,寻找一个比较合理的分类法是十分必要的。新中国成立后进行的探讨认为,以病因、病理变化为纲对内科疾病加以分类较为合适。以病因为纲,可将内科疾病分为外感疾病和内伤疾病两大类。外感疾病,是由外感六淫等邪气所致；内伤疾病是由情志刺激、饮食劳倦、起居失常，以及脏腑功能失调所产生的病理产物，如气血津液散布失常所生之痰浊、瘀血等引发。诚然，这两类疾病也是可以互相转化的。一些外感疾病可变为内伤疾病，内伤疾病使正气亏虚也易感受外邪，在病程的某一阶段可以变成外感疾病。按病理变化为纲可将内科疾病分为热病与杂病两大类。热病包括一切有热症而以六经、三焦、卫气营血为发生病理改变的病证；杂病包括以脏腑功能失调为主而产生的病证。

病因分类，突出了病因的特殊性，便于临床辨证求因，审因论治。病理分类反映了疾病病理变化的内在联系，有助于掌握疾病发生发展的规律。因为病理分类，主要是脏腑功能失调造成的，故可以进一步按五脏六腑进行分类。

病理分类法是在病因分类法的基础上进行的，是对病因分类的补充。因此，临床上可把这两种分类法结合起来，称之为外感热病与内伤杂病。

(一)外感热病的分类

外感热病，根据感受邪气的不同可分为伤寒与温病；温病又可分为温热病与湿热病。温热病包括了风温、春温、冬温、秋燥、温毒、温疫等；湿热病包括了湿温、伏暑、暑温等。按发病特点，温病又可分为新感温病与伏气温病两类。如风温、冬温、暑温、秋燥属新感温病，春温、伏暑则属伏气温病。

(二)内伤杂病的分类

内伤杂病分类的理论基础是脏象学说。人体是一个以脏腑为中心的有机整体，外联四肢百骸、五官九窍，以气血津液为物质基础，以经络为通路。因此，内伤杂病虽多，但其病理变化始终不离脏腑功能紊乱，经络通路障碍，气血津液生成运行输布失常。内伤杂症的分类，必须按照不同脏腑生理病理变化而分为肺系病证、心系病证、肝系病证、肾系病证、经络病证、气血病证和津液病证等所属病证。

现将内科常见病分类如下：

1. 外感病证：感冒、霍乱、疟疾。

2. 内伤病证

(1)肺系病证：咳嗽、喘证、哮证、肺痈、肺痿、肺胀、肺痨。

(2)脾胃病证：胃痛(附吐酸、嘈杂)、呕吐、呃逆、噎膈、腹痛、泄泻、痢疾、便秘、虫证。

(3)肝系病证：眩晕、中风、胁痛、黄疸、臌胀、痉证。

(4)心系病证：心悸、胸痛、失眠、多寐、癫狂、痫证。

(5)肾系病证：水肿、淋证、癃闭、遗精(附阳痿)、腰痛、耳鸣、耳聋。

(6)经络病证：痹证、痿证、头痛。

(7)气血津液病证：汗证、消渴、痰饮、积聚、内伤发热、虚劳、瘿气、血证、厥证、郁证。

第四节　治　疗　学

中医内科学的治疗学，其理论是严谨的，其方法是多样的。内容包括治疗原则和治疗方法。治疗原则可概括为整体论治、治病求本、动中施治等；治疗方法可概括为内治法和外治法两大类，其中各含有许多具体的方法。

成书时间较《内经》还早的《五十二病方》，即记载了汤液、醪醴等内治法和药浴、烟熏、蒸气、熏法、熨法、砭法、灸法、按摩法等外治法。《金匮要略》一书中的中药剂型已有汤剂、丸剂、散剂、酒剂、洗剂、熏剂、滴耳剂、吹鼻剂、灌鼻剂、软膏剂、肛门栓剂、阴道栓剂等。《伤寒论》还对服药法进行了深入的探讨。《理瀹骈文》对外治法作了比较全面的总结。所有关于治疗方法的改进，都旨在提高治疗效果，方便给药途径和减少毒副作用。

中药和方剂是内科治疗的主要手段，《神农本草经》收载药物 365 种，至《本草纲目》载药已达 1892 种，以后又经历代医家的努力，新的中药不断被发现和应用于临床，特别是新中国成立以来，医药学进入一个崭新的阶段，使用的中药已达 5000 种。另外，中药炮制方法的进步，也大大增强了药效，减轻了毒性。南北朝刘宋时期的《雷公炮炙论》，记载的炮炙方法有蒸、煮、炒、焙、炙、炮、煅、浸、水飞等 17 种。之后，加工炮炙方法不断增加，特别是新中国成立后，在剂型改革方面作了许多新的尝试，如片剂、冲剂、针剂等，更有利于临床应用。

方剂的组成是在中医药的理论指导下产生和发展的，《内经》之组方原则规定了君、臣、佐、使四项内容。成无己根据《内经》之旨，依病情轻重、病位上下、病势缓急、药味奇偶等，提出七方，即大、小、缓、急、奇、偶、复等 7 种类型的方剂。后《伤寒明理论》又按方剂的功效而确定 10 个分类，即宣、通、补、泻、轻、重、滑、涩、燥、湿。后世医家又不断补充，《医方集解》将方剂分类增至 21 种之多，即补养、发表、涌吐、攻里、表里、和解、理气、理血、祛风、祛寒、清暑、利湿、润燥、泻火、除痰、消导、收涩、杀虫、明目、痈疡、经产等，并附急救良方，这种分类法，有利于临床应用，且与中药分类也有联系，故为医家所欢迎。《医学心悟》遂在此基础上经过综合、归纳，结合病性而以八法概括之，即汗、吐、下、温、清、补、消、和，实为从繁就简、提纲挈领之分类法，故为后世医家所沿用。

方剂的产生和发展也是以提高临床疗效为基础的，《五十二病方》收载医方 280 多个，至宋代《太平圣惠方》广泛收集了前代方书和当时民间验方，集方达 16834 首，后《圣济总录》已逾 20000 首。《普济方》是我国现存最大的一部方书，载方已达 61730 首，可见中医方剂之宏丰。为了便于临床使用，对方剂进行筛选是必不可少的工作，《校正太平惠民和剂局方》曾根据当时临床需要，选列 297 首，后世的《医方集解》、《汤头歌诀》、《时方歌括》等书也都为了实用、诵读、记忆方便作了新的探索，因此，也具有很大的参考价值。

一、治疗原则

治疗原则，即治疗疾病的法则。它是按照整体观念和辨证论治精神制定的，对治疗过程中的立法、处方、用药等具有指导意义。其内容可概括为整体论治、治病求本、动中施治、医护结合和八法运用等。

(一)整体论治

由于人体的脏腑、经络以及形体诸窍构成一个完整的有机体，同时又与自然界保持密切联系。因此，人体任何局部的疾病往往影响到全身，治疗时单纯治疗局部是不够的，更应该注意整体，从调理整体达到治疗局部病变的目的。再者，治疗中还应该结合天时、地理、体质等因素通盘考虑，采取因时、因地、因人制宜的方法，才能获得更好的效果。

(二)治病求本

治病求本，是指针对发病的根本原因予以治疗。“本”和“标”是相对而言的，如就正邪而言正气是本，邪气是标；就疾病先后而言，旧病、原发病是本，新病、续发病是标。通过辨证分析能够认识疾病的本质，看出标与本，从而确定相应的治疗方法。运用治病求本这一法则，必须掌握“正治与反治”、“治标与治本”、“扶正与祛邪”以及“预防为主”等内容。

1. 正治与反治

(1)正治:是逆其证候性质而治的一种治疗法则,又称逆治。正治法适用于疾病的征象与本质相一致的病证。

(2)反治:是顺从疾病假象而治的一种治疗法则,又称从治。如"热因热用"治疗真寒假热证,"寒因寒用"治疗真热假寒证,"塞因塞用"治疗真虚假实证,"通因通用"治疗真实假虚证等。

2. 治标与治本:病变中常有主次标本的不同,治疗时也宜有先后缓急的区别,一般采取"急则治其标,缓则治其本"及标本并重则标本同治的原则。

(1)急则治其标:在疾病的过程中当标病甚急,如不及时解决,则危及患者生命或影响疾病的治疗时,必须抓紧时间,尽快解决标病。

(2)缓则治其本:在标病缓解之后或无明显危重症候的情况,可以针对发病的根本原因或原发疾病进行治疗。所以,此原则对慢性病或急性病的恢复期有重要意义。

(3)标本兼顾:标病本病并重之时,必须两者兼顾,而不能舍本治标或舍标治本,如益气解表法或表里双解法等。

标本的治疗法则,既有原则性,又有灵活性,但最终目的在于抓住疾病的主要矛盾,做到治病求本。

3. 扶正与祛邪:疾病的发生发展,就是正气与邪气相互斗争的表现,而治疗疾病就是扶助正气,祛除邪气,从而使病情逐渐好转,终至痊愈。

(1)扶正:即是扶助正气,增强体质,提高机体抗病能力。此法则适用于疾病过程中,以正气虚为主要矛盾,而邪气不盛的虚证。

(2)祛邪:即是用泻实之法祛除病邪,从而达到邪祛正安。此法则适用于以邪气盛为主要矛盾,而正气不衰的实证。

在具体运用扶正、祛邪时,还有先扶正后祛邪或先祛邪后扶正或扶正与祛邪兼用之别。先扶正后祛邪适用于正虚邪实而以正虚为主的情况,正气不耐攻邪,则当先扶正,待正气恢复后再攻其邪;先祛邪后扶正适用于正虚邪实,而正气尚能耐攻,或祛邪同时扶正反会助邪的情况,故先祛邪气,邪退正虚时再予扶正;扶正与祛邪兼用适用于正虚邪实,两者兼用则扶正不留邪,祛邪又不会伤正。

4. 预防为主:预防,是指采用一定措施,防止疾病的发生与发展,其内容包括未病先防和既病防变两个方面。

(1)未病先防:疾病的发生既然取决于正邪两个方面,因此,增强机体正气则能使邪不可干。正气的维护和增强主要依靠调摄精神,使情绪安定,气机调畅;锻炼身体,使体质增强,气血旺盛;保持生活起居的规律,养精蓄锐,以应付不断变化的不良刺激和损伤;另外,药物预防和人工免疫,以及讲究卫生,防止环境、水源和食物污染也很重要。

(2)既病防变:若疾病已经发生,则应早期诊断,早期治疗,以防止疾病发展和传变。

(三)动中施治

疾病发生以后,则多有好转或加重的变化,因此,必须用发展的观点,动态的观点进行观察和处理。在临证过程中,不仅需要掌握常法、主方,而且应该随病情的变化进行治疗,乃至方药的加减增损,不致于治疗疾病用一法一方守到底。

无论外感病或内伤病,都会形成一定的阶段,既要熟悉某一阶段的特点,又要知道其转化的规律,才能够知常达变,随证施治。

（四）医护结合

疾病的治疗效果，与调护有极为密切的关系，因此，在治疗疾病过程中，加强精神、饮食、起居、服药等方面的护理至关重要。在临床上，根据不同疾病的特点，在辨证施治的同时，采取必要的护理措施，以提高疗效。

二、八法运用

八法指临床上常用的汗、吐、下、和、温、清、补、消八种治法。

（一）汗法

本法是开泄肌腠，逐邪外出的一种治法。

适用范围：汗法除适用于一般外感病初期外，还适用于水肿和疮疡的初期，以及斑疹将透的阶段。

（二）吐法

是引导病邪或有毒物质，使之从口涌吐而出的一种治法。

适用范围：吐法适用于痰涎壅盛，食积胃脘不化，恶心欲呕，或误食毒物尚留胃中等疾病。

（三）下法

是攻逐体内积滞，通泄大便的一种治法。

适用范围：常用于邪在肠胃，燥屎内结，热结于里，以及水结，蓄血，痰滞，虫积等疾病。

（四）和法

是一方面祛邪，一方面扶正，达到祛邪而不伤正的一种和解治法。

适用范围：此法运用范围很广，如少阳证、太阳少阳及少阳阳明合病，肝胃不和，肝郁所致的月经不调，肝木乘土的腹痛泄泻等。

（五）温法

温法是祛除寒邪和补益阳气的一种治法，其主要作用在于回阳救逆，温中散寒，从而达到补益阳气而祛邪治病的目的。

适用范围：温法适用于寒邪留滞，或由热证转变为寒证的疾病。

（六）清法

清法是治疗一般热证的一种方法，有退热降火，保津除烦止渴的作用。

适用范围：凡热证，不论热在气分或营血，内伤或外感，只要里热炽盛，皆可用清法治疗。

（七）补法

是补益人体阴阳气血不足，或补益某一脏之虚损的一种治法。

适用范围：适用于正气不足，体力虚弱的病人，如气虚、血虚、阴虚、阳虚，以及正气虚弱而无力逐邪者。

（八）消法

包括消散和消破两个内容，其作用与下法相似又有不同。消法适用于食滞停积或慢性癥瘕积聚而又不宜攻下者，以渐消缓散的方法来达到治疗目的。

适用范围：适用于气、血、痰、食形成的积聚凝滞等疾病。

三、中医治疗方法

(一)内治法

用于内治法的剂型可有汤、散、丸、膏、丹、酒、片、颗粒、口服液、注射液等。

(二)外治法

用于外治法的方法可在贴、涂、敷、罨、熨、熏、浸、洗、擦、蒸、糁、扑、嚏、嗃、吹、吸、捏、塞、卧、枕、填、导、佩、刮痧、拔罐、按摩、灸法等。

以上就内科临床常用的内治法和外治法进行了简要介绍,只要正确使用和积极推广这些方法,定会提高治疗效果。

复习思考题

1. 试述陈言“三因学说”的内容及其对后世病因学说的影响。
2. 如何认识痰与瘀既是脏腑功能失调所产生的病理产物,又是病因?
3. 简述五脏辨证的主要证型。
4. 扼要陈述五脏病证各证型常用方剂。
5. 五脏病的病理如何掌握?
6. 如何认识气病分虚实?气机升降失调与脏腑有什么联系?
7. 出血、瘀血、血虚的病理变化是什么?
8. 风、火、痰、湿病理变化是什么?
9. 六经辨证的临床意义有哪几点?六经证的内容是什么?
10. 卫气营血和三焦两种病理如何在临床上运用。
11. 如何掌握和使用内治法和外治法?内伤杂病能用外治法吗?试举例说明之。

第三章　中医内科临证方法及病历书写

第一节　中医内科临证方法

内科学是临床各学科的基础。在内科学教学过程中，除了教授内科病证的辨证论治的理论知识、临床运用之外，非常重要的一个环节，就是教授临证方法。

临证方法，就是运用中医药学理论知识，对疾病进行诊断和治疗的方法。在中医临床上，一般概括为诊察、辨证、论治三个方面，它贯穿于诊治病人的全过程，既包涵医生诊治过程中的全部思维活动，也包括医生按规定书写完整病历的每一项内容，是医生理论知识与临床技能——基本功的真实反映。

临证的要求，是诊治迅速而正确，理法方药丝丝入扣，而且应使患者经治后获得疗效。因此，临证方法的训练、掌握、熟练，对每一位学生，都是必不可缺的。

一、诊　察

诊察的内容，主要是四诊，即望、闻、问、切。医生通过四诊，获得辨证所需的全部资料。资料内容应该包括患者的一般情况，如姓名、性别、年龄、籍贯、职业、工作单位、婚姻等，作为辨证需要，还应该了解患者性格、爱好、信仰、居住条件等。对于疾病，则要深入了解发病情况，最痛苦症状，诊治过程及疗效，以及患者就诊时的全部病症。中医的诊断与主诉有着非常密切的关系，所以，通过询问病史而确定主诉内容，即病人当下最痛苦的症状，最急需解除的病痛及其发生、延续的时间。同时，也应了解既往病史、家庭成员疾病或死亡情况、个人史、妇女的经带胎产史、药物过敏史等。然后通过望、闻、切诊进行查体，以发现阳性体征。随着科学进步，中医的望、闻、切的方法和内容，也逐步丰富和发展，如将纤维胃镜所看到的胃黏膜病变，已作为望诊的延伸，即胃镜像也在辨证时加以参考，其他像X线、B超、化验结果等也被中医所认识、所利用，丰富了中医四诊内容，提高了中医的诊治水平。

采集病史，要求全面、系统、确切、简明。所谓全面，就是耐心细致地了解疾病发生、发展的全过程，如起病原因，最初症状，诊断与治疗内容，效果如何，刻下最突出的症状是什么，以及既往患病情况等等。系统，就是将患者未加整理的病情，边问边思索，使之条理化，判断出该患者所得疾病是外感还是内伤，若是内伤杂病，还应判断其以心系为主，或心肝两系为主，或心肝脾三系为主等，必要时再追问病史，要求患者一五一十地介绍病情，同时医生也要防止主观臆测，或按书本知识引导患者叙述病情。所谓重点，就是把患者的没有条理的症状，经过医生头脑的思索、整理，有重点地书写在病历上。

查体，要求操作正规、轻柔、熟练。要反复训练，以中医望、闻、切诊为主，西医的望、触、叩、听为辅，西医为中医诊断服务。

二、辨　证

辨证，就是运用中医理论，对四诊所获得的资料，进行分析、综合、推理、判断，从而确定疾病的病位、病性、病机转化，最后得出病证名和证候名。

内科疾病包括外感病与内伤病两大类。中医在长期的发展过程中，形成了非常丰富的辨证方法。一般外感病常用六经辨证、卫气营血辨证或三焦辨证、内伤病常用脏腑辨证、气血辨证、风火痰湿辨证，但两者也是互相渗透的，并以脏腑的生理病理作基础，而且都以八纲作为总纲。

临证时如何分析病情，方法是多种多样的，在内科临证时，一般多采用综合分析的方法，即分析四诊所得到的资料，注意其主症的特异性，结合兼症，参考舌、脉等查体资料，用中医基础理论知识，从生理功能分析出病理变化，从而推断出疾病的病位、病性、病机转化等，最后确定诊断。

辨证的要求，应做到言之有理，理必有据，陈述简明，表达准确。在书写病历时，可以使用中医传统的四六句，也可以使用 1、2、3 逐点分析，最后得出结论。

诊断是辨证的结果，它包括二级诊断，一是病名或证名的诊断，其与主诉有非常密切的关系；一是证候的诊断，其内容既有病性又有病机转化，如病名、证名诊断为胃痛，证候诊断为脾胃不和、上热下寒等。

三、论　治

论治，是根据诊断，研讨、确定治疗方案、治则、治法、主方或基础方、药味组成、剂量、煎法、服法、调养宜忌等的过程。

治疗方案是论治的总体设计，如采用单一的中药，或中药配合针灸、按摩或食疗综合治疗；是用单一的攻法或补法，或先攻后补，或先补后攻，或攻补兼施，还可以有时间的初步安排等。治则即治疗原则，包括正治反治、标本缓急、脏腑补泻、三因制宜等。治法即具体治疗方法，如内治或外治，以及常用的十二法等。在治法的原则指导下，选取一张最合适的古方或自拟方作为主方，对初学者尤为必要，否则就会胡乱凑药，无章无法，影响疗效。有了主方后，根据病人的具体情况，加减用药以使之更适合本病的病情，临床经验越多加减也就越灵活，组成的方子也就贴切而有效。剂量也需根据古今经验而作调整，针对性也更强。煎法、服 法以及调养宜忌对治疗效果也至关重要，所以也是论治的组成部分，不可遗漏或疏忽。

论治的要求，要做到据证立法，以法选方，按方遣药，灵活变通，达到理法方药贯穿一致。

临证方法，是临床医生必须掌握的临床技能，只有反复训练，才能熟能生巧，达到提高疗效的目的。

第二节　中医内科病历的一般要求

中医病历是中医理论与临床实践紧密结合的医疗记录，它详细记载了整个疾病过程中病情演变、治疗方案及效果、各项检查、各级医师诊疗及会诊意见等内容，是正确进行辨证论治和推测疾病预后转归的重要依据，是医疗、教学、科研工作的宝贵资料，同时又可作为业务考核和行政、司法机关的重要参考资料。

加强对中医病历的管理，提高对中医病历的书写要求，是医院管理工作中的重要环节，也是提高中医临床诊断与治疗水平的重要措施；在教学医院，这又是教学过程中学生必须进行基本功训练的一项内容。

中医内科病历书写的一般要求归纳如下：

1. 一份完整的中医病历应包括社会部分、四诊检查、辨证论治三大项内容。按目前卫生行政部门的要求应有西医诊断的内容。

2. 中医病历的书写应以中医理论为指导，进行辨证论治，做到理、法、方、药完整统一，一般要求使用中医名词术语。

3. 病历格式中的各种项目应认真填写，完整无漏，应用钢笔书写，字迹工整，文字通顺，做到全面、系统、简练、准确、整洁。

4. 住院医师写的病历，由主治医师审阅，用铅笔修改并签名，修改过多时住院医师应重写。实习医师或进修医师书写的病历应由住院医师或主治医师用铅笔修改并签名，修改过多时应重写。

5. 住院病历(或住院志)应在 24 小时内完成，门诊病历要求当时完成。

第三节　内科住院病历书写格式及内容

一、格式与内容

姓名：	性别：
年龄：	籍贯：
民族：	婚姻：
住址：	发病季节：
入院时间	病史采集时间：
病史陈述者：	可靠性：

问诊：

主诉：病人自觉最痛苦的症状及其部位、性质、时间——即就医的主要原因。

现病史：围绕主症记述从发病至本次就诊时疾病的发生、发展及其演变的全过程。对于症状的描述要应用中医术语。对于诊疗经过应包括中、西医两方面的内容。

现在症：应详尽、确切地记载，作为当下辨证论治的主要依据。

既往史：记录一般健康状况和过去曾患过疾病的时间和治疗情况。

个人史：记录出生地、居留地、居住环境条件、生活和工作情况、饮食习惯、特殊嗜好。

经、带、胎、产史(女性患者)：记录月经初潮时间，周期，经量，色泽，性质，结婚年龄，孕产情况。

家族史：记录家庭亲属与本人生活密切相关的亲友的健康状况和发病情况，如亲属已死亡则记录其原因及年龄。

全身：包括神、色、形、态。

局部：头、面、毛发、五官、咽喉、颈、胸、腹、脊柱、腰背、四肢、爪甲、皮肤等，还有十四经脉循行部位的特殊情况。

排泄物：痰、呕吐物、汗、二便、涕、泪、体表分泌物等。

舌诊：详细记录舌形、舌质、舌苔的变化及舌下系带、舌背部的变化。

闻诊：

声音：发音、语音、呼吸、咳嗽、呃逆、呕吐、太息、呻吟、腹鸣等情况。

气味：口气、汗液、痰涎、呕吐物、二便等气味。

按肌肤：头、面、颈、胸、胁、腹部、躯干、四肢及压痛点。

切脉：必须详细记录寸口的脉象，包括左、右手，寸、关、尺各部分别记述。必要时描述三部九候的脉象。对于危重患者还应运用三部诊法，记录人迎、趺阳的脉象并注意胃、神、根的表现。

四诊摘要：

证候分析：辨病位、证候属性、病机转化。

中医诊断：归纳辨病与辨证，应包括主要病证和伴随病证。病名后的括号内写证候。

治则治法：包括治疗步骤的安排，具体治疗方法。

方药：主方：

药味：×××(包煎)　××(先煎)　××(后下)　××(烊化分冲)　×××　×××　×××　×××　×××　(分钟)

调护：包括给药、宜忌、食疗、起居等要求。

理化检查：物理检查及实验检查的阳性所见。

西医诊断：主要疾病与伴随疾病(期、型、性)。

诊断依据：

治疗安排：主要是支持疗法，对症处理和紧急处理。

医师签字

年　月　日　时　分

二、住院病历的具体要求

1. 社会部分的各自然项目应填写清楚。发病季节的记载是按照天人相应的理论，以便于总结发病与四时、节气的关系。

2. 四诊检查部分

(1)主症：要求记录病人自觉最痛苦的一个或几个主要症状，以及其部位、性质、时间，要体现出病人就医的主要原因。

(2)现病史：应围绕主症旁及兼症，记述从发病至本次就诊时疾病的发生、发展及其变化的全过程，包括起病情况，主要症状和特点，病情发展和演变，伴随的兼症，诊疗经过等。对于症状的描述还要应用中医术语。对于治疗经过应包括中西医药两方面的内容。

(3)既往史：个人史、经带胎产史、家族史的记录都应注意中医特点。如先天禀赋不足与家族史有关系者应详细的记载。

(4)望诊：应以舌诊为重点，舌形、舌质、舌苔的变化要详细地形容并记录。神与色重点观察颜面、五官的表现，对局部和排泄物的望诊所见也要重视。

(5)闻诊：闻声音和嗅气味，两方面的检查要全面记录。

(6)切诊：应以切脉为重点，必须详细记录寸口形象。必要时描述三部九候的脉象，对于重危患者还应运用三部诊法，记录人迎、趺阳脉象，并注意胃、神、根的表现，寸口脉象可按左、右手，寸、关、尺分别记述。

3. 辨证论治部分

(1)四诊摘要：应是四诊检查主要资料的摘要综合，尤其要详细记述入院当天的症状，应有概括性和系统性，能比较确切地反映病史的特点，为中医辨证与辨病提供依据。

(2)证候分析：将四诊所得的临床资料，可以主症、舌象、脉象为重点，按症状的内在有机联系进行分组，运用中医理论分析其产生的原因和病理机制。要求反映出病位、证候属性、病机转化、病势发展顺逆等方面的内容。要求做到言之有理，理必有据，陈述简明，表达正确。所谓言之有理，理必有据是指按照中医基础理论的辨证方法进行分析。

(3)中医诊断：归纳辨病与辨证，有几个就写几个，按主次进行排列，有病名的写病名，无病名的写主症，要写证候类型，诊断要采用两段或三段式如：

黄疸(占一行)

阴黄(另占一行向后错一个字)

寒湿瘀血内阻(另占一行)

(4)治则治法：依据辨证，进行立法，确定治则，注意写明标本先后，并包括诊疗步骤的安排。

(5)方药：有主方的应写方名，自拟方可不写方名，药味要求每行写四味药，药味右上角写煎法、服法、炮制要求等，右下角写明分量。药味排列要有章法，即按君、臣、佐、使及配伍关系写清。

(6)调护：服药和饮食的禁忌，配合哪些调养措施和饮食治疗要写清楚，并按照辨证施护的要求，重点提出住院期间，尤其是入院当时的护理要求，应分项写清。

三、内科住院病历举例

姓名：胡某某

年龄：45 岁　　　　性别：男

民族：满　　　　　籍贯：北京

职业：工人　　　　婚姻：已婚

住址：东城区东颂年 2 号

工作单位：北京客汽车改装公司四厂

入院时间：92、2、22　3：30/pm

发病节气：雨水前 3 天

病史陈述者：本人

病历采写时间：92、2、22，5：30/pm

可靠性：可靠

问诊：

主症：发热、恶寒、咳嗽 2 天，右胸掣痛半天。

现病历：患者缘于本月 20 日不慎衣着而始感头痛，连及巅面，鼻塞声重，时流清涕，微有咳嗽，恶寒重而发热轻、无汗出，自作“感冒”而服白药片(去痛片)效果不著，诸症依然，但仍坚持工作，未得将息。次晨症状加重，头痛连及项背，周身酸楚乏力，至下午 3 时许又突发寒战，咳嗽频作，痰黏而黄，涕浊，不欲饮食，便秘溲赤，急来我院急诊，查体温 39℃，被诊为“上感”，予“感冒冲剂”，“复方新诺明”口服及肌注“复方氨基比林”，且自服“A·P·C”后，濈然汗出，但身热不解。患者所苦有增无减，恶风怕寒，虽厚衣被而寒不减，气粗心烦，渴喜冷饮，入夜尤甚，今晨又觉右胸掣痛，不敢深息，咳吐暗红色痰，再来我院复诊，急查 T：39℃，WBC：29800/mm^3，N79％，L3％，胸透见右上叶大叶性肺炎征象，遂由急诊室收住我病区。

既往史：平素身体尚可，否认结核及其他传染病史，无慢性支气管炎史，无药物及食物过敏史。

个人史：出生北京，曾去过广东、东北、苏杭等地。住地无潮湿之弊，条件尚可，善食辛辣，嗜烟 10 余年，10 支/日，少量饮酒，性情较为开朗，善与人言谈，精神乐观。

婚姻史：29 岁成婚，配偶有咳嗽咯血史多年，反复发作；育一男一女，身体尚健。

家族史：其母年已七错，素体健康，其父因患“脑软化”而于 80 年故去。

望诊：

全身：神识清楚，精神倦怠，表情痛苦，面色萎黄，形体干瘦，双目有神，卧床懒动，体态自如。

局部：头发稀疏，间有花白，尚有光泽，目窠微陷，目珠不黄，白睛无红丝隐隐，瞳神等大等圆，鼻翼微有扇动，耳轮红润，无耳漏及生疮，唇色暗红干裂，牙齿垢黄，排列不整，左下大、磨齿各一枚缺如，无龋齿及齿衄。咽部色泽淡红，未见乳蛾肿大，颈部对称，柔软，无畸形，无瘿瘤及瘰疬，胸廓扁平，胸骨赤露，艰于呼吸，甚则用手紧箍胸膺，腹部松弛无膨隆，无青筋外露，脊柱平直，两侧对称，不向两侧弯曲，四肢不浮肿，无鹤膝及杵状指（趾），指（趾）甲润泽，皮肤润泽，无黄疸、斑疹、皮下结节、白痦及疖、痈、疔、疽。

排泄物：痰黄质黏稠，咳之易出，无血丝及包块；涕浊色白痰少；便秘 3 日未行，小便黄赤，周身时有汗出。

舌诊：舌体大小适中，质红苔黄微腻。舌下系带暗红，长短适中。

闻诊：

声音：声高有力，语音重浊，气粗息短，咳嗽偶作，咳声响亮，无郑声、浊语、谵语及呻吟声。

嗅：微有口臭，身有汗味，小便味臊。

切诊：

按肌肤：肌肤润柔，无凹陷，额、尺肤热甚，颈、腋、鼠蹊部无瘿瘤瘰疬。

按胸腹：虚里按之应手，动而不紧，和缓不急，右胸部及上腹部轻按则痛，甚则拒按，但无坚硬之癥积痞块。

切　脉

	寸	关	尺
左	弦滑略数	弦滑略数	弦细滑略数
右	浮略数	弦滑略数	弦滑略数

四诊摘要：

现症见发热恶寒，偶有寒战，周身酸楚，用发汗药则汗出，头痛连脑，鼻塞流涕，间有咳嗽，痰黄而黏，咳之易出，气粗微喘，右胸掣痛，深息加剧，渴喜冷饮，大便秘结已 3 日未行，小便短赤，舌红苔黄微腻，脉右寸浮略数，左弦滑略数。神志清楚，表情痛苦，神色倦怠，面色萎黄，形体干瘦，肌肤润泽，目窠微陷，白睛红丝隐隐，目珠不黄，鼻塞有扇动，唇色暗红干裂，牙齿黄垢，咽淡红，未见乳蛾肿大，声高语重，气粗息短，咳声偶作，微有口臭，周身有汗腥味，小便味臊，额及尺肤热甚，颈、腋、鼠蹊部无瘿瘤瘰疬，右胸及上腹部轻按则痛，甚则屏息拒按，但无坚硬积聚痞块，虚里按之应手，动而不紧，和缓不急。

证候分析：

患者形体瘦削，善食辛辣，脾胃素有蕴热，又时值早春，寒邪未尽，风气当令，患者不慎衣着，外感风寒之邪，肌表被束，卫阳不达，则见头痛、恶寒发热，周身酸楚不适；肺主宣发肃降，开窍于鼻，肺卫受邪，肺气郁闭不宣，又有痰热积肺，清肃之令失常，则见咳嗽鼻塞；肺与大肠相表里，肺气不宣，腑气不通，且肺胃内有壅热，津液受灼，水少舟停，则见大便秘结，小便短赤；舌红苔黄微腻，脉弦滑略数为内有痰热之象；右寸浮为表邪未尽之征。

纵观脉症，病位应在肺、胃、大肠，以实热为主，表里同病，属表邪未解，肺胃郁热，腑气不通之证。

中医诊断：风温

卫气同病

表寒里热

治则治法：疏风解表，清肺化痰，佐以通络止痛。

方药：①清解液　　60cc

5%G、N、S500cc/gttVst

②清开灵　　40cc

林格氏液　500cc/gttVst

③荆防败毒剂 2cc　im　st

④汤剂：以银翘散合麻杏石甘汤加减。

麻黄 3g、生石膏 30g(先煎)、连翘 10g、银花 10g、薄荷 5g(后下)、鲜芦根 30g、杏仁 10g、炒牛蒡子 10g、条黄芩 10g、全瓜蒌 30g、丝瓜络 10g，水煎服，当时急煎两付。

⑤针灸：取足太阳膀胱经、手阳明大肠经之穴为主，以疏风解表清热。

取穴：曲池双、合谷双、风门双、大椎，留针 20 分钟。

调护：宜保暖，避风寒，忌生冷，患者形体不健，需谨防高烧不退，气阴暴脱，且密切观察汗出、脉象、面色、呼吸之变化。

西医检查：

T：38℃；P：82 次/分；R：20 次/分；Bp：130/90mmHg

发育正常，营养中等，神清合作，皮肤黏膜无黄染，无溃疡、皮疹及疖肿，周身浅表淋巴结不大，头颅大小正常，面色稍暗，高热时红赤，双乳突及各副鼻窦无压痛，鼻翼微有扇动，鼻道轻度阻塞，有少量白黏分泌物，外耳道无异常分泌物，口腔黏膜正常，牙齿 3、4 缺如，咽部轻度充血，双腭扁桃体不大，颈软无抵抗，无颈静脉怒张及颈动脉异常搏动，气管居中，甲状腺不大，胸廓对称，呼吸运动基本均等，右胸第四肋中小水泡音，语音传导增强，左肺呼吸音略粗，但无明显干湿性啰音；心尖搏动在左第五肋间锁骨中线内 0.5cm，心界不大，心率 82 次/分，律齐，各瓣膜听诊区未闻及明显病理性杂音，腹软无压痛，肝脾肋下未及，莫非氏征(—)，脊柱四肢正常，生理反射存在，病理反射未引出。

化验室检查：WBC：29800/mm^3，N：97%，L：3%

胸透：大叶性肺炎(右上叶)

西医诊断及诊断依据：

诊断：大叶性肺炎（右上叶）

依据：①病史：发病急骤，病程 2 天；

②症状：发热恶寒，胸痛，咳嗽咯痰，气粗喘息；

③体征：右胸第四肋以上按语颤及语音传导增强，叩浊叩痛，中部可闻及中小水泡音。

④化验室检查：WBC：29800/mm^3，N：97%，L：13%。

⑤胸透：右上叶大叶性肺炎。

西医治疗：

支持疗法：

10%G·S	500cc	
5%G·N·S	1000cc	
5%G·S	1000cc	
Vitc	28	/V1 次/日

对症处理：必要时物理降温，酒精擦浴。

其他检查：①血 Rt　尿 Rt　便 Rt

②痰培养+药敏

③胸透，正位胸片。

记录人：×××

1982 年 2 月 22 日 17 点 20 分

第四节　内科门诊首次病历书写格式及内容

姓名：　　性别：

年龄：　　职业：

工作单位：　　就诊时间：

问诊：

主诉：

病史：

望、闻、切诊：

辨证分析：

诊断：（病名或证名后的括号内写证型）

治法

方药：（方名、药味及剂量）

医嘱：

体检及理化检查：

西医诊断：（有几个病写几个病，主要者先写）

医师签名：×××

年　月　日　时　分

复习思考题

1. 中医内科病历的一般要求是什么？
2. 如何掌握内科住院病历的内容？
3. 中医内科病历中哪些地方反映了中医特色？
4. 你对中医内科病历的格式有何认识和体会？
5. 中医内科门诊首次病历的格式和内容是哪些？

各　论

感　冒

〔概述〕

凡风邪侵袭人体所致，以鼻塞、流涕、喷嚏、头痛、恶寒、发热、全身不适等为主要临床表现的疾病，称之感冒。其病情轻者亦称“伤风”或“冒风”、“冒寒”；病情重者称为重伤风。在一个时期广泛流行，证候多相类似者，称为时行感冒。此病全年均发，尤以冬春季为多。因四季气候的变化和病邪有殊或体质强弱之异，感邪有轻重，在证候表现上分风寒、风热两大类，且有挟湿、挟暑及体虚感冒之别。

西医学中诊断的上呼吸道感染、流行性感冒可参考本篇辨证论治。

〔病因病机〕

感冒之病因，主要为感受风邪疫毒，尤在气候突变，寒暖失常，正气虚弱的情况下易发。

一、外感风邪疫毒：风邪虽为六淫之首，但于不同季节，往往随时气而侵入。如：冬季多属风寒，春季多属风热，夏季多挟暑湿，秋季多兼燥气，梅雨季节多挟湿邪。若四时之中气候失常，即春应温而反寒，夏应热而反冷，秋应凉而反热，冬应寒而反暖，亦能使风寒暑湿之邪，侵入人体发生感冒或引起时行感冒的流行。由此可见，外感风邪是感冒的主要原因，但风邪多合时气或非时之气及非时之气挟疫毒伤人为病。

二、正气虚弱，肺卫功能失常：若生活起居失常，寒暖不调或过度疲劳，皆使肌腠不密，肺卫调节功能失常，卫外不固，极易为外邪所侵为体虚感冒。且感邪性质与体质特点相关，阳虚之人易感风寒，阴虚之人易感风热、燥热。痰湿偏盛者易感外湿，湿热偏盛者易感受暑湿。

综上，感冒之病位在肺卫。风性轻扬，外邪侵袭，肺卫首当其冲，卫阳被遏，营卫失和，正邪相争则恶寒发热、头痛、身痛，肺失宣肃则鼻塞、流涕、咳嗽、咽痛。

由于感受四时之气的不同及禀赋素质的差异，故临床证候表现上有风寒、风热及挟湿、挟暑、挟燥、挟虚的不同，在病程中又可见寒与热的转化及错杂。

〔辨证论治〕

一、辨证要点

(一)辨风寒风热：风寒感冒者，多见于一般体质或阳虚体质，冬季为多，症见恶寒重，发热轻，头痛，身痛，鼻塞流清涕，口不渴，咽不痛不肿，咽痒，苔白，脉浮紧。风热感冒者，多见于一般体质或阴虚或阳盛之体，春季易发，以发热重，恶寒轻，鼻塞流黄涕，口渴咽痛，脉浮数为特征。

(二)辨兼挟症：挟湿者多见于梅雨季节，以身热不扬，头胀如裹，骨节疼痛，胸闷口淡或甜为特征。挟暑者，多见于长夏，以身热有汗，心烦口渴，小便短赤，苔黄腻为特征。挟燥者，多见于秋季，以身热头痛，鼻燥咽干，咳嗽无痰或少痰，口渴，舌红为特征。挟食者，多见于饱食过度，以身热脘胀纳呆，恶心腹泻，苔腻等为特征。

感冒病因病机示意图

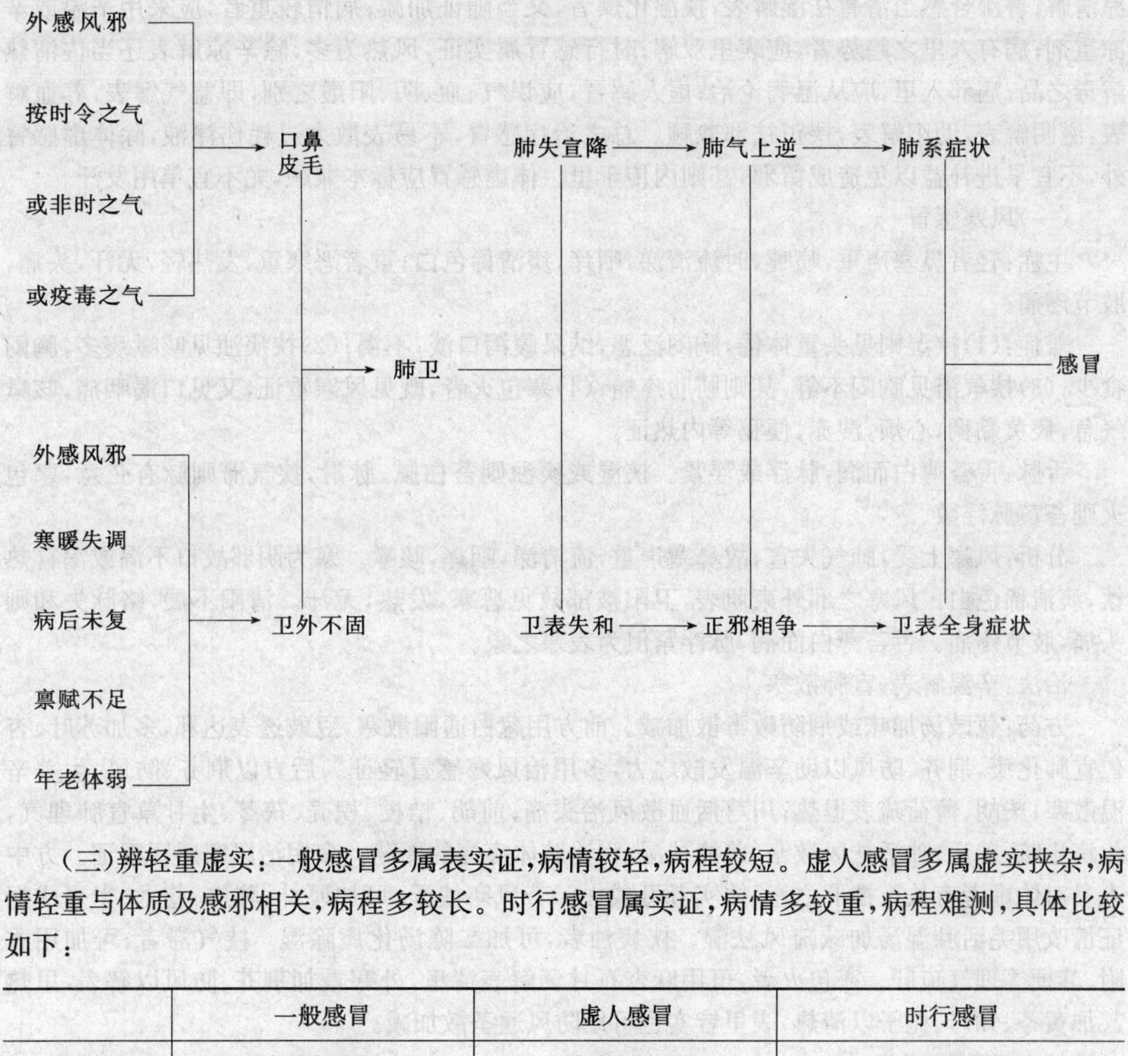

（三）辨轻重虚实：一般感冒多属表实证，病情较轻，病程较短。虚人感冒多属虚实挟杂，病情轻重与体质及感邪相关，病程多较长。时行感冒属实证，病情多较重，病程难测，具体比较如下：

	一般感冒	虚人感冒	时行感冒
年　龄	青壮年多见	中老年多见	任何年龄
体　质	形体壮实	形体虚弱	任何体质，尤虚人易感
慢性病	多无	多有	不一定
诱　因	寒温失调过度疲劳	稍不谨慎	时疫流行期，接触患病之人
证候特点	形实、邪实、症实、实证	虚实挟杂，寒热错综，病情较重不一	多实证，也有虚实相兼，病情较重
传染性	无	无	有

（四）辨感冒与伤寒、温病：感冒病情较轻，病变局限于肺卫。伤寒和温病的病情过重，发热

恶寒为其主症，感邪后有由表入里的传变过程，温病按卫气营血传变。

二、分型证治

感冒，邪在肺卫。一般感冒多实证，宜取解表达邪原则。风寒治以辛温发汗；风热治以辛凉清解；暑湿合感当清暑祛湿解表；挟湿化燥者，又当随证加减；病情较重者，应采用辛温或辛凉重剂；病有入里之趋势者，应表里双解；时行感冒属实证，风热为多，除辛凉解表还当佐清热解毒之品；病邪入里，应从温病论治；虚人感冒，应识气、血、阴、阳虚之别，即益气解表，养血解表，滋阴解表，助阳解表，扶正祛邪兼顾。总之治疗感冒，不易表散太过耗伤津液，除体虚感冒外，不宜早进补益以免造成留邪，甚则内传于里。体虚感冒应标本兼顾，尤不宜单用发汗。

（一）风寒感冒

主症：轻者鼻塞声重，喷嚏，时流清涕，咽痒，痰清稀色白；重者恶寒重，发热轻，无汗，头痛，肢节疼痛。

兼症：(1)挟湿则见头重体倦，胸闷泛恶，纳呆腹泻口淡，不渴；(2)挟痰浊见咳嗽痰多，胸闷食少；(3)挟气滞见胸闷不舒，甚则胁肋疼痛；(4)寒包火者，既见风寒重证，又见口渴咽痛，咳嗽气急，痰黄黏稠，心烦，溲赤，便秘等内热证。

舌脉：舌苔薄白而润，脉浮或浮紧。挟湿或痰浊则苔白腻、脉滑，挟气滞则脉有弦意，寒包火则苔黄脉浮数。

分析：风寒上受，肺气失宣，故鼻塞声重，流清涕，咽痒，咳嗽。寒为阴邪故口不渴或渴喜热饮，痰清稀色白。风寒之邪外束肌表，卫阳被郁故见恶寒，发热，无汗。清阳不展，络脉失和则头痛，肢节疼痛。舌苔薄白而润，脉浮紧俱为表寒之象。

治法：辛温解表，宣肺散寒。

方药：葱豉汤加味或荆防败毒散加减。前方用葱白通阳散寒，豆豉透表达邪，多加苏叶、杏仁宣肺化痰，荆芥、防风以助辛温发散之力，多用治风寒感冒轻证。后方以荆芥、防风、生姜辛温散寒；柴胡、薄荷疏表退热；川芎活血散风治头痛；前胡、桔梗、枳壳、茯苓、生甘草宣肺理气，化痰止咳；羌活、独活祛风散寒，兼能祛湿，为治肢体疼痛的要药。多用治风寒感冒重证。方中人参对体虚者有扶正祛邪之意，体实者可减去。若风寒挟湿，可加厚朴、陈皮、苍术、半夏或据证情改用羌活胜湿汤加减疏风祛湿。挟痰浊者，可加二陈汤化痰除湿。挟气滞者，可加用香附、苏梗等理气疏肝。寒包火者，可用麻杏石甘汤解表清里，外寒重加荆芥、防风以解表，里热甚加黄芩、知母、栀子以清热，表里皆实也可用防风通圣散加减。

处方举例：

豆豉 10g、苏叶 10g、荆芥 10g、防风 10g、桔梗 6g、白前 10g、川芎 10g、甘草 6g、杏仁 10g、枳壳 10g、生姜 10g

（二）风热感冒

主症：发热，微恶寒，汗出不畅，头痛，鼻塞涕浊，口干而渴，咽喉红肿疼痛，咳嗽，痰黄黏稠。

兼症：(1)风热重证或感受时疫之邪，可见高热不退，恶寒或有寒战，头痛，鼻咽干燥，口渴心烦。(2)风热挟湿可见头重体倦，胸闷，泛恶，小便赤。(3)夏令挟暑湿者可见发热较高，汗出而身热不退，身体沉重，口渴，小便短少或黄赤。(4)秋令挟燥邪者，可见口唇鼻咽干燥，口渴，干咳无痰或咳痰不爽。

舌脉：苔薄黄，脉浮数。若风热重证则舌红苔黄；挟湿苔黄腻；挟暑湿苔黄腻，脉濡数；挟燥邪舌红少津，脉略数。

分析：风热犯表，热郁肌腠，卫表失和，故身热，微恶风寒，汗出不扬。风热上扰则见头胀痛，风热之邪熏蒸则咽喉肿痛，咽燥口渴，鼻流浊涕。风热犯肺，肺失清肃，则咳嗽痰黏或黄。苔白微黄，脉浮数为风热侵于肺卫之征。

治法：辛凉解表，清肺透邪。

方药：银翘散加减。方中银花、连翘辛凉透表，清热解毒，薄荷、荆芥、豆豉疏风解表透邪外出，桔梗、牛蒡子、甘草宣肺祛痰，利咽消肿，竹叶、芦根甘凉清热，生津止渴。一般头痛者加桑叶、菊花等清利头目。咳嗽痰多加用杏仁、贝母、瓜蒌皮等止咳化痰。咽喉红肿疼痛甚加板蓝根、马勃、元参等清热解表利咽。风热重证或时疫外感，可在此方基础上加葛根以解肌；黄芩、石膏清热；知母、花粉生津、止渴。风热挟湿可在此方基础上加藿香、佩兰等以化湿。暑令挟暑湿者，可用新加香薷饮加减，并可据时令特点加鲜荷叶、荷梗、鲜藿佩、西瓜皮、六一散等清化暑湿。秋季挟燥邪者加杏仁、梨皮、瓜蒌皮；也可用桑杏汤加减以疏风清燥，肃肺养阴。

处方举例：

荆芥 10g、薄荷 6g（后下）、豆豉 10g、银花 10g、连翘 10g、桔梗 6g、甘草 6g、炒牛蒡子 10g、鲜芦根 30g、浙贝母 10g、杏仁 10g。

（三）体虚感冒

1. 气虚感冒

主症：恶寒发热，头痛鼻塞，咳嗽痰白，倦怠无力，气短懒言。

兼症：体胖多汗，面色不华，年老或素有喘证、胃脘痛等病。

舌脉：舌淡苔薄白，脉浮无力。

分析：气虚卫外不固，风寒束表，肺气不宣，故见表证。素体气虚体弱故见气短懒言，倦怠无力。舌脉为气虚，邪在卫表之象。

治法：益气解表。

方药：参苏饮加减。方中人参多用党参代；茯苓、甘草益气，扶正祛邪；苏叶、葛根疏风解表，前胡、桔梗、枳壳、半夏、陈皮宣肺理气，化痰止咳。若气虚较甚者，可加用黄芪，也可用补中益气汤加苏叶等益气升阳解表。若气虚自汗稍不慎易感外邪者，可用玉屏风散益气固表，止汗祛风。

处方举例：

苏叶 10g、党参 10g、茯苓 10g、甘草 6g、前胡 10g、桔梗 6g、枳壳 10g、半夏 10g、陈皮 10g、杏仁 10g、川芎 10g。

2. 阳虚感冒

主症：身热较轻，恶寒微重，头痛，身痛，面色发白，四肢不温，语声低微。

兼症：年老体弱或伴有长期五更泄泻，水肿，虚劳属脾肾阳虚者。

舌脉：舌质淡胖，苔薄白，脉沉无力。

分析：阳气不足，不能温养肌表，故有外寒症状，如语声低微，四肢不温，舌淡体胖，脉沉无力。感受风寒病邪后，表寒更为明显，故见寒多热少症状。风寒束表，阳气不展，络脉失和故头身疼痛。

治法：助阳解表。

方药：参附再造丸加减。方中以附子、桂枝助阳。气属阳，阳虚气也虚，故以人参、黄芪、炙甘草益气。羌活、防风、细辛解表散寒，本方助阳益气与疏表散寒并投使发汗而不伤正，补益而不恋邪。若恶寒无汗，阳虚的程度不太重者也可选用麻黄附子细辛汤加减。

处方举例：

附片 6g、桂枝 10g、党参 10g、生黄芪 15g、羌活 10g、防风 18g、细辛 3g、桔梗 6g、甘草 6g、杏仁 10g、白前 10g。

3. 血虚感冒

主症：头疼身热，微寒无汗，面色不华，唇甲色淡，心悸头晕。

兼症：产后或月经淋漓过多，肌衄、便血等出血病后。

舌脉：舌淡苔白，脉细或浮而无力。

分析：阴血亏虚故见头晕心悸，面色不华，唇甲色淡。血虚营卫不固，易感外邪而见头痛身热，微恶风寒，无汗等表证。舌质淡，脉细或浮而无力是血虚外感的征象。

治法：养血解表。

方药：葱白七味饮加减。本方用葱白、豆豉、葛根、生姜以解表，地黄、麦冬滋阴养血。养血而发汗，不致因发汗而伤阴血。若恶寒重，可加苏叶、荆芥，亦可用荆防合四物汤。热重加银花、连翘或黄芩，或用柴胡四物汤。出血未止，可用阿胶珠、藕节、白芨、三七等。

处方举例：

全当归 10g、地黄 10g、白芍 10g、川芎 10g、荆芥 10g、防风 10g、柴胡 10g、甘草 6g、杏仁 10g、葛根 10g。

4. 阴虚感冒

主症：头痛身热，微恶风寒，无汗或微汗，或寐中盗汗，头晕心烦，口渴咽干，手足心热，干咳少痰，或痰中带血丝。

兼症：阴虚体质或体弱病后而常有五心烦热、失眠、便秘等。

舌脉：舌嫩红少津，苔剥脱或无苔，脉细数。

分析：阴虚生内热，故见头晕心烦，手足心热；阴虚津少故口渴咽干，干咳少痰；由于素体阴虚，感邪后邪从热化故头痛身热，微恶风寒，常见风热之证。舌红苔剥或无苔，脉细数均为阴虚内热之象。

治法：滋阴解表。

方药：加减葳蕤汤化裁。方中玉竹滋阴生津以助汗源；葱白、豆豉、桔梗、薄荷发汗解表以疏散外邪；白薇清热和阴，清而能透；大枣、甘草甘润和中，可助玉竹之养阴。全方发汗而不伤阴，滋阴而不留邪。若表证较重，酌加荆芥、薄荷以祛风解表。咽干、咳嗽、咯痰不爽加牛蒡子、瓜蒌皮以利咽化痰。心烦口渴较甚，加竹叶、天花粉以清热除烦，生津止渴。

处方举例：

玉竹 15g、白薇 10g、麦冬 10g、沙参 15g、元参 12g、甘草 6g、桔梗 6g、玉蝴蝶 5g、炒牛蒡子 10g、芦茅根各 30g、荆芥 10g；

以上虚人感冒虽以气虚、阳虚、血虚、阴虚进行分类，但临床还可见气阴两亏、气血不足、阴阳俱虚等，需详细辨证，兼顾用药。

〔预防及护理措施〕

(1)保持室内空气新鲜，温度适宜。

(2)慎起居，适寒温，锻炼身体，增强体质。

(3)重症感冒有恶寒发热者，应卧床休息。时行感冒者应予隔离。

(4)注意观察患者的体温、出汗、脉象、舌苔等变化。

(5)多饮开水,饮食宜清淡,轻度发热时以素半流食为宜,热退后食荤半流食或普通饮食为宜。

(6)服用防治用药:

①冬春风寒当令季节,可用贯众、紫苏、荆芥各10g,甘草3g,水煎温服,连服3天。

②夏季暑湿当令季节,可用藿佩各10g,薄荷5g,煮汤以代饮料(鲜者用量可加)。

③如时邪疫毒盛行可用贯众15g,板蓝根(或大青叶)12g,生甘草3g,煎服日一剂;室内可用食醋熏蒸,每立方米空间用食醋5~10ml,加水1~2倍,稀释后加热熏蒸2小时,隔日一次做消毒,以防传染。

〔**典型病例分析**〕

案一:张××,男,成。

初诊:1955年2月25日。

恶寒发热,头痛骨楚,呕吐频发,苔薄腻,脉浮。新邪外受,湿热内蕴,胃失和降。先拟疏邪宣化为治。

处方:清水豆卷12g、带叶苏梗4.5g、薄荷叶2.4g(后下)、冬桑叶9g、炒杭菊4.5g、嫩前胡4.5g、象贝母9g、姜川连1g、甘露消毒丹12g(包煎),二剂。

二诊:

寒热渐退,头痛呕吐止,不能安寐,口苦未清。湿热未净,胃不和则卧不安也。转方安神和胃,而化湿热。

处方:辰茯神9g、炙远志3g、炒枣仁9g、淮小麦12g、水炒银柴胡3g、制半夏4.5g、酒炒黄芩4.5g、薄橘红4.5g、炒竹茹4.5g、北秫米9g(包煎)、炒香谷芽12g,二剂。

按:本例为外邪夹湿热,主法是解表退热,更用二陈、小柴胡法中的黄芩、半夏及泻心法中的姜川连、半夏等以内外同治,使湿热痰浊得以泄化,外邪无所依存,故能获得速效。透风或渗湿,可以孤立热势,缩短发热日程。

感冒属临床常见外感病。以鼻塞,流涕,喷嚏,咳嗽,头痛,恶寒发热,全身不适为主症。

病因为外感六淫,时行疫毒,于人体卫外功能减弱,不能调节应变之时,邪犯肺卫而致病。

辨证属表实,但据证情、病邪性质、禀赋体质、有风寒、风热、暑湿和体虚感冒之别。治疗以解表达邪为主,风寒宜辛温,风热应用辛凉,暑湿当清暑祛湿,体虚感冒则应标本兼顾,不可专行发散。大凡感冒皆不可发散太过,除体虚感冒亦忌补敛。

总之,临床治疗感冒应辨明寒热虚实,有无并发症及夹杂症,而相应治疗。

复习思考题

1. 试述感冒与伤寒、温病的区别。
2. 试述风寒、风热感冒的辨证论治。
3. 试述气虚感冒与阴虚感冒的辨证论治。

咳嗽

〔**概述**〕

咳嗽是肺系疾病的主要证候之一。既是具有独立性的证候,又是肺系多种疾病的一个症状。分而言之，有声无痰为咳，有痰无声为嗽，仅有声无痰则称干咳。因临床上多痰声并见，难以截然分开，故以咳嗽并称。

咳嗽的分类，历代所用名称甚多，现沿用明代张景岳之论将咳嗽分为外感、内伤两大类。

外感、内伤咳嗽，二者实有不同，应该严格区分。临证时要结合病史、病因、临床表现体征，及必要的理化检查进行分析。外感咳嗽多兼肺卫表证，内伤咳嗽则多有脏腑功能失调证。

本篇所论是以咳嗽为主要表现的病证，其他疾病兼见的咳嗽，可与本篇互参。久咳致喘，表现肺虚寒或寒饮伏肺等证者，应与喘证、痰饮等相参。

西医学诊断的上呼吸感染、急慢性支气管炎、肺炎、支气管扩张、肺结核、肺气肿、肺脓疡早期等以咳嗽为主症的疾病，皆可参考本篇辨证施治。

〔病因病机〕

咳嗽属肺系受病，肺气上逆所致。其病位主要在肺，与肝、脾、肾相关。

咳嗽的病因可概括为外感、内伤两大类，简述如下：

一、外感：六淫外邪，侵袭肺系。六淫之邪侵袭人体皆可引起咳嗽。但临床所见与风寒燥热关系最为密切。

肺主气，为五脏华盖，上连喉咙，开窍于鼻，司呼吸，外合皮毛，直接与外界接触。一旦遭受外邪侵袭，或从口鼻而入，或从皮毛而受，肺卫受侵，于是肺气壅遏不宣，清肃之令失常，则痰液滋生，阻塞气道，影响肺气之出入，引起咳嗽。因体质阴阳之偏，同时气候变化之异，人所受外邪亦有区别。风为六淫之首，其他外邪多随风邪侵袭人体，所以在临床上有风寒、风热、燥热等不同咳嗽。

二、内伤：脏腑功能失调。肺脏虚弱或其他脏腑有病累及于肺均可引起咳嗽。临床常见有以下几种病机：

(一)肺脏虚弱，肺阴亏耗，失于清润，气逆于上，引起咳嗽而痰少；肺气不足，清肃无权，主气无能，引起咳嗽气短。

(二)脾脏健运失常，脾失健运，饮食不能化为精微，反而酿成痰浊，湿痰上渍于肺，肺失宣降，肺气出入不利，遂即咳嗽。另脾肺为母子之脏，脾为后天之本，土虚不能生金，因脾虚亦致肺气不足，清肃无权而咳。

(三)肝火犯肺：肝脉布胁肋，上注于肺，肝气郁滞，日久化火，熏灼肺脏，炼津液为痰，阻碍肺气肃降，引起咳嗽。

(四)肾脏亏损：肾主纳气，为水脏，为气化之源，肾气衰弱，气失摄纳而上逆，气化无权，则水液不循常道，渍溢于肺，而生咳嗽。肺肾为母子之脏，肺肾之阴互滋，肾阴不足，阴虚火旺，更灼肺阴，虚火灼津成痰，更阻肺气肃降，而发咳嗽。

综上所述，咳嗽按病因不同分外感、内伤两大类。外感咳嗽，病位在肺，属邪实，为外邪犯肺，肺气壅遏不畅所致。若失治或治之不当，日久不愈，耗伤肺气、肺阴，可演变为内伤咳嗽。内伤咳嗽病位主要在肺，与肝、脾、肾关系密切。多属邪实与正虚并见，病理因素主要为“痰”与“火”。但痰有寒热之别，火有虚实之分；痰可郁而化火(热)，火能炼液灼津为痰。它脏及肺者，多因邪实导致正虚，如肝火犯肺则气火耗伤肺津，炼液为痰；痰湿犯肺者，多因脾失健运，水谷不能化为精微上输以养肺，反则聚为痰浊，上贮于肺，肺气壅塞，上逆为咳。若久延脾肺两虚，气不化津则痰浊滋生。甚则病延及肾，肺、脾、肾俱虚，影响气血之运行，如肺阴不足每致阴虚火炎，灼津为痰，肺失濡润，气逆作咳，或肺气亏虚，肃降无权，气不化津，津聚成痰，气逆于上而咳。再则内伤咳嗽患者，由于脏腑虚弱，营卫不固。易受外邪侵袭，而并有外感咳嗽，成为虚实夹杂之证。总之，咳嗽的病因病机虽有上述种种不同，但其发病之理均属肺失宣肃，肺气上逆。

〔辨证论治〕

一、辨证要点

（一）辨外感内伤：外感咳嗽多起病急，病程短，咳嗽之外兼表证，属实证，内伤咳嗽多起病慢，病程长，咳嗽之外兼脏腑内伤之证，属虚实夹杂之证。

（二）辨寒热虚实

1. 辨痰之有无、性状、色泽、痰质稀稠、量之多少、有无气味。

（1）干咳无痰属燥属火。

（2）有痰：痰少色白有稀泡沫属风燥伤肺或风寒伤肺；有黏泡沫属风热伤肺。痰少色黄黏稠属热伤肺（虚热或实热，内伤或外感）；黏块属痰热甚或津亏（内伤多）。痰多色白有水泡属风湿阻肺；清稀属寒痰水饮阻肺；黏稠属寒湿有化热之势。痰多色黄稀属湿热或风热；黏稠属热伤肺（虚热或实热）；脓样痰属火热伤肺（实热）。

（3）痰甜为脾热，痰酸辣为肝气犯肺，痰咸为肾虚水泛。

2. 辨咳嗽声音：咳声重浊多属风寒或挟湿；咳声粗亢多属风热；咳声嘶哑多属燥热；咳如串，阵作多属肝胆火旺；咳声如从瓮中出多属燥热风热；咳声不扬多属风寒；咳声低弱无力，时作时止，断续而咳多属内伤，肺阴不足或肺气虚弱。

3. 辨咳嗽发作时间：冬重夏轻，遇风冷加重，为寒为阳虚；夏秋加剧多为暑湿秋燥。上午咳多多胃中有火，多实热；午后咳多多阴虚；黄昏咳多多阴虚火旺，多火浮于肺；平旦咳多内有痰饮。咳嗽时间短，日夜不休为外感；久咳绵绵发作为内伤。

4. 辨咳嗽主要兼夹症：咳而喉痒多兼风邪。咳而多尿多兼肾气不固。咳而疲极兼气虚。咳声频连多为燥热或肝火。咳而兼表为外感。咳兼骨蒸潮热颧红为内伤阴虚火旺。

5. 咳嗽与感冒、痰饮、肺痨、肺痿的鉴别。

（1）外感咳嗽与感冒：外感咳嗽总以咳嗽为主症，而感冒则以肺卫表证为主症。

（2）内伤咳嗽与痰饮证、肺痨、肺痿：痰湿咳嗽当与饮证之饮犯胸肺、痰证之痰浊壅肺、脾虚痰盛区别，此三者病机虽同，但病情则有差别。饮犯胸肺，及痰浊壅肺的咳嗽症状远较痰湿咳嗽为重。饮犯胸肺，肺气上逆，咳嗽胸满，不能平卧，痰多白沫。实痰之痰浊壅肺可有热痰、湿痰、燥痰之不同，咳嗽喘促。虚痰之脾虚痰盛又以脾虚为主。肺虚咳嗽当与肺痨肺痿相别，严格讲肺痨、肺痿均属肺虚咳嗽之中，然肺痨咳嗽以咳嗽伴有消瘦、咳血、潮热、盗汗为特征，肺阴虚咳嗽不一定都是肺痨。肺痿更是一慢性过程，无论虚寒、虚热肺痿病情均较重。

二、分型证治

外感咳嗽多因风寒、风热犯肺，燥热伤肺致肺失宣肃，属实证，病位在肺，治宜疏散外邪，宣通肺气为主，邪去则正安，一般不宜过早使用滋腻、补益、收涩、镇咳之药以免碍邪。内伤咳嗽是由肺脏自病或其他脏腑病变涉及于肺而致肺气失于宣肃，属虚实夹杂，病位主要在肺，与肝、脾、肾关系密切。治以调整脏腑为主，如健脾、清肝泻火、养肺、补肾等。肝火、痰湿犯肺之咳嗽，常为虚中挟实之证，应根据标本缓急或标本兼顾，或治标为先。

咳嗽病因病机示意图

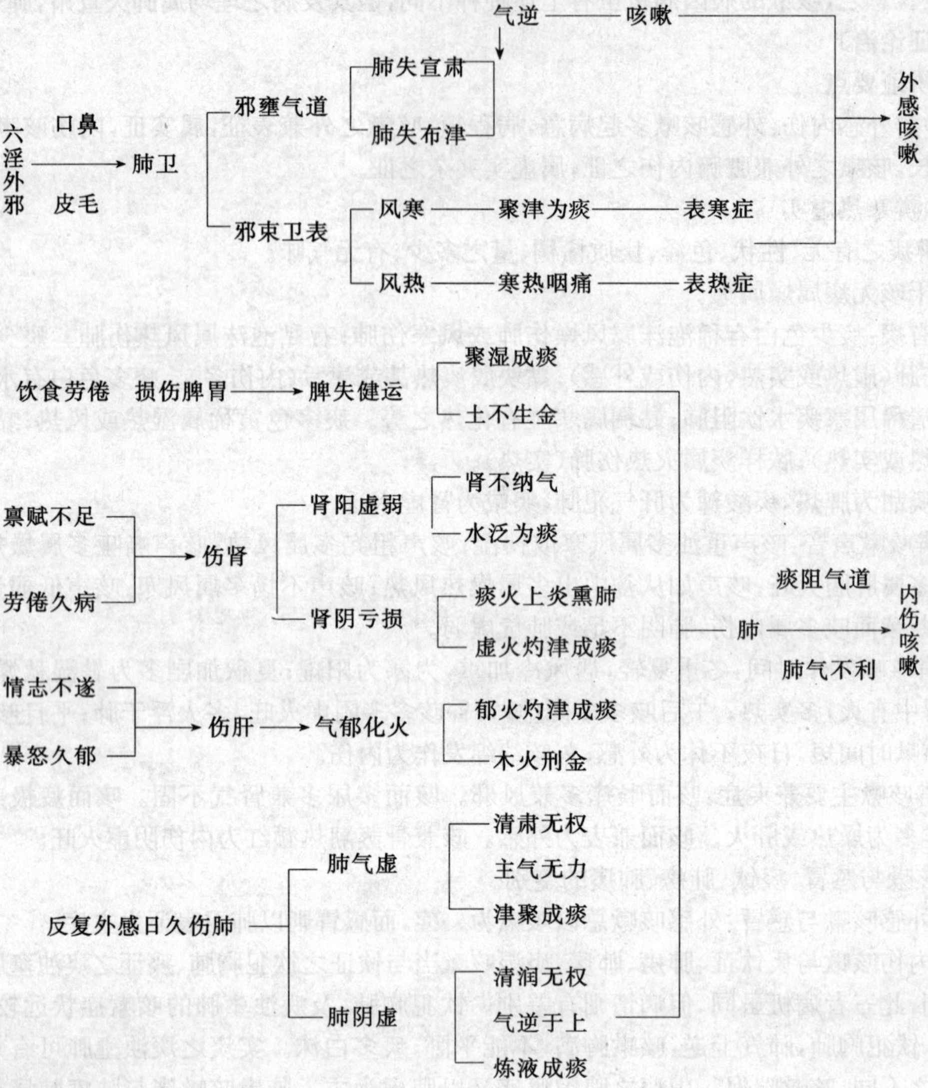

(一)外感咳嗽

1. 风寒咳嗽

主症:咳嗽新起,咳声重浊,痰稀色白。

兼症:多伴有头痛鼻塞,流清涕,骨节酸痛,恶寒无汗。

舌脉:舌苔薄白,脉浮。

分析:风寒犯肺,肺气壅塞不得宣通,故咳嗽新起,咳声重浊,痰稀色白,鼻塞清涕。寒主收引,风寒束于肌表,腠理闭塞,阻遏经络,故寒热无汗,头痛身楚。邪在肺在表,故舌苔薄白脉浮。

治法:疏风散寒,宣通肺气。

方药:三拗汤合杏苏散加减。前方麻黄、杏仁、甘草为宣肺止咳要药;后方苏叶、生姜疏散风寒,前胡、桔梗宣肺化痰利气,陈皮、枳壳、半夏、茯苓理气燥湿化痰。风寒重者加重麻黄用量以加强宣肺散寒之力。痰多加重陈皮、半夏。痰少加重桔梗、甘草，也可用金沸草散加减。若咳嗽咽疼，口干渴，痰浓难咯，咳嗽音嘎，身热较重，苔白腻或黄，脉浮数，此为风寒外束，肺热内郁(又称外寒内热咳嗽或寒包火咳)，可用麻杏石甘汤加味，或上方去生姜加桑白皮、牛蒡子、黄芩。

处方举例

炙麻黄 3～6g、杏仁 10g、苏梗 10g、生甘草 5g、桔梗 8g、前胡 10g、化橘红 10g、半夏 5g、枳壳 10g。

2. 风热咳嗽

主症：咳嗽新起，咳声粗亢，痰稠色黄。

兼症：多伴发热恶风、头痛、汗出、咽痛口渴。

舌脉：舌苔薄黄，脉浮数。

分析：风热犯肺，肺失宣肃故咳嗽新起，咳声粗亢。热邪灼津成痰故痰黏色黄。邪客皮毛故兼有恶风身热或头痛之证。肺热耗津故口渴咽痛。风热在肺在表则舌苔薄黄，脉浮数。

治法：疏风清热，宣肺化痰。

方药：桑菊饮加减。方中桑叶、菊花、薄荷辛凉解表而祛风热，杏仁、桔梗、生甘草开宣肺气，芦根清热生津。恶风加荆芥、防风以解表。肺热重加黄芩、生石膏以清热。咳重加牛蒡子、前胡加强宣肺之力。鼻衄加茅根、藕节以凉血。咽痛加牛蒡子、马勃、板蓝根以清热利咽。痰难出加冬瓜子、瓜蒌。又风热咳嗽兼见痰多，胸闷汗出，舌苔白腻中黄、脉濡数，此为风热挟湿伤肺，于桑菊饮中加苡仁、杏仁或少量厚朴宣肺化湿。风热咳嗽见病发暑天，咳嗽胸闷，心烦口渴，溺赤，舌质红苔黄，脉濡数，此为风热挟暑湿伤肺，宜清宣芳化，选用藿香、佩兰、前胡、六一散等疏风解暑药。湿重于热可化湿宣肺，以藿香正气散加减；热重于湿，可清热化湿以连朴饮或黄芩滑石汤加味。

处方举例：

荆芥 10g、薄荷(后下)5g、桔梗 10g、连翘 10g，牛蒡子 10g、前胡 10g、浙贝 10g、生甘草 5g，桑叶 10g、菊花 10g。

3. 燥热咳嗽

主症：咳嗽新起，咳声嘶哑或劈裂，干咳无痰或痰少黏稠难出。

兼症：多伴鼻燥咽干，或咳痰带血丝或咳引胸痛，或有恶风发热。

舌脉.舌尖红，苔薄黄而干，脉略数。

分析：本证常见于夏末秋初或秋季干燥季节，燥热伤肺，肺津受灼，肺气失宣故咳声嘶哑或劈裂，咽痒干咳无痰，鼻燥咽干，舌干少津。燥热伤肺灼津，肺失宣肃，气机不利则咳引胸痛。燥热伤及肺络，则痰中带血丝。

治法：清热润燥(轻宣滋润)。

方药：桑杏汤加味。方中桑叶轻清肺燥，杏仁润肺止咳，沙参、梨皮、栀皮生津润燥清热，辅以豆豉疏风宣肺，浙贝清肺化痰。可酌加瓜蒌、麦冬、苇茎等清润之品。若咳甚咽痒加前胡、蝉衣、桔梗、甘草以宣肺祛邪。若干咳不愈，舌红少津，形体消瘦，可用清燥救肺汤加减。热重加石膏、知母。咳血配止血药。若干咳少痰，咽干鼻燥，兼见明显恶寒发热，头痛无汗，舌苔薄白而干者，为凉燥伤肺(即风寒与风燥相结合)，可于上方中去栀皮、梨皮、贝母，或用杏苏散方加荆芥、防风、紫菀、款冬花散寒宣肺与润燥化痰并进。

处方举例：

桑叶10g、杏仁10g、沙参12g、前胡10g、炙杷叶10g、知母10g、贝母10g、生甘草5g、紫菀10g。

以上外感咳嗽诸证，如日久不愈，或愈而复发，喉痒咳嗽，咯痰不爽，咳甚则面红、呕吐，而表证不显著可用止嗽散加减。此方荆芥辛平散风，百部、白前、紫菀苦温而润以降肺气，甘草、桔梗利气化痰，以润咽喉。本方温凉并用，对余邪未清，肺气失于宣肃略兼痰浊者尤宜。

（二）内伤咳嗽

1. 痰湿犯肺

主症：久咳痰多，痰白而稠易出。

兼症：胸脘作闷或胃纳不振，神疲乏力，大便时溏。

舌脉：舌苔白腻，脉濡滑。

分析：脾失健运，痰湿内生，上渍于肺故咳嗽痰多，色白黏。痰湿内停，肺气失宣则腹脘作闷，苔白腻，脉濡滑。痰湿困脾则神疲乏力，大便时溏。

治法：健脾燥湿，化痰止咳。

方药：二陈汤加味。二陈汤为治湿痰之祖方，痰多脘闷可加苍术、厚朴、杏仁、苡仁健脾燥湿化痰；咳重可加麻黄、杏仁、苏子、白前宣肺降气；若脾虚明显，疲乏舌淡脉弱，可加党参、白术以六君子汤加减；咳嗽气逆明显可与三子养亲汤合方。本证易有寒化热化之变，如脾阳虚弱或过食寒凉，可寒化成为寒饮寒痰留伏之久咳。若过食辛热或感受热邪等因素，可致热化成为痰热郁肺之久咳。寒化则咳痰白稀，肢冷畏寒，便溏，面色青白，舌质淡，苔白腻水滑，脉弦迟，宜平胃散合二陈汤加减，或加细辛、干姜、五味子或苓桂术甘汤加味以温化痰湿，利气止咳。如寒痰内伏挟感风寒而见寒热头痛者，宜用小青龙汤解表温里，温化痰饮。热化则为痰热郁肺，咳痰黄黏或咯吐不爽或有腥味，咳嗽气息粗促，口苦口渴，舌苔黄腻，脉滑数，宜改用清金化痰汤以清热化痰止咳，本方清热化痰，药用桑白皮、黄芩、山栀、知母清泄肺热，贝母、瓜蒌、桔梗清肺止咳，麦冬、橘红、茯苓、甘草养阴化痰。

处方举例：

陈皮10g、茯苓10g、半夏10g、生甘草4g、杏仁10、厚朴6g、苡仁15g、苏梗子各10g，寒化加细辛3g、干姜6g、五味子5g，热化加黄芩10g、瓜蒌15g、山栀10g。

2. 痰热郁肺：

主症：咳嗽气息粗促，痰黄质黏。

兼证：咳引胸肋胀痛，口苦干渴，痰有腥臭味或血痰，或有身热。

舌脉：舌苔黄腻，脉滑数或弦滑。

证候分析：痰热壅阻肺气，肺失清肃，故咳嗽气息粗促，痰黄质黏。痰热郁蒸故痰有腥味。热伤肺络，气机不利，故胸肋胀疼或咳吐血痰。肺热内郁，则有身热，口苦干渴。舌苔黄腻，脉滑数均属痰热之象。

治法：清金化痰肃肺。

方药：清金化痰汤加减。本方化痰清肺，药用桑白皮、黄芩、山栀、知母清泻肺热，贝母、瓜蒌、桔梗化痰清肺止咳，橘红化痰理气，茯苓利湿，麦冬、甘草养阴润肺。痰黄稠如脓腥臭有味可加鱼腥草、金荞麦、连翘、冬瓜仁、苡仁等清热化痰。咳逆胸满，平卧咳甚可加葶苈子、风化硝泻肺逐痰。痰热伤津，口干渴、舌红可加配南沙参、天花粉、黛蛤散以养阴清热化痰。

处方举例：瓜蒌20g、黄芩10g、知贝母各10g、焦山栀10g、清半夏10g、胆星6g、桔梗6g、葶苈子10g、桑白皮10g。

3. 肝火犯肺

主症：咳嗽气逆，阵阵发作，干咳无痰或少痰，咳引胸胁痛。

兼症：面赤喉干，口干。症状随情绪波动增减。

舌脉：舌边红少津苔薄黄，脉弦数。

分析：肝气郁结化火，气火逆乘于肺，金虚不能制木，肺失清肃，乃成肝火犯肺之咳嗽，故常自觉气逆于喉而作咳嗽。肝火上炎故有面红。肺脉上连喉咙，火热伤津，故觉咽喉干燥。肝火灼金，炼液为痰，痰梗于喉则不易咳出。胁肋为肝经循行之区域，肝气不和，故咳引胁肋作痛。舌苔薄黄少津，脉弦数，为肝旺肺热津伤之象。

治法：清肺平肝，顺气降火。

方药：泻白散合黛蛤散加减。前方泻肺清热，后方清肝化痰。桑白皮清肺中郁热；地骨皮泻肺中伏火；粳米、甘草养胃和中以扶肺气；黛蛤散清泻肝火，清化老痰。临床可加青陈皮以顺气，黄芩、栀子以清热，大贝母、瓜蒌以化痰。

处方举例：

桑白皮10g、地骨皮10g、黄芩10g、瓜蒌15g、黛蛤散（包煎）12g、百部10g、山栀10g、生甘草5g。

4. 肺虚咳嗽

肺阴不足或肺气虚弱均可引起咳嗽。但气虚者，多气喘兼咳，详见“喘证”。这里只介绍肺阴不足引起的咳嗽。

主症：久咳，干咳少痰或痰中带血，午后潮热。

兼症：两颧红，手足心热，失眠盗汗，形疲身疲，心烦失眠。

舌脉：舌质红少苔，脉细数。

分析：肺阴亏虚，肺失滋润而生燥热，肺气上逆，故干咳少痰，口燥咽干。咳伤肺络，故痰中带血或咯血。阴虚火旺，故见午后潮热，颧红，手足心热，心烦失眠，夜寐盗汗。舌质红少苔，脉细数，均为阴虚有热之症。

治法：养阴清肺，化痰止咳。

方药：沙参麦门冬汤加减。方中沙参、麦冬、玉竹、天花粉养阴生津，润肺止咳；扁豆、甘草健脾补中。咳甚加杏仁、贝母止咳化痰。咯血加侧柏叶、仙鹤草、藕节、白芨、阿胶、参三七等以止血。午后潮热、颧红，可选用银柴胡、地骨皮、黄芩、白薇等清热除蒸。咳吐黄痰可加黄芩、知母、海蛤壳等清热化痰。若日久肺肾气阴两虚，咳而兼喘，当补肾纳气，加入熟地、山萸肉、五味子及人参、蛤蚧等。

处方举例：

沙参12g、麦冬10g、五味子6～10g、杏仁10g、炙杷叶10g、贝母10g、紫菀10g、炙甘草6g。

此外，内伤咳嗽日久，若确已邪势渐轻，肺气渐伤，在辨证论治的基础上，可酌加敛肺镇咳药如五味子、五倍子、诃子、罂粟壳等，此又名截咳。近年来通过慢性气管炎的防治研究，特别提出固本疗法，对内伤咳嗽反复发作，久治不愈或暂愈而易复发者，在其缓解期作长疗程的持续治疗，重点在补脾、补肾，能显著提高疗效，值得重视。

〔预防及护理措施〕

1. 详细、全面了解观察病人情况，辨明病因及诱因，分别处理。

2. 注意病室寒暖适宜，保持湿度，嘱患者慎起居、饮食，避外邪。根据体力情况，进行适当的锻炼。劝导病人戒烟。病室内禁止吸烟，加强通风换气，保持完全清新的空气。注意个人卫生，尤应保持口腔清洁。

3. 外感风热者，饮食应注意清淡，易消化。脾虚者更应注意饮食易消化，少用油腻辛辣之品，以免伤脾。肾虚寒者可多进牛、羊肉等温性补养之品。肺肾阴虚则可多给水果或用麦冬、沙参之类养阴之品泡水代茶。肝火旺者应劝其节情志。

4. 痰多者应尽量鼓励其将痰排出。咳出无力者，可翻身拍背等以助痰排出，必要时吸痰，但吸时要避免刺激或损伤咽部。切忌用峻猛之止咳药，使咳止而痰更难排出，以生变证。

5. 咳甚时，可采用下述方法帮助治疗：

(1)针刺。常用穴位：肺俞、列缺、天突、内关、足三里等。

(2)背部拔罐。

(3)梨一个去皮、心，加冰糖适量，也可以加贝母粉少许，蒸熟后服，此方化痰止咳，可以常服。

〔典型病例分析〕

案一：孙右　肺失展布。咳嗽痰稠，脉小弦，舌苔薄黄。先以泄化。

瓜蒌皮 6g、广郁金 4.5g、象贝母 6g、杜斗铃 4.5g、生紫菀 9g、胖大海 2 个、路路通(去刺)6g、生打代赭石 9g、苏半夏 4.5g、薄荷 0.3g、霜桑叶 6g。

二诊：痰热未清。咳嗽减而未除，经事逾期，腹部稍有膜胀，此气火上行致令经尚未行。舌根黄腻，脉则右弦。是宜柔肝泄降，化滞通经。

生玄胡 6g、四花青皮 4.5g、苏半夏 6g、当归尾 4.5g、生光桃仁 9g、泽兰叶 6g、楂肉炙 6g、生紫菀 9g、杜斗铃 4.5g、炒黑荆芥 4.5g、茺蔚子 9g、瓜蒌皮 6g。

三诊：经事未泻，腹胀已蠲，胃纳已醒，鼻流浊涕，脉右弦搏，舌心薄黄，是肺有郁热。再以毓阴培本，清肺治标。

炒萸肉 4.5g、甘杞子 6g、厚杜仲 6g、象贝母 3g、杜斗铃 3g、生桑白皮 6g、霜桑叶 6g、鲜竹茹 4.5g、荆芥炙 4.5g、生紫菀 6g、熟女贞子 12g、天台乌药 7.5g、泽兰叶 6g。

按：本案外无表证，而咳嗽痰稠，肺有郁热，属内伤咳嗽。先以泄化，宣肃肺气，后以毓阴培土。素体虚弱，故在病势减退、本虚邪微阶段，治以补泄兼施。(选自《医林荟萃》)。

咳嗽是肺系疾病的主要证候之一，分为外感、内伤两大类。外感为六淫犯肺；内伤为脏腑功能失调而致肺失宣肃，肺气上逆，发为咳嗽。

辨证首先应区分外感内伤。外感新病属于邪实，其病在肺，治应祛邪利肺；内伤久病多属邪实正虚，其病主要在肺而与肝、脾、肾相关，治应去邪止咳、扶正补虚，分别主次处理。

咳嗽的治疗，除直接治肺外，还应注意治脾、治肝、治肾等整体疗法。外感咳嗽一般均忌敛涩留邪，当因势利导，肺气宣畅则咳嗽自止。内伤咳嗽应防宣散伤正，须从调护正气着眼。

总之，咳嗽是人体祛邪达外的一种病理表现。治疗决不能单纯见咳止咳，必须按照不同的病因分别处理。一般而言，咳嗽轻重可以反映病邪的微甚，但某些情况下，因正虚不能祛邪达外，咳虽轻微，病情却重，应该警惕。

复习思考题

1. 如何区别外感咳嗽与内伤咳嗽。

2. 风寒咳嗽与风热咳嗽的区别及其辨证论治。

3. 常见内伤咳嗽有几种，怎样辨证论治。

4. 痰湿咳嗽与肺虚咳嗽的区别及其辨证论治。

哮　证

〔概述〕

哮证是一种发作性痰鸣气喘疾患，以喉中鸣响，呼吸急促困难，甚则喘息不能平卧为特征。

古代文献中多将哮证与喘证统属喘促一门不加区别。但二者性质实有不同，具体临床时应据病因、病理、临床表现特点辅之以必要的理化检查予以划分。临床上哮必兼喘，故一般通称“哮喘”，而喘未必兼哮。

西医学中支气管哮喘、喘息性支气管炎以及其他原因引起的哮喘，如心源性哮喘、嗜酸细胞增多症等，与本篇证候相类似者，均可参阅本篇辨证论治。

〔病因病机〕

哮证属于经常发作性的疾患，为宿痰内伏于肺，复加外感、饮食、情志、劳倦等因素，以致痰阻气道，肺气上逆而成。

一、外邪侵袭：外感风寒或风热之邪，未能及时表散，邪蕴于肺，壅阻肺气，气不布津，聚液成痰。此外，尚有某些体质、禀赋特殊者，吸入花粉、烟尘即影响肺气宣降，使津液凝聚，痰浊内蕴而发哮证。

二、饮食不当：贪食生冷，寒饮内停，或嗜食酸咸甘肥，积痰蒸热；或因进食海膻发物，而致脾失健运，饮食不归正化，痰浊内生，上干于肺，壅阻肺气，亦可致哮。

三、体虚病后，素质不强或病后体弱，如幼年患麻疹，顿咳，或反复感冒，咳嗽日久等，以致肺气耗损，气不化津，痰饮内生；或阴虚火旺，热蒸液聚，痰热胶固。素质不强者多以肝肾两虚为主；而病后导致者多以肺脾两虚、痰浊内蕴为主，又肝肾阴虚之体，内风易动，每致肝肺气机升降不利。

综上所述，哮证的病理因素以痰为主，痰的产生责之于肺不能布散津液，脾不能运输精微，肾不能蒸化水液，以致津液凝聚成痰，伏藏于肺，成为发病的“夙根”。此后如遇气候突变、饮食不当、情志失调、劳累、烟尘异味等多种诱因，均可引起发作。这些诱因每多互相关联，尤以气候为主。

哮喘的发作病机为内伏之宿痰，遇诱因引触，痰随气升，气因痰阻，相互搏结，壅塞气道，肺管狭窄，气管通畅不利，肺气宣降失常，停痰排化不能，而致痰鸣如吼，气息喘促。发作时的病理环节为痰阻气闭，以邪实为主。若病因感寒或素体阳虚，痰从寒化，属寒痰为患，则发为冷哮；病因于热或素体阳盛，痰从热化属痰热为患，则表现为热哮。此外，痰热内郁，风寒外束之寒包火证，在哮证中也不鲜见。若风邪明显作乱，或内风或外风可致成风哮。若因瘀血内停肺失宣降可成瘀血哮。若反复发作，寒痰每伤脾肾之阳，痰热耗灼肺肾之阴，则可从实转虚，在平时即可表现出肺、脾、肾脏气虚弱之候。肺虚不能主气，气不化津，则痰浊内蕴，肃降无权，并因卫外不固而反易受外邪的侵袭而发；脾虚不能化水谷为精微上输于肺，反而积湿生痰，上贮于肺，影响肺气升降；肾虚精气亏乏，摄纳失常，或阳虚水泛为痰或阴虚火旺灼液成痰，上干于肺而致肺气出纳失常，由于三脏相互影响，常可见肺脾气虚、肺肾阴虚、脾肾阳虚的证候。间歇期常感气短乏力，轻哮不止；一旦大发作，每易持续不解，邪实与正虚错综并见，脾肾两虚，痰浊壅盛；严重时，因肺不能朝百脉，不能调理心血的运行，命火不能上济于心，则心阳受累，也可发生喘脱危候。

哮证病因病机示意图

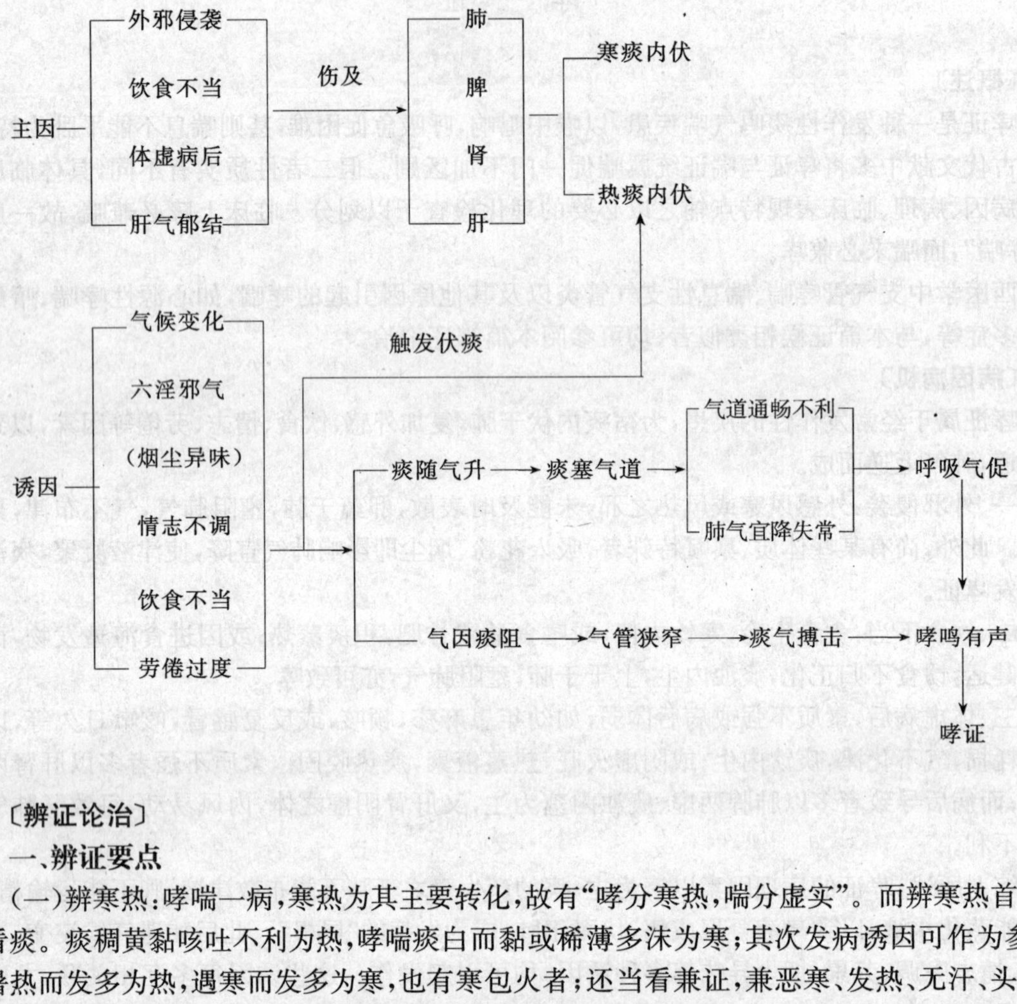

〔辨证论治〕

一、辨证要点

（一）辨寒热：哮喘一病，寒热为其主要转化，故有“哮分寒热，喘分虚实”。而辨寒热首先当要看痰。痰稠黄黏咳吐不利为热，哮喘痰白而黏或稀薄多沫为寒；其次发病诱因可作为参考，伤暑热而发多为热，遇寒而发多为寒，也有寒包火者；还当看兼证，兼恶寒、发热、无汗、头痛表寒者，多为冷哮或寒包火哮，夹头痛、咽痛、发热微恶风者多为热哮。

（二）辨虚实：从病理来看，新病多实，久病多虚；已发多实，未发以正虚为主。从病证来看，痰阻气壅，喉中响鸣，痰声漉漉，以咯出痰为舒，苔厚腻，脉弦滑为实；气机壅滞，胸憋满闷，胁肋胀痛，以呼出气为快，哮鸣声音细尖调高舌红苔薄，脉弦亦为实。自汗恶风，易于感冒，因气候变化而发作哮鸣，或面白神疲，食少脘痞，动则息促，腰酸肢软者为虚。

（三）辨风痰气血：风邪作乱之哮证，诱发哮证之因明确，起病急骤，多与体质禀赋有关。肝肾阴虚之体，风易内生；肺气不足，卫外不固之体，外风易入。

痰浊内伏之哮证，因有寒痰、热痰之别，进而发为寒哮、热哮。辨寒热部分已述及。

哮喘以气滞为主，多为外风或内风诱发之哮，怒郁后易发病，可见胸憋满闷，喉中鸣响，干哮无痰，胁肋胀痛，呼出为快，脉弦。

哮喘以血瘀为主，多哮证久发，缠绵难愈，面色晦黯，唇甲青紫，舌暗红或有瘀斑，胸胁疼痛。

（四）辨哮证与喘证：二者同有呼吸急促，临床上凭哮证的特点以与喘证区分。

1. 哮证喘息喉中痰鸣。喘是气息奔迫，主要在于气急；哮是气为痰阻，主要在于有声。

2. 哮证宿根可找，诱因可寻。而喘证无宿根，实喘有邪，邪去喘安；虚喘多为久病有脏虚特点。

3. 哮证具有发作性、反复性、顽固性的特点，而喘证则无此明显特征。

4. 哮证是一独立疾病，喘证可并发于多种急慢性疾病过程中。哮必兼喘，而喘未必兼哮，哮证久延，可发展为经常性的痰鸣气喘，可列为喘证范围。

二、分型证治：哮证已发，实证居多，以祛邪豁痰利气为主，随其病性寒热而施治。冷哮宜温化寒痰宣肺，热哮宜清化热痰肃肺，风邪诱发者重在祛风，瘀血阻络者重在活血。如久延兼虚者，又当适当兼顾。哮证未发，以扶正固本为主，区别脏腑之所属，了解肺、脾、肾所伤之主次，分别治以益肺、健脾、补肾。观其阴阳之偏虚，阳虚者应予温补，阴虚者则予滋补，以冀减轻、减少和控制哮喘发作。如寒热虚实错杂者，当兼以治之。

（一）已发

1. 寒哮

主症：喘息哮鸣，痰白而黏或稀薄多沫，胸膈满闷如窒，面色晦滞带青，口不渴或渴喜热饮。

兼症：天冷或受寒易发，头痛，发热，恶寒无汗或形寒肢冷。

舌脉：苔白腻或白滑，脉浮紧。

分析：寒痰留伏于肺，为诱因所触发，痰升气阻，痰气搏击而喘促哮鸣。肺气郁闭，不得宣畅，痰出不利而胸膈满闷如窒，咳痰白黏或稀薄多沫。阴盛于内，阳气不能宣达，故面色晦滞带青，形寒怕冷。阴寒内盛，尚未化热故口不渴而喜热饮，舌脉皆为内有寒痰之象。外寒易引动内饮，故天冷或受寒则发。头痛，发热，恶寒，无汗为表寒见证。

治法：温肺散寒，化痰利气。

方药：射干麻黄汤加减。药用射干、麻黄宣肺平喘，豁痰利咽；干姜、细辛、半夏温肺蠲饮降逆；款冬、紫菀、甘草化痰止咳；五味子收敛肺气；大枣和中。痰涌喘逆不得卧，可合三子养亲汤，也可加葶苈子泻肺降气涤痰。若表寒里饮，寒象较甚者，可用小青龙汤与杏仁、苏子、白芥子、橘皮等化痰利气。哮证剧甚，确属有沉寒痼冷顽痰不化者，可考虑在密切观察下服用砒剂如紫金丹以劫痰定喘，但砒易引起汞中毒，服用要非常小心，且服量要小，服用日期最好在5～7日之内。若寒哮发作频繁，病久虚实并见，上盛下虚，发时喉中痰鸣如鼾、声低，气短痰清，面色苍白，汗出肢冷，舌胖淡苔白，脉沉细者，当温阳补虚、降气化痰，用苏子降气汤配党参、胡桃肉、紫石英、沉香、诃子之类，肾阳虚明显者伍以附子、补骨脂、钟乳石等。

处方举例：

射干10g、麻黄5g、杏仁10g、苏子10g、橘皮10g、半夏10g、细辛3g、葶苈子10g、紫菀10g、款冬10g、甘草5g。

2. 热哮

主症：喘促哮鸣如吼，胸高气粗，咳呛阵作，痰稠黄胶黏，咳吐不利，烦闷不安，汗出面赤，口苦口渴喜饮。

兼症:头痛发热微恶风。

舌脉:舌苔黄腻,质红,脉滑数或弦滑。

分析:肺内素有郁热痰伏,外邪侵犯,肺失清肃,痰热壅肺,肺气上逆,痰气搏击,故喘促哮鸣如吼,胸高气粗,咳呛阵作。痰热交结,故咯痰黏浊稠厚,咯吐不利。痰热郁蒸则烦闷,自汗,面赤,口苦;病因于热,热灼津液故不恶寒而口渴喜饮。舌苔黄腻,脉滑数均是痰热内盛之征。痰热内蕴,外邪易从阳化热,故多有风热表证之见证。

治法:清热宣肺,化痰降逆。

方药:定喘汤加减。药用麻黄宣肺定喘,黄芩、桑白皮清热肃肺,橘红、半夏、款冬、苏子化痰降逆,白果以敛肺气,甘草和中。若寒邪外束,肺热内盛,可加生石膏,去白果以解肌清里。表寒重者酌配桂枝、生姜或以大青龙汤加减。肺气壅实,痰鸣息涌不得卧,加葶苈子、广地龙。热痰壅实,阻塞气道,气急欲死者,加吞猴枣粉。内热蕴盛,痰火熏蒸,舌苔燥黄者可加大黄、芒硝或用宣白承气汤加礞石滚痰丸通腑以利肺。痰黄黏稠难咯者酌配知母、海蛤粉、射干、鱼腥草、竹沥水等或合入千金苇茎汤、小陷胸汤以清化痰热。若病久热盛伤阴,虚中夹实,气急难续,呛咳盗汗,痰少质黏,形疲咽干,烦热颧红,舌红少苔脉细数者,当用麦门冬汤加沙参、五味子、贝母养阴清热,润肺化痰。若肾虚气逆,可配熟地、当归、山萸肉、紫石英、诃子等益肾纳气。

处方举例:

炙麻黄 5g、杏仁 10g、黄芩 10g、半夏 6g、瓜蒌 15g、生石膏(先下)20g、甘草 5g、葶苈子 10g、广地龙 10g、川贝母 10g。

3. 风哮

主症:哮喘骤然发作,干哮无痰或痰少难咯,胸膈满闷,诱因明确或为情志不遂,或嗅特殊气味而发病。

兼症:咽干口燥,面色潮红或萎黄不华,大便不爽。

舌脉:舌红少津,苔少或无苔,脉弦细。

分析:风善行而数变。外风始受于肺,内风始生于肝。或禀赋不足,卫外不固,外风易从肺入,致肺气失于宣肃。或素体阴虚血亏,肝风易从内动;或肝郁气滞,木郁化火生风,致使肝肺气机升降失常,肺失清肃。或外风,或内风,皆可致肺气不利,痰升气阻,痰气搏击而发哮鸣喘促,气机不利则胸膈满闷,甚则胸肋胀疼。阴血不足之体故面色萎黄不华,虚热灼津故咽干口燥,痰少难咯,虚火上炎则面色潮红。舌脉均为阴虚血亏之象。

治法:柔肝祛风利肺。

方药:过敏煎加减。方用柴胡舒肝解郁;防风祛除内外之风;乌梅、五味子、甘草酸甘化阴,养阴柔肝,熄除内风;杏仁宣肃肺气;苏梗、苏子理气降气平喘;地龙咸寒通络熄风。肝郁气滞明显加枳壳、赤芍,以取合四逆散之意加强疏肝理气之功。若诱因明确,起病骤急,证偏热,加僵蚕、蝉衣以解痉熄风,或合入杨栗山“升降散”以升降气机,熄风通络。若证偏寒可加全蝎、川芎以解痉熄风通络。若哮喘胸憋明显,哮鸣息粗,可加麻黄、葶苈子,取合三拗汤、葶苈大枣泻肺汤之意以宣降肺气平喘。若外寒内热即俗称“寒包火”,可加麻黄、生石膏,取合麻杏石甘汤之意以宣肺清热平喘。若有蛔虫内伏,也可先服乌梅丸汤驱虫安蛔,后再服此方。

处方举例:

柴胡 10g、防风 10g、乌梅 8g、五味子 6g、甘草 5g、杏仁 10g、苏梗子各 10g、地龙 10g。

4. 瘀哮

主症：哮喘久发，反复缠绵不愈，胸闷胁痛，爪甲青紫，面色晦黯。

兼症：急发常夹有口苦、咽干、便干、腹胀，女子多伴有月经不调或有轻度浮肿。

舌脉：舌紫暗或有瘀斑，脉沉涩。

分析：哮喘久发，肺气不利，肝肺气机不畅，气血失和，气滞则血瘀，瘀血内停，故哮喘爪甲青紫，面色晦黯，舌有瘀斑，脉涩，女子月经不调。瘀血内阻，少阳枢机不利，复感外邪，易成少阳、阳明实热夹瘀之症，故见咽干口苦，便干，腹胀。

治法：活血化瘀，降逆平喘。

方药：血府逐瘀汤加减。此方以四逆散、柴胡、枳壳、芍药、甘草疏理气机；桃红四物汤活血通络；桔梗、牛膝一升一降，通达气血。若肝血不足，脾湿内停，且痰浊瘀血互结，可用当归芍药散加苏梗、苏子、杏仁、地龙、麻黄等宣降肺气之品。若出现少阳、阳明实热夹瘀之象，可用大柴胡合桂枝茯苓丸方加减以通达少阳、阳明气血，使肺气宣畅。

处方举例：

当归 10g、川芎 10g、赤芍 10g、茯苓 12g、柴胡 10g、黄芩 10g、枳壳 10g、半夏 10g、酒军 4g、苏子 10g、杏仁 10g。

冷哮、热哮以痰分证；风哮虽风邪诱发，实以阴虚气滞为主；瘀哮是瘀血内阻，气滞血瘀，肺络失和。临床上，四种哮喘，各有主证，当细心审辨。因风邪、痰浊、气滞、血瘀易相合为病，故治疗上，既应针对主证之邪浊以立法处方用药，又应适当配伍祛除其他邪浊之品，即应当注意各证型相兼的治疗。

（二）未发

1. 肺虚

主症：自汗，恶风，常易感冒，每因气候变化而诱发，发前打嚏，鼻塞清涕，面色㿠白，咳痰清稀色白。

兼症：气短声低，或喉中常有轻度哮鸣。

舌脉：苔薄白，舌质淡，脉细弱或虚大。

分析：卫气虚弱，不能充实腠理，外邪易侵故自汗，恶风，常易感冒，每因气候变化而诱发，发前先见鼻塞流涕打嚏。肺虚不能主气，气不化津，痰饮蕴肺，故气短声低，咳痰清稀色白。面色㿠白，舌脉均为肺气虚弱表现。

治法：补肺固卫。

方药：玉屏风散加味。药用黄芪益气固表，白术、甘草健脾补肺，防风祛风以助黄芪实表固卫。若怕冷畏风明显，加用桂枝汤以桂枝、白芍、姜枣等调和营卫。若肺气阴两虚，咳呛，痰少而黏，口咽发干，舌质偏红者，用生脉散加北沙参、玉竹、黄芪等益气养阴，或用补肺汤以人参、黄芪补气，熟地、五味子养阴，紫菀、桑白皮化痰降气止咳。

处方举例：

生黄芪 12g、防风 8g、白术 6g、炙甘草 5g、党参 10g、麦冬 10g、五味子 10g、冬虫夏草 10g。

2. 脾虚

主症：平素食少脘痞，大便不实，易因饮食不当而诱发，倦怠气短。

兼症：食油腻易于腹泻，言语无力。

舌脉：苔薄腻或白滑，舌质淡，脉细弱软。

分析：脾虚健运无权，故少食脘痞，大便不实，常因饮食不当而诱发。中气不足，故倦怠气短，语言无力。苔薄腻或白滑，质淡，脉细软，皆属脾气虚弱之候。

治法：健脾化痰。

方药：六君子汤加减。药用党参、白术、茯苓、甘草健脾益气，陈皮、半夏理气化痰。若形寒肢冷便溏，痰白清稀为脾阳不振，加桂枝、干姜以温脾化饮。

处方举例：

党参15g、白术10g、茯苓10g、陈皮10g、半夏10g、甘草6g。

3. 肾虚

主症：平素短气息促，动则为甚，吸气不利，腰疲腿软，劳累后哮喘易发。

兼症：偏阳虚者畏寒肢冷，面色苍白，自汗。偏阴虚者颧红、烦热、盗汗。

舌脉：阳虚者苔白、质胖嫩，脉沉细。阴虚者舌红少苔，脉细数。

分析：久病肾虚，摄纳失常，气不归元，故短气，动则加甚，吸气不利。精气亏乏，则腰膝疲软，劳累易发。阳虚则见外寒之征，阴虚则有内热之候。

治法：补肾纳气。

方药：金匮肾气丸或麦味地黄丸，辨其阴阳予以选用。前方偏温肾助阳，后方偏益肾纳气。若阳虚明显加补骨脂、仙灵脾、仙芽、鹿角片或鹿角胶，阴虚去温补之品重用生地，加当归、女贞子、阿胶、龟板胶等。肾虚不能纳气明显者，可于上两方中加胡桃肉、冬虫草、紫石英，或用参蛤散配河车粉常服。

处方举例：

生熟地各12g、山萸肉10g、茯苓12g、当归10g、补骨脂10g、女贞子10g、陈皮10g、五味子8g、苏子10g。

肺虚、脾虚、肾虚虽有各自特点，但临床每多错杂并见，治疗时既应区别主次，又需适当兼顾。难以区分主次者，可平补三脏，又无论寒哮、热哮，经年累月，反复发作，缠绵不愈多夹瘀血，可酌加桃仁、川芎、当归、丹参等活血药，上述几方可配合应用。本证治疗上，除内服之外，尚有其他如外贴、中药气雾剂、针灸、割治、埋线、指压、单方、验方等方法，可在辨证论治的原则下选择应用。

（三）哮证危候—阳气暴脱，痰瘀闭窍

脉症：哮喘发病过程中，随见吐泻，筋惕肉瞤，面色青紫，神气倦怠，或烦躁昏昧，汗出如油，四肢厥冷，脉微欲绝，舌色紫暗，苔腻或滑。

分析：哮病久发，正气日虚，或因外邪急袭，闭郁肺气，阴阳格拒，而致阳气暴脱，痰瘀闭窍。

治法：回阳救逆，化痰治瘀。

方药：四味回阳饮加减。方用附子、干姜化浊阴以回阳，人参甘草益气固脱。面色青紫，舌紫者加桃仁、红花活血化瘀，神志昏昧加菖蒲、郁金、麝香少许以醒窍，阳气津液两脱者或用西洋参，或上方加山萸肉、麦冬、五味子。

〔预防及护理措施〕

1. 保持室内空气新鲜，阳光充足。寒哮病人尤应注意避免外感风寒，室温宜适当偏高些，热哮病人伴有发热要防止伤津耗气，室温宜偏低，空气要湿化。风哮瘀哮病人容易发生变证，如见张口抬肩，烦躁不安，面青唇紫，汗出肢冷，脉浮大无根或见结代者为心肾阳虚的喘脱危象，应积极抢救治疗。

2. 饮食宜清淡，避免过咸过酸，忌辛辣刺激食物，忌烟酒，慎戒异味、灰尘、海鲜等以杜 生痰之源。注意防止过劳，避免情志刺激。

3. 在病情观察中，要注意哮喘的诱发因素，发作时间，持续时间，发作时伴发的症状、体温、脉搏、痰液等情况。

4. 哮喘 发作有定时者，可在发作前 1～2 小时服药。发作时，病人应卧床，最好半卧位，必要时予吸氧。要保持呼吸道通畅，痰多者，应设法排痰。

5. 哮喘发作剧烈时，可酌情用下法止喘：

(1)洋金花烟雾吸入。

(2)针刺天突、膻中、气海等穴，寒证者可加用灸法。

(3)口服氨茶碱、喘息定等，慎用止咳及镇静剂。

6. 在哮喘缓解期应指导患者进行体育锻炼，增强体质。

〔典型病例分析〕

案一：陈某某，女，15 岁。

1976 年 7 月 12 日初诊：患者自 3 岁时即发哮喘，初起发作轻微，后来愈发愈频，以春夏为剧。发则气不接续，喘促痰鸣，不能平卧，不思饮食，常用氨茶碱、麻黄素等止咳平喘药等及青、链霉素等抗感染药才能缓解。连日外受风寒，哮喘又发，诊见张口抬肩，呼吸喘促，两肺哮鸣音及散在干湿性啰音，痰多而稠，颜面苍白，舌质红，苔黄腻，脉象细弦。

辨证：宿痰内伏，郁久成热，外寒相引，以致哮喘复作，系属肺寒膈热，本虚标实。

立法："急则治标"，先治以宣肺清热，止咳平喘。

方药：定喘汤加减。麻黄 10g、白果 3g(打)、黄芩 10g、苏子 10g、地龙 15g、杏仁 12g、款冬花 10g、川芎 10g、全蝎 5g。6 剂。

8 月 13 日二诊：服药后哮喘已缓解。一月来只发作一二次，程度较前减轻。发作时，服上药即平。唯动则气喘，汗多，不思饮食。"缓则治本"，当补肾纳气，益肺化痰平喘为法。

熟地 2g、五味子 5g、冬虫草 10g、紫河车 5g、甘草 5g、沉香末 1g(冲)、苏子 5g、川贝母 3g、党参 5g、麦冬 3g、煅牡蛎 12g。6 剂。

1977 年 9 月 6 日再诊：自诉发作时用初诊方，发作缓解后复诊方，交替服用近年余(有时中断或隔日 1 剂)哮喘基本控制。现咳痰不多，动则有轻度痰鸣气喘，一直没有大发作，能从事一般活动，嘱用复诊方加倍做丸药服用，以巩固之。

按：本例哮喘属发作期，肺寒膈热，本虚标实之证，系宿痰内伏，郁久化热，外寒相引所致。治疗上以宣肺清热，止咳平喘而治标为主，方以宣肺平喘、清热化痰之定喘汤去甘草、桑皮、半夏，加地龙、川芎、全蝎平喘解痉，全方既能清肺降气化痰，又能驱除宿饮。缓解时用熟地、五味子、紫河车、冬虫夏草之补肾纳气；党参、麦冬、贝母、苏子、沉香、甘草之益肺行气祛痰；少佐牡蛎以敛汗，从治本入手。这样标本缓急交替使用，从而使肺肾功能迅速得以恢复。

哮喘是一种发作性的痰鸣气喘疾患，以喉中哮鸣有声，呼吸急促困难为特征。病理因素以痰为主，因痰伏于肺，遇感诱发。发时痰阻气道，肺气失于肃降，表现邪实之征；如反复久发，气阴耗损，肺、脾、肾渐虚，则在平时表现正虚的情况。当大发作时可见正虚与邪实相互错杂。辨治原则根据已发、未发，分虚实施治。发时以邪实为主，当攻邪治标，分别寒热，予以温化宣肺或清化肃肺；病久发时虚实夹杂者，又当并顾。平时以正虚为主，当扶正治本，审察阴阳，分别采用补肺、健脾、益肾等法。

哮证必须注意寒热的相兼、转化、寒包火证、寒痰化热、热证转从寒化等情况。了解邪实与正虚的错杂为患，一般病史不长者，发作时以邪实为主；久病可兼虚象，平时则表现正虚为主。治当根据病的新久，发作与否，区别邪正缓急，虚实主次，加以处理。重视平时治本的措施，区别肺、脾、肾的主次，在抓住重点的基础上适当兼顾，因肾为先天之本，五脏之根，其中尤以补肾为要，精气充足则根本得固。

复习思考题

1. 何为哮证的辨证要点？急性期如何辨治？
2. 哮、喘两证如何鉴别？
3. 缓解期补肾的意义何在？

喘　证

〔概述〕

喘证是以呼吸急促甚或张口抬肩，鼻翼煽动或呼吸困难，动则加重为特征的病证。若喘促严重，持续不解，可发生喘脱。可见于多种急、慢性疾病过程中。

有关喘证，古代文献论述颇多，现代临床沿用《景岳全书·喘促》篇将喘证分为虚、实两大类。二者实有不同，临证时，应结合病史、病因、临床表现、体征及必要的理化检查严格予以区分。

西医学诊断的呼吸系统疾病如：喘息性支气管炎、肺炎、肺气肿、肺结核、尘肺、肺脓病、慢性肺源性心脏病以及由其他系统所造成的呼吸窘迫综合征、心源性哮喘、癔病等疾病过程中所出现的呼吸急促，呼吸困难，均可参照本篇辨证论治。

〔病因病机〕

喘证的成因虽多，但概括起来，不外外感与内伤两端，外感为六淫侵袭，内伤有饮食、七情、劳倦等方面。其病位主要在肺、肾，尚与肝、脾、心有关。病理性质有虚实两方面，有邪者为实，因邪壅于肺，宣降失司；无邪者属虚，因肺不主气，肾失摄纳。

一、外邪侵袭：以风寒风热最为常见。因重感风寒，邪袭于肺，内则壅遏肺气，外则郁闭皮毛腠理，肺卫为邪所伤，肺气宣降失常；或因风热犯肺，肺气壅实，甚则热蒸液聚成痰，清肃失司，以致肺气上逆作喘；或肺有蕴热，又为风寒束表，或表寒不解郁而化热，热为寒郁，热不得泄，皆能导致肺失宣降，气逆而喘。

二、痰浊壅盛：饮食不节，恣食肥甘生冷，或嗜酒伤中，脾失健运，积湿生痰或素体痰湿偏盛，是喘证产生的内在因素。脾为生痰之源，肺为贮痰之器，痰浊日盛，由中焦上干于肺，肺气壅阻，升降不利，发为喘促。若痰湿久郁化热，或肺火素盛，痰受热蒸，痰火受阻，痰壅火迫，清肃之令不行，肺气为之上逆而作喘，如复加外感诱发，可见痰浊与风寒邪热等内外合邪的复杂情况。

三、情志所伤：情志不遂，忧思气结，气机不利，肺气痹阻；或郁怒伤肝，肝气上逆于肺，肺气不得肃降，升多降少，气逆而喘。

四、肺肾虚弱：久咳伤肺或病久肺弱，肺之气阴不足，气失所主而短气喘促。若久病迁延不愈，由肺及肾，或劳欲伤肾，精气内压，肺之气阴亏耗，不能下荫于肾，肾之真元伤损，根本不固，则气失摄纳，上出于肺，出多入少，逆气上奔为喘。若肾阳虚衰，水无所主，干肺凌心，肺气上逆，心阳不振，而致喘者则属于虚中夹实之候。此外，中气虚弱，肺气失于充养，土不生金，亦可因气虚无力呼吸而喘。

综上所述，实喘为外邪、痰浊及肝郁气逆、瘀血阻络等壅阻肺气使之宣降不利；虚喘则为精气不足，肺肾出纳失常所致。其病位主要在肺肾，而与肝脾有关，严重时又常影响到心。因肺主气，司呼吸，外合皮毛，为五脏华盖，故外邪之侵袭，及他脏病气上犯，皆可使肺气失于宣降，呼吸不利，气逆而喘促。若肺虚则气失所主，亦可少气不足以息而喘。肾为气之根，摄纳失常，则气不归元，也可气逆于肺而喘。他如脾经痰浊上干，肝气逆乘于肺，以及中气虚弱等发生喘促也无不与肺有关。

喘证病因病机示意图

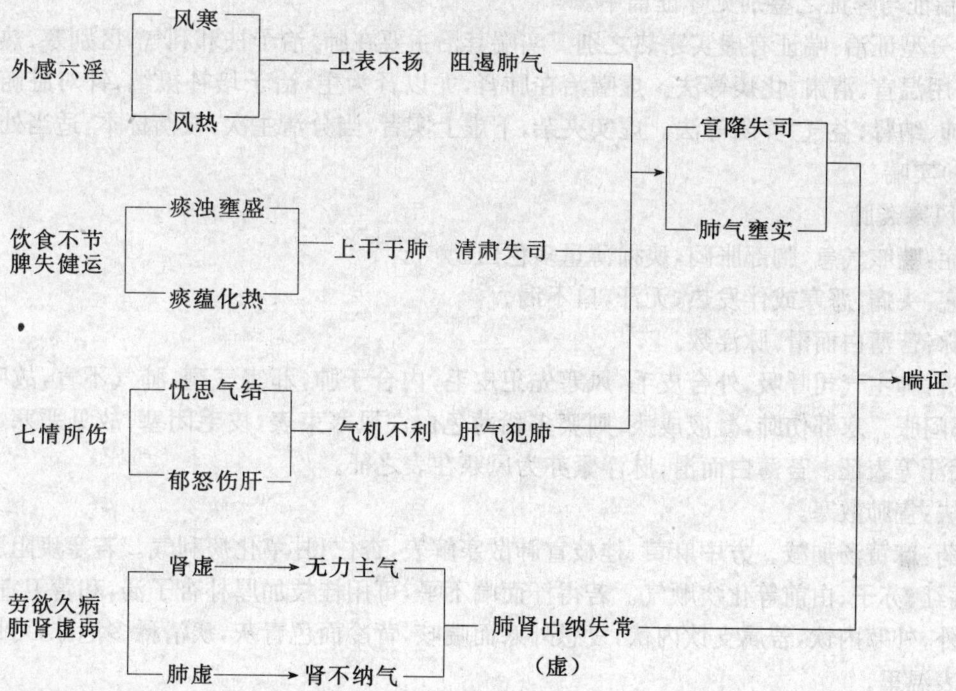

本证的严重阶段，不但肺肾俱衰，心阳亦同时受累，因心脉上通于肺，肺气治调心血之运行，宗气贯心肺而行呼吸，肾脉上络于心，心肾相互既济，心阳根于命门之火，故心阳的盛衰与先天肾气及后天呼吸之气皆有密切关系。一旦肺肾俱衰，则心气心阳亦弱，不能鼓动血脉，则心动急促，血行瘀滞，面色唇舌指甲皆发青紫，心气虚不敛心液，汗液大量外泄，出现喘汗致脱，亡阳竭阴的危局。

〔辨证论治〕

一、辨证要点

（一）辨虚实：辨虚实最为紧要。如误犯虚虚实实之戒，病情极易恶化。实喘呼吸深长有余，呼出为快，气粗声高，脉数有力。因于外感者发病骤急，病程较短，多有表证。因于内伤者病程多久，反复时作，外无表证，多有痰浊或痰热壅盛之表现，如胸中满闷等。或有郁怒伤肝之病因，喘促气憋，情志刺激而诱发。虚喘呼吸短促难续，深吸为快，气怯声低，脉微弱或浮大中空，一般病程较长，病势徐缓时轻时重，遇劳则甚。肺虚者喘促短气，自汗畏风，操劳后则喘；肾虚者静息时亦苦气息喘促，动则更甚，呼多吸少；若心气虚则喘息持续不已。

(二)辨寒热：喘证之寒热，舌红、脉数、小便往往不足为凭，关键是看舌苔与痰色性质。属寒者其痰清稀如水或痰白有沫，面色青灰，口不渴或渴喜热饮，苔白滑，脉浮紧或弦迟；属热者证见痰色黄，稠黏或色白而黏，咯吐不利，面赤，口渴引饮，舌质红苔黄腻或黄燥，脉滑数。

(三)辨喘证与气短、哮证

1. 喘证与气短：二者同为呼吸异常，但喘证是以呼吸困难，张口抬肩甚至不能平卧为特征，有虚实之别。气短亦即少气，即气虚不足、可见于各种急慢性疾病中，纯虚无实，主要表现为气息低微，说话或劳动时感觉气不够用，倦怠懒言，脉弱，多因中气不足、肺肾两虚所致，气短严重可造成虚喘。总之，气短可以是感觉，而喘证必须有形征可见。

2. 喘证与哮证之鉴别见哮证篇中。

二、分型证治：喘证有虚实寒热之别。实喘其治主要在肺，治予祛邪利气，区别寒、热、痰之不同，采用温宣、清肃、化痰等法。虚喘治在肺肾，尤以肾为主，治予培补摄纳，针对脏腑病机，采用补肺、纳肾、益气、养阴等法。虚实夹杂，下虚上实者，当分清主次，权衡标本，适当处理。

(一)实喘

1. 风寒袭肺

主症：喘咳气急，胸部胀闷，痰稀薄量多色白。

兼症：头痛、恶寒或伴发热，无汗，口不渴。

舌脉：苔薄白而滑，脉浮数。

分析：肺主气司呼吸，外合皮毛，风寒先犯皮毛，内合于肺，邪实气壅，肺气不宣，故喘咳气逆，胸部闷胀。寒邪伤肺，凝液成痰，则痰多稀薄色白。风寒束表，皮毛闭塞，故见恶寒，头痛，发热，无汗等表证。苔薄白而滑，脉浮紧亦为风寒在表之征。

治法：宣肺散寒。

方药：麻黄汤加减。方中麻黄、桂枝宣肺散寒解表，杏仁、甘草化痰利气。若寒痰阻肺可加半夏、橘红、苏子、白前等化痰顺气。若得汗而喘不平，可用桂枝加厚朴杏子汤，和营卫宣肺气。

另外，外寒内饮，若属支饮内伏，复感外寒而喘咳，背冷面色青灰，痰清稀多泡沫，可用小青龙汤发表温里。

处方举例：

麻黄 6g、杏仁 10g、桂枝 6g、甘草 5g、橘红 10g、半夏 8g、苏子 10g、茯苓 10g、白前 10g。

2. 风热犯肺

主症：喘促气急，甚则鼻翼煽动，痰黄黏稠难出。

兼症：胸痛烦闷，头痛身热汗出，口渴，便秘尿黄。

舌脉：舌苔薄白或黄，脉浮或滑数。

分析：风热犯肺，热盛气壅，肺失宣肃，肺气奔迫故喘促气急，甚则鼻翼煽动。热灼津液成痰，故痰黄黏稠难出。热盛伤津则口渴。痰热客阻胸中故烦闷或痛。身热汗出而头痛是里热盛而兼表邪。苔薄黄，脉浮数亦属风热在肺在表。

治法：清热解表，宣肺平喘。

方药：麻杏石甘汤加味。本方重用石膏清肺热，麻黄宣肺平喘，杏仁泄肺降气。肺热重可加黄芩、知母、鱼腥草，或加重石膏用量以清肺热。里实热结便秘者加凉膈散或用宣白承气汤泻火清金。风热表盛加银花、连翘解表清热。痰多喘甚加葶苈子、射干泻肺平喘。咳痰黄稠加瓜蒌、贝母清化肺热。

附：内热外寒者，即肺有郁热，风寒束表，或表寒未解，内已化热，热郁于肺，肺气上逆而喘逆息粗鼻煽，胸部胀痛，痰黄黏稠，仍可用麻杏石甘汤加味。有汗重用石膏，无汗重用麻黄。

处方举例：

麻黄 6g、杏仁 10g、石膏 30g(先下)、甘草 5g、黄芩 10g、瓜蒌 15g、连翘 10g、漏芦 10g、桔梗 6g。

3. 痰浊壅肺

主症：喘咳，痰多色白而黏，胸满窒闷。

兼证：纳呆口黏不渴，甚或呕恶。

舌脉：苔厚腻色白，脉滑。

分析：脾不健运，积湿成痰，痰浊壅肺，肺气失降，故喘满闷窒，胸盈仰息，痰多色白黏腻。痰湿蕴中，脾胃不和而见呕恶，纳呆，口黏，苔厚腻，脉滑。

治法：化痰降气。

方药：二陈汤合三子养亲汤加减。方中半夏、陈皮、茯苓健脾燥湿化痰，苏子、白芥子、莱菔子顺气降逆化痰。痰湿盛，胸闷纳呆明显可加苍术、厚朴等燥湿理脾行气。

处方举例：

陈皮 10g、半夏 10g、茯苓 12g、甘草 5g、炒苏子 10g、炒白芥子 6g、炒莱菔子 10g、厚朴 8g、杏仁 10g。

4. 痰热郁肺

主症：喘咳气涌，胸中烦热，胸部胀痛，痰多色黄黏稠。

兼症：渴喜冷饮，面红咽干，尿赤便秘或痰中夹血。

舌脉：苔黄腻，脉滑数。

分析：脾胃素有蕴热，或饮食厚味积热，或湿痰蕴久化热，或表邪入里化热，皆成痰热，郁结于肺，壅塞气道而见喘咳气涌。痰热郁蒸则胸中烦热，渴喜冷饮，痰黄黏稠，咽干面赤，苔黄腻脉滑数。热伤血络则见血痰。

治法：清泄肺热化痰。

方药：桑白皮汤加减。药用桑白皮、黄连、黄芩、栀子清泻肺热，贝母、杏仁、苏子、半夏降气化痰。身热者加石膏、知母。痰多黏稠加海蛤壳或黛蛤散。喘不能卧，痰涌便秘，酌加葶苈子、大黄、玄明粉。痰有腥味配鱼腥草、苡仁、冬瓜仁、芦根。

处方举例：

瓜蒌 18g、贝母 10g、苡仁 5g、黄芩 10g、葶苈子 10g、炒莱菔子 10g、桑皮 10g、冬瓜仁 10g、焦山栀 10g。

5. 气郁伤肺

主症：每遇情志刺激而诱发，呼吸短促，喘憋胸闷，咽中如窒。

兼症：常有失眠，心悸，胸闷胸痛。

舌脉：苔薄，脉弦。

分析：郁怒伤肝，肝气冲逆犯肺，肺气不降则喘促气憋，咽中如窒。肝肺络气不和而胸闷胸痛。心肝气郁则失眠心悸，脉弦。

治法：开郁降气平喘。

方药：五磨饮子加减，本方以沉香、木香、槟榔、乌药、枳壳芳香行气之品，开郁降气。宜劝慰病人心情开朗配合治疗；伴心悸失眠者加百合、合欢花、枣仁、远志等宁心安神；胸闷胀痛加旋覆花、香附。若气郁不舒，火气郁结上冲，喘促心烦者可用丹栀逍遥散去白术加郁金，清郁火畅气机；若气滞血瘀，喘咳胸闷刺痛，动则加重，肋下痞块，面色唇甲青紫，痰不多口不渴，舌紫暗或有瘀斑，脉弦涩或弦细可用血府逐瘀汤加减。此方用四逆散疏肝解郁，桃红四物汤养血活血，配以桔梗、牛膝取其升降之意。

处方举例：

柴胡 8g、枳壳 10g、白芍 10g、甘草 5g、焦槟榔 8g、香附 10g、苏梗子各 10g、合欢花 10g。

(二)虚喘

1. 气虚喘(肺脾气虚)

主症：喘促短气，言语无力，咳声低弱，咳痰稀薄，自汗畏风。

兼症：面色苍白，气少倦怠，食后脘胀，便溏或食后即便。

舌脉：苔薄白或薄白腻，舌胖边有齿痕，脉细弱。

分析：肺为气之主，肺气不足则喘促短气言语无力，咳声低弱。肺合皮毛，肺气虚弱，卫外不固故自汗畏风。脾虚有寒故咳痰稀薄。肺脾两虚脾不健运则食少倦怠，食后脘胀，便溏，或食后即便。舌苔薄舌体胖，脉弱也为肺脾气虚之象。

治法：健脾益肺。

方药：玉屏风散合六君子汤加减。方用参术芪益肺健脾，陈皮、茯苓、半夏健脾化痰，黄芪配防风益气固表。若咳痰稀薄，时觉形寒，为肺虚有寒可加干姜温中。大便溏可合人参苓白术散之意。若进食即便，便溏并有气坠感为中气下陷，可加用补中益气汤加减以升提下陷之气。

处方举例：

生黄芪 15g、防风 10g、白术 10g、党参 10g、陈皮 10g、茯苓 10g、半夏 10g、桔梗 6g、甘草 5g。

2. 阴虚喘(肺肾阴虚)

主症：喘促气短，动则加重，口咽发干，潮热盗汗，痰黏量少难咯。

兼症：面赤心烦，手足心热，腰酸耳鸣。

舌脉：舌红苔薄黄，脉细数。

分析：肺肾阴虚，气失主纳故喘促气短，动则加重。阴虚火旺则面赤心烦，手足心热。津不上乘故咽口发干。虚火灼津故痰黏量少难咯。腰为肾之府，肾开窍于耳，肾阴不足，清窍失养故腰酸耳鸣。舌红苔薄黄，脉细数为肺肾阴虚之征。

治法：滋肾养肺。

方药：生脉散合六味地黄丸加减。方以生脉散益气养阴，六味地黄丸合入五味子为都气丸滋肾纳气。偏肺阴不足，口咽干燥，面赤心烦，可加百合、南北沙参、玉竹等养阴清肺；偏肾阴虚，手足心热，潮热盗汗可加生龙牡以潜阳敛汗，退虚热。若真阴衰竭，阴不敛阳，气失摄纳，则喘急面红；咽干烦躁，汗出如油，舌红少津，脉细数为戴阳，可加重山萸肉，并加生龙牡、紫石英等潜镇药。

处方举例：

党参 10g、天麦冬各 10g、五味子 6g、生地 12g、女贞子 10g、山萸肉 10g、百合 10g、灵磁石

(先下)20g、陈皮 10g。

3. 阳虚喘(脾肾阳虚)

主症:喘促日久,呼多吸少,动则喘甚,气不得续。汗出肢冷,面浮胫肿,痰多清稀,面青唇紫。

兼症:腰酸神怯,面色皖白或黧黑,夜尿频多。

舌脉:舌胖淡,脉沉细无力或弦大无根。

分析:肾阳不足,气失摄纳,故喘促动则加重,气不得续。阳虚阴寒内盛,不能温煦,故肢冷神怯、面青。阳虚不固故汗出;阳虚不能化气行水则面浮胫肿,痰多清稀。舌胖淡脉沉细为阳气虚衰;脉弦大无根为虚阳外越。

治法:温阳补肾纳气。

方药:金匮肾气丸、参蛤散加减。前方温补肾阳,后方纳气归肾。若冲气上逆,脐下筑动,气从小腹上奔者加紫石英、磁石、沉香等镇纳。若阳虚停饮,上凌心肺而喘咳心悸或水泛肢肿,尿少,舌胖淡,脉沉细者,可用真武汤加桂枝、黄芪、防己、葶苈子、万年青根温肾益气行水。若喘咳痰多胸闷,动则尤甚,腰酸肢冷,汗出心悸,小便频数,舌苔腻,脉沉细或濡滑无力,此为痰气壅实于上,肾气亏损于下,为"上实下虚"之候,宜化痰降气,兼以温肾纳气,用苏子降气汤加减。

处方举例:

附片 6～10g、干姜 6g、白果 6g、五味子 6g、补骨脂 10g、茯苓 12g、党参 10g、苏子 10g。

(三)喘证危候

若喘逆甚剧,张口抬肩,鼻煽气促,端坐不能卧,心慌动悸,烦躁不安,面青舌紫,汗出淋漓,肢冷脉浮大无根或有歇止或模糊不清者,为心肾阳衰、肺气欲竭的喘脱危象,急宜扶阳固脱,潜镇肾气,可用参附煎汤送服黑锡丹、蛤蚧粉;若躁热颧红,汗出黏手为气阴俱竭,可去附子加西洋参、麦冬、五味子等益气养阴,汗多加龙牡敛汗固表。

〔预防及护理措施〕

1. 注意保持室内空气新鲜,阳光充足,温度、湿度适宜。室内禁止吸烟。患者吸烟应劝其戒除。嘱患者慎起居避六淫。

2. 饮食宜清淡,避免过咸、过酸,忌辛辣刺激食物,忌酒。

3. 病情观察中,应注意喘证的发作时间、持续时间、诱发因素、发作时伴随症状、体温脉搏、痰液等情况。

4. 喘证发作时,病人应卧床,最好半卧位,必要时给予吸氧。注意保持呼吸道通畅,痰多者应设法助痰排出,必要时吸痰。

5. 喘证发作剧烈时,可酌情用以下方法止喘。

(1)洋金花烟雾吸入。

(2)针刺天突、膻中、气海等穴。

(3)氨茶碱、喘息定等口服。慎用止咳剂或镇静剂。

6. 如发现病人久喘而有神志恍惚,烦躁不安或喘不能卧,面色青紫,吐大量泡沫痰者,可能为肺性脑病或心力衰竭,应予抢救。

7. 喘证发作平息,患者可进行活动时,应嘱其进行锻炼,以增强体质,有条件者,可学做呼吸操。

〔典型病例分析〕

案一：赵某某，女，56岁。

1972年6月15日初诊：多年咳喘，发作时不能平卧，不能安睡，喉中有痰声，早晚咳喘尤甚，近日咳喘发作，并有轻度浮肿。西医诊断为慢性喘息性支气管炎急性发作。舌苔薄黄，脉滑数。

辨证：痰热通肺，肺失宣利。

立法：宣肺定喘。

方药：麻黄15g、杏仁15g、黄芩15g、地龙15g、川芎5g、全蝎3g。3付。

6月19日二诊：服药后，咳喘大为减轻，已能平卧，夜寐亦安，浮肿逐渐消退，药中病机，稍轻其量，守方再进。

麻黄12g、杏仁12g、黄芩12g、地龙12g、川芎5g、全蝎3g。

连服3剂，咳喘近期控制，浮肿全消。

按：本例实喘系热性咳喘，痰热迫肺，肺失宣利，以致咳喘时发。肺闭宜开，痰热当清，方中用麻黄、杏仁宣肺定喘，清热不用石膏之辛寒，而用黄芩之苦寒，以清泻上焦实火及肺热，加入地龙更可发挥平喘作用，川芎、全蝎有活络镇痉作用。

喘证是呼吸困难，甚至张口抬肩，鼻翼煽动，不能平卧的一种病证，严重者可致喘脱。为外感六淫、内伤饮食、情志、以及久病体虚所致。其病位主要在于肺、肾，亦与肝、脾等脏有关。病理性质有虚实之分，实喘为邪气壅肺，气失宣降，治予祛邪利气，治重在肺；虚喘为精气不足，肺肾出纳失常，治予培补摄纳，治重在肺肾，而以肾为主。临床辨证实喘当区别寒热，虚喘需分清阴阳，以确定相应治疗。另外还应注意虚实、寒热的转化互见。对喘证危候，尤当重视急速处理。

复习思考题

1. 如何鉴别虚喘、实喘，试述各型的辨证论治。
2. 寒包火、上实下虚、喘脱如何辨治？
3. 如何理解喘证“在肺为实，在肾为虚”？

肺　　胀

〔概述〕

肺胀是多种慢性肺系疾病反复发作迁延不愈，肺脾肾虚损，而导致肺气壅滞，不能敛降的一种病证。临床表现为胸部膨满，喘咳上气，动后尤甚，胸闷胀满如塞，或伴痰多，心悸，烦躁，甚则面色晦黯，唇舌青紫，脘痞腹胀，颜面四肢浮肿，或发生喘脱等危候。本病病程缠绵，时轻时重，经久难愈。

肺胀的辨证，应首辨虚实标本，次辨证候轻重，并应注意与喘、哮、支饮的联系与区别。治疗上常分痰浊壅肺、痰热阻肺、肺肾气虚、阳虚水泛、痰浊蒙窍五型论治，尤应注意喘脱神昏等危候的预防及救治。

西医的多种肺系疾病，日久合并有肺气肿，甚或发展成慢性肺源性心脏病者，以及老年性肺气肿等，均可参照本篇辨证论治。至于肺性脑病，可按肺胀的危重变证进行相应的急救处理。

〔病因病机〕

一、病因：基本病因有二：一为久病肺虚，一为感受外邪。久病肺虚多由内伤久咳、支饮、哮喘、肺痨等肺系慢性疾患，迁延失治，反复发作，痰浊潴留，日久而致；在肺虚卫外不固的基础上，外邪每易反复乘袭，诱使本病发作。

二、病理：本病病理特点是正虚邪实，虚实夹杂。

（一）正虚主要指肺脾肾虚损，肺为娇脏，不耐邪侵，外合皮毛，开窍于鼻，若长期反复感受外邪，必致肺失宣降而发咳喘；其他慢性肺系疾患如久咳、支饮、哮喘、肺痨等，迁延失治，日久均可致肺虚。肺病久延，子耗母气，脾失健运，则可导致肺脾两虚。若先有脾运不健，停痰于肺，而使肺失宣降，致肺疾久发者，肺脾两虚更易出现。气主于肺而根于肾，金水相生，若肺虚日久，下及肾水，致成肺不主气，肾不纳气，呼多吸少之肺肾俱虚之证。若肾虚在先，如年老体弱、下元虚惫者，罹患肺疾，肺肾两虚更易出现。肺与心、肝有经脉相通，肺气佐心运行血液，肺降肝升共司气机升降，肺虚治节失职，久则病及于心，致心气虚、心阳虚，心阳又根于命门真火，若肾阳不振，更进一步导致心肾阳衰，可以出现喘脱等危候。病及于肝，气机升降不利，肝郁化火，更灼肺金，火郁化风，可见震颤、肉瞤，甚则抽搐等肝风内动之象。

（二）邪实方面：痰浊、水饮、气滞、血瘀常相互影响，兼见同病。痰浊的产生，可由肺虚不能化津，脾虚不能转输，肾虚不能蒸化而成。若复感风寒，可成外寒内饮之证；感受风热或痰郁化热，可成痰热证；痰热内郁，因热动风，也可见肝风内动；或因热动血，而见出血。如痰浊壅盛，阻塞气道，或肺虚不能吸清呼浊，浊邪害清，痰蒙神窍，则可发生烦躁、嗜睡、昏迷等变证。

痰、饮、水同出一源，皆属津液停积而成，又每可相互转化。如阳虚阴盛，气不化津，痰从阴化，为饮为水，饮留上焦，迫肺则咳逆上气。凌心则心悸、气短；痰饮困于中焦，则纳减呕恶，腹胀便溏；饮溢肌肤则为水肿尿少；饮停胸胁则为悬饮。

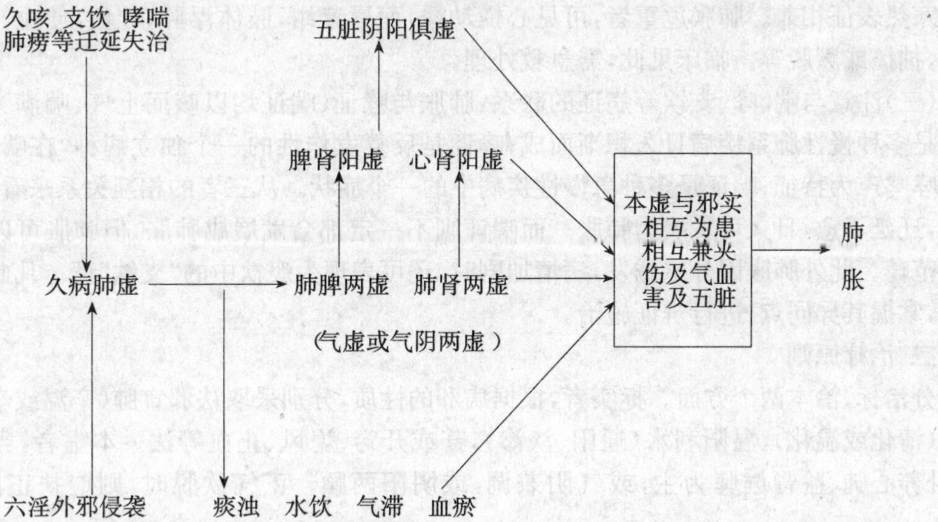

肺气壅滞或久病肺虚，不能治理调节心血的循行，心气、心阳虚衰，无力推动血脉，血流不畅，心血瘀滞，可见心悸，脉结代，唇甲青紫，颈脉动甚。心主血而肝藏血，心脉不利、肝失疏调，

血瘀胁下，则见癥积。肺脾气虚，气不摄血，可致咳血，吐血，便血等。

综上所述，肺胀病位在肺，而与脾、肾关系密切，后期累及心肝。病理性质多属正虚邪实，正虚在肺、脾、肾虚，早期多属肺脾气虚或气阴两虚；病情发展，可致肺、肾、脾、心阳虚，或阴阳两虚。邪实指痰浊、水饮、气滞、血瘀，四者可相互影响和转化，甚或错杂并见，相兼为患。且正虚与邪实多互为因果，如阳气亏虚，易感外邪，痰饮难蠲；阴虚内热者外邪、痰浊易从热化，故虚实之间常相兼并见，每致愈发愈频，甚则咳喘胸憋持续难解。

〔辨证论治〕

一、辨证要点

肺胀一病，是多种慢性肺系疾病积渐而成，以胸部膨满，喘咳上气，动则加剧，胸闷，痰多为其特点，因此仔细询问病史，详其望诊，再结合临床表现，一般不难诊断。辨证时，当掌握以下要点：

(一)辨虚实标本：肺胀总属本虚标实之证，但有偏虚偏实之不同。偏虚者当分清病位所在，五脏之中，何脏受损为主，是一脏虚弱，还是几脏相兼皆虚。肺虚特点是气虚、气阴两虚为主，还是阳虚为主。一般初起多为肺气虚，表现为咳喘短气，易受外邪侵袭；或肺气阴两虚，而见喘咳气短，痰少难咯，舌红，口咽干燥。渐成肺脾气虚，症见喘咳，胸脘胀满，痰多纳呆等；或肺肾两虚，而见呼吸浅短难续，声低气怯，张口抬肩，动则尤剧等。而后致心肾阳虚，易成喘脱之证；脾肾阳虚，易成阳虚水泛之证。偏实者需区别邪浊种类，如痰浊、痰热、水饮、气滞、血瘀等。若有水饮者，水气上逆，可见心悸，气逆浮肿，且胀欲脱；夹有痰浊者，痰浊凝滞可见痰黏难咯；夹有气滞者，气逆胸中，膨膨胀满更甚；夹有瘀血者，面色晦暗，唇舌紫暗，爪甲青紫。并当审有无外感之邪，若有外邪，必有寒热之表证，且肺胀诸症皆因之加剧。辨清正虚与邪实的标本主次，才能更好施治。

(二)辨证候轻重：肺胀若无外邪侵袭，仅见喘咳上气，胸闷胀满，动则加重，病情稳定，证候相对属轻；凡见鼻煽气促，张口抬肩，目胀欲脱，烦躁不安，痰多难咯，即表示病情加重。需注意有无寒热表证相兼。肺胀危重者，可见心慌动悸，面唇紫绀，肢体浮肿，吐血，便血，谵妄，嗜睡昏迷，抽搐或厥脱等。临床见此，需急救处理。

(三)注意与喘、哮、支饮等病证的联系：肺胀与哮证、喘证均以咳而上气、喘满为主症。但肺胀是多种慢性肺系疾病日久积渐而成；哮证是反复发作性的一个独立病种，在喘息之时，喉中有哮鸣声为特征；喘证是多种急慢性疾病中的一个症状。从三者的相互关系来看，哮证反复发作，迁延不愈，日久可发展为肺胀。而喘证则不一定都会发展成肺胀，但肺胀可以隶属于喘证的范畴。此外肺胀因外感诱发，病情加剧时，还可表现为痰饮中的"支饮"证。凡此俱应联系互参，掌握其异同点，进行辨证施治。

二、治疗原则

分治标、治本两个方面。标实者，根据病邪的性质，分别采取祛邪宣肺(辛温或辛凉)、降气化痰(清化或温化)、温阳利水(通阳、淡渗)，甚或开窍、熄风、止血等法。本虚者，当以补益肺脾、补养心肺、益肾健脾为主，或气阴兼调，或阴阳两顾。正气欲脱时，则应扶正固脱，救阴回阳。

三、分型论治

(一)痰浊壅肺

主症：咳喘痰多，色白黏或呈泡沫状。

兼症：短气喘息，稍劳即著，时易汗出，形寒怕风，脘痞纳少，倦怠乏力。

舌脉：舌质偏淡，苔薄腻或浊腻，脉小弦滑。

分析：肺虚脾弱，滋生痰浊，上逆于肺，则咳嗽，痰多色白黏腻；痰从寒化饮，则呈泡沫状。肺气虚弱，肃降无权，气机失畅，复加痰气交阻，故短气喘息，稍劳尤著。肺虚卫表不固则怕风，时易汗出。肺病及脾，脾气虚弱，健运失常，故见脘痞纳少，倦怠乏力。舌质偏淡，苔薄腻，脉小弦滑，是肺脾气虚，痰浊内蕴之象。

治法：化痰降气，健脾益肺。

方药：苏子降气汤、三子养亲汤、六君子汤加减。前二方功能降气化痰平喘，但苏子降气汤偏温，以痰湿壅盛，下元不足，上盛下虚相兼，寒痰喘咳为宜；三子养亲汤偏降气，化痰，消食，以肺实喘满，痰多涌盛，胸痞纳呆，痰多黏腻为宜。六君子汤健脾燥湿化痰，偏补，以脾虚兼有痰湿者为宜，也可作为症情稳定后的调治方。

加减：痰多胸满而不能平卧者，可加葶苈子以泻肺祛痰平喘；若痰从寒化为饮，又为外感风寒所诱发，喘咳痰多黏白泡沫，见表寒里饮证者，宜改用小青龙汤以解表化饮；若饮郁化热，烦躁而喘，脉浮，宜小青龙加石膏汤兼清郁热。

处方举例：

炙麻黄 4g、杏仁 10g、化橘红 10g、茯苓 10g、半夏 10g、苏子 10g、白芥子 3g、炒莱菔子 10g、生甘草 5g。

（二）痰热郁肺

主症：咳逆喘息气粗，痰黄，黏白难咯。

兼症：烦躁，胸满，或身热微恶寒，有汗或无汗，尿黄，便干，口渴。

舌脉：舌红苔薄黄或黄腻，脉数或滑数。

分析：痰浊内蕴化热，痰热壅肺，故痰黄，黏白难咯；肺热内郁，清肃失司，肺气上逆，则喘咳气逆息粗；痰热交阻胸中，故烦躁，胸满；热移大肠、膀胱，故见便干，尿黄。复感外邪，风热犯肺，故见发热微恶寒，有汗不多等表证。口渴，舌红，苔黄腻，脉滑数均为痰热内郁之象。

治法：清肺化痰，降逆平喘。

方药：越婢加半夏汤、桑白皮汤加减。前方宣肺泄热，用于饮热郁肺，外有表邪，喘咳上气，目如脱状，身热，脉浮大；后方清肺化痰，用于痰热壅肺，喘急胸满，咳吐痰黄，或黏白稠厚者。

加减：若痰热内盛，痰胶黏不易咯吐者，可加鱼腥草、瓜蒌皮、海蛤粉、风化硝等以清热化痰利肺；若肺气上逆，痰气交阻甚者，症见痰鸣喘息，不得平卧，可加射干、葶苈子等以泻肺平喘；若痰热伤津，口干舌燥，可加花粉、知母、芦根等以生津润燥；若见阴伤而痰量不多者，酌减苦寒之药物，加沙参、麦冬、元参等以养阴。

处方举例：

炙麻黄 3g、杏仁 10g、生石膏 30g(先下)、生甘草 5g、清半夏 6g、黄芩 10g、瓜蒌 30g(先下)、桑白皮 10g、贝母 10g。

（三）肺肾气虚

主症：呼吸浅短难续，动则喘促更甚。

兼症：喘甚则张口抬肩，倚息不能平卧，声低气怯，咳嗽，痰白如沫，咯吐不利，胸闷，心慌，形寒汗出。

舌脉：舌淡紫或舌淡而有瘀斑，脉沉细数无力，或有结代。

分析：肺为气之主，肾为气之根，肺肾两虚，不能主气、纳气，故呼吸浅短难续，张口抬肩，不能平卧，声低气怯。寒饮伏肺，肾虚水泛则咳痰色白如沫，咯吐不利。肺病及心，心气虚弱，故心慌动悸，形寒、汗出。肺失治节，气不帅血，气滞血瘀，则见舌淡或黯紫、脉沉细虚数或结代。

治法：补肺纳肾，降气平喘。

方药：平喘固本汤、补肺汤加减。前方补肺纳肾，降气化痰，用于肺肾气虚，喘咳有痰者；后方功在补肺益气，用于肺气虚弱，喘咳短气不足以息者。药用党参（人参）、黄芪、炙甘草补肺，冬虫夏草、熟地、胡桃肉、坎脐（或紫河车粉）益肾，五味子敛肺气，灵磁石、沉香纳气归元，紫菀、款冬、苏子、半夏、橘红化痰降气。

加减：若肺虚有寒，怕冷，舌淡，可加肉桂、干姜、钟乳石以温肺气；若兼有阴伤，而见低热，舌红苔少，可加麦冬、玉竹、生地等以养肺肾之阴；若肺肾阴虚，湿痰内盛，咳喘痰多呕恶者，可用金水六君煎加减，方中归地以滋阴，二陈汤以化痰；若气虚血瘀，见口唇指甲青紫，颈脉动甚，可加丹参、当归、桂枝、红花、苏木等活血通脉。

若见喘脱危象，汗出，肢冷，心悸气促，或烦躁不安，脉细欲绝，喘逆倚息不得卧，张口抬肩鼻煽者，急用参附汤送服蛤蚧粉或黑锡丹以补气纳肾，回阳固脱，待病情稳定后，可常服皱肺丸。

处方举例：

党参 10g、麦冬 10g、五味子 10g、生黄芪 12g、补骨脂 10g、熟地 12g、陈皮 10g、当归 10g、紫菀 10g、款冬花 10g。

（四）阳虚水泛

主症：喘咳上气，面目、下肢、甚则一身悉肿。

兼症：咳痰清稀，脘痞，纳呆，尿少，怕冷，心悸，腹部胀满或有水，面唇青紫。

舌脉：苔白滑，舌胖质黯，脉沉细。

分析：肺脾肾阳气衰微，肺无通降之力，脾乏转输之职，肾失蒸化之权，导致气不化水，水液停积，成痰成饮，水邪泛滥肌肤则面目肢体浮肿。水凌心肺故心悸，喘咳，咯痰清稀。水饮内停则脘痞腹胀纳呆。心阳被遏，阳虚血瘀则面唇青紫，舌质黯。肾阳不足，膀胱气化不利故尿少，怕冷。舌胖，苔白滑，脉沉细都是阳虚水停之征。

治法：温肾健脾，化饮利水。

方药：真武汤合五苓散加减。前方温阳利水，用于脾肾阳虚之水肿；后方通阳利水，配合真武汤可加强利尿消肿的作用。药用附子、桂枝温肾通阳，茯苓、白术、猪苓、泽泻、生姜健脾利水，赤芍同附子同用，能入阴破结。

加减：若水肿较甚，喘促加剧，可加葶苈子、沉香、万年青根等以泻肺定喘，强心利水；若血瘀甚，紫绀明显加泽兰、红花、桃仁、益母草以活血化瘀利水。

处方举例：

炮附片 10g、白术 10g、桂枝 10g、茯苓 30g、泽泻 15g、猪苓 15g、党参 10g、葶苈子 10g、益母草 15g、生姜 3 片。

（五）痰蒙神窍

主症：咳逆喘促，神志恍惚。

兼症：谵语，烦躁不安，撮空理线，表情淡漠，嗜睡，昏迷，或肢体瞤动，抽搐，咳痰不爽。

舌脉：苔白腻或黄腻，舌质暗红或淡紫或红绛，脉细数滑。

分析：痰迷心窍，蒙蔽神机，故见神志恍惚，谵妄，躁烦，撮空理线，嗜睡、昏迷。肝风内动则肢体瞤动，抽搐。肺虚痰蕴故咳逆喘促而咯痰不爽。苔白腻或淡黄腻，脉细滑数为痰浊内蕴之象。舌暗红或淡紫乃心血瘀阻之征；舌红绛为血分蕴热。

治法：降痰开窍，平肝熄风。

方药：选用涤痰汤加减，另服安宫牛黄丸或至宝丹。涤痰汤方中半夏、茯苓、橘红、胆星涤痰熄风；竹茹、枳实清热化痰利膈；菖蒲开窍化痰；痰盛正气未衰时方中人参、甘草可不用。本方具有涤痰开窍、熄风止痉之功，用于痰迷心窍，风痰内盛，神识昏蒙，嗜睡，痰多，肢体瞤动者最宜。至宝丹或安宫牛黄丸以清心开窍。

加减：若痰热内盛，身热，烦躁，谵语，神昏，大便秘结，苔黄腻者，可用凉膈散加天竺黄、竹沥等清化痰热等。方中大黄、朴硝有清下燥热之功；栀子、黄芩清热泻火；重用连翘清热解毒；配伍薄荷、竹叶清肺胃心胸之热；再以白蜜、甘草缓其急迫。总之本方"以下为清"。为了注意保存津液，还可在凉膈散基础上加用增液汤以通腑泄浊，肃降肺气。

若肝风内动，抽搐，可加钩藤、全蝎，另服羚羊角粉以平肝熄风。若血瘀明显，唇甲青紫，加丹参、红花、桃仁等活血通脉。

若皮肤黏膜出血、咯血、便血色鲜者，配清热凉血止血药，如水牛角、生地、丹皮、紫珠草等。

处方举例：

橘红 10g、半夏 10g、茯苓 12g、胆星 8g、菖蒲 10g、郁金 10g、连翘 10g、丹参 15g、枳实 10g、竹沥水 10g(兑入)。

本病的预后转归，与体质、年龄、病程及治疗的及时与否均有关系。一般说来，由于本病不单纯是一脏之病，病情比较复杂，多属积渐而成，病程缠绵，经常反复发作，难以根治。临证所见，尤其是老年患者，发病后若不及时控制，极易发生变端。如肺失治节而心血瘀阻，心慌悸动，脉促结；气不摄血而咳吐泡沫血痰，或吐血、便血；痰迷心窍则谵妄、嗜睡、昏迷，肝风内动而震颤、抽搐；或见喘肿，喘脱等危重证候。

〔预防及护理措施〕

在预防方面，主要是防止和彻底治疗引起本病的原发病。因此增强体质和抗病能力，是防治肺胀的根本方法。肺胀在发作期要及时控制症状，使其缓解，以免加重。在缓解期要扶正固本，增强正气。既病之人，更应注意保暖，秋冬季节，气候变化之际，尤需避免感受外邪。一经发病，立即治疗，以免加重。另外还需加强呼吸锻炼、太极拳、步行等，才能增进身体的健康；并应忌烟酒及辛辣、生冷、咸、甜之品。有水肿者应进低盐或无盐饮食。

〔典型病例分析〕

案一：娄某，男，61 岁。因咳嗽哮喘十余年，加重一月于 1972 年 12 月 1 日收入院。

现病史：患慢性咳喘 10 余年，冬重夏轻，反复发作，饮冷及暑气均易诱发本病。初用青链霉素、强的松、苯海拉明、麻黄素等药可获暂安，后药量渐大而效反差。近因天气寒冷病情加重，于 12 月 1 日因咳喘肢肿急入院。X 线检查：两肺纹理粗糙，透明度增强，右心扩大，横膈下移。诊为"慢性支气管炎、肺气肿、肺心病合并右心衰竭"。用以上西药无效，始改中药。

现症：端坐呼吸，咳嗽哮喘，张口抬肩，神志恍惚，两颊暗红，颈静脉怒张，口唇紫绀喉中痰鸣，周身凉汗，下肢浮肿，饮食难进。查肝下界剑突下 9 厘米，舌质青紫，苔薄白稍腻，脉虚大而数。

证属肾衰阳微，水气射肺凌心型肺胀、喘证。治宜补肾纳气，回阳固脱，用阳和汤加减。处方：麻黄 3g、熟地 18g、鹿角霜 12g、肉桂 10g、附子 10g、山茱萸 15g、硫磺 2g、钟乳石 12g、沉香 10g、龙骨 12g、牡蛎 12g、人参 6g、山药 12g、五味子 15g，一剂，急煎服。

二诊(12 月 2 日)：服后已能平卧，喘息已缓，冷汗已止，四肢转温，稍进稀粥。余证及舌脉同上。药之有效，上方 6g 人参加至 9g，续服二剂。

三诊(12 月 4 日)：患者精神复正，喘息已平，唇舌紫绀已减，颈静脉怒张好转，肝大稍减，舌青黯好转，脉已有根，仍予上方六剂。

四诊(12 月 11 日)：患者喘止，食欲增大、肢肿消退，体力渐复，并下床活动，口唇发绀消失，舌质淡红，苔薄白，六脉和缓，肝大缩小至剑突下一横指。症状基本消失，肿消阳复。考虑病久体弱，守原方倍量，炼蜜为丸(每丸重 9g，早晚各服 1 丸，连服 2 月)巩固疗效。药后即恢复轻微劳动。至今 9 年，每冬虽有咳嗽吐痰，但症状很轻。

按：本病属肺肾气衰，心阳欲脱之肺胀急证，尽管有咳嗽、喘息、水肿等复杂症状，但首宜温壮下元，益气固脱以救险情。故用甘温力宏之人参大补心脾肾之元气，以固后天；配附子、硫磺、钟乳石、肉桂大辛大热之品，可温壮肾阳；沉香纳气归肾，引气归元；龙骨、牡蛎、五味子平敛浮越之阳，尤用大量熟地，佐其大队温热之味，实有阴阳互根、阴中求阳之意；麻黄辛温，取其宣肺平喘之功而治其标，但用量要小。诸药配伍，上补心肺，下补肾命，中健脾土，不用利尿药则肿消，不用镇咳药则喘平。本方非独壮阳挽危于一时，更能补中健身，以消咳喘宿痰，实为制方之妙。(选自《河南省名老中医经验集锦·喘证》)

肺胀是由多种慢性肺系疾病反复发作，迁延不愈，后期转归而成。临床以喘咳上气，胸闷胀满，动后喘甚等为主症，病久或感受外邪使病情加重，可见面唇青紫，身肿，甚侧昏迷、抽搐以致喘脱等危重证候。根据其临床表现，与咳嗽、喘证、痰饮、心悸、水肿、喘厥、喘脱等证有关。

肺胀以久病肺虚为主，由于反复感邪，而使病情进行性加重。病位在肺，而与脾、肾关系密切，后期可及心、肝。病理性质多由气虚、气阴两虚发展为阳虚，在本虚的基础上，又形成痰浊、水饮、气滞、血瘀等病理产物。标本虚实相互兼挟或相互影响，最后因邪盛正虚、而发生诸端变证，甚或危及生命。

肺胀的辨证，首先要辨虚实标本，再辨证候轻重，并注意与喘、哮、支饮等证的联系互参。治疗当抓治标、治本两方面。感邪时偏于邪实，平时偏于正虚，据此有侧重地分别选用扶正与祛邪的不同治法。

临床常见痰浊壅肺、痰热阻肺、肺肾气虚、阳虚水泛、痰浊蒙窍等五个证候型，各证常可互相兼夹转化。临证既要掌握其各型证候特点，又要根据其错杂表现灵活施治。其中肺肾气虚、痰蒙神窍、阳虚水泛尤为危重，如不及时控制则预后不良。

老年、久病体虚的后期患者，每因感邪使病情恶化，但因正气衰竭，无力抗邪，正邪交争之象并不明显，故凡近期内咳喘突然加剧，痰色变黄，舌质变红，虽无发热恶寒表证，亦要考虑有外邪的存在。还应注意痰的色、质、量等变化，结合全身情况，综合判断，及时治疗。

复习思考题

1. 试述肺胀的概念。
2. 试述肺胀的发生基础及病理机制。怎样理解其本虚与邪实两个方面？
3. 临床常见肺胀的五个证型是什么？怎样辨证论治？哪些证型预后不良？

痰 饮

〔概述〕

痰饮是指水液在体内运化输布失常，停积于某些部位的一类病证。本病多由外感寒湿、饮食不节、阳气虚弱等原因，导致肺脾肾功能失常所引起，其中尤以脾阳不运为发病之关键。痰饮之为病，随处留积，走于肠间，则沥沥有声；留于胁下，则咳唾引痛；溢于四肢，则身体疼重；上迫于肺，则咳逆倚息，短气不得卧。

痰与饮同为水液输化失常的产物，然痰黏稠，饮清稀，饮积可以生痰，二者既有区别又有联系。痰饮并称实指饮证，其有广义、狭义之分。广义痰饮为诸饮之总称，包括《金匮要略》中所分的四饮，即痰饮、悬饮、溢饮、支饮；狭义痰饮为四饮中的一个证候。至于留饮、伏饮，则因饮邪留而不去、伏而不出而命名，包括在四饮之内。

早在《内经》即有"饮"、"积饮"之说，并指出水湿过盛，脾阳不运为本证的主要病理。张仲景首创痰饮病名，并列专篇对痰饮病的分类、证候、治法、方药进行了详细的论述，成为后世对痰饮病辨证论治的重要依据；特别是"病痰饮者，当以温药和之"的治疗大法一直被后世奉为治寒痰水饮的准绳。其后历代医家各有发挥，丰富和发展了本病的理论和治法。

饮证的病机关键为肺脾肾气化功能失调，病理性质总属阳虚阴盛，因虚致实。中阳素虚，脏气不足，为本病发生的内在病理基础。本病辨证当辨部位，分虚实，审兼夹证。并当鉴别痰、饮、水、湿的区别与联系，溢饮与风水之不同，支饮、伏饮与肺胀、哮症、喘症的关系。治疗总以温化为原则，当分标本缓急与表里虚实，分别采取相应的治疗。

西医的慢性支气管炎、支气管哮喘、渗出性胸膜炎、胃肠功能紊乱及不完全性幽门梗阻、肠梗阻等，在疾病的某些阶段，其临床表现与痰饮病相类似者，可参考本章进行辨证论治。

〔病因病机〕

饮证的成因为感受寒湿，饮食不当，或劳欲所伤。三者互为影响，致使肺脾肾的功能失调，三焦不利，水谷不得化为精微，输布周身，水湿停积而变生痰饮。

一、外感寒湿：凡气候湿冷，或冒雨涉水，经常坐卧湿地，水湿之邪侵袭卫表，卫外之阳先伤，肺气不得宣布，湿邪浸渍肌肉，由表及里困遏脾胃之气化功能，致水湿停滞，积而成饮。

二、饮食所伤：胃为水谷之海，脾司健运之职，暴饮过量之水，或有茶癖之人；或夏暑及酒后恣饮冷水，恣食生冷之物；因热伤冷，冷与热结，中阳暴遏，脾不能运，停而为饮。

三、劳欲所伤：水液属阴，全赖阳气以转输蒸化，劳倦、纵欲太过，或久病体虚，年高气弱，脾肾之阳不足，水液失于输化，亦能停而成饮，一旦伤于水湿，更易停蓄致病。

在正常生理情况下，水液的输化、排泄，主要依赖肺、脾、肾三脏的气化功能。肺居上焦，有宣化、通调水液的作用；脾居中焦有运化转输水谷精微的功能；肾处下焦，有温化蒸腾水液，分清泌浊的职责。通过肺的通调下降，脾的转输上行，肾的蒸化开阖以共同完成水液吸收、运行、排泄的整个过程。《素问·经脉别论》所说："饮入于胃，游溢精气，上输于脾，脾气散精，上归于肺，通调水道，下输膀胱，水精四布，五经并行。"即指出在水液代谢过程中，肺、脾、肾三脏为不可分割的三个环节。如三脏功能失调，肺之通调涩滞，脾之转输无权，肾之蒸化失职，则三脏相互影响，导致水液停积为饮，三脏之中，脾运失司，首当其要，因脾阳一虚，则上不能输精以养肺,水谷不从正化,反为痰饮而干肺,下不能助肾以制水,水寒之气反伤肾阳,由此导致水液内停中焦,流溢各处,波及五脏。

水液运行的道路为三焦,由于三焦外连躯壳,内及脏腑,贯通机体的内外上下,水谷精微必假三焦以布散于全身,所以三脏气化功能正常则三焦通利,否则三焦气涩,水道壅滞,不得宣行,也致水液停积为饮,流溢为害。故《圣济总录·痰饮统论》说:“三焦者,水谷之道路,气之所终始也。三焦调适,气脉平匀,则能宣通水液,行入于经,化而为血,灌溉周身;若三焦气塞,脉道壅闭,则水饮停积,不得宣行,聚成痰饮。”

综上所述,在各种内外因的作用下,肺脾肾气化功能失调,为饮证发生的关键所在。因肺脾肾三脏气化不行则三焦水道壅闭,蓄而成饮。

饮证论其病理性质总属阳虚阴盛,输化失调,因虚致实,水液停积为患。因水为阴类,非阳不化,若阳气虚衰,气不化津则阴邪偏盛,寒饮内停,故中阳素虚,脏气不足,实为本病发病的内在病理基础。饮证以寒证居多,间或有时邪与内饮相搏,或饮邪久郁化热,表现寒热错杂之候,究属少数。

痰饮病因病机示意图

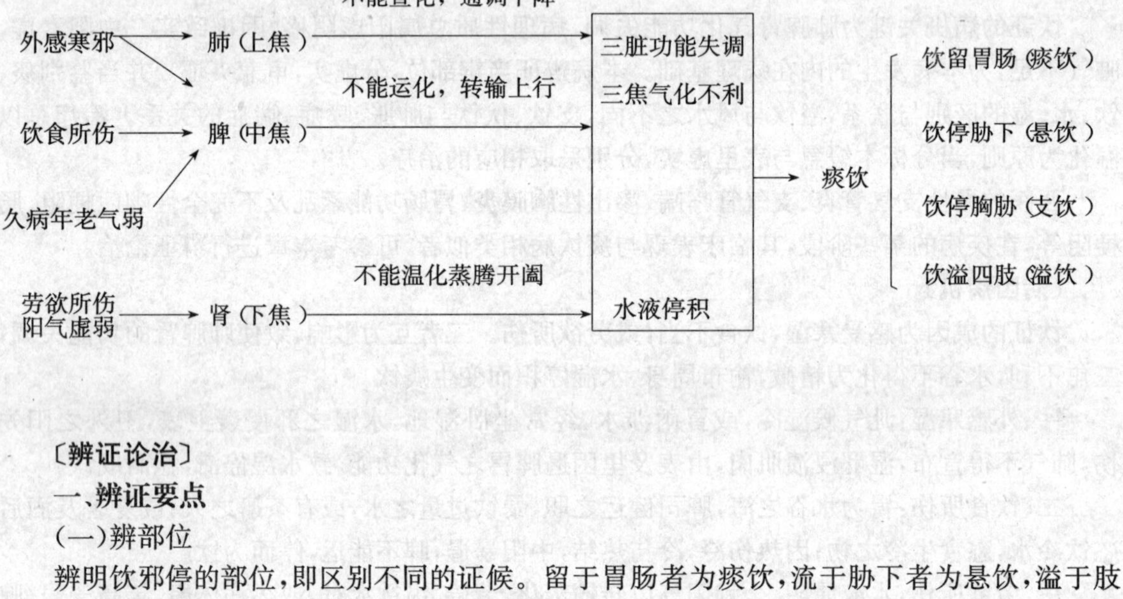

〔辨证论治〕

一、辨证要点

(一)辨部位

辨明饮邪停的部位,即区别不同的证候。留于胃肠者为痰饮,流于胁下者为悬饮,溢于肢体者为溢饮,聚于胸胁者为支饮。

(二)辨虚实

痰饮为有形之物,正气亏虚之处,即为饮邪停留之所,本虚标实为其病理基础,临床多见虚实相兼之候,应从起病新久、饮邪之盛衰、禀赋之强弱权衡虚实之偏胜,如新病饮盛为实,久病正虚、饮微为虚。

(三)辨兼夹证

痰饮虽为阴邪,寒证居多,但郁久也有化热者,当从口渴否、二便等症及舌脉来辨识有无夹热。初起若有寒热见证,多夹表邪,再当区分表寒表热,饮积不化,气机升降受阻,常夹气滞。饮聚日久,气滞血瘀或气虚血瘀,又可有夹瘀见症。

二、鉴别诊断

(一)湿、水、饮、痰的区别与联系

湿水饮痰四者同出一源,俱为津液不归正化,停积而成。分别言之,源虽同而流则异,其各有不同特点(相对的)。从自身形质言,饮为稀涎,痰多厚浊;水属清液,湿性黏滞而无定体。从病症言,饮之为病,多停于体内局部,如胃肠、胸胁、胁下、四肢等;痰湿为病,无处不到,变化多端;水之为病,可泛溢肌肤全身,多流聚于低下或松弛部位。从病理性质而言,饮主要因阳虚阴寒积聚而成;痰可有寒热之别,寒痰与水饮相类,而热痰则因热煎熬津液而成;水属阴类,又由于发病原因之不同而分阳水、阴水;湿为阴邪,可有寒热、表里之不同转化,故临床有寒湿、湿热,在表皮肤为患,在里脏腑气血为患。

合而言之,因四者源出一体,在一定条件下又可相互转化。

论其治疗,水饮一般都治以温运。至于合邪,则另当别论。痰、湿当先明其寒热,再以温化或清化,以图示之:

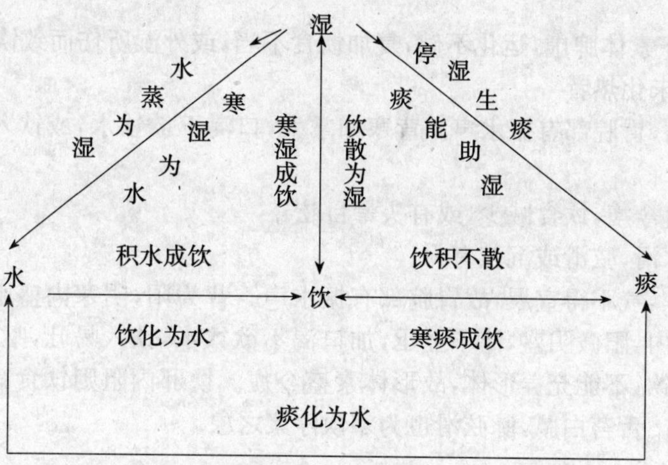

(二)溢饮与风水当互参

溢饮也可属水气病之类,如《医宗金鉴·金匮要略注痰饮咳嗽病》说:"溢饮者……即今之风水水肿病也。"但溢饮属水泛溢于四肢肌肤而成肿者,多伴有身体疼痛而沉重,肿以四肌明显,小便可自利,恶寒无汗,多伴有喘咳痰多白沫,胸闷等饮邪犯肺的表现,若内有郁热,表寒外束,则伴有咳喘发热烦躁。而风水泛溢,则眼睑浮肿为初,继而迅速溢及四肢、全身,小便不利,可伴有表寒、表热、表虚等不同见症。

(三)支饮、伏饮与肺胀、哮症、喘症的关系

肺胀在急性发病阶段可以表现支饮症候。喘证的肺寒、痰浊两类又常具支饮的特点。哮证的发作期与伏饮基本类同。如陈修园即认为"膈上伏饮,俗谓哮喘"。为此应对照互参。支饮与伏饮是从病理角度命名,而肺胀、哮、喘则根据病症特点为名,支饮、伏饮是肺胀、哮、喘的一个证候,或出现于病的某一阶段。肺胀病是肺系多种慢性疾病日久渐积而成;喘证可见于多种急慢性疾病的病程中;哮证是反复发作性病证。哮证、喘证、肺胀在发病中,又可以产生饮邪。

三、治则要点

1. 饮证总属阳微阴盛,本虚标实之候,治疗总以温化为原则。饮为阴邪,遇寒则聚,得温

则行，不仅阳虚饮邪不盛者应与温化，而在饮邪盛实而用逐饮、利水、发汗三剂时，亦均应佐以温药。

2. 治疗饮证还当分别标本缓急，根据表里虚实的不同，采取相应的处理。水饮壅盛者，祛邪治标；阳微气虚者，温阳治本。在表者宜温散发汗，在里者宜温化利水。正虚者宜补，邪实者当攻。如属邪实正虚，治当消补兼施。饮热相杂者又当温凉并用。

3.《医门法律·痰饮留伏论》提出虚实分治之法，可作为饮证辨治的要领，凡饮邪壅实者，根据饮停部位，分别治以攻逐、利水、发汗等法，因势利导，以祛除饮邪。阳虚饮微者，治以健脾温肾，阳气通则饮邪自化。即便实证，当饮邪基本消除后，如正气虚，亦需继用健脾温肾之剂，以固其本，饮邪久郁体内，易化热，夹气滞、血瘀，治当在温化中用清热、利气、活血化瘀之品。饮伏于内最易外感，当分清夹表寒、表热，夹表寒者宜加用温散，夹表热者宜加清解之品。

四、分型论治

(一)实证

1. 痰饮：多由于素体脾虚，运化不健，复加饮食不当，或外湿所伤而致饮留胃肠。

(1)饮停于胃，未化热者

主症：胸满脘痞，胃脘部有振水声。背寒如掌大，口渴不欲饮水，或饮入易吐，呕吐清水或稀涎。

兼症：形体素盛今瘦，饮食减少，或有头晕目眩。

舌脉：舌苔白水滑，弦滑或沉弦有力。

分析：饮停中焦，气不得宣展，故胃脘部有振水声。背为阳，阴寒内盛阳气不得外达，加背寒如掌大。饮伏于内，阳微阴盛，津不上承，加口渴不欲饮水，饮入易吐，呕吐清水或痰涎。水谷不化精微而成水饮，不能充养形体，故形体素盛今瘦。饮邪内阻则饮食减少。清阳不升，痰浊上犯则头晕目眩。舌苔白腻，脉弦滑也为寒饮停聚之象。

治法：温阳利水。

方药：以苓桂术甘汤为主方加味。方中桂枝、甘草、白术通阳运脾，茯苓淡渗除湿。

加减：呕吐者加半夏、生姜和胃降逆；头目眩晕者合泽泻汤渗湿升阳；胸脘痞满难忍者，或合枳术丸以下气开痞，或合平胃散以理气燥湿和胃。

处方举例：

茯苓20g、桂枝10g、苍术10g、生甘草6g、半夏10g、陈皮10g、生姜3片。

(2)饮停于胃肠，已化热者

主症：脘腹坚满而痛，自利，虽利心下续坚满，或水走肠间，沥沥有声，腹满，便秘，口干舌燥。

兼症：轻型所见诸症均可见。

舌脉：苔腻或白或黄，脉沉弦或伏。

分析：饮伏于胃肠，饮邪壅盛，故脘腹坚满而痛，虽利下而新饮又生，饮势不变，故虽下利而心下仍坚满。饮邪从胃下流于肠，则肠间沥沥有声。饮郁化热，大肠壅塞故腹满便秘，口干舌燥苔黄。舌脉亦为饮邪壅盛之征。

治法：攻逐水饮。

方药：分别选甘遂半夏汤或己椒苈黄丸治本。前方攻守兼施，因势利导，用于水饮在胃，取甘遂、半夏逐饮降逆；白芍、蜂蜜酸甘缓中，以防伤正；借遂草相反相激，祛逐留饮。后方苦辛宣泻，前后分消，用于水饮在肠，饮郁化热之证，药用大黄、葶苈、攻坚决壅，泻下逐水，防己、椒目辛宣苦泻，导水利尿。

加减：脘腹胀满甚者加枳实、厚朴以泻满。虽为饮邪壅盛，但不能徒快一时，攻逐太过，损伤正气。

处方举例：

水饮在胃：甘遂面冲服1～2g、半夏10g、白芍10g、蜂蜜兑入10g、甘草5g。

水饮在肠，饮郁化热：防己12g、川椒5g、葶苈子10g、生大黄3～5g、枳实6g、厚朴6g。

2. 悬饮：多因素体不强，或原有其他慢性疾病，肺虚卫弱，时邪外袭，肺失宣通，饮停胸胁。

主症：胸胁胀痛，唾咳呼吸及转侧时疼痛加重，病侧胸胁饱满。

兼症：多伴有寒热往来，身热起伏，或午后潮热，口苦咽干等，水饮留聚则可见胸闷不舒，呼吸不畅，或有闷咳等，日久或见有口干咽燥，潮热，盗汗，颧红，心烦，手足心热等。

舌脉：初期舌苔白或微黄，脉弦数。后期舌质偏红或暗，少苔，脉小数。

分析：胸胁受邪，肺气郁滞，气不布津，停而为饮，胸胁为气机升降之道，脉络受阻，故有胸胁胀痛，咳唾胸痛，呼吸不畅，或有闷咳等络气不和表现。肺居胸中，两胁为少阳经脉分布循行之处，邪犯胸胁，少阳枢机不和，则见寒热往来起伏，口苦咽干，饮郁阴伤或有午后潮热等。饮郁化热，阴伤肺燥，故见口干咽燥，潮热盗汗，颧红心烦等阴虚内热表现。舌脉也为饮停水结，气滞络阻或饮郁伤阴之象。

治法：泻肺降气，攻逐水饮。

方药：以椒目瓜蒌汤加减，配服十枣汤或控涎丹。前方以葶苈子、桑白皮泻肺逐饮，以苏子、瓜蒌皮、陈皮、半夏降气化痰，椒目、茯苓、生姜皮利水导饮，白蒺藜引药入两胁，且平肝以助肺降。十枣汤、控涎丹为攻逐水饮之剂，十枣汤力峻，体实证实、积饮量多、正气未衰者用之，取甘遂、大戟、芫花研面，大枣煎汤送下，空腹顿服。控涎丹药力较缓，反应较轻，系十枣汤去芫花加白芥子为丸，善去皮里膜外之痰水，有宣肺理气之功。后两方均宜从小量开始递增，连服3～5日，必要时停止2～3天再服。如呕吐、腹痛，腹泻过剧，即应减量或停服。

加减：若痰浊偏甚，胸部满闷，舌苔浊腻加薤白、杏仁宣化痰浊水饮；如水饮久停难去，胸胁支满，体弱，食少者，加苓桂术甘汤等通阳健脾化饮，不宜再予以竣攻。若正虚邪实，逐水同时可用葶苈大枣泻肺汤合三子养亲汤加味以降气祛饮。

悬饮初起伴有往来寒热等少阳枢机不利证，可以柴枳半夏汤加减，本方涤痰开结，和解清热，药用柴胡、黄芩和解清热，瓜蒌、半夏、杏仁化痰开始，枳壳、桔梗、赤芍理气和络，甘草调和诸药。

饮邪久郁，气机不利，而致络脉不和，见胸胁刺痛者，可用香附旋覆花汤，本方理气化痰和络，药用旋覆花、苏子、杏仁、半夏、苡仁、茯苓降气化痰，香附、陈皮理气解郁，刺痛甚加归须、赤芍、桃仁、红花、乳香、没药。水饮不降加通草、路路通、冬瓜皮等。

饮邪久停之后，气郁化热伤阴，出现阴虚内热见症时，可用泻白散合沙参麦冬汤，药用桑皮、地骨皮清肺降火，沙参、麦冬、玉竹、天花粉等养阴生津。潮热加鳖甲、功劳叶，咳嗽配百部、川贝母，闷痛甚加瓜篓、枳壳、郁金、丝瓜络，停饮未尽加牡蛎、泽泻，兼有气虚神疲者加太子参、黄芪、五味子。

处方举例：

川椒目50粒，瓜蒌15g、桑白皮10g、葶苈子10g、苏子5g、半夏5g、茯苓12g、橘红5g、白蒺藜10g、生姜3片。

3. 支饮：多由受寒饮冷，久咳致喘，迁延反复伤肺，肺气不能布津，阳虚不运，饮邪留伏犯肺。

主症：咳逆喘满不得卧，痰吐白沫量多，往往历年不愈，天冷受寒加重。

兼症：甚者伴有颜面、足踝浮肿，受寒引发时，或有寒热表证。

舌脉：舌苔白腻，脉弦紧。

分析：饮邪上逆犯肺，肺气不除，故咳喘不能卧，痰多白沫。饮邪恋肺，因而久病不愈。饮为阴邪故受寒每易诱发。水饮泛滥则面浮肢肿，伏饮因新寒触发，故见外寒束表之证。舌苔白腻或白滑，脉弦紧为寒饮内盛之征。

治法：温肺化饮。

方药：小青龙汤加减。本方有温里发表之功，用于支饮遇寒触发内饮外寒之证。药用麻黄、桂枝、干姜、细辛温肺散寒，半夏、甘草等化痰利气，佐以五味子、白芍，使散中有收。

加减：体虚表证不著者，可改用苓甘五味姜辛汤；饮多寒少外无表证，喘咳（盛）痰盛不得卧，可用葶苈大枣泻肺汤；痰多黏腻，胸满气逆配白芥子、莱菔子降气豁痰，或用桑苏桂苓饮以降气化痰，温阳祛饮，方用桑皮、苏子、半夏、大腹皮、杏仁下气，桂枝、橘皮温阳理气，猪茯苓、泽兰利水饮。

若饮邪入郁化热，正虚邪实，阳为阴遏，而见喘满胸闷，心下痞坚，烦渴，面色黧黑，苔黄而腻，脉沉紧，可以木防己汤行水散结，补虚清热。水邪结实者去石膏加茯苓、芒硝导水破结。

处方举例：

麻黄4g、桃杏仁各10g、桑白皮10g、苏子10g、桂枝3g、猪茯苓各10g、半夏8g、生甘草4g。

4. 溢饮：多因外感风寒，玄府闭塞，以致肺脾输布失职，水饮流溢四肢肌肤。

主症：身体疼痛而沉重，甚则肢体浮肿。

兼症：多兼有恶寒无汗，或喘咳痰多白沫，口不渴，胸闷。

舌脉：苔白，脉弦紧。

分析：水饮流溢四肢体表，则身体重疼浮肿。风寒束表故恶寒无汗。寒饮内伏，上逆迫肺，则喘咳，痰多白沫，胸闷，口不渴。苔白脉弦紧为表里俱寒之象。

治法：发表化饮。

方药：小青龙汤或麻杏苡甘汤加减。前方发表温里，后方解表祛湿去饮，也可用麻黄加术汤以解表健脾祛除水饮。

加减：若尿少可加茯苓、猪苓、泽泻等利水祛饮。若伴有发热、烦躁、苔白兼黄，为表寒外束，内有郁热，可加生石膏以清热；寒象不著，去干姜，细辛，处方改用大青龙汤或越婢加术汤以发表清里。表证不明显，肢疼胸闷，纳呆明显，可以神术散，本方为祛湿化饮和胃之剂。

处方举例：

桂枝6g、猪茯苓各10g、苍白术各10g、生苡仁20g、杏仁10g、生姜3片、泽泻10g、麻黄6g。

（二）虚证

1. 脾阳虚弱：多为脾虚，健运无力，又为外湿或饮食所伤而致，或饮邪经治后，衰其大半，正虚明显。

主症：胸胁支满，脘腹喜暖喜按，时时呕吐清水痰涎，心悸气短，头目眩晕。

兼症：背寒，胃中有振水声，呕逆喘满，或有晨起睑肿，午后下肢浮肿。

舌脉：苔白滑舌体胖，脉弦细而滑。

分析：脾不健运，正常水液失于输布，停留在胸胁则胸胁支满，停于胃肠则胃肠有振水声。呕吐清水稀涎，水饮上凌心肺则心悸气短；上犯清窍则头目眩晕。舌苔白滑，舌体胖，脉弦细而滑均为内有水饮，脾气虚弱，脾阳不振。

治法：温中健脾化饮。

方药：理中丸加味。若阳虚阴盛者，可加附子、吴茱萸、肉桂以温阳散寒；若呕吐稀涎量多，可合五苓散温阳化饮；若饮不明显，以脾虚为主，可服香砂六君子汤。

处方举例：

人参粉冲 3g、茯苓 10g、桂枝 10g、白术 10g、炙甘草 6g、法半夏 10g、化橘红 10g、肉桂 5g、干姜 6g、生姜 3 片。

2. 肾阳虚衰：多为年高或久病伤肾。

主症：怯寒肢冷，少腹拘急不仁，脐下惊动，气急短促，动则喘甚，呕而气怯，小便不利，足跗浮肿。

兼症：或呕吐涎沫而头目昏眩。

舌脉：苔白润或白腻，舌质胖大，脉沉细兼滑。

分析：久病及肾，肾不纳气，则喘促气短，动则为甚，肺脾气虚，痰饮内盛，故呕而气怯，痰多胸闷食少。肾阳虚弱不能温养形体则怯寒肢冷。肾虚气化无权，水饮停蓄于下焦故小便不利。少腹拘急不仁，或冲动为悸。饮溢于外则是肿，饮逆于上则呕吐涎而头目眩晕。舌胖苔白脉沉细而滑也属阳虚饮聚之象。

治法：温肾化饮。

方药：以真武汤合金匮肾气丸加减。二方均能温阳化饮。真武汤偏于脾肾双温，肾气丸偏于温肾，缓于图功，药用附片、肉桂、生姜温阳化饮，淮山药、白术、甘草补气健脾，茯苓、泽泻利水祛饮，熟地、山萸肉补肾纳气。

加减：食少配陈皮、半夏；若脐下悸动，呕吐涎沫而头昏目眩，是饮邪上逆，可加用五苓散化气行水。

处方举例：

肉桂 6g、附片 6g、熟地 10g、茯苓 10g、泽泻 15g、白术 10g、干姜 6g、山萸肉 10g。

《金匮要略》根据脉诊，推断痰饮病的预后，认为久病脉弱者，脉证相符可治；如脉反实大而数是正衰邪盛，属于危重之候；脉弦数亦为难治之症，因饮为阴邪，脉当沉弦，弦数乃脉证相反，这些在临床可作参考。

〔预防及护理措施〕

针对本病的发病原因，对本病的预防，要注意增强体质锻炼，提高抗病能力，居住地要保持干燥，避免湿邪侵袭，不恣食生冷，不暴饮暴食，保持脾胃功能的正常，得病后，要及时治疗，避风寒，慎起居，怡情志，以期早日康复。

〔典型病例分析〕

案一：邓某，女，48 岁，已婚。入院日期：1963 年 6 月 15 日。因浮肿气短半年，加重一周而入院。于 1961 年 1 月感冒后开始咳嗽气短，下肢逐渐浮肿，心下痞满，咳吐白痰，尿少。既往有八年慢性咳嗽史。脉弦细数，苔白唇色紫。西医诊为慢性肺源性心脏病。

辨证：心肾阳虚，水饮内停，痰湿阻遏，肺气壅塞。

治法：清宣肺金，降气化痰，温阳利湿。

方药：越婢汤合真武汤加减。

生石膏 12g、麻黄 3g、甘草 9g、云苓 12g、白术 9g、杭芍 9g、附子 6g、生姜 9g、大枣（擘）5 枚，车前子 15g、白茅根 30g、杏仁 9g。

上药服 3 剂后，尿量增加，每日达 1500～1900 毫升，下肢浮肿明显减退。服 5 剂后，浮肿不显，肝大回缩，咳嗽减轻，于上方加入厚朴 6g、陈皮 6g，气喘减，但有胸闷，故上方去白茅根、车前子、厚朴，加苏子 9g。再进 5 剂后，仍咳嗽未愈，乃肺气不宣所致，故改投宽胸理气清肺之法，方用厚朴麻黄加汤减，方药如下：

厚朴 6g、麻黄 3g、半夏 9g、杏仁 9g、甘草 9g、沙参 18g、小麦 30g、茯苓 9g、细辛 3g、五味子 6g、生姜 4.5g。

服上方后症状已大减。……病情稳定。（《赵锡武医疗经验》）

按：本例主症咳嗽气短，浮肿尿少，心下痞满，咳吐白痰，苔白唇紫，病属邪侵日久，肺脾肾三脏亏虚，重在肺肾阳虚，水湿不得宣化通利，水饮内停，痰湿壅肺，治重温阳利湿，宣肺行水，故用越婢汤合真武汤加车前子、白茅根、杏仁宣降肺气，温阳利水。药后尿量大增，浮肿明显消退，续以宽胸理气清肺之厚朴麻黄汤加味，重在降气化痰，前人所谓“积水成饮，饮凝成痰”。饮易行而痰难化，此案治疗掌握先易后难之原则，先化饮后祛痰，是切合本病病理特点的。

案二：王某某，男，45 岁。外感风寒，引动痰饮，肺气不宣，咳嗽胸痛，喘息不能平卧。舌苔薄腻，脉滑实。X 线胸部透视为“渗出性胸膜炎”。乃饮邪积于胸胁之间，证属悬饮，治拟疏风宣肺，攻逐水饮。

苏梗 10g、甜葶苈 15g、炙紫菀 5g、苏子 10g、桔梗 5g、杏仁 9g、竹茹 10g、陈皮 6g、制半夏 10g、茯苓 12g、吴萸 1.5g、瓜蒌仁 10g、蛤壳 30g、天将壳 10g、广郁金 10g、控涎丹 2g（包）。

服药 3 剂喘平，一月后再发，原方续服又效。（《黄一峰医案医话集》）

按：本案证属外感风寒，引动痰饮，肺失宣通，饮停胸胁之悬饮，以胸痛胁胀，咳时尤甚，喘息不能平卧，苔薄腻，脉滑实为主症。治疗舍十枣汤而以疏风宣肺攻逐水饮为法，汤丸并进，汤药以疏风宣肺以化痰饮，丸用控涎丹以攻逐水饮，是舍十枣汤之方而师其法，效其方而缓其势，而祛痰逐饮之功犹佳。

痰饮为内科大病之一，是由感受寒湿，饮食所伤，劳欲过度及阳气虚弱等原因，导致肺脾肾功能失常，水液不能输化，停积于某些部位而形成的病症。饮发于中，随处留积，走于肠间为痰饮，留于胁下为悬饮，上迫于肺为支饮，溢于四肢为溢饮。

临床辨证当辨清饮停部位，标实与本虚的主次及有无兼挟症。因痰饮总属阳虚阴盛、本虚标实之候，治疗当以温化为原则。若痰饮壅盛，其证属实，可采用攻下逐饮、理气分消等法以祛其邪，继则扶脾固肾以治其本；至于脾肾阳虚之微饮，则以扶正为首务，略参化饮之品。饮积日久，多有兼夹，有夹痰、夹热、夹气滞、夹血瘀、夹外感，当须辨明，分别施治。

痰饮的转归，主要表现为病由肺脾日久及肾，肾阳亏虚，开阖不利，水饮可凌心、射肺、犯脾。另一方面，痰饮多为慢性病，病程日久，常在寒热虚实之间相互转化，而且饮积生痰，痰瘀互结，病情更为缠绵，故宜早期治疗。

复习思考题

1. 痰饮的概念是什么？如何区分痰与饮？

2. 如何理解和掌握"病痰饮者，当以温药和之？"

3. 悬饮如何辨治？瓜蒌椒目汤组方原则是什么？

4. 小半夏加茯苓汤与苓桂术甘汤、甘遂半夏汤与己椒苈黄汤如何区别使用？

自汗、盗汗

〔概述〕

自汗、盗汗是指人体阴阳失调，营卫不和，腠理不固而引起的汗液外泄失常的病证。若清醒时汗出，动则尤甚者为自汗。若自汗只见于头部、或手、或足、或半身，为局部汗出。若寐中汗出，醒来自止者为盗汗。临床上，也有自汗、盗汗兼有者。

自汗、盗汗既可单独出现，也可在其他病证中伴见，本篇所讨论的内容是以自汗、盗汗为主症的病证。

西医学中的植物神经功能紊乱、甲状腺功能亢进、结核病、发作性低血糖、虚脱、休克及某些传染病等以自汗、盗汗为主要表现者，均可参考本篇辨证论治。

〔病因病机〕

汗证的发生，《内经》提出为"阳加于阴"和"腠理开"所致，这是其最基本的病理变化。后世医学将汗证按外感热病、内伤杂病、自汗、盗汗等分别论述。现将其归纳为营卫不和、阴虚火旺、邪热郁蒸，分述如下：

一、营卫不和：卫气有固护津液，不令其妄泄的作用，其为肺所主。若肺气不足，肌腠疏松，卫外而不固，故汗出。若风邪侵袭表虚之体，或湿邪留于肌肤，常使营卫不和，卫外失司，致汗出而恶风。

若阳气偏衰于人体一端，也致卫外功能障碍，常引起局部汗出。

二、阴虚火旺：心主血，肾藏精，精神过用，起居不慎，亡血失精致血虚精亏，虚火内生，阴津被扰不能自藏而外泄作汗。

若久患失眠之人，心血暗耗，人神被扰，以致阴阳不济，每遇情绪波动时，阳扰于阴，迫液外泄而汗出。

二、邪热郁蒸：风寒入里化热，或感受风温、暑邪，肺胃蕴热，热蒸津泄，则大汗出；若外感湿邪或饮食不节，湿浊化热，熏蒸津液，则汗自出，也可致局部汗出，或汗液发黄。

以上病理变化，可以单一出现，也可二者相兼，而且可以相互转化，使之错综复杂。

〔辨证论治〕

出汗是人体的一种生理现象，如穿衣过厚、天气炎热、过饮热汤、劳动奔走或服发散药等均可致汗出，其量不多，人体无明显不适，均属正常。发汗法又是驱邪的一种方法，外感病邪气在表，常需通过发汗以祛邪疗病。缘汗为心之液，精气所化，所以不可过泄，太多则伤正气而为病。

一、证候鉴别

临床上，汗证除自汗、盗汗最为常见以外，还有脱汗、战汗、黄汗，其表现各异，治疗与转归亦不相同，因此应该加以鉴别，以免贻误病情。

(一)脱汗：亦属自汗，具体特点为病情危笃之时，或通身大汗淋漓，或汗出如油，伴见肢冷脉微，呼吸低微，反应迟钝等症，古人亦称绝汗。与自汗相比，其性质远属严重，为阴竭阳脱之象。

(二)战汗：但见虚人外感病中，患者先作寒战，尔后汗出，是人体正气拒邪外出的表现。正气盛则战后汗出，脉静身凉而病向愈；否则，战而无汗或战而汗出，脉不静或脉微弱等皆预后欠佳，甚至汗出太过而转变成脱汗。

(三)黄汗：汗色发黄而染衣是其特点，常伴有身重倦怠，肢体浮肿，状如风水，口渴不欲饮，舌苔黄腻，脉沉滑，乃湿热熏蒸或湿邪郁于肌表所致。

二、辨证要点

汗证当分虚实，辨寒热。所谓虚实之分，应正邪合参，邪气甚多实，或在表，或在里，或为寒，或为热；正气衰则虚，或气虚，或血虚，或阴虚，或阳虚；正衰邪盛则虚实夹杂。所谓寒热之辨，乃阳气衰则寒，阳气盛则热。

三、分型证治

自汗、盗汗之发，或因外感，或因内伤，二者皆可为病。然外感之汗虽为邪气在表所致，但表邪一般停留短暂，旋即入里，或化热，或损阴，或伤阳，其病理机转与内伤雷同。自汗虽多以阳气虚常见，但也需辨别其虚或实，或寒或热；盗汗虽以虚热多见，然气虚、阳虚、湿热亦间而有之。

自汗、盗汗病因病机示意图

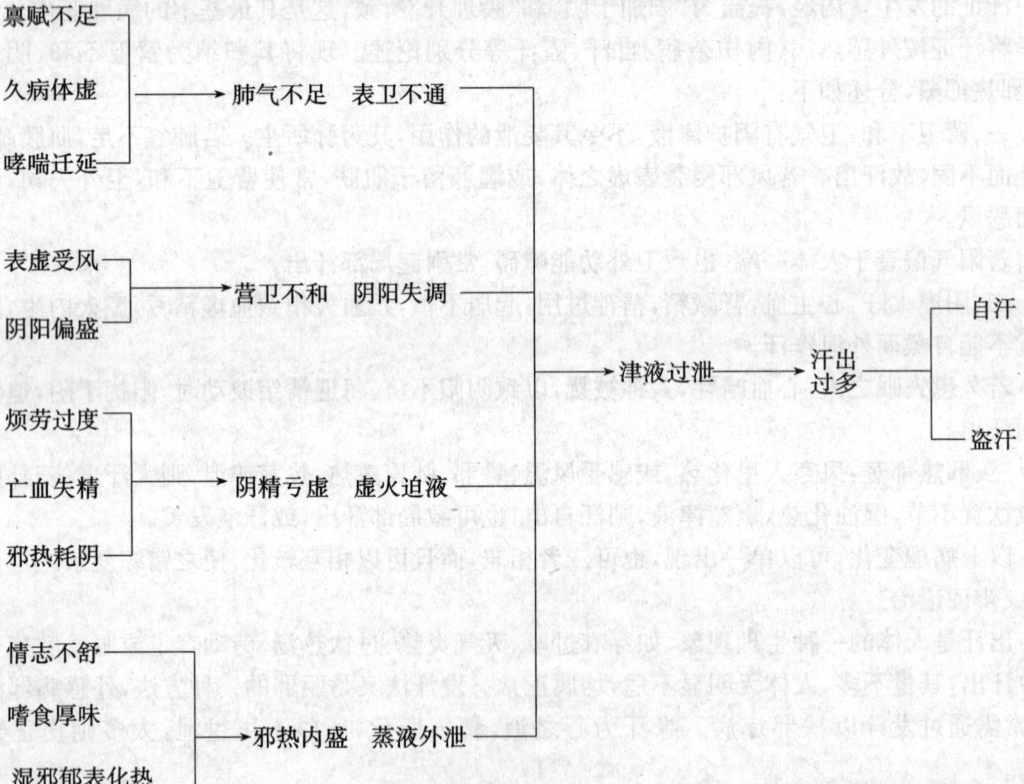

治疗原则，当遵虚者补之，脱者固之，实者泄之，热者清之，寒者温之之旨，汗出过多还可配合外用药扑之。

（一）营卫不和

主症：时时汗出，或但见头、手、足或半身汗出，微恶风、反复发作。

兼症：周身酸楚、疼痛，或微发热，头痛。

舌脉：舌淡红，苔薄白，脉浮缓。

分析：体弱之人，风邪外束，营卫失和，腠理不固，汗出恶风，周身酸痛。邪正相搏，故发热头痛。脉浮缓，苔薄白为风邪在表之象。

治法：疏风解表，调和营卫。

方药：以桂枝汤为主。方中桂枝解肌发表，白芍和营敛阴，桂枝、白芍同用调和营卫以使腠理固密。佐以姜、枣、草和中。若汗多身重，苔白腻为挟湿之象，可加防风、豆卷祛风化湿，湿化则阳气通达，卫表自固。若风热犯肺，肺卫失和，症见发热汗出，咽痛而咳，又当辛凉清解为治，宜桑菊饮加元参、银花等。若暑热伤气，汗出口渴者，宜以白虎汤辛凉重剂加鲜荷叶、西瓜翠衣等清暑泄热。

另外，临床上常见久患失眠之人，每遇情绪波动之时常易自汗出，为心之阴阳失调所致，经云："损其心者，调其营卫。"治宜桂枝加龙骨牡蛎汤。

处方举例：

桂枝 10g、白芍 10g、生姜 3 片、大枣 7 枚、炙甘草 6g、防风 6g、清豆卷 10g、白术 10g。

（二）肺气不固

主症：咳嗽、吐泻等久病体虚之人，汗出时作，动则益甚。

兼症：面色萎黄不华，纳少不馨，神疲乏力，易患感冒。

舌脉：舌淡红，苔薄白，脉细弱。

分析：肺主皮毛而司卫外，咳喘日久伤及肺气，肌表不实，皮毛不固，腠理疏松，稍一活动则自汗出，动则气耗，气不摄津，故汗出益甚。子盗母气，脾肺气虚，则面色萎黄不华，纳少不馨，神疲乏力。肺气不足，卫外不固，故易于感冒。舌淡红，脉细弱为气虚之象。

治法：益气固表。

方药：玉屏风散加味。方中黄芪宜生用，益气固表止汗；白术健脾化湿以实表；防风走表而助黄芪固表之功和白术化湿之力。出汗者可加麻黄根、浮小麦、糯稻根、煅牡蛎、煅龙骨、瘪桃干以止汗敛阴；气虚甚者加党参、黄精、五味子以益气固摄；若手足等局部汗出，缘于脾主四肢，气虚不能达于四末，气不摄阴者，宜用黄芪建中汤以温中补虚，固表止汗。

处方举例：

生黄芪 30g、炒白术 12g、防风 6g、麻黄根 10g、糯稻根 10g、煅牡蛎 30g（先下）、煅龙骨 30g（先下）、党参 10g、炙甘草 6g。

（三）阴虚火旺

主症：寐则汗出，或者白昼也阵阵汗出。

兼症：多见于久咳虚喘之人，虚烦少眠，形体消瘦，骨蒸潮热，五心烦热，女子月经不调，男子梦遗。

舌脉：舌嫩红少苔，脉细弦。

分析：肺痨久咳，或生活失宜，亡血失精，阴血亏耗，虚火内炽，迫液外泄，故见寐则汗出，或白昼也阵阵汗出，形体消瘦，骨蒸潮热，五心烦热。热扰神明，则虚烦少寐。阴虚火旺，相火妄动，故女子月经不调，经水量多，男子梦遗。脉象细弦，舌红少苔，亦为阴精衰少而有虚火之象。

治法：滋阴降火，敛液止汗。

方药：轻者用当归六黄汤化裁。方中丹参可易当归，合生地、熟地以滋阴养血，并需重用二地以制阳光；黄连、黄芩以清心肺之火，因其味苦而燥，故虚火甚对此二味用量宜小；黄柏泻相火而坚阴；黄芪益气固表，以其气随汗泄而散故也。若属久病肺肾阴亏者，可用麦味地黄丸加龙骨、牡蛎、糯稻根以滋阴敛汗。骨蒸潮热者加知母、地骨皮、青蒿、龟板、鳖甲以滋阴除蒸。

处方举例：

生黄芪 15g、生熟地各 10g、黄柏 10g、丹参 20g、黄连 5g、黄芩 10g、五味子 10g、浮小麦 30g、煅龙牡各 30g、山萸肉 10g。

（四）热淫于内

主症：自觉胸中烦热，蒸蒸汗出。或但头汗出，或手足汗出。

兼症：口渴或口黏，喜冷饮，发热或烦闷不宁，或便干不畅。

舌脉：舌红苔黄厚少津或黄腻，脉滑数或洪大。

分析：邪气入里化热，或湿邪郁而化热，或过食肥甘，滋生湿热，或肝郁化火等而致肺胃蕴热，热蒸液泄，汗出过多，胸中烦热，或头汗出，或手足汗出。热邪伤津，故口渴喜冷饮。湿热熏蒸则口黏不爽，饮冷而不欲咽。热扰心神，故烦闷不宁。表邪未解，故或发热。热结腑实，故便干不畅。舌红苔黄厚少津，脉洪大，为热感津伤之象；舌红苔黄腻，脉滑数为湿热蕴积之象。

治法：清胃泄热，或清化湿热。

方药：清胃泄热，方以白虎汤为主。方中生石膏清热除烦，知母清热护阴，佐以粳米、甘草养胃和中。若汗出口渴明显，加鲜芦根、花粉、石斛等清热生津之味。热结便秘，当釜底抽薪，可用小承气汤为治。清化湿热，方用龙胆泻肝汤或四妙丸。前方以龙胆草、黄芩、栀子、柴胡清肺泻热，泽泻、木通、车前子清利湿热；当归、生地滋阴养血和营。后方以黄柏、苍术、栀仁清化下焦湿热为主，故下肢及会阴部汗出过多者，用之尤宜，或加牛膝引药下行。若湿热中阻，症见胸脘痞闷而汗出者，可加黄连、厚朴以清化湿热。

处方举例：

生石膏 30g(先下)、知母 10g、鲜芦根 30g、天花粉 10g、元参 10g、栀子 10g、碧桃干 10g、生甘草 6g。

〔预防与护理措施〕

1. 汗证患者所处的环境温度很重要，阳盛者宜居偏凉处，阴盛者宜居偏暖处。

2. 患者情绪宜安定，勿过激；失眠严重者宜练习内养功，排除杂念，争取睡好。

3. 饮食宜清淡，过于辛辣、厚味之味宜少食。

4. 体虚者，应适当加强锻炼，增强体质，天气变化时，宜注意增减衣被。

5. 汗出过多者，宜避风寒，防止感冒；勤换衣被；汗后宜用温水擦身，或用止汗粉扑身，注意安静休息，适当多饮水或淡盐水。

6. 汗出太多时，宜防变成脱汗。或及时服用生脉散或参附液，以预防之。

〔典型病例〕

案一：俞某某，女，72 岁。

自觉胃脘内阵发性烘热，热气外窜，随即汗出浸衣，日数次发，睡眠欲醒时尤易发作，汗后畏冷，口干不渴，轻微咳嗽，饮食、二便皆可。病起于月前肺炎之后，现胸透已趋正常，唯遗此恙。前医用参、麦、五味、龙、牡及玉屏风之类未效。脉寸尺沉细，两关洪数，舌红苔黄腻，此由病后湿热未清，郁遏肺胃，治宜清泄肺胃郁热。处方：

冬瓜仁 9g、苡仁 12g、杏仁 6g、苇根 18g、竹叶 6g、煅石膏 9g、知母 3g、枇杷叶（炙）6g、荷叶 6g、粳米 12g。两剂。

再诊：服药后自觉热气下行，一直窜至小腿而有蚁行感，汗出减少，醒后亦未见大汗出，口仍觉干有甜味，胸膺微闷。脉弦滑有间歇，舌质红，黄腻苔减。湿热下移，肺胃未和，仍宜清宣，因势利导之。处方：

冬瓜仁 9g、苡仁 12g、杏仁 6g、芦根 12g、竹叶 6g、生石膏 9g、茵陈 6g、豆卷 9g、防己 5g、姜黄 5g、通草 3g。三剂。

三诊：服药后，热平汗息，口干亦减，饮食、二便俱正常。脉左弦数有力，右略缓，舌质正仍有薄黄腻苔，乃余热未清之象，宜调和肺胃续清湿热。处方：

茯苓皮 9g、杏仁 6g、桑皮 6g、豆卷 9g、黄芩 3g、茵陈 9g、姜黄 3g、滑石 9g、通草 3g、苡仁 12g。连服三剂，诸状悉平，一切正常。

按：本例为肺炎后，湿热余邪，逗留肺胃，遏郁不解，热迫汗出……蒲老以竹叶石膏清阳明伏热，合苇茎汤并以杏仁易桃仁，疏利肺气，加荷叶宣肺启胃，服两剂后汗出减少，自觉热气下行，两腿有蚁行感。蒲老认为：熟石膏清里力强，但失辛散之力，故郁热从里而下趋，二诊改用生石膏加茵陈、豆卷、防己、通草清利湿热，因势利导，服两剂后热平汗止。经治此例，深知治病求本之必要。观其前用参麦五味及玉屏风均为止汗之品，而汗出不止，知其药证不合，后用清热利湿，而邪去自汗方止。于斯益信辨证求因的重要。（上二案选自《蒲辅周医案》）

自汗、盗汗是人体阴阳失调，营卫不和，腠理开阖不利而致津液外泄的病证，为临床所常见，虽自汗属阳气虚多见，盗汗以阴虚内热居多，但临床上也不尽然，常需辨证论治方能药到病除。实证以肝火、里热、湿热为主，虚证以营卫不和，阴虚失业、阴虚火旺、肺气不足为主。治疗以调和营卫、清热泄火、清化湿热、益气固表、滋阴降火、温阳敛汗为法。汗为心液，精气所化，汗出过多则正气必伤，故治疗汗证要抓住病机，采取积极措施，内外合治，调整机体之阴阳，祛除病邪，使之病除汗止。

复习思考题

1. 自汗、盗汗、脱汗、战汗、黄汗的概念是什么？
2. 试述自汗、盗汗的病因病机。
3. 自汗、盗汗的证治规律是什么？
4. 汗证如何调养、护理？

血　证

〔概述〕

血证有广义与狭义两种解释。广义血证泛指一切血的病证，如血虚、血瘀、出血等；通常所说血证多为狭义，即各种出血病证的统称。凡由机体内在病理变化，而致血液不循常道，外溢于上下诸窍或渗出于肌肤所形成的疾患称为出血，也称血证。根据出血部位及症状，血证又有多种命名，在内科范围内常见的有咳血、吐血、衄血（鼻衄、齿衄、肌衄又名紫斑）、尿血、便血等。

《内经》对血的生理、病理已有较深刻认识；在有关篇章里记载了衄血、咳血、呕血、溺血、便血等病证，并论述了出血病因及部分血证的预后。《金匮要略》记载的治疗吐血、便血的泻心汤、柏叶汤、黄土汤、赤小豆当归散等方剂和《备急千金要方》记载的治疗血证的犀角地黄汤等方剂一直沿用至今。《诸病源候论》、《济生方》及《平治荟萃》对血证的病因病机都有较详细的论述。《景岳全书》将血证病机概括为"火盛"与"气伤"甚为精辟。《血证论》是论血证的专著，对血证病因病机、辨证施治等方面论述甚为全面，所提出的"止血、消瘀、宁血、补虚"治血四法，已成为通治血证大纲。

血证的范围相当广泛，现代医学中许多急、慢性疾病，如各种急、慢性血液病，各脏腑的感染、结核、肿瘤，多种原因造成的肝病、胃病、肾病、肺系病及心血管疾病等所引起的出血，均属本病范畴。由于大出血易造成厥（窒息）、脱（休克）之患，因此血证有时是内科急症，临床更需重视。

〔病因病机〕

血生成于脾，藏受于肝，总统于心，输布于肺，化精于肾，即血赖五脏的功能作用以生成、调节、输布于全身，气与血相互为用，循环运行于经脉之中，环流不息营养脏腑、四肢、百骸，维持生命的正常活动。当感受外邪，酒热辛辣无度，情志过极，劳倦体虚等病因导致脉络损伤或血液妄行时，形成血液溢出脉外，就会出现血证。血证属热者居多，其病位当随其出血部位及特点，从相关脏腑求之。现简述如下：

一、感受外邪：由于外邪侵袭，损伤脉络或热邪迫血妄行而致出血。其中以感受风热、燥、火阳邪为多，也有初感风寒，入里化热而致者。如邪热犯肺，伤及肺络，迫血上逆则致咳血，鼻衄；温热疫毒之邪，热伤营血，迫血妄行而致各种衄血；湿热之邪侵及肠道则致便血。

二、饮食所伤：饮酒嗜辛辣肥甘厚味无度，易使胃肠蕴积湿热，熏灼血络，迫血妄行而致吐血、衄血、便血等症；也可由于饮食不节，损伤脾胃，脾胃虚弱，失其健运统摄之职，则血不循经，血溢脉外，而发吐血、便血、衄血、尿血。

三、情志过极：七情太过，五志化火，则火动于内，气逆于上，迫血妄行而成血证。如郁怒伤肝，肝气郁结，横逆犯胃，损伤胃络而致吐血；气郁化火，肝火犯肺，血随火升则致咳血、衄血；忧思扰心，心火内炽，下移小肠，下注膀胱则生尿血。

四、劳倦过度：心主神明，神劳伤心；脾主肌肉，体劳伤脾；肾主藏精，房劳伤肾。所以劳倦过度损伤心、脾、肾之气阴。若损于气，则气虚不能摄血，血无所归，血液外溢而形成吐血、便血、衄血；若损伤于阴，则阴虚火旺，虚火迫血妄行，虚火灼伤脉络而致尿血及衄血多种。

五、热病或久病之后：热病或久病导致血证的机理主要有三个方面。一是热病、久病使阴津、阴血耗伤，以致阴虚火旺，迫血妄行而致出血；二是热病、久病使正气亏损，以致气虚不摄，血溢脉外而出血；三是根据初病在气，久必及血之理，病久邪气入络，使血脉瘀阻，血行不畅，血不循经而致出血。

总之，导致血证的病因，外感多是风热燥火阳邪为患，亦有湿热疫毒或阴邪入里化热；内伤不外饮食不节，情志过极，劳倦太过及热病、久病之后。血证的病机主要有火盛、气伤、瘀血三类。火盛则火热熏灼，损伤脉络或迫血妄行；气伤则气不摄血，血溢脉外；瘀血则脉络瘀阻，血不归经。火盛有实火及虚火之分。外感风热燥火邪气，湿热内蕴，气郁化火等，均属实火，而阴虚火旺之火则属虚火。气伤之中，又有仅见气虚及气损及阳，阳气亦虚之别。瘀血可由气虚、热结、气滞、寒凝、跌仆损伤等多种原因形成，而且离经之血便是瘀，因此瘀血多是病理产物，更可使出血加剧。在疾病过程中，火热、气伤、瘀血三者既有区别，又有联系，还可以相互转化。血证的病性，有虚实之分，由内外邪实火盛所致者属实证，气滞、寒凝、热结致瘀之瘀血出血者，也属实证；由阴虚火旺及气虚不摄，正气虚损所致者属虚证。实证和虚证虽各有不同的病因病机，但在疾病发展变化的过程中，常易发生由实证向虚证的转化。如病始为火盛气逆，迫血妄行，但在反复出血之后，则会导致阴血亏损，虚火内生；或因出血过多，血去气伤，气虚阳衰，虚不摄血，于是疾病逐渐由实向虚演变。因此，阴虚火旺，气虚不摄既是出血的后果，又是导致继续出血的病机。又如，出血之后，离经之血留积体内，蓄结为瘀血，瘀血不去，妨碍新血的生成，影响气血的正常运行，致使出血加重或反复不止，也导致疾病由实转虚或虚中夹实。血证的病位，常随出血部位、临床表现及病史而异，就是同一部位的出血，证候不同，病变脏腑亦不同。一般认为，属实火者，病变多在肺、胃、心、肝、肠及膀胱；属虚火者，病位以肝肾居多，也有在肺及胃者；属气虚者，病位多在脾、肾。

血证病因病机示意图

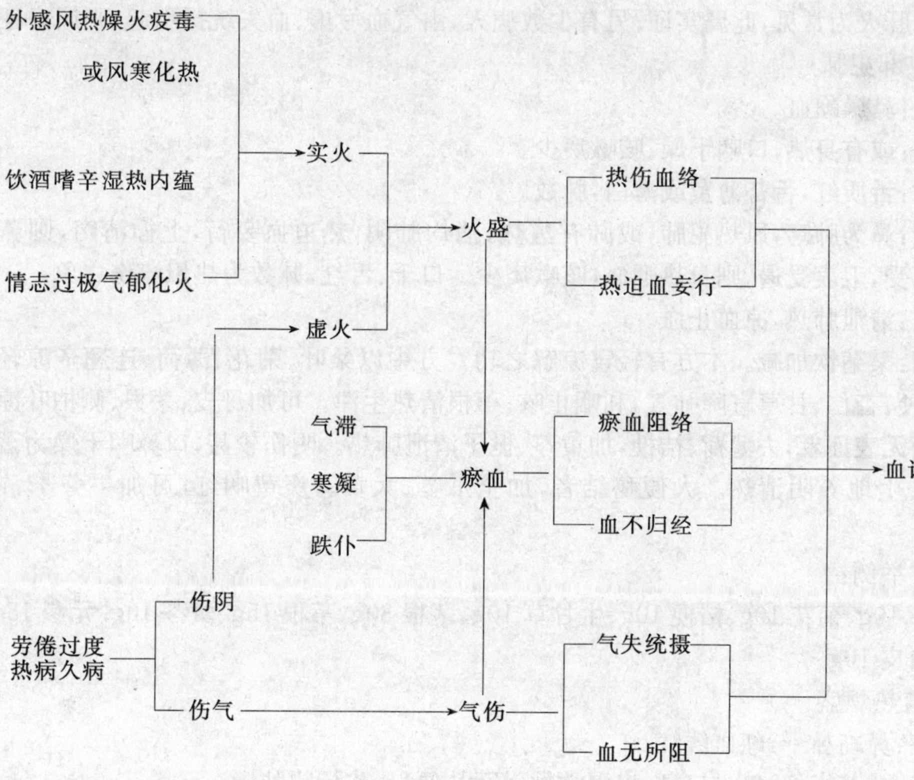

〔病证论治〕

一、辨证要点

对于血证，首先应辨清出血的部位及脏腑病位。例如同属鼻衄，其脏腑病位有在肺、在胃、在肝的不同，应根据病史、临床表现及脏腑经络关系等加以辨识。其次应辨清证候的虚实，病邪病机的种类，以及病情的轻重缓急，通过对临床上出血部位、血色、血量及所见舌、脉、症的分析，一般不难辨出。

二、治疗大法

治疗血证，应针对各种出血的病因及损伤脏腑的不同，结合证候的虚实及病情轻重而辨证施治，灵活掌握止血、治因、固本三大原则，从治血、治气、治火三方面入手，分清主次，选方用药。止血，就是根据病情选用适宜、适量的止血药，以达止血之功，是治疗血证的目的，也是急则治标之法。尤其是急性大出血，止血常为首选原则。治因，就是对出血的病因进行针对性治疗，是治本之法。如虚则补之，实则泻之，热则清之，瘀则化之；固本，就是复旧，出血之后，气血必虚，故于止血、治因之后，视其所虚而补益。补益之法，或从调治后天入手，补中益气；或从滋补先天着眼，滋补肝肾，此为善后、收功之法。治血包括止血与治因两方面内容，如清热止血，凉血止血，收敛止血或活血止血。在血证之中，由于以热迫血妄行者最多，所以凉血止血药相应应用较多。治火与治气基本属治因范畴。治火，实火当清热泻火，虚火当滋阴降火；治气，实证当清气降气，虚证当补气益气。

三、分型论治

(一)鼻衄

鼻中出血谓之鼻衄，是血证中最常见的一种。鼻衄多由火热迫血妄行所致，其中尤以肺热、胃热、肝火为常见，此属实证；另有少数病人，由气血亏虚、血失统摄引起，则属虚证。

1. 热邪犯肺

主症：鼻燥衄血。

兼症：或有身热，口咽干燥、咳嗽痰少。

舌脉：舌质红，舌苔薄黄或薄白，脉数。

分析：鼻为肺窍，风热犯肺，或肺有蕴热，消灼肺阴，热迫血妄行，上循清窍，则鼻燥鼻衄。若风热上受，卫表受遏，则身热咽痛，咳嗽痰少。口干、舌红，脉数为热炽津伤之象。

治法：清泄肺热，凉血止血。

方药：桑菊饮加减。本方有轻宣凉解之功。方中以桑叶、菊花、薄荷、连翘辛凉轻透，宣散风热；桔梗、杏仁、甘草宣降肺气，利咽止咳；苇根清热生津。可加丹皮、茅根、侧柏叶凉血止血。肺热盛而无表证者，去薄荷、桔梗，加黄芩、栀子清泄肺热。阴伤较甚，口鼻咽干燥为著者，加元参、麦冬、生地养阴清热。大便秘结者，加全瓜蒌、大黄。痰黄咽红，可加牛蒡子、银花散风解热。

处方举例：

桑叶 10g、菊花 10g、桔梗 10g、生甘草 10g、茅根 30g、苇根 15g、黄芩 10g、元参 15g、侧柏叶 10g、桑白皮 10g

2. 胃热炽盛

主症：鼻衄鼻干，衄血鲜红。

兼症：或兼齿衄，口干口臭，口渴欲饮，烦躁，便秘，或牙龈肿痛。

舌脉：舌红苔黄，脉数。

分析：足阳明胃之经脉上交鼻頞，牙龈为阳明经脉所过之处，胃火上炎，则口鼻干燥，口臭，齿龈肿痛。热伤血络迫血妄行，则鼻衄，齿衄，血色鲜红。胃火消灼津液，则口干鼻干，口渴引饮，大便秘结。胃热扰心，则烦躁不安。舌红苔黄，脉数均为胃热炽盛之象。

治法：清胃泻火，凉血止血。

方药：玉女煎加减。本方有清胃滋阴之功。方中生石膏清胃泻火；知母、麦冬、地黄养阴清热；牛膝引血下行。原方熟地滋阴腻胃，改用生地兼能凉血止血；为加强凉血止血之功，可加茅根、大蓟、小蓟、藕节、侧柏叶等药。热势盛者，加山栀、丹皮、黄芩清热泻火。热盛便秘者，加生大黄通腑泻热。阴伤较甚，口渴，舌红少苔，脉细数者，加天花粉、石斛、玉竹养胃生津。胃火炽盛而无津伤者，可用三黄石膏汤加减治之。

处方举例：

生石膏 30g(先下)、黄连 6g、黄芩 10g、知母 10g、丹皮 10g、生地 10g、茅根 30g、牛膝 10g、麦冬 10g。

3. 肝火上炎

主症：鼻衄，头痛，目眩，口苦。

兼症：目赤耳鸣，烦躁易怒。

舌脉：舌红苔薄黄，脉弦数。

分析：肝郁化火，火热迫血上溢清窍，故致鼻衄。肝火上扰清窍，故致头痛，目眩，耳鸣，口苦。肝开窍于目，肝火上乘，故两目红赤。烦躁，舌红苔黄，脉弦数为肝火内盛之象。

治法：清肝泻火、凉血止血。

方药：龙胆泻肝汤加减。本方有泻肝胆实火，清三焦湿热之功。方中以龙胆草、黄芩、山栀清肝泻火为主；泽泻、木通、车前子清利湿热；柴胡以疏肝解郁；生地、当归、甘草滋阴养血和中，诸药伍用泻中有补、清中有养，使火泻湿清而阴血不伤。可酌加白茅根、蒲黄、大蓟、小蓟、丹皮、藕节等凉血止血。肝火炽盛者，耳鸣烦急，目赤头痛可加夏枯草、青黛以清肝凉血。若阴液亏耗，口鼻干燥，舌红少津，脉细数者，可去车前子、泽泻、当归，酌加玄参、麦冬、女贞子、旱莲草以养阴清热。

4. 气血亏虚

主症：鼻衄，血色淡红。或兼见齿衄，肌衄。

兼症：面色㿠白，夜寐不宁，神疲乏力，头晕心悸。

舌脉：舌质淡，脉细无力或呈芤脉。

分析：气虚不能统摄血液，故致鼻衄，甚或齿衄、肌衄。气血亏虚，失于温煦濡养，脑海失养则头晕耳鸣。心失所养则心悸眠差。四肢百骸失养则神疲乏力。血虚不能上荣于面则面色㿠白。气血不足。血脉不充则衄血淡红，舌质亦淡，脉细无力或芤。

治法：补气摄血。

方药：归脾汤加减。本方有益气养血摄血，心脾共补之功。方由四君子汤、当归补血汤加龙眼肉、酸枣仁、远志、木香、生姜、大枣而成。意在益气以生血，气旺以摄血，是治疗心脾不足，气血虚弱，脾不统血的常用方剂。可酌加仙鹤草、阿胶、茜草等药加强止血作用。

处方举例：

党参 10g、白术 10g、炙黄芪 15g、茯神 10g、当归 10g、远志 10g、酸枣仁 10g、阿胶 10g(烊化)、炙甘草 10g、木香 6g、仙鹤草 12g。

对以上各种证候的鼻衄，除内服汤药治疗外，在鼻衄当时，可酌情配合局部用药，以利及早止血。外用药可选用；(1)云南白药外敷出血局部；(2)用棉花蘸青黛粉塞入鼻腔止血；(3)用湿棉条蘸塞鼻散(百草霜 15g、龙骨 15g、枯矾 60g，共研极细末)塞鼻止血；(4)鲜小蓟叶洗净揉碎塞鼻止血；(5)棉花蘸血余炭塞鼻。

（二）齿衄

齿龈出血称为齿衄，又称牙衄、牙宣。因手阳明大肠经入下齿龈，足阳明胃经入上齿龈；肾主骨，齿为骨之余，故齿衄主要与胃肠及肾的病变有关。多由胃火炽盛或阴虚火旺所致，前者属实热，后者为虚火。

1. 胃火炽盛

主症：齿衄血色鲜红，齿龈红肿疼痛。

兼症：头痛，口臭，大便秘结。

舌脉：舌红，苔黄，脉洪数。

分析：胃火炽盛，循阳明经脉上熏，以致齿龈红肿疼痛，络损血溢则齿龈出血。胃热上蒸则头痛，口臭。热结阳明则大便秘结。苔黄，脉洪数，为阳明热盛之象。

治法：清胃泻火，凉血止血。

方药：加味清胃散合泻心汤加减。加味清胃散有清胃降火，凉血止血之功。方中生地、丹皮、犀角（可用水牛角代）清热凉血；黄连、连翘清热泻火；升麻引经，清热解毒；当归、生甘草养血和中。合用泻心汤以增强其清胃泻火的作用。可酌加白茅根、大蓟、小蓟、藕节以凉血止血。齿龈化脓者，可加银花、公英、地丁以加强清热解毒。胃火炽盛，口渴欲饮者，加生石膏、知母以甘寒清气。

处方举例：

生地12g、丹皮10g、生石膏30g（先下）、知母10g、黄芩10g、黄连6g、酒大黄5g、升麻6g、生甘草6g、连翘10g

2. 阴虚火旺

主症：齿衄血色淡红，龈肿齿摇不坚。

兼症：反复迁延，常因受热或烦劳诱发，或伴有手足心热。

舌脉：舌红苔少，脉细数。

分析：肾主骨，齿为骨之余，肝肾阴虚，相火上浮，热迫血行，则致齿龈出血，齿摇不坚。烦劳或受热，可致阴虚加重，故易诱发齿衄。手足心热，舌红苔少，脉细数均为阴虚火动之象。

治法：滋阴降火，凉血止血。

方药：滋水清肝饮合茜根散加减。滋水清肝饮由六味地黄丸与丹栀逍遥散合方化裁而成，重在补养肝肾，滋阴降火。其中六味地黄丸药物三补三泻、三阴并治以补益肝肾为主；丹栀逍遥散去白术、煨姜、薄荷，加酸枣仁，旨在养肝凉血清热。茜根散中黄芩、甘草清热和中；茜根、侧柏叶凉血止血；生地、阿胶滋阴养血，凉血止血。两方合用共奏滋阴降火，凉血止血之功。若肾阴亏虚，腰酸潮热，还可合入二至丸以助滋补肝肾之力。

处方举例：

生地15g、山萸肉10g、山药10g、丹皮10g、泽泻10g、女贞子10g、旱莲草12g、侧柏叶12g、茜根12g、阿胶10g（烊化）

（三）紫斑（肌衄）

血液溢出于肌肤之间，皮肤出现青紫斑点或斑块的病症，称为紫斑，亦称肌衄或葡萄疫。紫斑由热入营血，血热妄行而引起者，属实证；由阴虚火旺，虚火伤络，或气虚不摄，血不循经而引起者，属虚证。

1. 血热妄行

主症：皮肤出现青紫斑点或斑块，起病急暴突然。

兼症：可伴有鼻衄、齿衄、便血、尿血，或有发热、口渴、便秘。

舌脉：舌红，苔黄，脉弦数。

分析：热毒壅盛，热入营血，迫血妄行，血出于肌腠之间，则见青紫斑点或斑块。热毒灼伤鼻、齿龈、肠、胃等处之脉络，则伴见鼻衄，齿衄，便血，尿血。内热郁蒸则发热，热盛津伤则口渴、便秘。舌红，苔黄，脉弦数，均为实热之征象。

治法：清热解毒，凉血止血。

方药：犀角地黄汤加减。本方有清热凉血散瘀之功。方用犀角（水牛角代）、地黄清热解毒，滋阴凉血；丹皮、赤芍清热凉血，活血散瘀。此方为治疗热在血分、血热妄行所致各种血证之常用有效方剂，可合用十灰散凉血止血。热毒炽盛而发热、口渴者，加生石膏、知母、焦山栀或冲服紫雪丹以加强清热作用。热壅胃肠，气血郁滞，症见腹痛、便血者，可加用白芍、生甘草、制香附、地榆、槐花以缓急止痛，凉血止血。大便秘结者，加大黄、瓜蒌。邪热阻滞经络，兼见关节肿痛者，加秦艽、桑枝、木瓜、金银藤以通经活络。

处方举例：

水牛角 30g、生地 12g、赤芍 10g、丹皮 10g、生石膏 30g（先下）、知母 10g、山栀 10g、侧柏叶 10g、生甘草 6g

2. 阴虚火旺

主症：皮肤青紫斑点或斑块，时发时止。

兼症：常伴鼻衄，齿衄或月经过多，颧红，心烦，手足心热，口渴，潮热，盗汗。

舌脉：舌质红，苔少，脉细数。

分析：阴虚则火旺，火旺则更宜伤阴，虚火伤及脉络，血溢皮下肌肤，而致肌衄或他处出血。每因烦劳或受热而诱发加重，故时发时止。水亏不能济火，心火扰动，故心烦。虚火内蒸，则见五心烦热，潮热，颧红。虚火迫津外泄，则见盗汗。阴津不足，故口渴咽干。舌红，苔少，脉细数为阴虚火旺之象。

治法：滋阴降火，宁络止血。

方药：茜根散加减。本方有滋阴清热、凉血止血之功。阴虚较甚者，酌加龟板、玄参、女贞子、旱莲草等养阴清热。对于本证候中属肾阴亏虚而火热不甚，症见腰膝酸软，头晕乏力，手足心热，舌红少苔，脉沉细数者，可用六味地黄丸滋补肾阴，加茜草根、紫草、侧柏叶、仙鹤草等凉血止血。

处方举例：

生地 12g、山萸肉 10g、女贞子 10g、旱莲草 10g、丹皮 10g、泽泻 10g、茜草根 12g、侧柏叶 12g、知母 10g

3. 气虚不摄

主症：皮肤青紫斑点或斑块，色泽淡暗，反复出现，迁延不愈。

兼症：头晕目眩，食欲不振，神疲乏力，面色苍白或萎黄。

舌脉：舌质淡，舌体胖，苔薄白，脉细弱。

分析：气虚不能摄血，故肌衄反复发作，久病不愈。气虚不能帅血运行而血瘀，故血色淡暗。气血亏耗，筋脉百骸失于濡养，故神疲乏力，头晕目眩面色无华。脾气虚不能健运，故食欲不振。舌质淡，舌体胖，脉细弱均为气血亏虚之象。

治法：补气摄血。

方药：归脾汤加减。用归脾汤补益心脾，益气摄血。酌情选加仙鹤草、棕榈炭、三七、蒲黄炭、茜草根、血余炭等收敛止血，化瘀消斑。脾虚清浊不分，大便溏泻者，可加用山药、莲肉、芡实等健脾涩肠。兼有肾气不足而见腰膝酸软者，可加菟丝子、山萸肉、续断以补益肾气。若肾阳不足，形寒畏冷者，可加仙茅、肉桂等温阳益肾。

处方举例：

党参 10g、黄芪 15g、白术 10g、当归 10g、茯苓 10g、仙鹤草 20g、三七粉 3g（冲）棕榈炭 10g

以上鼻衄、齿衄、紫斑统属衄血。血自流出谓之衄，衄血乃泛指鼻、齿龈、耳、肌眼及肌肤等部位的出血，依其出血部位不同，命名各异。但要注意某些医书所言衄血，有的仅指鼻衄。

鼻衄、齿衄、肌衄的病因病机，虽以热迫血妄行为多，然气血亏虚、气不摄血亦不少见，必须辨清虚实。因热出血，实热多由肺热、肝火、胃火及热入营血而引起；虚热多由阴虚所致。因于虚者，初起常为气血不足，渐致脾肾两虚。肺热者多兼有鼻干咽燥及咳嗽，治当清泄肺热，凉血止血，多以桑菊饮加减。胃火者，多兼有口渴口臭、苔黄、脉洪数，治当清胃泻火，凉血止血，多用玉女煎、三黄石膏汤化裁。肝火者，多兼头晕头胀目眩、口苦易怒，治当清肝泻火，凉血止血，多以龙胆泻肝汤加减。热入营血者，以多部位出血为常见，或伴见发热，治当清热解毒，凉血止血，常用犀角地黄汤加减。阴虚火旺者，多兼有五心烦热、头晕耳鸣、潮热盗汗，治当滋阴降火，凉血止血，可以滋水清肝饮合茜根散加减治之。气虚不摄者，多兼有神疲乏力，心悸气短，食欲不振，治当补气摄血，多用归脾汤加减。此外鼻衄、齿衄还可配合局部外用药治疗。

（四）咳血

血由肺系而来，经气道咳嗽而出，或痰中带有血丝，或痰血相兼，或纯血鲜红，间夹泡沫，均称为咳血，亦有称为嗽血者，近又称咯血，即血经喉咽咯出。

咳血总因肺络受伤所致。因肺为娇脏不耐寒热，肺位为脏腑之华盖，肺主宣发、肃降，喜润恶燥，喜清恶浊，故常易受邪侵袭。邪气犯肺，使肺失清肃则咳嗽，损伤肺络，血溢脉外，则为咳血。病位主要在肺，连及肝、肾。临床上主要分燥热伤肺、肝火犯肺、阴虚肺热三型，分别以清热润肺、宁络止血，或清肝泻肺，凉血止血、或滋阴润肺，宁络止血为治疗大法。

1. 燥热伤肺

主症：咽痒咳嗽，痰中带血，血色鲜红，血量不多。

兼症：口干鼻燥，或兼有身热、微恶风寒、鼻塞头痛等表热症。

舌脉：舌红少津，苔薄黄，脉数。

分析：感受风热燥邪，损伤于肺，使肺失宣肃，肺络受损，则咳嗽咽痒，痰中带血，血色鲜红。燥热伤津，则口干鼻燥。风热燥邪外客，卫表失和，则有身热，微恶风等表热症。舌红少津，苔薄黄，脉数，均为燥热伤津之象。

治法：清热润肺，宁络止血。

方药：桑杏汤加减。本方清宣凉润，方中以桑叶、栀子、豆豉清宣肺热；沙参、梨皮养阴清热；杏仁、浙贝润肺化痰止咳。可加白茅根、侧柏叶、茜草、藕节凉血止血。兼有发热、头痛、咳嗽、咽痛、脉浮数等外感风热表证时，加银花、连翘、牛蒡子、菊花等以辛凉解表，清热利咽。肺热内盛者，咳嗽痰黄、咳血量多，酌加生石膏、黄芩、桑白皮、知母以清肺泻热。燥热伤津较甚者，可加麦冬、元参、天花粉、苇茎等以养阴润肺。

处方举例：

桑叶 10g、杏仁 10g、南沙参 15g、知贝母各 10g、黄芩 10g、山栀 10g、桑白皮 10g、侧柏叶 12g、茅根 30g

2. 肝火犯肺

主症：咳嗽阵作，痰中带血或纯血鲜红。

兼症：烦躁易怒，口苦咽干，胸胁胀痛，症状常随情绪变化而波动。

舌脉：舌质红，苔薄黄，脉弦数。

分析：情志不遂或暴怒伤肝，肝郁化火，上逆犯肺，使肺失清肃，肺络受损，故咳嗽、咳血，且病情随情志而变化。肝之脉络布于胁肋，肝火偏亢，脉络壅滞，故胸胁胀痛。肝火上炎，故口苦，烦躁易怒。舌质红，苔薄黄，脉弦数，为肝火亢盛之象。

治法：清肝泻肺，凉血止血。

方药：泻白散合黛蛤散加减。泻白散清泻肺热，止咳平湍；黛蛤散清肺泻肝，凉血化痰。两方合用，以桑白皮、地骨皮清泻肺热；海蛤壳清肺化痰；青黛清肝凉血；甘草、粳米养胃和中，使清肝泻肺而不伤正。可酌加生地、旱莲草、茅根、大小蓟、藕节等凉血止血。肝火亢盛，头晕目赤、心烦易怒者，加丹皮、栀子、黄芩清肝泻火。若咳血量较多，纯血鲜红，可用犀角地黄汤加三七粉、白皮粉、大黄粉冲服，以清热泻火，凉血止血。

处方举例：

桑白皮 10g、地骨皮 10g、黛蛤散 12g（包煎）、黄芩 10g、丹皮 10g、藕节 10g、焦山栀 10g、白茅根 30g

3. 阴虚肺热

主症：咳嗽痰少，痰中带血或反复咳血，血色鲜红。

兼症：口干咽燥，颧红，潮热盗汗。

舌脉：舌质红瘦，苔薄黄，脉细数。

分析：肺肾阴亏，虚火内灼，肺失清肃，故咳嗽痰少或干咳，咳声短促。火热灼肺，损伤肺络，虚火灼津成痰，故痰少而黏，痰中带血或反复咳血，血色鲜红。阴虚津乏，不能上润咽喉，故口干咽燥。阴虚火旺，则颧红、潮热、盗汗、舌红瘦、苔薄黄、脉细数。

治法：滋阴润肺，宁络止血。

方药：百合固金丸加减。本方滋阴润肺，金水并调。方中以百合、麦冬、元参、生熟地滋阴清热，润肺生津；当归、白芍柔润养血；贝母、甘草化痰止咳。原方中有桔梗，同其性升提，于咳血不利，在此宜去。多加入侧柏叶、藕节、茅根、白芨等药，或合用十灰散以凉血止血、收敛止血。反复咳血及咳血量多者，可加阿胶、龟板胶、三七粉养血止血。阴虚内热较甚，潮热、颧红者，可加青蒿、鳖甲、地骨皮、白薇等清退虚热。盗汗严重，可加糯稻根、浮小麦、五味子、牡蛎等以收敛止汗。

处方举例：

百合 20g、生地 12g、麦冬 10g、元参 10g、白芍 10g、地骨皮 10g、贝母 10g、侧柏叶 12g、茅根 20g、白芨 10g

（五）吐血

血由胃系而来，经呕吐从口而出，甚则倾盆盈碗，血色红或黯红，常夹有食物残渣，称为吐血，亦称为呕血。《医碥·吐血》说："吐血即呕血，旧分无声曰吐、有声曰呕。"

因吐血与咳血二者均是血经口而出，故应注意鉴别。一般来说，咳血之血色鲜红，常混有泡沫痰涎，血来自肺系。咳血之前多有咳嗽、喉痒、胸闷等症状。较大量的咳血之后，可见痰中带血数天。而吐血多血色紫黯，常夹有食物残渣，血来自胃系。吐血之前多有胃脘不适或胃痛、恶心等症状。吐血之后无痰中带血，但大便多呈黑色。

吐血以肝胃蕴热、迫血妄行所致为多，也有脾胃虚寒、气不摄血而成。病性多属实证热证，尤其是虚寒为本，实热为标之证更多见，属虚证寒证者少。病位主要在胃、肝、脾。临床上主要分胃热壅盛、肝火犯胃和气虚血溢三型，分别以清胃泻火、化瘀止血，或泻肝清胃、凉血止血，或健脾益气、摄血止血为治疗大法。

1. 胃热壅盛

主症：脘腹胀闷，甚则作痛，吐血色红或紫黯，常夹有食物残渣。

兼症：口臭，便秘或大便色黑。

舌脉：舌红，苔黄腻，脉滑数。

分析：胃为水谷之海，为多血多气之府，主受纳，腐熟水谷，通降为顺。酒食无度，致胃失和降，胃中积热，气血不和，故脘腹胀闷，甚则作痛。热伤胃络，迫血妄行，故吐血色红，或瘀久而出色呈紫黯。胃气上逆，故呕血挟食。胃中食积化腐，故口臭。胃热耗津，故大便秘结。血随糟粕而下，则使大便色黑。舌红，苔黄腻，脉滑数为内有积热之象。

治法：清胃泻火，化瘀止血。

方药：泻心汤合十灰散加减。泻心汤有苦寒清胃泻火之功。《血证论·吐血》说："方名泻心，实则泻胃"，方由黄芩、黄连、大黄组成。十灰散凉血止血、兼能化瘀，止血而无凝滞留瘀之弊；大黄因其苦寒沉降，峻下实热，荡涤胃肠，为治胃有实热而吐血的要药；白芨苦甘涩而微寒，收敛止血，消肿生肌，是治吐血、咳血的常用药。两药既可配伍在汤药中，又可研末单用。胃气上逆而致恶心呕吐者，加旋覆花、代赭石、竹茹以和胃降逆。胃失和降，脘腹胀闷较甚或胀痛者，可加枳壳、陈皮、或炒川楝、元参等以理气和胃止痛。

处方举例：

黄连 6g、黄芩 10g、侧柏叶 12g、荷叶 12g、枳壳 10g、竹茹 10g、焦三仙各 10g、大黄粉 3g(冲)、白芨粉 6g(冲)、三七粉 3g(冲)

2. 肝火犯胃

主症：吐血色红或紫黯。

兼症：心烦易怒，寐少梦多，口苦胁痛。

舌脉：舌质红绛，脉弦数。

分析：气郁化火，肝火横逆犯胃，胃络损伤则吐血，色或红或紫黯。肝火上炎，则口苦、胁痛、易怒。肝火扰心，心神不安，则心烦，少寐多梦。舌红绛，脉弦数为肝火亢盛、耗伤胃阴之象。

治法：泻肝清胃，凉血止血。

方药：龙胆泻肝汤加减。本方主清肝胆湿热，在此应用必须视症而加减。可加茅根、藕节、旱莲草、茜草、白芨，或合用十灰散以凉血止血。如暴吐血、血出如涌者，也可用犀角地黄汤调服三七粉、白芨粉、大黄粉服之，以清热凉血，化瘀止血。

处方举例：

龙胆草 6g、黄芩 10g、焦山栀 10g、丹皮 10g、茅根 30g、大小蓟各 10g、三七粉 3g(冲)、

白芨粉 6g(冲)、旱莲草 12g

3. 气虚血溢

主症:吐血缠绵不止,时轻时重,血色淡黯。

兼症:面色苍白,心悸气短,神疲乏力。

舌脉:舌质淡,脉细弱。

分析:脾气亏虚,血失统摄,血溢脉外,故吐血缠绵不止,时轻时重,血色淡黯。脾气已虚,复又出血,气随血去,以致气血两虚,心失所养则心悸气短;面失所荣则面色苍白;筋脉肢体失于濡养则神疲乏力。舌质淡,脉细弱为气血亏虚之象。

治法:健脾益气,摄血止血。

方药:归脾汤加减。可酌加乌贼骨、仙鹤草、白芨、炮姜炭等温经固涩止血药。若气损及阳,脾胃虚寒,症见肢冷、畏寒、便溏者,可改用《金匮》柏叶汤合理中丸治之。方中党参、白术、甘草健脾益气以摄血;艾叶、炮姜炭温经止血;侧柏叶凉血清降,折其逆上之势;童便化瘀止血,用以替代古方中所用之乌梅汁。两方合用,有益气摄血、温中止血之效。若出血过多,气随血脱,症见面色苍白、四肢厥冷,汗出、脉微者,应急服独参汤益气固脱,此乃"有形之血不能速生,无形之气所当急固"之意。如汗出,肢冷尤甚者,为气脱亡阳,可再加用附片,名参附汤以回阳救逆。

处方举例:

党参 10g、白术 10g、黄芪 15g、当归 6g、炙甘草 6g、茯苓 10g、炮姜炭 10g、乌贼骨 12g、白芨粉 5g(冲)

(六)便血

血从肛门排出体外,无论在大便前,或大便后下血,或单纯下血,或与粪便混杂而下,均称为便血,亦称下血、泻血。

历代医家论便血,有远血、近血、肠风、脏毒之分。以血在便后来者为远血,其病变部位多在小肠、胃,而距肛门远;以血在便前来者为近血,其病变部位多在结肠、直肠或肛门,而距肛门近。以血清而色鲜者为肠风;血浊而色黯者为脏毒。临床上以血在便前、便后分血来之近远并不可靠,而且在不少情况下,血和大便混杂而下,难于分辨其前后。而便血的颜色,可作为诊断便血部位的参考。一般情况下,便血色鲜红者,其来较近;便血色紫黯者,其来较远。便血应与赤痢鉴别,便血者以血便为主,多无腹痛及里急后重;赤痢者以便下脓血为主,赤多白少,或纯下赤冻,常有腹痛及里急后重。

便血总由胃肠之脉络受损所致。临床上主要有肠道湿热和脾胃虚寒两类,分别以清化湿热、凉血止血,或健脾温中、养血止血为治疗大法。

1. 肠道湿热

主症:便血鲜红。

兼症:大便不畅或稀溏,或有肛门灼热,腹痛,口苦。

舌脉:苔黄腻,脉濡数或滑数。

分析:湿热蕴结肠道,灼伤肠道脉络,以致便血。肠道传化失常,则大便不畅或稀溏。肠道气机失和,则腹痛。湿热上蒸则口苦,湿热下注则肛门灼热。苔黄腻,脉濡数或滑数均为湿热内蕴之象。

治法:清化湿热,凉血止血。

方药：地榆散或槐角丸加减。两方均有清化湿热，凉血止血之功。前者清化湿热之力较强，后者兼能养血行气活血。地榆散以地榆、茜草凉血止血；黄芩、黄连、山栀清热燥湿，泻火解毒；茯苓淡渗利湿。槐角丸以槐角、地榆凉血止血；黄芩清热；防风、积壳、当归疏风利湿，养血活血。临床上便血量多，可酌加白芨、三七、侧柏叶等以凉血止血。若便血日久，失血过多，营阴已亏而湿热未清，症见心中烦热，舌红苔黄，脉细数者，可加白芍、阿胶、生地炭以养血敛阴，和营清热。

处方举例：

地榆 15g、槐角 10g、茜草 10g、焦山栀 10g、茯苓 10g、炒枳壳 6g、黄连 6g、白芨粉 5g、三七粉 3g

2. 脾胃虚寒

主症：便血紫黯，甚则黑如柏油。

兼症：腹部隐痛，得热痛减，面色不华，神倦懒言，大便溏薄。

舌脉：舌质淡，脉细弱。

分析：脾胃虚寒，中气不足，统血无力，血溢肠内，随大便而下，故便血，血色紫黯，甚至色黑。中焦虚寒，寒凝气滞，气机失和，故腹部隐痛绵绵，得热痛减。脾失健运，气血乏源，故面色不华，神倦懒言，舌淡，脉细弱。

治法，健脾温中，养血止血。

方药：黄土汤加减。本方有健脾温中，养血止血之功。方中以灶心土温中止血为君药；辅以白术、附之温阳健脾；佐以生地、阿胶养血止血，且制术、附之温燥，黄芩苦寒坚阴，起反佐作用；使以甘草调中。诸药合用，刚柔相济，温阳止血而不伤阴，滋阴养血而不碍脾。临床应用此方时，若虑附子大辛大热、走而不守，可用炮姜炭替之，取其守而不走，温中止泻，兼能止血。可酌情加用白芨、乌贼骨以收敛止血。三七、花蕊石以活血止血。阳虚较甚，畏寒肢冷者，可加鹿角霜、炮姜、艾叶等温阳止血。

处方举例：

灶心土 30～60g(另包)、炮姜炭 10g、白术 10g、生地 10g、阿胶 10g(烊化)、黄芩 10g、黄芪 15g、当归 10g、炙甘草 6g、乌贼骨 12g、白芨 10g

先用灶心土煎汤，取汁，以其代水再煎煮余药。

(七)尿血

小便中混有血液，甚或有血块的病症称为尿血，亦称溲血、溺血。随出血量多少的不同，而使小便呈淡红色、鲜红色或茶褐色。

尿中有血，应区分尿血与血淋两种情况。凡排尿不痛或痛不明显者称为尿血；尿血而兼小便滴沥涩痛者称为血淋。尿血的病位主要在膀胱与肾脾。其主要病机为热伤脉络及脾肾不固。而热伤脉络之中又有实热和虚热之分。属实热者治以清热泻火、凉血止血，属虚热者治以滋阴降火、宁络止血。脾肾不固之中又有脾虚及肾虚之别。脾虚者治以补脾摄血，肾虚者治以补益肾气、固涩止血。

1. 下焦热盛

主症：小便热赤，尿血鲜红。

兼症：心烦口渴，面赤口疮，夜寐不安。

舌脉：舌红，脉数。

分析：热邪盛于下焦，故小便热赤；热伤血络，热迫血妄行，血渗膀胱，故尿血鲜红。热扰心神则心烦，夜寐不安；火热上炎，则面赤口疮，热伤津液则口渴。舌红，脉数为热盛之象。

治法：清热泻火，凉血止血。

方药：小蓟饮子加减。本方有清热利尿、凉血止血之功。方中以小蓟、生地清热凉血止血；辅以蒲黄、藕节止血消瘀；佐以滑石、通草、淡竹叶、山栀清热利小便，当归活血和营；使以甘草和中缓急。若心火偏旺，移热小肠、膀胱而小便灼热、口渴心烦者，可加用木通、黄连或黄柏以苦寒泻火，夜寐不安可加用琥珀粉 1～2g 以镇心安神，行血消瘀。

处方举例：

生地 12g、大蓟 12g、山栀 10g、小蓟 12g、木通 6g、淡竹叶 10g、生甘草 6g、茅根 30g、蒲黄炭 6g

2. 肾虚火旺

主症：小便短赤带血。

兼症：头晕耳鸣，消瘦神疲，颧红潮热，腰膝酸软。

舌脉：舌质红，脉细数。

分析：肾阴亏虚，虚火内炽，灼伤脉络，则小便短赤带血。肾阴亏损，髓海不足，则头晕耳鸣。肾虚失养则消瘦神疲，腰膝酸软。阴虚火旺，虚火上炎则颧红潮热。舌质红，脉细数为阴虚火旺之象。

治法：滋阴降火，凉血止血。

方药：知柏地黄丸加减。本方有滋阴降火之功。方中以六味地黄丸滋补肾阴，“壮水之主，以制阳光”；知母、黄柏滋阴泻火。可加旱莲草、龟板以滋阴止血，加大小蓟、地榆、蒲黄、藕节等凉血止血。

处方举例：

生地 15g、山萸肉 10g、旱莲草 30g、女贞子 10g、丹皮 10g、泽泻 10g、知母 10g、黄柏 6g、大小蓟各 10g、茅根 30g

3. 脾不统血

主症：久病尿血，血色淡红。

兼症：面色不华，体倦乏力，气短声低，常兼多部位衄血，如齿衄、肌衄、鼻衄等。

舌脉：舌质淡，舌体胖，脉细弱。

分析：脾气亏虚，统血无力，血不循经，故尿血、血色淡红，甚则兼鼻衄、齿衄、肌衄。脾虚运化失职，气血生化乏源，则面色不华，纳少神倦乏力，气短声低。舌质淡、舌体胖、脉细弱为气血亏虚之象。

治法：补脾摄血。

方药：归脾汤加减。可加熟地、阿胶、仙鹤草等养血止血。如有气虚下陷，症见大便溏泻，小腹坠胀，气短懒言者，可合用补中益气汤加减，以健脾益气升阳。

处方举例：

党参 12g、黄芪 15g、当归 10g、白术 10g、茯苓 10g、陈皮 10g、仙鹤草 15g、炙甘草 6g、紫河车粉 3g(冲)

4. 肾气不固

主症：久病尿血，血色淡红，小便频数。

兼症：头晕耳鸣，精神困惫，腰脊酸痛，夜尿频多。

舌脉：舌质淡，脉沉弱。

分析：劳倦或久病及肾，肾气不固，封藏失职，血随尿出，故久病尿血，血色淡红。肾司二便，肾主温化，肾气亏虚，气化失常，则小便频数，夜尿频多。腰为肾之府，脑为髓海，肾虚失于濡养，故腰脊酸痛，头晕耳鸣，精神困惫。舌质淡，脉沉弱为肾气虚衰之象。

治法：补益肾气，固摄止血。

方药：无比山药丸加减。本方有补肾固摄之功。方中以熟地、山药、山萸肉、淮牛膝补肾益精。肉苁蓉、菟丝子、杜仲、巴戟天温补肾阳。茯苓健脾，五味子、赤石脂益气收敛固涩。可加仙鹤草、侧柏叶、地榆、蒲黄炭等收敛或行血止血。若肾虚精关不固而遗精、滑精者，可加金樱子、牡蛎、芡实等收敛固涩。若腰脊酸痛、肢冷畏寒神怯者，可加生鹿肉、狗脊、补骨脂等温补督脉肾经。

处方举例：

熟地 15g、山药 12g、山萸肉 10g、补骨脂 10g、菟丝子 12g、巴戟天 10g、杜仲 10g、茯苓 10g、仙鹤草 15g、三七粉 3g(冲)

〔预防及护理措施〕

对于血证，应根据体质特点、每次发病诱因、常发血证部位及发病时的证候特点来进行预防。如热迫血妄行者，当忌食辛辣烟酒等动火之品，注意保持情绪稳定，精神愉快，以防肝火内炽，并应及时治疗外感，以防热入营血。因于阴虚火旺出血者，当注意生活起居、劳欲适度，以防耗伤肝肾之阴。因气虚不摄出血者，当特别预防感冒，注意加强饮食调养，以保脾胃运化正常，亦忌忧思恼怒，劳倦过度。

血证的护理措施主要有如下几点：

1. 注意出血部位及血量、血色、舌、脉、精神、面色、有无汗出、四肢温度等特点，以观察病位、病性及病情轻重。

2. 若出血量多，出血势急，或忽多忽少而日久，症见面色㿠白，精神疲困或神志恍惚，汗出肢冷，为血脱之象，当以急救止血。

3. 上窍出血，或咳、或吐、或衄，需安慰病人，精神勿紧张，尽量让体位适宜血液外出。切忌仰卧或仰面，或用毛巾等堵塞血道，以防瘀血滞塞气道，发生窒息而厥。若有血呛气道之表现，则当拍背、引吐等以使血出。

4. 居室宜空气新鲜，温度适合，以预防外感。一般饮食宜清淡，若气血已虚，脾肾不足，宜加强食补，并注意精神、起居的调养。

5. 随各种血证而进行辨证、辨病施护。

〔典型病例分析〕

案一：尿血。

谌某某，男，35 岁，湖南省计委干部。

初诊：1980 年 1 月 9 日。

因外出劳累，血尿月余，经×院 X 线照片、膀胱镜检、静脉肾盂造影、细菌培养等检查，未见异常，经治疗无效，而转服中药。

诊时：尿血如前，腰部灼热，神疲乏力，心烦少寐，口干喜饮，大便微溏，无浮肿，无尿频、尿急、尿痛及中断现象，舌质红，苔薄淡黄，脉细弦。小便化验：红细胞＋＋＋＋，白细胞 0—1，蛋白微量。尿血多系热结下焦,迫血妄行所致,然本例由气阴俱伤引起,治宜益气养血,清热凉血,化瘀止血,标本兼顾,宗小蓟饮子加减,处方:

黄芪 15g、白芍 12g、小蓟炭 10g、生地黄 20g、木通 10g、当归 10g、黑栀仁 10g、蒲黄炭(包)10g、茯苓 12g、白茅根 15g、藕节炭 10g、血余炭 5g、甘草梢 5g。服 5 剂。

二诊:1980 年 1 月 14 日。

药后尿血大减,小便检查:红细胞 0～3,余症依然。继服原方 5 剂。

三诊:1980 年 1 月 20 日。

尿血全止,小便化验恢复正常。仅诉左侧腰痛灼热,活动后加重,易疲劳,小溲黄。舌、脉如前。此气阴待复,治宜益气养阴,处方:

黄芪 15g、知母 10g、生地黄 20g、丹皮 10g、黄柏 10g、泽泻 10g、淮山药 15g、山茱萸 6g、茯苓 12g、白茅根 15g、川续断 12g、核桃肉 15g。再服 5 剂,诸症全瘥。

按《素问·气厥论》篇云:"胞热移于膀胱,则癃溺血。"《金匮要略》云:"热在下焦者,则尿血。"可见下焦湿热是尿血常见的原因,当属实证范畴。但本案尿血量多,且时间已久,故无"尿路刺激症",乃气阴俱伤,与纯系湿热殊异,证属虚实夹杂。治以标本兼顾,方以小蓟饮子去滑石、竹叶之甘寒滑泄,加茅根、血余炭清热凉血、化瘀止血,加黄芪、白芍配合当归益气滋阴。尤其生地黄一味,用量颇重,既能凉血止血,又能滋阴养血。全方共收清热化瘀、益气养阴之功。(选自《疑难病中医治疗》)

案二:便血。

毛某某,男,18 岁。胃脘痛已十载,每逢冬春则发作,一周来胃脘疼痛夜间较剧,反酸泛恶,便血色黑,苔白质淡,脉细。脾虚生寒不能摄血,肝虚生热不能藏血,统藏失职,血不归经,下渗大肠则为便血,拟《金匮》黄土汤,刚柔温清和肝脾以止血。

党参 12g、炒白术 9g、熟附片(先煎)9g、熟地 12g、炒黄芩 9g、阿胶 9g(烊化)、仙鹤草 30g、灶心土(包)30g。服四付,大便潜血阴性。

按:便血有远近之分,又 有寒热之别。患者胃痛七载,夜间较剧,又见便血色黑,脾胃虚寒之症也。平时又见恶心泛酸,乃肝热之象。虚寒挟热,寒重热轻,故用金匮黄土汤,刚柔相济,温中寓清,有温阳而不伤阴、滋阴而不碍阳之特点,辨证确切,药效卓著。(选自《张伯臾医案》)

案三:咳血。

陈某某,男,42 岁,农民。1977 年 6 月 29 日诊治。患者原有慢性咳嗽病史 10 年余。间断咳血多次,曾先后大咯血五次,每次咳血 100～200ml。近经温州××医院支气管碘油造影,确诊为右肺广泛性柱状支气管扩张。长期服用抗生素、祛痰剂、止血药无明显疗效,因不适于手术治疗,而来我院诊治。患者近因饮酒后咯血盈口,五天来连续每日咯吐鲜血数口,胸闷,咳嗽阵作,口干口苦,多汗,便结如羊矢,舌红苔黄腻而糙,脉来弦数。脉证合参,良由肠胃积热,气火上炎气道引动营血妄行。治宜清胃泄火,降气止血。处方:

焦山栀、桑白皮、生侧柏各 9g,黄芩 8g,白芨、生大黄(后下)各 10g,白茅根、生赭石(先煎)各 30g

服上方三剂,咯血辄止,大便通润,脉象弦缓。因腑气下行,肝火亢逆之势已平,故予清金益阴、保肺宁络之品调理自安。至今未再发作。

按:张景岳认为:"血动之由,惟火与气"。唐容川认为:"气为血帅,血随气来运行……"。故气逆咯血之证,不外乎热,由于阳明胃腑多气多血,且六腑以通为补,气火以降为顺。本案酒后胃中积热，气火上炎，遂令络血外溢，故用大黄亦必辅生赭石，以抑其上逆之凶势，助其下降之力，则血随气降，自无溢出之虞矣！（选自《新中医》1986年3期）

案四：鼻衄。

马子施鸣玉，鼻衄如注，一切止衄疗法并无一应。切其脉虚大而缓，面色痿黄而胖。如其四肢酸软、浑身倦怠懒于言动而嗜卧者，匪朝夕也。询之果然。而衄起之故，缘自钟溪归家，一路逆风操舟尽力，不及达岸即衄，至今第四日矣。余曰：此人中气大亏，本不足以摄血，而复因劳力太甚，重伤胃络，胃络阳络也，阳络伤则血出上窍，胃脉络鼻，所以血自鼻孔出也。乃用补中益气汤加炒黑干姜一剂而衄止。复去干姜加白芍、五味子守服数剂，而从前的倦懈怠懒言嗜卧等症渐除。（《潜村医案》）

按：出血多属实热，本例病人鼻衄如注，前医用一般清热凉血常规疗法无效。《张氏医通》说："衄血，脉……大而虚者，为脾虚不能统摄。"本例病人素有肢软、倦怠、嗜卧等症，知是素体脾虚，又因劳累太甚而诱发鼻衄。后医接诊时，根据患者体质及诱发原因，并结合面色萎黄、神倦乏力、舌体胖大，脉虚大而缓等症，通过全面辨析，诊为中气已伤，气伤则血无所主，溢于鼻窍，发为衄血，治以补中益气，气足则血自止。

案五：吐血。

杨某某，男，28岁。嗜酒，有失眠史，愈失眠则愈纵饮。一日，忽感膈间痞闷，气上冲咽喉，顷刻吐血不止，面色苍白，精神困乏。诊视脉弦大且数，舌苔淡黄。此阳明胃络出血，"阳络伤则血上溢"。患者饮酒过度，湿热伤胃，胃气以降为顺，"酒性大热有毒，气味俱阳"。伤酒太甚，胃中湿热挟冲脉之气载血上行。"冲为血海，隶于阳明"，一旦阳明的阳旺无制，则血涌如潮不可遏止，法当清胃降冲，导下解醒。

生地炭15g、侧柏炭13g、白茅根15g、京赤芍10g、牡丹皮10g、枳椇子10g、雪藕节10g、清童便1杯；

复诊：一日二剂，连服二日，吐血止，自汗失眠，脉显浮芤。脱血后，心脾失养，拟用归脾法，俾血有所归，心有所养。

炙黄芪13g、潞党参10g、蒸于术10g、当归身10g、炒枣仁10g、抱茯神10g、炙远志3g、广木香2g、龙眼肉10g、炮姜炭1g、炙甘草3g；

按：本例患者，吐血来势急骤，血量大。在急剧清胃降冲止血后，暴露了心脾血亏的脉证。故治标为急，而治本亦不宜缓。不然，脱血之后，元气随之衰竭。方用归脾汤加入姜炭1克意义何在？因为阴血大损，虚阳无以收敛，表现在脉象弦大且数转变为浮芤，故用极少量姜炭，变辛热为苦温，收摄虚阳于甘温归脾剂中，取效尤捷。虽呕以后严禁饮酒，如不自觉守禁，必成痨损。（《李聪甫医案》）

血证总由外感、内伤的多种原因引起，而基本病机可归纳为火热熏灼，气虚不摄和瘀血阻络三类。火有实火、虚火之分。实火多是肺热、胃热、肝火、心火、肠道湿热及血分热炽；虚火多为肝肾阴虚火旺，或肺、胃阴伤火盛。气虚之中有气虚及气损及阳之别。气虚以肺、脾、肾气虚为主，阳虚多为脾阳虚或脾肾阳虚。瘀血以气滞、气虚、寒凝、热结、离经之血所成为多。血证证候不外虚实两端，一般由火热亢盛所致者属实证，由阴虚火旺及气虚不摄所致者属虚证。治疗血证应掌握止血、治因、固本三原则，从治血、治气、治火三方面入手。实火当清热泻火，虚火当滋阴降火；气实宜清气降气，气虚宜补气益气。止血即针对出血对症治疗，根据病因病性酌情配伍收敛止血，凉血止血，温经止血或祛瘀止血的方药，以图止血。若出血暴急量多，当权衡病势病情，或直折其火，或急固其脱。灵活运用对症与对因治疗是提高疗效的关键。血证的预后，主要和三个因素有关，一是引起血证的原因，一般因于外感者易治、内伤者难治，新病初发者易治、久病屡发者难治。二是与出血的急缓和出血量的多少有关。出血量少，势缓者病轻，血出急迫、量多者病重，要警惕由大量出血，而造成气随血脱的危急重症。三是与兼见的症状、脉象有关。出血而伴见发热、咳喘、烦躁不安，或汗出、肢冷等症状，脉见洪大数疾者难治。出血之后，每因出血而致体虚，应针对气虚、阴虚、血虚之侧重，进行适宜的调治。并从生活起居、饮食情志等多方面注意以预防复发。

复习思考题

1. 试述血证的病因病机？
2. 试述血证的辨治要点？
3. 简述衄血，咳血，吐血，便血及尿血的分型论治？
4. 如何在血证的治疗中选用泻心汤、玉女煎、犀角地黄汤、归脾汤、小蓟饮子、地榆散。
5. 试述吐血一病中治肝、治胃、治脾的临床见症特点。
6. 如何鉴别脾胃虚寒和湿热蕴蒸引起的便血？并说明其不同治法和主方。

心　悸

〔概述〕

心悸包括惊悸与怔忡，是指病人自觉心中悸动，惊悸不安，甚则不能自主；或同时见有脉象的相应变化，如疾、数、促、结、迟等脉单独或相兼出现的一种病证。临床一般多呈阵发性，每因情志波动或劳累而发作，也间有久发不止者。

惊悸与怔忡既有区别又有联系，临床上可从病因，病情，主证，病性等方面区别二者之不同；可从二者的相互转化和影响来理解其密切的联系。

心悸以病人自觉心中跳动，惊惕不安，不能自主为主证，常兼见少寐多梦，头晕目眩，胸闷喘憋，心痛，脉迟，数或结代；病位在心，可累及脾、肾、肝、肺；病机多为本虚标实，虚为气、血、阴、阳亏损；实为气、瘀、痰、饮阻滞心脉，病情一般较重，甚者可发生厥逆、汗多、脉微、神昏等心阳欲脱之心悸危候。

据本病的临床证候表现，西医之各种原因引起的心律失常，如心动过速、心动过缓、早搏、心房颤动与扑动、房室传导阻滞、束支传导阻滞、病态窦房结综合征、预激综合征、心力衰竭、心肌炎、心包炎以及部分神经官能症等，有本病表现者，可参考本篇辨证治疗。

〔病因病机〕

心悸的形成，与精神因素、体质因素、浊邪因素有关。精神因素主要指惊恐、郁怒；体质因素主要为心血不足，肾阴亏陨，阳气虚衰；浊邪因素不外痰、火、水、饮、瘀血、气滞作乱。三种因素多相互影响，相互作用而致心悸发生。

临 床常见心悸的病因病机有以下几点：

一、心虚胆怯：由于禀赋不足，或后天失养，平素心虚胆怯之人，突受惊恐，如耳闻巨响，目睹异物，或遇险临危，致心惊神慌不能自主，渐到稍受惊恐即心悸不已，而成本病。此外如大怒伤肝，大恐伤肾，怒则气逆，恐则精却，阴虚于下，火逆于上，亦可动撼心神，而发惊悸。又有痰热内蕴，复加郁怒，胃失和降，痰火互结，上扰心神，而致心悸发生。

心悸病因病机示意图

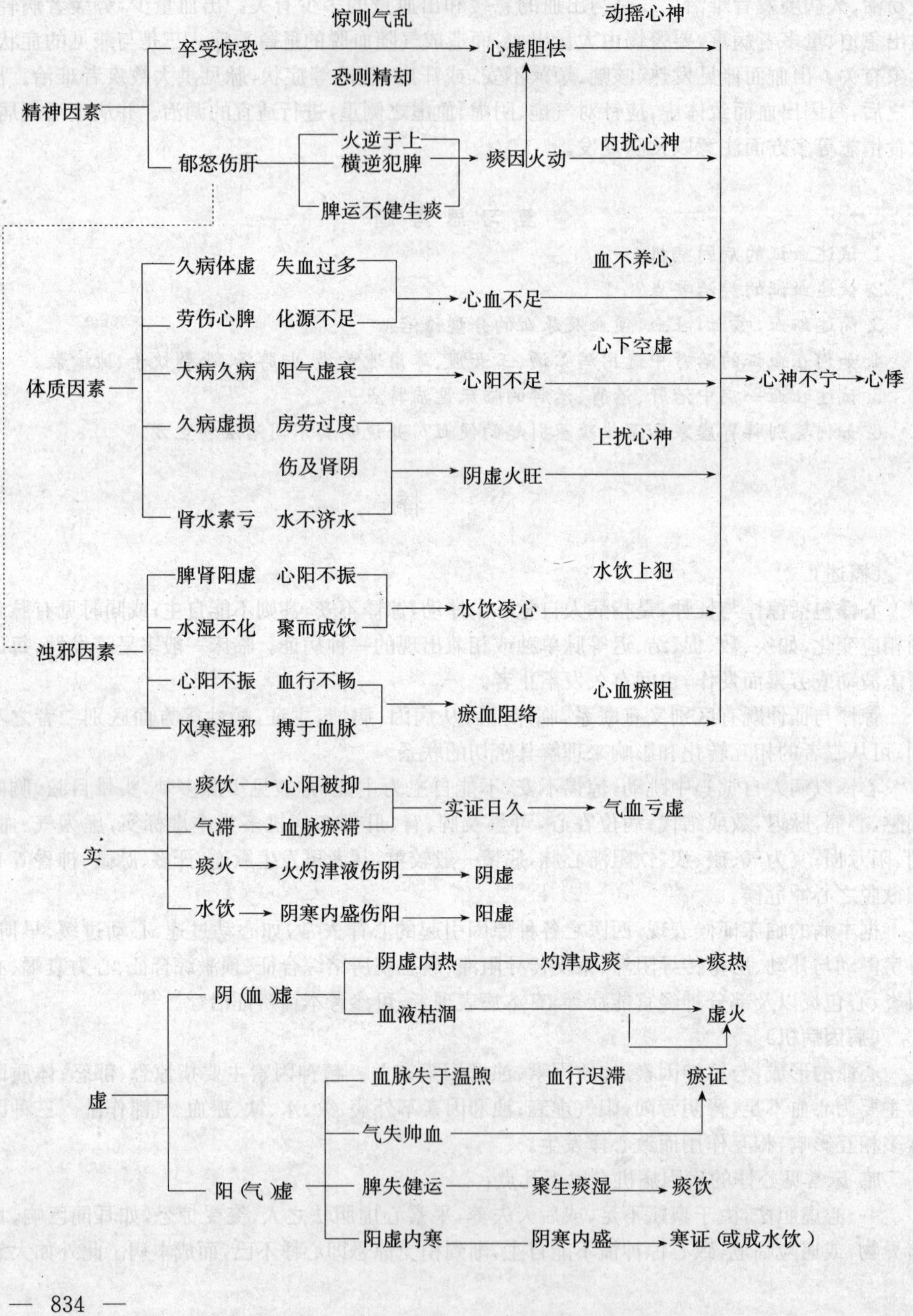

二、心血不足：心主血，血赖心气的推动才能运行周身，荣养脏腑四肢百骸，心脏亦有赖于血液的濡养。心藏神，心血充足，心有所养，则神有所藏，而无惊悸怔忡之症。若禀赋不足，脏腑虚损；或病后失于调养，或思虑过度，劳伤心脾，或脾胃虚衰，气血生化无源，或失血过多等，均可导致心血亏虚，心失所养，不能藏神而发为心悸。

三、阴虚火旺：久病体弱，或房劳过度，久病虚损，或遗泄频繁，胎产过多，伤及肾阴，或肾水素亏之人，水不济火，虚火妄动，上扰心神，而致心悸。

四、心阳不足：心之阳气，有维护心脏正常生理功能，鼓动血液运行，并能资助脾肾之阳的作用。若心阳不振，心气不足则无以鼓动血液的运行，心失温养而作悸。

五、水饮凌心：脾肾阳虚，不能蒸化水液，水湿停聚为饮，饮邪上犯，心阳被抑，或心阳不足，气化失利，水液不得下行，停于心下，而致心悸，亦即《伤寒明理论·悸》篇所说："其停饮者，由水停心下，心生火而恶水，水既内停，心不自安，则为悸也。"

六、瘀血阻络：瘀血阻滞心络而致心悸，其原因主要有二：一由心阳不振，血行不畅心脉受阻，一由痹证日久发展而来，此因风寒湿邪搏于血脉，内犯于心，血行不畅致心脉痹阻，引起惊悸怔忡。正如《素问·痹论》所说："脉痹不已，复感于邪，内舍于心"及"心痹者，脉不通，烦则心下鼓。"《医宗必读·悸》解释说："鼓者，跳动如击鼓也。"

综上所述，心悸的病位在心，而与脾、肾、肝、肺密切相关，病理特点为心神不宁。病因病机概括而言，不外虚实两方面：虚者正气虚也，即人体阴、阳、气、血亏损，使心失所养，失却主血脉、主神明的功能；实者为气、痰、饮、瘀阻滞心脉，使心气被抑，血脉运行障碍，虚实可以互相兼夹和转化，如实证日久，正气亏虚，可见有阴、阳、气、血亏损。而虚证又往往夹有实象，如阴虚可以生内热，灼津成痰，故阴虚常夹痰热。阳虚水湿不能运化聚生痰饮，水饮内停，水气凌心，故阳虚常夹痰饮，气血虚则血脉运行不利，又可导致血瘀之症。痰火内盛，火灼津液伤阴可致阴虚，水饮内停，阴寒内盛，伤阳可致阳虚。虚实夹杂与转化的规律，在辨证论治过程中，应当引起注意。

〔辨证论治〕

一、辨证要点

（一）辨标本虚实：本虚当审心之气、血、阴、阳，哪方面虚甚；标实当视痰、饮、水、火、瘀血，何邪为主，这主要通过心悸特点及脉象和脉证合参来辨别。

1. 心悸特点：虚者若心气虚、心阳虚则见空虚而悸，短气，活动后加剧。心血虚，心阴虚则见虚烦而悸，思虑劳神后加剧。实者如痰火扰心，常见心悸烦躁，胸中烦热，少眠乱梦等热象。痰气上逆则见心悸易惊，胸满胁胀。饮邪上犯之心悸多为惊而眩晕，胸闷、喘憋或有水肿。瘀血阻络之心悸则心悸惕惕，多兼心痛或胸痹，唇舌紫暗或有瘀斑。

2. 脉象和脉证合参：数脉，滑数有力为痰火内盛，细数无力为阴虚火旺。迟脉，主寒证，沉迟无力多属阳虚内寒。

结代脉：促、结、代三种脉象单独或两种相合出现，通常统称为结代脉，偶见于正常人情绪激动、悲伤时，短时间内即可消失。心悸病人出现结代脉，多因气血不足，心血痹阻而致，若见于心悸危重阶段，则为心气衰败之象。结代脉渐渐恢复正常搏动，是心气恢复之征，结代脉加重渐趋停止，并见神昏抽搐等证，为心气欲绝之险候。

由于心悸一证，本虚标实夹杂者甚多，心气虚、心阳虚多伴有瘀血、水饮；心血虚，心阴虚多夹有虚热或痰火。故辨证时还当注意虚实二证的相兼与夹杂。

(二)辨心悸的轻重与危候:若因外来因素而诱发,心悸阵作,时间较短,且可自行缓解者,病情较轻。若无外因诱发,心悸持续,稍活动则加重,或伴喘憋,水肿,心痛,肢冷,眩晕者,病情重。若怔忡,大汗淋漓,四肢厥冷,唇口青紫,呼吸微弱,脉微欲绝,甚则神昏者为心阳衰微欲脱的危证。

(三)辨惊悸与怔忡的区别与联系

1. 二者的区别:惊悸与怔忡同属一类疾病但二者尚有区别。一般认为,怔忡每由内因引起,并无外惊,自觉心中惕惕,稍劳即发,病来虽渐,但全身情况较差,病情较为深重;惊悸则相反,常由外界刺激或受惊恐、恼怒而发病,发则心悸,时作时止,病来虽速,但全身情况较好,病势浅而短暂。

惊悸与怔忡辨别表

	惊　　悸	怔　　忡
病　因	多因外受惊恐恼怒而发(平素心虚胆怯)	多遇内因所成(素体脏腑亏虚),久病遇劳即发
病　情	病浅易治,可自行缓解	病深难治,常持续发作
主　症	心卒动而不宁	心中躁动不安
病　性	实中带虚(多痰火为患,心虚胆怯)多功能性	多为虚证,虚中夹实(多气血不足,心血瘀阻)多器质性
治　则	以镇惊为主	以补虚为主

2. 二者的联系:一方面,惊悸日久可以发展为怔忡;另一方面,怔忡患者又易受外惊所扰,而使动悸加重。

二、分型证治

心悸一病病变部位主要在心,证候特点是虚实相兼,以虚为主,故补虚是治疗本病的基本治则,当视气血阴阳亏虚之不同,分别选用益气、养血、滋阴、温阳等法,以求阴平阳秘、气血运行调畅。本病的邪实以痰火、水饮、瘀血最为常见,治宜分别采取化痰清火、化痰涤饮、活血化瘀等法。虚实兼夹者,病情较为复杂,当分清主次缓急,相应兼顾,补虚与补邪并施,或有所侧重。因心中悸动不安为本病主要临床症状,故又常在补虚及祛邪基础上,酌情配伍镇心安神或养心安神的方药。

(一)心虚胆怯

主症:心悸,善惊易怒。

兼症:坐卧不安,少寐多梦。

舌脉:舌苔薄白或如常,脉象虚数,结代或弦滑促。

分析:惊则气乱,心神不能自主而致心悸。心不藏神,心中惕惕,则善惊易恐,坐卧不安,少寐多梦。脉虚数、结代或弦滑促为心神不安,气血逆乱之象。本型病情较轻者,时发时止,重者怔忡不宁,心慌神乱,不能自主。

治法:镇惊定志,养心安神。

方药:选用安神定志丸加琥珀、磁石、朱砂。用龙齿、琥珀、磁石以镇惊宁心,朱砂拌茯神、菖蒲、远志以安神定志,人参(可用党参代)益心气。若心气虚不明显者不用人参;若惊悸心虚胆怯可加炙甘草以补益心气;心阴不足加柏子仁、五味子、酸枣仁以养心安神收敛心气;若心悸而烦，喜惊痰多，食少泛恶，舌苔黄腻，脉象滑数者，是痰热内扰，胃火和降，心神不安之故，可用黄连温胆汤以清痰热，和胃降浊，痰热清则心自安。方中也可加入枣仁、远志等以安神养心。

处方举例：

磁石(先下)30g、菖蒲10g、远志10g、茯神10g、丹参10g、太子参12g、炙甘草8g、生龙牡(先下)各15g、朱砂(分冲)0.5g。

(二)心血不足

主症：心悸，头晕乏力。

兼症：面色无华，神疲倦怠。

舌脉：舌质淡红，脉象细弱。

分析：心血不足，心失所养，故而心悸。心血亏虚，不能上营于脑，故而头晕。心主血脉，其华在面，血虚故面色无华。血亏气弱故倦怠神疲。舌为心之苗，心主血脉，心血不足，故舌质淡红，脉象细弱。

治法：补血养心，益气安神。

方药：归脾汤加减。方中当归、龙眼肉补养心血；人参、黄芪、白术、炙甘草益气健脾，以资生血之源；酸枣仁、茯神、远志安神定志；再辅木香行气，使之补而不滞。

加减：若见心动悸而脉结代者，为气虚血少，血不养心所致，宜用炙甘草汤益气养血、滋阴复脉。方中炙甘草甘温复脉，以利心气；人参、大枣补气益胃；桂枝、生姜辛温通阳；地黄、阿胶、麦冬、麻仁滋阴补血，以养心阴。诸药相配，能使气血充盈，则心动悸、脉结代之症可解。若热病后期，损及心阴而致心悸者，可用生脉散益气养阴，本方人参补益元气、麦冬养阴，五味子收敛耗散之肺气，三药合用，有益气养阴之功。

处方举例：

党参10g、炙黄芪12g、白术8g、当归10g、茯神10g、远志10g、麦冬10g、五味子8g、炙甘草20g。

(三)阴虚火旺

主症：心悸不安，心烦少寐。

兼症：手足心热，腰酸耳鸣，头晕目眩。

舌脉：舌质红，少苔或无苔，脉象细数。

分析：肾阴不足，水不济火，以致心火内动，扰动心神，故心悸而烦，不能安眠。阴虚于下，则见腰酸；阳扰于上，则眩晕耳鸣，手足心热。舌质红，脉细数，皆为阴虚火旺之征。

治法：滋阴清火，养心安神。

方药：天王补心丹或朱砂安神丸加减，二方同为滋阴养血、清心安神之剂。前方宜于阴虚而火不甚旺者，方中生地、元参、麦冬、天冬等以养阴清热；当归、丹参补血养心；人参补益心气；朱砂、茯苓、远志、枣仁、柏子仁安养心神；五味子收敛心气；桔梗引药上行，以通心气。朱砂安神丸对虚烦咽燥、口干口苦等热象较著者相宜，方中朱砂重镇安神，当归、生地养血滋阴，黄连清心火以安神。诸药相伍，有泻心火、养心阴、补心血、宁心神四种功效，为治疗心神不安、烦躁心悸的常用方药。

加减：若阴虚火旺而兼五心烦热，梦遗腰酸者，为阴虚相火妄动之故，可用知柏地黄丸化裁，以滋阴降火。

处方举例：

麦冬 10g、五味子 10g、生地 12g、沙参 12g、元参 12g、丹参 12g、太子参 10g、苦参 10g、炙甘草 8g。

(四)心阳不足

主症:心悸不安,胸闷气短。

兼症:面色苍白,形寒肢冷。

舌脉:舌质淡白,脉象虚弱或沉细而弱或沉迟、结、代。

分析:久病体弱,损伤心阳,心失温养,故心悸不安。胸中阳气不足,故胸闷气短。心阳虚弱,血液运行迟缓,肢体失于温煦,故形寒肢冷,面色苍白。舌质淡白,脉象虚弱,或沉细而弱,或沉迟、结代,均为心阳不足,鼓动无力之征。

治法:温补心阳,安神定悸。

方药:桂枝甘草龙骨牡蛎汤加味。方中桂枝、甘草温补心阳,龙骨、牡蛎安神定悸。可加人参、附子以温阳益气。

加减:若病情严重,汗出肢冷,面青唇紫,喘憋不能平卧者,上方重用人参、附子,加服黑锡丹以回阳救逆。当知此为心阳欲脱之危候,若心中空虚而悸,脉沉迟,形寒肢冷尤甚,此为心肾阳气皆虚,阴寒内盛,可用麻黄附子细辛汤加党参、炙甘草治之。

处方举例:

附片 6g、桂枝 10g、黄芪 12g、黄精 12g、炙甘草 10g、生龙牡各 15g、人参粉(冲)3g(或党参 10g)、当归 10g、干姜 6g。

(五)水饮凌心

主症:心悸胸憋,喘咳浮肿。

兼症:眩晕肢冷,胸脘痞满,小便短少,渴不欲饮,恶心吐涎。

舌脉:舌苔白滑,脉象弦滑。

分析:水为阴邪,赖阳气化之,今阳虚不能化水,水邪内停,上凌于心,故见心悸。阴邪乘于阳位,故见胸憋。水饮凌心犯肺,故见喘咳。气化不利,水液内停,则渴不欲饮,小便短少或下肢浮肿。阳气不能达于四肢,不能充于肌表,故形寒肢冷。水饮中阻,清阳不升,故见眩晕。气机不利,故胸脘痞满。舌苔白滑,脉象弦滑,亦为水饮内停之象。

治法:振奋心阳,化气行水。

方药:苓桂术甘汤加减。方中茯苓淡渗利水,桂枝、甘草通阳化气,白术健脾祛湿。

加减:水饮上逆,恶心呕吐者,加半夏、陈皮、生姜以和胃降逆。如肾阳虚衰,不能制水,水气凌心症见心悸喘咳,不能平卧,小便不利,浮肿较甚者,宜用真武汤加减,以温阳行水。如心脾阳气虚弱,水饮停聚,水气凌心,症见 心悸水肿,倦怠乏力者,可用春泽汤加减,此方药物即五苓散加人参,具有益气健脾、化气行水之功。

处方举例:

党参 12g、炮附子 6g、桂枝 10g、茯苓 20g、猪苓 15g、泽泻 12g、白术 10g、赤芍 10g、炙甘草 5g、苏子 6g、生姜 3 片。

(六)心血瘀阻

主症:心悸不安,阵发心痛。

兼症:胸闷不舒,唇甲青紫。

舌脉:舌质暗紫或有瘀斑,脉结代或涩。

分析：心主血脉，心脉瘀阻，心失所养，故心悸不安；血瘀气滞，心阳被抑，则胸闷不舒；心络瘀阻，络脉挛急，则心痛时作。脉络瘀阻，故见唇甲青紫，舌质紫暗，或有瘀斑，脉涩或结代，皆为瘀血蓄积、心阳阻遏之征。

治法：活血化瘀，理气通络。

方药：桃仁红花煎加减。方中桃仁、红花、丹参、赤芍、川芎活血化瘀，元胡、香附、青皮理气通脉，生地、当归养血和血。

加减：可加入桂枝、甘草以通阳气，加龙骨、牡蛎以镇心神，诸药合用，使心络通畅，则悸痛自止。若痰瘀闭阻者，症兼见痰多泛恶，纳呆，脘痞，舌苔厚腻，脉滑，可合入瓜蒌薤白半夏汤以宽胸化痰。

处方举例：

丹参 15g、赤芍 10g、川芎 10g、红花 10g、瓜蒌 20g、薤白 6g、半夏 10g、党参 10g、郁金 10g、元胡 10g。

总之，心悸是病人自觉心中悸动，甚则不能自主的病证，有惊悸、怔忡之区别。在临床上大致分为心虚胆怯、心血不足、阴虚火旺、心阳不足、水饮凌心、心血瘀阻六个类型，每个类型各有特点，临证时应详细辨别，随证施治，方可取得应有疗效。

〔**预防及护理措施**〕

1. 保持心情愉快，避免情志内伤。惊悸、怔忡每因情志内伤，恐惧而悸发。经常保持心情愉快，则可避免情志为害，减少发病。

2. 饮食有节，起居有常。平素饮食不宜过饱，宜少食辛辣油腻食物，生活要有一定的规律。要保证一定的休息和睡眠，注意劳逸结合。

3. 注意寒暑变化，避免外邪侵袭。防止因感受风、寒、湿、热等外邪，而诱发心悸，或使病情加重。

4. 轻症患者若可作适当的体力活动，以不感觉劳累为限度，应避免剧烈活动及强体力活动。重症患者若平时即觉心悸、气短较甚，甚至面浮肢肿，脉象结代，则应卧床休息。

5. 药物治疗十分重要，治疗过程中应坚持服药，症状缓解后，亦当遵医嘱服药巩固一段时间。

〔**典型病例分析**〕

案一：陈某某，男，50 岁。患高血压病 20 年，近五、六年头晕目眩，心慌加重。检查：心率 58 次/分，血压 170/100mmHg，形体肥胖，口唇发绀，肺(—)，心尖搏动约在左锁骨中线外 1.5cm，有抬举性搏动，心律绝对不齐，心尖部可闻及收缩期雷鸣样杂音，脉搏短绌。西医诊断：①高血压病Ⅲ期；②高血压性心脏病；③冠心病合并心房纤颤；④心衰Ⅱ°。经西药较长期治疗，无明显好转。后因活动而突发胸闷气促，张口抬肩，头晕跌仆，额汗淋漓，经西医抢救，病情仍危笃。请肖医师诊治，症见心悸不安，头晕目眩倦怠卧床，语音低怯，面白无华，唇干寐差，脉迟结代。辨证为心阳不振，气阴两虚，治宜温通心阳，益气养阴。处方：制附片 9 克，肉桂 4 克，麦冬 12 克，党参 20 克，五味子 9 克，制黄精 15 克，上方化裁续服，复诊时病情减轻，早搏消失，心慌诸症悉除，精神好转，能短途步履。(《江西中医药》1983：2)

按：此案为心悸阴阳俱虚型。心阴素虚，心神失养，故心慌心跳，头晕寐差；心阳不振无力鼓动脉道，故胸闷心悸，脉迟结代。方用党参、五味子、麦冬益气养阴，生津复脉；附子、肉桂大辛大热，补命火以助以阳；黄精味甘纯正，补脾阴，益中气，润五脏，为滋阴益气之佳品。全方温阳益气而不伤阴，滋阳养心而不腻胃，配伍严谨，药少力专。

心悸是病人自觉心慌，心跳不能自主的病证，有惊悸、怔忡之别。病因主要是体质素虚（久病或先天所致的气血阴阳亏虚或脏腑功能失调）、情志所伤以及外邪侵袭。此三者互相影响，互为因果，有主有从，其中体质因素是发病的根本。本病病位在心，但亦常与其他脏腑有密切关系，其病理变化不外虚、实两端，虚为气、血、阴、阳的亏虚，而致心失所养；实则多为痰饮内停，瘀血阻络，以致心脉不畅，心神不宁。虚实两者常互相夹杂。虚证之中，常兼痰浊、水饮或瘀血为患；实证之中，则多有脏腑虚衰的表现，且随着病情的变化，虚实可以互相转化，或由实转虚，或因虚致实。

本病的辨证，首先当从心悸的特点和脉证的不同辨标本虚实，次辨心悸的轻重与危候，第三要辨惊悸与怔忡的区别与联系。

本病临床上主要分为心虚胆怯、心血不足、阴虚火旺、心阳不足、水饮凌心、心血瘀阻六型，治法不外乎镇、养、化、温。心虚胆怯治宜镇惊定志，养心安神。心血不足治宜补血养心，益气安神；阴虚火旺治当滋阴降火，养心安神；心阳不足治宜温补心阳，安神定悸；水饮凌心者治当振奋心阳，化气行水；心血瘀阻者又宜活血化瘀，理气通络。因本病以心中悸动不安为主症，所以不论哪型心悸，均应适当配伍养心安神或重镇安神之品，但重镇安神药一般不宜久用。

本病初起，病情较轻，正虚不甚，治疗较易；若病久失治或误治，多个脏腑受累，正虚邪实夹杂者，病情较重，治疗较难，常可出现心肾阳气虚脱之危候，当及时抢救。

复习思考题

1. 试述心悸的病因病机。
2. 试述惊悸与怔忡的区别与联系。
3. 临床上常见的六个心悸类型是什么？怎样辨证论治？

胸　痹

〔概述〕

痹者闭也，胸痹为胸中气血闭阻之意，是以胸部闷痛，则甚胸痛彻背，短气、喘息不得卧为主症的一种疾病；轻者仅感胸痛如窒、呼吸不畅，重者则见胸痛心悸，严重者心痛彻背，背痛彻心，手足青冷。

胸痹应与胃痛、胸痛相鉴别。可通过疼痛部位、伴随症状、心电图、X线及其他理化检查来鉴别。

胸痹病位在心、肺，发病与肝、脾、肾有关，病因主要有寒暑外袭、情志、饮食、劳倦、亡血失精。病机特点为本虚标实，本虚为五脏气血阴阳亏虚，标实责之气滞血瘀、痰凝、寒盛、热壅。基本病机为心脉不充或心脉闭阻所致气滞血瘀。随着病情发展，可出现真心痛、厥脱、心悸、喘咳、肢肿等心肾阳气虚衰之危候。

西医冠状动脉粥样硬化性心脏病、心绞痛、心肌梗塞以及心包炎等疾病而致的心前区疼痛，其临床表现与本病特点相符者，可参照本病辨证论治。

〔病因病机〕

胸痹的病位在心、肺。胸为心、肺之所居，心主血、肺主气，心肺协调，气血才能正常运行，其发病与肾、肝、脾诸脏的盛衰也有密切关系。若素体胸阳不振，脏腑功能低下，阴阳气血失调，外邪乘虚侵袭，或饮食不节、思虑过度、痰湿痹阻、经脉失和，均可引起胸痛。其病因病机归纳如下：

一、寒暑犯心：素体心气不足或心阳不振，复因寒邪直中，寒凝胸中，胸阳不展，心脉痹阻，乃发胸痹，故患者每于气候突然转冷，则易于卒然发生心痛。本为阳虚，包括心气虚、心阳虚，以及脾、肾的阳虚；标为寒盛，两者当有主次之分，宜详辨。另外，酷暑炎热，犯于心君，耗伤心气，亦可导致血脉运行不畅而心痛。

二、七情内伤：由于忧思恼怒，气机郁滞，气血运行不畅，心脉瘀阻则致心痛；情志不遂，气机不利，则津液凝聚为痰，或气郁日久化火，火能煎熬津液成痰。痰阻脉络，气血瘀滞，或痰瘀交阻，胸阳不展，心脉痹阻，均可发为胸痹。

三、饮食失节：过食肥甘厚味，或辛辣炙煿之品，或嗜酒成癖，以致脾胃损伤，运化失健，水谷不化精微而成痰浊，痰阻脉络，则气滞血瘀，心脉不畅而成胸痹。

四、气血不足：思虑劳倦，损伤心脾，或大病之后，正气不复，脾胃虚弱，运化无权，气血化生乏源，气血亏虚，心失濡养，或亡血之人，气血过耗、不能养心，心脉不充血液涩滞，均可引起胸痹。心之气血不足，日久不复，可致心阳不足，阳气不振，鼓动无力，清阳失展，血行迟滞，发为心痛。心之气血不足，日久也易引起阴血亏乏，心脉失于濡养，拘急而痛。

五、肝肾亏虚：多育或失精，损伤肾气，或年过五旬，天癸渐衰。肝肾同源，阴精不足，则不能滋养五脏之阴，而致心阴亏损，血脉枯涩而致胸痹心痛。若阴虚火旺，虚火上炎，也可燥伤心阴，可使心脉枯涸而成心痛。

总之，胸痹的发生，以本虚标实为多，标实则责之气滞、血瘀、痰凝、寒盛、热壅等；本虚则当分心气虚、心血虚、心阳虚、肝肾阴虚、脾肾阳虚及肺气虚等。上述病理变化，可单一为病，也可二者、三者相兼为害。

胸痹病因病机示意图

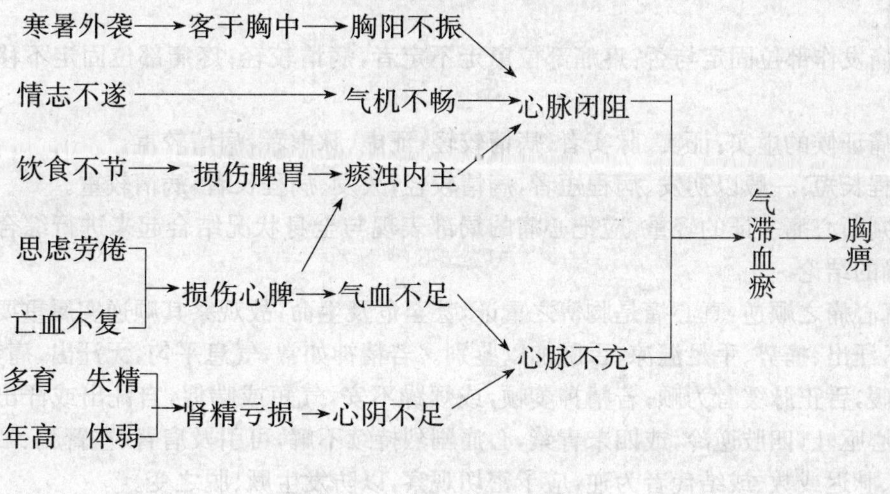

胸痹若治疗不及时，则可以变生多种疾病。如瘀血闭阻心脉，阳衰阴盛，则心胸卒然剧痛，

持续不止，而成真心痛；如心脉痹阻不通，阴阳过耗而离绝，也可成脱证；如心之气血不足，心失所养，可见心动悸、脉结代；如心、脾、肾阳虚，水邪泛滥，上逆凌心射肺，可出现咳喘、肢肿等症。

〔辨证论治〕

一、辨证要点

（一）辨虚实、分主次：本病证以本虚标实为多，虚则分心气虚（包括肺气虚）、心血虚、心阳虚、脾肾阳虚、肝肾阴虚，虚者为本；实可见气滞、血瘀、痰凝、寒盛、热结，实者为标。胸痹而见虚证、虚脉者，以虚为主，治从其本；胸痹而见实证、实脉者，以实为主，治从其标。

（二）辨疼痛性质：胸痹心痛，在临床上可见到闷痛、刺痛、灼痛、绞痛、隐痛等。

闷痛：闷重而痛轻，时作时休，与情绪变化有关者，多为气滞；若闷痛并作，身胖痰多，阴天易作，苔腻者，多为痰凝；若胸中隐痛而闷，稍劳则重，气短乏力，易汗出者，多为心气不足；若胸中隐痛而闷，亡血或经后而发，心悸少寐，舌淡者，多属心血亏虚。

刺痛：胸中作痛，状若锥刺，固定不移，舌质紫黯，或有瘀斑、瘀点，或舌下筋脉青紫者，多属血瘀。但血瘀常因多种原因所致，故当结合具体病情，全面考虑而定。

灼痛：总由火热所致，每宜分其虚实。若胸中灼痛，心烦躁扰不宁，夜难成寐，口干而苦者，多属实火；若胸中灼痛而闷，痰稠色黄，苔黄腻者，多属痰火；若胸中灼痛不剧，伴五心烦热，眩晕，心悸，舌红体瘦少苔者，多属阴虚有火。

绞痛：疼痛如绞，突然发作，遇寒则发，得冷则剧，多伴畏寒肢冷，胸闷如窒，为寒凝心脉所致；若有阳虚见症，畏寒踡卧，舌淡而胖者，多属阳虚内寒。另外，这种剧烈的心痛也常因劳累过度，七情喜怒，过食饮酒等等因素而诱发，故当随证审视而定属性，不可为“寒”所囿。

隐痛：胸中疼痛隐隐而作，劳后易发，气短神疲者，多属气虚，也属阳虚；若胸中隐痛而烦，头晕耳鸣者，又属阴虚。

（三）辨病势轻重、顺逆

1. 辨轻重：一般情况下，病势的轻重应以疼痛为标志，判断可遵以下几点：

（1）心痛发作次数：发作频繁者重；偶尔发作者轻。

（2）每次心痛发作的持续时间：瞬间即逝者轻；持续时间长者重；若持续时间达数小时，或数天者更重。

（3）心痛发作部位固定与否：疼痛部位窜走不定者，病情较轻；疼痛部位固定不移者，病情较重。

（4）心痛证候的虚实：证实、脉实者，病情较轻；证虚、脉虚者，病情较重。

（5）病程长短：一般以初发、病程短者，病情较轻；久发、病程长者，病情较重。

总之，判断心痛一证的轻重，应把心痛的局部表现与全身状况结合起来进行综合分析，才能得出正确的结论。

2. 辨真心痛之顺逆：真心痛是胸痹之重证，甚至危及生命，故观察其顺逆实属重要，一般从神志、气息、汗出、痛势、手足温凉、舌脉加以鉴别。若精神如常，气息平匀，无汗出，痛势轻而短暂，手足温暖，舌正脉缓者为顺；若精神萎顿，或烦躁不安，气短或喘促，自汗出或汗出如油，心悸慌乱，恶心呕吐，四肢逆冷，或四末青紫，心痛剧烈持续不解，可引及肩背、左臂臑、咽喉、脘腹等处，舌紫、脉迟或数、或结代者为逆，应予密切观察，以防发生厥、脱之变。

二、胸痹与胃痛、胸痛的鉴别

胸痹：疼痛以胸部为主，多伴有胸痛彻背，心悸气短，喘息不得卧的症状。配合心电图及其他理化检查,更易证实。

胃痛:疼痛部位以鸠尾下为主,多伴有嗳气,吞酸,脘满或胀,与饮食有密切关系。配合X线钡餐造影或纤维胃镜,更易证实。

胸痛:疼痛部位与胸痹相近,但不尽在左胸,多属肺病所致,疼痛持续不解,常与咳嗽或呼吸有关,多伴有咳喘、咯吐痰涎,或寒热等,配合X线或其他理化检查,多易证实。

三、治则要点

本病的治疗原则应先治其标,后顾其本;先从祛邪入手,然后再予扶正;若标不重,而正已虚时,当补消兼施,标本兼顾;若正气衰败已显时,又当扶正救脱为先。祛邪治标之法常以活血化瘀、辛温通阳、泄浊豁痰、理气宽胸、清热通腑为主;扶正固本常用温中助阳、益气养阴、补益气血、滋养肝肾等法。

四、分型证治

(一)心血瘀阻

主症:胸部刺痛,固定不移,入夜更甚。

兼症:心悸不宁,平素胸部憋闷,以手按摩则舒。

舌脉:舌质紫黯,或有瘀斑、瘀点,或舌下筋脉青紫,脉象沉涩。

分析:气郁日久,瘀血内停,络脉不通,故见胸部刺痛。血脉凝滞,故痛处固定不移。血属阴,夜亦属阴,故入夜痛甚。瘀血阻塞,心失所养,故心悸不宁。气血阻滞于胸,故平素胸部憋闷,以手按摩则能助气血运行,故可缓解。舌质紫黯,或有瘀斑、瘀点,或舌下筋脉青紫,脉象沉涩,均为瘀血内停之候。

治法:活血化瘀,通络止痛。

方药:以血府逐瘀汤加减。方中当归、赤芍、川芎、桃仁、红花等均为活血祛瘀之品,柴胡疏肝,枳壳理气,一升一降,调理气机,取气为血帅,气行则血行之意。若胸痛甚者,可配加降香、田三七、郁金、元胡以活血理气止痛。若胸部憋闷明显者,可加旋覆花、瓜蒌皮、青皮等宽胸理气之品;若心悸不宁甚重时,可加生龙骨、生牡蛎、代赭石等镇心安神。

若血瘀轻者,则可改用丹参饮为治。方中丹参活血化瘀,能治血瘀作痛;檀香温中理气,兼治心腹诸痛;砂仁温胃畅中,能疏散胸中郁闷,三药相伍配用,能活血化瘀,理气止痛。

处方举例:

全当归10g、京赤芍12g、川芎10g、丹参20g、三七粉(冲)3g、炒枳壳10g、降香6g、红花6g、瓜蒌皮15g、代赭石(先下)20g。

(二)痰浊壅塞

主症:胸闷如窒而痛,或痛引肩背。

兼症:形体肥胖,痰多脘闷。

舌脉:苔浊腻,脉滑。

分析:痰浊壅肺,胸阳失展,故胸闷如窒而痛。痰浊阻滞脉络,故痛引肩背。脾主肌肉与四肢,痰浊困脾,脾气不运,故形体肥胖,痰多脘闷,肢体沉重。痰浊壅肺,气机闭阻不畅,故气短喘促。苔浊腻,脉滑,也为痰浊壅阻之象。

治法:通阳泄浊,豁痰开结。

方药:瓜蒌薤白半夏汤加味。方中瓜蒌开胸中痰结;半夏化痰降逆;薤白辛热通阳,豁痰下气。本方如再加入苏子、苏梗、枳壳、陈皮、白蔻仁、茯苓等理气化痰、通阳散结之品,效果更佳。

若症见胃脘痞闷，恶心纳呆，口黏而苦，苔腻而黄，为湿热中阻，胃气上逆，可选用小陷胸汤或黄连温胆汤，以清化湿热，心胃同治，也可收效。

若痰浊与血瘀同时并见，苔腻而舌黯或有瘀斑者，宜通阳豁痰与活血化瘀法并用，临证时根据两者的偏盛而有侧重。

处方举例：

全瓜蒌 30g、薤白 10g、半夏 10g、炒陈皮 10g、茯苓 15g、苏梗 10g、炒枳壳 10g、白蔻仁 6g、川芎 10g、草红花 10g、降香 6g。

(三)阴寒凝滞

主症：胸痛彻背，背痛彻胸，感寒痛甚，往往遇寒而发，起病急骤。

兼症：胸闷气短，心悸，重则喘息，不能平卧，面色苍白，四肢厥冷。

舌脉：舌淡红苔白，脉沉细而紧。

分析：诸阳受气于胸中而转行于背，寒邪内侵，客于胸中，致使阳气不展，气机阻痹，故见胸疼彻背，背痛彻胸，感寒则痛甚，往往遇寒而发，起病急骤。胸阳不振，气机受阻，故见胸闷气短，心悸，甚则喘息不能平卧。阳气不足，故面色苍白，四肢厥冷。舌苔白，脉沉细，均为阴寒凝滞，阳气不运之候。

治法：辛温通阳，开痹散寒。

方药：瓜蒌薤白白酒汤加枳实、桂枝、附子、丹参、檀香。方中桂枝、附子、薤白辛温通阳，开痹散寒；瓜蒌、枳实化痰散结，泄满降逆；檀香理气温中；丹参活血通络。若痰湿内盛，胸痹伴有咳唾痰涎，可加生姜、橘皮、茯苓、杏仁等以行气化痰。

若症见心痛彻背、背痛彻胸，痛剧而无休止，身寒肢冷，喘息不得卧，脉象沉紧，此为阴寒极盛乃胸痹之重证，宜用乌头赤石脂丸合苏合香丸以芳香温通而止疼痛。方中蜀椒、干姜温中散寒，附子、乌头以治心痛厥逆，赤石脂在此用以养心气，合苏合香丸同用以温开止痛。临床附子与乌头同用者较少，故可去乌头加肉桂其效更佳，现在常用的冠心苏合丸即从苏合香丸化裁而来。

处方举例：

全瓜蒌 30g、薤白 10g、桂枝 10g、食醋 20g(另兑)、生姜五片、炒陈皮 10g、炒枳壳 10g、丹参 30g、檀香 6g、砂仁 5g、制附片 6g。

(四)心肾阴虚

主症：胸中隐隐灼痛，时作时休。

兼症：心悸盗汗，心烦不寐，腰酸膝软，头晕耳鸣。

舌脉：舌质红，体瘦，或有瘀斑，脉弦细或细数。

分析：病延日久，阴血暗耗，血脉不充，血行滞涩，故见胸中隐痛。阴虚则火旺，虚火内扰，故也可见胸中灼痛，但不似实火之重。虚火扰心，故心悸时作，心烦不寐。阴不敛阳，或(阴)虚火迫液外泄，而见盗汗。肾阴亏损，筋脉失养，故腰酸膝软。阴虚阳亢，故头晕耳鸣。舌质红，体瘦，或有瘀斑，脉弦细或细数，均为阴血亏虚，心脉瘀阻，心失濡养之象。

治法：滋阴益肾，养心安神。

方药：左归饮加减。方中熟地、山茱萸、杞子滋阴益肾；淮山药、茯苓、甘草健脾以助生化之源。若心阴亏虚而见心悸、盗汗、心烦不寐者，可加麦冬、五味子、柏子仁、酸枣仁等以养心安神，麦冬可以重用。若胸闷而痛者，可加当归、丹参、川芎、郁金等以养血通络；若阴虚阳亢而见头晕目眩、舌麻肢麻、面部烘热者，可酌加制首乌、女贞子、钩藤、生石决明、生牡蛎、鳖甲等滋阴潜阳。

处方举例：

生熟地各10g、山萸肉10g、丹皮10g、泽泻10g、茯苓15g、天麦冬各10g、丹参20g、五味子6g、女贞子10g、旱莲草10g、三七粉3g(分冲)。

(五)气阴两虚

主症：胸闷隐痛，时作时止。

兼症：心悸气短，倦怠懒言，面色少华，头晕目眩，遇劳则甚，大便或秘、或溏。

舌脉：舌偏红或有齿痕，脉细弱，或结代。

分析：胸痹日久，气阴两虚，气虚则脉络不利，血行不畅，气血瘀滞，故见胸闷隐痛，时作时止。气阴两虚，心脉失养，故见心悸。气虚故见短气，倦怠懒言，面色少华。阴虚阳亢故见头晕目眩。虚不耐劳，故遇劳则甚。气阴两虚，偏于气虚，运化无权，故便溏；偏于阴虚，大肠干燥，故便秘。舌偏红或有齿印，脉细弱，或结代均为气阴两虚之征。

治法：益气养阴，活血通络。

方药：生脉散合人参养营汤加减。方中人参、黄芪、白术、茯苓、甘草健脾益气，以助生化气血之源；麦冬、地黄、当归、白芍滋阴养血；远志、五味子养心安神。若脉结代，心动悸，为气虚血少，血不养心所致，可合炙甘草汤以益气养血，滋阴复脉。若心阴亏虚较甚，症见心胸灼痛，心悸心烦，失眠盗汗，面赤便秘，舌红少苔，脉细数或结代等，可用滋阴养血，活血清热之天王补心丹加减。方中以生地、玄参、天冬、麦冬滋阴而泻虚火；人参、炙甘草、茯苓益心气，也寓有从阳引阴之意；柏子仁、枣仁、远志、五味子养心安神，化阴敛汗；丹参、当归身养心活血而通心脉；桔梗、辰砂为引使之品，全方能使心阴复、虚火平、血脉利而使心胸灼痛得解。若心胸灼痛甚者，应择丹皮、赤芍、凌霄花、郁金等性凉微寒的活血之品。若胸闷胸痛，可加丹参、三七、益母草、郁金、五灵脂、降香以活血通络。

处方举例：

人参粉3g(分冲)、麦门冬10g、五味子10g、丹参20g、赤白芍各10g、炙黄芪15g、全当归10g、熟地10g、三七粉3g(分冲)、生龙牡各30g、茯苓15g、丹皮10g；

(六)阳气虚衰

主症：胸闷隐痛，偶尔绞痛，甚则胸痛彻背，遇冷则心痛加剧。

兼症：心悸气短，汗出乏力，畏寒肢冷，腰膝冷痛，面色苍白，唇甲淡白或青紫。

舌脉：舌质淡白或紫暗，脉沉细或沉微欲绝。

分析：阳气虚衰，胸阳不运，气机痹阻，血行瘀滞，故胸闷隐痛；阳虚生内寒，寒凝心脉，不通则痛，故心痛遇冷则加剧，甚则胸痛彻背。心阳不振，故心悸气短，阳虚则卫外不固，故汗出乏力；脾肾阳衰，故畏寒肢冷，腰膝冷痛，面色苍白，唇甲淡白或青紫。舌淡白或紫黯，脉沉细或沉微欲绝，均为阳气虚衰，瘀血内阻之象。

治法：益气温阳，活血通络。

方药：参附汤合右归饮加减。方中人参大补元气，附子、肉桂温肾助阳，熟地、山萸肉、杞子、杜仲补肾益精。若见面唇青紫，大汗出，四肢厥冷，脉沉微欲绝者，乃心阳欲脱之危候，可重用红参(或别直参)、附子，并加用龙骨、牡蛎以回阳救逆固脱；若阳损及阴，阴阳两虚者，可再加麦冬、五味子以温阳滋阴并用。若肾阳虚衰，水气凌心，症见心悸，喘促，不能平卧，小便减少，肢体浮肿者，可用真武汤加汉防己、猪苓、车前子以温阳行水。

处方举例：

人参粉 3g(分冲)、炮附子 6g、肉桂粉 3g(分冲)、茯苓 15g、生龙骨(先下)30g、生牡蛎(先下)30g、补骨脂 10g、白术 10g、赤白芍各 10g、三七粉 3g(分冲)、仙灵脾 10g。

〔预防及护理措施〕

一、预防

1. 注意调摄精神，避免情绪波动。情志异常波动如忧思恼怒等，可致气机郁滞血行不畅，心脉瘀阻而致心痛。因此，保持心情愉快，避免过于激动喜怒或思虑无度，这对预防心痛的发生、发展是很重要的。

2. 注意生活起居，寒温适宜。气候的寒暑晴雨变化，对心痛的发生、发展有明显影响，如寒邪直中，胸阳痹阻，或暑热犯心，耗伤心气，均可致心脉痹阻而发心痛。因此，平素注意生活起居，做到寒暖适宜对预防心痛的发生是十分重要的。

3. 注意饮食调节，避免膏粱厚味，并注意纠正偏食。中医认为，过食肥甘、膏粱厚味易产生痰浊，阻塞经络，痰湿壅阻，脾失健运，气机不畅，易致心痛。近年来的病因调查中也得出喜食肥甘者其发病率高于一般人群，同时偏嗜咸食者，亦可导致心痛的发生。因此，平素饮食注意调节是十分重要的。另外，酒烟等刺激之品对于脏腑功能亦有影响，应予禁止。

4. 注意劳逸结合，坚持适当的体育锻炼。过劳易耗伤心及其他脏腑的气血阴阳；好逸则易致气血停滞，对心痛都不利。因此注意劳逸结合，坚持适当的体育锻炼，可预防或减少心痛的发作。

二、护理

1. 使病人情志舒畅，建立战胜疾病的信心，减轻思想负担，不致过于紧张，以利于气血畅达，脏腑功能协调。

2. 引导病人循序渐进地适当活动，如散步、打太极拳等，以利于康复。

3. 饮食上避免过食肥甘，禁酒，宜少食多餐。

4. 心痛发作时要心情平静，勿惊慌躁动，应立即服用速效止痛药物，防止痛情发展。

5. 疼痛缓解后亦不能过饱过劳。

〔典型病例分析〕

案一：蒋某某，男，48 岁。患左胸痹痛已四、五年，经某医院确诊为冠心病，冠状动脉供血不足，多次检查心电图异常，唇舌青暗，面色暗黑，心烦寐少，脉律不齐，长期口干饮少，大便不畅，经诊为心络瘀阻，投旋覆花汤加减：

旋覆花(包)15g、茜草 9g、红花 9g、青葱管 15g、瓜蒌仁 12g、丹参 15g、赤芍 15g、川芎 9g、降香 9g、琥珀末 1.5g(睡前吞服)。

服五剂后，左胸胀痛减轻，续用上方达 3 个月余，症状基本消失，乃改用原方制成丸药善后，服 1 年余，心电图基本正常，现已正常上班工作，三、四年来未见复发。(《中医内科新论》)

按：本案面、舌、唇、脉均为瘀血所致。心烦寐少，为心络瘀阻，心神失养。口干饮少即瘀血证的“但欲漱水不欲咽”，盖瘀血内留而不上承，故口干，瘀血属阴，阴蓄于内而有余，故不欲饮水。大便不畅为瘀阻气滞，大肠传导不利所致。《金匮》旋覆花汤由旋覆花、新绛、青葱管组成。清代医家叶天士喜用此方治疗久病入络之胁痛，常收捷效。本例以旋覆花汤加减，方中除有诸活血药化瘀通络外，更有旋覆花、青葱管、瓜蒌仁、降香等以宣降肺气，通利大肠，辛香灵动，气行则血行，从而有助于心络瘀血的活化，药证相符，故效如桴鼓。

胸痹为临床常见病、多发病，其临床特征为胸部闷痛，甚则胸痛彻背，短气，喘息不得卧等。其病因与寒暑外袭，饮食不节，情志失调，思虑劳倦，多育失精，亡血不复，以及年高体弱，大病久病之后，正气亏虚有关。其病机总属本虚标实，本虚为阴阳气血亏虚，标实为阴寒、痰浊、血瘀交互为患。临床上应与胃痛、胸痛相鉴别，辨证上应辨虚实、分主次，辨心痛的性质和病势的轻重顺逆。本病的证候大致可分为心血瘀阻、痰浊壅塞、阴寒凝滞、心肾阴虚、气阴两虚、阳气虚衰六型，总属实证和虚证两大类。实证宜用活血化瘀、辛温通阳、泄浊豁痰等法，治标为主；虚证当补养扶正为主，或滋阳益肾，益气养阴，温阳补气，但虚实多相互夹杂和转化，故当按虚实的主次缓急而兼顾同治，并配合运用有效成药，每可取得较好的效果。对于真心痛的治疗，关键在于防脱防厥，要抓住病情的细微变化，一旦见有厥脱先兆，即须用药救治于厥脱之先。

本病只要积极治疗，并善摄养，大多能得以控制和缓解。本病的预防，须注意调摄精神，起居有节，调节饮食，劳逸结合等诸方面，且应持之以恒。

复习思考题

1. 胸痹的概念是什么？
2. 如何掌握胸痹发生的病理变化的标本内容及其关系？
3. 治疗胸痹的方法，如何掌握治标、治本的原则和具体方法？
4. 如何鉴别胸痹的轻重与顺逆？
5. 治疗胸痹的中成药有哪些？

不　寐

[概述]

不寐即一般所谓的“失眠”，古称“不得卧”、“不得眠”或“目不瞑”。“不寐”之名始见于《难经》，是指以经常不能获得正常睡眠为特征的一种病证。其临床表现因证情轻重之别，而有以下几种情况：初就寝即难以入寐，称为入寐困难；寐而易醒，醒后不能再寐，称为寐而早醒；寐而不酣，或时寐时醒，或伴恶梦，称为寐而不实；甚者可整夜不能入睡，称为彻夜不寐。若因一时情志影响，如兴奋、恐惧、思虑、悲伤等，或环境影响，如四周吵闹、灯光明亮等引起的暂时性失眠，经除去诱因或安静休息后能很快好转，且无其他兼证者，不属病态。若因某些疾病如发热、咳喘、疼痛等引起的不寐，应先治原发病，病除而眠自安，切不可舍本求末。每日睡眠时间因人而异，如睡眠时间虽少，但精力体力不减，且无任何不适，亦不可视为病态。不寐一证，既可单独出现，也可兼见头痛、眩晕、心悸、健忘等症，临床诊治时应与相关病证联系互参。

不寐应与“不得卧”相鉴别。“不得卧”是指患者因疾病所苦，不能躺下，与“不寐”有明显不同。

本病预后大多较好，唯严重不寐而精神失常者，须防发生意外。

西医学的神经官能症、高血压、脑动脉硬化、贫血、肝炎、更年期综合征以及某些精神病等，凡有不寐表现者，均可参考本篇辨证施治。

［病因病机］

不寐的病因与情志所伤、劳逸失调、饮食不节及素体虚弱、或久病未复等因素有关。主要病机为思虑劳倦，伤及心脾，阳不入阴，心肾不交；气郁化火，肝阳扰动；心胆气虚，心神不安；食滞痰热，胃气不和，以上种种皆可扰动心神而致不寐，临床证候有虚有实，并可由实致虚，由虚转实，以及虚实夹杂。

不寐病因病机示意图

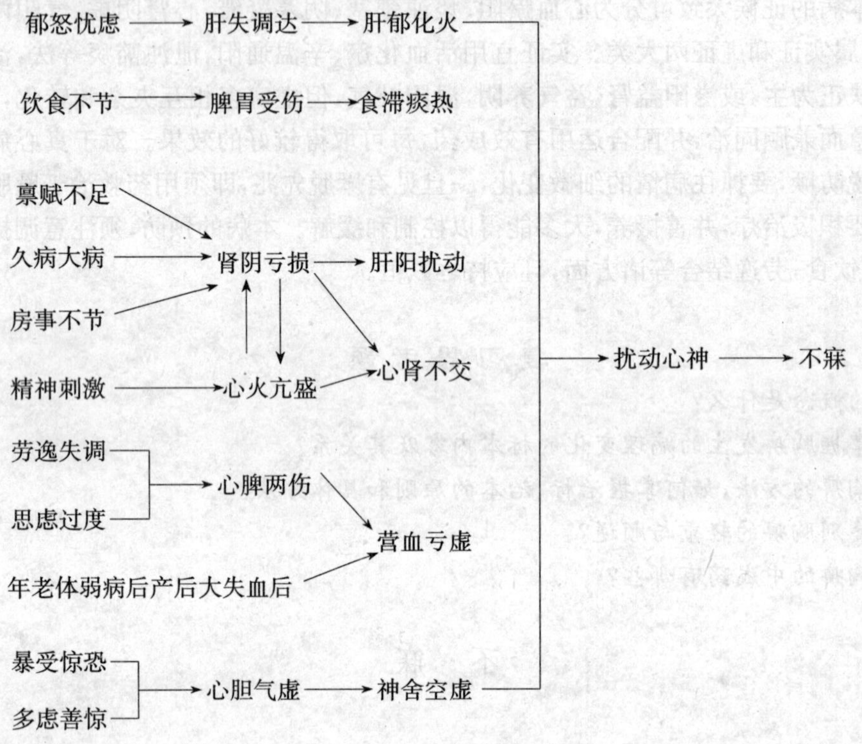

一、情志所伤：郁怒忧虑，肝失调达，气郁不舒，郁而化火，火性炎上，扰动心神，神不得安则不寐；或五志过极，亦能化火，心火内炽不能下交于肾，心肾失交，心火亢盛，热扰神明，神志不宁，因而不寐；或暴受惊恐，情绪紧张，终日惕惕，渐至心虚胆怯，神无所依，则心神不安而不寐；或思虑太过，劳伤心脾，心伤则阴血暗耗，神不守舍，脾伤则纳少迟消化源不足，营血亏虚，心失所养，均致不寐。

二、饮食不节：嗜食辛辣煎炸、肥甘油腻或暴饮暴食，饮食不节，肠胃受伤而宿食停滞，酿成痰热，壅遏于中，则胃气不和，痰热上扰而眠不得安。

三、素体虚弱，或久病、大病之后：禀赋不足，年老体弱，病后未复，皆可伤肾，肾阴耗伤，不能上奉于心，水不济火，则心阳独亢，神志不宁而不寐，此为心肾不交所致不寐。还有，由于病后、产后、大失血后以及素体虚弱、年迈之人，心血不足，血不养心以致心神不安而成不寐，若平素体弱，心虚胆怯之人，卒受惊恐，则心气更虚，神无所附而不寐。可见因虚而易惊，因惊又复虚，二者可互为因果，均能导致不寐。

四、劳逸失调：过劳则耗气，过逸则脾弱，脾弱气虚，运化无权，水谷精微不能化生气血，以致血虚不能养心，心神不安而不寐。又性欲不节，房事无度耗伤肾精，精少阴虚，不能上承于心，则心火独亢，心肾不交而不寐。

综上所述，不寐的原因虽多，总不外先天禀赋薄弱与后天失养两类，诸多病因导致脏腑功能紊乱，气血、阴阳失调，而致心肝火旺，痰热上扰，心肾不交，营血不足，心胆气虚，扰动心神而不寐。病位主要在心，涉及脾、肾、肝、胆、胃。由于神明被扰有营血不足、精血内耗、心胆气虚与痰火亢盛、邪气内扰之别，故不寐可分虚实两类，其中虚者居多、实者少见，久病之后，多虚实夹杂，互为因果，形成顽固性的不寐。

〔辨证论治〕

一、辨证要点

1. 分析不寐特征：一般入睡困难者，多属有火，火有实火、虚火之分。寐而不实者，多属虚实夹杂；寐而易醒，多属于虚，常为心脾两虚；彻夜不寐者，可虚可实。

2. 辨别虚实：久病者多虚，多属阴血不足，责之心脾肝肾，以气血亏虚和阴虚火旺为多见；新病者多实，多属邪火内扰，责之心脾肝胃，以肝郁化火和食滞痰热、胃府不和为多见。实证日久，气血耗伤，可转为虚；虚证也可兼实，逐成虚实夹杂之证。

3. 治疗应以补虚泻实、调整阴阳为原则：不寐属虚者，补其不足，益气养血，滋补肝肾；属实者，泻其有余，消导和中，清化痰火；虚实夹杂者，补泻兼顾。另外，除针对病因以治本外，还可酌加养心安神之品以治其标，提高疗效。

二、分型论治

(一)实证

1. 肝郁化火

主症：不寐，入睡困难，恶梦纷纭。

兼症：性急易怒，目赤口苦，口渴喜饮，不思饮食，溲赤便秘。

舌脉：舌红，苔黄，脉弦而数。

分析：本证因抑郁、恼怒伤神，肝失条达，气郁化火，上扰心神而致不寐。因火为阳邪，火热内炽，阳不入阴，则就寝不易入睡。待至子亥时辰，为昼夜阴气之最，阳始入阴而神安；虽已入寐，但心肝火旺，时扰神明而恶梦纷纭。肝火偏旺，火性炎上，则性急易怒，目赤口苦。肝气犯胃，则不思饮食。肝火乘胃，胃热则口渴喜饮。溲赤便秘，舌红苔黄，脉象弦数均为热象；热盛阴伤则舌红，胃中有热则苔黄，肝火旺盛则脉弦数。

治法：疏肝泻热，佐以安神。

方药：龙胆泻肝汤加味。方中龙胆草、黄芩、山栀清肝泻火；泽泻、木通、车前子清利肝经湿热；柴胡疏畅肝胆之气，并作引经药；当归、生地养血益阴以和肝，与清热药相配伍是寓泻中有补，疏中有养，既防泻火药苦燥伤阴，又防肝胆火盛灼伤阴液；甘草和中缓急。可加磁石、龙骨、龙齿、珍珠母以滋阴潜阳，重镇安神。如胸闷胁胀，喜叹息，加郁金、香附、白芍三类疏肝调气。如脘闷纳呆、嗳气呃逆，加代赭石、佛手、香缘、枳壳疏肝和胃。

处方举例：

龙胆草 9g、黄芩 10g、柴胡 10g、白芍 10g、山栀 9g、郁金 10g、香附 10g、陈皮 10g、珍珠母(先下)30g、生龙牡(先下)各 30g、生地 10g。

2. 痰热内扰

主症：不寐，入睡困难，寐而不实，常有饮食不节作为诱因。

兼症：头重目眩，痰多胸闷，恶食嗳气，心烦懊侬。

舌脉：苔黄腻，脉滑数。

分析：本证多因饮食不节，宿食内停，食滞脾伤，健运无权，积湿生痰，痰郁生热，宿食痰热壅遏中焦，则痰多胸闷。痰热上扰，心神不宁，则心烦懊侬，难于入寐，寐亦不实，且随饮食不适而加重。痰热阻遏，清阳被蒙，则头重目眩。痰食停滞，气机不畅，胃失和降，则恶食嗳气，吞酸呕恶。苔黄腻，脉滑数为痰热、宿食内停之象。

治法：化痰清热，和中安神。

方药：温胆汤加黄连、山栀。温胆汤即二陈汤加竹茹、枳实、生姜、大枣而成，方名温胆，实为清胆和胃，除痰止呕。方用半夏、陈皮、茯苓、枳实理气化痰，和胃降逆；黄连、山栀、竹茹清心降火；茯苓还可宁心安神。如痰食阻滞，胃中不和，可酌情合用半夏秫米汤，或保和丸，或枳实导滞丸，以消导和中。其中半夏秫米汤能益阴和胃安神，保和丸或枳实导滞丸能消积和胃，清利湿热。如食积不化明显，加槟榔、焦三仙、莱菔子、鸡内金等以消积化痰。如痰热较重而大便不通，可用礞石滚痰丸或加大黄、瓜蒌以降火泻热，逐痰安神。如心悸惊惕不安，可加珍珠母、龙齿、龙骨、磁石之类以镇惊定志。

处方举例：

茯苓 15g、橘红 10g、半夏 10g、竹茹 10g、枳实 10g、黄连 6g、山栀 12g、秫米 10g、焦三仙各 10g、瓜蒌 20g；

（二）虚证

1. 阴虚火旺

主症：心烦不寐，入睡困难。

兼症：心悸不安，五心烦热，头晕耳鸣，腰膝酸软，健忘梦遗，口干津少。

舌脉：舌质红，脉细数。

分析：心为阳脏，居上焦，性属火；肾为阴脏，居下焦，性属水。“心肾相交”即心火下降于肾，使肾水不寒；肾水上济于心，使心阳不亢，此为“水火既济”。若肾阴不足，不能上济以滋心阳，则心肝火旺，虚火扰神，故心烦不寐，心悸不安。肾精亏耗，髓海空虚，则头晕耳鸣，健忘。肾虚，腰府失养，则腰膝酸软。心肾不交，精关不固，则梦交遗精。五心烦热，口干津少，舌质红，脉细数，均为阴虚火旺之象。

治法：滋阴降火，养心安神。

方药：黄连阿胶汤、朱砂安神丸、天王补心丹等随证选用。此三方均为清热安神之剂，黄连阿胶汤和朱砂安神丸重在滋阴降火，天王补心丹重在滋阴养血兼清热。黄连阿胶汤，方用黄连、黄芩清心火，除烦热；阿胶、白芍、鸡子黄滋阴养血，安心神，一清一滋，使心肾得交，水火相济，则心烦不寐自愈。朱砂安神丸，取朱砂微寒，“重可镇怯”，清热镇心安神为主药；辅以黄连清心泻火；佐以当归、地黄滋阴养血；使以炙甘草养胃和中，调和诸药，意在清心安神。上二方方义相似，朱砂安神丸制成丸药，便于服用，但因朱砂主要成分为硫化汞，不宜久服多服，以防汞中毒。天王补心丹中以生地、玄参滋阴清热为主药；辅以丹参、当归补血养心，党参、茯苓益心气，柏子仁、远志安心神；佐以天冬、麦冬滋阴清热，五味子、酸枣仁敛心气；使以桔梗载药上行，朱砂为衣，入心安神，诸药共奏滋阴安神之功。当阴虚血少，而火盛不甚时选用为宜。可加牡蛎、磁石、珍珠母等重镇安神药，使阳升得平，阳入于阴则寐。阴虚火旺，心肾不交者，可用六味地黄丸或麦味地黄丸合交泰丸治之，取六味地黄丸或麦味地黄丸滋养肾阴或益心肾，交泰丸清心火，引火归源。

处方举例：

黄连 6g、黄芩 10g、阿胶 10g(烊化)、白芍 12g、生地 12g、麦冬 12g、五味子 6g、莲子心 3g、生牡蛎(先下)30g、生甘草 6g。

2. 心脾两虚

主症：多梦易醒，夜寐不实。

兼症：心悸健忘，头晕目眩；肢倦神疲，饮食无味，面色少华。

舌脉：舌质淡，苔薄白，脉细弱。

分析：心主血，藏神；脾主运化，为生血之源。思虑过度，劳逸失调，则心脾两伤，营血不足，心失所养，则心悸健忘。阴不敛阳，神不守舍，则寐而不实。劳逸思虑不独耗血，亦伤心脾之气，而致阳气亦虚，常于子夜之后，阳气升动之时，阳出于阴而醒。所以本证特点是初寝能寐，寐中多梦，寐而易醒。血少不能上奉于脑，气弱清阳不能上升，则头晕目眩；血虚不能上荣于面，则面色少华，舌质淡红。气虚脾运力薄则纳食无味。气血亏虚，则肢倦神疲，脉象虚弱。

治法：补养心脾，以生气血。

方药：归脾汤加减。本方有益气健脾，养血宁心之功。方用人参、白术、黄芪、甘草补气健脾为主，使脾胃强健，气血自生；辅以当归滋阴养血，血充神安；佐以茯神、枣仁、龙眼肉、远志养心益脾，安神定志；木香理气醒脾，使之补而不滞；姜、枣为使，调和营卫；诸药相合，重在益气生血，养心安神。如心悸气短较重，可加熟地、白芍、阿胶以养心血；若失眠多梦较甚，可加五味子、柏子仁以养心安神；还可加龙齿、龙骨、牡蛎、珍珠母以镇静安神。如脾虚湿停，脘闷纳呆，腹胀便溏，舌苔滑腻者，加茯苓、半夏、陈皮、厚朴以健脾理气化湿。若心脾气血亏虚较甚者，可合用养心汤，养心汤中除用五味子、柏子仁加强养心安神作用外，更在大队补气养血药中，配伍少量肉桂，以温宣阳气，鼓舞气血之生长。

处方举例：

党参 10g、白术 10g、炙黄芪 12g、当归 10g、茯神 10g、木香 6g、炒枣仁 15g、远志 10g、首乌藤 30g、炙甘草 6g、龙眼肉 10g、陈皮 10g。

3. 心胆气虚

主症：不寐多梦，易于惊醒。

兼症：胆怯心悸，遇事善惊，神疲体倦，自汗少气。

舌脉：舌质淡，脉弦细或细弱。

分析：肝与心为母子之脏，二者互为影响，胆附于肝，与肝相表里，故惊恐伤胆，致胆气虚，胆夺心气，心气亦虚；而心气虚，不济于胆，亦致胆气虚。胆虚则胆怯善惊，心虚则心悸不寐，故心胆气虚，可见不寐多梦，易于惊醒，醒后心中惕惕然。神疲体倦，自汗少气均为气虚之象。舌质淡，脉弦细或细弱为气血不足之征。总之，心胆气虚之不寐，有因虚而惊和因惊而虚之不同，两者常互为因果，治疗时亦需兼顾。

治法：益气镇惊，安神定志。

方药：安神定志丸加味。方用人参益气、龙齿镇惊为主药，伍以茯苓、茯神、菖蒲、远志补气益胆，宁心安神。如胸闷气短，畏寒肢冷，为心气心阳俱虚者，加桂枝、炙甘草以补心气，温心阳。如虚烦不眠，为血虚阳浮者，宜用酸枣仁汤以养血安神，清热除烦，方用酸枣仁养肝血、安心神，川芎调畅气血、疏达肝气，茯苓、甘草宁心，知母清热除烦。对本型中气血亏虚较重者，依其气、血亏虚之不同，酌选安神定志丸合桂枝甘草汤，或合酸枣仁汤。

处方举例：

党参10g、茯神10g、生龙齿(先下)30g、菖蒲10g、桂枝6g、炙甘草6g、炒枣仁15g、远志10g、知母10g。

此外，若病后虚烦不眠，形体消瘦，面色皖白，倦怠神疲，舌淡，脉细弱，或年老体虚，夜寐早醒而无虚烦之证者，多属气血不足，治宜养血安神，可用归脾汤调治。如病后血虚肝热而不寐，宜用琥珀多寐丸，或酸枣仁汤加生石决明、龙齿、牡蛎之类治之。如心肾不交，虚阳上扰，可用交泰丸，方中黄连清火为主，反佐肉桂之温以入心肾，取其引火归元之意。一般不寐多梦，心悸不安者，在辨证治疗的同时，均可酌加对症治疗的安神药，如平肝潜阳、镇静安神之龙骨、龙齿、磁石、珍珠母，镇心安神之朱砂，安神定惊之琥珀，养心安神之酸枣仁、柏子仁、首乌藤。

〔预防及护理措施〕

由于本病属于心神的病变，故尤应注意精神方面的调摄，应喜怒有节，心情舒畅；既病之后，应注意了解病人的精神状况，消除其顾虑，减少或避免精神刺激。睡前忌饮酒、饮浓茶、禁吸烟，宜用温水洗脚。居处环境噪音太大，常可影响入睡而酿成不寐，故应设法避免或消除噪音。

不寐病人，每日应参加适当的体力劳动，加强体育锻炼，增强体质，促进身心健康。平日注意生活规律，按时作息，养成良好的睡眠习惯。

不寐病人的服药方法很重要，为了使中药达到安神的目的，一般早晨和上午不服药，只在午后或午休及晚上临睡前各服一次。对于严重不寐或同时具有精神失常的不寐患者，要注意安全，以防发生意外。

〔典型病例分析〕

案一：徐某某，壮年。因操劳忧虑，心神交瘁，久之酿成失眠，往往通宵不能合目。西药治疗可取眠数小时，然梦魂颠倒，醒后益增疲乏。今岁入夏以来，失眠变本加厉，历经医治罔效，自8月14日起至今已3夜未睡，头脑懵懵，衣不知热，食不知味……面虽皖白而神采飞扬，谈笑自若，双目隐隐现红丝，脉象两关均弦长，舌边有青纹。方药：

桃仁12g、红花9g、当归9g、川芎9g、淮牛膝9g、参三七9g、大生地9g、柴胡6g、京赤芍9g、炒枳壳6g、炙甘草3g。

一剂后即夜卧贻然，连服15剂，未见再发。后此二月，复来求治，言旬日来又苦失眠，但不若前次之甚。……两关仍弦，依然实证也，因有头痛目赤、胁胀痛等肝火上炎症象，改用龙胆泻肝汤。方药：

黄芩9g、龙胆草4.5g、生地9g、泽泻9g、车前子9g、生甘草3g、柴胡6g、黑山栀9g、当归6g、木通9g。

上方共服5剂而夜眠全安，肝火上炎症象亦除。(孙幼立整理：范文虎先生失眠医案一则。《中医杂志》7,15,1963)

按：患者忧思操劳过度，气机郁结日久，血行瘀滞，瘀血不去，气郁化热，瘀热扰心，故失眠难寐。瘀血内阻，现于肝窍，故双目隐隐见红丝，脉象两关均弦长，舌边有青纹。故投以血府逐瘀汤加参三七活血化瘀而获效。复诊时证见肝火上炎之象，此乃柯韵伯所言，“肝火旺，则上走空窍，不得睡”，改用龙胆泻肝汤清肝泻火，药证相符，起效霍然。

不寐，即失眠，多由情志所伤，饮食不节，劳逸失调，或病后体虚等原因所致，按其病机可分肝郁化火、痰热内扰、阴虚火旺、心脾两虚、心胆气虚五型。本病病位主要在心，影响到肝、胆、脾、胃、肾，基本病机是阳盛阴虚，阴阳失调，神明被扰。由于心神被扰的原因有正虚邪实之分，故不寐的辨证，首先应分辨虚实。因气血不足、精血内耗者为虚，因于痰火亢盛、食滞内扰者为实。一般虚证多见，实证少见，也有的虚实并见。治疗以补虚泻实，调整阴阳为原则，酌情选用疏肝泻热、滋阴降火、交通心肾、补益心脾、益气镇惊及化痰泻热等法。

复习思考题

1. 简述不寐的病因病机。

2. 试述阴虚火旺和痰热上扰之不寐的主症、治法和方药。

郁证

〔概述〕

郁证是由于情志不舒，气机郁滞所引起的疾病的总称。所谓郁，指滞而不通，涩而不畅，不得发越之意，既包含病因，又囊括病机。郁证既是一个病因病机学概念，又是一种综合病证，临床表现错综复杂。因此，广义讲，凡因外感六淫，内伤七情等诸郁引起的脏腑机能失和，气血津液运行紊乱，失其畅通调达，气、血、痰、火、湿、食等病理产物壅塞郁结所产生的病证皆称郁证。狭义的郁证，指由于情志不舒，气机郁滞所引起的性情抑郁，情绪不宁，悲伤善哭，胸胁胀痛，咽中如有异物梗阻等复杂症状的一类病证。

早在《内经·六元正纪大论》就提出了五郁，首创五郁治则，即"木郁达之，火郁发之，土郁夺之，金郁泄之，水郁折之"。认为百病皆生于气，五脏皆可发生郁证，并把情志不舒看作郁证发病的重要原因之一。《金匮要略》记载了郁证的多种多样的临床表现及行之有效的治疗措施。北宋代陈言在《三因方》中提出七情致郁学说，为后世"郁不离乎七情"奠定了理论基础。

元代朱丹溪首倡"六郁"之说，即气、血、痰、热、湿、食，而六郁以气郁为先，相因为病，创越鞠丸疗诸郁，以香附开郁利气为主。明代张景岳从广义概念出发，认为有"因病而郁"和"因郁而病"，较前人更为深入。至清代叶天士强调"七情之郁居多"，病变涉及肝、胆、心、脾，治疗当分气血新久，以苦辛凉润宣通为要，不可辛散破气，注意精神调护，这一理论迄今仍有重要指导意义。

西医学中的神经官能症、癔病、更年期综合征等，凡有郁证表现者，皆可参考本篇进行辨证治疗。

〔病因病机〕

郁证的发生，多由谋虑不遂，忧思气结，郁怒不解等情志所伤，致肝气郁结，失其条达，进而导致五脏气机不和。主要病变在肝、脾、心三脏及气血失调。

一、郁怒不畅，肝失条达，气失疏泄，而致肝气郁结。气郁不得发越，日久化火；气郁日久，则血行不畅，可致血瘀。若肝郁及脾，或思虑不解，劳倦伤脾，则脾失健运，蕴湿生痰，痰气互结，而致气滞痰郁；气滞不通，湿浊难化，而成湿郁；食滞不消，则成食郁。于是诸郁随之而起，气、湿、痰、食郁，蓄积日久，皆可化热，郁热不得宣泄，终成热郁。

二、情志不遂，肝郁抑脾，一是脾失健运，纳少迟消，生化乏源，则气血不足，心脾两虚，心神失养；二是心脾既虚，久郁化火，热灼阴血，累及于肾，则阴虚火旺，由此发展而成种种虚损之候。

总之，郁证的发生，主要因郁怒、思虑、悲哀、忧愁七情之所伤，导致肝失疏泄，脾失健运，心神失常，脏腑阴阳气血失调而成。初病在气，气失调畅，再由气及血，影响五脏，气血不畅，进而导致湿、痰、热、食诸郁相继出现或相兼为病，多属实证；诸郁又反果为因加重了气机的郁滞。气郁日久，损伤气血，由实转虚，可致心脾俱亏、阴虚火旺等病证，甚至由此可发展成虚劳。

郁证病因病机示意图

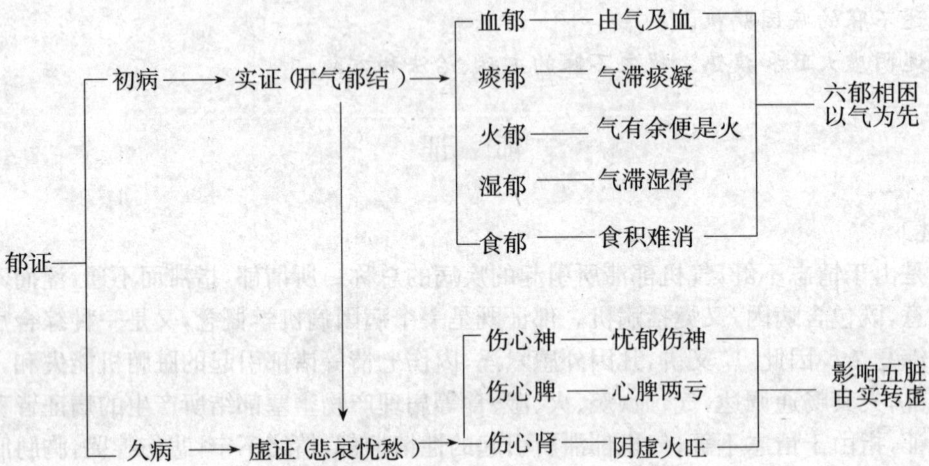

〔辨证论治〕

一、辨证要点

1. 由于郁证是情志不舒，气机郁滞所致，故本病起因每有精神刺激，七情所伤，其中由郁怒所致病者最多，由忧思悲恐致病者亦多。

2. 抓住主症，辨清虚实：郁证早期肝气郁结，或挟痰湿、食积、热郁，多为实证；久病由气及血，由实转虚；临床所见虚实夹杂最多。其次，应根据临床表现及病之新久，辨病在气或在血，是单郁或诸郁兼见。

3. 郁证的临床特点：因病始于气分郁结，故常以肝气郁结的症候为主要表现；或隐晦内蓄，迟留不发，变化多端，错综复杂；亦有自觉痛苦万分，莫可名状，但医者检查却无客观体征。另有药误失治，百病丛生。沉疴难起，终成"疑难杂病"，临证须审因辨治，溯本求源。

二、治疗原则

治疗郁证的总则是疏通气机，即"木郁达之"。早期疏理气机对防止病情发展及变生他证具有重要意义。属实者，治以舒肝理气为法，酌配行血、化痰、利湿、清热、消食之剂；属虚者，治以益气补血、滋阴养心诸扶正之品。

三、分型论治

（一）实证

1. 肝气郁结

主症：胸胁脘腹胀闷疼痛，病无定处。

兼症：常伴精神情绪变化，精神抑郁，情绪不宁，常喜太息，善怒易哭，得嗳气、矢气为快；或伴脾胃不和，纳少腹胀，恶心呕吐，大便失常；或有月事不行。

舌脉：舌苔薄白或薄腻脉弦或弦滑。

分析：肝经布胸胁，挟胃，抵少腹，故肝失疏泄，气机不利，病现胸胁脘腹胀闷疼痛，因气则走窜不定，痛无定处。气滞血瘀，脉络失和，则疼痛加重。闷多因湿滞所致，常在胀后发生或与胀并见。情志所伤，肝失条达，故情绪不宁，精神抑郁；常喜太息，善怒易哭，得嗳气及矢气胀痛可减，气滞暂缓，故以其为快。若肝木乘土，犯胃伤脾，胃失和降，脾失健运，则纳少腹胀，恶心呕吐，大便失常。若气郁及血，气滞血瘀，冲任不和，则女子月事不行。肝郁不舒则脉弦，苔薄白；兼湿郁，则脉弦滑，苔白腻。

治法：疏肝理气解郁。

方药：柴胡疏肝散加减。本方有疏肝理气，活血止痛之功，方中柴胡、枳壳、香附疏肝行气解郁；川芎、芍药、甘草和血行血止痛；柴胡配芍药，一散一敛，调理气机，柴胡苦平入肝，解郁而治在气分；白芍酸苦微寒亦入肝，柔肝缓急而治在血分，二药为伍，气血兼顾，相得益彰。可加郁金、青皮、佛手、香橼以增强解郁之力。如嗳气频作，胸脘满闷，加旋覆花、代赭石、苏梗、陈皮以平肝和胃，降逆止呕。如食滞胀满，纳少脘闷，加神曲、山楂、麦芽、莱菔子、鸡内金以消食化积。如腹胀便溏，舌苔薄腻或白腻，加苍术、茯苓、厚朴以健脾除湿。如胸胁胀痛不移，或月事不行，脉象弦涩，加当归、益母草、丹参、桃仁、红花以活血化瘀。

由于六郁为病，首因气郁，故在治疗期间，可以常服或配服越鞠丸，以行气解郁治气郁为主，兼顾血、痰、湿、食、火诸郁，为通治六郁之剂。

治疗肝气郁结，可依据胀痛之轻重、所在之部位，测知气郁程度，适当选用疏肝理气药。如胀轻者，治宜调气舒气，可用香橼、佛手、绿萼梅；如胀而不甚者，治宜行气理气，可用香附、陈皮、郁金、川楝子、枳壳、青皮、厚朴、木香；如胀甚且痛者，治宜行气破气，兼以活血，可用枳实、沉香、檀香、降香、红花、丹参。因理气药物多辛温香燥，气郁日久又易化火伤阴，故临证治疗常用辛平不燥之香橼、佛手、木蝴蝶之类，或苦味性寒之郁金、川楝子、元胡、槟榔。另外，还应结合兼证，加减施治。

处方举例：柴胡10g、白芍10g、枳壳10g、香附10g、郁金10g、川芎6g、佛手10g、苍术9g、焦三仙各10g。

2.气郁化火

主症：胸胁胀闷疼痛，性情急躁易怒。

兼症：头痛耳鸣，面红目赤；或口干而苦，嘈杂吞酸，大便秘结。

舌脉：舌质红，苔薄黄，脉弦数。

分析：肝气郁结，气滞血瘀，不通则痛，故胸胁胀闷疼痛。气郁化火，肝火上炎，故性急易怒，头痛耳鸣，面红耳赤。肝火犯胃，故口干而苦，嘈杂吞酸，大便秘结。舌质红，苔薄黄，脉弦数均为肝火有余之象。

治法：清肝泻火，解郁和胃。

方药：丹栀逍遥散合左金丸。丹栀逍遥散乃逍遥散加丹皮、栀子，有疏肝解郁清热、健脾养血之功；左金丸有泻肝和胃之效。其中逍遥散用柴胡、白芍、薄荷疏肝解郁；白芍、当归养血柔肝；白术、茯苓、甘草、煨姜健脾和中；加丹皮、栀子清肝泻火凉血。左金丸用黄连清心胃之火，法取实则泻子，少佐吴萸开郁和胃。如口苦苔黄，大便秘结，加龙胆草、大黄泻火通便。如肝火亢盛，头胀头痛，烦躁暴怒，大便干结，用丹栀逍遥散加当归龙荟丸治之。

处方举例：柴胡 9g、白芍 12g、薄荷(后下)6g、当归 10g、茯苓 12g、丹皮 9g、栀子 9g、黄连 6g、吴萸 2g、郁金 10g。

3. 气滞痰郁

主症：咽中不适，有异物感，咯之不出，咽之不下，胸中窒闷。

兼症：胸胁胀闷疼痛。

舌脉：舌苔白腻，脉象弦滑。

分析：情志不舒，肝郁乘脾，脾失健运，痰湿内生，痰气胶结于胸咽，故觉咽部不适，似物梗塞，咯之不出，咽之不下，俗你“梅核气”。此症常随情志变化而增减。肝失条达，气失舒展，故胸中窒闷，胸胁胀闷疼痛。苔白腻，脉弦滑为痰气互结之征。

治法：化痰利气解郁。

方药：半夏厚朴汤加减。本方有解郁降逆，化痰开结之功。方用半夏、厚朴、生姜辛以散结，苦以降逆；配茯苓健脾化痰；配苏叶解郁和血。可加香附、枳壳、佛手、香橼理气开郁；加苏梗、苏子、旋覆花、代赭石化痰降逆。如兼见口干口苦，呕恶烦急，舌苔黄腻，为痰郁化热，用温胆汤加黄芩、贝母、瓜蒌皮、香附、郁金、苏梗之类，化痰清热，疏理气机。

处方举例：旋覆花(布包)15g、苏梗 10g、香附 10g、黄芩 10g、茯苓 15g、代赭石(先下)30g、半夏 10g、厚朴 9g、枳壳 9g、陈皮 10g。

(二)虚证

1. 忧郁伤神

主症：悲忧善哭，如神灵所作，时欠时伸。

兼症：神情恍惚，心神不宁。

舌脉：舌质淡，苔薄白，脉弦细。

分析：忧郁不解，抑郁过度，则心气耗伤，营血暗损，致心神失养，而见精神失常，如心神不宁，悲伤欲哭，不能自主，呵欠频作等言行改变。此即《金匮要略》所谓“脏躁”证，多发于女子。舌质淡，苔薄白，脉弦细，为气郁血虚之象。

治法：养心安神。

方药：甘麦大枣汤加味。方中甘草和中益气缓急；小麦味甘微寒，养心气安心神；大枣甘平质润，补中润燥，三药合用甘润滋养，缓急和中，养心安神。可加柏子仁、酸枣仁、茯神、合欢花等加强药力。如心悸不安，五心烦热，或虚烦不寐，加阿胶、龙齿、牡蛎、珍珠母、生铁落以养心肝之阴，重镇安神；亦可用加味甘麦大枣汤治之，即甘麦大枣汤加芍药、紫石英，此方出自《妇科辑要》，寓芍药、甘草酸甘化阴，柔肝缓急；紫石英镇心安神。如性情急躁易怒，眩晕耳鸣，加生石决明、代赭石、白蒺藜，以平肝潜阳。

处方举例：炙甘草 12g、浮小麦 30g、大枣 7 枚、炒枣仁 20g、茯神 15g、白芍 10g、合欢花 10g、生龙齿(先下)30g、生牡蛎(先下)30g。

2. 心脾两虚

主症：多思善虑，心悸胆怯。

兼症：少寐健忘，面色不华，头晕神疲，食欲不振。

舌脉：舌质淡，脉细弱。

分析：劳心思虑，耗伤心脾，气血两虚。心失所养，心夺胆气，神不内守，则心悸胆怯，少寐健忘；中土不健，脾胃不和，气血乏源，则食欲不振，面色不华。头晕神疲，舌质淡，脉细弱。

治法：健脾养心，益气补血。

方药：归脾汤加减。本方由四君子汤、当归补血汤加龙眼肉、酸枣仁、木香、远志、生姜、大枣而成，有健脾养心，益气补血之功，为治心脾两虚之常用方，旨在健脾益气以生血，气旺血生以养心，可加郁金、香附、合欢花等解郁安神之品，亦可加香橼、佛手、绿萼梅等以舒肝和胃。

处方举例：太子参 15g、黄芪 10g、炒白术 10g、茯神 15g、当归 10g、炒枣仁 15g、龙眼肉 10g、木香 4g、炙甘草 6g、郁金 10g、佛手 10g、大枣 5 枚。

3. 阴虚火旺

主症：眩晕耳鸣，心烦易怒，心悸少寐。

兼症：腰酸遗精，或月经不调。

舌脉：舌质红，脉弦细数。

分析：素体阴虚，或肝气郁结，气郁化火，灼津伤阴，致脏之营阴不足，阴虚火旺，虚阳不浮，则眩晕耳鸣，心烦易怒。阴血亏耗，心神失养，则心悸少寐。肾阴不足，腰府失养则腰酸。相火扰动精室，精关不固，则遗精。肝肾失养，冲任空虚，则月经不调。舌质红，脉弦细数，为阴虚火旺之象。

治法：滋阴清热，镇心安神。

方药：滋水清肝饮加减。本方由六味地黄丸加当归、白芍、柴胡、山栀、酸枣仁而成，有滋阴清热，柔肝安神之功。方中六味地黄丸滋阴补肾，壮水制火；柴胡、白芍、当归疏肝养肝柔肝，丹皮、山栀清肝泻火；更用酸枣仁养心安神。可酌加珍珠母、磁石、生铁落、生龙齿、生牡蛎等药，重镇安神，平肝潜阳。如腰酸遗精者，加龟板、知母、芡实、金樱子益肾固精。如月经不调加香附、郁金、益母草以解郁调经。

处方举例：生地 12g、山萸肉 10g、山药 12g、丹皮 9g、女贞子 10g、旱莲草 30g、柴胡 4g、白芍 10g、山栀 9g、茯神 15g、珍珠母（先下）30g。

〔预防及护理措施〕

1. 本病除药物治疗以外，尚须配合精神疗法。医务人员要关心病人痛苦，作好思想工作，让病人树立乐观主义精神，正确对待疾病，保持心情舒畅，有利于疾病恢复。必要时可配合暗示疗法。

2. 加强身体锻炼，适当配合气功、太极拳等辅助治疗，可收事半功倍之效。

〔典型病例分析〕

案一、高某，男，40 岁。4 个月前，因故发怒后突感胸闷憋气，头晕目眩，继而晕厥，少顷即复。以后即经常发生胸闷憋气，常牵及背部出现酸痛等症，且多与情绪波动有关。西医诊为“可疑冠心病”。近日复因恼怒而发病，前症发作较频，并右胁胀痛。察之面色微暗，唇有瘀色，舌稍胖边有齿痕，脉弦。方老诊为胸痹类证。定位在肝，证属肝郁气滞挟瘀。治以疏肝解郁，行气活血，经以治脾以治其未发，拟加味丹栀逍遥散方：

丹参 30g、当归 12g、赤白芍各 12g、柴胡 10g、茯苓 30g、苍白术各 10g、甘草 6g、生姜 6g、薄荷（后下）3g、姜黄 10g、郁金 10g、川芎 10g、香附 10g、枳壳 10g、陈皮 10g。

二剂后诸症大减，但午后至夜仍偶感胸闷，于前方加党参 15g、黄芪 30g，继服四剂而愈。（王克勤《辽宁中医杂志》1985(10)：37）

按：该病者因于恼怒，暴怒伤肝，肝气暴张，气阻胸膈不得发越，故胸闷憋气；血随气升，并走于上，则头晕目眩，甚而为厥为仆，少顷气血平复，得以缓解。发病与精神不调有关，当属肝郁，且由气及血，面黯唇瘀是其明证，故用疏肝解郁、行气活血之剂效。肝旺克土，脾虚而舌胖有齿痕，加参芪以培补中土。

郁证是由于情志不畅，气机郁滞所引起的一类病证。病因为恼怒、忧虑、多思、悲哀等七情所伤，病机为情志不舒，肝失条达，肝气郁结。病始为气郁，渐可致痰郁、湿郁、食郁、热郁及血郁，日久脾虚，心神失养，肾阴不足，终致脏腑阴阳气血失调。郁证分虚实两大类，初起多实，治宜疏肝理气解郁为主，酌配清热、化痰、除湿、消食、活血之法；久病多虚，治宜益气补血养心为主，酌伍健脾、滋阴、安神之品。在运用理气药时，应注意此类药物虽能理气开郁，但多为香燥辛温之品，若郁而化火，或久病伤阴者，自当慎用。而香橼、佛手、绿萼梅、木蝴蝶之类，药性平和，理气而不伤阴，无论新病久病，病之寒热皆可选用。在辨证治疗时要抓住主症，结合病史、病程，辨其属虚属实，在气在血，偏寒偏热，以及病与何脏有关，以确定治法方药。用药宜轻灵，苦辛凉润宣通，勿投敛涩呆补、重浊滋腻之品。其次，本病要重视精神调摄，保持乐观情绪，树立战胜疾病信心。

复习思考题

1. 何谓郁证？临床特点是什么？
2. 试述郁证的病因病机。
3. 谈谈六郁的关系及对临床的指导意义。
4. 郁证的治疗原则是什么？对郁证怎样辨证论治？

癫　狂

〔概述〕

癫证与狂证都是精神失常的疾患。癫证以精神抑郁，表情淡漠，沉默痴呆，语无伦次，静而多喜为特征，多由痰气郁结，蒙蔽心神所致。狂证以精神亢奋，狂躁刚暴，喧扰不宁，毁物打骂，动而多怒为特征，多由痰火壅盛，迷塞心窍所致。二者在临床上能互相转化，难以截然分开，故癫狂常并称。

癫狂相当于现代医学精神系统疾病中各种类型的精神病，包括器质性及功能性者，凡见有上述表现者，均可参考本节所述内容进行辨证施治。

〔病因病机〕

癫狂发生的原因，在外多因六淫邪气内侵，跌打损伤。在内总与七情内伤密切相关，或以思虑过度，所欲不遂，或以悲喜交加，或以恼怒惊恐，皆能损伤心脾肝胆肾，导致脏腑功能失调，阴阳失于平秘，进而气滞、痰结、实火、血瘀导致心神失养，脑髓失充，而滋生精神失常诸般症状。可是狂证属阳，癫证属阴，由于证候的差异，病因病机也有所不同。兹从阴阳失调、情志抑郁、痰火上扰、气血凝滞、六淫外感、跌打损伤等几个方面对本病的病因病 机分别加以叙述。

一、阴阳失调：历代医家多以阴阳失去平衡立论来说明阴阳的盛衰是癫狂发病的重要原因。“阴平阳秘，精神乃治”，阴阳互相协调，才能维持正常的精神活动，如果这种正常的平衡受到破坏，精神就会出现异常，发生癫狂。外感六淫邪气，内为七情所伤及不内外因，皆可使阴阳失去相对的平衡。除了外感邪气引起人体的阴阳失调产生癫狂外，内伤七情也可引起阴阳的损伤。

阴阳的偏盛与偏衰，其表现的症状是不一样的。通常认为，狂是由于阳偏亢，而癫则由于是阴偏盛。《脉经》记有“阴附阳则狂，阳附阴则癫”。朱丹溪则认为“癫属阴，狂属阳”。

二、七情内伤：七情内伤是癫狂发病的重要原因之一。《内经》把人的情感活动分属五脏，并指出情志过极可以使脏气受损，进而导致正常生理功能的紊乱，引起癫狂。由于情绪不稳，或强烈的情绪刺激，七情过极则可损伤五脏，五脏受损，则不能发挥正常的生理功能，而出现诸多病理变化，导致心神失养，或病邪内扰。由于恼怒惊恐损伤肝肾，或因喜怒无常，忧思伤脾，致使心脾俱伤，肝肾不足，心阴耗损，则脑髓不充，神明失养，导致神态失常，情绪改变和行为的异常，以及记忆障碍，智力衰退；心阴不足，心火暴张，则可见狂言乱语，吵骂不休，赤身露体，逾垣上屋。如因所欲不遂，思虑过度，损伤心脾，心伤则神耗，脾虚则气血不得生化，终致心血虚，心神失养，而出现神无所主。

三、痰迷心窍：由于痰浊上扰清窍，以致心窍蒙塞，心神不明，神志错乱，狂躁不宁或则沉默寡言，痴呆不聪，发为癫狂。祖国医学历来重视痰在癫狂病发病中的作用。孙思邈提出癫与“痰热相感而动风”有关，及至金元时代，刘完素、张子和及朱丹溪等明确提出了痰在癫狂病发病中的病理作用。若因长期的精神因素造成气机不畅，肝郁累脾，健运不利使痰涎内生，则可形成气郁痰结。若脾气虚弱，清浊升降失常，阴浊蕴结成痰，是属气虚痰结。无论气郁痰结还是气虚痰结，总由“痰迷心窍”而发病。若因五志之火不得宣泄，炼液成痰，或肝火乘胃，津液被熬，结为痰火，或痰结日久，郁而化火，总因痰火上扰，心窍被蒙，神志遂乱可发为狂证。

四、火邪乘心：狂证多因火邪乘心而发。按经络的循行是胃络上通于心，是阳明热盛，上扰心窍，致心神昏乱则精神失常诸症发生。综观胃、肝、胆三经实火上升扰动心神皆可发狂证。若狂病日久，或经治火势渐衰而痰浊留恋，可转变为癫证。

五、气血瘀滞：由于气血瘀滞，使脑气与脏腑之气不相顺接而发狂。早在《内经》中就已提出“血”与“神”的关系，有“血者神气也”，“血有余则怒，不足则恐”。说明血与精神活动密切相关。李梴提出“血迷心包”而致狂发，清代医家王清任则明确提出癫狂是由于“气血凝滞”引起的。在其所著《医林改错》一书中，记有自创癫狂梦醒汤治疗本病。如因气血凝滞而致脑髓失养或因血瘀气滞在脑，使脏腑化生的气血不能正常地充养元神之府，或因血瘀凝滞脉络，气血不能上荣于脑髓，则可造成灵机记性混乱，神志失常发为癫狂。

综上所述，癫狂一证的基本病因病机改变，是以阴阳失调，七情内伤，痰气上扰，气血凝滞为主要因素。如因忧思不解，或因悲喜过度，或因惊恐恼怒而致心肝脾肾诸脏受损，肝肾阴伤，则水火不济，心火亢盛，肝气郁结，郁久也可化火，火邪上扰心神。或因肝郁失于条达，木克脾土，致使脾失健运，湿浊不化内聚痰涎，以致痰火互结，郁于胸膈，上蒙心窍则神明逆乱。或因气郁血凝，心神失养，从而导致机体阴阳偏胜，正常的功能紊乱，因而出现阳气盛的躁狂不宁，阴气盛的沉默少语，神情呆滞。

此外，张仲景《伤寒论》尚有蓄血发狂的记载，应属血瘀一类；《医学正传》又说：“癫为心血不足”，可见血虚也可致病。再者，癫狂证的发生与先天秉赋密切相关，若秉赋不亏，体质强壮，阴平阳秘，虽受七情刺激也只是短暂的情志失畅；反之秉赋素虚，遇有惊骇悲恐，意志不遂，则常由七情内伤，阴阳失调而发病。至于秉赋不足又往往是家族性的，故本病患者的家族往往也有类似的病史。

对同一患者而言，其致病原因也可以是多种因素相互影响，这一点尤应注意。

〔辨证论治〕

癫狂为一组以精神异常为主要临床表现的疾病。人的精神活动为心所主，与肝胆密切相关，亦与脾肾有内在联系，脏腑功能正常，“阴平阳秘，精神乃治”。癫狂一证，其主要病因病机为七情内伤，气机不畅，痰火内生，阴阳失调，其病变在肝胆心脾，以心为主。由于病邪的阴阳属性不同，体质的强弱各异，因而临床表现有癫狂之分。区分癫证、狂证最为重要，为辨证的关键。癫证表现为精神抑郁、沉默痴呆，行动迟缓；狂症表现为喧扰打骂，狂躁不宁，行为亢奋多动。二者在临床表现上不同，但也是互相联系，不能截然分开。癫证日久可气机郁滞，内生痰热而转化为狂症；狂症日久，正气大伤，邪从阴化也可转化为癫证。有时癫狂互见，错综复杂。癫狂证在初发病时多为实证，以邪实为主，如病情延误日久不愈，正气渐衰，或气血不足，或阴阳俱虚，或虚实夹杂，尤应细辨。

癫狂病因病机示意图

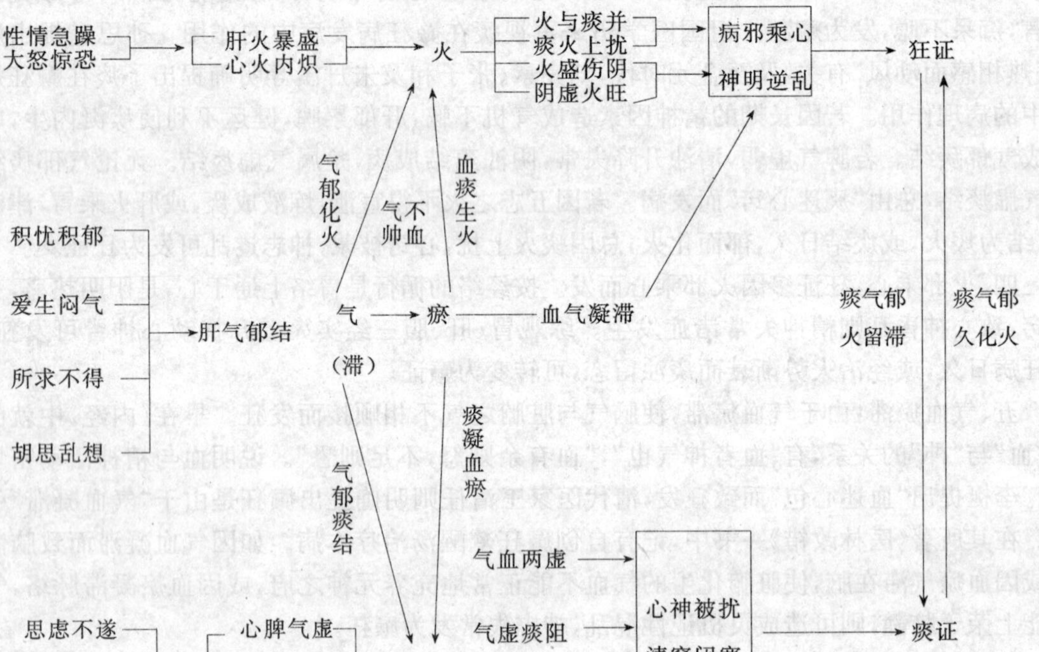

癫狂的发生，总由七情内伤，阴阳不得平衡，或气并于阳，或血并于内而发病，因而治疗总则应该调理阴阳，使之归于平衡。癫症多因痰气郁结而致气机不畅，或因心脾两虚而致心神失养，治疗总以理气开郁、化痰开窍、补益心脾、养血安神等法为主。狂症或为痰火上扰，或为火盛伤阴，邪盛而正气不衰，治疗之法，重在祛邪，泻火涤痰、滋阴降火为常用之法，用药亦多竣猛，务使病人安静为要。至于挟有瘀血内阻，又当重在活血祛瘀。癫狂日久，正气已伤，或见虚实挟杂，则应扶正为主或者攻补兼施。尤其要注意恢复期的调理和治疗，避免诱因，防止病情复发。

癫证多喜多虚，为重阴之病，主于气与痰，治疗以解郁化痰、宁心安神、补养气血为主要原则。狂证多怒多实，为重阳之病，主于痰火、瘀血，治疗宜先夺其食，或降其火，或下其痰，后期应予滋养心肝阴液，以清虚火。概言之，癫证与狂证总因七情内伤，使阴阳二气虚实不调，或气并于阳，或血并于阴而发病，故治诊原则应该以调理阴阳，使之归于平衡。

一、癫证

(一)痰气郁结

主症：精神抑郁，表情淡漠，沉默寡言，神情呆滞，或多疑多虑，哭笑无常，语无伦次。

兼症：喃喃自语，喜怒无常，不思饮食。

舌脉：舌淡苔白腻，脉弦滑。

分析：因思虑太过，所欲不遂，所求不得，使肝气被郁，失于条达，疏泄不利，木克脾土，脾失健运而生痰浊。痰浊内盛，阻蔽神明，故出现抑郁，呆滞，语无伦次等症。因痰扰而心神昏乱，故见喜怒无常。又因痰浊中阻，故不思饮食。舌脉皆为气郁痰结之征。

治法：疏肝解郁，化痰开窍。

方药：选用逍遥散合涤痰汤加减。药用柴胡疏肝解郁，配白芍养血柔肝，可加香附、郁金以增强理气解郁之力，其中茯苓、白术可以健脾利湿化浊。但是本方重在舒肝解郁，化痰之力弱，故宜并用涤痰之剂。涤痰汤为二陈汤增入胆星、枳实、人参、菖蒲、竹茹五味药，二陈汤为化痰的基本方剂。菖蒲合郁金可以开窍，枳实配香附可以理气，人参可不用。

如神思迷惘，表情呆滞，言语错乱，瞪目不瞬，舌苔白腻，乃心窍为痰浊蒙塞，心神失用，治宜豁痰宣窍，理气散结，先用苏合香丸芳香开窍，继用四七汤加胆星、菖蒲、郁金、远志之类，以行气化痰。

若胸膈痰浊壅盛，而形体壮实，脉滑大有力者，可先用三圣散涌吐痰涎，方中瓜蒂、防风、藜芦三味，以藜芦药性猛悍，虽有毒性，但劫夺痰浊速效可以愈病。吐后如形神俱乏，应及时调养饮食。本法重在祛邪，易伤正气，不可久用。此外痰浊壅盛而体质强健者，还可用控涎丹，下其顽痰，使从大便排除。

若兼失眠易惊，烦躁不安而神志昏乱，舌苔转为黄腻，舌质渐红者，系痰气郁结化热，痰热互结，上扰心神，治当清化痰热，清心开窍，可用温胆汤送服至宝丹。如逐渐出现高声吵闹不休，毁物伤人，则为火盛欲狂的征象，当从狂证论治。

处方举例：

当归 10g、白芍 10g、茯苓 30g、郁金 10g、柴胡 9g、白术 12g、半夏 10g、陈皮 9g、胆星 10g、枳实 9g、菖蒲 10g、竹茹 6g。

(二)气虚痰结

主症：情感淡漠，不动不语，甚则呆如木鸡，目瞪如愚，傻笑自语，思维混乱，甚则目妄见，耳妄闻，自责自罪。

兼症：面色萎黄，便溏溲清。

舌脉：舌质淡，舌体肥，苔白腻，脉滑或脉弱无力。

分析：癫病日久，正气自虚，脾失健运，痰浊益甚。一方面因痰结日甚则心神被蒙也日重，故情感淡漠而呆若木鸡，目瞪如愚，甚至灵机混乱，幻觉症状出现；另一方面是痰浊渐耗阳气，脾气日衰，故面色萎黄，便溏溲清诸症可见。舌脉皆由气虚痰结而成。

本证如经及时治疗，积极调养，投以益气涤痰之品，使痰浊渐化，正气渐复，则经较长时间治疗之后可以向愈，但较痰气郁结证易于复发。本证如迁延失治或调养不当，是气愈虚而痰愈盛，又痰愈深而症愈重，故终日灵机混乱，日久不复而成废人。

治法：益气健脾，豁痰宣窍。

方药：选用四君子汤合涤痰汤加减，药用参、苓、术、草四君子益气健脾为扶正培本之法。再予半夏、胆星、橘红、枳实、菖蒲、竹茹涤除痰涎，可加远志、郁金既可理气化痰，又可辅助菖蒲宣开心窍。若神思迷惘，表情呆钝症情较重，是痰迷心窍亦深，治宜温开，可用苏合香丸，每服一丸，日两次，以豁痰宣窍。

处方举例：

党参10g、白术10g、茯苓30g、半夏10g、陈皮9g、枳实10g、菖蒲12g、竹茹6g、远志10g、郁金10g。

（三）心脾两虚

主症：病程漫长，迁延日久，病势缓，面色苍白不华，少动懒言，神思恍惚，心悸易惊，善悲欲哭，妄想妄见妄闻，言语混乱无序，记忆力衰退。

兼症：夜寐梦多，不思饮食，便溏。

舌脉：舌质淡，体胖大有齿痕，舌苔薄白，脉细弱无力。

分析：癫病迁延日久，中气渐衰，气血生化乏源，可见面色苍白，肢体困倦，甚至疲惫不堪之象。由心血内亏，心神失养，可见神思恍惚，心悸易惊，记忆力衰退诸症。气血俱虚，神明失养，灵机混乱，故可出现幻觉，妄闻妄见。本证总因癫证日久，心脾两虚，血少气衰，心神失养所致。舌脉是气血俱衰之征。

治法：健脾益气，养心安神。

方药：选用养心汤加减。方中人参、黄芪、甘草补脾气，当归、川芎养心血，茯苓、远志、柏子仁、酸枣仁、五味子宁心神，更有肉桂引药入心，共奏养心安神之功。若兼畏寒蜷缩，卧姿如弓，小便清长，下利清谷，属肾阳不足，应加入温补肾阳之品，如补骨脂、巴戟天、肉苁蓉等，也可改拟右归饮加减。

处方举例：

人参6g、黄芪20g、炙甘草10g、当归10g、川芎6g、茯苓30g、远志10g、柏子仁6g、酸枣仁10g、五味子12g、肉桂3g、郁金10g。

二、狂证

（一）痰火扰心

主症：起病急骤，常先有性情急躁，头痛失眠，两目怒视，面红目赤，突然狂暴无知。情感高涨，言语杂乱，逾垣上屋，气力逾常，骂詈叫号，不避亲疏，或毁物伤人，或哭笑无常，登高而歌，弃衣而走，渴喜冷饮，便秘溲赤。

兼症：昼夜不眠，不食。

舌脉：舌质红绛，舌苔黄腻，脉象弦滑或滑数有力。

分析：暴怒伤肝，肝阳暴张，阳热火盛，鼓动阳明痰热，上扰清窍，故先见性情急躁，头痛失眠。清窍被蒙，则神明昏乱，症见狂暴无知，言语杂乱，骂詈不避亲疏。四肢为诸阳之本，阳盛则四肢实，实则登高逾墙上屋而气力超常。舌绛苔黄腻，脉弦滑而数，皆属痰火壅盛，且有伤阴之势。以火属阳，阳主动，故起病急骤而狂暴不休。

治法：泻火逐痰，镇心安神。

方药：选用泻心汤加味，送服礞石滚痰丸。方中大黄、黄连、黄芩苦寒直折，可泻心肝胃三经之火邪；重加知母，滋阴降火且能维护阴液；佐入生铁落镇心安神。其煎煮方法，先下生铁落，煎20分钟，数沸之后，入知母再煎15分钟，令汤沸起，再入三黄，煎2～3分钟，汤数沸后，即可滤出药汁温服。礞石滚痰丸药用青礞石、沉香、大黄、黄芩、朴硝。本方逐痰降火，药性猛悍，服量每次不宜大于10克，每天二次随汤药冲送内服。待痰火渐退时，礞石滚痰丸也可改成包煎，用量也可渐减为3～5克。

如属阳明热结，症见神志昏乱，谵语烦躁，面赤腹满，便秘燥结，舌苔焦黄起刺或焦黑燥裂，舌质红绛，脉滑实而大，宜先用大承气汤荡涤秽浊，清泻胃肠实火，急下存阴。如见烦渴引饮，则加石膏、知母以清热。其症重者，可酌用龙虎丸，方剂组成有牛黄、巴豆霜、辰砂、砒石。服后往往吐泻交作，故只可暂用，以能荡涤火实热为限，若多服必损伤肠胃，耗伤正气。

若经用逐痰泻火之后，神志转清，但痰火未尽，症见心烦失眠，哭笑无常者，可用温胆汤送服朱砂安神丸化痰安神；若火势渐衰而痰浊难除，神情痴呆，其状如癫，即可按癫证论治。

处方举例：

青礞石30g、代赭石30g、生石膏20g、生大黄(后下)10g、黄芩12g、莲子心6g、沉香6g、夜交藤30g、丹皮12g。

(二)阴虚火旺

主症：狂病日久，病势转缓，精神疲惫，情绪不稳，紧张焦虑，心悸易惊，时而躁狂，烦躁不眠，五心烦热。

兼症：形体消瘦，小便短赤，大便秘结。

舌脉：舌质红，少苔或舌光无苔，脉细数或弦细数。

分析：狂证躁动日久，必致气阴两伤，气不足则精神疲惫，阴伤火旺，扰动神明，则时有躁狂，终因正气已伤，故仅有时躁狂而不能持久。本证主要因阴伤而虚火旺盛，扰动心神，故症见情绪焦虑，多言善惊，烦躁不眠形瘦面红等。舌质红，脉细数也为阴虚内热之象。

若及时给予确当的治疗，使内热清则阴液渐复，病情可向愈发展。如治疗失当，火越旺则阴越伤，阴越亏则火越亢，进而躁狂之症时隐时发，时轻时重。另一方面按“火与元气不两立”的说法，火邪除了伤阴也能耗气，终致气阴两衰，其证迁延不愈，灵机昏乱而预后不良。

治法：滋阴降火，安神定志。

方药：选用二阴煎加减，送服定志丸。方中生地、麦冬、玄参养阴清热，黄连、木通、竹叶、灯心泻热清心安神，可加白薇、地骨皮清虚热，茯神、炒枣仁、甘草养心安神。定志丸药用人参、茯神、石菖蒲、远志、甘草，其方健脾养心，安神定志，可用汤药冲送，也可布包入煎。

处方举例：

生地30g、麦冬10g、五味子12g、元参10g、木通3g、竹叶6g、白薇10g、茯神30g、地骨皮10g、炒枣仁10g、炙甘草10g、生牡蛎(先下)30g。

(三)血气凝滞

主症：情绪躁扰不安，恼怒多言，甚则登高而歌，弃衣而走，或目妄见，耳妄闻，或呆滞少语，妄思离奇多端，常兼面色暗滞，胸胁满闷刺痛，心悸，或妇人经期腹痛，经血紫暗有块，或有头部跌打损伤。

兼症：头痛或头胀。

舌脉：舌质紫暗有瘀斑，舌苔薄白或薄黄，脉弦细或沉弦。

分析：气为血帅，气行则血行，气滞则血凝。如因气血凝滞，精气不得上承，则心神失养。本证由血气凝滞使脑气与脏腑之气不相连接而成，若瘀兼实热，苔黄，脉弦数者多表现为狂症。

若瘀兼虚寒，苔白、脉沉弦而迟者多表现为癫证，但是无论属狂属癫均以血瘀气滞为主因。

如给予活血化瘀行气的药物治疗，血瘀指征不断改善，则癫狂症状也可逐渐好转，其证可以痊愈。若瘀血日久不已，久瘀致虚，则预后较差。

治法：活血化瘀，兼以行气。

方药：选用癫狂梦醒汤加减，送服大黄䗪虫丸。方中重用桃仁合以赤芍活血祛瘀，还可加丹参、红花、水蛭以助活血之力，柴胡、香附理气解郁，青陈皮、大腹皮、桑皮、苏子行气降气，半夏和胃，甘草调中。如久瘀内有蕴热用木通加黄芩以清之；如兼寒加干姜、附子助阳温经。大黄䗪虫丸药用大黄、黄芩、甘草、桃仁、杏仁、芍药、地黄、干漆、虻虫、水蛭、蛴螬、䗪虫。其功用可祛瘀生新，攻逐蓄血。治疗本证需要时间较长，至少服药半年以上，每服4克，日服三次。

处方举例：

桃仁10g、赤芍12g、半夏6g、丹参30g、红花6g、郁金10g、香附10g、元胡10g、甘草6g。

〔预防及护理措施〕

癫狂一证，除了要积极进行治疗外，合理调护亦十分重要。癫狂证是一种以精神和行为紊乱异常的病症。罹患此病，则患者生活、学习、工作都很困难，而且给社会和家庭都带来很大负担，本病又易于复发，因此，对于急性病人，在经过治疗症状得到控制后，还应预防复发。其中调情志、戒郁怒，宁心守志，保持乐观向上的精神是非常重要的。精神饱满，心情舒畅，维持人体正常的阴阳平衡，"阴平阳秘，精神乃治"。还要注意起居饮食，少食辛热厚腻之品，以免湿浊邪热内蕴而致痰涎滋生，脾胃受损。还应避免跌打损伤，血瘀内阻。

在护理方面，首先是正确对待病人的各种病态表现，不应讥笑、讽刺病人，要尊重、关怀病人。对于轻症病人，可采取心理治疗。对其不合理的要求要耐心解释，对于其合理的要求要尽量满足。对于重症病人发生的打人、骂人、自伤、毁物等症状，要采取相应措施，注意安全，防止意外。对于拒食病人应找出原因，根据其特点进行劝导、督促、喂食或鼻饲，以保证营养。对有自杀、杀人企图或行为的病人要严格注意，专人照顾，并将危险品如刀、剪、绳、药品等藏起来，并注意预防投河、跳楼、触电等意外行为。

〔典型病例分析〕

案一：有一姜姓妇女，年四十有五，平素即心胸狭窄，多疑善虑，夫妻感情不好，因丈夫长期在外，回家后疑其有外遇，而打骂她，在一次剧烈的生气之后，突然该妇人两目直视，不言不语，不饮不食，继而大喊大叫，逾垣上屋，哭笑无常，当着众人面即脱衣服，打人毁物，三四个年轻力壮的男人竟难以制止她，就诊时上述狂暴症状已减轻许多，检查时面红目赤，舌红苔黄，便秘，诊断为狂症，乃肝郁痰火扰心所致。遂耐心开导患者，且告诉家人正确对待患者，多予体贴、关怀，不要增加其精神负担，处方予丹栀逍遥散加减煎汤冲服礞石滚痰丸，一日二丸，药后便秘得通，精神渐趋安定，连服十余剂，基本恢复正常。

按：此患者年届四十以上，平素夫妻感情不和，心情抑郁，肝气不舒，后因连续吵闹生气致肝郁化火犯脾，脾失健运而生痰，肝郁痰火上犯心窍，神明被蒙而发狂，出现狂症。诸般表现可知病在心、肝、脾三脏，治疗应泻火除痰，健脾安神，予丹栀逍遥散调理肝脾、清泻肝火，礞石滚痰丸清火涤痰，二方合治，正合病机，连服十余剂后痰热得除，气郁得舒，加之情志调护，渐恢复常人。

癫和狂都是精神失常的疾患，癫狂二者临床表现不同但又能互相转化，不能截然分开。癫以静默为主，多喜多虚，主为痰气郁结，治宜解郁化痰，宁心安神，补养气血，逍遥散、涤痰汤、养心汤为其常用方剂。狂以躁狂为主，多怒多实，主为痰火上扰，治宜降火逐痰，镇心安神，滋养肝肾，常选用礞石滚痰丸、龙虎丸、安神定志丸、二阴煎等治疗。现代医学的精神系统疾患而见有这类表现者可参考癫狂辨治。

复习思考题

1. 癫狂是一个病吗？两者有什么异同？

2. 癫狂的基本病因是什么？

3. 癫狂应该怎样治疗？狂证的治疗原则是什么？

4. 如何正确掌握和运用攻下、涤痰、探吐方药来治疗癫狂？

痫　证

〔概述〕

痫证是以突然仆倒，昏不识人，口吐涎沫，两目上视，肢体抽搐，或口中如做猪羊叫声，移时苏醒为主要临床表现的一种发作性疾病。痫证具有以下两方面特定的临床表现：(1)出现神志异常的肢体抽搐。(2)本病为发作性，起病急速而移时清醒，醒后一如常人，但常反复发作。

〔病因病机〕

本病《素问》称为巅疾，可理解为病变部位在巅顶，是属于脑髓的病变。本证主要是由于情志失调，先天因素，饮食不节，劳逸失度，跌打外伤，或患他病之后，造成脏腑功能失调，气机逆乱，痰浊阻滞，风痰互结，内风煽动所致。诸种原因之中，尤以痰邪作祟最为主要。

一、情志失调：七情之中与痫证发病最为相关的是惊恐。惊与癫痫发作的关系有两方面，一是因惊而心神失守，如突然感受大惊大恐，其他强烈的精神刺激也可以作为诱因，致使癫痫发作。再则惊恐则脏气不平，进而气机逆乱损伤脏腑，肝肾受损则易致阴不敛阳，而阳化风动，脾胃受伤则精微不布，痰浊内聚，一遇诱因，痰浊或随气逆，或随火炎，或随风动，蒙塞心神清窍，窜扰经脉，阻碍气血流通，致使突然昏仆，神识昏蒙，筋脉拘急，抽搐不止。

小儿脏腑娇嫩，元气未充，神气怯弱，易受惊恐而发病。

二、先天因素：痫证之发病，常始于幼年，这与先天因素密切相关，《内经》即认为本病是一种先天性疾病。《活幼心法》一书继承《内经》“母孕大惊子发癫疾”之说，对本病的先天因素进一步做了阐述：“胎病者，因未产前腹内受惊，或为七情所阻致伤胎气，儿生百日内有者是也。”母体突受惊恐，导致气机逆乱，还可导致母体精气耗伤，影响胎儿的正常发育，因而出生后极易发生痫证。

三、其他：六淫邪气侵袭，饮食失调，或头脑外伤及患有其他疾病之后，均可致脏腑受损，积痰内伏，遇有气恼劳作过度，生活起居失于调摄，遂致气机逆乱而触动积痰，痰浊之邪上扰心窍，神明闭塞，经脉壅滞，发为痫证。

综上所述，本病的发生，主要责之于肝气郁结，惊恐伤肾等精神因素，或饮食不节脾胃受伤，或先天禀赋不足而生后未能及时调治。总之由脏腑功能失调引起的痰火壅盛、气血逆乱、内风动越是本病的主要病因。论其病位，主要在肝、脾、肾三脏，尚涉及心脉胆络。至于病机转化，一般不越惊、痰、火三字范围。若惊恐伤及肝肾，肝肾阴亏不能敛阳而生热，热极可动内风；

又火热之邪煎熬津液而生痰；或饮食不节，脾胃受伤，健运不利以致精微不布，痰浊内聚；还有气郁化火，火邪灼阴，肾精耗伤，精不化血，血虚势必引动肝风，这都是癫证发作的病理基础，但应强调内伏之积痰至为重要。倘若人身没有积痰内伏，虽遇惊恐，或有内风，但患病而不作痫；如有积痰内伏，遇情志郁结或劳累过度等诱因，一旦触动内伏之积痰，致使气机逆乱，风阳挟痰上扰，壅闭经络，阻塞心窍则突然昏仆，抽搐发作而病癫痫。叶氏阐明了本病之所以是发作性疾患，其原因是诱因触动积痰则发，正气恢复即止。此见解对本病治疗和预防均有重要的指导意义。

痫证病因病机示意图

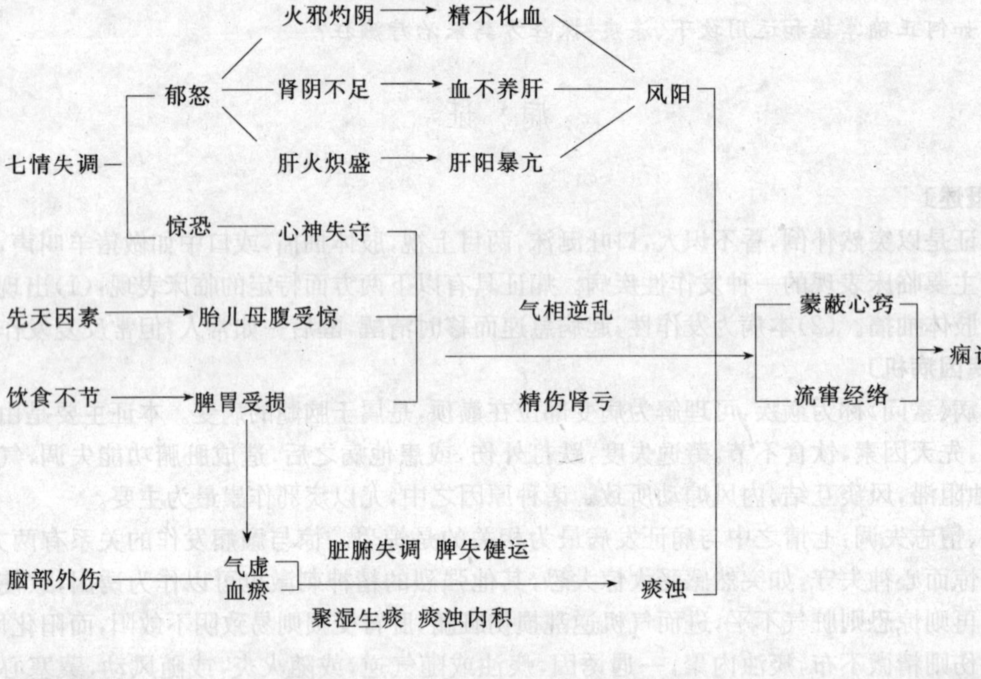

〔辨证论治〕

痫证有其特定的发病形式和临床特点，但由于病人的年龄和体质不同、致痫原因的差异、病程长短和发作次数等各方面的差别，在发病的症状和间歇期的表现也就错综复杂。因此临证时，应抓住要点，区别发作期还是间歇期，把握阳痫和阴痫两个总纲，再据舌脉症进行辨证论治。

在发病形式上，本病具有突然性、短暂性和反复性三大特点。突然性指起病急，多突然而发，也有部分病例于发病前数小时或数天，先出现精神紧张、易急烦躁等前驱症状，临近发病之前也有先觉眩晕头痛、肢体麻木、胸闷欠伸者，但为时极短。短暂性指发作时间短，一般自开始发作至意识清楚历时数分钟，也有突然意识丧失几秒钟即神志转清者。反复性是指反复发作，但其发作间歇的长短和发作频率的高低因病情轻重和发作形式的不同而有区别。

阳痫是偏于实热的一种证候，病人一般体质较好，发作急骤，卒倒号叫，抽搐吐涎，牙关紧闭，两目上视，脉象弦数或弦滑。阴痫是偏于虚寒的一种证候，病人一般体质较弱，或癫痫频发，正气渐衰而痰结不化，发作时症见面色苍白，呆滞无知，不动不语，脉象沉弦或沉滑。在癫痫的发作期主要是通过发痫时的症状表现和舌象、脉象，以辨别阳痫、阴痫而确定治疗法则。

至于癫痫间歇期，常见脾虚痰盛，或有肝火痰热，或有肝肾阴虚的表现。痫证频发，久治不愈，则气血不调，肾命虚衰，导致髓海不足，而见智力衰退出现痴呆，即王肯堂所说的“志愚”。也可因痫发抽搐不止，痰涎壅滞，气机阻塞而致阴阳离绝，危及生命。但应指出，有些病例可以在间歇期毫无自觉症状可寻。对无自觉症状的病人应注意了解发痫时的舌、脉、症状的表现，特别是自发病至就诊时在发病形式上有何变化。追访病史时应注意起病时的原始原因，如外伤病史、温热病史等，患病以后体质、智力的变化，重视就诊时舌象、脉象的观察。一般根据这些临床材料进行辨证论治。

在痫证发作时，还必须注意与中风、痉证等进行区别。癫痫与中风虽同有昏仆，然癫痫仆地有声，神昏片刻即醒，醒后如常，可以再发；中风仆地无声，神昏需辗转救活或可逐渐清醒，醒多有半身不遂、偏身麻木诸症存在。癫痫与痉证虽均有四肢抽搐拘急，然而癫痫发后四肢软倦，短时间神志转清，不伴发热；痉证发时多身强直、角弓反张，不易清醒，常伴发热。

痫证是一发作性疾病，具有突发性、反复性和一过性的特点，因而在治疗上也应区分发作期和间歇期，根据病因的不同表现，采用不同的治法。

一、发作期证治

(一)阳痫

主症：常先有头晕头痛，胸闷欠伸等先兆症状，旋即昏仆倒地，不省人事，两目上视，口唇青暗，牙关紧闭，颈项侧扭，手足搐搦，或四肢抽掣，或喉中痰鸣，或口吐涎沫。

兼症：发作时可有类似猪羊的叫声，甚则二便自遗。发作停止后，渐渐苏醒，除感疲乏无力外，饮食起居如常。

舌脉：舌苔白腻或黄腻，脉弦滑或弦数。

分析：头晕头痛，胸闷欠伸，仅有片刻，旋即神昏，此为风痰上逆的前驱表现。神昏仆地是因内风挟痰横窜，气血逆流于胸中，心神被蒙之故。口唇青暗为风痰痰热闭塞心胸，阳气受遏，血行瘀阻而致。两目上视，牙关紧闭，颈项侧扭，手足搦搐或四肢抽掣皆由内风窜扰筋脉所成。腻苔主湿盛，淡黄腻苔为内蕴痰热，其脉是属风痰内盛之征。惟风痰聚散无常，故时常发作而醒后一如常人。

治法：清化痰热，熄风定痫。

方药：清热镇惊汤化裁，用汤药送服定痫丸。药用生石决明、紫石英、龙胆草、山栀、木通、生大黄、干姜、柴胡、麦冬、天竺黄、胆南星、远志、菖蒲、明天麻、钩藤。方中生石决明平肝熄风，紫石英镇心定惊，龙胆草泻肝经之实火，与山栀、木通同用有通达三焦利湿之效，用生大黄泻热，反佐干姜苦辛并用以和胃降逆，又有助于天竺黄、胆南星清热豁痰，远志、菖蒲逐痰开窍，天麻、钩藤熄风止痉，柴胡一味可为引经药又可疏气解郁，配用麦冬既可防胆草等苦药伤阴，兼可安神。

处方举例：

生石决明(先下)30g、紫石英 15g、龙胆草 10g、生大黄 6g、胆南星 10g、天竺黄 10g、钩藤 30g、天麻 10g、菖蒲 10g、远志 9g、柴胡 6g、麦冬 10g、山栀 6g、木通 3g。

若治疗措施确当，痫止后再予丸药调理数月，有数年或十数年癫痫未再发作的病例。如调治不当，或经常遇有惊恐、劳累、饮食不节等诱因的触动，致使频繁发作，进而正气渐衰，湿痰内盛，则可以转变为阴痫。临床上遇阳痫初发或病程在半年以内者，治疗护理尤当精心，以防止痫证的频繁发作。

(二)阴痫

主症:发痫时面色晦暗萎黄,手足清冷,双眼半开半阖而神志昏愦,偃卧拘急或抽搐时发,口吐涎沫。

兼症:发作时一般口不啼叫,或声音微小。也有的仅表现为呆木无知,不闻不见,不动不语,频频发作。醒后全身疲惫无力,逐渐恢复。

舌脉:舌质淡苔白腻,脉沉细或细滑。

分析:本证儿科多见,常因慢惊之后痰迷心窍而成,成人则因阳痫病久,频繁发作使正气日衰,痰结不化而逐渐演变而来。阴痫病在里属脏病,主在脾肾而先后天俱受损,一则气血生化乏源,再则命火不足气化力薄,水寒上泛,故发痫时面色晦暗萎黄,手足清冷。湿痰上壅扰乱神明,又因心胸阳气虚衰有败脱之象,故两眼半开半闭而神志昏愦。《内经》有"风胜则动","四肢为诸阳之本"之说,可见风阳亢盛则抽掣搐搦亦剧,且因血不养筋,筋脉燥涩仅有暗煽之虚风,故偃卧拘急或抽搐时发;口吐涎沫可资证明内伏痰湿壅盛,随气逆而涌出。口不啼叫或声音微小是虽有积痰阻窍,然而正不胜邪之故。仅表现为呆木无知的病位主在心肾,以心主血、肾主髓,若心血不济、髓海空虚之人,遇有痰浊上蒙清窍则神明丧失,舌脉所见均属阳虚痰湿内盛之候。

治法:温脏除痰。

方药:选用五生丸以二陈汤送服。五生丸药用南星、半夏、川乌、白附子、黑豆等量,姜汁糊丸,每服 6 克至 10 克。方中南星、半夏、白附子均辛温,皆可除痰;半夏入脾胃兼以降逆散结;南星入肺、肝、脾,兼以祛风解痉;白附子主入胃,祛风痰而逐寒湿;川乌为大辛大热之品,温脾肾,助气化而能驱散沉寒结滞;黑豆一味补肾而利湿。总观五生丸以温脏除痰为主治,再予二陈汤加减以理气化痰,辅助丸药之药力。

还有因内热蒸表,汗出当风,风邪聚于肌腠而营卫之行涩,风邪干扰心营而血壅不行,血脉即乱,神气不定,因致发痫者,治当祛风除痰,可用化风锭,每服 1～2 丸。

有因惊怖所触,惊则气乱,神出舍空,遂致发痫者,痫发时吐舌急叫,面色乍白乍红,痫止时惕惕不安如人将捕之状,脉象虚弦。治当镇惊安神,可服金箔镇心丸,每服 1 至 2 丸。

处方举例:

胆南星 10g、半夏 10g、橘红 9g、茯苓 30g、僵蚕 10g、生姜 10g、白附子 6g。

阴痫证情虽重,若调养治疗得当,于痫止之后,先予调脾胃,和气血,健脑髓,兼或顺气涤痰,活血祛瘀,以攻补兼施之法,若能奏效,使患者体质渐复则癫痫也能缓解。

对于阳痫频发,虽经多方治疗不效者,多见渐而昏痴健忘,最终难以胜任原来的学习和工作。也有个别病例,于发痫时突然痰涌喉间而窒息,不及抢救致阴阳离绝而死亡。

二、间歇期证治

间歇期依据临床表现和舌脉的不同,可分为脾虚痰盛、肝火痰热、肝肾阴虚、肝风痰浊四种证候类型。现分述如下:

(一)脾虚痰盛

主症:神疲乏力,身体瘦弱,眩晕时作,面色不华,食欲不振,大便溏薄。

兼症:恶心泛呕,或胸脘痞闷,或咯白痰。

舌脉:舌质淡,苔白腻,脉濡滑或细弦滑。

分析:脾虚失于运化,以致生化乏源,气血不足,因而神疲乏力,身体瘦弱,面色不华,脾不健运，湿浊内停，聚浊成痰。积痰内伏日久，脾土更伤。脾虚则痰浊益甚，中焦为痰浊壅塞，则食欲不振。升降失常，则恶心泛呕。气机不畅，则胸脘痞闷。大便溏薄、咯痰皆为脾虚痰盛的表现。舌质淡是脾虚，苔白腻是痰湿之征象。

治法：健脾化痰。

方药：六君子汤加减。方用党参、茯苓、白术、炙甘草健脾益气；半夏、陈皮和胃化痰浊。若痰多可加南星、瓜蒌；呕恶者可加竹茹、旋覆花；便溏者可加薏苡仁、白扁豆；还可选用菖蒲、远志、僵蚕以除痰浊，宁心神；若痰黄量多，舌苔黄腻者可改用温胆汤加减。

处方举例：

党参10g、茯苓15g、白术10g、炙甘草10g、半夏9g、陈皮6g、南星6g、炒苡仁20g。

(二)肝风痰浊

主症：在发作前常有眩晕、头昏胸闷、乏力等先兆表现，亦有并无明显先兆而突然发病的。病发时突然跌倒，神识不清，抽搐吐涎。也可仅有短暂意识不清，或精神恍惚而无抽搐发作。

兼症：或发作时有尖叫声，二便失禁，咯痰。

舌脉：舌质红或暗红，苔腻，脉弦滑。

分析：眩晕时发，胸闷乏力等表现，均为风痰上逆的前兆症状。肝风内动，风痰互结，风痰上扰心神，心窍蒙塞则痫证突发，神识不清。肝风内扰，脾失健运，痰浊内生，痰随风动，上涌而吐涎沫，苔腻，脉弦滑均是肝风挟痰浊之象。

治法：涤痰熄风，开窍定痫。

方药：定痫丸加减。本方组成为天麻、川贝母、胆星、半夏、陈皮、茯苓、茯神、丹参、麦冬、远志、菖蒲、全蝎、僵蚕、琥珀、辰砂，用竹沥、甘草、姜汁熬膏，和药为丸，如弹子大，辰砂为衣，每服一至三丸。方中天麻、全蝎、僵蚕以平熄肝风而止抽搐；川贝、胆星、半夏、竹沥、菖蒲以化痰开窍降逆气；琥珀、茯神、远志、辰砂以镇心安神而能定惊；茯苓、陈皮以健脾理气；丹参、麦冬以理血育阴；姜汁、甘草可以温中和胃。

处方举例：

天麻10g、胆南星10g、半夏9g、茯神20g、石菖蒲10g、远志10g、僵蚕9g、全蝎6g、竹沥水(另兑)20ml。

(三)肝肾阴虚

主症：痫证频发，日久则正气大伤，平素记忆力差，神思恍惚，面色晦暗，头晕目眩，两眼干涩。

兼证：健忘失眠，腰酸腿软，大便干燥。

舌脉：舌质红，苔少，脉细数。

分析：癫痫频发的病人多气血先虚，久病及肾，肝肾同源，血虚日重势必耗用肾精，精血同源故也。肾精不足，髓海空虚则可见神思恍惚，面色晦暗，健忘等。目为肝窍，若血虚液燥则两目干涩，血虚肝旺故头晕目眩。肾开窍于耳，又肾主腰，故肾精虚衰则耳轮焦枯不泽，腰酸腿软。舌质脉象为精血不足之征。

治法：滋补肝肾，养心安神。

方药：左归丸加减。方中熟地、山药、山萸肉、龟板胶、枸杞子以滋养肝肾；可加用牡蛎、鳖甲以滋阴潜阳；柏子仁、磁石、辰砂宁心安神；贝母、天竺黄、竹茹清热除痰；如心中烦热重者加竹叶、山栀、莲子心等以清心除烦；大便干燥者加元参、当归、火麻仁以滋液润肠。

处方举例：

熟地30g、山药10g、山萸肉10g、枸杞子12g、牡蛎(先下)30g、柏子仁10g、磁石(先下)30g、川贝母10g、天竺黄10g、竹茹6g、莲子心3g、山栀6g。

(四)肝火痰热

主症：发作时昏仆跌倒，四肢抽搐，口吐涎沫，或有吼叫。平时性情急躁易怒，心烦气急失眠，头昏头痛。

兼症：口干口苦，便秘，咯痰不爽。

舌脉：舌质红，苔黄腻，脉弦滑数。

分析：肝火上炎，清窍被扰故见头晕头痛，肝气不舒，气机失于条达，则情绪急躁，火扰心神则心烦；火升风动，煎熬津液，结而为痰，风痰互结，阻塞清窍则突然昏仆跌倒，神志丧失；风性主动，则四肢抽搐不止。舌质红、苔黄腻、脉弦滑，均为肝火痰热内盛的征象。

治法：清肝泻火，化痰开窍。

方药：龙胆泻肝汤合涤痰汤加减。方中龙胆草、黄芩、栀子、木通等清肝泻火，又能利湿；半夏、橘红、胆星、菖蒲等化痰开窍，还可随证加用石决明、钩藤、鲜竹沥、天竺黄、地龙等泄热熄风、化痰通络镇痉；心烦甚可加莲子心；若痰火壅盛，大便秘结可加大黄，亦可并用竹沥达痰丸。

处方举例：

龙胆草10g、黄芩10g、栀子9g、木通6g、半夏6g、胆星10g、菖蒲10g、钩藤30g、生石决明(先下)30g、天竺黄10g。

此外，有因头部外伤后而发痫者，或痫病久发，屡有突然仆倒，头颅着地受伤，或痫证频发抽搐不止者，均可见有血瘀的表现。如头晕头痛，肢体麻木，胸闷刺痛，舌质紫暗或舌边有瘀点瘀斑，脉沉弦。在治疗方面应注重活血化瘀，再加入顺气开痰疏肝之品，一般可选用通窍活血汤加减。

〔预防和护理措施〕

癫痫的预防包括两个方面，一是对已知的致病因素和诱发因素的预防，以及增强体质的有关措施。在这方面最重要的是保持精神愉快情绪乐观，避免一切精神刺激，悦养性情。生活宜规律化，做到起居有节，注意保持二便通畅。应适当参加文娱活动和体育锻炼，但不可过劳，保证充足的睡眠。对久病体质差者加强营养也很重要；二是加强间歇期的治疗，防止癫痫的频繁发作，延长发作的间歇时间，这也是预防的一个重要方面。

本病的护理工作非常重要，首先对病情观察要认真仔细，应重视神志的变化，持续的时间和证候表现以及舌象、脉象、饮食、睡眠和二便情况，为辨证论治提供可靠的资料。对频繁发作的住院病人，要加用床挡等保护装置，以免发作时从床上跌下。有义齿者应取下。发作时应用裹纱布的压舌板放于上下磨牙间，以免咬伤舌头。神志失常者，应加强护理，以免发生意外，对病痫日久频繁发作的危重病人，于发作时特别应注意保护呼吸道通畅，以免发生窒息死亡。饮食宜清淡，多吃青菜，或选用山药、苡米、赤豆、绿豆、小米煮粥，可收健脾化湿的功效。

〔典型病例分析〕

案一：李某，男，14岁，1985年5月6日就诊。

自幼患有癫病，每隔一至数月发作一次，常因惊吓或紧张诱发，发作前自觉胸中堵闷头晕，随之大叫一声，昏仆倒地，不省人事，四肢抽搐，牙关紧闭，有时甚至咬破舌头，口吐涎沫。发作持续约5～6分钟，渐渐苏醒，自觉疲乏无力，不发作时起居饮食如常。多处求医服药，未获良效。近年来记忆力减退，学习成绩明显下降，神疲懒动，舌苔白腻，脉弦滑而缓。治拟顺气化痰，熄风定痫：

胆南星10g、天竺黄10g、远志10g、菖蒲6g、生石决明(先下)30g、紫石英15g、天麻10g、钩藤30g、茯苓30g。

上方送服定痫丸，于发作期服用。

间歇期治拟健脾化痰，以六君子汤加减：

太子参15g、茯苓30g、白术10g、半夏6g、生苡仁30g、陈皮10g、南星6g、甘草6g。

上方送服定痫丸，每日2次，每次1丸。

如此治疗，二年未发。后因报考高中，复习紧张后发作一次，时间较前缩短，3分钟即清醒，继续调治，至今未作。

按：本例痫证，为肝风内动，风痰互结，风痰上扰心窍，心窍蒙塞所致。病久正气不足，脾土受伤，健运失司，痰湿益盛。故治疗始终以化痰为主，发作期则侧重熄风定痫，间歇期注重健脾化湿，使痰无所生，痫证难发。然体内积痰难以清除，遇诱因则易复发。

癫痫是一短暂性发作性脑系疾病，中医对本病历代论述颇多，其病机后世医家多强调积痰内伏，每由情志不遂或劳累等因诱发，以致气逆，风阳挟痰上扰，阻塞清窍而发病。痫病初发多为实证、阳证，当以熄风涤痰为主；痫病既久，多为阴证、虚证，当以益气、育阴、养血为主，本病发作期，总以定痫治标为先，而休止期以调补气血，强键脾胃，滋养肝肾为主。

复习思考题

1. 痫证有什么临床特征？

2. 怎样理解痫证的病因和病机？

3. 痫证的治疗原则是什么？常见的痫证有哪几种证候类型？怎样进行治疗？

胃　痛

〔附：吐酸、嘈杂〕

〔概述〕

凡由于脾胃受损，气血不调所引起的胃脘部疼痛，称之胃痛，又称胃脘痛。胃脘部一般系指上、中、下三脘部位，或指两侧肋骨下缘联线以上至鸠尾形的梯形部位。

古代文献中常以心痛取代胃痛，二者实有不同，应该严格区分。临证时，从病因、临床表现、体征及必要的理化检查，是不难分清的，这对治疗和预后都是极为重要的。

胃痛以各种性质的胃脘部位的疼痛为主症，往往兼见胃脘部痞满、胀闷、嗳气、吐酸、倒饱、纳呆、胁胀、腹胀等症。常反复发作。久治难愈，甚至可见吐血、黑便、呕吐、关格等证。

西医学诊断的急慢性胃炎，消化性溃疡，胃神经官能症，胃癌以及部分肝、胆、胰疾病，均可见胃脘部位疼痛，可参考本病加以辨证论治。

〔病因病机〕

胃痛初发多属实证，其病主要在胃，间可及肝；病久常见虚证，其病主要在脾；亦有虚实夹杂者，或脾胃同病，或肝脾同病。古人常说："实则阳明，虚则太阴。"对胃痛也是如此。

胃痛的常见病因，可概括为病邪犯胃，饮食不节，情志不畅，脾胃虚弱等几个方面，简述如下：

一、外邪犯胃：外邪之中以寒邪最易犯胃，夏暑之季，暑热、湿浊之邪也间有之。邪气客胃，胃气受伤，轻则气机壅滞，重则和降失司，而致胃脘作痛。寒主凝滞，多见绞痛；暑热急迫常致灼痛；湿浊黏腻，常见闷痛。

二、饮食不节：胃主受纳，开窍于口。若纵恣口腹，饥饱失调，寒热不适，偏嗜烟酒，或过用伤胃药物，均可伐伤胃气，气机升降失调而作胃痛。目前，临床上以过食肥甘及烟酒最为常见，厚味及烟酒皆湿热之性，停于胃腑伤津耗液为先，久则损脾。

三、情志不畅：情志所伤，使肝脾功能受到影响，也能引起胃痛。如气郁恼怒则伤肝，肝气失于疏泄条达，横犯脾胃，而致肝胃不和或肝脾不和，气血阻滞则胃病；忧思焦虑则伤脾，脾伤则运化失司，升降失常，气机不畅也致胃病。

四、脾胃虚弱：劳倦太过，失血过多，或久病不愈，伤及脾胃；或身体素虚，脾胃不健，运化无权，升降转枢乏力，气机阻滞而致胃病；若中气下陷者，病情可进一步加重；若脾胃阳虚，阴寒内生，脉络失于温养，则拘急而痛。若胃病日久，阴津暗耗，胃失濡养，气机失调，也致胃病。

胃痛病因病机示意图

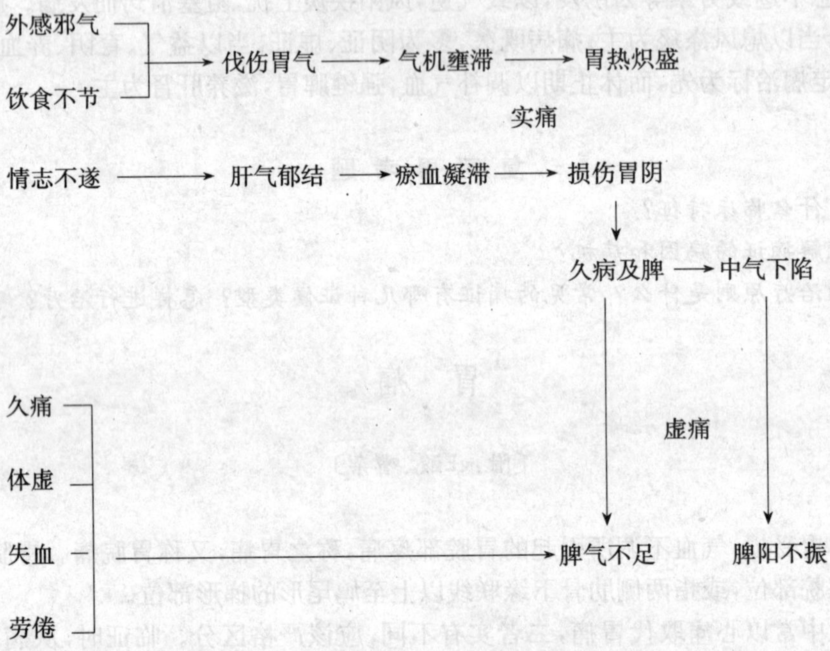

综上所述，胃痛与胃、肝、脾关系最为密切，初起病位主要在胃，间可旁及于肝；病久则主要在脾，或脾胃同病，或肝脾同病。胃为阳土，喜润恶燥，主受纳、腐熟水谷，以和降为顺。胃气一伤，初则壅滞，继则上逆，此即气滞为病。其中首先是胃气的壅滞，无论外感、食积均可引发；其次是肝胃气滞，即肝气郁结，横逆犯胃所造成的气机阻滞。气为血帅，气行则血行，故气滞日久，必致血瘀，也即久病入络之意。另外，“气有余便是火”，气机不畅，蕴久化热。此火也有单纯在胃或同在肝胃之说。火能灼伤阴津，或血脉瘀阻而新血不生，阴血虚少也有胃阴不足或脾胃阴虚或肝胃、肝脾阴虚的不同。胃病延久，内传于脾，脾属阴土，喜燥恶湿，主运化，输布精微，以升为健。故脾气受伤，轻则中气不足，运化无权；继则中气下陷，升降失司；再则脾胃阳虚，阴寒内生，胃络失于温养。总之，胃痛病因虽有上述种种不同，病理尚有虚实寒热、在气在血之异，但其发病原理确有共同之点，即所谓“不通则痛”，若胃痛失治误治，血络损伤，则可见吐血，便血等证。

〔**辨证论治**〕

一、辨证要点

1. 辨寒热：外受寒凉或过食生冷而发病或加重，胃中绞痛，得温熨或饮热汤则痛减，口淡不渴或渴饮而不欲咽者属寒；胃中灼痛，痛势急迫，得冷饮或冷熨而痛减，口干渴或口苦者属热。

2. 辨虚实：凡属暴痛，痛势剧烈，痛而拒按，食后痛甚或痛而不移，痛无休止者属实；若疼痛日久或反复发作，痛势绵绵，痛而喜按，得食痛减或劳倦加重，休息后减轻者属虚。壮年新病者多实；年高久病者多虚。补而痛剧者为实，攻而痛甚者为虚。

3. 辨气血：从疼痛的性质而言，若以胀痛为主，伴有嗳气者属于气滞；痛如针刺或刀割或伴吐血、黑便者属于血瘀。从疼痛的部位而言，若以游走不定、攻冲作痛者为气滞；痛处固定或扪之有积块者为血瘀。从病程而论，初病多在气，久病多入血。

4. 辨在胃、在肝、在脾：在胃多属胃病初发，常因外感、伤食所引起，症见胃脘胀痛、闷痛，嗳气倒饱，痛无休止，大便不爽，脉滑等。

在肝多属反复发作，每与情志不遂有关，胃脘胀痛连及胁肋，窜走不定，太息为快，脉弦等。

在脾多属久病，胃中隐痛，饥时为甚，进食可缓。劳倦则重，休息则轻。面色萎黄，疲乏无力，大便溏薄，脉缓等。

(五)辨胃痛与真心痛

胃痛：多有胃病史，除胃脘部疼痛外，尚伴有嗳气、泛酸、纳食不馨、大便不调等症，结合上消化道钡餐造影，胃镜等检查多可明确诊断。

真心痛：多有心脏病史，除心窝部疼痛外，多见于中年以上之人，常伴有胸闷憋气，心慌气短，头晕耳鸣，唇甲紫黯，脉结代等症，结合心电图及生化检查多可确诊。

二、分型证治

胃痛，初病在气，实证居多，病位有在胃在肝之别。其中受寒、冒暑、伤食、积热易伤胃，使胃气壅滞，甚至不降反逆；情志不遂易损肝，肝气郁结则横逆犯胃，致肝胃气滞。气滞郁久化热或久痛入络。胃病失治误治，病位由胃及脾，脾病以虚证居多，虚中夹实间而有之。脾病或见脾气虚弱，或见中气下陷，或见脾阳不振。故胃痛的治疗，治胃以理气和胃通降为主，依病因之异，或散寒，或祛暑，或消食，或清热，或化瘀，分别施治。治肝以疏肝解郁为主，化热则清肝，入络则行血，阴伤则滋养。治脾以健脾益气为主，下陷者升提，阳虚者温补。若临证之时，见肝胃、肝脾或脾胃同病者，又当权衡标本轻重，辨证施治。

(一)胃气壅滞

1. 寒邪犯胃

主症：突然发作，疼痛如绞，得温熨或饮热汤则痛减。多有受寒或过食生冷病史。

兼症：恶寒或畏寒，遇寒痛甚，口不渴，喜饮热汤。

舌脉：舌淡红，苔薄白，脉浮紧或紧。

分析：突受寒邪直中或过食生冷之物。寒邪客气，寒主收引凝滞，阳气被遏而不展，故胃痛如绞。寒得温则散，故胃痛得热熨或饮热汤则减。阳气郁遏，故恶寒或畏寒，口不渴，饮则欲饮热汤。苔薄白，脉浮紧或紧，均为寒盛之象。

治法：温中散寒，和胃止痛。

方药：轻症可用热熨胃脘部，或热服姜葱汤，或艾灸中脘、足三里等即能止痛。重者以良附丸加味治之。方中以高良姜温中散寒，香附行气止痛；或再加荜澄茄、桂枝、荜拨、生姜、川椒等以增强散寒止痛之力。若兼外感，症见恶寒身痛等，可加苏叶、豆豉、葱白等以辛温疏解，或合用香苏散以疏 表散寒止痛。若因夏日露宿，感受阴暑而致胃痛时，应加香薷、藿香、佩兰等以芳化和中。

处方举例：

高良姜 10g、制香附 10g、苏叶 10g、炒陈皮 10g、生姜 3 片、荜澄茄 10g、焦三仙各 10g、半夏 10g、茯苓 10g。

2. 饮食停滞

主症：胃脘闷痛，得嗳气或矢气则舒。

兼症：嗳腐倒饱，胃中掣胀，饥时稍舒，进食加重，甚则呕吐不化之物，吐后胃舒痛减，或大便不爽。

舌脉：舌苔白厚或腻，脉滑。

分析：饮食不节，伐伤胃气，受纳腐熟失司，食滞气结，故胃脘闷痛；得嗳气或矢气，气机宣畅，得呕吐则食积有减，故闷痛稍缓。食滞于中，蕴而化热则嗳腐倒饱，大便不畅。舌苔白厚或腻，脉滑均为食积之象。

治法：消食导滞，和中止痛。

方药：保和丸合香苏散加减。方中保和丸以二陈汤和中降逆、消痞除满，合神曲、谷麦芽、山楂消食导滞。香苏散以苏梗、陈皮、香附理气和胃降逆，再加连翘以清除食积所化之热。若胃痛明显，可加枳实、厚朴、莱菔子、大腹皮、槟榔等以宽中下气。若食积化热，腑气不通者，可合小承气汤以通腑泻热，或改用枳实导滞丸化裁也可。

处方举例：

苏梗 10g、制香附 10g、炒陈皮 10g、半夏曲 10g、茯苓 10g、焦三仙各 10g、焦槟榔 10g、莱菔子 10g、连翘 10g。

（二）肝胃气滞

主症：胃脘胀痛，连及两胁，攻撑走窜，每因情志不遂而加重。

兼症：喜太息，不思饮食。

舌脉：舌苔薄白，脉弦滑。

分析：肝气郁结，横逆犯胃，肝胃气滞，故胃脘胀痛。气病多游走不定，胁为肝之分野，故胃痛连胁，攻撑走窜，每因情志不遂而加重气机不畅，故以太息为快。胃失和降，受纳失司，故不思饮食。舌苔薄白，脉弦滑为肝胃不和之象。

治法：疏肝和胃，理气止痛。

方药：柴胡疏肝散加减。此方以四逆散气血双调，使肝体得养，肝用自如，气血调畅，再加用川芎以调血中之气，香附以理气中之血，青皮、陈皮以调肝理气，从而达到调和肝胃，消胀止痛之效。还可加郁金以疏肝解郁。若疼痛严重时，宜加元胡、川楝子以理气和血止痛，若气郁化热，宜加山栀、丹皮、蒲公英以疏气泄热。由于肝乃体阴用阳之脏，调气之品不宜过用香燥。

处方举例：

醋柴胡10g、炒枳壳10g、赤白芍各10g、制香附10g、青陈皮各6g、焦三仙各10g、旋覆花(包)10g、广郁金10g、川芎6g、元胡10g、炒川楝10g。

(三)肝胃郁热

主症：胃脘灼痛，痛势急迫。

兼症：嘈杂泛酸，口干口苦，渴喜凉饮，烦躁易怒。

舌脉：舌红苔黄，脉弦滑数。

分析："气有余便是火"，肝胃不和，气机郁滞，久而化热。热积中州，故胃脘灼痛，痛势急迫。若肝热犯胃，则症见脘胁烦痛，泛酸嘈杂，烦躁易怒。热邪灼津，故口干口苦而喜凉饮。舌红苔黄、脉弦滑数，亦为肝胃蕴热之象。

治法：清肝泄热、和胃止痛。

方药：肝热移胃者用化肝煎加减。胃热伤津明显者用白虎汤加味；胃肠蕴热，腑气不通者用泻心汤加减。

目前，临床上所见烟酒太过，实是引起胃痛的重要因素，而烟酒之品皆属火热之品，烟偏燥热，酒偏湿热；烟酒过用则致胃中积热，症见胃中烧灼作痛，治疗时宜清胃与生津或清胃与除湿合参。

另外，邪热蕴久则可成毒，热毒伤胃，在胃镜下可见胃黏膜充血、水肿，甚至糜烂、渗血、溃疡，此时治疗宜适用蒲公英、连翘、金银花、虎杖、生苡仁、土贝母等药以清热解毒，对胃病治疗有积极意义。

处方举例：

川贝母10g、青皮6g、山栀10g、蒲公英15g、香橼皮10g、佛手10g、炒川芎10g、黄连5g、吴茱萸3g、天花粉10g。

(四)瘀血阻滞

主症：胃脘疼痛，状如针刺或刀割，痛有定处而拒按。

兼症：病程日久，胃痛反复发作而不愈，面色晦黯无华，唇黯；女子月经愆期，色黯。

舌脉：舌质紫黯，有瘀点、瘀斑，脉弦或涩。

分析：胃乃多气多血之腑，气为血帅，气行则血行，气滞则血瘀。或吐血、便血之后、离经之血停积于胃，也成瘀血。瘀血停胃故疼痛状如针刺或刀割，固定而不移，拒按。瘀血不净，新血不生，故面色晦黯无华，口唇紫黯，女子则可见月事不调，愆期色黯。舌质紫黯，或有瘀点、瘀斑，脉弦或涩，也是血脉瘀阻之象。

治法：理气治血、化瘀止痛。

方药：失笑散合丹参饮。两方均系瘀血胃痛常用方。若缘气滞而致血瘀，气滞仍明显时，宜加理气之品，但忌香燥太过。若血瘀而兼血虚者，宜加四物汤等养血活血之味。若血瘀而兼脾胃虚衰者，宜加炙黄芪、党参等健脾益气以助血行。若瘀血日久，血不循常道而外溢出血者，应参考吐血、便血篇处理。

处方举例：

炒灵脂10g、生蒲黄(包煎)10g、丹参20g、檀香6g、砂仁5g、制香附10g、炒陈皮10g、三七粉(分冲)3g、延胡索 6g、川芎 6g。

(五)胃阴不足

主症:胃脘隐痛或隐隐灼痛。

兼症:嘈杂似饥,饥不欲食,口干不思饮,咽干唇燥,大便干结或腑行不畅。

舌脉:舌体瘦,质嫩红,少苔或无苔,脉细而数。

分析:胃属阳土,喜润恶燥,气郁化热,热伤胃津,或瘀血积留,新血不生,均可使胃阴不足。阴津亏损则胃络失养,故见胃脘隐痛,若阴虚有火,则可见胃中灼痛隐隐。胃津亏虚则胃纳失司,故嘈杂似饥,知饥而不能受纳。阴液亏乏,津不上承,故咽干唇燥。阴液不足则肠道干涩,故大便干结或腑行不畅。舌体瘦舌质嫩红,少苔或无苔,脉细而数,皆为胃阴不足而兼虚火之象。

治法:养阴益胃,和络止痛。

方药:养胃汤合芍药甘草汤加减。若气滞仍著时,宜加佛手、香橼皮、玫瑰花、代代花等轻清畅气而不伤阴之品;胃病较甚时加金铃子散合用,止痛而不化燥。津伤液亏明显时,可加芦根、天花粉、乌梅等以生津养液;大便干结者,加火麻仁、郁李仁、瓜蒌仁等润肠之品。若兼肝阴亦虚,症见脘痛连胁者,可加白芍、枸杞、生地等柔肝之品,或用一贯煎化裁治之。

处方举例:

沙丹参各 15g、天麦冬各 10g、玉竹 15g、生甘草 6g、佛手 10g、香橼皮 10g、炒川楝 10g、乌梅 6g、火麻仁 15g、玫瑰花 6g。

(六)脾胃虚寒

主症:胃脘隐痛,遇寒或饥时痛剧,得温熨或进食则缓,喜暖喜按。

兼症:面色不华,神疲肢怠,四末不温,食少便溏,或泛吐清水。

舌脉:舌淡而胖,边有齿痕,苔薄白,脉沉细无力。

分析:胃病日久,累及脾阳。脾胃阳虚,故胃痛绵绵,遇寒或饥时痛甚,得温熨或进食则缓,喜暖喜按。脾为气血生化之源,化源不足则气血虚弱,机体失养,故面色不华,神疲肢怠。脾主四肢,阳气既虚不达四末,故四肢不温。脾虚不运,转输失常,故食少便溏。若脾阳不振,寒湿内生,饮邪上逆,则见泛吐清水。舌淡而胖,边有齿痕,苔薄白,脉沉细无力亦为脾胃虚寒之象。

治法:温中健脾。

方药:黄芪建中汤加减。若阳虚内寒较重者,也可用大建中汤化裁,或加附子、肉桂、荜拨、荜澄茄等温中散寒;兼泛酸者,可加黄连汁炒吴萸、煅瓦楞、海螵蛸等制酸之品。泛吐清水时,可与小半夏加茯苓汤或与苓桂术甘汤合方为治。

若仅见脾胃虚弱,阳虚内寒不明显时,可用香砂六君子汤调治;兼见血虚者,也可用归芪建中汤治之。若胃脘坠痛,证属中气下陷者,可用补中益气汤化裁为治。

临床上胃强脾弱,上热下寒者也不少见,治疗时,可选用半夏泻心汤、连理汤或温脾汤等化裁。

处方举例:

炙黄芪 30g、炙桂枝 10g、炒白芍 15g、炙甘草 6g、生姜 3 片、大枣 7 枚、饴糖(烊化冲)30g、荜澄茄 10g、当归 10g。

附一、吐酸

吐酸,即泛吐酸水,或口中发酸,临床上当有寒热之分,肝胃之别。高鼓峰在《医家心法·

吞酸》中精辟地指出："凡是吞酸，尽属肝木曲直作酸也。河间主热，东垣主寒；毕竟东垣言其因，河间言其化也。盖寒则阳气不舒，气不舒则郁而为热，热则酸矣；然亦有不因寒而酸者，尽是水气郁甚，熏蒸湿土而成也，或吞酸或吐酸也。又有饮食太过，胃脘填塞，脾气不运而酸者，是沸郁之极，湿热蒸变，如酒缸太热则酸也。然总是木气所致。"不难看出，吐酸一证，与肝胃相关，然酸总为肝味，故治之当以从肝而论为根本。兹分述之。

热证：多由肝郁化热，横逆犯胃所致。《内经》云："诸呕吐酸，皆属于热"。症见泛吐酸水，心烦易怒，咽干口苦，不思饮食，舌边尖红、苔黄，脉多弦滑。治宜泄肝和胃，方用左金丸加味。

处方举例：

黄连 6g、吴茱萸 3g、煅瓦楞 15g、乌贼骨 15g、川贝母 6g、山栀 10g、青皮 6g、连翘 10g、焦三仙各 10g。

寒证：多由脾胃虚寒所致。症见泛吐酸水清稀，脘闷纳呆，饮食不慎则益甚，胃脘喜暖喜按，四肢不温，疲倦无力，大便溏薄，舌淡苔白滑，脉象细弦。治宜温中健脾、抑肝和胃，方用香砂六君子汤合吴茱萸汤化裁。

处方举例：

党参 10g、茯苓 15g、炒白术 12g、砂仁 6g、木香 10g、半夏 10g、炒陈皮 10g、生姜 3 片、吴茱萸 5g、厚朴 10g、藿香 10g。

附二、嘈杂

嘈杂，是指胃中饥嘈，胸膈懊侬而不可名状而言。临证时常有胃热、胃虚、血虚之别。兹分述如下。

胃热：嘈杂而兼见胸闷痰多，心烦少寐，口干喜冷饮，嗳腐吞酸，舌红、苔黄、脉象弦滑或滑数。治宜清热和中，方用黄连温胆汤加减。

处方举例：

黄连 6g、清半夏 10g、炒陈皮 10g、茯苓 15g、竹茹 6g、枳实 10g、生甘草 6g、山栀 10g、焦三仙各 10g。

胃虚：嘈杂而兼见口淡无味，食后脘胀，神疲肢倦，舌淡、苔薄白，脉细弱。治宜健脾和胃，方用香砂六君子汤加减。

处方举例：

砂仁 6g、木香 10g、党参 15g、茯苓 15g、炒白术 10g、半夏曲 10g、炒陈皮 6g、鸡内金 10g、枳实 10g。

血虚：嘈杂而兼见面白无华，心悸头晕，少眠多梦，形体消瘦，肌肤不泽，舌淡，脉细治宜补养气血，方用归脾汤化裁。

处方举例：

炙黄芪 20g、党参 15g、当归 10g、茯苓 15g、白芍 10g、白术 10g、龙眼肉 10g、炙甘草 6g、木香 6g、远志 10g、生龙骨(先下)30g、生牡蛎(先下)30g。

〔预防及护理措施〕

1. 实证胃痛的发生与感受外邪，特别是受寒，饮食不节，情绪过激以及烟酒过度关系密切。因此，为了预防发作，应注意气候变化，尤其突然转寒时，注意增减衣服，免遭外邪侵袭；饮食宜清淡、半流质、易消化、不凉不热及八分饱；保持情绪稳定和乐观。虚证胃病的发生与体弱、脾胃不健的关系尤为重要，因此，宜劳逸结合，避免过劳过虚。

2. 若胃痛剧烈难忍，胃脘拒按，或伴有寒战高热，大汗出或汗出如油，面色苍白，四肢发冷，应嘱患者保持镇静、卧床休息，并及时报告医生。

3. 胃痛而呕吐，便血或便秘者，应按血证或便秘及时处理，血止、便通后再治胃病，或胃痛自除。

4. 注意鉴别胃病、真心痛，属真心痛者按其诊治规律处理，以防误诊。

〔典型病例分析〕

案一：田某某，男，27岁，工人。

以胃脘痛伴呕吐、便血3天，经急诊入院。患者有胃病史六、七年，平时胃脘疼痛，饭前为甚，进食稍缓，泛酸，每作皆对症处理，从未系统诊治。3天前因吃肉较多，至当晚下半夜胃中痛甚，呕吐食物夹有鲜红或黯红血块，腹泻一次为柏油样便，遂来我院急诊室留观。在留观中又呕血、便血各二次，量较多，血色素降至6.9g，遂收入病房。当时患者胃脘痛甚，胀满不舒，口干口渴，稍恶心，头晕心悸，面唇发白，脉象弦细滑数，舌胖而淡、苔薄黄。入院后急查胃镜，见十二指肠球部与降部交界处后壁有一1.8×0.7cm大小溃疡，中心凹陷，有白苔覆盖，正中有新鲜渗血，另外胃角下有一陈旧性溃疡瘢痕。证属胃病日久，脾气亏虚，运化失司，加之饮食不当，食滞气结，蕴而化热，热迫血络而外溢。故急用白芨粉、大黄粉冲服以凉血活血止血。汤药则标本兼顾，拟方如下：炙黄芪20g、炒赤芍12g、全当归10g、连翘10g、生甘草5g、炒五灵脂10g、生蒲黄10g、三七粉（分冲）3g、乌贼骨15g、代赭石（先下）20g、党参10g。药进一剂则疼痛缓解。至第二日便通，一日三次，晨为柏油样，午则色变浅，至晚上已见黄色。便潜血也转阴性。以上药为基础，随症加减，如泛酸加左金丸，血虚加阿胶、首乌、胎盘糖衣片，恶心加二陈等调治2月余，复查胃镜，十二指肠球部溃疡已愈合，尚留有小片状浅表糜烂，血色素升至113g/l，遂出院门诊调治。

按：此例胃痛，病程较长，病情也较复杂，虚实错综、寒热相见，如胃脘疼甚，胀满不舒，恶心皆属气结气逆之虚象；如胃痛以饭前为甚，进食能缓解，头晕心悸，面唇发白，舌胖而淡均属脾虚之象；如口干口渴、苔薄黄则属热象；如舌胖而淡等也属寒象。治疗时必当攻补兼施，寒热并调，法遵益气活血解毒而治之，故胃痛药进辄止；呕血、便血也不3日停止；巨大溃疡则二月余方获愈合。（本案录自《北京中医学院学报》85,4）

胃痛，其病位初病在胃，久病及脾，与肝也有密切关系。本病初发，无论外邪侵犯、饮食所伤，或肝气郁结，均可以使胃气受伤。其中外邪与饮食可直接伤胃，轻则使胃气壅滞，重则胃失和降而致气机上逆。肝气郁结，横逆犯胃，往往肝胃同病而致肝胃气滞。若此时未能掌握住病机，失治误治，则气滞化热或久病入络致瘀。邪热则伤阴津，瘀血不化则新血不生，病渐转虚，胃阴亏虚者常见。胃病日久，病由胃及脾，病性由实转虚或虚实夹杂。脾虚又当有脾气不足、中气下陷、脾胃虚寒之别，区分论治。

胃痛治疗，虽遵“通则不痛”之旨，但具体方法迥异。治胃以理气和胃通降为主，依病因不同，或散寒、或祛暑、或消食、或清热、或消瘀；若胃阴已伤，则又当生津养阴以益胃，治肝以疏肝理气为主，化热则佐以清肝，入络则行血。治脾以健脾益气为主，下陷者则佐以升提，虚寒者佐以温补。若虚实夹杂、寒热并见者，又当标本兼顾。

当前临床上，胃痛以实证、热证多见，虚实寒热错杂次之，纯虚证较少。

调护得当，对胃痛的预后极为重要。

吐酸，多与胃痛同时出现，若以吐酸为主时，当以吐酸作为病证辨治。吐酸有寒热的偏盛，病位也有责之肝与责之胃之差异。热证多由肝郁化热，胃失和降所致，治宜泻肝和胃；寒证多以脾胃虚寒为本，治宜温中和胃。

嘈杂，以似饥非饥，胃中不舒为主症，也多在胃痛转化中出现。常分为胃热、胃虚、血虚三个类型进行辨证论治。

复习思考题

1. 胃痛与哪些脏腑关系最密切？其病理变化是什么？
2. 如何区别胃气壅滞与肝胃气滞两型胃痛的证治？
3. 胃痛由实转虚，由气及血以及寒热转化的临床特点，治法及方药是什么？
4. 吐酸的病理特点是什么？
5. 嘈杂如何辨证论治？

呕　吐

〔概述〕

凡因胃失和降，气逆于上引起胃中之物上逆，经口而出，谓之呕吐。前人以有物有声谓之呕，有物无声谓之吐，其实，呕与吐往往同时发出，难以截然分开，故一般通称为呕吐，另外，常将有声无物谓之干呕，无声无物谓之恶心，症状虽有差异，但病理与呕吐相同，只是轻重有别，治疗亦可互参，故予一并讨论。

呕吐，有时又是人体排出胃内有害之物的保护性反应，属生理现象，临证时，故应明确加以区分，不可混淆。

西医学的多种疾病，如神经性呕吐，急慢性胃炎，幽门痉挛或不全梗阻、胆囊炎、急慢性胰腺炎及某些慢性肾功能不全等，表现以呕吐为主等，均可参考本证进行辨证论治。

〔病因病机〕

呕吐的发生，总由胃气上逆所致。胃主受纳，其气以和降为顺，若邪气扰胃或胃虚失和，气逆于上，则引起呕吐。

脾与胃互为表里，为气机升降之枢纽。脾主运化，以升为健，若脾失健运，清气不升，影响胃气不行，失其和降反而上逆，也可作呕吐。

此外，呕吐与肝、肺二脏功能失调也有关系。肝属春木，主升发疏泄；肺归秋金，司治节肃降。肝肺之气，左升右降，协助脾胃和调气机升降。若肝气怫郁，横逆犯胃，则可挟持胃气上逆作呕；若肺失宣肃，虽易作喘作咳，甚则也常影响胃之和降，肺胃之气同时上逆，而致呕咳或呕喘并作。现将呕吐的病因病机概括如下：

一、外邪侵扰：外感六淫及秽浊不正之气，从口鼻而入，侵犯胃腑，使胃气不降，反而上逆，可致呕吐。此外，外邪客肺，肺失宣肃，亦可引动或挟持胃气上逆，而发生呕吐。

二、饮食不节：恣食生冷肥甘及不洁之物，戕伤胃气而致食停不化，胃气不能下行，甚则上逆为呕。若脾胃素虚，运化无权，水谷不化精微而成痰饮，停痰留饮积于中州，气机升降失司，痰饮上逆，亦作呕吐。

三、情志不遂：恼怒伤肝，肝失条达，横逆犯胃，胃气上逆而为呕吐。此外，忧思伤脾，脾失健运，食停难化，胃失和降，亦可发生呕吐。

四、脾胃虚弱：劳倦过度，久病失养，耗伤中气，或年高体弱之人，脾运不健，以致水谷转输无力，清浊相混，升降失司，气逆而作呕。此外，脾胃阴亏，艰于润降，气逆于上亦易致吐。

总之，呕吐一证，其病位在胃，病机关键为胃气上逆。外感六淫，内伤七情，饮食不节，劳倦过度，以及久病、年高、体弱，引起胃气上逆，则可发生呕吐，究之临床，初病缘于邪气所干，病情多属实证；久病多为脏腑功能失调，病情属虚者多，且有阴、阳之别；病情反复，缠绵不愈者，则多虚实挟杂、寒热错综。

呕吐病因病机示意图

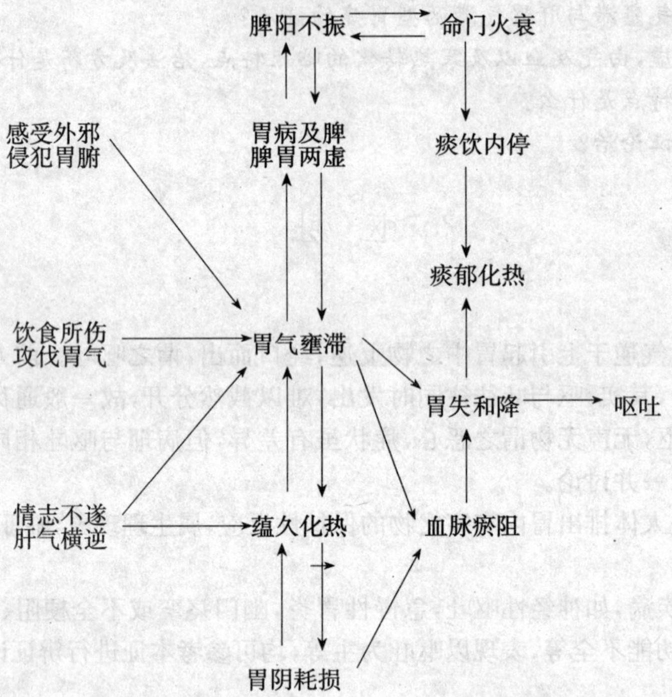

〔**辨证论治**〕

呕吐一证，首当辨其虚实。一般而言，实证发病急、病程短，呕吐症状重而持续，多由外邪犯胃、饮食伤胃、肝气挟持或肺失宣肃，令胃气上逆使然；虚证发病缓，病程长，多反复发作，呕吐症状轻而间断，多以脾胃虚弱为由，与命门火衰也有密切关系。

呕吐既是一个病证，但在某种情况下，又是人体排出胃内有害物质的保护性反应，而吐法也是一种治病手段，临证时，须加详辨。

一、实证

（一）外邪犯胃

主症：突然呕吐，来势急暴，与感受外邪有明显关系。

兼症：感受风寒则恶寒重，发热轻，头痛身痛；感受风温则发热重，微恶风，咽痛口干；感受暑湿则面垢肢怠，胸脘痞闷，纳呆泛呕，口黏便溏，或有低热。

舌脉：舌淡红，苔或薄白，或薄黄，或白腻，脉象或浮紧，或浮滑数，濡滑。

分析：外邪客胃，气机壅滞而失于和降，浊气上逆，故突然呕吐，来势急暴，且与外感邪气有明显关系。若系风寒束于肌表，营卫失和，故见恶寒发热，头痛身痛；若系风温上受，客于肺胃，气失肃降，故咽痛口干，发热恶风；若系感受暑湿之邪，阻于上中二焦，气机不利，故胸脘痞闷，纳呆泛恶，面垢肢怠。苔薄白，脉浮紧为感受风寒之象；苔薄黄，脉浮滑数为感受风温之象；苔白腻，脉濡滑为感受暑湿之象。

治法：疏邪解表，化浊和胃。

方药：香苏散加味。方中苏叶功专疏表和胃，为辛温解表之润剂。陈皮理气和胃降逆。香附调理胃中气血。甘草和中。四药相合，共奏疏表和中，理气降逆之功。

风寒重者，加豆豉、生姜、防风以增加辛散之力；风热重者，加荆芥、薄荷、芦根以助清解之势；暑湿所伤者，加鲜藿香、鲜佩兰、鲜荷叶、西瓜翠衣、六一散等以芳化解暑。邪传少阳，胆胃气逆，症见心烦喜呕，可与小柴胡汤或蒿芩清胆汤合方化裁为治。若邪客阳明，症见口干口苦而喜冷饮，或食入即吐，心烦、便秘、小溲短赤，舌红、苔黄少津，宜清胃降逆，用大黄甘草汤或泻心汤化裁。若咳喘甚而致呕吐者，乃肺胃气逆不降，宜加金沸草、枇杷叶等肺胃同治。呕吐严重而不能进药者，可用鲜生姜涂舌面，或少饮鲜姜汁，或玉枢丹半锭研磨冲服。若夹有食滞者，症见呕吐酸腐者，可加谷麦芽、山楂以消导之。

处方举例：

苏叶梗各 10g、炒陈皮 12g、制香附 10g、姜半夏 10g、茯苓 15g、生姜 3 片、谷麦芽各 10g、炒山楂 10g、炙杷叶 10g、鲜藿佩各 10g。

(二)饮食停滞

主症：呕吐酸腐，得食则甚，吐后反快。

兼症：脘腹胀满，嗳气厌食，甚则疼痛拒按，大便或溏或秘。

舌脉：苔白厚或腻，脉滑。

分析：饮食不节，食滞中州，蕴而化热，胃失和降而反逆，故呕吐酸腐，吐后反快，得食则剧。食停不化，阻碍气机，故脘腹胀满，嗳气厌食，甚则疼痛拒按。食滞于中，传导失常，故大便或溏或秘。苔白厚或腻，脉滑均为食积内停之象。

治法：消食化滞，和胃止呕。

方药：保和丸加味。方中山楂、神曲、麦芽、炒莱菔子消食化滞，和胃下气。陈皮、半夏、茯苓理气和中，降逆止呕。连翘能清食积蕴久之热。因肉食之积者，重用山楂；因米食之积者，重用谷芽，因面食之积者，重用麦芽、炒莱菔子；因酒食陈腐之积者，重用神曲。若舌苔转黄，食积化热明显者，可加黄芩、黄连或山栀以清胃泄热。若大便秘结或溏泻不爽者，加槟榔、大黄以消导之。

若为误食不洁、腐败食物，脘腹疼痛欲吐者，病发之初，当因势利导，用盐汤等探吐，使毒物尽快吐出，而后给予安胃和中之剂以善其后，若食入延久，则当泻下通腑，使毒物从大便排出。

处方举例：

半夏曲 10g、炒陈皮 10g、茯苓 15g、生姜 3 片、炒山楂 12g、神曲 10g、炒谷麦芽各 10g、炒莱菔子 10g、连翘 10g、炒黄芩 10g、刀豆子 15g。

(三)痰饮内停

主症：恶心，呕吐痰涎清水，或咳吐痰涎，其色或白或黄。

兼症：素体肥胖或消瘦，好食肥甘或纳食少馨，饮食后胃中不舒，甚则胃中有振水声，头晕心悸。

舌脉：舌淡红，苔白腻或水滑或微黄，脉细滑。

分析：脾运失司，水谷不化精微而聚生痰饮，停于中州，胃失和降而上逆，故恶心，呕吐痰涎清水，形体消瘦，纳食少馨。饮食无地再受，故纳后胃中不舒，以吐为快。亦有形体肥胖，素嗜肥甘者，均系湿重痰盛之征，辨证时亦当参考。饮停于胃中，故动作时可闻及振水声。痰饮上犯，清阳不展，则头晕心悸。苔白腻，或水滑，脉细滑，均为饮邪内停之象。若化热则可见薄黄苔。

治法：温化痰饮，和胃降逆。

方药：小半夏汤合苓桂术甘汤。方中半夏、生姜化痰消痞，和胃降逆。茯苓、桂枝、白术、甘草温化痰饮。饮消气调，升降有序而无偏逆，呕吐何生？若痰多胸脘痞满明显，可加陈皮、枳壳，利气化痰之力增强。若痰郁化热，壅阻于胃，升降不利，清浊相混，症见恶心，呕吐，目眩头晕心悸者，可用黄芩温胆汤合加味泽泻汤化裁以清胆和胃，化痰消痞，降逆止呕。若咳喘太甚而致呕吐者，可加苏子、莱菔子、旋覆花、枇杷叶等以肃降肺胃之气。若饮邪化热，胃阴已伤者，症见呕吐黄绿苦水，口干而不欲饮，苔薄黄少津，也可用甘遂半夏汤增减而治。

处方举例：

清半夏 10g、生姜 3 片、茯苓 15g、炒陈皮 10g、炒白术 10g、桂枝 6g、炙甘草 6g、炒苏子 10g、泽泻 15g。

(四)肝气犯胃

主症：呕吐酸苦，嗳气频作，得嗳则舒。

兼症：胸胁满痛，烦闷不舒，脘痞纳呆，每因情志不遂时，症情加重。

舌脉：舌边红，苔薄腻，脉弦滑。

分析：肝气怫郁，横逆犯胃，肝气挟持胃气上逆，故呕吐酸苦。酸苦之味乃肝胆郁结化热所致，即所谓“邪在胆，逆在胃”之意。肝胃气逆，故嗳气频作，嗳出则气郁得泻，故嗳气则舒。肝气郁结，气机不畅，络脉失和，故胸胁满痛。气郁日久化热，故烦闷不舒。舌脉亦为肝胃不和，郁而化热之象。

治法：疏肝理气，和胃降逆。

方药：四七汤合左金丸化裁。方中紫苏和胃下气止呕，厚朴理气宽中，半夏、茯苓、生姜和胃降逆止呕。黄连、吴萸辛开苦降，肝胃同治，以制酸止呕。若呕吐酸苦明显，也可用柴参温胆汤变化而治。若热象较著，舌红苔黄者，也可加黄芩、竹茹、山栀以清肝降火。若兼见口苦嘈杂便秘者，可加大黄、枳实以泄热降逆。若气郁日久，血运不畅，症见舌黯有瘀斑者，也可加赤芍、炒五灵脂、生蒲黄等化瘀之品。

处方举例：

全紫苏 10g、姜半夏 10g、厚朴花 6g、茯苓 10g、炒陈皮 12g、旋覆花(包)10g、炒黄芩 10g、钩藤 10g、黄连 6g、吴萸 3g、炒枳壳 10g。

二、虚证

(一)脾胃虚寒

主症：久吐或反复呕吐，或过劳或饮食不慎则恶心呕吐，或呕吐清涎。

兼症：面色萎黄，倦怠乏力，大便不实，或面色㿠白，四肢不温，喜暖畏寒，大便稀溏。

舌脉：舌质淡，苔薄白，脉沉细弱。

分析：久病、重病之后，脾胃虚弱，甚则中阳不振，运化无权，气机升降失司，故每遇过劳或饮食不慎，脾胃再伤，升降逆乱，上逆泛呕作吐。脾虚不运，水饮内停则呕吐清涎。中虚不复，病情迁延或反复发作，中气不足，气血化生乏源，故面色萎黄，倦怠乏力。若中阳虚衰，阳气失其温煦之能，故面色㿠白，四肢不温，喜暖畏寒。脾阳亏虚，运化不健，故大便不实，甚则稀溏。舌脉也为脾胃阳虚之象。

治法：温中健脾，和胃降逆。

方药：砂半理中汤加减。方中党参、白术、甘草健脾益气，干姜温中散寒，半夏、砂仁化痰理脾，降逆止呕，诸药相合，共奏温中健脾和胃止呕之功。

若呕吐清水不止，再加生姜、吴萸以温中散寒化饮。若呕吐不止，嗳气频作，可加旋覆花、代赭石以加强降逆止呕之力。呕吐久作，时发时止，舌胖淡脉沉迟，是属脾胃虚甚，应加灶心土、肉豆蔻以温中健脾止呕。若呕吐而苔见薄黄，脘腹隐痛而大便不实，脉细滑者，症属脾胃不和，上热下寒之象，也可予半夏泻心汤意化裁为治，以调和脾胃，寒热并治。若见呕吐日久，在脾阳虚之见症外，更有腰膝冷痛，阴囊湿冷，脉沉细而迟等，为脾肾阳虚，当加炙附子、肉桂、沉香、丁香等温补脾肾以止呕；若在此基础上，恶心呕吐频作，舌苔黄厚而腻，脉沉细无力，为脾肾阳虚，水湿不化，蕴而生热，本虚标实之象，当用温脾汤标本兼顾，补泻并施。

处方举例：

砂仁 5g、姜半夏 10g、党参 15g、炒白术 12g、淡干姜 10g、炙甘草 6g、炒陈皮 10g、茯苓 15g、灶心土(先煎代水)30g。

(二)胃阴不足

主症：呕吐反复发作，或时作干呕。

兼症：胃中嘈杂，似饥而不欲食，口燥咽干，饮水而不欲咽。

舌脉：舌嫩红少津，苔花剥或无苔，脉细略数。

分析：胃为阳土，喜润恶燥。热病之后，或气郁化火，或过用温燥之品，致津液耗伤，胃失濡润，气失和降、故上逆而呕，反复发作，或时作干呕。阴虚火旺，扰动胃府，故胃中嘈杂，似饥非饥，不欲饮食。胃阴不足，津液无以上承，故口燥咽干。舌嫩红少津，苔花剥或无苔，脉细略数，也为胃中阴津损伤而生虚热之象。

治法：滋养胃阴，降逆止呕。

方药：麦门冬汤加减。方中人参、麦冬、粳米、甘草等以滋养胃阴，半夏、竹茹降逆止呕。余热未清者加鲜芦根、连翘、薄荷等清热生津。若胃阴大亏，舌红者，可加石斛、生地、沙参等甘寒养阴之品。若肺胃同病，气逆不降者，可加枇杷叶、旋覆花，肺胃同治。阴伤肠燥而见大便干结者，加火麻仁、瓜蒌以润燥通便。

处方举例：

沙参 15g、麦冬 10g、石斛 10g、清半夏 10g、竹茹 6g、鲜芦根 30g、炙杷叶 12g、刀豆子 15g、佛手片 10g。

〔预防及护理措施〕

1. 呕吐患者的病情轻重不一。轻者，适当控制饮食，去除诱因，即可缓解；重者，应当仔细诊治，防止意外发生。

2. 呕吐时，一般应使患者安静、镇静，重者应卧床休息。呕吐发作时，头应低位或偏向一侧，轻拍其背部，以防吐物吸入气管。

3. 呕吐止后，饮食宜清淡，温凉适度，切忌生冷油腻之品。以全流或半流饮食较好，更宜少食多餐，以免再犯。

4. 止呕中药汤剂，也宜少量频服，以免引起进药也吐。

5. 若在呕吐剧烈时，见到高烧，头痛剧烈；神志烦躁或嗜睡、神昏；吐物中有血，且血量较多；脘腹痛症、拒按，无大便或矢气者，当及时诊治原发病证、积极救治。

6. 若呕吐严重，口舌干燥，肌肤失润，弹力减弱，目凹神疲者，宜及时补液。

7. 为预防呕吐，可配合针刺。

〔典型病例分析〕

案一：张某某，男，35岁，教师。

胃病史四年余。近二月胃病频频发作，进食后尤甚，伴腹胀，傍晚尤甚，直至吐尽方舒。前医因视其为朝食暮吐，诊为脾胃虚寒，先后用理中汤、大半夏汤治疗月余不效。查体见胃中可闻及明显振水音，舌淡、苔薄白，脉弦。钡餐检查诊为“十二指肠球部溃疡，幽门不完全性梗阻”。因虑及前医温补止呕不效，当属气结血凝，气机失调，胃气上逆使然。遂拟调气和营，缓急止呕为治，处方：川芎6g、当归9g、芍药20g、甘草6g，二剂后呕停，又三剂，诸症消失。

按：患者朝食暮吐，吐尽方舒，当属脾胃虚寒，温运无力所致。然前医温之无效，知其虚寒为假，实乃血行不畅，瘀于下脘，阳气不得宣达为真，故用芎、归、芍和血行瘀，血行而气舒，再佐以甘草和中，固护胃气。气血调畅，升降有序，则呕止病除。前曾读广东名老中医刘赤选医案，也有用失笑散加芍药、山楂治疗本病之验，同属此理。（录自《中医杂志》1990年第6期）

呕吐的发生，当责之胃气上逆，治则以和胃降逆为基本大法，临证时，首须分清虚实。实证呕吐，病程较短，呕吐持续而剧烈，每易见邪实之象，如外邪犯胃者，常兼见表证；饮食停滞，则呕吐酸腐，口臭厌食；肝郁犯胃，则呕吐酸苦，脘部胀痛连及胁肋；痰饮内阻，则呕吐痰涎清水或稠痰。虚证呕吐，病程较长，反复发作，常因饮食不慎或小劳即发，多见于病后或体弱之人；呕吐时作时休，呕也不剧，每易见正虚之证。如脾虚呕吐，则面色萎黄，神疲乏力；阳虚呕吐，则面色㿠白，畏寒肢冷；阴虚呕吐，则虚烦嘈杂，似饥而不能纳。治疗上，实证呕吐当以祛邪为主，邪去则呕吐自止；虚证呕吐治宜扶正为主，正复则呕吐自愈。

复习思考题

1. 如何看待呕吐应止与不应止？
2. 试述呕吐的病理变化，怎样认识本证与胃、脾、肺、肝、肾的关系？
3. 如何鉴别痰饮内停与脾胃虚寒两证型呕吐？
4. 呕吐的常见证型的辨治是什么？

泄　泻

〔**概述**〕

泄泻，是指排便次数增多，粪质清稀，甚至如水样，或便下完谷不化而言。泄之与泻，略有不同，泄指大便溏薄而势缓，泻为大便清稀而直下，故统称泄泻。本病证一年四季均可发生，但以夏秋季节为多见。

本证首见于《内经》，称之为“泄”，且有飧泄、濡泄、洞泄、溏泄及注泄等名称，论其病因病机或言风，或言湿，或言寒，或云热或曰清气在下……。《难经》指出："泄凡有五"。汉唐时代称为"下利"，宋代以后统称"泄泻"，《医宗必读》总括治泄有九法：即淡渗、升提、清凉、疏利、甘缓、酸收、燥脾、温肾、固涩。《景岳全书》对泄泻的分型以暴泻、久泻为纲，认为"泄泻之因，惟水、火、土三气为最"，"泄泻之本，无不由于脾胃"，对泄泻的辨治具有重要的指导意义。

西医学中凡因胃、肠、肝、胆、胰腺等消化器官发生功能性或器质性病变引起的腹泻，如急慢性结肠炎、肠结核、结肠过敏等以及其他系统某些病变引起的腹泻，均可参考本证进行辨证论治。

〔病因病机〕

泄泻的主要病变部位在脾胃与大小肠，以脾为主。其致病原因，有感受外邪，饮食所伤，肝郁乘脾，脾胃虚弱及肾阳虚衰，其病理关键，是脾胃功能障碍。其病因虽多，但以湿邪为发病的主要因素，且有寒湿、湿热之分；湿往往挟风、暑、食，故前人云"无湿不成泄"。脾胃功能障碍是多种原因引起的，有外邪影响，脾胃本身虚弱，肝脾不和及肾阳不足等，均可导致脾胃运化功能失常，而发生泄泻。

一、感受外邪：引起泄泻的外因有风、寒、暑、湿、热诸邪，尤以湿邪为主，脾喜燥而恶湿，湿性濡润最能引起泄泻，《难经》所谓"湿多成五泄"，外邪亦可直接客于胃肠，使脾胃运化功能障碍，水谷不化精微而变为湿浊，下流于肠，发生泄泻。临床上湿邪多挟风、寒、暑、热伤于胃肠，由于病人体质及兼夹邪气不同，故转归不尽相同，湿邪若兼风、兼寒，伤于人则多转化为寒湿；湿邪若兼暑、兼热，伤于人则易转化成湿热。

二、饮食所伤：暑热时节，恣食生冷，或误食不洁之物，损伤脾胃；饮食过量，宿食内停；或嗜食肥甘，运化不及，呆胃滞脾，使脾胃受戕。脾胃既伤，传导失职，升降失调，而成泄泻。若脾胃素虚，运化力弱，饮食稍有不慎，更易发生泄泻。

三、肝郁乘脾：肝气不舒，气机不畅，最易影响脾胃运化，脾失健运，水谷精微不归正化，反为湿浊，下降成泻。亦有脾胃素虚之体，复因忧思恼怒，精神紧张，则肝气怫郁，横逆犯脾，运化失常，清浊相混，而成泄泻。

四、脾胃虚弱：脾主运化，胃主受纳，若饮食不节，劳倦内伤，久病体弱，久泻伤正，均可使脾胃虚衰，运化无权，既不能受纳腐熟水谷，又不能运化转输精微，以致水反成湿，谷反为滞，清浊不分，混杂而下，遂成泄泻。

五、肾阳虚衰：脾之所以能运化水谷，全赖肾阳之温煦；况肾司二便，大便的通导调节关系于肾。若久病体弱，年老阳衰或亡血，失精，生育过多，均可致肾阳虚衰，脾失温煦，运化失常，阴寒内生，清气沉降，水湿下注，则生泄泻。

综上所述，脾虚湿盛是导致本证发生的重要因素。外因以湿邪关系为最，湿邪侵入，困阻中阳，损伤脾胃，无以行运化之权，则水谷清浊不分，混杂而下，酿成泄泻。内因多系脾虚，脾虚则无力运化，水谷不化精微反变湿浊，清气不升，浊液下流，混杂而下，发生泄泻。其他疾病所引起的泄泻也多在脾虚的基础上发生。脾虚失运，可造成湿盛，而湿盛又可影响脾的运化，故脾虚与湿盛互相影响，互为因果，亦是泄泻发生、发展、缠绵难愈的根本原因。肝气乘脾，或脾虚及肾，一旦肾虚进一步加重者脾虚失运的程度，故泻难平复。

〔辨证论治〕

一、辨证要点

本病的辨证临床上一般以暴泻、久泻为纲，虚实寒热为目。实证有寒湿、湿热、伤食三类；

虚证有脾肾之分；虚实挟杂多见于肝气乘脾。

（一）辨虚实：起病急、病程短，泻下次数频繁，腹痛拒按，泻后痛减，多属实证；起病缓，病程长，泻泄呈间歇发作，腹痛喜按，其痛不甚，便后痛重者，多属虚证。

泄泻病因病机示意图

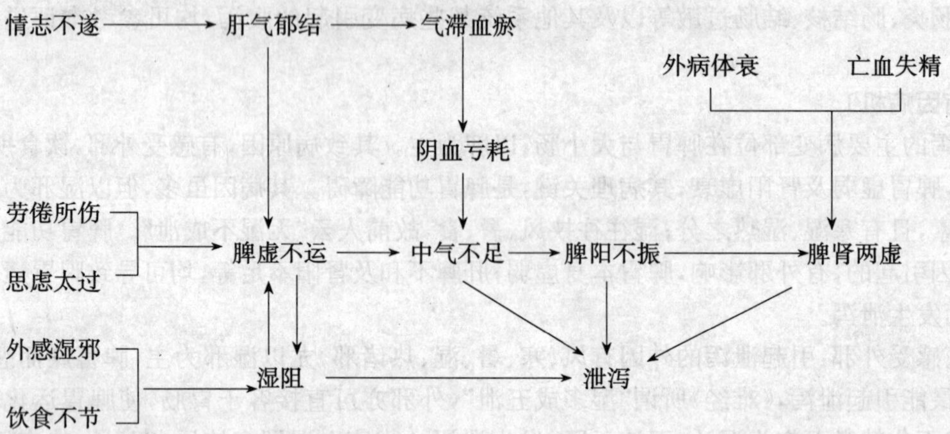

（二）辨寒热：见下表。

	寒　证	热　证
大便性状	鸭溏清冷，或泻下如水，甚则完谷不化	来势急迫，大便黏稠色黄，肛门灼热
腹　痛	腹中雷鸣切痛，温熨之则缓	腹中灼痛，痛泻陈作
口　渴	口不渴，饮热汤则痛减	烦渴喜冷饮
小　便	清白	短赤
舌　象	质润苔白	质红苔黄、
脉　象	沉紧	滑数

（三）辨大便色质：大便色黄褐，黏秽而臭，肛门灼热，多属湿热；大便青灰或青黑，便下清稀或如水样，秽腥而臭不著者，多属寒湿；大便溏垢，黏滞不爽，臭如败卵，挟有食物残渣者，多为伤食。便下溏薄，其色正常，时作时止，每因情志因素而作者多属肝气乘脾。大便不实，时溏时泻，其则挟有不消化之食物，累劳及进食后加重者为脾虚；便下色白质清，甚则完谷不化，多在五更作泻者为肾虚。

二、泄泻与痢疾的鉴别

鉴别 病名	病　位	脓血便	排　便	腹　痛	大便常规 WBC＋RBC	病　理	危证
泄　泻	脾（中焦）	无	通　畅	腹痛肠鸣	＜15 个	温盛与脾虚	少见
痢　疾	肠（下焦）	有	滞下不爽 虚坐努争	腹痛较重 痛痢交作	＞15 个	邪客肠道，气血 相搏化腐成脓	易见

泄泻与痢疾，两者均多发于夏秋季节，病因为感受外邪，内伤饮食，痢疾早期为表现为泄

泻，泄泻失治，误治亦可能转成痢疾。

三、治疗原则

暴泻以邪实为主，治当祛邪为先，利湿燥脾为法，挟表者宜疏散，挟热者宜清利，挟食者宜消导；久泻以正虚为多见，治宜扶正为先，健脾温阳为法，兼理肝肾。若虚实兼挟，寒热并见者，又当标本兼顾，寒热并调。此外急性泄泻不可骤用补涩，以免恋邪而致病情缠绵难愈；慢性泄泻不宜分利太过，惟恐损正伤阴而终致难愈。

四、分型论治

(一)暴泻

1. 寒湿泄泻(或风寒泄泻)

主症：发病急暴，大便清稀甚则如水样，痛泻阵作，肠鸣漉漉。

兼症：多见风寒挟湿之表证，如恶寒发热，头重体倦，周身酸痛，脘闷纳呆，口淡不渴，或口黏不爽等。

舌脉：苔薄白或白腻，脉濡缓或浮紧。

分析：外感风寒或寒湿之邪，客于肠胃，或过食生冷黏腻及不洁之物，戕伤胃肠，升降失调，清浊不分，传导失司，湿浊下注，故大便清稀，甚如水样，发病急暴。寒主收引，湿性濡润，寒湿内盛，阻滞气机故痛泻阵作，水湿下注则肠鸣漉漉。风寒挟湿，侵袭肌表，卫阳被遏，故发热、恶寒、头重身痛。湿阻中焦则脘闷纳呆泛呕，口淡不渴或口黏不爽。风寒外束，故苔薄白，脉浮紧。若寒湿客中，则可见苔白腻，脉濡缓。

治法：解表散寒，化浊利湿。

方药：胃苓汤合藿香正气散加减。

藿香正气散专主湿浊之气客于肠胃，方用藿香辛温散寒，芳香化浊为主药；苍术、茯苓健脾除湿；厚朴、大腹皮理气散满，疏利气机；紫苏、白芷解表散寒。平胃散为化湿和中之良剂。五苓散利水渗湿，导湿浊之邪从小便而出，所谓“治泄不利小水，非其治也”；湿为阴邪，寒湿明显时，方中桂枝可温通阳气以化湿浊。若风寒客胃，腹痛明显者，也可选用正气天香散合胃苓汤为治。

风寒之邪较重加淡豆豉、防风以增强温散风寒之力；若缘过食生冷油腻之物者加焦三仙、鸡内金以消食导滞；泻下如水，腹痛较剧，频频登厕者，可用周氏回生丹，每次十粒，日二次。

处方举例：

藿香 10g、苏叶 10g、苍术 10g、白蔻仁(后下)5g、陈皮 10g、半夏 10g、厚朴 10g、大腹皮 12g、生姜 5g、五苓散(包煎)1 袋。

2. 湿热泄泻(或暑湿泄泻)

主症：腹痛即泻，泻下急迫，或泻而不爽，粪色黄褐，质地稠黏，气味臭秽。

兼症：肛门灼热，心烦口渴，小便短赤。

舌脉：舌质红，苔黄腻，脉滑数或濡数。

分析：夏秋之间暑湿较盛，或因恣食肥甘厚味，湿热蕴积，伤于肠胃，传导失常，故发生泄泻。湿性下趋，热性急迫，湿热下注，故腹痛而泻，泻下急迫。湿性黏腻，最易阻滞气机，则泻下不爽。湿热炽盛，浊邪下注故粪色黄褐，气味臭秽，肛门灼热。湿热久羁，则心烦口渴，小便短赤。舌苔黄腻，脉象濡数或滑数均为湿热内盛之征。

治法：清热利湿。

方药：葛根芩连汤加减。

方中葛根解肌清热，升清止泻，一般煨用力强；芩连苦寒，清热燥湿，善能止泻。生甘草甘缓和中，配滑石名六一散，解暑除烦。临证遇湿重者加苡仁、茯苓、木通之类以助利湿，使湿热分消；热盛者可加银花、连翘、大黄以解毒；挟食者加神曲、麦芽、山楂以消导；暑热象著时加藿香、佩兰、鲜荷叶、扁豆花以解暑清热。

治疗湿热泄泻，当辨别湿多抑或热多。湿多者，用药则偏重于祛湿利尿，热多者，用药应偏重于清热，使湿热分利。

若病发于盛暑之季，泻如米泔、烦渴、尿赤、自汗、面垢，舌苔薄黄，脉象濡数者，治宜清暑化湿，方用新加香薷饮合六一散或香连丸。

处方举例：

葛根10g、炒黄芩12g、黄连6g、生甘草6g、滑石块10g、生苡仁15g、通草10g、车前草20g、焦三仙各10g、木香10g。

3. 伤食泄泻

主症：腹痛即泻，粪便臭如败卵，泻后痛减。

兼症：脘腹痞满，嗳腐倒饱，不思饮食。

舌脉：苔厚腻垢浊，脉滑。

分析：饮食不节，宿食内停，阻滞肠胃，传导失常，故腹痛而泻。食宿不化，浊气上逆则嗳腐倒饱，下注则泻下臭如败卵，泻后浊气下流故泻后痛减。食滞中焦，气机失畅，则脘腹痞满，甚则作痛；胃失和降，脾失健运则不思饮食。苔厚腻垢浊，脉滑皆为食积之征。

治法：消食导滞。

方药：保和丸加减。

本方消食导滞，和中化湿，为治疗食积的主要方剂。其中，神曲、麦芽、山楂、莱菔子消食下气除满，陈皮、半夏和胃降逆，茯苓理脾化湿，连翘味苦微寒，善清食积蕴久滋生之热毒。

若因过食辛甘炙煿之品，症见苔黄脉滑者，当清热燥湿，可加黄芩、黄连。如由过食寒凉之物，而见苔白脉缓者，宜合平胃散增强苦温燥湿之力。食积过重，脘腹痞满，泻下不爽者，可因势利导，"通因通因"，改用枳实导滞丸，此方以大黄、枳实为主，推荡积滞，使邪有所出路，达到邪祛而正安。

处方举例：

半夏曲10g、炒陈皮10g、茯苓15g、焦神曲10g、焦谷芽10g、炒麦芽10g、焦山楂10g、莱菔子(炒)10g、连翘10g、炒白术10g、木香10g。

(二)久泻

1. 脾虚泄泻

主症：大便不实，时溏时泻，每因稍进油腻或劳累之后，则便次增多，甚则挟有不化之物。

兼症：面色萎黄，肢倦乏力，或形体消瘦，纳食不馨，脘腹痞闷不舒，肠鸣。

舌脉：舌淡，体胖，苔薄白，脉细弱。

分析：脾胃久伤，中气虚弱，运化无权，清气下陷，水谷不化，清浊不分，下降作泻，故大便不实，肠鸣漉漉。稍进油腻或小有作劳，脾气更伤，则泻下加重，便次增多，甚有挟有不化之物。脾胃既虚，化源不足，气血不足，故面色萎黄，肢倦乏力，久而形体消瘦。脾胃虚弱，消化迟缓，故纳少不香；气弱行缓，故脘腹痞闷不舒；舌淡胖，苔薄白，脉细弱，均为脾胃虚弱之象。

治法：健脾益气。

方药：参苓白术散加减。

本方以四君子汤为基础，补气健脾，扁豆、山药、莲子肉，炒苡仁化湿理脾，加砂仁醒脾开胃，陈皮行气和中，桔梗上浮以升下陷之清气，是治疗脾虚湿泻的常用方。

若久泻不愈，中气下陷而兼有脱肛者，可用补中益气汤，益气升提，健脾止泻，若泄泻日久，气阴两伤而湿浊未净，舌体瘦质嫩红，苔薄黄腻者，可加石榴皮、五倍子、山楂等酸收之品。但要注意：选用健脾益气不宜温燥，益胃养阴不宜滋腻，清热化湿不宜苦寒，淡渗利湿不宜太过，即养阴不助湿，利湿不伤阴，清热不伤中。久泻脾虚，湿浊内停，蕴而化热者，可加苦参、黄柏、樗根白皮等清热化湿之品。若脾阳已衰，阴寒内盛，腹中冷痛雷鸣，手足不温者宜用附子理中汤加吴萸、肉桂以温中散寒。

处方举例：

党参 10g、茯苓 15g、炒白术 12g、炒扁豆 15g、淮山药 10g、炒陈皮 10g、煨木香 10g、炒苡仁 15g、桔梗 3g、砂仁 g、莲子肉 10g。

2. 肝气乘脾

主症：每因情绪不宁之时即发生腹痛泄泻，便后腹痛略减，再痛再泻。

兼症：平时情志不畅，多愁善感，易于紧张或激动，胸胁胀闷，嗳气少食，口苦吞酸，面黄肌瘦，神疲乏力。

舌脉：质淡红，苔薄白或薄黄，脉弦细。

分析：情志不遂则肝气怫郁，疏泄不利，横逆犯脾。脾病则运化无权，升降失常，清浊不分，混杂而下，故腹痛作泻；泻后肝气暂疏，气机稍畅，故泻后疼痛略减，再郁则再痛，再痛而再泻，如此痛泻交作，久泻伤脾，气血不足，故形瘦面黄，神疲乏力。肝体阴用阳，血虚则肝失柔养，气失条达，常易郁结，故情绪易于波动，胸胁痞闷不舒。肝气犯胃则嗳气少食，口苦吞酸。舌质淡红，脉象弦细亦为肝旺脾虚之象。

治法：抑肝扶脾。

方药：痛泻要方加减。

方中白芍味酸入肝，柔肝以缓急；防风为疏散之润剂，可散肝而不伤正，风能胜湿，用之又可理脾化湿。白术健脾，脾旺则湿化而泻止。再用陈皮理气和中，四药相合，能调达肝气，升运脾气，共奏抑肝扶脾之效。

若肝阴不足者可加五味子、五倍子、木瓜酸敛柔肝；脾气不健者可加茯苓、扁豆、淮山药以益气健脾；情绪不宁者，可加绿萼梅、郁金、合欢花、生龙牡以解郁安神。

处方举例：

炒白芍 12g、防风 6g、炒白术 10g、炒陈皮 10g、炒山楂 15g、乌梅 5g、炙甘草 5g、茯苓 15g、炒扁豆 15g、淮山药 10g、绿萼梅 10g。

3. 肾阳虚衰

主症：五更作泻，大便溏薄，甚则完谷不化，泻后则安。

兼症：脐腹隐痛，畏寒，肠鸣，形寒肢冷，腰酸冷痛，男子阳痿，阴囊湿冷，女子月事愆期量少。

舌脉：体胖质淡，苔白水滑，脉沉迟。

分析：久病失养，肾阳虚衰，不能温煦脾土以助运化，又值五更时分，阳气未复，阴寒极盛，故五更作泻，甚则完谷不化，泻后则安。脾肾阳虚，阳气不振，内不得温养脏腑，故脐腹畏寒，疼痛，肠鸣；外不能温养经脉，故腰膝冷痛，形寒肢冷，男子阳痿，阴囊湿冷，女子冲任虚寒故月经愆期量少。舌胖而淡，苔白水滑，脉象沉迟，均为阳虚阴盛之象。

治法：温肾健脾。

方药：四神丸加味。

方中补骨脂温补命门之火以止泻，肉蔻、吴茱萸暖脾散寒，五味子收敛止泻，姜枣健脾和中。若脾阳不振明显者，合附子理中汤以增强温补脾肾之力。命门火衰突出者，可加巴戟天、益智仁、肉桂以图温肾。年高体衰，久泻不止而致中气下陷者，可合补中益气汤以升清阳；若久泻无度，大便失禁者，可加桃花汤以固涩止泻。亦有因久泻，脾肾阳衰，无力推动气血运行，而见阳虚血瘀之象者，可合少腹逐瘀汤为治。

处方举例：

补骨脂 10g、肉豆蔻 10g、吴茱萸 5g、五味子 10g、党参 15g、茯苓 15g、炙附片 6g、炮姜 6g、炒白术 12g、煨木香 6g、台乌药 10g。

〔预防及护理措施〕

1. 注意饮食卫生，不吃腐馊变质食物。

2. 开展爱国卫生运动，消灭苍蝇，加强水源管理，不喝生水，生吃瓜果要洗烫，要养成饭前便后洗手的良好习惯。

3. 泄泻病人要给予流质或半流质饮食，忌食辛热炙煿肥甘厚味。若暴泻耗伤胃气，可给予淡盐汤、饭汤、米粥等以养胃气。若属虚寒泄泻，亦可给予淡姜汤饮之，振奋脾阳，调和胃气。久泻病人应避免过劳及精神刺激，注意保暖，防止受寒。

4. 药粥。

〔典型病例分析〕

案一：薛立斋治进士刘华甫，停食腹痛，泄黄吐痰，服二陈山栀黄连枳实之类，其症益甚。左关弦紧，右关弦长，乃肝脏克脾土，用六君加木香治之而愈。若食已消而泄未已，宜用异功散以补脾胃，如不应，用补中益气汤升发阳气。凡泄痢色黄，脾土亏损，其气下陷，必用前汤加木香豆蔻温补；如不应，当补其母，宜八味丸。(《名医类案·第四卷·泻》)

按："服二陈山栀黄连枳实之类，其症益甚"，"停食腹痛，泄黄吐痰"似痰热郁滞而实非也。究其因，实由脾胃亏损、脾虚肝旺，即"肝木克脾土"也，治当实脾为主，脾旺则不受邪，补脾用六君，加木香以理气止痛，温中和胃，药症相应，效如桴鼓。

泄泻是以大便次数增多，粪质清稀，甚至如水样为特征的病证。其主要病理因素为湿，发病关键在于脾虚湿盛。湿有内外之分，外因为气候湿盛，内因为脾失健运，二者之间常相互影响。病机为脾运不健，小肠受盛，大肠之传导失职，则水反为湿，谷反为滞，清浊不分，合污而下，故成泄泻。

泄泻的病变部位，主要在脾胃大小肠，亦与肝肾有关。其辨证首当分清虚实寒热。急性暴泻多为热证或实证；慢性久泻多属虚证或寒证；肝气乘脾多为虚实夹杂证。治疗原则，总以运脾祛湿为大法，分清暴泻、久泻及寒热虚实之偏盛，灵活立法遣方。此外在治疗过程中，还须注意饮食、情志、保暖及休息等护理措施。

复习思考题

1. 如何理解脾虚与湿盛在泄泻发病过程中的重要意义。
2. 泄泻的分型有几种？其证治如何？
3. 怎样鉴别泄泻与痢疾？
4. 久泻即可伤脾阳，亦可伤脾阴，临床上应如何区别处理？
5. 久泻气阴两伤而湿热未净，治疗时应注意哪几点？
6. 固涩药与酸收药在治疗泄泻过程中如何使用？
7. 食积在暴泻与久泻中如何认识和处理？
8. 肝木乘脾之泄泻，肝阴未伤与已伤如何区别处理？

痢　疾

〔概述〕

痢疾是以腹痛，里急后重，便下赤白脓血为特征的病证。一年四季均可发病，而以夏秋季节为多见。

《内经》称本病为“肠澼”，《难经》谓之“小肠泄”、“大瘕泄”，在《伤寒论》中有“热利下重”之白头翁汤证，虚寒“下利便脓血”之桃花汤证及久痢寒热错杂乌梅丸证。《诸病源候论》有赤白痢、血痢、脓血痢、热痢等名称。并以病程较长者称为久痢，时愈时止者称为休息痢，《千金方·热痢第七》指出：“大凡痢有四种，谓冷、热、疳、蛊。冷则白，热则赤，疳则赤白相杂……蛊则纯痢瘀血。”宋以前的方书还有称为“滞下”的。金元时代已认识到本病有传染性，故有时疫之名。如《丹溪心法》指出：“时疫作痢，一方一家，上下传染相似。”

西医学的急慢性细菌性痢疾，阿米巴痢疾以及某些结肠病变以脓血便为主症者可参考本病辨证论治。

〔病因病机〕

本病多由外受湿热、疫毒之气，内伤饮食生冷，损伤脾胃与肠而成。

一、感受外邪：夏秋之交，暑热湿浊及疫毒之邪，客于胃肠，湿蕴热蒸，气血壅滞，进而化腐成脓，便下赤白脓血，而成湿热痢或疫毒痢。另外，寒湿之邪内侵胃肠，或痢疾日久，脾胃俱伤，运化障碍，湿浊内生，从阴化寒，与气血相搏而便下白冻，成为寒湿痢。一般认为，伤于气分则为白痢，伤于血分则为赤痢，气血俱伤则为赤白痢。

二、饮食内伤：饮食不节，过食肥甘厚味，或误食腐馊不洁之物，损伤肠胃，酿生湿热，湿蕴热蒸，气血凝滞，化为脓血，则成湿热痢，若湿热内郁不清，伤及阴血，而成阴虚痢；若其人恣食生冷瓜果，胃肠受损，湿浊内停，致寒湿食积壅塞肠中，气机受阻，气滞血瘀，与肠中腐浊之气相搏结，化为脓血而成寒湿痢。若其人脾胃素虚，复感寒湿之邪，或热痢过服寒凉药物，转成虚寒痢。

上述病因，虽有外感与饮食之分，但常互相影响，内外交感而发病。

本病病位虽然在肠，但与胃密切相关，如湿热、疫毒之气，上攻于胃，或久痢伤正，胃虚气逆，则呕恶不食，而成为噤口痢。痢疾迁延，正虚邪恋，则成久痢或休息痢。痢久不愈，或反复发作，则胃病及脾，甚则及肾，脾肾俱伤而致下痢不止。

总之，本病的发生与感受外邪及饮食不节有关，其病位在肠。湿热、疫毒、寒湿及食积等壅滞于肠中，气血与之相搏结，使肠道传导失司，脉络受伤，气血凝滞，腐败化为脓血而痢下赤白；气机阻滞，腑气不通则腹痛，里急后重。

痢疾病因病机示意图

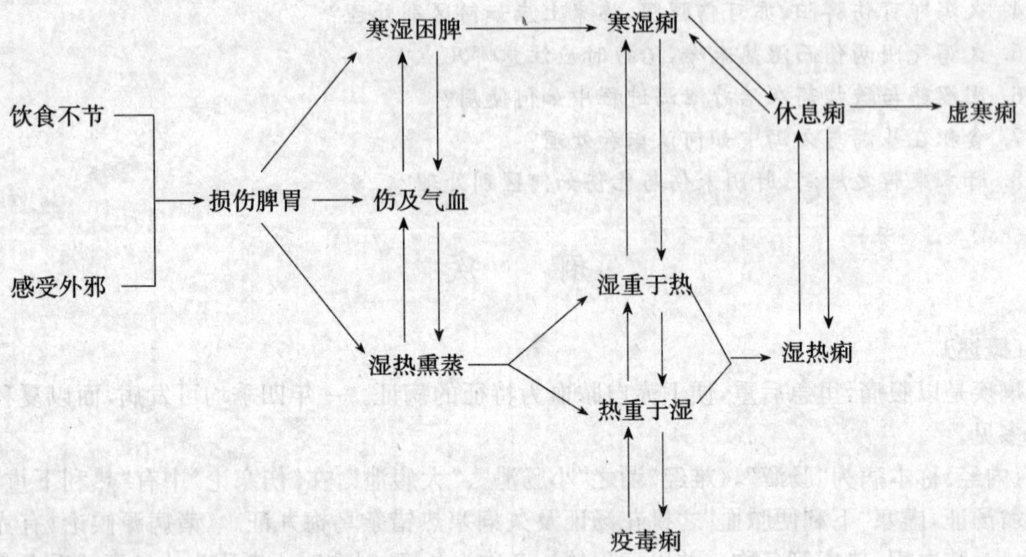

〔**辨证论治**〕

一般来说，初痢多实，宜通宜导；久痢多虚，或虚中挟实，宜补宜涩，或攻补兼施。赤痢其病在血，治宜凉血和血，重用血药；白痢其病在气，治宜行气化湿，重用气药。古有“无积不成痢”与“和血则便脓自愈，调气则后重自除”之说，所以，在各型痢疾的治疗中，均应在辨证论治的基础上加用消导及调气、和血药。痢疾初期，以湿热居多；久病之后，脾气渐伤，则易从寒化，始终以固护胃气为本，故俗称“见痢莫治痢，提防伤胃气”。

(一)湿热痢

主症：下痢赤白，以赤为主，肛门灼热，腹痛，里急后重。

兼症：脘闷纳呆，口黏泛恶，小便短赤。

舌脉：舌质红，苔黄腻，脉滑数。

分析：湿热之邪壅滞肠中，脉络受伤，与气血搏结，化为脓血，故下痢赤白；血络受损，故下痢以赤色为主。气机阻滞则腹痛。湿热挟积欲从便出而反不能出，故里急后重。胃失和降，故脘闷纳呆，口黏泛恶。湿热下注，则肛门灼热，小便短赤。舌脉均为湿热蕴蒸之象。

治法：清热化湿解毒，佐以调气行血导滞。

方药：芍药汤加减。

方中黄芩、黄连清热化湿以解毒；芍药、当归、甘草行血和营，缓急止痛。木香、槟榔行气导滞，即所谓“行血则便脓自愈，调气则后重自除”。少用肉桂反佐，以助行血和营之功。大黄泻实热、导积滞、凉营血。

若挟食滞，加山楂、神曲、枳实以消食导滞。若表证较重。依感受邪气之不同，可加荆芥、薄荷、苏叶、豆豉、藿香、佩兰等以疏散表邪。若表邪未解而里热已盛，则宜解肌清热，用葛根芩连汤。如表邪已解，痢犹不止者，可用香连丸以治之。

若热势较重，下痢赤多白少，或纯下赤痢，发热较高，口渴饮冷，舌红苔黄，脉滑数者，可用白头翁汤加清热解毒药，如银花、蒲公英、马齿苋、赤芍、甘草、枳实心解毒和营，行气导滞。

处方举例：

炒白芍 15g、全当归 10g、生大黄 5g、黄连 5g、炒黄芩 10g、木香 10g、焦槟榔 10g、炒山楂 10g、生甘草 6g。

（二）疫毒痢

主症：发病急骤，壮热烦躁，下痢鲜紫脓血，腹痛如绞，里急后重。

兼症：口渴饮冷，头痛，神志昏蒙，甚则昏迷痉厥。

舌脉：舌质红绛，苔黄燥，脉滑数。

分析：外感疫毒之邪，毒邪暴盛，则发病急骤，壮热不寒；热毒熏灼肠道，损伤气血，故便下鲜紫脓血；肠道气机逆乱，故腹痛如绞，后重难忍。热盛则津伤而口渴饮冷，热毒上扰清空，故头痛；热扰营心，则烦躁；热毒蒙闭清窍则神志不清，昏迷；热盛动风，故痉厥抽搐。舌脉亦为热毒炽盛之象。

治法：清热，凉血，解毒。

方药；白头翁汤加味。

方中白头翁清热凉血，为治痢之要药，黄连、黄柏清热解毒，坚阴止痢，秦皮清热化湿，可加银花、连翘、赤芍、丹皮、地榆以增强解毒凉血止痢之功。如见高热神昏者，为热毒深入营血，加水牛角 30～60g；另服紫雪丹或安宫牛黄丸以清营凉血，开窍醒神。如见痉厥抽搐者，为热毒引动肝风，加钩藤、羚羊角粉、全蝎、蜈蚣以镇肝熄风。

若见面色苍白，四肢厥冷，汗出喘促，脉细弱者，为邪盛正衰，正不胜邪，阳气欲脱之内闭外脱证候，应急服参附汤以回阳救逆，不能口服时，可以鼻饲给药，并配合针灸治疗。脱证解除后，仍按原证治疗。若病情危重时，则中西医结合紧急抢救。

处方举例：

白头翁 10g、黄连 6g、炒黄芩 10g、秦皮 10g、银花 10g、连翘 10g、炒山楂 15g、地榆 10g、马齿苋 15g。

（三）寒湿痢

主症：下痢赤白黏冻，白多赤少，或纯为白冻，腹痛，里急后重。

兼症：头身重困，中脘饱闷，饮食乏味。

舌脉：舌质正常或稍淡，苔白腻、脉濡缓。

分析：寒湿滞留肠中，伤及脂膜，故下痢赤白黏冻，白多赤少，或纯为白冻。腑气不和，传导失职，则腹痛，里急后重。寒湿中阻，运化失司，故头身重困，中脘痞闷，饮食乏味。苔白腻，脉濡缓均为寒湿之象。

治法：温化寒湿，佐以行气。

方药：胃苓汤加味。

方中苍术、厚朴、陈皮燥湿运脾，行气散满；合五苓散以温化寒湿。可酌加当归以和血，木香、槟榔行气散寒止痛。若兼外湿，头重身困，加羌活、防风以祛风胜湿；若寒湿盛者，加炮姜以增强散寒之力，或加茯苓、车前子等利湿之品。若寒湿久积不化，脾阳已伤，则当温中健脾，用理中汤加味治疗。

处方举例：

苍术 10g、厚朴 10g、干姜 6g、乌药 3g、木香 10g、焦槟榔 10g、全当归 10g、炒山楂 15g、炒陈皮 10g、生甘草 6g、五苓散(包煎)6g。

四、虚寒痢

主症：痢久不已，时轻时重，下痢稀薄，带有白冻，便下不爽，甚则滑脱不禁，小腹隐痛。

兼症：身倦乏力，畏寒肢冷，食少神疲，口淡不渴。

舌脉：舌质淡，苔薄白，脉细弱。

分析：久痢不愈，脾肾俱伤，寒湿滞留肠中，故久痢不已，下痢稀薄；中气下陷则滑脱不禁；气机不畅，故小腹隐痛，便下不爽；脾阳不振，运化失司，故身倦乏力，畏寒肢冷，食少神疲，口淡不渴，淡苔薄白，脉细弱均为脾胃虚寒之象。

治法：温补脾肾，涩肠固脱。

方药：真人养脏汤加减。

方中党参益气健脾，肉豆蔻、干姜、肉桂温补脾肾，诃子、罂粟壳涩肠固脱，木香行气止痛，白芍、甘草和血缓急止痛。

若中气下陷，滑泻脱肛者去木香，加黄芪、升麻；畏寒肢冷明显者加吴萸、附子；挟有积滞，大便不爽者去诃子、罂粟壳，加山楂、槟榔。

处方举例：

党参 10g、炒白术 10g、煨豆蔻 10g、炮姜 6g、肉桂 3g、白芍 10g、木香 10g、诃子 6g、炒山楂 15g、甘草 6g、灶心土(先煎代水)30g。

(五)休息痢

主症：下痢时发时止，日久不愈，发则下痢脓血，腹痛，里急后重。

兼症：食欲不振，倦怠乏力，甚则形体消瘦。

舌脉：舌质淡，苔腻，脉弱。

分析：病久正虚，脾胃虚弱，湿热留恋不净，每因饮食不慎或受凉而诱发，正气恢复时则病轻痢止。脾气不足则食欲不振，倦怠乏力；化源不足，气血虚少，故形体消瘦。湿热转甚则下痢脓血，腹痛，里急后重。舌脉均为正虚而湿浊不化之象。

治法：健脾益气与清热化湿交替使用。

方药：发作时，连理汤加减；平时，六君子汤加减。方中理中汤温中健脾，黄连清肠中湿热余邪；合而治之，标本兼顾。可酌加当归、赤芍、地榆以和营；木香以调气。如湿热较重者，亦可用芍药汤加减为治。痢疾缓解后，平时可服六君子汤以健脾和胃。加黄连清余热以巩固疗效。

若脾阳不振，肠中寒积不化，遇寒即发，下痢白冻，倦怠少食，舌淡苔白脉沉，可用温脾汤加减以温中散寒，消食导滞。

处方举例：

党参 10g、炮姜 10g、炒白术 12g、炙甘草 6g、黄连 5g、当归 12g、木香 9g、炒山楂 15g。

(六)阴虚痢

主症：痢下赤白脓血，黏稠如胶，量少难出，虚从努争，脐下急痛。

兼症：心烦，口干，午后低热，神疲乏力。

舌脉：舌红少津，苔少或花剥，脉细数。

分析：痢久不愈，湿热伤阴，遂为阴虚痢。阴血亏虚，湿热熏蒸，化腐成脓故便下脓血，黏稠如胶;阴亏于下,湿热交阻,余邪不尽故虚坐努争,脐下急痛;阴津耗伤则心烦,口干,低热;脾虚气弱则神疲乏力。舌红苔少脉数均为一派阴虚之象。

治法:养阴清热止痢。

方药:驻车丸加减。

方中黄连清热止痢,当归、阿胶养阴和营,热著者可去炮姜。阴伤甚者宜加白芍、甘草、乌梅炭以酸甘化阴,和营止痛,或加熟地,麦冬滋阴生津。痢下血多,加丹皮炭、地榆凉血止血;泻痢日久,滑脱难禁者可加石榴皮、诃子肉收敛止痢。阴虚而挟有湿热,养阴有碍祛湿,祛湿反伤阴血,清热苦寒有败胃化燥之弊,治疗颇难。可使用李中梓提出的酸收法,药如:五倍子、石榴皮、黄柏等标本兼顾。

处方举例:黄柏 10g、乌梅 6g、五倍子 6g、焦山楂 10g、石榴皮 10g、生白芍 10g、生甘草 6g、煨樁 5g。

此外,下痢不能进食,或呕而不能食者,称为"噤口痢",其证当分虚实。实证多由湿热疫毒蕴积肠中,上攻于胃,胃失和降所致,症见胸闷,呕逆,口秽纳呆,舌苔黄腻。治宜苦辛通降,泄热和胃,用开噤散加减,多次徐徐咽下或鼻饲给药以解毒降逆。倘汤剂不受,可先用玉枢丹磨汁少量与服。若呕吐频繁,舌红绛而干,脉细数者,乃胃之气阴耗伤较甚所致,可于方中酌加人参、麦冬、沙参、五味子等以益气养阴。虚证多由素体脾胃虚弱或久痢致虚,胃气上逆所致,症见呕恶不食,或食入即吐,口淡不渴,舌淡脉弱,治宜健脾和胃为主,方用六君子汤加砂仁、石菖蒲、姜汁以醒脾开胃。

〔预防及护理措施〕

1. 注意饮食卫生,不食生冷、油腻、不洁及变质食物。

2. 顺应气候变化,纳凉取暖皆应适宜;保持心情舒畅。

3. 夏秋季节,常食生大蒜可预防之。

4. 注意饮食调配,《千金要方》指出:"凡痢病,通忌生冷酢滑,猪鸡鱼油,乳酪酥干,脯酱粉咸,所食诸食,皆须大熟烂为佳,亦不得伤饱,此将息之大经也。"

〔典型病例分析〕

案一:奚某某,女,46 岁,农民。1970 年 7 月 2 日就诊。患者昨日中午憎寒热壮,今晨恶心呕吐,腹痛且下痞赤白脓冻,有里急后重感,日行 10 余次,脘痞满,口渴引饮,肢体酸痛,苔白中黄腻,脉滑数。体温 39.2℃。大便常规:脓细胞(++),红细胞(+++),大便培养两次均有痢疾杆菌生长。中医辨证属风热外侵,湿热积滞内阻,肠腑传导失司而为疫毒痢,选用"救绝神丹":当归 30g、白芍 30g、飞滑石 30g、生甘草 5g、花槟榔 10g、炒莱菔子 10g、炒枳壳 6g、广木香 3g、薤白头 10g,1 剂热退痢止,3 剂告愈。细菌培养三次转阴。(许绳学:治痢古方"救绝神丹",《上海中医药杂志》。1989:(3):34)

按:古方"救绝神丹"近人治痢颇佳,具和血调气,宽肠利湿,解毒利窍之功,适用于湿热在肠,而热邪不甚,气血失和,水湿壅塞之泄痢。蒲辅周先生说:"在临床上用古方救绝神丹治疗休息痢效果较好。其方以当归、芍药为主,槟榔、木香、莱菔子、枳壳为辅,甘草和中解毒为佐,薤白通阳利水为使,滑石利窍以导邪外出。痢疾大伤元气者,因里急后重、出汗使脾胃受伤而气血两虚。此方重用归芍调和肝脾,甘草和中解毒,佐使协合,痼疾往往根治。"痢疾是以腹痛,里急后重,痢下赤白脓血为特征。发病机理乃病邪与气血相搏于肠道,以致肠中脂膜与血络受伤,腐败化为脓血或赤白黏冻,遂成痢疾。其病因为外受湿浊、疫毒之气,内伤饮食生冷,损伤脾胃与肠腑，多发于夏秋季节。

痢疾的辨证宜分清寒热虚实。一般而言，暴痢多实，久痢多虚。实证又有湿热痢与寒湿痢的不同，而以湿热痢较为多见。疫毒痢来势急骤，病情严重，宜及早图治。虚证有阴虚痢与虚寒痢区别。若下痢不能进食，或呕不能食，称为噤口痢。由湿热疫毒上攻或胃虚气逆所致，亦属危急之证，必须高度重视。至于休息痢有时发时止的特点。

关于本病的治疗，应依其证候的寒热虚实而定。一般新感暴痢多为热证、实证，治当以祛邪为主，湿热痢治宜清热化湿，佐以调气行血；疫毒痢治宜清热凉血解毒，神昏者兼以清心开窍，惊厥者加凉肝熄风之品；寒湿痢治宜温化寒湿。久痢多为虚证、寒证，治当扶正为先，痢疾日久，伤及阴血者，治宜养阴清肠；肝脾虚寒，关门不固者，宜温补脾肾，佐以固涩；休息痢宜温中清肠，佐以调气化滞。但不论虚证、实证，皆可以辅以调气和血之品，兼积滞者则需消积导滞。此外，在痢疾的病变过程中，绝不可忽视顾护胃气这一环节。

复习思考题

1. 你对痢疾的源流认识如何？
2. 痢疾的主要病因是什么？为什么说其发病关键在于肠中积滞？
3. 痢疾的发病特点是什么？什么样的情况下运用“逆流挽舟”之法？
4. 湿热痢与疫毒痢的关系是什么？如何处理？
5. 湿热未净而阴血已伤的久痢应如何处理？注意点有哪些？
6. 久痢与瘀血有何关系？
7. 在痢疾的治疗中如何使用固涩药？

便　秘

〔概述〕

便秘，是指大便秘结不通而言。其内容包括三个方面，即或大便干结，或排便间隔时间延长，或大便虽不干而排便困难。

西医学的习惯性便秘，肠神经官能症，结肠、直肠以及肛门炎症等疾病所引起的便秘，年老体弱引起的排便无力而致的便秘，药物引起的便秘，以及其他各种急慢性疾病中所见到的便秘均可参阅本篇进行治疗。

〔病因病机〕

饮食入胃，经过胃的受纳、腐熟，脾的运化、转输，其精微被吸收，所剩糟粕最后由大肠传送而出，成为大便。便秘的发生，主要是由于大肠传导功能失常，粪便在肠内停留过久，水份被吸收，从而粪便过于干燥、坚硬所致。常见的便秘病因病机为：燥热内结，津液不足；情绪波动，气机郁滞；劳倦内伤，气血不足；年高体衰，阴寒凝结等，皆能使胃肠功能发生障碍，传导不畅而产生便秘。现就便秘病因病机分述如下：

一、肠胃积热：凡阳盛之体，或恣饮酒浆，过食辛辣厚味，或过服辛热温补之品，以致热毒蕴盛；也有热病之后，余热不清而留恋于肠胃，耗伤津液，导致肠道燥热。另外，肺燥肺热下移于大肠，也可以导致肠道燥热，燥热伤津，以致肠道干涩燥结，形成热秘。

二、气机郁滞：因于忧愁思虑，情志不舒，或久坐少动，往往引起气机郁滞；也有由于外科手术后的肠粘连，或金创跌仆损伤胃肠，或肺失宣降，大肠气机不畅，均可使肠胃通降、传导功能失常，因之糟粕内停，不能下行，造成大便秘结。

三、气血阴津亏虚：劳倦、饮食内伤脾胃，化源不充，气血亏虚，或大病、久病、产后以及年高体衰之人，气血两虚。也有病中过用汗、下之剂，耗伤阴津，或亡血失精、生育不节，损伤气血阴精。气虚则大肠传送无力；血虚、津少、精亏则不能滋润大肠，肠道干槁，便行艰涩。若阴损及阳，阴阳两虚，则不能腐熟水谷，化生津液，滋润肠道，都能使大便排出困难，而致虚秘。

四、阴寒凝滞：年高体弱，或久病不复，真阳亏损，阳气不运，则阴邪凝结；也有平素脾虚之人，久食生冷之物，或过用苦寒之剂，伐伤阳气，而致脾肾阳衰，温煦无权，阴寒内结。寒凝气滞，使肠道传送无力而大便艰难，此即寒结便秘，或者称为冷秘。

综上所述，便秘虽属大肠传导失职，但与肺、脾、肾也有非常密切的关系。肺与大肠相表里，气热肺燥，肺失宣降，往往使大肠传导失常而致便秘；脾主运化，职司水谷精微的吸收、转输，脾病则气血乏源，转输不利，糟粕内停，而致便秘；肾司二便、主开阖，内寄元阴元阳，肾虚则或阴亏肠燥，或阳衰寒凝，传导失常而形成便秘。

便秘病因病机示意图

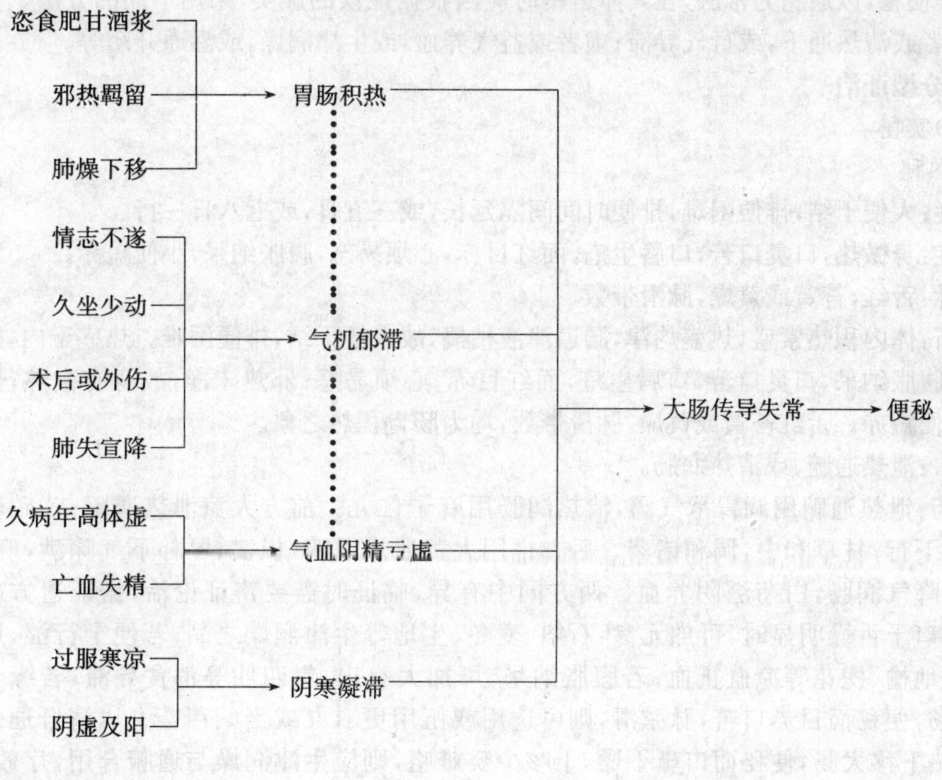

〔**辨证论治**〕

便秘的临床表现为大便燥结，排便间隔时间延长，经常三五日或七八日才一次，个别病人甚至更长。或者虽然次数不减，但是粪质干燥坚硬，排出困难。或时有便意，大便并不干，只是排出不畅，或临厕努挣，不能顺利排出。便秘日久，常常引发其他症状，如腹中胀满、甚至疼痛，恶心，嗳气，食欲不振，头昏脑胀，睡眠不安，心烦易怒等症。

一、辨证要点

(一)辨虚实:按照便秘的发病原因及临床表现,归纳为实秘与虚秘两类。实秘一般起病急,病程短,症状虽重,但治疗后容易收效。虚秘一般起病缓,病程长,症状虽轻,但治疗后不易收效。实秘有燥热与气滞之分;虚秘有气虚、血虚及阳衰之别。热秘以大便干结、排便间隔时间延长及排便困难为特征;气秘以大便干结或不干结,欲便不得,排出不畅为特征;气虚以虽有便意,临厕努挣乏力为特征;血虚以便次正常,大便燥结如球,排便困难为特征;阳虚以便质未必干结,但大便艰涩、排出困难为特征。

(二)辨良性、恶性:便秘的发生,究其病理变化,有功能性与器质性之不同,一般通过望诊、问诊、切脉等可以区分,在临床上,借助X线钡餐造影,乙状结肠镜或纤维结肠镜,更容易加以明确。在器质性病变中,更需要进一步区分良性病变与恶性病变。良性病变大多患者年龄较轻,病程短,便秘不甚严重,全身虚衰及脏腑功能障碍的症状也不明显;恶性病变则多数患者年龄较高,病程长,便秘严重或时轻时重,全身虚衰及脏腑功能障碍的症状也较明显。有条件时,借助理化检查,有助于鉴别。区分良性病变与恶性病变,对治疗效果和预后的估计关系密切。

二、治则要点

治疗便秘,以通腑为常法,在具体运用时应当根据证候的虚实,采用不同的方法。其治疗大法,实者或清热通下,或行气导滞;虚者或益气养血,或生津润燥,或温通开闭等。

三、分型证治

(一)实秘

1. 热秘

主症:大便干结,排便困难,排便时间间隔延长,或三五日,或七八日一行。

兼症:身微热,口臭口苦,口唇生疮,面红目赤,心烦易怒,腹胀纳呆,小便短赤。

舌脉:舌红,苔黄或黄燥,脉滑带数。

分析:体内积热素盛,热盛灼津,肠道津液枯槁,故大便干结,排便困难。热盛于内,腑气不通,故见腹胀纳呆,口臭口苦,口唇生疮,面红目赤,心烦易怒;邪热未净,故身有微热;热移膀胱,则小便短赤。舌红苔黄或黄燥,脉滑带数,均为肠胃积热之象。

治法:泄热通腑,或清热润肠。

方药:泄热通腑用调胃承气汤,清热润肠用麻子仁丸。前方大黄泄热通腑;芒硝软坚散结,导便下行;甘草和中,调和诸药。后方也用大黄泄热通腑,枳实、厚朴下气除满,麻仁、杏仁、白密降气润肠,白芍滋阴养血。两方同中有异,临证时需要辨证论治,据证遣方。若热盛伤津,口干舌燥明显时,可加元参、石斛、麦冬、生地等生津润燥之品;若便干行涩,肛裂出血,可加地榆、槐花等凉血止血;若腹胀纳呆,可加大腹皮、焦四仙等消食导滞;若缘于肝热移于胃肠,便秘而目赤口苦,脉弦滑,则可选用或伍用更衣丸或当归芦荟丸以清肝通便。若肺中燥热下移大肠,便秘而口鼻干燥,干咳少痰难咯,则应生津润燥与通腑合用,疗效较好,如瓜蒌、山栀等。

泄热通腑法,是治疗热秘之常法,但不可过用或久用,否则易苦寒伤胃,故使用时应中病即止,再以养阴润肠之剂调之。

处方举例:

熟大黄9g、火麻仁10g、杏仁10g、枳实10g、大腹皮10g、焦四仙各10g、生甘草6g、蜂蜜

30g(冲)、清半夏 10g、炒陈皮 10g。

2. 气秘

主症:大便干结或不干结,欲便不得,排出不畅,每于情绪不好时便秘加重。

兼症:嗳气频作,胸胁痞满,腹中胀痛,喜太息或矢气后稍宽。

舌脉:舌红,苔薄白腻或薄黄腻,脉象弦。

分析:肺肝为气机升降之路,肺有邪客则气闭而失于宣降,肝因情伤则气郁而失于疏泄。气机郁滞,大肠传导失司,故大便排泄不畅,欲便而不行。肺肝不和,故胁肋痞满,嗳气频作,嗳出或矢气则舒,腹中胀痛。苔薄白腻,脉弦为气机郁滞之象,若有化热之势则舌苔转黄。

治法:顺气行滞。

方药:六磨汤为主方。方中枳实下气宽胸,引肺气下行;木香理气和中,调理中焦气机;乌药行气散满,治在中下焦;沉香芳化降气,槟榔下气消胀;用大黄泄热通腑。若腑气渐通,肝气未舒时,可用柴胡疏肝散调理。若气郁化热,症见口苦咽干,苔黄,脉数时,可加芦荟、黄芩、栀子等泄肝通腑。若由于肺气闭阻者,当从宣降肺气入手,可加杏仁、瓜蒌皮、葶苈子等泻肺通便之品;若由于手术或外伤所致者,则应加桃仁、红花、赤芍、三七等活血化瘀之药调理之血;若在中风、偏瘫中兼见便秘者,可用搜风顺丸调治。

处方举例:

炒枳实 10g、广木香 10g、台乌药 12g、沉香粉 3g(分冲)、熟大黄 5g、焦槟榔 10g、杏仁 10g、柴胡 10g、赤芍 10g、青陈皮各 6g。

(二)虚秘

主症:虽有便意,临厕努挣乏力,排便艰涩不畅,便质一般并不干结。

兼症:年高体弱,或久病之人,面黄肌瘦,神疲气怯,短气,便后更甚。

舌脉:舌淡,苔薄白,脉细弱。

分析:肺脾气虚之人,因肺主气,与大肠相表里,肺气虚则大肠传导无力,故排便艰涩不畅,便不干而难于排出。肺气虚则卫外不固,腠理疏松,故排便努挣时易于汗出短气。脾主运化,为后天之本,脾虚不运,气血乏源,故面黄肌瘦,神疲气怯。排便之后,气随便泄,故气短神疲等症见加重。舌淡,苔薄白,脉细弱,也为肺脾气虚之象。

治法:健脾益气。

方药:黄芪汤为主方。方义重在益气助运,方中黄芪为健脾益气之要药,甘草补虚和中,以助黄芪补气之力;陈皮理气和胃;火麻仁、白蜜润肠通便。若补气乏力不足,可加党参、黄精等,若气虚下陷,肛门坠迫,屡欲登厕而虚坐努挣不下,可加升麻,柴胡等,升举清气以降浊;若肺气虚明显,则久咳气喘可合用生脉散,或参蛤散;肾为气之根,气虚久治不愈,当从肾治,可用大补元煎加味。

处方举例:

炙黄芪 30g、党参 10g、黄精 30g、炒陈皮 10g、火麻仁 15g、白蜜 30g(冲)、炙甘草 6g、炒枳实 10g、台乌药 10g、广木香 10g。

2. 血虚

主症:大便燥结如球,便次虽然正常,但排便不畅。

兼症:头眩心悸,少眠多梦,面色、唇爪白而无华。

舌脉:舌淡,苔薄白,脉象细软。

分析：血虚津少，不能滑润肠道，故大便燥结如球，排便不畅；血虚则清空失养，故头目眩晕；血不养心，心神不宁，故心悸，少眠多梦；血脉不充，则唇爪及面色白而无华。舌淡，苔薄白，脉象细软，均为血虚脉不充之象。

治法：养血润燥。

方药：润肠丸为主方。方中当归、生地补血养阴；桃仁、火麻仁润燥滑肠；枳壳破气下行，五药共用，以补血润下。若出现五心烦热，口干津少，舌红光无苔或花剥，为阴血亏虚，当以滋阴增液为主，可于上方加用玄参、麦冬、生首乌等；若血虚夹瘀，舌淡而黯或有瘀斑，可用通幽汤养血活血，润燥通便。若兼见腰脊痠软，经少色淡，也可加制首乌、肉苁蓉、胡桃肉等补肾益阴之品；若经常便燥而秘，可常服五仁丸以润肠通便，缓图调治。

处方举例：

当归 10g、生地 10g、熟地 10g、桃仁 10g、砂仁 3g、火麻仁 10g、炒枳实 10g、生首乌 10g、胡桃肉 10g、赤芍 10g、生甘草 6g。

3. 冷秘

主症：大便艰涩，难以排出，便质或干或不干。

兼症：面色㿠白，畏寒肢冷，腹中冷气攻痛，肠鸣，或腰脊冷痛，小便清长。

舌脉：舌质淡胖，苔白润，脉象沉迟而弱。

分析：脾肾阳衰，阴寒内生，留于肠胃，阴气固结，阳气不运，致使肠道传送无力而大便艰涩，便质虽然不硬，但难以排出。阳气虚衰，不达四末，故面色㿠白，畏寒肢冷，或腰脊冷痛。阴寒凝滞于腹中，故腹中冷气攻痛，肠鸣。阳气不足，膀胱虚寒，水不化气，故小便清长。舌淡而胖，苔白润，脉象沉迟而弱，均为阳衰阴盛之象。

治法：温通开秘。

方药：剂川煎为主方。方中当归、肉苁蓉、牛膝滋补精血，润肠通便；升麻升清气以降浊气；枳壳下气行滞；可加用肉桂、乌药温通气机；减去泽泻利湿实便之弊。或加用胡桃肉、首乌等补肾养血润肠。若阴寒较甚，也可配合服用半硫丸，每次 6g，日二次，以增强温通寒凝、开闭散结之力。平时，也可以常服右归丸或金匮肾气丸等温补肾阳，温通开秘，对于此型便秘有效。

处方举例：

全当归 10g、肉苁蓉 15g、胡桃肉 10g、首乌 10g、肉桂 6g、乌药 10g、枳实 10g、牛膝 12g、升麻 5g、半硫丸(包煎)9g。

关于便秘的治疗，除了内服中药外，尚有外导之法。脐中给药，以及其他多种方法，如针灸、按摩等也可以配合使用；单方、验方也往往获得较好功效，如番泻叶、草决明、生白术、莱菔子等。另外，还可以采用食饵疗法，如黑芝麻、胡桃肉、松子仁等分，研细，稍加白蜜冲服，对于阴血不足的便秘有效。此外，对习惯性便秘，如保持精神的舒畅，进行轻微活动，以及饮食的调整和定时登厕等，均有利于便秘的治疗。至于热病之后，或患其他之病者，由于水谷少进而不大便的，不必急于通便，只须扶养胃气，使饮食渐增，则大便自能正常。

〔预防及护理措施〕

1. 起居有时，培养每日定日排便的习惯。

2. 饮食有节，宜多吃蔬菜及粗粮，忌食辛辣、刺激性之食物。

3. 虚者应加强腹部功能锻炼，以助排便。

〔典型病例分析〕

案一：林某某，女，29岁，1984年9月13日诊治。

患者自去年9月始发便秘，每登厕努责艰行，需服大黄泻下，经查为"陈旧性肛门裂"，一年来，多方医治罔效。

刻下症：纳谷不香，食后嗳噫食气，大便结硬如羊矢，三天来欲便不得，性情急躁，盗汗，口咽干燥，舌质红，苔剥，脉弦细稍数。

中医诊断：便秘。

证属：阴虚津亏，大肠气滞。

治则：滋阴润燥，行滞通便。

方药：增液汤合六磨汤化裁。

生地18g、玄参12g、麦冬12g、沉香1.5g(冲)、乌药6g、木香6g、槟榔9g、大黄(制)9g、枳壳10g、决明子20g。

服药两剂，翌日畅便五次，食嗳减少，食纳增馨，余症皆得改善。续进三剂，大便即趋正常，予滋阴润燥之品以善其后。

按：本案乃患者情志失和，肝脾不调，气机壅滞，日久化火伤阴而致便秘。药用生地、麦冬、玄参养阴润燥，增水行舟；木香、乌药、沉香调节气机以解郁；大黄、槟榔、枳壳下气行滞，更加一味决明子，助大便下行而病愈。(池绳业·便秘《新中医》1987；(1)：18)

便秘是临床上常见病，是由多种原因引起的，在临床上应当根据发病原因和临床表现分辨虚实论治。实秘有热秘、气秘之分，虚秘有气虚、血虚、冷秘之别。治疗大法则因证而施，热秘宜泄热通腑或清热润肠；气秘宜顺气行滞，从肝、从肺论治；气虚宜益气润肠；血虚宜养血润燥，兼阴虚者又当滋养阴血以润肠；冷秘宜温阳开闭等。上述诸秘，有时单一独见，有时相兼并见，故各种治法应随证灵活运用，如气秘延久则化热，气秘与热秘同时并见，治疗时行滞与泄热同用；气虚失治、误治往往导致阳虚，如脾肾阳衰，治疗时就当益气、温阳同用等等。因此，便秘的治疗虽以通腑为常法，也应根据不同的病因病机与临床证候，采用不同的治疗方法。除上述内治法外，其他如导法、脐中给药、针灸、按摩等，也可随证配合使用，增强疗效。

复习思考题

1. 便秘的病机是什么？
2. 便秘常分哪几型？其证治规律如何掌握？
3. 便秘的辨证要点是哪些？如何识别引起便秘的恶性病变特点？
4. 便秘的简便疗法有哪些？

胁　痛

〔概述〕

凡以肝胆受损，气血不调所引起的一侧或两侧胁肋部位疼痛为主要表现的病症，称为胁痛。临床上多兼见有胃脘胀痛、胁下痞块、癥瘕。

西医中的肝胆疾病，如急慢性肝炎，肝硬化，胆道感染，胆囊炎，胆结石，干性或渗出性胸膜炎，肋间神经痛，肋软骨膜炎等，以胁痛为主要症状的，即可参考本病辨证论治。

〔病因病机〕

肝居胁下，其经脉布于两胁，胆附于肝，其脉亦循于胁，故胁痛之病主要责之于肝胆。又因肝藏血，主疏泄，性喜条达，胆内藏胆汁，又称“中精之府”。古人说：“肝之余气，溢于胆聚而成精汁”，胆汁也随肝气而疏泄，所以情志失调，肝气内郁，或气郁日久，气 滞血瘀，瘀血停积，或精血亏损，肝阴不足，络脉失养，或脾失健运，湿热内郁，疏泄不利等均可导致胁痛，其具体病因病机分述如下：

一、肝气郁结：情志抑郁，或暴怒伤肝，肝失调达，疏泄不利，气阻络痹而致胁痛。

二、瘀血停着：气郁日久，血流不畅，瘀血停积，胁络不畅，出现胁痛，或强力负重，跌仆损伤，胁络受伤，瘀血停留，阻塞胁络，致使胁痛。

三、肝胆湿热：外湿内侵，或饮食所伤，脾失健运，痰浊中阻，土壅木郁，气郁化热，湿热郁结于肝胆脾胃，肝胆失其疏泄、条达，导致胁痛。

四、肝阴不足：久病体虚或劳役过度，精血亏损，肝阴不足，血虚不能养肝，使络脉失养亦能导致胁痛。

五、饮停胁下：水饮停积于胸胁，络脉受阻，肝肺气机升降不利，也致胁痛。

六、邪郁半表半里：外邪不解，郁于半表半里，少阳胆气不利，也致胁痛。

综上所述，胁痛的病变主要在肝胆，内伤、外感均可致胁痛，就其病因病机来说，又与脾、胃、肺、肾有关。因肝胆之气失于疏泄条达，不但可以乘脾犯胃，并可循经侮肺，以致肝肺升降失常。又因肝肾乙癸同源，可因肾阴不足不能养肝而致肝虚胁痛。本篇主要讲前四种胁痛。在病证方面胁痛有虚有实而以实证为多见。实证以气滞、血瘀、湿热为主，三者又以气滞为先；虚证多属气血亏虚；此外，实证日久，化热伤阴，致肝肾阴虚，亦可出现虚实并见。

胁痛病因病机示意图

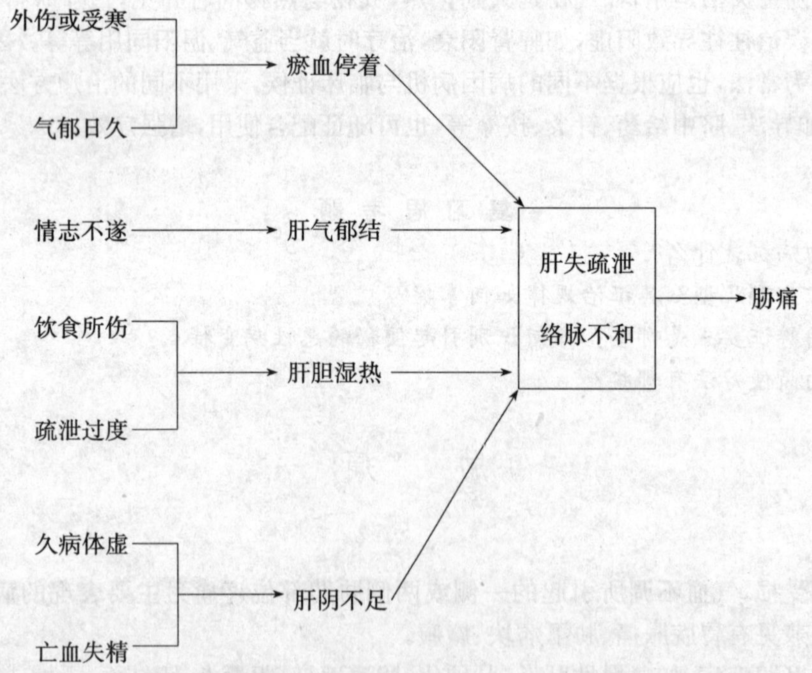

〔辨证论治〕

一、辨证要点

1. 辨表里：即内伤外感。外感胁痛起病较急，大多属湿热病邪侵犯肝胆，临床多有表证，发热恶寒，并伴有呕吐、黄疸等，脉浮数或弦数，舌红苔腻或黄或白；内伤胁痛，起病较缓，无寒热出现。胁痛一病，里证多而表证少。

2. 辨寒热：胁痛体虚形寒，口淡无味，舌淡苔白，喜着厚衣，痛处得热则减，天寒易加重，脉弦迟沉涩者，属寒证。体壮面红，口苦，舌红，苔黄或黄腻，灼热喜凉爽，痛处得热则剧，喜着薄衣，或喜袒襟露怀，天热易加重，脉弦数洪促者属热证。

3. 辨气血：新病多气，久病则入血，疼痛游走不，定忽左忽右，倏聚倏散，痛无定处。胀痛主属气滞。痛有定处，午后或夜间加重，唇舌有瘀斑为血瘀，痛多胀少或只痛不胀，刺痛不移或有外伤史当属血瘀。

4. 辨虚实：新病痛剧体壮，脉弦大有力，痛处拒按为实；久病体虚，绵绵隐痛，脉虚细沉弱无力，痛处喜按为虚。但临床上往往虚实互见，既有湿热又有血虚或兼有瘀血内停。因此须注意其标本先后，孰轻孰重，以决定相应治则或统筹兼顾。

二、鉴别诊断

作为痛证，胁痛应与胃脘痛、胸痹相鉴别，这从疼痛部位一般不难区别。胁痛主要痛在两胁，有胀痛、刺痛、灼痛、隐痛之区别，或可触及癥瘕或痞块，或曾有悬饮，疼痛发作与进食油腻有关，疼痛剧者常辗转反侧，且喜变换体位。胃脘痛以剑突下胃脘部疼痛明显，虚痛喜暖喜按，实痛拒按，多伴有呕吐吞酸等；胸痹则痛在胸，甚则彻背，偶在左胁，痛则不敢活动，闷痛为主，多伴有心悸气短等。

胁痛、胃脘痛、胸痹鉴别简表

鉴别＼病名	胁　痛	胃脘痛	胸　痹
部　位	一侧或两侧胁肋部位	胃脘部	胸骨后或左前胸，偶或连及左胁肋、左肩臂
特　点	以胀痛、刺痛、隐痛、灼痛、绞痛为多，痛剧欲变动体位	以胀满、刺痛、痞满为主，虚痛喜按，实痛拒按	以闷痛为主，痛时不欲变动体位
伴随症	有的有胁下痞块、癥瘕、或有悬饮	多伴有呕吐恶心，吞酸等	多伴气短、胸闷、手足发凉、心悸等
诱　因	与外感、饮食、七情有关	多与饮食、情志、受凉有关	多与过饱、情绪变动有关
病　史	肝胆病史	脾胃病史	心脏病史
放射部位	右肩背	正后背	左肩背

三、治则要点

胁痛的治疗，根据“痛则不通，通则不痛”的理论，灵活应用疏肝、泻肝、柔肝之法以使肝气疏泄条达，肝络和畅，肝经湿热清除，肝阴不亏，肝络得养，则胁痛自然会消除。

四、分型论治

(一)肝气郁结

主症:胁痛以胀痛为主,走窜不定,疼痛每因情志之变动而增减。

兼症:常兼有胃脘胀满,胸闷不舒,嗳气频作。

舌脉:苔薄,脉弦。

分析:肝气失于条达,阻于胁络,故见胁肋胀痛。气属无形,时聚时散,故疼痛走串不定。情志变化与气之郁结关系极为密切,故疼痛每与情志的变动有关,气机不畅故胸闷不舒;肝气横逆,常易侵犯脾胃,故食少嗳气,胃脘胀满。脉弦为肝郁之象。

治法:疏肝理气。

方药:柴胡舒肝散加减。方中柴胡疏肝,枳壳、香附、陈皮理气,川芎活血,芍药、甘草缓急止痛。胁痛重酌加青皮、川楝子、郁金、元胡以加强理气止痛的作用;气郁化火,见胁 肋掣痛,心急烦躁,口干口苦,溲黄便秘,舌红苔黄,脉弦数,去川芎加丹皮、栀子、黄连、川楝子、元胡等以清肝理气,活血止痛;若气郁化火,进而伤阴,症见隐痛不休,遇劳则剧,头晕,心烦,睡眠欠佳,舌红,苔黄少津,脉细弦,可去川芎加丹参、首乌、枸杞子、丹皮、山栀、菊花等,滋阴清热,兼疏肝气;肝气横逆,脾失健运而见胁痛,伴肠鸣腹泻者可加白术、茯苓、苡仁、扁豆健脾止泻。胃失和降,症见恶心呕吐者加旋覆花、代赭石、半夏、生姜和胃止呕。

处方举例:

柴胡 10g、炒枳壳 10g、炒赤芍 10g、甘草 6g、青皮 6g、陈皮 10g、川芎 10g、制香附 10g、郁金 12g、元胡 6g、炒川楝 10g。

(二)瘀血停着

主症:胁痛如刺,痛处不移,入夜更甚。

兼症:胁肋下或见癥块。

舌脉:舌质紫暗,或有瘀斑,脉象沉涩。

分析:肝郁日久,气滞血瘀,或跌仆损伤致瘀血停着,痹阻胁络,故疼痛如刺,痛有定处,入夜痛甚。瘀结所积,积久不散,则渐成癥块。舌质紫暗、瘀斑,脉沉涩均为瘀血内停之征。

治法:祛瘀通络。

方药:旋覆花汤加减。方中新绛可以茜草代替,以活血痛络;旋覆花理气止痛,可酌加郁金、桃仁、归尾、元胡等以加强理气活血之力。也可用血府逐瘀汤化裁治之。瘀血较重,或为外伤所致,可用复元活血汤以活血祛瘀,疏肝通络,方中大黄、桃仁、红花、山甲破瘀行滞,当归养血行瘀,柴胡调气散结,引药直达胁下。若胁下有癥块,而正气未衰者,可加三棱、莪术、地鳖虫等破血消坚之药,亦可口服鳖甲煎丸。

处方举例:

柴胡 10g、赤白芍各 10g、当归尾 10g、桃仁 10g、红花 10g、炙山甲 10g、莪术 6g、川芎 g、郁金 12g、元胡 6g、三七粉 3g(分冲)。

(三)肝胆湿热

主症:胁肋闷痛。

兼症:胸脘闷,纳呆,恶心呕吐,目黄或身黄或伴有寒热,小便涩滞不爽,或有呕吐蛔虫。

舌脉:舌苔黄腻,脉弦数。

分析:湿热蕴结于肝胆,肝络失和,胆不疏泄,故胁痛口苦。湿热中阻,以致胸脘满闷纳呆,恶心呕吐。肝开窍于目，肝火上炎故目赤。湿热交蒸，胆液不循常道而外溢故见目黄身黄。湿热下注膀胱则尿黄，或有尿涩痛不爽。湿热之邪郁于肝胆，少阳不和故有寒热。舌苔黄腻，脉弦数，均是肝胆湿热之征。

治法：清热利湿。

方药：龙胆泻肝汤加减。方中以龙胆草泻肝胆湿热，柴胡疏达肝气，黄芩、栀子清热泄火，木通、泽泻、车前子清利湿热。胁痛重可加金铃子散，青皮、郁金、半夏以疏肝和胃，理气止痛。若发热黄疸者，加茵陈、黄柏以清利湿热除黄。若疼痛加剧，呕吐蛔虫者，先以乌梅丸安蛔，继则除蛔。若湿热煎熬，结成砂石，阻滞胆道，症见胁痛连及肩背者，可加金钱草、海金砂、郁金及硝石矾石散等以利胆排石。若热盛伤津，大便秘结，腹部胀满者，可加大黄、芒硝及泄热通便。

处方举例：

柴胡10g、龙胆草10g、黄芩10g、山栀10g、郁金12g、金钱草30g、赤芍12g、木通5g、土茯苓30g、半夏10g、青皮10g。

（四）肝阴不足

主症：胁肋隐痛，绵绵不休。

兼症：口干咽燥，心中烦热，头晕目眩，潮热盗汗，五心烦热，腰酸乏力。

舌脉：舌红少苔，脉细弦而数。

分析：肝郁日久化热，耗伤肝阴，或久病体虚，精血亏损，不能濡养肝络，故胁肋隐痛，其痛绵绵不休。阴虚内热故口干咽燥时觉烦热。甚则潮热盗汗，五心烦热。精血亏虚不能上荣，清窍失养则头晕目眩。舌红少苔，脉细弦而数，均为阴虚内热之征。

治则：养阴柔肝。

方药：一贯煎为主方加减。方以生地、杞子滋养肝肾，沙参、麦冬、当归养阴柔肝，川楝子疏肝理气止痛，并可酌加合欢花、玫瑰花、白蒺藜等以舒肝调气。心中烦热，加酸枣仁、炒栀子以清热安神。头晕目眩，加黄精、女贞子、菊花以益肾凉肝。

处方举例：

沙参15g、丹参30g、麦冬10g、生地10g、枸杞10g、炒川楝10g、元胡6g、绿萼梅10g、生白芍10g、炙甘草6g、玫瑰花10g。

〔预防及护理措施〕

1. 保持精神乐观，戒烦躁，禁忧郁。
2. 饮食有节，少食辛辣、海腥、油腻厚味之品，不饮酒。
3. 起居有时，注意个人卫生，防止外邪入侵。
4. 配合指针、按摩。
5. 适当运动、增加气血流通。

〔典型病例分析〕

案一：冯某某，男，54岁，干部。

主诉：胁痛反复发作3年余。

病史：1960年患肝炎，经治疗后基本痊愈，但在工作劳累、气候异常、情志失宁的情况下，胁痛时有发作。近3年来，发作较频，甚至影响工作和睡眠，曾服保肝药及疏肝理气中药未效3，且疼痛不断增剧，精神负担颇重，纳谷不香，形体消瘦。

刻下症：皮肤干燥，面色黧黑，形体瘦弱，纳谷不香，口干苦，大便干，胁下疼痛，舌质红，苔薄黄，舌中有裂纹，脉弦细。

中医诊断：胁痛（肝郁阴虚）。

治则：养阴疏肝。

方药：一贯煎化裁。

当归10g、白芍10g、枸杞10g、生地10g、郁金10g、川楝子10g、白蒺藜10g、北沙参15g、麦冬15g、制首乌15g、女贞子15g、旱莲草15g。

服上方5剂后，胁痛显著减轻，饮食进步；继服5剂后，胁痛完全消失，饮食正常。

按：患者平素肝气不舒，肝郁化火伤阴，再加上服用一些理气温燥之品更使阴伤，故治疗当养阴与疏肝兼顾，药用当归、白芍、枸杞、生地、白蒺藜、北沙参、麦冬、制首乌、女贞子、旱莲草补血养肝肾之阴而调肝，辅以郁金、川楝子疏肝而不使阴伤，故使病愈。（章真如　加味一贯煎治疗阴虚胁痛《新中医》1984·（2）：25）

胁痛是临床常见病，其病位主要在肝胆。形成本病的原因，不外内伤外感。临床辨证应结合兼证，分清内伤、外感，在气、在血，虚、实、寒、热。气滞、血瘀、湿热而致胁痛多为实证，肝阴不足而致胁痛多为虚证。虚证与实证并不是单一不变的。如病起气滞为主，日久常可导致血瘀，血瘀或湿热为主，又可兼有气滞。实证化热伤阴，或虚证兼有气滞，常可虚实并见。故辨证时应全面分析。

治疗上，依据以通为主的原则，实证采用理气、化瘀、清热、利湿等法；虚证滋阴柔肝为治，同时适当加入理气之品。但理气不宜过分辛燥，以免更伤其阴，可选辛平调气之品。对于各种兼证可参阅其他各篇予以论治。

复习思考题

1. 如何掌握胁痛病机特点？气与血、虚与实如何辨证？
2. 试述肝郁气滞、瘀血停着、肝胆湿热、肝阴不足四型胁痛的证治。
3. 治疗胁痛，如何理解“通则不痛”？

黄　疸

〔附：萎黄〕

〔概述〕

黄疸是以目黄、身黄、小便黄为主要特征的病证。古代又称为“黄瘅”，一般将其分为阳黄、阴黄和急黄三种，以阳黄多见，且其中一部分具有传染性。

中医学的黄疸与西医学中的黄疸含义相同，所以传染性肝炎、胆囊炎、胆道疾患、肝硬变、溶血、急性或亚急性黄色肝萎缩、钩端螺旋体病等所出现的黄疸，均可参阅本篇辨证论治。

〔病因病机〕

黄疸的病因有内外两个方面，外因主要为感受外邪或饮食不节所致，内因多与脾胃虚寒、内伤不足有关，而内外二因又多有关联。现分述如下：

一、感受外邪：外感湿热、疫毒，从表入里，郁而不达，内阻中焦，脾胃运化失常，湿热交蒸于肝胆，不能泄越，以致肝失疏泄，胆汁外溢，浸淫肌肤，下流膀胱而见身目小便俱黄。若湿热疫毒过盛,伤人后病势暴急,或具有传染性,很快表现出伤及营血的严重现象,称为急黄。

二、饮食所伤:饮食不节,饥饱失常,或嗜酒过度,贪食肥甘油腻,皆能损伤脾胃,以致运化功能失职,湿浊内主。若素体阳气内盛,湿易化热而成湿热,熏蒸于肝胆,胆汁不循常道,浸淫肌肤而发阳黄;若饮食不节,寒凉太过损伤脾胃阳气,或素体脾胃虚寒,脾不健运,所生湿浊则易从寒化,而成寒湿阻滞中焦,胆汁受阻,不得正常输泄,溢于肌肤而发阴黄。

三、劳倦内伤:劳伤太过,脾胃虚弱,可以产生黄疸,主要分以下两个方面:一为脾阳受损或脾胃虚寒,不能健运水湿,湿从寒化,以致寒湿阻于中焦,胆液排泄受阻,溢于肌肤而发为阴黄,此乃脾虚寒湿内盛所致;二为脾虚不能化生气血,气血亏虚,血败而不华色,从而产生黄疸,此证乃因虚而发黄,故又称为虚证黄疸,简称虚黄。

四、砂石、虫体阻滞胆道:由于体质的特异性,或湿热煎熬结成砂石,留于胆府,阻于胆道,或由于湿热内郁,脾胃功能失调,蛔虫不伏于肠而乱窜,阻于胆道,迫使胆汁外溢而成黄疸。

五、积聚日久不消:瘀血阻滞胆道,胆汁外溢而产生黄疸。

黄疸病因病机示意图

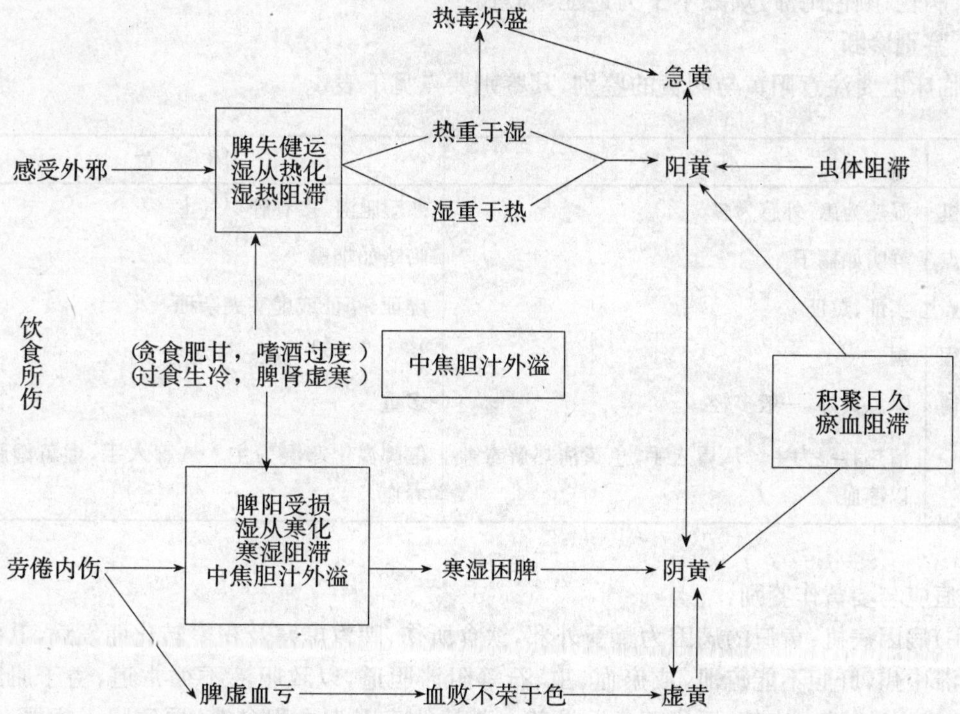

总之,黄疸的发生,病机关键是湿邪为患,且有湿热与寒湿之不同。从脏腑来看,主要累及脾胃肝胆,且往往由脾胃涉及肝胆,脾主运化而恶湿,无论湿邪自外感受或由饮食不节,湿自内生,均首先是脾胃功能受损。脾失健运,湿邪阻滞中焦,脾胃升降失常,脾气不升则肝气郁结不能疏泄,胃气不降则胆汁的输送排泄失常。湿邪阻遏,导致胆液不循常道渗入血液,溢于肌肤而发黄。阳黄与阴黄的不同点在于阳黄之人阳盛热重,平素胃火偏旺,湿从热化而致湿热阻滞为患,由于湿和热常有所偏盛,故阳黄病机上有湿重于热或热重于湿之别。火热极盛谓之毒,如热毒壅盛,邪入营血,内陷心包,多为急黄。阴黄之人,阴盛寒重,平素脾阳不足,湿从寒化而致寒湿为患;同时阳黄日久,或用寒凉之药过度,损伤脾阳,湿从寒化,也可转化为阴黄。此外,因砂石、虫体阻滞胆道而发黄者，病一开始即见肝胆症状，表现也常以热为主，属于阳黄范围。积聚日久不消，瘀血阻滞胆道成黄者，多随体质寒热而转化为阴黄或阳黄。

〔辨证论治〕

一、辨证要点

(一)首先确诊是否是黄疸：目黄是诊断黄疸的主要依据。因此临床 上要做好望诊，望目睛气轮有无黄染，望全身皮肤色泽，望小便颜色。

(二)辨别黄疸的性质：主要从以下方面进行。

1. 从发病时间及病程长短来辨别：阳黄起病急，病程短；阴黄起病缓，病程长；急黄起病急骤，变化迅速。

2. 从黄疸的色泽来进行辨别：阳黄黄色鲜明，属热证实证；阴黄色晦暗或黧色，属虚证寒证；急黄身黄如金，属热毒炽盛，后期气阴耗伤，也会出现虚实夹杂之证。

(三)辨别黄疸的病势轻重：主要以观察黄疸的色泽变化为标志。

如黄疸逐渐加深，提示病势加重；黄疸逐渐浅淡，表明病情好转，黄疸色泽鲜明，神清气爽，为顺证，病轻；颜色晦滞，烦躁不宁为逆证，病重。

二、鉴别诊断

在临床上要注意阳黄与阴黄的鉴别，其鉴别要点见下表。

	阳　黄	阴　黄
病因病机	湿热为患，外感为多	寒湿阻滞，多有脾胃气虚
黄色特点	鲜明如橘子	晦暗如烟熏
证候特点	实证、热证	虚证、寒证或虚实夹杂证
病　程	短	长
病　情	除急黄外，一般多轻	多重
治　疗	清热利湿为主。从胃入手，急黄清热解毒兼以凉血	健脾温化寒湿为主。从脾入手，虚黄健脾益气养血

黄疸应与萎黄作鉴别：

(一)病因病机：黄疸的病因为感受外邪，饮食所伤，脾胃虚寒及积聚转化而发病，其病机为湿邪阻滞中焦，肝胆不能疏泄，或瘀血、虫、石等阻滞胆道，以致胆液不循常道，溢于肌肤而发黄，或脾虚血败，败血内停，不华于色而发黄。萎黄的病因为虫积食滞，导致脾土虚弱，水谷不能化生精微而生气血，或失血、病后血气亏虚，气血不足，肌肤呈黄色。

(二)主症：黄疸以目黄、身黄、小便黄为主症，随着湿热、寒湿和瘀血内阻的不同病机，黄色可出现鲜明晦暗的不同。萎黄的主症是两目和小便均不黄，肌肤呈淡黄色，干萎无光泽，且常伴有眩晕、耳鸣、心悸、少寐等症状。

三、治则要点

因为黄疸由湿得之，因此去湿利小便是治疗黄疸的基本法则，利小便为湿邪开导出路，使湿邪从小便而去，属利湿之法。利湿法主要有淡渗利湿，清热利湿，温阳利湿。治疗黄疸，祛湿退黄常用利湿、化湿和泄湿三大方法。化湿即温阳化湿、清热化湿、芳香化湿，使湿邪从中焦而化；泄湿即通腑泄湿、通瘀泄湿，使湿邪从大便泄出。临床上，根据黄疸的不同性质，而分别用不同祛湿方法。阳黄主要用清热利湿，必要时配用通腑泻下；阴黄主要用温阳化湿，有的也酌配益气养血或疏肝血等法；急黄属阳黄范围，因毒热炽盛，邪入营血，又当以清热解毒，凉营开窍法。

四、分型论治

（一）阳黄：阳黄主要有三型，但总不离湿热。

1. 热重于湿

主症：身目俱黄，黄色鲜明如橘子，有光泽，小便短少色黄。

兼症：多发热口渴，心烦，腹满，恶心欲吐，口干而苦，大便秘结。

舌脉：舌苔黄腻，脉弦数。

分析：湿热蕴蒸，胆汁外溢肌肤，因热为阳邪，故黄色鲜明。湿热内盛，热邪偏重，热耗津液故发热口渴。膀胱为湿热所扰，气化不到，故小便短少色黄。阳明热盛故大便秘结，腑气不通故腹部胀满。湿热熏蒸，胃浊和胆汁上逆，故心烦，恶心欲吐，口干而苦。舌苔黄腻，脉弦数均为肝胆脾胃湿热内盛之征。

治法：清热利湿，佐以泄下。

方药：茵陈蒿汤加味。方中茵陈为清热利湿除黄之要药，用量宜偏重，30～50g，栀子能清利三焦湿热，大黄降泄瘀热。茵陈配栀子可使湿热从小便而出，茵陈配大黄可使瘀热从大便而解。可酌加猪茯苓、车前子、滑石等渗湿之品，使湿热之邪从二便而去。恶心欲吐，心中懊憹，可加黄连、竹茹、橘皮等清火降逆止呕。右肋疼痛较甚，可加柴胡、郁金、川楝子、元胡等疏肝理气止痛。脘腹胀满，可少加枳实、厚朴或藿香、佩兰。

如因砂石内阻胆道，症见右胁疼痛，牵引肩背，或有恶寒发热，大便色淡灰白，可用大柴胡汤加茵陈、郁金、海金砂、鸡内金、金钱草以利胆排石，清热退黄。

若黄疸突然出现，时寒时热，疼痛时发时止，痛有钻顶感，呕吐蛔虫，则为虫体阻于胆道所致，可用乌梅丸合茵陈、山栀以安蛔止痛，利胆退黄。热偏重者可去附子、桂枝，少用川椒、干姜，重用黄连、黄柏；无虚象去党参、当归，一般可加川楝子、槟榔、使君子等以驱虫，行气止痛。

处方举例：

茵陈 30g、山栀子 10g、生大黄 6g、板蓝根 15g、秦艽 10g、猪苓 15g、泽泻 15g、生甘草 6g、蒲公英 15g、陈皮 10g、半夏 10g。

2. 湿重于热

主症：身目俱黄，但黄不如热重者之鲜明。

兼症：发热不扬，头重身困，口淡不渴，胸脘痞闷，食欲减退，腹胀，厌油腻，恶心欲吐，大便溏垢。

舌脉：舌苔厚腻微黄，脉弦滑或濡缓。

分析：湿遏热壅，胆汁不循常道，溢于肌肤，故身目俱黄。因湿重于热，湿为阴邪，故黄色不如热重者鲜明。湿盛故发热不扬。湿热内阻，清阳不得发越故身困头重。口淡不渴，胸脘痞闷，食减，厌油腻，恶心欲吐，腹胀便溏均为湿困脾土，脾胃功能减退所致。舌苔厚腻微黄，脉弦滑或濡缓，为湿重热轻之征。

治法：利湿化浊，佐以清热。

方药：茵陈五苓散加减。方中以茵陈为主药，以清热利湿退黄，配五苓散温阳化气利湿，使湿从小便而去；若湿热并重，可用甘露消毒丹治疗，方用黄芩、木通、滑石苦寒清热化湿，以藿香、蔻仁等芳香化浊之品以宣利气机而化湿浊。呕吐加陈皮、半夏化湿和胃降逆；灼腹胀加木香，大腹皮等下气消胀。

阳黄初起见表证者，宜先用麻黄连翘赤小豆汤以解表消热利湿。若湿热不得透泄，发热不退者，可加用栀子柏皮汤以增强泄热利湿作用。若在阳黄病程中见阳明热盛，灼伤津液，积滞成实，大便不通，宜用大黄硝石汤以泄热去实，急下存阴。

处方举例：

茵陈 30g、猪苓 15g、茯苓 15g、白术 10g、泽泻 10g、半夏 10g、陈皮 10g、竹茹 10g、白蔻 6g、藿香 10g、大腹皮 10g。

3. 毒热炽盛(急黄)

主症：发病急骤，黄疸迅速加深，其色如金。

兼症：高热烦渴，胁痛腹满，神昏谵语，或见衄血、便血，或肌肤出现瘀斑，舌质红绛。

舌脉：舌质红绛，苔黄而燥，脉弦滑数或细数。

分析：湿热夹毒，热毒炽盛，故发病迅速，高热口渴，热毒迫使胆汁外溢肌肤，则黄疸迅速加深，身目俱黄，其色如金。热毒内盛，气机失调则胁痛腹满；热毒迫血妄行，则见衄血便血，或肌肤出现瘀斑。舌质红绛，苔黄而燥脉，弦滑数或细数为肝胆热毒内盛之象。

治法：清热解毒，凉血开窍。

方药：犀角散加味。方中犀角为解毒凉血之要药，配黄连、栀子、升麻则清热解毒力更大，茵陈清热退黄，可酌情加用大青叶、银花、连翘等清热解毒，生地、丹皮、玄参、石斛等药以增加清热凉血之力。

加减：神昏谵语可配服安宫牛黄丸或至宝丹以凉开透窍；如衄血、便血或肌肤瘀斑重者，可酌加地榆炭、柏叶炭凉血止血之品；如小便短少不利，或出现腹水者，可加木通、白茅根、车前草、大腹皮等清热利尿之品。

处方举例：

犀角粉 1.5g(分冲)、黄连 6g、山栀子 10g、茵陈 45g、大青叶 10g、银花 10g、连翘 15g、生地 15g、丹皮 10g、元参 15g。

(二)阴黄

1. 寒湿阻遏

主症：色黄晦暗如烟熏。

兼症：神疲畏寒，食少纳呆，脘闷腹满，大便不实，口淡不渴。

舌脉：舌质淡，苔白腻，脉濡缓或沉迟。

分析：寒湿阻滞脾胃，阳气不宣，胆汁外溢，因寒湿为阴邪，故黄色晦暗，或如烟熏。湿困脾土，脾阳不振，运化功能失常则见纳少、脘闷、腹胀、大便不实、口淡不渴等症。阳所不足，气血亦虚故畏寒神疲。舌淡苔腻，脉濡缓或沉迟，多阳虚湿浊不化，寒湿留于阴分之象。

治法：健脾和胃，温化寒湿。

方药：茵陈术附汤加味。方中茵陈、附子温化寒湿而退黄，白术、干姜、甘草健脾温中，并可加郁金、川朴、茯苓、泽泻等行气利湿之品。

加减：若腹胀苔厚者，去白术、甘草，加苍术、厚朴以燥湿消胀；皮肤搔痒者加秦艽、地肤子祛风止痒。

处方举例：

茵陈 30g、制附片 6g、白术 10g、干姜 10g、半夏 10g、陈皮 10g、茯苓 15g、川朴 10g、木香 10g、白蔻 6g、苍术 10g。

2. 瘀血停积

主症：身目发黄而晦暗。

兼症：皮肤可见蛛纹丝缕，面色青紫晦滞，胁下有癥块且疼痛不舒，固定不移，大便偏黑。

舌脉：舌质青紫或瘀斑，脉弦涩或细涩。

分析：瘀血停积，胆汁运行受阻，故身目发黄。瘀血内阻，新血不能营养头面，故面色青紫晦暗。瘀血留滞于胁下，气血流通受阻，故胁有癥块而疼痛，皮肤有蛛纹丝缕。便黑及舌脉变化均为瘀血之征。

治法：活血化瘀退黄。

方药：膈下逐瘀汤加减。方中桃仁、红花、牡丹皮、五灵脂活血化瘀，当归、川芎养血行血，元胡、乌药、香附行气活血止疼，并宜加用茵陈退黄。或服用硝石矾石散以化浊祛瘀软坚，并可配服逍遥散以疏肝扶脾。若脾虚明显者可配合香砂六君子汤以健脾和胃。若黄疸日久不退，两胁下痞块明显，湿浊蕴聚，可成积聚或臌胀。

处方举例：

全当归 10g、川芎 10g、赤白芍各 10g、桃仁 10g、红花 6g、丹皮 10g、茜草 10g、茵陈 30g、生蒲黄（包煎）10g、制香附 10g、郁金 15g。

3. 脾虚血亏（虚黄）

主症：面目、肌肤发黄，色淡无华，小便赤黄，或以夜间为著。

兼症：神疲乏力，四肢酸软，心悸气短，纳呆便溏，懒言声怯，夜寐不安。

舌脉：舌质淡，苔薄白，脉细弱。

分析：脾胃虚弱，运化无权，气血化源不充，血败而不华色，不能荣养内外，故面目肌肤发黄，色淡而少光泽，小便黄赤，或以夜间为著。脾气不足则神疲乏力，四肢酸软，气短懒言。血虚则不能养心，心神不宁则心悸，夜寐不安。脾虚运迟则纳呆便溏。舌淡苔薄白，脉细弱，也是脾虚血亏之征象。

治法：健脾温中，补养气血。

方药：小建中汤加味。方中桂枝宜蜜炙，以健脾温中，配合姜枣辛甘相合而生阳；白芍滋养阴血，与甘草同用酸甘化阴。桂枝、白芍相伍调和阴阳，中州化源充盛；饴糖缓中健脾。从而使脾胃健旺，气血滋生，黄疸得以消退。若气虚明显时，可加黄芪、党参；血虚明显时，可加当归、地黄、阿胶、旱莲草等；阳虚明显时，桂枝改为肉桂，也可加干姜等。

处方举例：

炙桂枝 10g、白芍 12g、炙甘草 10g、生姜 3 片、大枣 7 枚、饴糖 30g（烊化冲）、炙黄芪 20g、全当归 10g、阿胶 10g（烊化）、旱莲草 10g、党参 10g。

附：萎黄

萎黄一证，与黄疸有所不同，其主要症状为两目不黄，周身肌肤呈淡黄色，干萎无光泽，小便通畅而色不黄，倦怠乏力，眩晕耳鸣，心悸少寐，大便溏薄，舌淡苔薄，脉象濡细。

本病是由于虫积食滞导致脾胃虚弱，水谷不能化精微而生气血，气血衰少，既不能滋润皮肌肌肉，又不能营养脏腑，以致肌肤萎黄无光泽。此外，失血过多，或大病之后，血亏气耗，以致气血不足而发本病，临床亦属常见。

治疗上主要是调理脾胃，益气补血，可选用黄芪建中汤或人参养营汤之类。由钩虫病引起者，还应给予驱虫治疗。

〔预防及护理措施〕

1. 注意休息，黄疸未退以卧床为主。

2. 饮食有节，忌油腻、海腥发物及辛辣刺激性食物。禁饮酒。

3. 有传染性者，应注意隔离，防止毒邪外传。

4. 精神乐观，情绪稳定，积极配合治疗。

〔典型病例分析〕

案一：雷某某，女，20岁，工人。

4个月以前，始发热恶寒，恶心呕吐，不思饮食，口苦而干，渐至身目、小便皆黄如橘色，经某医院诊为“急性传染性肝炎”，住院四个月，给予栀子、黄柏、龙胆草等苦寒之品，黄疸稍退，但腹胀，乏力，体瘦，遂来门诊求治。

刻下：面色萎黄，体瘦，神疲畏寒，两胁胀痛，腹胀痞满，目微黄，大便稀溏，舌苔白腻，脉左关弦大，右关沉迟无力。

理化检查：麝香草酚浊度试验：15u，麝香草酚絮状试验：＋＋＋，谷丙转氨酶：300u。

中医诊断：黄疸（肝气乘脾，寒湿阻遏）。

治则：健脾疏肝，温中和胃，佐以利湿。

处方：党参12g、白术12g、云苓12g、陈皮9g、良姜9g、生山药12g、砂仁6g、茵陈10g、橘叶9g、白芍12g、玄胡12g、甘草5g。

二诊：上方服10余剂，症状显著减轻，黄疸消失。此后，以健脾和胃疏肝之法，调理三个月，复查肝功能四次，渐次正常。

按：本病由阳黄过服苦寒之品，损伤脾阳，迁延日久所致。辨证属肝气乘脾、寒湿阻遏之阴黄，治当健脾疏肝，温中和胃，佐以利湿。药用茵陈主黄疸而利湿，良姜、砂仁温中散寒，白芍、玄胡、橘叶舒肝理气止痛，诸药合用共奏健脾疏肝、和胃利湿之效而使症减。黄疸退后，继用健脾和胃、疏肝之法调理三个月而病愈。（《许玉山医案》）。

黄疸一病，以目黄、身黄，小便黄为特征。目睛气轮色黄是诊断本病的关键。其发病总与感受外邪、饮食不节、脾胃虚寒、瘀血、砂石、虫体阻滞胆道和内伤不足有关。但主要的是湿邪为患，多侵犯肝胆脾胃诸脏腑。

临床上要注意鉴别阳黄与阴黄、虚黄与萎黄。阳黄与阴黄均以湿邪为患，阳黄属实证、热证，阴黄属虚证、寒证或虚实夹杂证。但阳黄与阴黄之间不是绝对的，可以相互转化。虚黄与萎黄皆属虚证，虚黄以目黄、身黄、小便黄为主症，萎黄两目和小便均不黄，可供鉴别。

治疗上去湿利小便是治疗本病的重要原则。可根据黄疸的性质加配清化或温化，以及泄下及健脾养血、活血等剂。凡病之初起，治疗及时而恰当者，预后良好。若迁延日久，反复发作，气滞血瘀，胁下癥块，正虚邪实者，多缠绵难治。急黄者是黄疸危候，应积极抢救。黄疸消退后，不可骤然停药，应根据病证，适当服用调理脾胃之品以做善后。

复习思考题

1. 黄疸的概念是什么？以哪一症状为黄疸的主要特征？
2. 临床上目前如何对黄疸进行分类？
3. 虚黄与萎黄如何区别？
4. 黄疸的病机变化与哪种邪气关系最密切？与哪些脏腑有关？
5. 试述阳黄、急黄、阴黄的证治规律。

积　聚

〔概述〕

积聚是腹内结块，或胀或痛的病证。积和聚在病情轻重与病机变化上不尽相同，积者有形，固定不移，胀、痛均有定处，病属血分，乃为脏病；聚者无形，聚散无常，胀、痛均无定处，病属气分，乃为腑病。

一般说，聚病较轻，为时尚暂，故易治。积病较重，为时较久，积而成块，故难治。

在文献中，又有癥瘕之名，大抵属于积聚之类，积与癥、聚与瘕均为同一类疾病。此外，文献记载的"癖块"、"痃癖"、"痞块"，按其病机与症状，均可归入积聚的范围。

西医学的胃肠功能紊乱、不完全性肠梗阻、幽门梗阻、肝脾肿大、内脏下垂、肠结核、腹腔肿痛等，均可参考本证进行辨证论治。

〔病因病机〕

积聚的发生，有一逐渐发生、发展的过程，多因情志不遂，饮食所伤，淫邪所客以及病后体虚，或黄疸、胁痛、疟疾等证失治、误治而致经久不愈，引起肝脾受损，脏腑失和，气机阻滞，瘀血内停，或兼痰湿凝滞，而成积聚。积聚的发生主要关系到肝、脾两脏。一般而言，聚证以气机阻滞为主；积证以瘀血凝滞为主，但两者都可兼挟痰湿。气血相关，气滞日久，可致血瘀，瘀血不消，亦必阻滞气机。故积与聚既有区别，亦有联系，聚证延久，常致积证；积证不化，每多胀痛，积、聚同病。另外积聚日久，肝脾功能障碍，则可导致正气亏虚。故本证一般初病多实，久病多虚，或虚实夹杂。兹就其病因病机分述如下：

一、情志不遂，气滞血瘀：忧思恼怒，肝脾受损。肝伤则气机不畅，气为血帅，气滞日久则致血脉瘀阻，日积月累，气血凝滞，而成积聚；脾伤则运化失司，水谷不化精微而成痰浊，痰浊阻塞血脉，则血液行涩，痰瘀互结，搏于腹中则致积聚。

二、饮食不节，滋生痰浊：由于饮酒太过，或嗜食肥甘厚味，煎炸辛辣之品；或饮食无制，饥饱不调，起居无常，使脾胃受损，运化之职失司，以致湿浊内生，凝结成痰。痰阻气机，气血失和，气、血、痰互相搏结，阻于腹中，结成积聚。

三、邪气所客，留着不去：寒邪或湿热等外邪侵犯机体，客于腹中，留而不散，蓄久成聚，聚之致积。

四、黄疸、胁痛、疟疾、感染血吸虫等，每因湿浊蕴结，气血不和，导致肝脾不和，气滞、血瘀、痰凝相互影响，胶结不化，搏结腹部而成积聚。

总之，本病证的病因虽多，但其病位主要责之肝、脾，病理变化与气滞、血瘀、痰凝三者密切相关。同时，本病证的形成与正气的强弱也有密切关系。一般初病，多以气滞、湿阻、血瘀为患;久病,多为痰瘀互结、正气亏虚为害。若肝脾统藏失职,或瘀热灼伤血络,可致出血;若湿热蕴积中焦,熏蒸肝胆,可出现黄疸;如水湿停留,则可出现腹满水肿等症。

〔辨证论治〕

积聚之证,起病多缓,发展亦慢,且与黄疸、胁痛、疟疾、虫证、臌胀等证互相联系,互相转化。就积聚本身而言,初病为聚,尚属无形,延久成积,病已成形,两者亦难绝对分开,故每以积聚并称。临证时应根据病史长短、证候特点、病理变化,宜将其分为初、中、末三期进行辨证施行。在辨证时,宜辨其偏于气滞,或偏于血瘀,或偏于湿阻、食积,或偏于痰凝,或偏于正虚。并应结合积聚部位,或在腹,或在胁下确定病位,从脏腑特点予以考虑。

一、辨证要点

(1)辨初、中、晚三期:积聚初起,肝脾同病,每致气滞、血瘀、湿阻停积。停积于腹部,脾胃所属,以气滞、食积、湿阻为主;停积于胁下,肝脾所属,以气滞、血瘀为主。病至中期,气滞血瘀,湿聚成痰,气、血、痰三者凝结成块,亦可结于腹中或结于胁下。病至晚期,邪势未衰,正气已伤,正虚邪恋,为本虚标实之证。

(二)辨在气、在血,属湿、属痰、属虚:本病证之初,多先见气滞,以胀痛为主,时聚时散,病无定处。病久入络,症见血瘀,痛有定处,触有包块,质地多硬。脾病易生湿浊,脘腹痞闷,纳呆便溏,面色晦暗,肢体疲困。湿聚日久,凝结成痰,或咯吐可见,或肿胀有形,质地钝厚,触之活动。邪气羁留日久,正气耗伤,或气阴虚,或气血虚,或阳气虚,表现有异。

积聚病因病机示意图

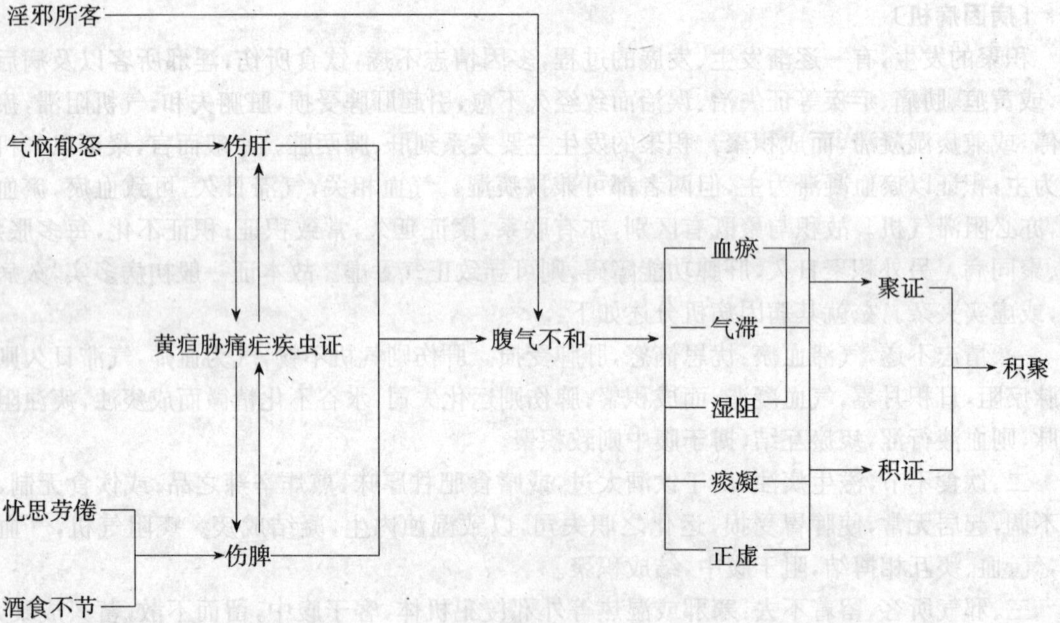

二、积聚与痞证、臌胀的鉴别

积聚以腹内有结块,或胀或痛为特点,聚者聚则成形,散则无迹;积者有形可循,长久不消。

痞证为患者自觉脘腹堵闷不舒,始终无形迹可及。痞虽有虚实之分,当以食前、食后测之,食前饥时痞满者为虚,食后饱时痞满者为实。

臌胀以腹胀大，皮色苍黄，腹皮脉络暴露为特征。臌胀虽有气臌、血臌、水臌、虫蛊之分，总以腹中有振水声，或腹部按之如囊裹水所独具，并且每为积聚失治、误治后演变而成。

三、治则要点

（一）根据积聚在临床上变化规律，其初起常以气滞、食积、血瘀、湿阻为患，治当宜行气、消导、活血、化湿为主；中期常以气结、血瘀、痰凝为患，治当宜行气、化瘀、消痰为主；晚期常见邪盛正衰，治当宜扶正祛邪，攻补兼施为法。

（二）积聚日久，损伤气血，故在治疗上要始终注意保护正气，攻伐之药用之不宜太过，以免伤正。

（三）聚轻而积重。聚证病在气分，治重调气；积证病在血分，治重活血。聚证之时当抓紧治疗，尚易取效，由聚成积，终属难治。

四、分型证治

（一）初期

主症：腹中胀痛，气聚攻窜，可随情绪变化而聚散。

兼症：纳呆恶心，甚则呕吐痰涎，便秘行涩，或胁下胀闷不舒。

舌脉：舌质黯，苔白腻，脉象弦滑。

分析：气血不和，运行滞涩，结于腹中，故腹中胀痛，气聚攻窜。情志不遂则气机不利，故症情加重，情志舒畅则气通而散。肝脾俱伤，运化失司，湿浊内生，阻碍气机升降，故纳呆恶心，甚则呕吐痰涎，便秘行涩，或见胁下胀闷不舒。气血不畅，则舌黯；湿浊内停则苔腻；脉象弦滑，亦为肝脾不和之象。

治法：理气活血，化湿消聚。

方药：木香顺气散加减。方中诸多理气药，疏理上中下三焦气机。枳壳偏上焦，木香、陈皮、青皮偏中焦，川楝子、乌药偏下焦，气机转动，则胀痛得消，气聚能散。川芎为血中气药，香附为气中血药，两者相合，调和气血。砂仁、苍术化湿醒脾。少佐肉桂辛热助通，能使聚消痛止。若胁下胀闷较重，为肝气郁结较甚，也可加柴胡、赤芍、郁金或片姜黄，以加强疏肝理气之力，或以柴胡疏肝散化裁为治。若呕吐痰涎较多，为痰饮不化，可合小半夏加茯苓汤，或合苓桂术甘汤为治；痰饮化热，可合甘遂半夏汤为治。若口干而苦，舌边尖红，苔薄黄而腻，加左金丸以泄肝清热。若食滞、湿阻，腑气不通，也可选用六磨饮，方以大黄、枳实、槟榔化滞通腑；沉香、木香、乌药通利气机。若挟痰浊阻滞，也可配合用半夏厚朴汤治之，方中厚朴、紫苏行气宽中，半夏、茯苓化痰散结，则瘕聚可散。若病情迁延，瘀血明显，舌黯而有瘀斑，也可与失笑散化裁为治。若病程日久，肝旺脾虚，神疲便溏，也可加党参、白术以益气补脾。

处方举例：

炒枳壳 10g、广木香 10g、青陈皮各 6g、乌药 10g、川芎 10g、制香附 10g、清半夏 10g、苍术 10g、砂仁 3g、厚朴 10g、炒赤芍 12g。

（二）中期

主症：腹中积块，固定不移，胀痛有定处。

兼症：面黯形瘦，纳少痰黏，时有寒热，肌肤甲错，女子或有经闭。

舌脉：舌青紫，或有瘀斑，苔腻，脉弦滑或细涩。

分析：气聚日久，渐成积证，气滞、血瘀、痰凝结于腹中，故腹中积块，固定不移，胀痛有定处。肝脾不和，气血行涩，运化失健，化源不充，故面黯形瘦，纳少痰黏，肌肤甲错。气结血瘀，营卫失和，故时有寒热。肝郁血瘀，则女子经闭。舌青紫而有瘀斑，脉细涩均为血瘀气结之象。苔腻为痰浊内停；脉弦滑则为肝脾不和之征。

治法：行气活血，化痰消积。

方药：膈下逐瘀汤加减。方中桃红四物汤去生地，加丹皮，增强养血活血、散结消积之力；五灵脂去瘀止痛，枳壳、乌药调理气机；香附、延胡索入血行气以止痛，使气行则血行，以助祛瘀之力；并可加半夏、土贝母、橘红、茯苓、三棱、莪术，增强化痰消积之功。

若积聚兼见寒热、身痛、苔白、脉浮等症，乃外有风寒之邪，宜予宣表理气，通滞消积。可用五积散，本方汇集解表、散寒、祛湿、化痰、行气、利水、活血、通络、温中、止痛之药于一炉，对于积聚初起又兼外感，气机不利所导致的表里同病，多样病邪阻于腹中的证候，能使其表里同治，诸邪得以消散，对于积聚而病机比较复杂者，尤为适宜。

若气滞血阻较甚，兼有寒象者，也可用大七气汤，方中青皮、陈皮、桔梗、香附、藿香行气散结，桂心、三棱、莪术温通血络，软坚散结。

若积块坚硬作痛拒按，可吞服鳖甲煎丸以化瘀软坚止痛；若妇女经闭不行，肌肤甲错，可吞服大黄䗪虫丸以破瘀消积通经。以上二方，可与六君子汤间服，以补益脾胃之气，为攻补兼施之法。在此阶段，气结血瘀痰凝较重，积块肿大渐增，坚硬、疼痛者，还可以用虫类破瘀消积之品，如䗪虫、鼠妇、蛴螬、鳖甲、牡蛎、海藻等治之，以增加疗效。

若积块肿大，灼热作痛，舌红、苔黄，也可加用清热解毒药，如连翘、蒲公英、半枝莲、白英、白花蛇舌草等，也有积极意义。痰浊较重，可加生苡仁、瓜蒌、土贝母、半夏、黄药子等消痰散结之品。

处方举例：

全当归 10g、赤白芍各 10g、川芎 10g、桃仁 10g、草红花 6g、三棱 6g、莪术 6g、青陈皮各 10g、丹皮 10g、土贝母 10g、清半夏 10g、茯苓 15g。

(三)晚期

主症：积块坚硬，长久不消，疼痛逐渐加剧，正气渐衰。

兼症：面色萎黄或黧黑，饮食锐减，肌肉瘦削，神疲肢怠，口舌干燥，五心烦热，或心悸不宁，少寐多梦，或畏寒肢冷，便溏溲清。

舌脉：舌体瘦、嫩红少苔，有瘀点，舌淡紫而胖，苔薄腻，脉象弦细或沉细。

分析：积块日久，痰瘀阻滞，故坚硬渐增，长久不消，疼痛日益加剧。中气大伤，运化无权，故饮食锐减，形体瘦削，神疲肢怠。若气阴两虚，故见口舌干燥，五心烦热；若气血俱虚，故见心悸不宁，少寐多梦；若阳气已衰，故见畏寒肢冷，便溏溲清。舌体瘦、嫩红少苔，有瘀点，脉弦细为气阴两虚夹瘀之象；舌淡紫而胖，苔薄腻，脉沉细，为气血俱虚或阳气大衰而夹瘀之征。

治法：扶正祛邪。

方药：八珍汤合化积丸化裁。前方用四君、四物以大补气血；后方用香附、苏木、五灵脂理气化瘀；用三棱、莪术、阿魏、海浮石等软坚散结。两方合用，扶正祛邪，标本兼顾。

若气阴两虚，而见虚火明显时，可将八珍汤易为益胃汤加太子参、黄精等益气养阴。若阳气已衰，阴寒内生，可合附子理中汤化裁为治，增强温中健脾之力。若脾弱胃强，脾寒胃热，口苦苔黄，便溏脉弱时，也可用半夏泻心汤或温脾汤化裁，进行调治。若久病及肾，阴阳两虚，腰膝酸软，头晕目眩，畏寒蜷卧者，当阴阳双补，选用补天大造丸与化积丸，交替服用。

积证不论病程长短，均可配合外治法，目前临床上一般采用阿魏膏或水红花膏，有助于消积散瘀。

处方举例：

人参粉 3g(冲)、茯苓 10g、炒白术 10g、全当归 10g、赤白芍各 10g、川芎 10g、三棱 6g、莪术 6、制香附 10g、炒五灵脂 10g、生蒲黄(包煎)10g、三七粉 3g(分冲)。

〔预防及护理措施〕

1. 情绪稳定，戒烦躁，忌忧郁，禁恼怒。

2. 饮食有节，禁食辛辣，肥甘厚味，煎炸之品，不饮酒。

3. 注意个人及户外卫生，以防外邪内侵。

4. 积极治疗黄疸、胁痛、癥瘕、血吸虫等病。

〔典型病例分析〕

案一：陆某某，女，40 岁，1976 年 7 月 7 日初诊。

患者几个月前忽然发现左小腹长出一小包块，并逐渐胀大，现已有鸡蛋大小。刻下症见：乏力，动则气短不续，两胁及小腹两侧胀痛，饮食甚少，大便稀溏，一日二三次，频频嗳气，自汗怕冷，舌淡少苔，脉弦细。

中医诊断：癥瘕(肝郁脾虚)。

治则：疏肝理气，温阳健脾。

方药：

柴胡 9g、白芍 12g、枳壳 9g、香附 9g、党参 9g、白术 9g、茯苓 9g、小茴香 6g、厚朴 9g、木香 6g、金铃炭 12g、甘草 3g。

二诊：上方服四剂后，嗳气减轻，饮食增加，时转矢气，上方加荔枝核、橘核。

三诊：八剂后，左小腹包块全部散去，自觉全身有力，以后又继服数剂，饮食渐正常，无短气、自汗、怕冷等感觉，以后随访未再发作。

按：本病腹部包块属癥瘕范畴，辨证属肝气乘脾，肝郁脾虚，治宜疏肝理气，温阳健脾，治当用柴胡、白芍、枳壳、香附、金铃炭疏肝理气，用党参、白术、茯苓、甘草补脾，用小茴香、厚朴、木香以温通少腹，并酌加荔枝核、橘核以增强驱散少腹包块之力，诸药协同，使肝郁得解，脾虚得健而使病去。(《李斯炽医案》)。

积聚是指腹内出现结块，或胀或痛的一种疾病。积者有形，固定不移，疼痛有一定之部位；聚者无形，聚散无常，疼痛没有固定的部位。形成积聚的病因主要归之于情志不遂，饮食不节，邪气客居，以及黄疸、胁痛、疟疾，感染血吸虫等。其发病主因气滞、血瘀、痰结所致，而正气亏虚则是其发病的内在因素。

临床上应注意本病与痞证、臌胀之鉴别。痞证以患者自觉脘腹堵闷不舒，始终无形迹可及为特征。臌胀则以腹胀大，皮色苍黄，腹皮脉络暴露为特征，并且每为积聚失治、误治后演变而成。

治疗上，聚证以理气为主，积证以理血为主，并分早、中、末三期分而治之。临证时常用化瘀散结的药物，以消除其实。但积聚形成，正气必虚，往往虚中挟实，实中挟虚，因此治实应当照顾虚的一面，补虚应当注意实的一面。如果需要用攻法，则不可滥用攻伐的药物，否则积聚虽然渐消，但脾胃损伤，正气衰惫，反而引起严重后果。所以，治疗中必须正确处理“正”与“邪”，“攻”与“补”之间的关系。或先攻后补，或先补后攻，或寓补于攻，或寓攻于补，随证施治，灵活运用，使正气渐复，邪气渐衰，促进疾病向好的方面转化。

复习思考题

1. 积聚的概念是什么？它和癥有什么关系？

2. 积聚的病机关键是什么？与哪些脏腑关系最密切？

3. 试述积聚证治规律。

4. 试述积聚与黄疸、胁痛、臌胀等病证的关系。

臌　胀

〔概述〕

臌胀是以腹部胀大如鼓，或腹部中空外急，击之如鼓而得名。临床上以腹胀大，皮色苍黄，腹皮青筋暴露，胁下或腹部痞块，四肢枯瘦为特征。本病在古代文献中名称繁多，如水蛊、蛊胀、膨脝、蜘蛛蛊、单腹胀等。前人根据其病因、病机及临床表现分为气臌、血臌、水臌、虫臌等。本病反复迁延，久治难愈，晚期可见吐血，便血，昏迷等症。

西医的肝硬化腹水主要见于本病。此外，结核性腹膜炎、腹腔内肿瘤等病而出现腹水，类似臌胀的证候时，可参考本篇进行辨证施治。

〔病因病机〕

臌胀的发生，其来势缓慢，故致病之因虽与酒食不节、情志所伤、血吸虫感染等有关，但它的直接原因，当责之于黄疸、胁痛、积聚等病证失治、误治之后，迁延日久，使肝、脾、肾三脏功能失调，气、血、水瘀积于腹内，以致腹部日渐胀大，而成臌胀。

一、直接原因

黄疸、胁痛、积聚等病迁延日久，而成臌胀。

黄疸的病理变化以阳黄、阴黄二者为多，阳黄总因湿热及湿热夹毒阻滞中焦，而致气机升降失常，肝脾不调。阴黄是由寒湿阻遏或瘀血内停，或脾虚血亏所致。寒湿阻遏或瘀血内停，均使中焦气机升降枢纽失常，湿浊不化，而致肝脾俱伤。脾虚血亏，运化失职，而致湿浊内主，气机失调，亦致肝脾俱损。肝脾俱伤，若治疗不当，迁延日久，伤及于肾，肾失开合，水湿内停，气、血、水互结，终成臌胀。

胁痛的病机可归纳为瘀血停着，肝气郁结，肝胆湿热及肝阴不足。前三者可致肝失疏泄，气机不畅，日久肝气犯脾，脾失健运，湿浊内生，若治不及时，累及于肾，终至肝、脾、肾俱伤，气、血、水互结而成臌胀。肝阴不足，一方面，肝脉失养，络脉不和，气机不利，进一步犯脾而致肝脾不调；另一方面，肝阴伤日久伤及肾阴，肝肾阴虚，若治疗不当，最终亦致肝、脾、肾俱伤，气、血、水互结而生臌胀。

积聚的主要病理表现是肝脾受损，脏腑失和，气机阻滞，瘀血内停，或兼痰湿凝滞，食积内阻，若治疗失宜，迁延日久，病及于肾，肾开合不利，水湿内停，最终气、血、水互结而成臌胀。

二、诱发原因

(一)情志不遂：忧思恼怒，肝失调达，气阻络痹而致胁痛；肝伤气滞日久，则致血脉瘀阻，日积月累，气血凝滞，而成积聚。胁痛、积聚迁延日久则成臌胀。

(二)饮食不节：由于饮酒太过，或嗜食肥甘厚味，使脾胃受损，运化失职，湿浊内生，湿邪阻滞中焦，胆汁被阻不循常道，浸淫肌肤而发黄疸。此外，湿浊内生，凝结成痰，痰阻气机，气血失和，气、血、痰互相搏结，阻于腹中，结成积聚。黄疸、胁痛迁延日久可成臌胀。

（三）血吸虫感染：虫阻脉道，肝脾气血失和，脾伤运化失健而致痰浊内生，日久，气滞、血瘀、痰凝互相影响，胶结不化，搏结腹部而成积聚，积聚日久又可发为臌胀。

在臌胀形成之后，若不注意调畅情志，注意饮食，或复感血吸虫，则可使臌胀进一步加重。

在臌胀形成过程中，气滞、血瘀、水停互为因果，是邪实的主要内容。正虚是气滞、血瘀、水停发展的必然趋势。所涉及的脏腑主要是肝、脾、肾。其病的性质是实中夹虚，虚中有实，虚实挟杂，而形成本虚标实之证。

〔辨证论治〕

一、辨证要点

臌胀为本虚标实之证，其标实又有气滞、血瘀、水停的侧重，而本虚也有脾气虚、气阴两虚、脾阳虚、脾肾两虚、肝肾阴虚的不同。因此，其主症虽然都以腹大如鼓，胀满不适为主，但临床表现尚有差异。偏于气滞，兼症常有两胁胀满，善太息，嗳气，或得矢气后腹胀稍缓，口苦脉弦等；偏于血瘀，兼症常有四肢消瘦，腹皮脉络显露，胁下或腹部痞块，面色黧黑，面颊、胸臂血痣或血缕，肌肤甲错不润，朱砂掌，唇及爪甲色黯舌边尖瘀点，瘀斑等；偏于水停，兼症常有腹胀之形，如囊裹水，或腹中有振水音，周身困乏无力，溲少便溏等；偏于脾气虚，兼症常有面色萎黄，神疲乏力，纳少不香，舌淡，脉缓等；偏于气阴两虚，兼症除有脾气虚的症状外，还可见口干不欲饮，知饥而不能纳，形体消瘦，五心烦热，肌肤槁热，舌红舌体瘦少津等；偏于脾阳虚，兼症常有面色苍黄，畏寒肢冷，大便溏薄，舌淡体胖，脉沉细无力等；偏于脾肾阳虚，兼症除有脾阳虚证外，还可见腰膝冷痛，男子阴囊湿冷，阳痿早泄，女子月经衍期，量少色淡等；偏于肝肾阴虚，兼症常有头晕耳鸣，腰膝痠软，心烦少寐，颧红烘热，齿鼻衄血，舌红少苔，脉弦而细等。

二、臌胀与水肿的鉴别

臌胀与水肿的晚期鉴别甚难，早期尚能鉴别清楚。现将臌胀、水肿早期的鉴别归纳如下。

病名 区别	鼓　　胀	水　　肿
肿　　胀	腹大坚满，四肢不肿或枯瘦	颜面、四肢肿胀，腹平而软
兼　　症	腹皮脉络显露，颈，胸血痣，吐血，便血，黄疸，发热，烦躁，神昏	胸闷，心悸，气喘，恶心，呕吐，烦躁，嗜睡
病　　位	肝、脾、肾	肺、脾、肾
病　　机	气滞、血瘀、水停、正虚互结于腹	水湿泛滥，溢于肌肤
治　　则	理气消胀，活血化瘀，利湿逐水，扶正固本	发汗、利尿，攻逐、健脾、温肾，化瘀
常用方剂	木香顺气丸，中满分消丸，调营饮	越婢加术汤，疏凿饮子，五苓散，参苓白术散

三、治则要点

对于臌胀的治疗，应按照气滞、血瘀、水停、正虚的不同侧重，在理气消胀、活血化瘀、利尿逐水、扶正培本诸法中化裁，早期以祛邪为主，中期和晚期均宜攻补兼施，中期以利水消胀为目的，晚期以防治严重兼症为重点。

四、分型证治

臌胀的证治，根据病程和正邪关系，分为初期、中期、晚期。一般发病初期，多肝脾失调，气滞、血瘀、湿阻互结于腹；由于初期失治误治，正气渐伤，转入中期，正虚而邪盛；至晚期，正气渐衰，各种严重兼症相继出现，病理变化错综复杂。

臌胀病因病机示意图

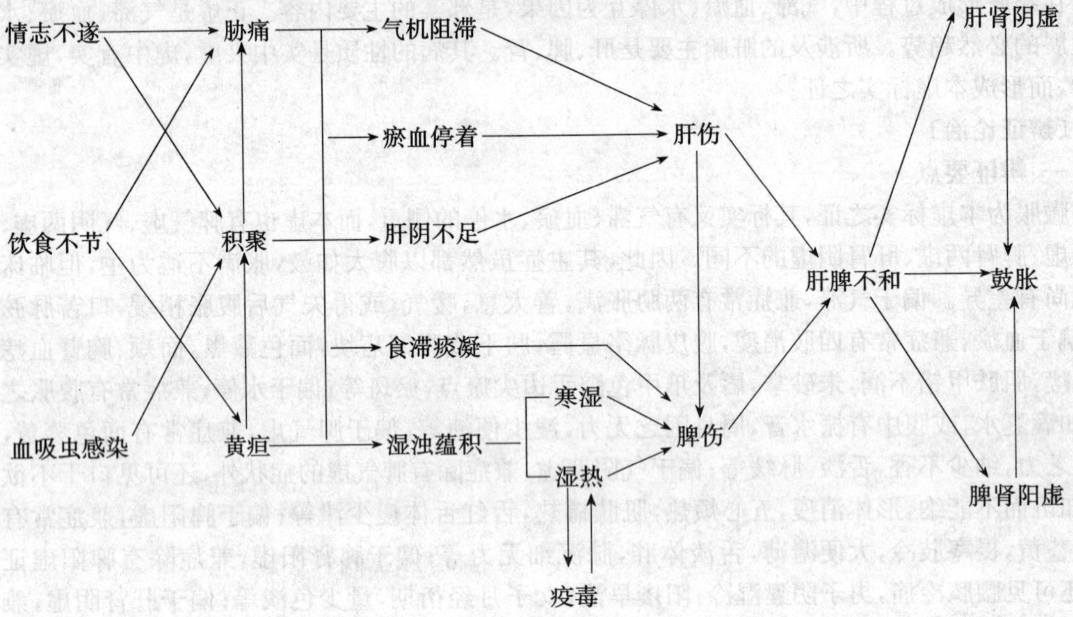

(一)早期证治

主症：腹大胀满，叩之如鼓，持久不减。

兼症：胁下胀满或疼痛，纳少不香，食后脘腹胀满益甚，以嗳气或矢气为快，肢体沉困乏力，小便短少。

舌脉：舌质黯，或有瘀点，苔白腻，脉弦滑。

分析：黄疸、胁痛、积聚等病证失治或误治，以致肝脾不和。肝气郁滞，脾运不健，使气滞不畅，血脉瘀阻，湿浊停留而充塞于腹中，故腹大胀满。因气滞血瘀偏重而湿浊尚轻，故腹胀而叩之如鼓。由于病之根深势笃，故持久不减。肝失条达，经气痹阻，故胁下胀或疼痛。脾胃不健，纳运失司，故纳少不馨，食后脘腹胀满益甚，嗳气或矢气后气机稍动，故自觉为快。气壅湿阻，水道不利，故肢体沉困乏力，小便短少。舌黯或有瘀点，苔白腻，脉弦滑，也是气血瘀滞，湿浊蕴积之征。

治法：理气和血，行湿散满。

方药：以木香顺气散为主方。方中枳壳、木香、青皮、陈皮、川朴、乌药上中下三焦气机一起疏理，再配合香附、川芎、桂心气血并调，以期气血调畅而消腹胀；苍术、砂仁理脾行湿以散满；甘草和中。

假若胁下胀满或疼痛明显时，可加柴胡、郁金、延胡索、苏木等疏肝理气止痛之品。若胁下痞块，痛如针刺，可加赤芍、丹参、三棱、莪术、生牡蛎等活血行瘀、软坚散结之品。若纳食少馨，食后腹脘胀满，可加保和丸或越鞠保和丸包煎，以消食导滞。若肢体沉困，小便短小，可加车前子、泽泻、猪苓、茯苓等化湿利水药物。若腹胀明显时，也可加黑白丑、大腹皮、莱菔子、薤白等以下气除满消痞。

处方举例：

炒枳壳10g、木香10g、青皮6g、陈皮10g、厚朴10g、台乌药10g、制香附10g、川芎6g、苍术10g、砂仁3g、大腹皮子各10g。

（二）中期证治

主症：腹大坚满、撑急，动之有振水声，或按之凹陷。

兼症：面色苍黄无华，神疲肢怠，脘腹痞胀，不敢进食，口渴不欲饮，颈部、面颊或胸背部散在红痣血缕，腹皮脉络怒张，手掌赤痕，大便或秘或溏，小便短少。

舌脉：舌质淡胖，有齿痕，或紫黯，或有瘀斑，舌苔厚腻，脉细滑。

分析：臌胀迁延，气、血、水蓄积腹中日趋严重，故腹大坚满撑急，昼夜不休，痛楚难忍；水湿停蓄腹中，故动之有振水声，或按之凹陷。病邪之羁，肝脾肾败伤，故面色苍黄无华，神疲肢怠。脾胃不运，气机转枢不利，则脘腹痞胀，不敢进食，进食则痞胀益甚。水湿不化，水精不布，故口渴不欲饮，大便或秘或溏，小便短少。血脉瘀阻，故面颊、颈部或胸背部散在红痣血缕，腹皮脉络怒张，手掌赤痕。舌质淡胖，有齿痕，或紫黯，或有瘀斑，舌苔厚腻，脉细滑为肝脾肾三脏功能失调，正气败伤，气、血、水邪势盛之象。

治法：扶正行气，化瘀利水，标本兼顾。

方药：扶正消鼓方（自拟方）。方中黄芪、黄精用量宜大，健脾益气以扶正。虽然肝脾肾三脏俱伤，治当从后天脾胃调治入手，以资化源。木香、大腹皮、大腹子、抽葫芦行气消胀，兼可利水；益母草、泽兰、水红花子活血祛瘀，也兼除湿；白术、猪苓、茯苓、车前子或草，专司利水除湿。诸药相合，扶正祛邪，标本兼顾，以期消除胀满。

假若腹水明显，舌苔白腻，可加干姜、桂枝，或肉桂、附子振奋脾阳；也可再加泽泻、赤小豆、防已等增强除湿利尿之力。若湿蕴化热而发黄，则应加茵陈、土茯苓、金钱草等清利湿热之品，若小便赤涩不利，可加滑石、通草、蟋蟀粉利窍行水。若气阴两虚，舌质嫩红，可加沙参、玉竹、麦冬以养阴益胃。若气血两虚，舌淡，心悸少寐，可加当归、首乌、阿胶等以养血宁心。若湿浊中阻，胃失和降，恶心呕吐，可加半夏、陈皮、生姜、竹茹等和胃降逆。若湿浊化热，可加黄芩、黄连等清化中焦湿热，黄柏、山栀等清利下焦湿热。若腹水胀满太甚，伴见喘促不宁，可加麻黄、杏仁、桔梗以宣肺利水，或桑白皮、葶苈子泻肺利水，或枇杷叶、瓜蒌皮润肺利水。

若腹水严重，常法治疗不效时，也可以选用攻逐利水的方法。使用这一治法，应该掌握如下原则：(1)腹水严重，腹胀撑急难忍；(2)患者当能承受攻逐之力，脾肾未败；(3)中病即止，或腹水退其七、八即止；(4)攻逐之后，注重调理脾胃，以巩固疗效。常用方剂以舟车丸、十枣汤化裁为用。

处方举例：

炙黄芪30g、黄精30g、木香10g、大腹皮10g、抽葫芦20g、益母草12g、水红花子20g、猪苓20g、茯苓20g、车前草30g、泽兰叶10g。

（三）晚期证治：包括邪气未净，而以正虚为主，以及出现昏迷、吐血、便血等合并症。

1. 正虚邪恶

主症：腹大胀满不舒，早宽暮急，神倦懒动，气短声怯，骨瘦如柴。

兼症：面色苍黄或皖白，或腰膝冷痛，畏寒肢冷，男子阳痿，女子停经，或五心烦热，肌肤甲错，头晕耳鸣，少寐盗汗等。

舌脉：舌淡苔白，脉沉细，或弱，或弦。

分析：气、血、水停留日久，脾肾败伤，无以化气，进一步加重水湿的蓄积，故仍见腹大胀满不舒，随正气消长而有早宽暮急的变化。正气亏虚，则神倦懒动，气短声怯。化源不充，精血难生，则骨瘦如柴，面色苍黄或㿠白。若偏于脾肾阳虚，阳衰阴盛，故腰膝冷痛，畏寒肢冷，男子阳痿，女子停经，舌淡胖，脉沉细无力。若偏于肝肾阴亏，阴虚火旺，故五心烦热，肌肤甲错，头晕耳鸣，少寐盗汗，舌嫩红而胖，脉沉细而弦。

治法：温补脾肾，或滋补肝肾。

方药：温补脾肾以附子理中丸合济生肾气丸化裁，滋补肝肾以麦味地黄丸为主。附子理中丸以温中健脾，振奋中阳为主，济生肾气丸以温肾助阳，化气行水为主。脾肾阳虚者，两方可以交替服用。麦味地黄丸能补养肝脾肾之阴。

正虚为主，治疗时只宜缓图，不可求其速效，更不能以治标法投之，再伤正气。正虚也可变为本虚标实之证，又当以中期之法处理。

处方举例：

炙附片 6g、炮姜 5g、党参 10g、生熟地各 10g、山萸肉 10g、茯苓 15g、泽泻 10g、丹皮 10g、炒白术 10g、淮山药 10g。

2. 吐血、便血

主症：轻者呕吐时，物中夹有鲜血或血块，或大便色黑；重者吐血盈碗盈盆，或大便黯红而溏薄。

兼症：口干而苦，胃脘灼热，肠鸣腹胀或心悸气短，汗出肢冷，舌红，或红中黄，或舌淡，脉弦滑而数，或沉细而数。

分析：肝脾不和，中焦气机壅滞蕴久化热，热迫血络，故吐血，便血，口干而苦，胃脘灼热，肠鸣腹胀。若气随血耗，气血不足，故心悸气短，汗出肢冷。舌红苔黄，脉弦滑为热盛于中之象；舌淡，脉沉细而数，为气血耗伤之象。

治法：泄热宁络，凉血止血，气血耗伤者合益气固脱为法。

方药：大黄白芨粉凉开水调为糊状，慢慢吞服。药用大黄粉 2g、白芨粉 6～9g，一日 2～3 次。若吐血、便血来势猛烈，病位在贲门上下者，可先将三腔管送入胃中，令胃囊充气，再吞服大黄白芨粉半次量，然后将食管囊充气，以增强止血功效。

假若气血耗损，汗出肢冷时，于上方加人参粉 3g，以益气固脱，或服黄土汤。

处方举例：

大黄粉 2g、白芨粉 6g、三七粉 3g。

凉开水调成稀糊状，缓缓吞服，2～3 次/日。

3. 昏迷

主症：先见烦躁不宁，逐渐嗜睡，终至昏迷；或先语无伦次，逐渐嗜睡，终至昏迷。

兼症：脘闷纳呆，恶心呕吐，腑行不畅。

舌脉：舌红苔黄腻，或舌淡红，苔腻，脉滑。

分析：湿热蕴积，蒙闭心包，故先烦躁不宁，逐渐嗜睡，终至昏迷。舌红，苔黄腻，脉滑，也是湿热之象。若为痰湿壅盛，蒙闭心包，故先见语无伦次，逐渐嗜睡，终至昏迷。舌淡红苔腻，也是痰浊之象。中焦气机不利，胃失和降，故脘闷纳呆，恶心呕吐，腑行不畅。

治法：醒神开窍。

方药：湿热蒙闭心包者，用局方至宝丹，研化，吞服或鼻饲，以清热凉开透窍。痰湿蒙闭心包者，用苏合香丸，研化，吞服或鼻饲，以芳香温开透窍。

在有清开灵注射液时，也可用清开灵 20ml 与 5%葡萄糖盐水 200ml 一起静脉点滴，每日1～2次。清开灵治疗湿热蒙闭心包者最佳。

处方举例：

局方至宝丹 1 丸研化，鼻饲，2 次/日。

〔预防及护理措施〕

1. 注意休息，病重者以卧床休息为主。

2. 饮食有节，宜低盐饮食，禁食海腥、生冷、油腻、辛辣刺激性食物，以及油炸、粗糙、坚硬类食物。忌饮酒、少吸烟。

3. 保持情绪稳定，消除恐惧心理，增强治疗信心。积极治疗积聚、黄疸、胁痛等病。

4. 注意气候寒湿变化，防止正虚邪侵。

〔典型病例分析〕

案一：任某某，男，44 岁。

主诉：反复发作腹胀满、小便少近二年。

病史：患者自 1973 年 10 月始患“黄疸性肝炎”，曾在传染病医院住治疗，效果不显，出院后渐出现腹胀满，小便少，1977 年 7 月前来就诊。

刻下症：腹大坚满，青筋暴露，形体消瘦，面色黧黑，口燥心烦，鼻齿出血，小便短赤，颈项前胸有蛛丝赤缕。舌质红绛少津，无苔，脉细数。

检体：心肺（－），颈项、前胸可见蛛蜘痣，肝下界剑突下 2.5cm，脾胁下 3.5cm，腹围 84cm，移动性浊音（＋），可见肝掌。

理化检查：(1)肝功能：黄疸指数 21 单位，谷丙转氨酶 120 单位。(2)血清总蛋白：7.8%，白蛋白：3.79g%，球蛋白：4.01g%。

中医诊断：臌胀（肝肾阴虚、水停中焦）。

西医诊断：肝硬化。

治则：滋养肝肾、软坚化瘀利水。

处方：自拟方。

当归 24g、川芎 12g、赤芍 15g、女贞子 24g、玉竹 18g、生地 12g、莪术 12g、牡蛎 30g、柴胡 15g、板蓝根 30g、玄参 15g、丹皮 15g、猪苓 15g、泽泻 18g、茵陈 30g、甘草 10g。

二诊，上方服 40 余剂后，诸症大减，查肝功能：黄胆指数 3 单位，血清总蛋白：8.1g%，白蛋白：4.63g%，球蛋白：3.47g%，腹围减至 74cm。给予滋养肝肾、顾扶脾气之品：

当归 24g、杭芍 24g、熟地 24g、山药 30g、女贞子 30g、玉竹 24g、黄精 18g、党参 24g、沙参 15g、麦冬 15g、玄参 15g、茯苓 12g。

三诊，上方加减又服近 60 剂，患者面色由黧黑转黄，蜘蛛痣消失，饮食增加，二便正常，舌质稍红，苔薄白，脉细有力，肝未触及，脾仍肿大，以后随访未复发。

按：本案为臌胀重症，阴虚挟湿，本虚标实，治疗以扶正祛邪为原则，滋阴养血而不碍胃，清热祛邪而不伤正。方中当归、赤芍、柴胡调肝养活血活血，女贞子、玉竹、丹皮、生地、玄参滋阴凉血，板蓝根、茵陈清热利湿，莪术、牡蛎、赤芍破积软坚化瘀。共服 40 余剂，诸症大减，惟精神不佳，故继用党参、茯苓、山药益气健脾，当归、赤芍、玉竹、女贞子、熟地、麦冬、黄精、玄参养血活血柔肝。又服近60剂，病近愈出院。(河南省卫生厅《河南省名老中医经验集锦》)。

臌胀，其病位初在肝脾，日久伤肾。其主要病理机制为气、血、水互结，肝、脾、肾俱伤。病初，黄疸、胁痛、积聚等病失治、或误治，以致肝脾不和，气滞湿阻，寒湿或湿热困脾。中期，肝脾益伤，累及于肾，形成气滞、血瘀、水停，肝肾阴虚或脾肾阳虚等本虚标实之证。晚期，气、血、水停留日久，肝肾、脾肾之虚益甚；在此基础上又可合并昏迷、吐血、便血等症。

臌胀之治疗，依据标、本、虚、实之不同，而区分论治。病初，以邪实为主，正气未衰，重在驱邪，或行气祛湿，或温中化湿，或清热利湿，使肝脾得调，水去胀消。中期，邪伤正气，在祛除气滞、血瘀、水停的同时，当顾护正气，或兼温补脾肾，或兼滋养肝肾。晚期，以正虚为主，邪气留连，并可出现并发症，较为难治，预后不良。此时治虚为主，但只宜缓图，兼有标实，当予兼顾。针对昏迷、吐血、便血等并发症，当醒神开窍，凉血止血，予以积极抢救。

复习思考题

1. 臌胀的病机变化应如何认识？
2. 试述臌胀的常见证型证治规律。
3. 如何掌握逐水法在臌胀治疗中的使用要点？
4. 臌胀平时应如何进行调护？

头　痛

〔概述〕

头痛是指由于外感或内伤等原因引起的，以头部疼痛为主症的病证。可有急慢之分，全头或局部之异。头痛可见于多种急慢性病症之中，本篇将讨论的头痛，是内科病范围内，以头痛作为主要症状者。若属某一疾病过程中所出现的兼症，不列入本篇讨论的范围内。

头痛之因多端，但不外外感与内伤。其治疗，大抵外感头痛以疏风散邪为主，内伤头痛以平肝、清火、化痰、祛瘀、滋阴、养血、补气等法为主。

头痛可见于西医学之内、外、神经、精神、五官等各科疾病中。在内科临床上，若感染性发热性疾病、高血压病、颅内疾病，神经官能症等以头痛为主要症状时，可参考本篇进行辨证论治。

〔病因病机〕

头为“诸阳之会”、“清阳之府”，又为髓海之所在，凡五脏精华之血，六腑清阳之气，皆上注于头，若气血充盈，阴阳升降有序，外无非时之感，则头爽而神慧。若六淫之邪外袭，或直犯清窍，或循经络上干；或痰浊、瘀血痹阻经脉，阻折清阳；或气重清阳不升；或血虚清窍失养；或肝肾阴亏，虚火上扰；或情志怫郁，日久化火，肝阳上亢等，均可导致头痛的发生。其病因虽多，归纳起来不外外感、内伤两端。现分述如下：

一、外感头痛：多因起居不慎，腠理不密，风、寒、暑、湿、火等外邪自肌表或口鼻乘虚而入，客于经脉，循经上犯巅顶，清阳之气被阻遏，气血凝滞，而致头痛。六淫之中，以风邪为首，所谓“伤于风者，上先受之”，“巅高之上，唯风可到”，头痛之发，每为风邪夹时邪而相合成病。若风挟寒邪，寒凝血涩，络道不畅而为头痛；若风夹热邪，风热上炎，侵扰清窍而为头痛；若风夹湿邪，蒙蔽清窍，清阳不展而致头痛。

二、内伤头痛："脑为髓之海"，主要依赖肝肾精血及脾胃运化水谷精微，输布气血以濡养，故内伤头痛，其发病与肝、脾、肾三脏有密切关系。因于肝者，或肝阴不足，虚阳偏亢；或肝气郁结，日久化火，上扰清空而为头痛。因于脾者，或脾虚化源不足，气血亏虚，气虚则清阳不升，血虚则清窍失养皆致头痛；或脾失健运，痰浊内生，阻于中州则气机升降不利，浊阴不降，清窍被蒙而致头痛。因于肾者，多缘于亡血失精，而致髓海空虚，或偏于肾阴不足，水不涵木，风阳上扰；或偏于肾阳虚衰，清空失于温养，亦有阳衰内寒自生，而致清阳阻遏者，皆可导致头痛。凡头痛经久不愈，其痛如锥如刺，则因久痛入络，血瘀络痹之故。

此外，外伤跌仆，络脉瘀阻，不通则痛，亦可引起头痛。

头痛的病因病机示意图

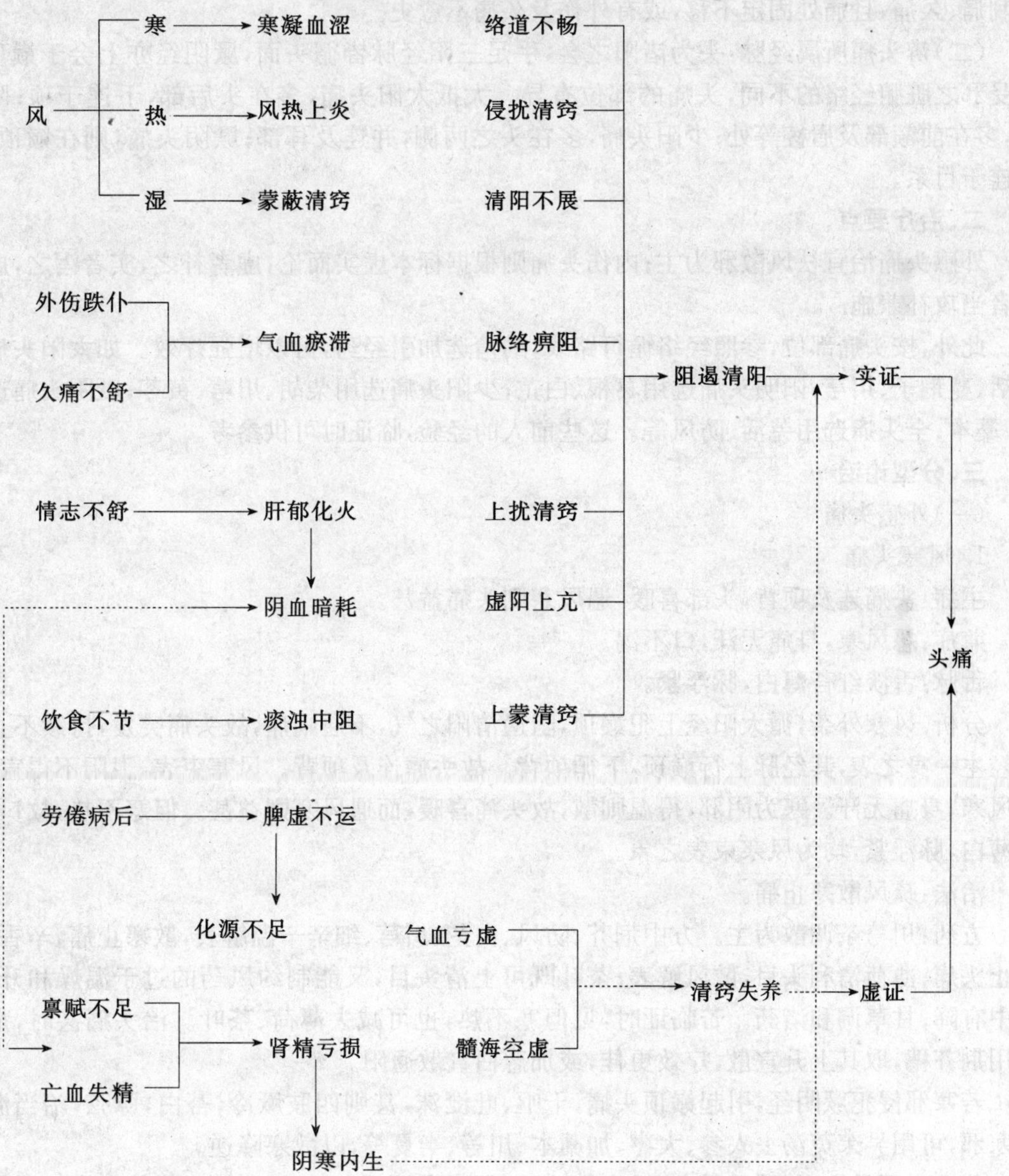

〔辨证论治〕

一、辨证要点

(一)辨头痛之外感、内伤:外感头痛一般发病较急,病势较剧,多表现为掣痛、跳痛、灼痛、胀痛、闷痛等,疼痛持续,昼夜不止,每因感受外邪而发病或加重。临证时,还应辨清邪气属性,或风、或寒、或湿、或暑、或火等。其中暑与火皆属热,其性相似。

内伤头痛一般起病缓慢,痛势较缓,多表现为隐痛、空痛、昏痛等,疼痛间作,时轻时重,时发时止,劳则加剧,休息则减。其性有虚有实,虚中夹实也不少见。临证时,应辨清气虚、血虚、精亏、肝阳、虚阳、痰浊、瘀血等。大抵气虚头痛多见隐痛,遇劳则发;血虚头痛多为头空而痛,出血后加重;精亏头痛亦头空而痛,较血虚者更甚,且伴目涩羞明,腰膝酸软;肝阳头痛多头胀而痛,目赤口苦;虚阳头痛多头晕且痛,耳鸣如蝉;痰浊头痛多昏蒙而痛,恶心纳呆;瘀血头痛多为刺痛、久痛,且痛处固定不移,或有外伤及久痛不愈史。

(二)辨头痛所属经脉:头为诸阳之会,手足三阳经脉皆循头面,厥阴经亦上会于巅顶。由于受邪之脏腑经络的不同,头痛的部位有异。大抵太阳头痛,多在头后部,下连于项;阳明头痛,多在前额部及眉棱等处;少阳头痛,多在头之两侧,并连及耳部;厥阴头痛,则在巅顶部位,或连于目系。

二、治疗要点

外感头痛治宜祛风散邪为主;内伤头痛则根据标本虚实而论,虚者补之,实者泻之,虚实夹杂者当攻补兼施。

此外,按头痛部位,参照经络循行路线,酌情选加引经药,可以增强疗效。如太阳头痛选用羌活、蔓荆子、川芎;阳明头痛选用葛根、白芷;少阳头痛选用柴胡、川芎、黄芩;厥阴头痛选用吴萸、藁本;全头痛选用羌活、防风等。这些前人的经验,临证时可供参考。

三、分型论治

(一)外感头痛

1. 风寒头痛

主症:头痛连及项背,头部喜暖,遇风寒则头痛益甚。

兼症:恶风寒,身痛无汗,口不渴。

舌脉:舌淡红苔薄白,脉浮紧。

分析:风寒外袭,循太阳经上犯巅顶,阻遏清阳之气,不通则痛,故头痛突发,持续不止。太阳经主一身之表,其经脉上行巅顶,下循项背。故头痛连及项背。风寒束表,卫阳不得宣达,故恶风寒,身痛无汗。寒为阴邪,得温则散,故头痛喜暖,而遇风寒则益甚。但寒不热,故口不渴。苔薄白,脉浮紧,均为风寒束表之象。

治法:疏风散寒止痛。

方药:川芎茶调散为主。方中荆芥、防风、白芷、川芎、细辛辛温解表,散寒止痛,辛香上窜,尤止头痛;薄荷清利头目,散风解表;茶叶既可上清头目,又能制约风药的过于温燥和升散,使升中有降;甘草调和诸药。若临证时,见但寒不热,也可减去薄荷、茶叶。治头痛甚时,荆芥应改用荆芥穗,取其上升宣散,疗效更佳,或加葱白宣散通阳。

若寒邪侵犯厥阴经,引起巅顶头痛,干呕,吐涎沫,甚则四肢厥冷,苔白,脉弦,治当温散厥阴寒邪,可用吴茱萸汤去人参、大枣,加藁本、川芎、半夏等,以散寒降逆。

若命火不足之人,再受风寒,后头痛甚,可用麻黄附子细辛汤以温经散寒止痛。方中细辛既散太阴肺之游风，又散少阴肾之伏风，乃引十二经之风寒出表，为止寒痛之圣药。

处方举例：

川芎 10g、羌活 10g、荆芥穗 10g、防风 10g、细辛 3g、甘草 6g、葱白 6g、白芷 10g。

2. 风热头痛

主症：头痛而胀，甚而头痛如裂。

兼症：发热恶风，面红目赤，咽喉肿痛，口干欲饮。

舌脉：舌红，苔黄少津，脉浮数。

分析：风热、暑热或火邪伤人，或从肌表而入，或从口鼻而入，热性炎上，上扰清窍，故头痛且胀，甚则其痛如裂，面红目赤。咽喉乃肺之门户，为热邪熏蒸，故肿痛。热盛津伤，故口干欲饮。舌红，苔黄少津，脉浮数，乃风热伤于肺卫之象。

治法：疏风清热。

方药：芎芷石膏汤为主。方中川芎、白芷、菊花、石膏相伍，疏散风热以止头痛。该方中藁本、羌活偏于辛温，热盛者不宜，可去，再加桑叶、薄荷以辛凉清解。若为暑热所伤，宜加鲜佩兰、鲜荷叶以清暑泄热。若为火热所伤，宜加黄芩、山栀、连翘以泻热解毒。

若热盛津伤，口干欲饮明显，可加鲜芦根、元参、天花粉等生津止渴。若面红目赤明显，可加龙胆草、木贼草以清肝泻热。若咽喉肿痛明显，可加板蓝根、金银花、蒲公英以清热解毒。

若热结腑实，头痛如裂，大便秘结者，可加山栀、大黄、元明粉等以泻热通腑。也可与黄连上清丸同用，该方苦寒降火，釜底抽薪，使邪有出路，头痛可止。

处方举例：

川芎 10g、白芷 10g、生石膏（先下）30g、菊花 10g、桑叶 10g、薄荷（后下）6g、炒黄芩 10g、金银花 10g、连翘 10g、桔梗 6g、生甘草 6g。

3. 风湿头痛

主症：头痛而沉，遇阴雨天加重。

兼症：肢体困乏，胸闷纳呆，口黏不爽，小便不利，大便或溏。

舌脉：舌苔白腻，脉濡。

分析：风湿外浸，卫阳被遏，邪气上蒙清窍，故头痛而沉，遇阴雨天则湿浊更甚，故头痛也剧。卫阳不得宣通，故肢体困乏。湿浊阻于中州，纳化不运，故胸闷纳呆，口黏不爽。湿浊内停，不能分清泌浊，故小便不利，大便或溏。苔白腻，脉濡均为湿浊偏盛之象。

治法：祛风胜湿。

方药：羌活胜湿汤为主方。方中羌活、独活、川芎、防风、蔓荆子、藁本等辛温而散，祛风以除湿，乃风能胜湿之意。若属暑湿之邪伤人，宜加藿香、佩兰、六一散等芳香解暑之品。若湿浊中阻，也可用藿朴夏苓汤与上方同用。

处方举例：

羌活 10g、川芎 10g、蔓荆子 10g、苍术 10g、藿香 10g、佩兰 10g、防风 10g、藁本 6g、荷叶 10g。

（二）内伤头痛

1. 肝阳头痛

主症：头痛且胀，每遇恼怒后加重；多见偏头痛。

兼症：面红耳赤，口苦咽干，胁肋胀痛，心烦易怒，眠差多恶梦。

舌脉：舌边尖红，苔薄黄，脉弦滑有力。

分析：恼怒伤肝，气郁化火，肝阳上亢，循经扰动清窍，故头痛且胀，气恼后加重。厥阴经脉循行头侧，故多见偏头痛。气火上炎，故面红目赤，口苦咽干。厥阴经脉布两胁，故肝气不舒则胁肋胀痛。心肝火旺，神明被扰，故心烦易怒，眠差多恶梦。舌边尖红，苔薄黄，脉弦滑有力，均为火盛阳亢之象。

治法：平肝潜阳。

方药：以天麻钩藤饮为主。方中天麻、钩藤、生石决明以平肝潜阳；黄芩、山栀以清泄肝火；牛膝、桑寄生、杜仲补肝肾、强腰背，且能引药及邪热下行；夜交藤、茯神养心安神；益母草应以茺蔚子取代，意在活血通络以止头痛。若风阳上扰，头痛且晕，可加菊花、白蒺藜平肝熄风。若肝火旺盛，面红目赤，心烦易怒，宜加龙胆草、夏枯草、羚羊粉等。若火旺灼阴，已见肝肾阴亏者，可加生地、白芍、女贞子、旱莲草等滋养肝肾。

处方举例：

天麻 10g、钩藤 10g、生石决明（先下）30g、黄芩 10g、山栀 10g、川牛膝 10g、茺蔚子 10g、赤白芍各 10g、菊花 10g、龙胆草 6g。

2. 肾虚头痛

主症：头脑空痛，烦劳则重，眠后则轻。

兼症：神倦乏力，头晕耳鸣，腰膝酸软，遗精带下，心悸少寐。

舌脉：舌嫩红少苔，脉细无力。

分析：肾主藏精、生髓，脑为髓海。肾精亏虚，髓海不足，故头痛空痛。烦劳则伤肾，故空痛益甚；眠卧则精复，故空痛减轻。肾虚则精血不足，不能上荣于脑，脑海空虚，故眩晕耳鸣，神倦无力。腰为肾府，肾虚则腰膝酸软。肾虚精关不固而遗精，带脉不束而带多。精血亏耗，神明失养，故心悸少寐。舌嫩红少苔，脉细无力，亦为肾精不足之象。

治法：益肾生精。

方药：大补元煎为主。方中熟地、山萸肉、山药、枸杞子滋补肝肾；人参大补元气；当归养血补血；杜仲益肾强腰。若头痛著者，也可加川芎、细辛活络止痛，若偏于肾阳虚衰，头空痛而畏寒，遇寒则重，面白肢冷，舌淡，脉沉细而缓，可用右归丸化裁以温肾助阳，填补精血。

若头脑空痛，时发时止，或痛减未净者，可常服杞菊地黄丸，平补肝肾，潜镇浮阳。

若头痛而虚眩，也可加生龙骨、生牡蛎以镇潜浮阳。

处方举例：

熟地黄 12g、山萸肉 10g、枸杞 10g、鹿角胶 10g（烊化）、龟板胶 10g（烊化）、菟丝子 10g、川芎 6g、细辛 3g、桑寄生 30g、炒杜仲 12g。

3. 气虚头痛

主症：头痛绵绵，劳累则重。

兼症：面色萎黄，形体消瘦，身倦乏力，口淡乏味，纳少不馨，大便溏薄。

舌脉：舌淡而胖，苔薄白，脉细弱无力。

分析：脾主升清，若脾虚则升降失司，清阳不升，浊阴不降，清窍不利，故头痛绵绵。劳则气伤，每遇劳累则头痛发作或加重，休息后则减轻。中虚不运，阳气不能达于四肢百骸，故面色萎黄，形体消瘦，身倦乏力。脾胃不健，纳化无权，故口淡乏味，纳少不香，大便溏薄。舌淡而胖，苔薄白，脉细弱无力，亦为脾弱气虚之象。

治法：健脾益气，升举清阳。

方药：顺气和中汤为主。方中以补中益气汤作基本方，以健脾益气，升举清阳；加蔓荆子、川芎、细辛以祛风止痛。补中有散，标本兼顾，常可获效。若兼见血虚之症，则应气血双补，与四物汤合方化裁。若脾虚不运，痰浊内生，则宜于上方加化痰之品，攻补兼施。

处方举例：

党参 10g、炙黄芪 15g、炒白术 10g、柴胡 10g、升麻 6g、川芎 10g、蔓荆子 10g、细辛 3g、茯苓 15g、炙甘草 6g。

4. 血虚头痛

主症：头空痛，以眉楞骨痛较多，出血后痛重。

兼症：面色不华，神疲乏力，心悸不宁，女子经少色淡。

舌脉：舌淡，苔薄白，脉细弱。

分析：血虚清窍失养，故头空而痛，或以眉棱骨痛较多。出血之后，血虚益甚，故头痛亦甚。血不上荣于面，故面色不华。血不养筋，故身疲乏力。心主血，血虚则心神失养，故心悸不宁。血少则冲任不充，故经少色淡。舌淡苔薄白，脉细弱，也为血虚之征。

治法：养血补血。

方药：以加味四物汤为主。本方即四物汤加菊花、蔓荆子、黄芩、甘草而成。方中当归、地黄、白芍养阴补血；川芎、蔓荆子、菊花清头目以止痛；甘草和中，兼调和诸药。无热象者，黄芩可省去。若兼有气虚之症，如神疲乏力，稍劳则剧者，也可与举元煎合方化裁治之。若属虚血不足，症见血虚浮之象，如头晕耳鸣、腰膝酸软者，可于本方减川芎用量，加用何首乌、枸杞子、阿胶、女贞子等滋阴养血之品。若血虚兼血瘀之征，症见痛久不愈，发黯有瘀斑等，也可佐以活血祛瘀之品，如茺蔚子、川芎等。

处方举例：

何首乌 12g、枸杞子 10g、当归 10g、赤白芍各 10g、川芎 6g、熟地黄 10g、砂仁 3g、蔓荆子 10g、菊花 10g、钩藤 10g。

5. 痰浊头痛

主症：头痛而昏蒙。

兼症：胸腔满闷，纳呆恶心，呕吐痰涎。

舌脉：舌苔白腻，脉滑或濡滑。

分析：饮食不节，脾运不健，滋生痰浊，困阻中州，气机升降失司，浊阴不降，清窍被遏，故头痛而昏蒙。痰浊中阻，故胸脘满闷。胃失和降，故纳呆恶心，甚则呕吐痰涎。舌苔白腻，脉滑或濡滑，均为痰浊不化之征。

治法：理脾化痰，散浊降逆。

方药：半夏白术天麻汤为主。本方为二陈汤变方。方中二陈祛湿化痰，痰浊消散，升降方能有序；白术理脾化湿以清其源；天麻化痰熄风以止头昏痛；姜枣和中。诸药相合，使浊阴得降，清空自爽，头痛则止。若湿浊夹暑，可加省头草、藿香、荷叶以祛暑散浊。若头痛甚，可加祛风药，以风能胜湿也，药如白蒺藜、蔓荆子、羌活等。若湿浊不化，阻于中焦明显时，可加苍术、厚朴、白蔻等和中化浊、宣畅气机。

若痰浊郁久化热，痰热上扰，症见头痛而胀闷，心烦少寐，舌苔黄腻，脉滑数者，宜于上方去白术，加竹茹、枳实、黄芩或黄连、山栀等清化痰热。

若痰瘀互阻，蒙闭清窍，则头痛昏蒙益甚，经久难愈，宜痰瘀同治，方可收效。

处方举例：

半夏10g、炒陈皮10g、天麻10g、白术10g、荷叶10g、省头草10g、白蒺藜10g、蔓荆子16g、茯苓10g、生姜3片。

6. 瘀血头痛

主症：头痛经久不愈，痛处固定不移，状如针刺，或钝痛，或有头部外伤史。

兼证：面色晦黯无华，神情呆滞，夜寐不安；或有外伤瘢痕。

舌脉：舌质紫黯，或有瘀斑、瘀点，脉细或涩。

分析：头部外伤，或久痛入络，瘀血内停，脉络不畅，不通则痛，故头痛经久不愈，痛处固定不移，状如针刺，或钝痛。血瘀不能荣于面，故面色晦黯不华。血瘀神明失养，故呆滞不灵，夜寐不安。舌质紫黯，或有瘀斑、瘀点，脉细或涩，均为血瘀不畅之象。

治法：活血化瘀，通络利窍。

方药：通窍活血汤为主。方中桃仁、红花、川芎、赤芍活血化瘀；麝香、葱白、生姜温通经络，其中麝香香窜，止痛效果尤佳，但药源较紧，必要时可用含有麝香的中成药替代。还可加茺蔚子、郁金、菖蒲、细辛、白芷以理气活血，宣窍止痛。

若瘀痛日久，气血不足者，宜加当归、首乌、黄芪、党参以补气养血，助气血运行。若头痛甚剧，可加虫类搜剔通络之品，如全蝎、蜈蚣、地鳖虫、蕲蛇、地龙等，但要中病即止，不宜大量或久服。若头痛顽固，确有死血内停者，也可加水蛭、鬼见羽等以逐瘀活血。

若血瘀气滞，积久化热，症见心烦少寐，舌红而干者，可加芥穗、夏枯草、青蒿以清气分郁热，或加丹皮、丹参、白头翁等以清血分伏热。若瘀血头痛，缘于受寒所得，遇寒则更甚者，可加桂枝、细辛温经散寒以通络。

若属血瘀与痰浊互结，阻于清窍而头痛者，治宜活血祛瘀与除湿化痰合用，上方可与导痰汤、牵正散等化裁。

处方举例：

茺蔚子12g、川芎10g、赤芍10g、地龙10g、桃仁10g、红花10g、钩藤10g、菖蒲6g、细辛3g、郁金10g、葱白6g。

此外，临床上尚有一些特殊类型的头痛，也应掌握其辨治规律。如：

(1)“雷头风”：本病特点是头痛如雷鸣，头面起核或肿痛红赤，多因湿热酒毒挟痰上冲所致。治以清热解毒，除湿化痰，方用清震汤加味。若热毒明显，可与普济消毒饮合方化裁为治。

(2)偏头风：本病又称偏头痛。其特点是疼痛部位在一侧或两侧，暴发而剧烈，或痛连于目、齿，痛止如常人，多系肝经风火上窜所致。治宜平肝祛风通络以止痛，常用菊花、天麻、川芎、白芷、蔓荆子、钩藤、全蝎、地龙等药。若肝火偏亢，可加山栀、黄芩、龙胆草、丹皮等药。若痰多络阻者，可加半夏、南星、竹沥水、生姜汁或白芥子等。若久病入络，可加化瘀通络之品，如赤芍、桃仁、红花、穿山甲、川芎等。

〔预防及护理措施〕

1. 外感头痛多因感受外邪所致，故平时宜起居有常，及时增减衣物，注意身体锻炼，增强体质，以免受邪发病。

2. 内伤头痛，应注意颐养性情，情绪宜安定，保证足够睡眠，饮食宜清淡。久病年高体弱之人，注意节劳节欲。

3. 头痛剧烈者，宜卧床休息，环境宜清静，光线宜柔和。宜禁烟酒，避免情绪刺激。饮食也应忌辛辣、厚味等刺激伤胃动火之品。

4. 有条件者，可配合推拿、按摩、或针刺等辅助疗法。

〔**典型病例分析**〕

案一：刘某某，男，38岁。

经常头痛，目眩，心烦，已数年之久，性情急躁，记忆力显著减退，小便微黄，大便如常，食纳尚佳，脉象浮取微浮，沉取弦细有力，舌红边缘不齐，苔黄微腻。属肝胆火旺兼外感风邪，宜清热降火为主，佐以养阴祛风。处方：桑叶6g、菊花6g、僵蚕6g、刺蒺藜10g、川芎5g、藁本6g、丹皮5g、炒栀子6g、龙胆草5g、玄参6g、甘草3g、荷叶10g、石决明(煅)15g、木通5g。服三剂。

复诊：头痛消失，但有时头晕，脉转弦细缓已不浮，舌苔减少，余症同前，拟滋阴养血兼调肠胃，以丸药缓图。处方：

当归尾10g、川芎10g、白芍12g、干生地18g、丹参10g、炒栀子10g、玄参12g、菊花15g、地骨皮15g、蒺藜15g、决明子(炒)15g、石斛15g、肉苁蓉15g、胡麻仁(炒研)15g、黑芝麻(炒研)15g、建曲30g、制香附30g，共研为细末，和匀，炼蜜为丸，每丸重9g，每日早晚各服一丸，细嚼，白开水送下，连服两料，诸症悉平。嘱其颐养性情，勿使肝胆相火再炽。

按：朱丹溪“五志烦劳，皆属于火”之说，在临床上是屡见不鲜的。本例患者情志过急，水不足以濡之，肝胆火旺，又兼风邪，风火相煽，故头痛、目眩、心烦、尿黄、脉弦细有力，乃虚中有实之象。采用清热降火，养阴去风，虚实互治，先以汤剂折其既燃之势，继以滋水濡养、丸剂缓图养其已平之火。虚实缓急，各有次第，故获痊愈。(录自《蒲辅周医案》)。

头痛为临床上常见病证，病因不离外感、内伤两途，辨证的关键为分清外感、内伤及辨别虚实。外感头痛，一般以风邪致病为主，但多有风寒、风热(或暑热、火)、风湿相夹。内伤头痛，多因脏腑气血功能失调，与肝、脾、肾三脏关系最为密切。外感头痛多实证；内伤头痛以虚证多见，但也有实证或虚中夹实证。对于头痛的治疗，外感头痛以祛风散邪为主，根据兼夹，随症加减。内伤头痛，以调和脏腑功能为主，虚则补之，实则泻之。如肝阳当以平肝潜阳，痰浊当以化痰散浊，瘀血当以活血化瘀随证参治；虚实挟杂则攻补兼施。由于头痛病情复杂多变，因此必须分清主次，结合病因及病机变化、证候特点进行辨证论治。并注意头痛部位，结合经络循行加用引经药物，方能提高疗效。且忌头痛医头，只重视止痛药物的堆砌，而忽略整体辨证。除药物治疗以外，还可以根据病情，配合针灸、推拿、外治等治疗，疗效更佳。

复习思考题

1. 试述头痛的病因病机。
2. 试述外感头痛的证候及其辨治规律。
3. 试述内伤头痛的证候及其辨治规律。
4. 常用治疗头痛的引经药是什么？

眩　　晕

〔概述〕

眩晕是目眩与头晕的统称，目眩是指眼花或眼前发黑，视物模糊；头晕是指感觉自身或周围景物旋转，站立不稳。二者常同时并见，故称之眩晕。轻者闭目即止，重者如坐车船，甚至不能站稳，或兼见恶心、呕吐、汗出、昏倒等症。

内伤、外感均可引发眩晕，其病机与风、火、痰、虚、瘀关系密切。

西医学中的多种疾病，如耳源性眩晕、脑性眩晕，以及高血压、低血压、贫血、神经官能症等，以眩晕为主要表现时，均可参考本病进行辨证论治。

眩晕病因病机示意图

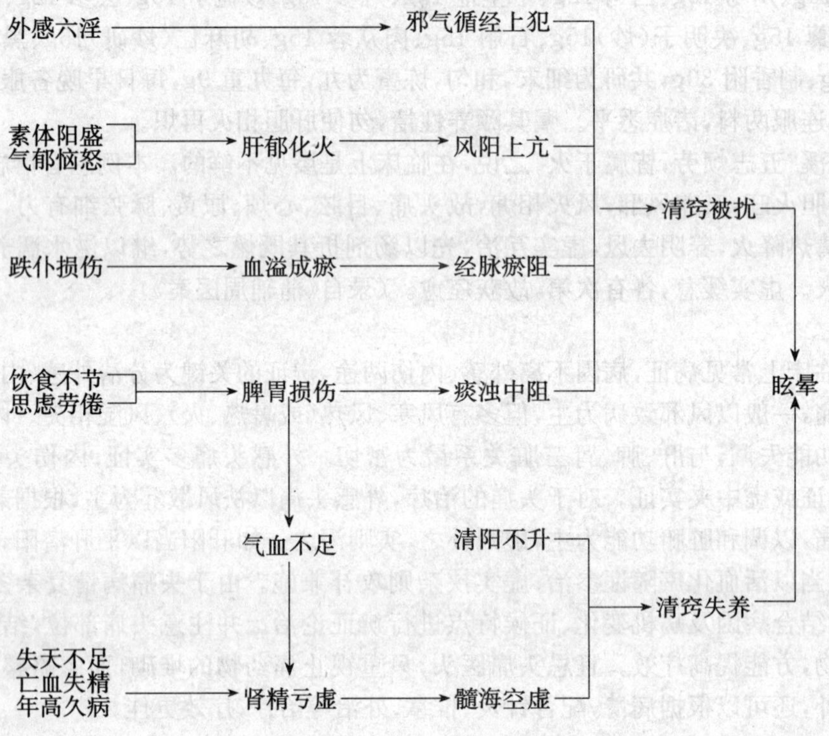

〔病因病机〕

本病的发生，多与肝阳上亢、肾精不足、气血亏虚、痰浊中阻、瘀血停留等有关，一般以虚者多，现将其分述如下：

一、肝阳上亢：肝为风木之脏，体阴而用阳，其性喜升发、疏泄。若素体阳盛，心肝火旺，易致风阳上扰，而生眩晕，此其一，为纯实之证。若素体阴虚，水不涵木，虚风内动，上扰清空，亦致眩晕，此其二，为虚中夹实。

二、肾精不足：肾为先天之本，内寄元阴元阳，主藏精生髓。若先天不足，年高久病，亡血失精，则肾精亏损，髓海不充，脑失滋养，上下俱虚，遂致头晕目眩。

三、气血亏虚：脾胃为后天之本，气血化生之源。若饮食不节，思虑劳倦，损伤脾胃；亦有脾胃素弱，或久病致虚之人，脾胃不健，纳化失司，水谷不化精微，气血乏源。气虚则清阳不升，浊气不降，清浊相混，清空失养而致眩晕；血虚则不能化精生髓，上奉清窍，更易使肝失柔养，而致虚风内动，上扰清空亦致眩晕。

四、痰浊中阻：体素肥胖，嗜食酒肉，戕伤脾胃，健运失司，聚湿生痰，痰阻中州，气机升降不利，痰湿蒙闭清窍，则头昏且眩晕；若痰浊不化，郁而化热，则痰热上扰，眩晕更甚。

五、瘀血停留：跌仆坠损，头脑损伤，血溢成瘀，阻滞经脉，清窍失养，发为眩晕。瘀血不去，新血难生，可进一步加重清窍失养，而使眩晕更甚。若血瘀阻于清窍，窍闭不聪，头痛眩晕而生。若血瘀津凝，而致痰瘀互阻于清窍，使眩晕缠绵难愈。

六、感受外邪：头为诸阳之会，十二经脉与奇经八脉都与头部有联系，若六淫之邪或从皮毛，或从口鼻侵袭人体，邪气循经上扰巅顶，清窍被扰，则可发生眩晕。六淫之中以风、暑、湿、火为害最甚。若邪传入半表半里，或入里化热等，邪气亦能循经上干清窍而致眩晕。

眩晕的病因，可单一致病，亦可相互转化，二者或三者共同致病。如气血两虚可致眩晕，但由气血两虚源于脾虚，脾虚也可生湿成痰，痰浊往往加重眩晕。再加肾精不足可致眩晕，但肝肾同源，肾精不足而肝失滋养，可致肝风内动，风阳上扰，也使眩晕尤甚。临证时宜注意详辨。

〔辨证论治〕

一、辨证要点：

1. 辨内伤、外感：眩晕之发，内伤、外感皆可为病，外感者多有感邪之病史，症状除眩晕外，多有明显表证，且起病急，传变快。邪气之属性也当细辨或风、或寒，或暑、或湿、或火。邪若传里，又当辨其居于少阳或阳明。内伤者多以肝肾、脾胃损伤为主，肝伤则阴血衰少，阴不潜阳，虚阳上扰；或肝郁化火，风火相煽，肝阳上亢；肾伤则元精亏虚，髓海不足；脾胃伤者运化无权，化源乏竭，气血两虚，清窍失养。内伤虽以虚为主，但亦兼有内生风、火、痰、瘀之变。

2. 辨虚实：眩晕之虚实中以虚者多。虚实之辨，当从主症、兼症、舌脉合参。虚者多头脑空虚，头重脚轻，不能自主，多兼肝、肾、脾胃虚弱之症，舌或瘦、或胖、或嫩红而光、或淡，脉沉细、或虚弦。实者多头脑昏蒙、胀痛，多兼表证，或痰浊、或瘀血、或肝火之症，舌或红、或黯而有瘀点、瘀斑，苔多厚腻，色黄、少津等。若虚实挟杂者，则症状错杂，临证时当以详辨。

3. 辨标本缓急：眩晕以内伤者多，内伤中又多以虚实挟杂者为突出，因此，临证时，宜分辨其标本，治疗时才能分清缓急。一般以正虚为本，邪实为标。邪实者，或风、或痰、或瘀、或火，若其邪盛明显时，当先祛邪为急；正虚者，或阴血衰少，或元精亏虚，或气血不足，若其正虚明显，而邪气不著时，治当缓图。兼有而无偏盛、偏虚者，则当兼顾之。

二、治疗要点

外感眩晕以祛邪为先，在表者按其风、寒、暑、湿、火之性而疏解之；半表半里者当和解之；在里者当清泄之。内伤眩晕，当分清虚实而治之，虚者补之、填之、滋之、温之，视其虚之地而施之。实者，火盛阳亢则镇之、清之；湿阴痰凝则化之、消之；瘀血阻络则散之、搜之。虚实互见者，则当攻补兼施，或先攻后补，或先补后攻。

三、分型证治

眩晕，虽可见于外感、内伤，然外感眩晕之证治，已见于《伤寒论》、《温病学》之中，且与本书中的“感冒”、“外感头痛”等内容相似，故可互参，本篇不再重述。在此仅对内伤眩晕加以归纳，分述如下：

(一)肝阳上亢

主症:头胀而眩晕,因烦劳或恼怒而加剧。

兼症:偏头痛,烦急易怒,面目红赤,口苦恶心,少寐多梦,耳鸣如潮。

舌脉:舌质红,苔黄糙,脉弦。

分析:烦劳恼怒,肝郁化火,风阳上扰清空,故头胀而眩晕,面红目赤,偏头作痛,烦急易怒,耳鸣如潮。肝热挟持胃气上犯,故口苦恶心。热扰神明,故少寐多梦。舌红,苔黄而糙,脉弦,均为肝热化火,风动阳亢之象。

治法:平肝潜阳,清火熄风。

方药:天麻钩藤饮加减。方中天麻、钩藤、石决明平肝潜阳以降上扰之风阳;山栀、黄芩清肝泄火以除风阳妄动之源;益母草、牛膝相得益彰,使上逆之血气下行,潜藏于肝而不使其升动;再佐以杜仲、桑寄生补肝肾以固其本;夜交藤、朱茯神交通心肾以安神定志。若眩晕不止,有增无减,则应加菊花、夏枯草、决明子、罗布麻叶等平肝潜阳、熄风止眩之品。若肝火过盛,躁扰不宁者,应加龙胆草、生地、玳瑁、寒水石等清泄肝火,必要时也可使用羚羊角,以增加清肝熄风之力,若药源紧张时用水牛角代替,用量宜大。若肝肾阴虚明显时,宜加二至丸合用以增强滋养之力。若出现手足震颤、筋惕肉瞤等虚风欲动症状时,加龙骨、牡蛎、龟板、鳖甲等镇肝熄风之品。若火结肠燥、大便不通者,又当加当归龙荟丸或搜风顺气丸等以泻肝通腑,切不可登圊过久或用力太甚。

若症见眩晕,如坐舟中,精神不振,腰膝酸软,目涩羞明,男子梦遗,女子月经不调,脉弦细而滑,舌嫩红而光,苔少或无苔,属肝肾虚亏,虚阳上扰,治宜育阴潜阳,可选用大定风珠化裁。药后若诸症减轻,则宜于平时常服杞菊地黄丸,以滋养肝肾,巩固疗效。

处方举例:

明天麻 10g、钩藤 12g、生石决明(先下)30g、菊花 10g、夏枯草 10g、黄芩 10g、山栀 10g、牛膝 15g、灵磁石(先下)30g、生代赭石(先下)30g、桑寄生 20g。

(二)气血两虚

主症:眩晕,劳倦易发或加重。

兼症:面色苍白无华,唇甲淡,神疲乏力,纳呆少馨,心慌气短,眠差多梦。

舌脉:舌质淡,苔薄,脉细弱。

分析:气虚则清阳不升,血虚则脑失所养,劳倦则伤心脾,气血益虚,清窍失养,故可发 眩晕或使其加重。血虚则心神失养,其华不荣,故心慌不宁,眠则多梦,面色苍白无华,唇甲亦淡。气虚则脾失健运,故神疲乏力,气短,纳呆少香。舌质淡,苔薄,脉细弱,均是气血两虚之象。

治法:健脾益气,养心补血。

方药:归脾汤加减。方中以健脾益气为主。缘于脾为气血之化源,脾健则能正常运化,气血自然而充盈,故以参、芪、术、草、姜、枣甘温健脾益气;当归甘辛温养血生血,共同达到补养气血之目的。茯苓、枣仁、龙眼肉、远志养心宁神,木香理气醒脾,以防益气养血药之壅滞气机,使化源健运,利于气血之化生。若食少便溏,脾胃虚弱明显时,应加砂仁、菖蒲、莲子肉、扁豆、山药,或木香宜煨、当归宜酒炙,以使增强健脾和胃之力。若胃纳尚可,血虚更甚者,应加白芍、阿胶、首乌等养血生血之品;若脾阳不足,畏寒肢冷者,更宜加炮姜、炙桂枝温中健脾之品。若中气下陷,头空而晕,气短乏力,脱肛,站则加重,卧则稍缓者,可以补中益气丸包煎同服。

处方举例：

党参10g、炙黄芪20g、酒当归10g、炒白芍10g、阿胶10g(烊化)、炒白术10g、煨木香6g、茯苓15g、远志10g、龙眼肉10g、煨葛根10g。

(三)肾精亏耗

主症：眩晕，神疲健忘。

兼症：精神萎靡，目涩羞明，腰膝酸软。偏于阴虚者，五心烦热，盗汗梦遗，月经提前，舌质嫩红少苔，脉弦细；偏于阳虚者，形寒怕冷，腰膝冷痛，阳痿阴冷，舌质淡，脉沉细无力。

分析：肾虚精亏，髓海不足，清空失养，故头晕目晕，神疲健忘，精神萎靡。肝主目，肝肾同源，精血不充，故目涩羞明，腰膝酸软。阴虚多虚火，相火妄动，故五心烦热，盗汗梦遗，月经提前。舌质嫩红少苔，脉弦细，也属阴虚火旺之象。肾阳虚则命火衰，阳气不能内暖五脏，外不充肌肤，故形寒怕冷，腰膝冷痛，阳痿阴冷。舌质淡，脉沉细无力，亦为命门火衰之象。

治法：偏阴虚者，养阴益肾；偏阳虚者，温肾助阳。

方药：养阴益肾，用左归丸为主；温肾助阳，用右归丸为主。两方中熟地黄、山萸肉、山药、枸杞子、菟丝子补肾填精；鹿角胶为血肉有情之品，补益精血。左归丸中还配合龟板胶滋养阴血，以敛浮阳；牛膝益肾强筋、引药下行归肾。右归丸还配合杜仲补肝肾，强筋骨；当归养血补血，精血同源，血生则精旺；肉桂、附子温肾助阳，更助填精补髓之品发生功效。

若阴虚火旺明显时，也可加知母、黄柏清泄相火，或加生龙骨、生牡蛎潜镇浮阳，若服药后碍胃，可加砂仁、陈皮等理脾和胃，以消滋腻。若阴阳俱虚，治宜平补，可加巴戟天、仙茅、仙灵脾等。若眩晕明显时，可加灵磁石、代赭石等重镇潜阳。

处方举例：

偏肾阴亏者：生熟地各10g、山萸肉10g、枸杞子10g、生白芍12g、女贞子10g、旱莲草10g、桑寄生20g、怀牛膝10g、生龙骨(先下)20g、生牡蛎(先下)20g、龟板胶10g(烊化)、杭菊花10g。

偏于肾阳虚者：熟地黄12g(砂仁2g拌)、山萸肉10g、枸杞子10g、菟丝子10g、炒杜仲12g、巴戟12g、仙茅10g、炙附片6g、鹿角胶10g(烊化)、灵磁石(先下)20g、明天麻10g。

三、痰浊中阻

主症：眩晕而头昏蒙。

兼症：形体肥胖，嗜食肥甘，胸脘痞闷，纳呆恶心，肢体沉困。

舌脉：舌苔白腻，脉濡滑。

分析：胖人多痰湿，加之嗜肥甘，助湿生痰，痰浊中阻，气机升降失司，浊气不降，上蒙清窍。清气不升，清空失养，故眩晕而头昏蒙不爽。中焦气机壅滞，甚则上逆，故胸脘痞闷，纳呆恶心。痰湿困脾，阳气不展，故肢体沉困。舌苔白腻，脉象濡滑，亦为痰湿内蕴之象。

治法：祛湿化痰，理脾定眩。

方药：以半夏天麻白术汤加减。方中二陈汤为基础，祛湿化痰，和胃降逆以消痰浊；白术为理脾化湿之药，天麻熄风定眩。诸药相合，痰浊得化，升降有序，则眩晕自止。若眩晕较甚，属风痰上扰者，可加白僵蚕、胆南星以熄风化痰。若痰浊壅盛，可加炒苏子、竹茹、枳实以化痰降浊，或加旋覆花、枇杷叶以降气祛痰。若眩晕与恶心、呕吐并重，可加钩藤、赭石、泽泻以加强熄风镇逆、祛湿化痰之力。若头晕、目眩、耳鸣并见者，可加菖蒲、郁金以化痰开窍之品。若脘闷纳呆者，可加莱菔子、蔻仁、砂仁开胃理脾之品。

若痰郁化火，而见头目胀痛，心烦易怒，眩晕随情绪波动而增减，口苦泛呕，少寐梦魇，舌苔黄腻，脉弦滑者，宜用温胆汤加黄连、黄芩、钩藤、天麻以化痰泄热，熄风止眩。

处方举例：

清半夏10g、炒陈皮10g、茯苓15g、竹茹10g、炒枳实10g、炒白术10g、钩藤12g、明天麻10g、远志10g、砂仁5g、代赭石（先下）20g。

（五）瘀血阻络

主症：头部外伤后，或久治不愈之眩晕。

兼症：头痛而固定，或刺痛，病情反复发作，常法治疗不效，面唇发黯，眠差健忘，神倦心悸。

舌脉：舌质紫黯，或有瘀点、瘀斑，脉弦滑或细涩。

分析：外伤头部，血溢络阻，或眩晕日久，常法不效，久病入络。血瘀络阻，清窍失养，神机不灵，故眩晕顽固，头痛如刺而有定处，眠差健忘。瘀血不去，新血不生，心神失养，故心悸神疲。舌质黯，或有瘀点、瘀斑，脉弦滑或细清，均为血瘀络阻之象。

治法：祛瘀通络，活血通窍。

方药：以通窍活血汤加减。方中赤芍、川芎、桃仁、红花活血祛瘀；老葱、麝香通阳醒窍，姜、枣调理脾胃，同时使上药不致伤胃。若头部瘀血明显者，还可加茺蔚子、穿山甲、全蝎、蜈蚣等活血通络。若情志不遂，肝郁气滞而见胸胁疼痛，喜太息等，可加柴胡、枳壳、郁金以疏肝解郁。若兼气虚，症见身倦乏力，汗多恶风者，可加生、炙黄芪，党参等健脾益气。若兼阳虚寒盛，症见畏寒肢冷，遇寒病甚者，可加炙附子、桂枝等温阳活血。若兼阴虚，症见骨蒸劳热，肌肤甲错者，可加丹皮、知母、黄柏、生地等滋阴退热。

处方举例：

川芎10g、茺蔚子10g、炒赤芍12g、全蝎粉3g（分冲）、蜈蚣2条、全当归10g、桃仁10g、红花10g、葱白2寸、钩藤10g、天麻10g。

〔预防及护理措施〕

1. 环境宜安静、舒适，避免噪音，光线宜柔和。眩晕发作时，患者宜静卧、少动，尤其不宜过于旋转体位。

2. 患者心情宜愉快，避免精神不良刺激，以解除或减少忧虑、恐惧等情绪。

3. 饮食宜清淡，痰湿胜者尤其要注意。虚者进补，也宜少食多餐，循序渐进，不可暴饮暴食。

4. 眩晕严重时，伴有剧烈呕吐，眼颤肢麻，神志模糊，血压不稳等，应及时请医生诊治，以免耽误病情。

〔典型病例分析〕

案一：薛某某，男，59岁。

时发眩晕10余年。发时如立舟车，恶心呕吐，以春发为多，失眠多梦，纳差，腹胀嗳气，口干喜热饮，时有手指颤动，大便秘结时夹稀水，小便正常，肝稍肿大，肝功能正常。脉寸尺弦细，两关弦大而空；舌淡红无苔，边有齿痕。诊断为美尼尔氏综合征。属阴虚阳浮，治宜益阴潜阳，兼调脾胃。处方：

红参30g、茯神30g、山萸肉60g、枸杞30g、肉苁蓉60g、淮山药90g、黄精60g、炙龟板（打碎）120g、黑芝麻（炒香）90g、灵磁石（打）60g、珍珠母（打）60g、潼蒺藜60g、砂仁（打）15g、白术30g、广陈皮15g、莲子肉（打）60g、龙眼肉30g。

上药浓煎三次，去渣再浓缩，加蜂蜜为膏，每早晚各服10g，温开水冲服。感冒时停服。

上药约服3个月，头晕已消失，胃口渐好，停药后腹胀痛、食纳减退等阴虚脾弱、肠胃失调之证再发，于上方加减再进一料而资巩固。

按：本例属阴虚脾弱，虚阳上逆，兼脾胃失调。采用滋补肝肾，益阴潜阳，兼调和脾胃，药中病机而收功。又因病程迁延，反复发作，治当缓图，故拟膏方调治，也属相宜。（录自《蒲辅周医疗经验》）。

眩晕是临床上的常见病证，病情有轻重之别，轻则一时头晕目眩，稍静自止；重则天旋地转，呕吐不食，烦躁难寐。病机虽较复杂，但归纳起来，不外风、火、痰、虚、瘀五个方面，其可单纯致病，亦可二者三者共同发病，如肝肾的阴亏挟有肝阳上亢，痰浊与瘀血互结，相互为患引发眩晕等等。在临床上以虚证及虚中挟实者多，单纯实证者较为少见。治疗当遵实者泻之，虚者补之，本虚标实者攻补兼施。然急者多实，可选用平肝、熄风、潜阳、清火、化痰、祛瘀等法；缓者多虚，当用补气养血、健脾、柔肝、益肾等法。或一法独进，或数法同治，随病情虚实而设。

中年以上之人，若眩晕频发，缘于肝肾多虚，易于引动肝风，病情严重者可卒然晕倒，有发展成中风之可能，故应积极调治。平时宜节食肥甘醇酒辛辣，戒恚怒，远房事，注意劳逸结合，适当进行体力活动。病重者可学练习养功，遵医嘱服药调治。

复习思考题

1. 试述眩晕的病理。
2. 怎样理解肝、脾胃、肾在眩晕发病中的意义。
3. 试述眩晕常见证型的证候特点，及其相互间的关系。
4. 试述眩晕常见证型的治法方药。
5. 如何认识眩晕与中风的关系。

中　风

〔概述〕

中风又名“卒中”，是以突然昏仆，不省人事，半身不遂，偏身麻木，言语不利或不语，或未经昏仆而以半身不遂，口舌歪斜为主要临床表现的一种病证。由于本证多具有起病急，来势快，证候多，变化迅速，且有昏仆、抽引等临床表现，与“风”善行数变的特征相似，因而古代医家就从广义上来认识和研究这种病，采用中医常用的取类比象法，把具有上述特点的一组病称之为中风。后世医家沿用这种病名，对本病认识不断完善，创立了独特的中风病病因病机学说，积累了丰富的防治中风病的经验。

中风病具有上述特定的临床表现，与《伤寒论・辨太阳病》篇所说“太阳病，发热汗出恶风脉缓者，名为中风”的太阳中风表证是根本不同的，《伤寒论》中所说“太阳中风”，是属于外感表证，也即我们现在通常所说的“伤风”“感冒”一类的病，与本节我们所要讨论的中风病名同而实异，在阅读古代文献时尤应注意，以免混淆。

现代医学之脑出血，闭塞性脑血管病，以及瘤形卒中，各种颅内动脉炎而以上述特征为主要表现者，可属本病范畴而参考辨证论治。

〔病因病机〕

中风的发生，主要在于患者平素阴阳失调，气血亏虚，加之失于调养，忧思恼怒，或饮食失节，或房室所伤，或劳累伤正，外受时邪，以致气血运行受阻，肌肤筋脉失于濡养，以致阴陷于下，肝阳暴张，阳化风动，气血逆乱，挟痰挟火，窜扰经脉，蒙塞心窍，而突然发生昏仆，半身不遂，形成上实下虚，阴阳互不维系的危重证候。其病机转化迅速、多变，兹分述如下：

一、正气不足，络脉空虚，风邪入侵。外风是六淫邪气之一。风邪从皮毛侵入，或逗留于肌肉腠理之间，或游走于经络之中，多因正气不足、腠理不密、卫外不固，风邪乘虚而入，伤于经络，肌肤失于濡养；或因平素痰浊内盛，外风引动痰浊流窜经络。其风邪中人较浅，多以阳经、头面受病为主，因此临床见证主要是口眼㖞斜，或肌肤不仁、半身不遂。

二、过度烦劳，病后体虚，年老体衰，阴阳失调，内风煽动。过度烦劳，可动越阳气，使阳气升窜而化风。过度烦劳，还可耗损精血，久病之后或年老体衰，均因精血不足，肝肾阴亏，肝失所养，肝阳亢盛。而在阴阳严重失调之情况下，加以情志过激，或嗜酒劳累及气候变化等诱因作用下，致使阴亏于下，阳亢于上，阳化风动，气血上冲，心神昏冒而发为中风。此为内风。内风煽动之时，必气火俱浮，迫血上涌，也可兼挟痰浊瘀血窜扰经络上壅清窍，更为甚者，气之与血并走于上，而迫血离经，终成大厥。本病由内风煽动而成者最多，其病情益重。

中风病的病因病机示意图

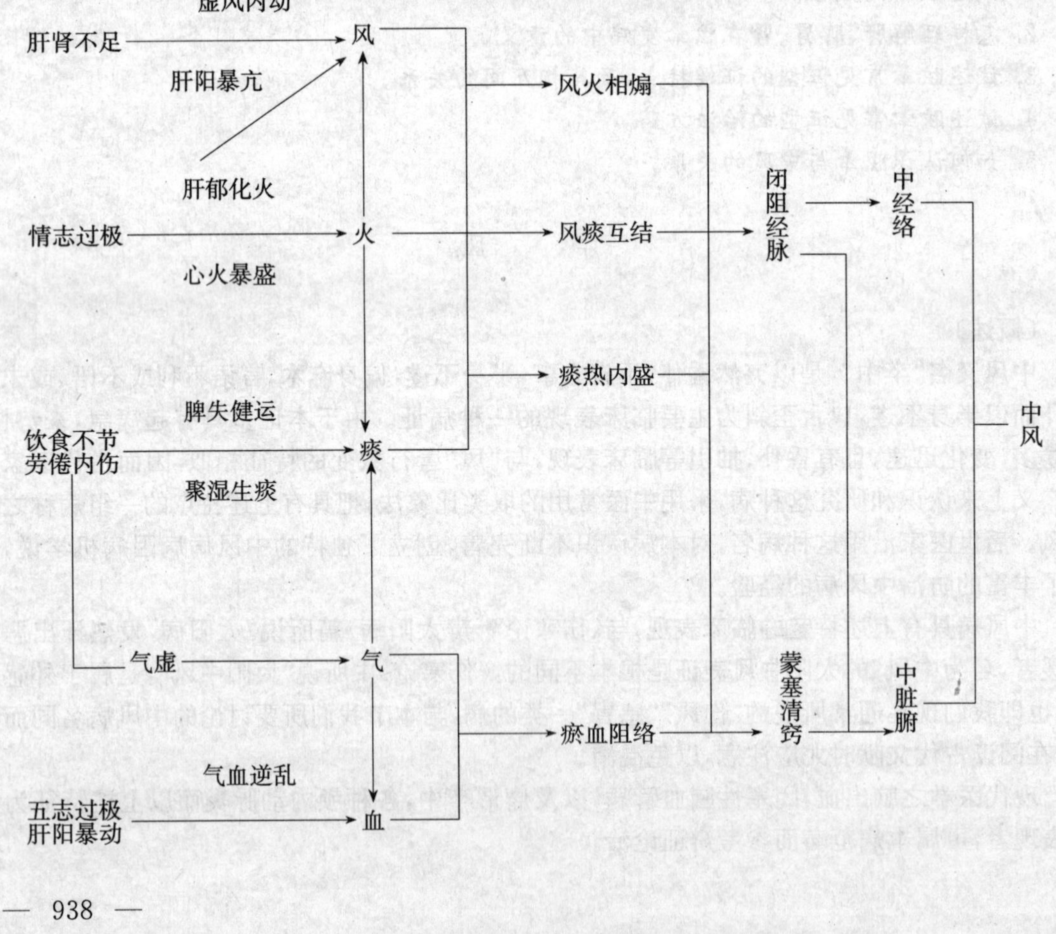

三、饮食不节，劳倦内伤，脾失健运，聚湿生痰，痰郁化热，阻滞经络，蒙蔽清窍；或肝阳素旺，木克脾土，脾失运化，内生痰浊；或内火炽盛，炼液成痰，以致肝风挟痰火，窜扰经络，蒙蔽清窍而猝仆昏迷，㖞僻不遂。总之，此乃脾失运化内生痰浊。而痰又分湿痰、热痰和风痰，而且可以互相转化。

四、五志过极，心火暴盛，风火相煽，或肝郁气滞，气滞血瘀；或暴怒伤肝，肝阳暴动。凡此种种，均易引起气血逆乱而致心神昏冒猝倒无知，发为本病。临床所见，暴怒伤肝引发本病者最为多见。因暴怒之下，顷刻之间肝阳暴张，气血俱浮，迫血上冲于脑，气血并行于上，则大厥之候突发。平素情绪紧张，忧思过度，性情暴躁者又均易患本病。

综上所述，中风病虽然病理机制比较复杂，但其病理变化不外风、火、痰、气、血、虚六端。风有外风、内风之不同；火有心火、肝火之别；痰有风痰、湿痰、热痰之异；以及气虚、气滞、气逆、血虚、血瘀、阴虚等，但总以血瘀为最多；气虚、脾虚、肾虚，而肝肾阴虚为形成本根本；内风、痰浊、瘀血常相互兼挟而发病。

有外邪侵袭而发病者称外风，又称真中风或真中，无外邪侵袭而发病的称为内风，又称类中风或类中。本病初期虽因病位浅深、病情轻重的不同而分为中经络和中脏腑，但其基本病理转化则是一致的。

〔辨证论治〕

中风的发生，虽有多种原因，但总的病理变化在本为阴阳偏胜，气血逆乱；在标为风火相煽，痰浊壅塞，瘀血闭阻；形成本虚标实，上盛下虚的复杂证候。但由于正邪双方强弱不同，个人体质阴阳偏盛之异，因而病情有轻重，病位有深浅，证候有寒热虚实，病势有顺逆的不同。在这错综复杂的环境中，如何正确辨证，关键在于掌握临床辨证要点。

辨病位浅深和病情轻重：中风急性期大抵可分为中经络和中脏腑两类证候。中络是以肌肤麻木、口舌㖞斜为主症，其麻木多为偏身或一侧手足，此证邪浅病轻。中经是以半身不遂，口舌歪斜，偏身麻木，言语蹇涩为主症，无昏仆，此证比中络为重。在临床上常将中络与中经归为一种，统称中经络。中腑是以半身不遂、口舌歪斜、偏身麻木、言语蹇涩而神志不清为主症，但其神志障碍较轻，一般属意识蒙眬或昏昏多睡。中脏是以突然昏仆而半身不遂，其神志障碍重，甚至完全昏迷无知，或以九窍闭塞突出，目不能眴、言语蹇涩或不语、吞咽困难、尿闭便秘。亦可见目合手撒、二便自遗。此证邪中最深，病情最重。中腑中脏因二者皆有神志障碍，难以决然分开，故常并为一种，统称中脏腑。从病情来看，中经络、中脏腑都属于急性期的见证。若病情超过半年以上仍有症状，则属中风后遗症。

辨闭证和脱证：中脏腑主要表现为神志障碍伴半身不遂、口舌歪斜及言语蹇涩或不语，但又有闭证脱证的区别。闭证是邪闭于内，症见牙关紧闭，口噤不开，两拳握固，大小便闭，肢体强痉，多属实证。治疗宜以祛邪为先。由于引起闭证的病邪不同，因而闭证又分有阳闭和阴闭。由于闭证时患者神志障碍，因此阳闭与阴闭的分辨，常以舌诊、脉诊为重要依据。脱证是阳气散脱于外，症见目合口张，鼻息低微，手撒遗尿，这是五脏真阳之气衰微欲绝的表现，多属虚证，治宜扶正固脱。

辨病势的顺逆：中风病急性期多变化快，但其变化有顺逆的不同。辨别病势的顺逆，掌握病势发展趋向，有助于判断预后。一般讲，神志的变化是辨别病势顺逆的重要标准。先中脏腑，如神志渐渐清醒，半身不遂等症状未再加重或有恢复者，病由中脏腑向中经络转化，病势为顺；若神昏偏瘫诸症加重或有波动，多由痰热内盛或正气不足而成，在中风急性期最为多见，其病势发展尚属顺境。如见呃逆频频，或突然神昏，四肢抽搐不已，或腹背灼热而四肢逆冷，或呕血便血，均属变证，乃病势逆转。

中风应与痫证、痿证、厥证相鉴别。

痫证虽有突然昏仆、肢体抽搐。但多为时短暂，移时苏醒，醒后如常人，无半身不遂、口舌歪斜、言语不利等表现。且痫证为一反复发作的疾病，常有多次相似发作病史可寻，可资鉴别。

痿证也可有肢体瘫痪，活动无力。但痿证一般起病缓慢，表现为双下肢瘫者多见，也可为四肢瘫，常有肌肉瘦消。

厥证亦可表现为突然昏仆，不省人事，可伴四肢逆冷，一般常在发后短期内苏醒，醒后无偏瘫、口舌歪斜、言语不利等表现。

中风属本虚标实之证。在本多为肝肾不足、气血虚衰；在标为风火相煽、痰浊壅盛、气机逆乱、瘀血闭阻。由于病位有浅深，病情有轻重，标本虚实也有先后缓急之差异，所以临床上常将中风分为中经络、中脏腑和后遗症来进行辨证论治。

一、中经络

（一）络脉空虚，风邪入中

主症：外受风邪，突然口眼㖞斜；或平素常有头晕，突然偏身麻木，肌肤不仁；或见言语不利，口角流涎，甚则半身不遂。

兼症：或有头痛鼻塞，恶寒发热，关节酸痛等症。

舌脉：舌苔薄白或薄黄，脉象浮紧或弦细。

分析：由于正气不足，卫外不固，或劳作汗出，皮毛开泄，或迎风而卧，风邪则乘虚入中经络，引起气血痹阻，运行不畅，则筋脉失于荣养，又因风邪伤人，上先受之，头为诸阳之会，位置最高，故风邪入中，多见口眼㖞斜。如遇痰湿内盛之体或素患内风之人，则外风入里，引动痰邪，或外风引动内风，而至内外合邪，风痰互结，窜扰经脉，可以导致半身不遂，言语謇涩，或风痰走窜络脉，气血运行不畅，而致营卫失用，则可有肌肤麻木不仁。风邪外袭，营卫不和，则有恶寒发热，关节酸痛等症。苔薄白，脉浮弦为表邪入里之证。若脉见弦细则又为气血不足之象。

治法：祛风通络，养血和营。

方药：大秦艽加减。本方乃是以解表散风药为主，配合养血、活血、清热之品组成。以秦艽为君药，祛风散邪，兼通经络，羌活、防风散太阳经之风邪，白芷散阳明经风邪，细辛、独活搜少阴经之风邪。因发表散风之药其性多燥，故配用白芍敛阴养血，地黄、川芎、当归等养血和营。复用白术、茯苓、甘草等健脾益气，共成养血益气散风，为扶正祛邪之剂。风为阳邪，入里最易化热，加入黄芩、石膏。若经治疗，口眼㖞斜，肢体麻木诸症不减，多因湿痰瘀血阻滞脉络，可加丹参、鸡血藤等活血之品，增强祛瘀通络之力，加白芥子、白附子、全蝎等，祛风痰，通脉络，散经络之顽邪。如兼有风热表证，可去羌活、防风、当归等药，加桑叶、菊花、薄荷等疏风清热之品。如有颈项强紧拘急麻木等症，则可加葛根、桂枝以疏风解肌。如呃逆痰盛，苔白腻者，可去地黄、白芍、当归，加半夏、南星、橘红以燥湿化痰。

如仅见口眼㖞斜而半身不遂等症，则可用牵正散加荆芥、防风、白芷以散风祛邪，加红花以活血祛瘀。

处方举例：

秦艽 6g、防风 10g、白芍 10g、黄芩 6g、地龙 10g、川芎 9g、茯苓 15g、白术 6g、当归 10g、丹皮

10g、全蝎 3g、甘草 6g。

(二)肝肾阴虚,风阳上扰

主症:平素头晕目眩,头痛,耳鸣,少眠多梦,腰酸腿软,突然手足沉重麻木,半身不遂,口舌歪斜,言语蹇涩,或舌强不语。

兼症:口干,平素便干便秘,小便黄。

舌脉:舌质红,苔黄,脉弦细数或弦滑。

分析:由于素体肝肾阴虚,肝阳偏亢,阴阳失调,精亏于下,阳浮于上,血菀气逆,形成上盛下虚,因而头晕头痛,耳鸣目眩。乃因肾藏精,主骨髓通于脑,肾开窍于耳,肝开窍于目,肝肾不足,髓海不充,耳目失养。少眠多梦,腰酸腿软,总因心肾不济,肾虚引起。有的还可出现面部烘热,心中烦闷,急躁易怒,走路头重脚轻等阴虚阳亢的症状。肝阴不足,肝阳失于制约而亢盛乃至肝风动越。风为阳邪,若肝风挟痰上扰,或挟瘀血流窜经络,故而突然发生口舌歪斜,言语蹇涩,半身不遂等证。从脉象看,弦主肝风,滑为痰湿,如弦细而数者,乃肝肾阴虚而生内热,邪热内扰,更灼阴液而致风阳浮动。舌质红为阴伤内热,舌苔腻是兼有痰湿,苔黄是化热的表现。

本证无神志障碍而以半身不遂为主,此属中经,常于起病后一周之内,变化较多。如能及时治疗,调理得当,则内风平熄,病情逐渐趋于平稳,痰浊化,内火清,瘀血祛,则偏瘫、言蹇渐减,病情好转,预后较好。如逢重证,或病后失于调治,或者服用助阳生热之品,而致内风动越不止,则在病后一周内,常见病势渐渐恶化,偏瘫加重,进而神志转为不清,遂成中脏中腑。特别要注意的是,对于素有肝肾阴虚、内风时动之人,尤宜悉心调养,切忌忧思恼怒。如因暴怒,则致肝阳暴张,风阳聚起,引起痰浊,迫血上逆,终成大厥危候。

治法:育阴潜阳,镇肝熄风。

方药:镇肝熄风汤加减,方中白芍、玄参、天冬、龟板滋养肝肾之阴,柔肝熄风;生龙骨、生牡蛎、代赭石镇肝潜阳,降逆平冲,配天麻、钩藤、菊花,增强平肝熄风之力。重用牛膝辅以川楝子引血下行,合茵陈、麦芽清肝解郁,助胃和中。痰热盛者,去龟板、天冬等滋腻之品,加胆南星、竹沥清痰热。心中烦者,加黄芩、栀子、生石膏,清热除烦。头痛重者可加生石决明、夏枯草潜阳熄风。失眠多梦者,加珍珠母、龙齿、夜交藤、茯神以镇静安神。还可酌情加用通窍活络的药物,如菖蒲、远志、地龙、红花、鸡血藤等。

处方举例:

天麻 10g、钩藤 30g、菊花 6g、白芍 12g、玄参 12g、地龙 6g、牛膝 10g、生牡蛎(先下)30g、生地 20g、栀子 6g、代赭石(先下)30g、天冬 10g。

(三)风痰上扰,痰热腑实

主症:突然口舌歪斜,半身不遂,偏身麻木,痰涎壅盛,大便秘结。

兼证:或头晕,舌强语蹇,或脘腹胀满,或发热。

舌脉:舌质红,舌苔黄或黄厚而腻,脉弦滑,或弦滑数。

分析:平时饮食不节,肥甘厚味过多,克伤脾胃,嗜酒过度,内生湿热,或因劳倦内伤致脾失健运,聚湿生痰,痰湿之邪,郁久化热,若因忧思恼怒,内风骤起,内风挟痰热闭阻经脉,则突发半身不遂,口角歪斜。痰热之邪阻于中焦,传导功能失司,升清降浊失常,导致腑气不通而便秘。清阳之气不升,浊气上冲于脑则头晕。风痰之邪阻于舌本,气血不得通畅,则可引起舌强语蹇。本证亦可因瘀血阻滞,经脉不通,致使脏腑功能失调,痰热内生而成内风挟痰热瘀血之候。舌苔黄、黄腻,脉弦滑均为痰热内盛的表现。

本证临床实为多见，虽属中经络，但痰热内盛或腑气不通，痰热内闭日久者，亦可见意识蒙眬思睡等心神被蒙的表现，如不及时的治疗，则痰热日盛，内闭心窍，可发展成为中脏腑的闭证。因此也可以认为本证介于中经络和中脏腑之间。治疗方面，可以通腑化痰为先，一旦腑气得通，继之可用清热化痰通络之剂，痰热已化，则宜活血化瘀通络为主，以期半身不遂诸症得以恢复。

治法：化痰通腑。

方药：星蒌承气汤加减。其药用胆南星、全瓜蒌、生大黄、芒硝。方中胆南星、全瓜蒌清化痰热；生大黄、芒硝通腑导滞。本方是由承气汤变化而来，如便秘日久，腹满腹胀甚者，亦可在前方加入枳实、厚朴等理气之品，如服药后大便通畅，则腑气得通，痰热亦减，神志障碍及偏瘫常可有一定的好转。如一剂之后，大便未通或腑气不畅，可再服。大黄芒硝的用量为 10 克左右。不可通泻过度，以免损伤正气。对于气阴两伤又有痰热积滞者，治宜攻补兼施，宗增液承气之意，于上方之中加入生地、玄参、麦冬养阴润燥之品。若因下之润泄不止，乃正气大伤，不可再下。腑气通后，予以清热化痰，活血通络之剂，药用胆南星、全瓜蒌、丹参、赤芍、鸡血藤等。头晕者，加钩藤、菊花、生石决明等药。

处方举例：

全瓜蒌 30g、胆南星 10g、生大黄（后下）10g、芒硝（分冲）10g、菖蒲 10g、天竺黄 10g、丹参 20g。

二、中脏腑

中脏腑是中风的危急重症。一是起病时即表现为突然昏仆，不省人事，肢体瘫痪；还有的是从中经络变化而来。中脏腑根据临床表现的不同又分闭证与脱证。二证治疗方法决然不同，临证时尤宜细察。现分别讨论：

（一）闭证：闭证的主要症状是突然昏仆，不省人事，牙关紧闭，口噤不开，两手握固，肢体强痉，二便闭塞不通。

由于引起中风的原因不同，病人体质的强弱各异，虽同为邪闭心窍，但临床见证不一，因此闭证又分为阳闭、阴闭二种。

1. 阳闭

主症：除具有突然昏仆，不省人事，牙关紧闭，口噤不开，两手握固，肢体强痉，二便闭塞等闭证的主要见症外，还兼有颜面潮红或面赤身热，痰涎壅盛，呼吸气粗，躁动不安。

兼症：肢体抽动，呃逆。

舌脉：舌质红，苔黄腻，脉象弦滑有力。

分析：由于平素肝阳偏亢，遇有情志相激，肝阳暴张，阳升风动，血随气逆上涌，挟痰挟火，上蒙清窍，心主不明则突然昏仆，不少人事。阳闭证是风火内闭，痰热互结，阻闭心窍，闭阻经脉引起的。因此还可见到面赤、潮红、身热、躁动等火热之邪为害的见证。舌红，舌苔黄腻，脉象弦滑有力等皆为内风痰火的征象。

阳闭为中风的危急重症，邪盛而正气未败。如能及时救治，病邪得去，心窍开，则神志可逐渐清醒，预后一般较好。待神志完全清楚，仅遗有半身不遂，言语障碍等症，则由中脏腑转为中经络，可望逐渐恢复。若神昏日久，或因正不胜邪，若因失治和误治，则可由闭证转为脱证。此乃风火痰热灼伤阴津耗伤正气引起，是病势逆转的表现。如因邪热内闭气血，阴阳离绝，变证亦多，吐血、呕血、便血、抽搐不止，或腹背灼热而四肢逆冷，均属于预后不良。

治法：辛凉开窍，清肝熄风。

方药：先鼻饲或灌服至宝丹以辛凉开窍，继服羚羊角汤，清肝熄风，育阴潜阳，方中羚羊角、菊花、夏枯草清肝熄风，白芍、龟板、石决明滋阴潜阳，生地、丹皮清热凉血，加牛膝、益母草引血下行。若痰多昏迷者加竹沥水、胆南星、天竺黄以豁痰开窍。若见肢体抽搐者，加全蝎、蜈蚣、僵蚕等熄风解痉。口臭、腹胀、便秘者加大黄、枳实、芒硝泻热通腑。呕血、便血者，可加竹茹、黄芩、生地榆、白芨粉。身热者可加生石膏、知母。

处方举例：

菊花 6g、夏枯草 10g、白芍 10g、生地 30g、丹皮 12g、生石决明（先下）30g、菖蒲 10g、生大黄（后下）6g、羚羊粉（分冲）1g。

2. 阴闭

主症：除具有突然昏仆，不省人事，牙关紧闭，口噤不开等闭证的主要见症外，还有面白唇暗，静卧不烦，四肢欠温，痰涎壅盛等表现。

兼症：腹胀满，自汗出。

舌脉：舌质暗或淡，苔白腻，脉象沉滑或缓。

分析：本证易发于阳虚之人。由于平素阳虚阴盛，脾肾不足，心阳虚衰，运化失常，而致湿浊内停，如因情志不遂，内风窜扰，风挟湿浊痰邪上塞清窍，湿浊痰邪其性属阴，邪从阴化而成阴闭之证，湿浊痰邪阻滞阳气，阳气不得温煦，故见面白唇暗，四肢不温，静卧不烦等症。舌苔白腻，脉象沉滑而缓，皆主痰浊闭阻。

阴闭也是中风的危急重症。如经及时有效的治疗后，神志逐渐清醒，亦可转为中经络，预后尚好。如阴邪盛，阳气衰，正气终不可复，则易转为脱证，实难救治。阴闭日久，气机不得运化，痰湿之邪郁久亦可化热而转为痰热内闭的阳闭证。

治法：辛温开窍，豁痰熄风。

方药：急用苏合香丸灌肠或鼻饲，辛温开窍。继服涤痰汤加味。涤痰汤是由燥湿化痰理气和中之剂二陈汤加减变化而成。其中陈皮、半夏燥湿化痰，竹茹、茯苓和湿化痰，枳实降气和中，菖蒲、南星豁痰开窍，加天麻、钩藤、僵蚕平肝熄风。如挟有瘀血阻络，加丹参、川芎、地龙等，增强活血祛瘀通络之力。

处方举例：

半夏 10g、陈皮 10g、茯苓 20g、竹茹 6g、枳实 9g、菖蒲 10g、远志 10g、胆星 6g、僵蚕 9g；送服苏合香丸。

（二）脱证

主症：突然昏倒，不省人事，目合不开，呼吸微弱，四肢瘫痪，肢体汗出不止。

兼症：舌卷囊缩，脉微欲绝。

分析：阳气是人体内脏腑功能活动的动力，是生命的根本。中风脱证是阳气衰微到了极点，阴阳有离决之势，因而出现目合、口开、呼吸微弱等症，这些表现皆为五脏之气衰微欲绝的表现。心气衰则脉微欲绝；肺气衰则呼吸微弱；舌卷舌痿，汗出不止亦为心气衰败的重要见证；二便自遗是肾气衰的表现。阴衰于内，孤阳欲脱，实为中风危候。

脱证常由闭证转化而来。其主要矛盾是邪盛而正气虚，治疗上当以扶正为主。若经急救治疗后，出现闭证的表现，或闭脱诸症互见，则又当扶正祛邪。

治法：益气回阳，扶正固脱。

方药：参附汤加味。方中人参大补元气，附子回阳救逆。汗出不止者可加黄芪、牡蛎、五味子以敛汗固脱。

经过治疗，阳气回复之后，如症见面赤足冷，虚烦不宁，脉弱或浮大无根，是由于真阴亏损，虚阳浮越所引起的。真阴亏于内，虚阳浮于上，此时虚阳上浮欲脱，因此宜用地黄饮子以峻补其阴，温补肾阳，以达到阴阳双补的目的。方中熟地、麦冬、石斛、巴戟天、肉苁蓉、山萸肉、五味子补肾益精，滋阴敛液，附子、肉桂温肾扶正，摄纳浮阳，远志、菖蒲豁痰开窍。

处方举例：

制附片 10g、人参 10g、五味子 12g、黄芪 20g、麦冬 10g。

闭脱二证，因正邪双方强弱不同，病邪的阴阳属性的差异，因此临床表现不同。一般而言，闭证在中风起病时和急性期比较多见。脱证少见，多难救治。闭证和脱证也可互相转化，但有时亦可出现二者兼见的情况。在治疗上，闭证以祛邪开窍治标为主，脱证以扶正固脱，救急为先。如为闭脱互见，又当分清主次，标本兼顾，扶正祛邪。

三、后遗症

中风起病急躁，在急性期病情变化多端，经积极有效地治疗后，病情可逐渐平稳，半身不遂，言语障碍诸症也可逐渐恢复。但是一些病人由于邪气盛，正气衰，急性期和恢复期虽经多方治疗，而一些症状常难以消除，往往遗有半身不遂，言语不利或失语，情志异常，痴呆等后遗症。对后遗症的治疗除在辨证论治的原则指导下，随证加减用药外，常须结合活血、化瘀、通络、益气等法则灵活用药，还应配合针灸按摩以及加强功能锻炼，以提高疗效。对后遗症的治疗，一方面是促进功能的恢复；另一方面是预防短期内复中，对于神志失常、痴呆及抽搐发作，可按癫狂、痴呆及痫证进行辨证论治。现就半身不遂和言语不利的辨证论治分述于下：

(一)半身不遂

1. 气虚血瘀，经脉阻滞

主症：肢软无力，偏枯不用，面色萎黄，神疲乏力，或见肢体麻木，口舌歪斜。

兼证：纳少便溏，语言不利。

舌脉：舌紫暗或有瘀斑，苔白，脉细涩或重按无力。

分析：中风日久，正气大伤。气虚不能运血，气不能行，血不能荣，气血瘀滞，经脉痹阻因而引起肢软无力，偏枯不用。肢体麻木皆因气虚血瘀，经脉不得通利引起，舌紫有瘀斑均为血瘀的佐证。

治法：益气活血通络。

方药：用补阳还五汤加减，方中重用黄芪益气；当归、赤芍、川芎、桃仁、红花活血化瘀；地龙通经活络；共成益气活血。若兼见言语不利，加半夏、菖蒲、远志以祛痰利窍。兼口舌歪斜者，加白附子、僵蚕、全蝎以祛风化痰。兼有心悸心阳不足者，加桂枝、炙甘草益气温阳；兼肢体麻木者，可加木瓜、伸筋草、防己等舒筋通络，半夏、南星、陈皮、茯苓理气燥湿祛风痰之邪。小便失禁者，可加桑螵蛸、益智仁温阳补肾。肢体软弱无力者加川断、桑寄生、杜仲、牛膝等壮肾强筋骨。如因病久，血瘀症重，还要酌加水蛭、穿山甲等破血通络之品。

处方举例：

黄芪 30g、桃仁 6g、红花 6g、丹参 20g、地龙 10g、赤芍 12g、当归 10g、半夏 10g、茯苓 30g。

2. 阴虚阳亢，脉络瘀阻

主症：中风日久，半身不遂，患肢强痉僵硬拘挛，关节屈伸不利，头晕头痛，颜面潮红，耳鸣如蝉。

兼症:烦躁不安,言语不利,肢体麻木。

舌脉:舌红苔黄,脉弦有力。

分析:肝肾不足,阴不敛阳,肝阳上亢,火升风动,气血冲逆于上,因此面红、火疼、头晕、耳鸣诸症随作,筋脉失于濡养,脉络为瘀血所阻,因此半身不遂,患肢强痉拘挛,关节不利。舌红苔黄,脉弦均为阳亢之征。

治法:平肝潜阳,熄风通络。

方药:镇肝熄风汤或天麻钩藤饮加减。天麻钩藤汤中,天麻、钩藤、石决明平肝降逆;寄生、杜仲补肾;益母草、茯神、夜交藤养血安神;牛膝引气血下行;山栀、黄芩清热;还可加生地、白芍、麦冬等滋阴潜阳;木瓜、伸筋草等舒筋通络;丹参、丹皮、红花等活血祛瘀通络。

处方举例:

天麻 10g、钩藤 30g、石决明(先下)30g、桑寄生 12g、杜仲 10g、益母草 15g、生地 20g、白芍 10g、代赭石(先下)30g、山栀 6g、丹参 15g、牛膝 10g。

(二)言语不利

1. 风痰阻络

主症:舌强语蹇,甚则舌卷难以伸出,言语困难,或吞咽困难,或痰多痰稠,咯吐不利,肢体活动不利,或肢体麻木。

兼症:头晕头痛,肢体颤抖。

舌脉:舌红而暗,苔白腻或黄腻,脉象弦滑。

分析:舌为心之苗,言语的表达与心神和舌体的运动密切相关。心神蒙塞则言无所出,舌强、舌卷、活动不灵,亦可出现语言不利。心、肝、脾、肾之经络皆络于舌,心脉系于舌根,肝脉循喉咙之后上入颃嗓,脾脉连舌本散舌下,肾脉循喉咙挟舌本。因此,言语不清,舌瘖不语是风痰、瘀血阻滞舌本脉络所引起。

治法:祛风除痰,宣窍通络。

方药;解语丹加减。方中天麻、全蝎、胆南星等平肝熄风祛痰;天竺黄、远志、菖蒲、郁金、木香等宣窍利气通络,以丸、散之剂调服为宜。

处方举例:

天麻 10g、全蝎 6g、胆南星 10g、菖蒲 10g、远志 10g、天竺黄 10g、木香 6g、郁金 9g、半夏 10g、地龙 10g、丹参 30g、赤芍 10g。

2. 肾虚精亏

主症:舌瘖失语,腰膝酸软无力,心悸气短。

兼症:二便失禁,头昏眼花

舌脉:舌质瘦小或舌卷,苔白,脉沉细。

分析:中风日久,经脉不利,气血失于运达,因而久病及肾,而致肾虚精亏,精气不能上承。

治法:滋阴补肾利窍。

方药:地黄饮子加减。还可加杏仁、桔梗等利窍开瘖。

如因肾虚肝旺,肝阳上亢,挟有风痰阻滞,又宜平肝潜阳,化痰开窍。可选用天麻钩藤饮或镇肝熄风汤加菖蒲、远志、胆南星、天竺黄等化痰开窍之品。如兼见心烦失眠,可加珍珠母、琥珀以安心神。

处方举例：

熟地30g、肉苁蓉20g、山萸肉12g、石斛15g、五味子10g、菖蒲10g、远志10g、珍珠母(先下)30g、丹皮12g、丹参20g、天麻10g、茯苓20g。

(三)口眼㖞斜：如单纯遗有口眼㖞斜者，多由风痰阻络而成。风痰瘀血阻滞经络，气血不得通利，天长日久，则筋脉因失濡养而致拘急。治疗宜祛风除痰，活血通络。常用牵正散加减。方中白附子祛风除痰、镇痉、通络；僵蚕、全蝎化痰、熄风、解痉；如兼有口眼瞤动，加天麻、钩藤、石决明等平肝熄风，加白芍、木瓜柔筋通络。

处方举例：

白附子6g、全蝎6g、僵蚕6g、天麻10g、川芎10g、木瓜30g、赤芍10g。

〔预防及护理措施〕

1. 预防

(1)加强先兆症状的观察。中风虽然起病急骤，但实际上其病理变化是一个慢性发展过程，在未发病之前，常有先兆症状。清·王清任《医林改错》记录了34种中风前驱症状：有偶尔一阵头晕者，有耳内无故一阵风响者，有无故一阵眼前发直者，有睡卧口流涎沫者，有平素聪明忽然无记性者，有两手长战者，有胳膊无故发麻者，有肌肉无故跳动者，有眼无故抽筋者……。中风的预防，确应从慎起居，调情志，节饮食三方面着手。所谓慎起居，不仅生活要有规律，注意劳逸适度，更重要的是中老年人应重视体育锻炼，使气机和调，血脉流畅，关节疏利，防止本病的发生；所谓调情志，是指要经常保持心情舒畅、情绪稳定，避免七情所伤。情志过极，常为中风诱因，因此，调情志，戒郁怒，甚为重要。节饮食是指饮食要以清淡为主，避免肥甘厚味之品，切忌嗜烟酗酒，亦不可食之过饱。

(2)加强对先兆症状的早期治疗。若见眩晕、耳鸣、肉瞤、抽搐等症，为肝阳偏亢，肝风欲动之象，予平肝熄风之钩藤、菊花、白蒺藜、牡蛎、白芍等药；若见肢体麻木，沉滞者，为脉络气血痹阻，予活血通络之丹参、赤芍、桃仁、红花、鸡血藤等药。

(3)关于复发问题：中风经积极治疗后可以恢复，但易于复发。若复发再次中风称复中。由此说明中风易于复发，而且复发后病势必加重，甚至有生命危险，因此应当认真预防。

2. 护理

中风急性期，重症病人多有五不会，即翻身、咳嗽、说话、进食、大小便均不能自主。要严密观察，精心护理，积极抢救以促进病情自愈，减少并发症、后遗症。

(1)认真观察病情的变化，是判断病情顺逆的重要环节。如患者神志变化，由昏迷转清醒者为顺，反之为逆。其他可对抽搐发作次数的多少、发作形式及时间，戴阳、呕血、便血等症状表现仔细观察、记录。脉证的变化，对判断顺逆很重要。本病如阳闭之证，脉来沉迟或见代脉，是有暴亡之可能；后遗症的半身不遂，本属气虚脉缓者，骤然脉弦劲而数，多有复中的可能，所以在护理上均应细察。

(2)饮食宜忌：中风病的饮食原则以清淡为宜。尤其在急性期，重症吞咽不能者可鼻饲混合奶、蔬菜汁。切忌肥甘厚味、辛辣刺激之品，肥甘厚味而碍胃生湿化痰，辛辣之品有动火之虞，对病情不利。此外，酗酒可加重或诱发中风，应忌酒。

(3)预防褥疮：中风急性期卧床不动最易发生褥疮，护理上尽做到勤翻身，对神昏者要定时检查皮肤，衣褥床单要干燥，平整，柔软，受压部位皮肤发红者应用手掌揉擦，或用红花酊外擦，以疏通经络，促进血液循环。

(4)功能锻炼：鼓励和辅导病人进行功能锻炼，是中风恢复期和后遗症期护理工作重点，对瘫痪肢体不能自主运动时，应进行按摩，加强被动运动，以促进血脉流通，防止关节挛缩，加快恢复。患者能自主活动者，应根据其活动程度指导锻炼。对中风不语者，应耐心教病人发音，逐步恢复语言功能。

〔典型病例分析〕

案一：余某某，男性，64岁，工人，于1984年7月9日入院。

患者素体肥胖，平时经常头晕，高血压病史十余年，两天前在劳动时突然跌倒，左侧肢体瘫疲，神志欠清，急诊入院。当时症见神识迷蒙，重咳偶醒，舌强言蹇，左侧半身不遂，口舌歪斜，大便三日未行，舌暗红少津，苔微黄而腻，脉弦滑大，左大于右，投星蒌承气汤加味：

全瓜蒌30g、胆南星6g、天竺黄6g、丹皮10g、丹参30g、芒硝（冲）6g、生大黄（后下）10g、菖蒲6g。

二剂后便出黏臭大便六七次，泻后神志转清，脉仍弦滑，余症同前；改投清热化痰活血通络之剂：全瓜蒌15g、胆南星6g、天竺黄6g、丹参30g、丹皮10g、鸡血藤30g、酒军6g。

进12剂后黄厚苔化，言语较前较清，患侧肢体略能抬举，再进活血祛瘀，化痰通络之剂，于上方中加重活血通络之品，随症化裁。服二十余剂后可由人搀扶行走，语言流利，病人转针灸科恢复治疗。

按：本例发病时证属痰热腑实，风痰上扰症，风火挟痰浊上蒙清窍阻塞脉络，故见神志迷蒙，言语蹇涩，半身不遂等症，经化痰通腑治疗后，腑气通，痰热减，神志转清，证由中腑转为中经，再予清热化痰、活血通络之剂，痰热瘀血渐消，病情好转。可见抓住辨证要点，对症治疗是本例奏效的关键。

中风病为临床常见病多发病，因其急性期病变快、变化多、死亡率高，有的虽经积极救治，度过了急性期，又常遗有半身不遂，言语不利等症，有的甚至终身致残。其发病原因虽有多种，但其根本在于脏腑功能失调，阴阳偏胜。如由经络空虚，外邪入中经络引起者，称为真中；类中是由于风阳扰动，气血上逆，挟痰挟火，流窜经脉，蒙塞清窍而成。在临床分证时，则依据有无神识障碍分为中脏腑和中经络。中经络者又分为外风入中和内风所伤两类，外风入中多无先兆，而兼外感表现，治宜扶正祛邪，疏风解表，和营通络。中脏腑表现为神识昏蒙，但有闭脱之分。闭证又按痰火和痰湿的不同而分为阳闭和阴闭，二者各具特点。在治疗上，阳闭宜辛凉开窍，清肝熄风；阴闭则宜辛温开窍，除痰熄风。至于脱证，乃因元气衰微，阴阳将欲离绝，治宜急救，以益气固脱为先。

中风急性期后，经适当调理，常可逐渐康复，但也有不少患者留有后遗症，应积极治疗半身不遂。如属气虚血瘀，经脉不通，当以益气活血通络为主；如为肝阳亢盛，瘀阻脉络者，治以平肝潜阳，熄风通络；语言不利，又有风痰阻络，肾虚精亏的不同，当随证或祛风除痰或补肾填精。若因痰热阻滞所致，又应清热化痰利窍，祛瘀通脉。中风又易复发，预防调理甚为重要，应注意在出现先兆症状时，即应认真治疗，防止卒中发生。

复习思考题

1. 中风有哪些主要临床特征？

2. 中风的基本病因有哪些？其具体病理变化是什么？

3. 中经络与中脏腑的主要区别是什么？怎样进行辨证治疗？

4. 中风闭证与脱证的急救措施有哪些？

5. 中风病人应当怎样调护？

水　肿

〔概述〕

水肿是指体内水液潴留，泛滥肌肤，引起眼睑、头面、四肢、腹背、阴囊甚至全身浮肿的一种病证。严重者可伴胸、腹腔积水，甚至变生它病，威胁生命。

本病在《内经》中称"水"，根据不同的症状分为"风水"、"石水"、"涌水"等。并详细描述了水肿的病因、病机、分类。治疗上提出攻逐、发汗、利小便三种方法。《金匮要略》称为"水气病"，并设专篇进行论述，从病因脉证而分其为"风水"、"皮水"、"正水"、"石水"、"黄汗"；又按五脏证候特点分其为心水、肝水、肺水、脾水、肾水，且指出应根据水肿的不同部位，采用不同治法，即"腰以下肿当利小便，腰以上肿当发汗"。

《丹溪心法》将水肿分为阴水与阳水两大类，切合实用。宋元以后，对病机认识有了较大的发展，强调肺脾肾三脏气化功能失调在水肿发病中的重要作用，治疗由祛邪改为健脾、补肾、温阳，及攻补兼施等法，至此成为一完整的理论体系。

西医学的急慢性肾炎、充血性心力衰竭、内分泌失调及营养障碍等所出现的水肿皆可参考本病进行辨证施治。

〔病因病机〕

水液在人体的正常运行，有赖于肺气的通调，脾气的转输，肾气的开阖，从而使三焦发挥决渎职能，膀胱气化畅行，小便通利。反之，凡影响肺脾肾三脏调节水液代谢功能，致三焦决渎无权，膀胱气化不利，水液运行障碍，停聚泛滥发为水肿。

引起水肿的病因，有外感和内伤两类。因于外感者，以风寒、湿致病为多；因于内伤者，以饮食、劳倦、房劳及体虚致病为多。

一、风邪外袭，肺失通调：肺主宣发，为水之上源，外合皮毛，主一身之表，风寒或风热，外袭肌表，肺失宣降，不能通调水道，下输膀胱，以致风遏水阻，风水相搏，流溢肌肤，发为水肿。

二、水湿浸渍，脾失健运：脾主运化，喜燥恶湿，居住潮湿、阴冷或冒雨涉水，则寒邪水湿内侵；或平素酒食不节，生冷太过，则湿蕴于中，脾为湿困，健运失司，以致清阳不升，浊阴不降，水湿内停，泛滥肌肤，而成水肿。若水湿下去，久郁化热，湿热交蒸，膀胱气化失常，亦成水肿。

三、湿热疮毒，内侵脾肺：肌肤疮疡痒疹，留恋不愈，风毒湿热郁遏体表，内归肺脾，导致水液代谢受阻，外溢为肿。

四、饮食劳倦，伤及脾胃：脾主运化，胃主受纳。饮食失调，饥饱无常，必致脾胃受伤；劳倦过度，则脾虚气耗，健运失司，土不制水，湿停水聚，而致水肿。又脾虚生化乏源，气血虚弱，气不化水，遂成虚肿。

五、房劳多育，内伤肾气：肾藏精，为先天之本；又主水，为气之根。禀赋不足，或房劳多育，耗伤肾气，肾虚则不能化气行水，水液停聚，外溢肌肤，形成水肿。

水肿病因病机示意图

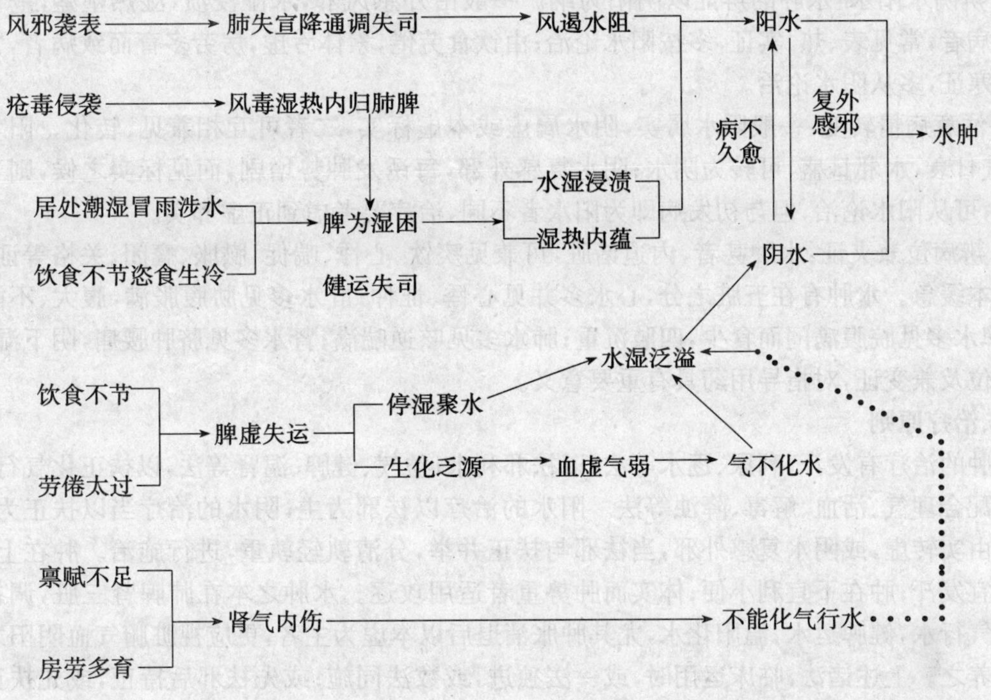

总之，水肿发生的病因为：外感风邪，内舍于肺，肺失通调，肌肤疮疡痒疹，未能清消，疮毒内归脾肺；外居湿地，冒雨涉水，水湿之邪内侵，或平素饮食不节，贪食生冷，致脾为湿困而失健运；湿热久羁，或湿郁化热，使湿热内盛，中焦不得升降而三焦壅滞；饮食不节，劳倦太过，伤及脾胃而运化无权；房劳过度，生育不节内伤肾元而气化不行。以上各种病因，有外感，有内伤，因外感而致者，多为阳水，因内伤而生者，多成阴水。其可以是单一原因发病，也可兼杂致病，且阴水、阳水并非一成不变，可以相互转化。如阳水久延不愈，水湿浸渍，留恋不去，以致正气日衰，脾肾阳虚，使病情更为缠绵，转为阴水；反之，阴水复感外邪，肺气失宣，使肿势突然增剧，则当以阳水论治，先治其标。阴水感邪，出现阳证，不能理解为病情由重转轻，乃正虚邪盛，病情更为复杂。水肿的病理变化主要在肺脾肾三脏，肺失通调，脾失转输，肾失开阖，全身气化功能障碍，导致水液潴留，泛滥成肿；三者之间，又相互联系，相互影响。如肾水上泛，凌心犯肺，致肺气不降，水道不通，使肾气更虚，水邪更盛；相反，肺经受邪而传入肾经时，亦能引起同样结果。肾虚不能温煦脾土，致脾失健运，水湿停聚则湿更困脾；脾气益虚，气血乏源，血不化精，肾精亏乏，不能主水，水肿更甚。三脏之中，以肾为本，以肺为标，以脾为制水之脏，实为治疗水肿的关键所在。此外，瘀血阻滞，伤及三焦水道，使水肿顽固难愈；水肿久延，肾元衰竭，浊邪上犯或肝风内动，可产生脱变，预后多属不良。

〔辨证论治〕

水肿初起，大都从眼睑部开始，继则延及头面、四肢、腰腹及全身。也有从下肢开始，然后渐及全身者。轻者仅见颜面、下肢等局部水肿，严重者周身俱肿，甚至腹满胸闷，心悸气喘，不能平卧。在治疗方法上如《素问·汤液醪醴论》说："平治于权衡，去菀陈莝……开鬼门，洁净府。"迄今仍有重要的临床指导意义。

一、辨证要点

1. 辨阴水阳水：水肿的辨证以阴阳为纲。一般由外感风邪，水湿浸渍，湿热壅盛，疮毒内侵而致病者，常见表、热、实证，多按阳水论治；由饮食劳倦，素体亏虚，房劳多育而致病者，常见里、虚、寒证，多从阴水论治。

2. 注意病情转变：一般阳水属实，阴水属虚或本虚标实，二者可互相兼见、转化。阳水迁延，正气日衰，水邪日盛，可转为阴水；阴水复感外邪，每诱发肿势增剧，而见标实之候，则当治标为急，可从阳水论治，但与初发病即为阳水者不同，治疗要考虑到正虚邪实。

3. 辨病位兼夹证：水肿甚者，内迫诸脏，可兼见痰饮、心悸、喘促、臌胀、癃闭、关格等证，应分清标本缓急。水肿有在五脏之分，心水多并见心悸、怔忡；肝水多见胁腹胀满，腹大、不能自转侧；脾水多见脘腹满闷而食少，四肢沉重；肺水多见咳逆喘满；肾水多见脐肿腰痛，阴下湿冷。明其病位及兼变证，对指导用药具有重要意义。

二、治疗原则

水肿的治疗有发汗、利尿、逐水等法，以祛邪利水；益气、健脾、温肾等法，以扶正化气行水；另外可配合理气、活血、解毒、降浊等法。阳水的治疗以祛邪为主，阴水的治疗当以扶正为先；若阳水由实转虚，或阴水复感外邪，当祛邪与扶正并举，分清孰轻孰重，进行施治。肿在上，有表证者宜发汗；肿在下宜利小便；体实而肿势重者适用攻逐。水肿之本在肺脾肾三脏，调补内脏可益气行水，健脾运水，温阳化水，尤其肿胀消退后以本虚为主者，更应视脏腑气血阴阳之亏损以补养之。上述诸法，临床运用时，或一法独进，或数法同施；或先祛邪后持正，或先扶正后祛邪，或正邪兼顾，依病情而择之。

三、分型论治

(一)阳水

1. 风水泛滥

主症：水肿先从眼睑开始，继则四肢、胸背、腹部及全身皆肿，来势迅速，以头面肿为剧，皮肤鲜泽光亮而薄，按之凹陷易于恢复，小便不利。

兼症：多有恶寒发热，肢节酸重，或咳嗽气喘，或咽喉疼痛，乳蛾红肿。

舌脉：偏于风寒者，舌苔薄白而滑，脉浮滑或紧；偏于风热者，舌质红，苔薄黄，脉浮滑数。如水邪泛溢，肿势较重，可见脉沉。

分析：肺主宣发，外合皮毛；主肃降，通调水道。风邪外袭，肺气失宣，不能通调水道，下输膀胱，故小便不利，水聚泛滥肌肤发为水肿。风为阳邪，其性轻扬，善行数变，风水相搏，推波助澜，故水肿起于面目，迅速波及肢体。风邪为患，其病在表，正气尚盛，阳气通达，故皮肤鲜泽光亮而薄，按之凹陷容易恢复。邪客肌表，卫阳被遏，营卫不和，则发热恶寒，肢节酸重。外邪犯肺，肺气失宣，或水气凌肺，肺失宣降，皆可见咳嗽气喘。风热上扰则咽喉肿痛。苔薄白而滑，脉浮滑或紧，为风水偏寒。舌质红，苔薄黄，脉浮数，是风水偏热。肿势严重，阳气被遏，则见沉脉。

治法：疏风清热，宣肺行水。

方药：越婢加术汤加减。方中麻黄散风宣肺，行水消肿；石膏清肺泄热；白术健脾利水；生姜、甘草、大枣调和营卫；诸药配伍使肺气宣通，肺热清泄，水湿下行，风水自退。如热重尿少，可重用石膏，加鲜茅根、赤小豆以清热利尿。如表邪甚而偏寒者，少用或去石膏，加羌活，防风以疏风散寒解表。若咽喉红肿疼痛，加板蓝根、桔梗、射干、牛蒡子以清热毒、利咽消肿。若热盛伤阴,烦热口渴,舌红少津,加玄参、芦根、知母以滋阴清热;若咳喘痰多,加杏仁、桔梗、前胡宣肺止咳,甚则加桑白皮、葶苈子、苏子泻肺平喘。

若表证渐解,身重水肿不退,可按水湿浸渍治法,用五苓散、五皮饮等方,以通阳利水,健脾化湿。若汗出恶风,身重浮肿,为卫阳已虚,宜防己黄芪汤加减,助卫气以行水湿。

处方举例:

麻黄 6g、生石膏 15g、白术 12g、赤小豆 30g、桔梗 9g、车前子(包煎)30g,生姜 4g、炙甘草 4g。

(二)水湿浸渍

主症:全身水肿,下肢尤甚,按之凹陷,小便短少。起病较缓慢,病程较长。

兼症:身重困倦,胸闷腹胀,纳呆泛恶。

舌脉:舌苔白腻或白滑,脉沉缓。

分析:居住潮湿,或冒雨涉水,衣着湿冷,或贪食生冷,水湿内侵,困阻中土,则脾失健运,水湿停聚;水湿内聚,三焦决读失司,膀胱气化不利,故小便短少。水湿之邪与日俱增,浸渍肌肤,壅塞不行,故全身肢体浮肿,肿势日甚,按之没指。湿为阴邪,其性黏腻,不易骤化,故疾病缠绵,经久难愈。湿停中焦,胃失和降,故纳呆泛恶。脾为湿困,阳气不得舒展,故胸闷腹胀,身重困倦。舌苔白腻或白滑,脉沉缓,为湿困之象。

治法:通阳利水,健脾化湿。

方药:五苓散合五皮饮加减。方中白术、茯苓皮、猪苓、泽泻甘淡渗湿,通利小便;桂枝辛温通阳,使气化而水行;生姜皮辛散水气;陈皮、大腹皮行气化湿;桑白皮肃降肺气,通调水道;白术、茯苓、陈皮健脾化湿;诸药合用有通阳化气行水,健脾化湿消肿的功能。如上半身肿甚而咳喘气逆者,加麻黄、杏仁以宣肺平喘;甚者加葶苈子泻肺平喘,利水消肿。如口淡神疲,脘闷腹胀,纳呆泛恶,舌苔白厚,为湿阻中焦,胃失和降,可加厚朴、苍术即胃苓汤意,使脾健而湿化。气行而水行。下肢肿著,可加车前子、抽胡芦利水消肿。

处方举例:

茯苓皮 30g、桑白皮 10g、猪苓 15g、泽泻 15g、炒白术 10g、桂枝 6g、生姜皮 6g、厚朴 6g、砂仁 3g。

(三)疮毒内侵

主症:身患疮疡,或咽喉肿痛溃烂,眼睑浮肿,延及全身,小便不利。

兼症:恶风发热,或身痒。

古脉:古质红,苔薄黄,脉浮数或滑数。

分析:肌肤乃肺脾所主之域,疮疡痒疹,治疗不当,湿毒未能及时清解消散,内归脏腑致脾不能运化水湿,肺不能通调水道,故小便不利。风毒在表,肺气不利,营卫不和,则恶寒发热;湿浊内聚、风水相捕,故肿起眼睑,延及全身。舌质红、苔薄黄,脉浮数或滑数,是风邪夹湿毒所致。

治法:宣肺解毒,利湿消肿。

方药:麻黄连翘赤小豆汤加减。方中麻黄、杏仁宣肺行水;桑白皮、赤小豆清热利湿消肿;连翘清热解毒消痈,生姜、大枣、甘草调和营卫。若脓毒甚者加五味消毒饮以加强解毒消痈之力;若湿盛而糜烂者,加苦参、土茯苓清热燥湿;若风盛而瘙痒者加白藓皮、地肤子祛风止痒;大便不通,加大黄、芒硝通腑泄浊。

处方举例：

炙麻黄5g、连翘15g、赤小豆30g、土茯苓30g、野菊花10g、地丁10g、银花10g、车前草15g、通草6g、白芷10g。

(四)湿热壅盛

主症：全身水肿，皮肤绷紧光亮，肿势多剧，小便短赤，大便干结。

兼症：烦热口渴，脘腹胀满。

舌脉；舌苔黄腻，脉沉数或滑数。

分析；感受湿热或水湿之邪，郁而化热，淫溢于肌肤、经络之间，故遍身水肿而皮肤润泽绷紧光亮；湿热壅盛，故肿势多剧；湿热熏蒸，三焦气化不利，气机升降失常，故小便短赤，胸脘腹胀；热盛灼津，故烦热口渴，小便短赤；传导失常则大便干结。舌苔黄腻，脉沉数或滑数均为湿热壅盛之象。

治法：分利湿热。

方药：疏凿饮子加减。本方能攻逐水湿，具上下表里分消之功，使蓄积之水从二便排出，热清水去，肿势自退。方中羌活、秦艽疏风透表，使在表水气从汗而解；商陆、椒目、赤小豆、泽泻、木通通利二便，使在里之水从下而去；大腹皮、槟榔行气利水，气行则水行。此为治水肿属表里俱实，湿热壅盛，遍身水肿的一般泻剂，如腹大胀满，二便涩少，可合用已椒苈黄丸以助攻泻之力，使水从大便下泄。若肿势严重，兼见胸满气粗，咳喘不能平卧，脉弦数有力，为水在胸中，上迫于肺，肺气不降，宜泻肺行水为主，可用五苓散、五皮饮等方合葶苈大枣泻肺汤，以泻胸中之水气。

处方举例：

商陆6g、茯苓皮30g、大腹皮15g、泽泻10g、车前子(包煎)30g、防风6g、赤小豆30g、川椒目6g、防己10g、槟榔10g。

二、脾阳不振

主症：身肿腰以下为甚，按之凹陷不易恢复。

兼症：面色萎黄，脘闷腹胀，纳减便溏，神倦肢冷，小便短少。

舌脉：舌淡体胖，苔白滑或白腻，脉沉缓或沉细无力。

分析：饥饱劳役，年高体弱，久病体虚，致中阳不足，脾失健运，气不化水，水湿潴留，故小便短少；水湿沉降，泛滥下焦，故水肿腰以下为甚，按之凹陷不起；脾阳不振，运化无权，故脘闷腹胀，纳少便溏；脾气不足，卫阳亦虚，气无华色，故神倦肢冷，面色少华。舌淡体胖，苔白滑或白腻，脉沉缓或沉细无力，为脾阳不振，津液不化，水湿停聚之象。

治法：温阳健脾，行气利水。

方药：实脾饮加减。方中茯苓、白术健脾利湿；附子、干姜温运中阳，以化水湿；佐以大腹皮、木香、木瓜行气利水；厚朴、草果燥湿行气；甘草、大枣补脾和中。诸药共凑温阳健脾，行气利水。如水湿过重，加桂枝、泽泻、猪苓助膀胱气化以利小便。气虚息短加党参、黄芪以补脾胃之气；若脘闷呕恶，舌苔白厚腻，加苍术、佩兰、藿香以健脾燥湿，芳香化浊。

处方举例：

茯苓30g、苍白术各10g、干姜6g、制附片6g、木香10g、厚朴10g、草果10g、大腹皮12g、木瓜10g、泽泻10g。

（二）肾阳衰微

主症：水肿日久，反复迁延，腰以下肿甚，按之凹陷不起，尿量减少或反增多。

兼症：面色灰滞或㿠白，腰痛酸重，四肢厥冷，怯寒神疲，甚者心悸气促。

舌脉：舌质淡胖，苔白，脉沉细或沉迟。

分析：肾主水，三焦气化赖肾阳温煦、蒸腾。若禀赋不足，或久病失养，或水肿迁延不愈，均可耗伤肾气，致肾阳不足，气化不利而水液停留，游溢肌肤，发为水肿。腰膝以下，肾气主之，故肾阳衰微，阴盛于下，则腰以下肿甚，按之凹陷不起。肾司二便，与膀胱相表里，肾阳不足，膀胱气化不利，则尿量减少；肾关不固，开多阖少，则尿反增多。腰为肾之腑，肾虚水气内盛，则腰痛酸重。肾虚火衰，不能温养肢体，故四肢厥冷，怯寒神疲。阳气不能温煦于上，则面色㿠白，阴寒内盛，气血凝滞，则面色晦暗。水邪上逆，凌心射肺，则心悸气促。舌淡体胖，苔薄白，脉沉细或沉迟，为肾阳衰微，水湿内盛之象。

治法：温肾助阳，化气行水。

方药：济生肾气丸或真武汤加减。肾为水火之脏，内寄元阴元阳，由于阴阳互根，故善补阳者，必于阴中求阳，前方用六味地黄丸滋补肾阴；附子、肉桂温肾助阳、化气行水；与六味地黄丸相伍，能补水中之火，温肾中之阳；车前子利水消肿。后方附子温肾助阳以消阴翳；白术、茯苓以健脾行水；生姜以温散水寒之气；白芍调和营阴以利水行。前方适用于肾阴阳两虚，以阳虚为主，水邪内停；后方为脾肾阳衰，阴寒内盛，水邪内停。如虚寒过甚，可加葫芦巴、巴戟天等温补肾阳，以助气化；如肾虚不固，小便清长量多，去泽泻、车前子加补骨脂、益智仁、巴戟天以温固肾阳，如喘息气短，呼多吸少，动则益甚，汗出肢冷，为水邪凌肺、肾不纳气，加人参、五味子、蛤蚧、煅牡蛎或吞服黑锡丹以助阳纳气，防喘脱之变；如心悸胸闷，唇舌紫绀，脉虚数或结代，为水邪上逆，心阳被遏，心血瘀阻，宜重用附子，加桂枝、炙甘草、丹参、红花以温阳化瘀；如头重呕恶，神倦思睡，甚至神昏，口有尿味，病情严重，为湿浊上蒙清窍，宜温脾汤合平胃散加藿香、佩兰以温阳泻浊，和胃降逆；或用制附子合大黄、黄连、半夏以解毒降浊。如病久不愈，复感外邪，肿势增剧，发热恶寒，无汗，应按风水论治，但不可过用表散之剂，宜顾护正气，扶正祛邪。病延至后期，肾阳虚衰，阳损及阴，致肾阴亏虚，证见水肿缠绵，头晕乏力，腰酸遗精，口干咽燥，烦热盗汗，舌红少苔脉细数，治宜补肾阳、滋肾阴，兼利小便以祛水邪，可加大补元煎，然滋阴不可过于凉腻，防碍水邪，利水不可太甚，免伤阴津。

处方举例：

熟地 10g、茯苓 30g、制附片 9g、山药 10g、白术 10g、白芍 10g、炙甘草 6g、肉桂 6g、益母草 30g、泽泻 12g。

另外，对于水肿的治疗，常配合活血化瘀法。如《血证论》说："瘀血化水，亦发水肿，是血病而兼水也。"血行水亦行。故治疗水肿尤其常法罔效而有瘀血证候者，加用益母草、泽兰、桃仁、红花能加强利尿消肿的作用。

〔预防及护理措施〕

1. 注意忌盐。《世医得效方》："凡水肿唯忌盐"。故水肿初期，应进无盐饮食；待肿势渐退，逐步改为低盐，最后改为普通饮食。

2. 禁食生冷、油腻、辛辣及酒酪等刺激性食物，宜食富有营养又容易消化吸收的食物。

3. 调摄寒温，避免外邪入侵；戒暴怒、节情志，树立战胜疾病信心，戒房劳及勿过劳，以防重伤精气，加重病情。

4. 及时治疗疮毒，皮疹，咽烂，防止疮毒内攻。

5. 病情严重，应密切注意病情变化，预防喘脱、动风，扰神蒙心等变证发生。

〔典型病例分析〕

案一：张某，男，15 岁，住院号 1382。

1983 年 11 月 26 日入院。10 天前感冒头痛，发热恶寒，咽喉肿痛，面目、全身浮肿 4 天。诊见：面目浮肿，目不能启，腹部胀大，下肢微肿，溺短赤，畏寒项强，身倦神差，咳嗽痰清，纳差食少，苔薄白，脉浮缓。

本例风邪外袭，郁遏化热，水热互结，风水相搏，壅塞肺气，宣降失司，治节无权，致三焦气化不利，水邪不能下输膀胱，水湿泛滥横逆而为全身水肿。治宜宣肺发表，利水消肿，拟方：

麻黄 12g、石膏 50g、苍术 12g、大枣 25g、云苓 15g、泽泻 15g、猪苓 15g、车前子（包煎）25g、白茅根 25g、夏枯草 15g、益母草 15g、防己 25g、甘草 6g。

服上方 6 剂，尿量增加，水肿消失。原方出入续服 10 剂告愈，尿检正常。随访 5 月，未见复发。（《四川中医》，1985(6)：24）

按：本案病因外邪，病位在肺，风水泛滥，肿势为面目浮肿甚于下肢，病程四天，四诊所见，病属风水，病机为肺失宣降，故选用越婢加术汤加减宣肺行水而愈。

水肿是指体内水液潴留，泛滥肌肤，甚至停留胸腹腔为主要症状的一类病证。其病因外感内伤皆有，每因风邪外袭，水湿浸淫，湿热疮毒内盛，以及饮食劳倦，房劳多育而致肺失通调，脾失转输，肾失开阖，水湿潴留，泛滥肌肤乃成。其病与肺脾肾三脏关系密切，而三脏中又以肾最为重要。

水肿辨证以阴阳为纲，凡由风水泛滥，水湿浸渍，湿热疮毒壅盛所致者，多为阳水，属实，病在肺脾；由脾阳不振，肾阳衰微所致者，多为阴水，属虚，病在脾肾。但临证时，常是阴阳错杂，虚实互见，必须注意其转化。水肿的治疗方法，有发汗，利尿、逐水及健脾、温肾、降浊、化瘀等法；阳水证以发汗，利小便为主，湿浊壅结，大便不通，可暂用攻下逐水，病缓即止，以免伤正。阴水证以温化为主，其中脾虚者，温脾实土；肾虚者，温肾助阳。若虚实夹杂者，当攻补兼施，或先标后本。一般水肿消退后，常见虚象，应根据脏腑气血阴阳之不足予以调补。

至于水肿预后，凡起病不久，或由于营养障碍所致的浮肿，只要及时治疗，预后较好；病起日久，反复发作，正虚邪恋，则缠绵难愈。如肿势较甚，症见心悸、唇绀、气急喘促不能平卧，或唇黑、缺盆平，脐突，足不平，背平，或恶心呕吐，口有尿味，神志昏蒙，或头晕头痛，肢体振颤甚至抽搐，或尿闭，衄血、尿血、便血、均属病情危笃，预后不良。

另外，本病注意禁盐，避免食辛辣厚味，防止感冒及过劳，方可使其不致复发。

复习思考题

1. 简述肺、脾、肾三脏功能障碍在水肿发病中的重要意义。

2. 水肿病的辨证要点及常见治则是什么？怎样运用之？

3. 阴水、阳水的特点是什么？如何辨证论治？

4. 水肿的预后如何？

5. 水肿病人怎样调摄？

淋　　证

〔附:尿浊〕

〔概述〕

淋证是以小便频数短涩,滴沥刺痛,欲出未尽,小腹拘急,或痛引腰腹为特征的病证。

淋证之名,首见于《内经》。《金匮要略》称本证为"淋"、"淋秘",指出淋病以小便淋沥不爽,尿道刺痛为特征。其"小便如粟状"系言一者尿道如有粟粒阻塞,引起涩痛难忍;再者为尿中排出结石,状如粟粒。此乃对中医淋证特征的生动描述。《中藏经》已认识到淋征属于一种全身性的病证。诸如五脏不通,六腑不和,三焦痞涩,营卫耗失等均可致淋,又根据病因及临床表现不同,提出淋有冷、热、气、劳、膏、砂、虚、实八种,使淋证临床分类始具雏形。《外台秘要》具体指出五淋的内容为:"集验论五淋者,石淋,气淋,膏淋,劳淋,热淋也。"临床沿用迄今,惟内容略有不同,一般分为气、血、石、劳、膏五种。有关本病的病机,丹溪认为属热,河间指出与气血郁结有关;《景岳全书》则言其有"为寒为热为虚",较为完备。治则方面,《丹溪心法·淋》,《金匮翼》提出的治疗方法,对临床具有重要指导意义。

西医学的泌尿系感染,泌尿系结石,肿瘤,前列腺疾病以及乳糜尿等病出现淋病证状者,皆可参考本病进行辨证施治。

〔病因病机〕

淋证的主要病因是湿热蕴结于下焦。《金匮要略·五脏风寒积聚病脉证并治》认为是"热在下焦"。《丹溪心法·淋》说:"淋有五,皆属乎热。"《诸病源候论·淋病诸候》进一步提出"诸淋者,由肾虚而膀胱热故也"。由此说明淋证初起,多属湿热蕴结膀胱,日久则由实转虚,或虚实挟杂。

兹根据历代医家论述,将淋证的病因可归纳为以下三方面:

一、膀胱湿热:湿热多受自于外,亦可由内而生,感于外者,或因下阴不洁,秽浊之邪侵入膀胱;或由其他脏腑邪热传入膀胱,如心火炽盛,移热小肠,下注膀胱。生于内者,多因嗜食辛热肥甘之品,或饮酒成癖,酿成湿热,流注膀胱,气化失司,水道不利,发为淋证。若小便灼热刺痛者为热淋;若膀胱热盛,热伤脉络,迫血妄行,小便涩痛有血,则为血淋;若湿热下注,膀胱气化不利,清浊不分,脂液不循常道,随小便而出,小便如脂如膏,则为膏淋;若湿热蕴结,煎熬尿液,尿中杂质结为砂石,则为石淋。总之,热、血、膏、石诸淋多因膀胱湿热而致。

二、脾肾亏虚:久淋不愈,湿热耗伤正气,或年老,久病体弱,劳累过度及房室不节,均可导致脾肾亏虚,脾虚则中气下陷,肾虚则下元不固,因而小便淋沥不已。肾为先天之本,脾为后天之本,二者相互资生,相互促进,故脾虚可致肾虚,肾虚亦可致脾虚。脾肾亏虚。外邪易于侵袭膀胱,罹患淋证;而淋病之后湿热伤及脾肾,使病情缠绵难愈。可见脾肾亏虚与膀胱湿热皆是淋证发生的重要病因。若遇劳即加重者,则为劳淋。若中气不足,气虚下陷者,则为气淋。若肾气亏虚,下元不固,不能摄约脂液,脂液下泄,尿液浑浊,如脂膏者,则为膏淋。若肾阴亏虚,阴虚火旺,虚火灼络,尿中挟血者,则为血淋。

三、肝郁气滞:恼怒伤肝,气滞不宣,气郁化火,或气火郁于下焦,膀胱气化不利,则少腹作胀,小便艰涩而痛,余沥不尽,发为气淋,此属气淋之实证。中气下陷所致气淋,属气淋之虚证。

综上所述,淋证的病因以膀胱湿热为主,病位主要在膀胱与肾,且和肝脾有关,病机主要是湿热蕴结下焦，膀胱气化不利。病初多为邪实，久病则由实转虚；如邪气未尽，正气已伤，则虚实夹杂。

淋证病因病机示意图

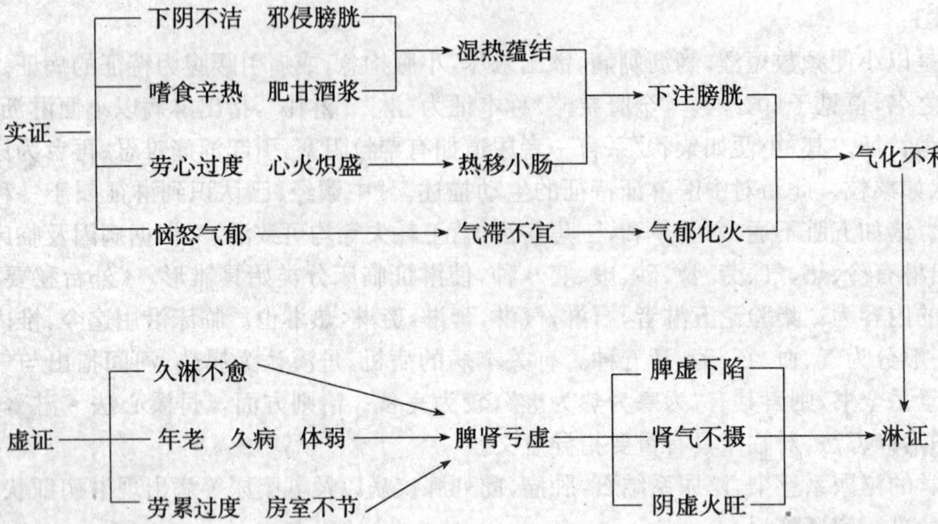

〔辨证论治〕

一、辨证要点

1. 辨明淋证类别：小便频数短涩，滴沥刺痛，欲出未尽，小腹拘急，或痛引腰腹，为诸淋共有的症状；但各种淋证，又各具特征。石淋以小便排出砂石为主证；膏淋以小便浑浊如米泔水或如脂膏为主证；血淋以溺血而涩痛为主证；气淋以少腹满痛或坠胀，小便艰涩疼痛，尿有余沥为主证；热淋以小便灼热刺痛为主证；劳淋以小便淋沥不已，遇劳即发或加重为主证。

2. 审察证候虚实：淋证在区别各种不同类型基础上，还需审察证候虚实，辨证以病因，病程，局部及整体症状，小便色泽及性状为依据。一般初病或在急性发作阶段属实，以膀胱湿热，结石结聚，气滞不利为主；久病多虚，病在脾肾，以脾虚、肾虚、气阴两虚为主。尿灼热刺痛明显，溲浊色赤，而无脏腑阴阳虚弱者多实；尿灼热刺痛不著，溲清色淡，而兼脏腑阴阳虚亏者多虚。同一种淋证，由于病因病机不同，有虚有实。如石淋因湿下注，灼尿成石者为实；因久病伤阴，或脾肾亏虚者为虚，膏热淋因湿热下注，气化不利，脂液失于约束，症见尿浊，热涩疼痛者为实；因久病肾虚，下元不固，症见淋如脂膏，形瘦神疲，腰酸膝软者为虚。血淋因湿热下注，热伤血络，症见尿热涩痛，尿色深红者为实；因阴虚火旺，迫血妄行，尿痛涩滞不甚，尿色淡红，腰膝酸软者为虚。

3. 注意标本缓急：淋证可由实转虚，或因虚致实，或虚实互见；同时各种淋证之间，也可互相转化或并存。因此，临证时要辨清标本缓急，才能分明主次，确定治则。如初病石淋，多系湿热下注，煎熬尿液，结为砂石，标本皆实；日久不愈，耗伤气阴，可见阴虚或气虚之证。逐渐由实转虚，而呈本虚标实。又如劳淋，多系脾肾两虚，若复感外邪，湿热之邪侵入膀胱，则发热淋；常现本虚标实之候，根据急则治标，缓则治本的原则，当先清利湿热，治标治热淋，再乎扶正补虚，治本治劳淋。

4.类证鉴别

(1)癃闭:癃闭以排尿困难,小便量少甚至点滴全无为特征,其小便量少,排尿困难与淋证相似;但淋证尿频而疼痛,每日排尿总量多为正常,癃闭则无尿痛,每日排尿总量低于正常,严重时,小便闭塞,无尿排出。

(2)尿血:血淋和尿血都是尿中混有血液,或伴有血块夹杂而下,甚至溺出纯血;不同的是尿痛的有无,尿血多无尿痛,而血淋常尿痛难忍。

(3)尿浊:膏淋和尿浊都是小便混浊,白如泔浆;不同的是尿浊不伴尿痛涩滞感,而膏淋则有。

二、治疗原则及禁忌

实则清利,虚则补益,虚实夹杂则补虚泻实,是治疗淋证的基本原则。实证以膀胱湿热为主者,治宜清热利湿;以热伤血络为主者,治宜凉血止血;以结石结聚为主者,治宜通淋排石;以气滞小便不利为主者,治宜利气疏导。虚证以脾虚为主者,治宜健脾益气;以肾虚为主者,治宜补虚益肾。

淋证的治法,古有忌汗,忌补之说,如淋证确有外感诱发,或复感新邪,症见恶寒、发热、鼻塞流涕、咽痒者,可适当配合疏风解表之剂,表里同治。至于淋证忌补之说,是指实热之证而言,诸如脾虚中气下陷,肾虚下元不固,自当运用健脾益气,补肾固涩等法治之,不必拘泥。

三、分型论治

(一)热淋

主症:小便短数,灼热刺痛,尿色黄赤。

兼症:少腹拘急胀痛,或腰痛拒按,或有寒热口苦,恶心呕吐,或大便秘结。

舌脉:苔黄腻,脉濡数。

分析:湿热蕴结下焦,膀胱气化不利,是热淋的主要病机,故见小便短数,灼热刺痛,尿色黄赤。湿热蕴滞,气机失宣,则少腹拘急胀痛;湿热之邪侵犯于肾,故腰痛拒按;湿热内蒸、邪犯少阳,则寒热起伏,口苦呕恶,甚则波及大肠而见大便秘结。苔黄腻、脉濡数,均为湿热之象。

治法:清热利湿通淋。

方药:八正散加减。本方清热泻火,利尿通淋,为热淋常用之方。方中瞿麦、萹蓄、木通、车前子、滑石以通淋利湿,清热利窍;大黄、山栀、甘草梢清热泻火,导热下行。若大便秘结,腹胀痛者,可重用生大黄,加枳实以通腑泄热。若见寒热口苦,呕恶者,可合小柴胡汤以和解少阳。若腰痛甚者,加牛膝以补肾活血,利尿通淋而止痛;若湿热伤阴,或素体阴虚而病热淋,症见舌红少苔,脉细数者,用猪苓汤加白茅根育阴、利尿、通淋。

处方举例:

瞿麦 10g、萹蓄 10g、车前草 30g、木通 6g、山栀 10g、生川军(后下)6g,六一散(包)10g,虎杖 15g。

(二)石淋

主症:尿中时挟砂石,小便艰涩,或排尿时突然中断,尿道刺痛窘迫,尿色黄赤,甚则带血。

兼症:伴少腹拘急,或腰腹绞痛,牵引少腹,连及会阴。如病久不愈,血尿不止,或砂石不去,可见神疲乏力,腰酸隐痛,手足心热。

舌脉:初病苔薄黄,脉弦或弦数;病久舌红少苔,或质淡边有齿印,脉细数或细弱。

分析:湿热下注,尿液煎熬,结为砂石,而成石淋,砂石不能随尿排出,则小便艰涩,尿时疼痛;如砂粒阻塞尿路,则尿时突然中断,并因阻塞不通而致尿道刺痛,窘迫难忍;砂石损伤脉络,则尿中带血，甚至尿血。砂石闭阻，膀胱气化不利，气滞不行，则少腹拘急，腰部绞痛，并牵引少腹、会阴。初起湿热邪盛，正气未损，则苔薄黄，脉弦或弦数；久则气虚阴伤，则神疲乏力，腰酸隐痛，手足心热，或舌红少苔，脉细弱或细数。

治法：清热利湿，通淋排石。

方药：石韦散加味。本方有清热利尿，通淋排石之功，由石韦、冬葵子、瞿麦、滑石、车前子五药组成，其清热作用逊于八正散，利尿通淋之功优于八正散。为增强清利、排石消坚的作用，可加金钱草、海金砂、鸡内金、鱼脑石等药。腰腹绞痛者，酌加赤白芍、甘草、乳香、没药、沉香以解痉缓急，行气活血止痛。若兼发热，加蒲公英、连翘、黄柏以清热解毒。如尿中带血，加大小蓟、生地、地榆、茅根以凉血止血。如大便秘结，加生大黄以泻火通便。如石淋日久，正气已虚，虚实夹杂者，治当标本兼顾。偏于气血虚者，合用八珍汤；偏于肾阴虚者，合用六味地黄丸；偏于肾气虚者，合用《济生》肾气丸。

处方举例：

石韦 30g、冬葵子 12g、瞿麦 10g、滑石 12g、车前子（包煎）15g，鸡内金 30g、海金砂 12g、金钱草 30g。

（三）气淋

1. 实证（气郁淋）

主症：小便涩滞，少腹满痛。

兼症：胸胁苦满。

舌脉：苔薄白，脉沉弦。

分析：肝主疏泄，其经脉循少腹，布胸胁，络阴器。若情志怫郁，肝失条达，则少腹、胸胁胀满。气结不行，膀胱气化不利，则小便涩滞。肝郁不舒，脉多沉弦，苔薄白，若气郁血瘀，则舌质暗。

治法：理气和血，利尿通淋。

方药：沉香散加味。方中沉香、橘皮利气；当归、白芍柔肝和血；佐以石韦、滑石、冬葵子、王不留行利尿通淋；甘草调和诸药兼清热；诸药配合具有理气和血利尿通淋之功。胸胁胀痛者，加元胡、川楝子、青皮以疏肝理气。小腹胀痛者，加乌药、香附、木香以理气止痛。如胸胁少腹刺痛明显，舌暗有瘀斑者，加赤芍、红花、泽兰、川牛膝、益母草以活血行瘀利尿。

处方举例：

白芍 15g、当归 12g、青陈皮各 10g、石韦 30g、沉香粉 1g（冲），滑石 10g、牛膝 12g、冬葵子 10g。

2. 虚证

主症：少腹坠胀，空痛喜按，溲频尿清，余沥难尽。

兼症：面色㿠白，神疲乏力，大便溏泄。

舌脉：舌质淡，脉虚细。

分析：脾主升运，其经脉循腹部，若病久不愈，或过用苦寒疏利之剂，则耗伤中气。中气不足，气虚下陷，则少腹坠胀，空痛喜按；气虚不能摄纳，则溲频尿清，余沥难尽。脾虚失运，生化乏源，则面色㿠白，神疲乏力，大便溏泄，舌淡、脉虚细。

治法：补中益气。

方药：补中益气汤加减。方中黄芪补中益气升阳为主药；党参、白术、甘草补脾益气为辅；

佐以当归养血和营，陈皮理气化滞；使以升麻、柴胡协同参、芪升举清阳。如神疲乏力明显，重用参、芪，加山药、黄精以益气；如面色萎黄，头晕心悸，加白芍、熟地以养血；如腰膝酸软隐痛，加牛膝、杜仲、枸杞子以补肾。

处方举例：

黄芪 15g、党参 10g、白术 10g、炙甘草 6g、当归 10g、陈皮 10g、升麻 6g、柴胡 4g、乌药 6g、沉香粉 1g(分冲)。

（四）血淋

1. 实证

主症：小便频急，热涩刺痛，尿色红赤，或夹血块、血丝。

兼证：小腹胀满疼痛。或见心烦。

舌脉；舌苔黄，脉滑数。

分析：湿热下注膀胱，热伤血络，而致血淋实证。心火炽盛，移热小肠，热迫膀胱，血热伤络，则血与溲俱下而尿色红赤，或夹血块、血丝。湿热蕴结下焦，血块阻塞尿道，则小便频急，热涩刺痛。湿热下注，气机不畅，气滞不行，则少腹胀满疼痛。心火扰神，则心烦。舌苔黄，脉滑数，均为实热征象。

治法：清热通淋，凉血止血。

方药：小蓟饮子合导赤散。方中小蓟、生地清热凉血止血；蒲黄、藕节止血消瘀；滑石、木通、竹叶、山栀清热利湿，清心除烦；当归、甘草和营养血，缓急止痛；诸药合用，有清热通淋，凉血止血之功。若血多痛甚者，配伍琥珀粉、三七粉冲服以化瘀通淋止血。

处方举例：

小蓟 30g、生地 30g、山栀 10g、藕节 15g、滑石 12g、炒蒲黄 10g、木通 6g、竹叶 6g、白茅根 30g、琥珀粉 3g(分冲)。

2. 虚证

主症：尿色淡红，涩痛不著。

兼症：腰膝酸软，神疲乏力。

舌脉：舌红少苔，脉细数。

分析：病延日久，湿热伤阴，肾阴不足，虚火灼络，络伤血溢，则尿色淡红，尿痛涩滞不著。肾阴亏耗，则腰酸神疲。舌红少苔脉细数，为阴虚有热之象。

治法：滋补肾阴，清热止血。

方药：知柏地黄丸加味。用六味地黄丸滋补肾阴，知柏清热止血，加旱莲草、女贞子、阿胶滋阴凉血止血。若出血不止，加侧柏叶、白茅根、仙鹤草以止血。

处方举例：

生地炭 30g、茯苓 12g、山药 12g、山萸肉 10g、丹皮 10g、黄柏 6g、知母 10g、旱莲草 30g、侧柏叶 10g、阿胶 10g(烊化)。

（五）膏淋

1. 实证

主症：小便混浊如米泔水，置之沉淀如絮状，上有浮油如脂，或夹有凝块，或混有血液，尿道热涩疼痛。

兼症：口干咽燥，或口渴而不欲饮。

舌脉：舌质红，苔黄腻，脉濡数。

分析：湿热蕴结下焦，膀胱气化不利，清浊不分，脂液失于约束，则小便混浊如米泔水，尿道热涩疼痛。热伤血络则尿中夹有血块、血液。热盛则口干咽燥，湿阻则口渴而不欲饮。舌质红，苔黄腻，脉濡数，均为湿热之征。

治法：清热利湿，分清泄浊。

方药：程氏萆薢分清饮加减。方用萆薢、菖蒲分清泌浊；黄柏、车前子清热利湿；茯苓、白术健脾除湿；莲子芯、丹参清心除烦，活血通络，诸药配伍，使清浊分，湿热除，络脉通，脂液重归其道。如小便黄赤，热涩痛甚者，加滑石、木通以清利湿热。如少腹胀，尿涩不畅者，加乌药、青皮以行气消胀。如小便夹血者，加小蓟、藕节、白茅根以清热凉血止血。如日久湿热渐退，或热去湿留，逐致脾肾两虚，治宜温肾利湿，分清祛浊，选用《丹溪心法》萆薢分清饮治之。

处方举例：

萆薢24g、菖蒲10g、车前子（包煎）10g、土茯苓15g、黄柏10g、莲子心12g、丹参12g、白术10g、泽兰10g、甘草4g。

2. 虚证

主症：病久不已，或反复发作，淋出如脂，涩痛不著。

兼症：形体消瘦，腰酸膝软，头昏乏力。

舌脉：舌质淡，苔白腻，脉沉弱。

分析：久病迁延，反复不愈，湿热渐退，正气转虚，肾虚则下亢不固，脂液下泄，故淋出如脂，形体消瘦，腰酸膝软，头昏乏力。舌质淡，苔白腻，脉沉弱，为湿停肾虚之象。

治法：补肾固涩。

方药：膏淋汤加减。方中地黄、芡实益肾；党参、山药补脾；龙骨、牡蛎、白芍收敛固涩。若兼脾虚中气下陷者，合用补中益气汤。肾阴阳两虚者，合用《金匮》肾气丸。

处方举例：

熟地10g、山药15g、芡实12g、党参12g、煅龙牡（先煎）各30g、茯苓12g、菟丝子10g、桑螵蛸12g。

（六）劳淋

主症：小便赤涩不甚，溺痛不著淋沥不已，时作时止，遇劳加重或诱发。

兼症：神疲乏力，腰膝酸软。

舌脉：舌质淡，脉细弱。

分析：诸淋日久，或过服寒凉，或久病体虚，或劳伤过度，以致脾肾两虚；湿浊留恋不去，气化不利，故小便赤涩不甚，溺痛不著却淋沥不已，逢劳即作。脾肾气虚，故神疲乏力，腰膝酸软，舌淡脉细弱。

治法：健脾益肾。

方药：无比山药丸加减。本方双补脾肾，兼能利湿。方中山药为主，既补脾肾，又益气阴；茯苓健脾、熟地、山萸、巴戟天、肉苁蓉、菟丝子、杜仲、牛膝、五味子益肾固涩；佐泽泻利湿。如脾虚气陷，少腹坠胀，小便涩滞，可合用补中益气汤以益气升陷。如肾阴亏虚，低热颧红，五心烦热，舌红少苔脉细数，去巴戟天、肉苁蓉、加女贞子、旱莲草滋阴补肾；虚热明显者，合知柏地黄丸以滋阴降火。如肾阴虚衰，肢冷，夜尿多，加益智仁、覆盆子、鹿角粉以温肾固涩。

处方举例：

山药30g、熟地12g、五味子10g、山萸肉12g、茯苓12g、肉苁蓉10g、菟丝子12g、杜仲10g、牛膝12g、泽泻10g。

以上各种淋证，虽各具特点，但彼此之间又有一定关系。从临床表现看，可以某一种淋证为主，也可两种或三种淋证互见。如热淋、血淋并见，或石淋并发热淋、血淋。从转归看，有虚实之间的转化，也有诸淋之间的转化，如气淋、血淋、膏淋之实证，可转化为虚证；其虚证又可因复发、加重而表现为实证。又如实证之热淋、气淋、血淋可转化为虚证之劳淋；而虚证之劳淋，也可转化为实证之热淋、气淋、血淋；当湿热未尽，正气已伤，处于实证和虚证移行过度时，或虚证由于邪实而见实证时，表现为虚实夹杂。因此，临床要灵活掌握。

淋证的预后，常与其类型、病情轻重和治疗是否及时彻底有关。一般淋证初起，多可治愈，如血淋、气淋、膏淋早期若能积极、适当地治疗，并注意调养，均能痊愈，而不致转成慢性。若诸淋失治、误治或缺乏系统治疗，常迁延难愈，或反复发作，终成劳淋，而较难治愈。劳淋每因病程长，病势缓，症状轻，时作时止，而忽视长期治疗，日久气血阴阳俱亏，转成虚劳；或气化不利，水液潴留，发为水肿；若水毒浊邪上逆，中阻蒙窍，可致咳喘、心悸、呕恶、嗜睡、神昏等恶变。

〔预防及护理措施〕

1. 增强人体正气，防止情志失和，消除各种外邪入侵和湿热内生的有关因素，如忍尿、过食肥甘、纵欲过劳、外阴不洁等。

2. 注意妊娠及产后卫生，对预防子淋及产后淋的发生有重要意义；积极治疗消渴、痨瘵等肾虚疾患，也可减少淋证的发生。

3. 多喝水，饮食宜清淡，忌肥甘香燥、辛辣之品。注意适当休息，保持心情舒畅。

4. 禁房事。

附：尿浊

尿浊以小便混浊，白如泔浆，排尿时并无疼痛为主症。

本病的发生，多因饮食肥甘，脾失健运，酿湿生熟，或病后湿热余邪未尽，下注膀胱，清浊不分，而致小便混浊；或病久脾肾两伤，脾虚气陷，肾虚不固，精微脂液下流，以致尿浊。如湿热灼络，络伤血溢，则尿浊夹血；如脾虚不摄，或肾阴亏损，虚火伤络，则尿浊亦夹血。适逢贪恣油腻肥甘，或劳欲过度，可使尿浊加重，或引起复发。病位主要在脾、肾、膀胱。初起以湿热为多，属实，治宜清热利湿；病久则脾肾虚亏，治宜培补脾肾，固摄下元；虚实夹杂者，应予兼顾正邪。兹分述如下：

1. 湿热下注

主症：小便混浊呈乳白色，或夹凝块，上有浮油，或带血色，或夹血丝、血块，每因过食肥甘油腻而加重。

兼症：胸满口渴，但不欲饮，或尿道有热涩感。

舌脉：苔黄腻，脉濡数。

分析：由于过食肥甘，湿热内生，下注膀胱，不能分泌清浊所致。

治法：清热化湿

方药：程氏萆薢分清饮加减。

2. 脾虚气陷

主症：尿浊反复发作，日久不愈，小便混浊如白浆，劳累或过食油腻则发作或加重。

兼症：小便坠胀，尿意频作，神疲乏力，面色无华。

舌脉：舌质淡，脉虚弱。

分析：久病不愈，脾虚气陷，精微下注所致。

治法：健脾益气，升清固涩。

方药：补中益气汤加减。可加山药、芡实、白果以健脾益肾固摄。如气虚不振，尿浊夹血者，加三七、藕节收涩止血。如肢冷便溏者，加炮姜炭、补骨脂温脾补肾止泻。

3. 肾虚不固

主症：尿浊迁延不愈，小便混浊如凝脂或胶冻，腰膝酸软。

兼症：偏肾阴虚者，头晕耳鸣，烦热口干；偏肾阳虚者，面色㿠白，形寒肢冷。

舌脉：偏肾阴虚者，舌质红，脉细数；偏肾阳虚者，舌质淡，脉沉弱。

分析：病延日久，肾气亏虚，封藏不固，精脂下流所致。

治法：偏肾阴虚者，滋阴益肾；偏肾阳虚者，温肾固涩。

方药：偏肾阴虚者，用知柏地黄丸合二至丸为主；偏肾阳虚者，用右归丸加味。

〔典型病例分析〕

案一：宋某某，女，35 岁，干部。

小便短赤带血约半年，感冒后加重，尿频且痛，有灼热感，腰酸背困，少腹满急，有下坠感，脉数无力，经多次治疗，屡愈屡发，因来就诊。辨证：下焦湿热之血淋。立法：清热利湿，凉血止血。

银花 25g、生地 12g、瞿麦 12g、木通 10g、车前子（包煎）12g、黄柏 6g、萹蓄 12g、泽泻 10g、海金砂 10g、甘草梢 9g、竹叶 10g。

二诊：服药 6 剂，小便短赤带血及灼热疼痛好转，但腰痛不已。又加补肾壮腰之剂。

赤茯苓 12g、泽泻 10g、萹蓄 12g、栀子炭 6g、阿胶 12g（烊化）、川断 12g、生地炭 10g、杜仲炭 8g、竹叶 9g、甘草梢 9g。

上方调理一个月，病愈。随访两年，情况良好。（《许玉山医案》）

按：本案血淋患者，肾虚下焦有热，湿热熏灼膀胱，迫血妄行，则尿血。络伤血溢，瘀热互结，阻于尿道，气化不利，故尿频疼痛灼热，小腹满急，有下坠感。病历日久，肾阴亏耗，故腰酸背困，脉数无力。治当急则治标为主，清热利湿，凉血止血；待湿热势退，继以补肾凉血止血之品医之，标本兼顾，扶正祛邪，月余病愈。

淋证是指小便频数，滴沥刺痛，欲出未尽，小腹拘急，或痛引腰腹的病证。其病因以膀胱湿热为主，病位在肾与膀胱，初起多为实证，久病由实转虚，亦可呈虚实夹杂。临床症状有两类：一类是膀胱气化失司引起的症状；另一类是不同病因所引起的各种淋证的特殊症状。前者是诊断淋证的依据，后者是区别不同淋证的特征。同时还要与癃闭、尿血、尿浊相鉴别。

淋证分为热淋、石淋、气淋、血淋、膏淋与劳淋六种，在辨证时，要注意辨明淋证的类别，审察证候的虚实、标本缓急，并结合病程、体质等条件立法处方，进行针对性治疗。初起实证以湿热蕴结下焦，膀胱气化不利为主，治宜清热利湿通淋，佐以行气；虚证以脾肾亏虚，膀胱气化无权为主，治宜培补脾肾；虚实夹杂者，治宜标本兼顾。并根据各种淋证特点，参以止血、排石、泌别清浊等法。至于前人关于治疗淋证的忌补、忌汗之说，应做具体分析，不可一概而论。

各种淋证彼此之间又有一定的关系，表现在转归上，一是虚实的相互转化，在不同淋证之间和同一淋证本身都存在这种情况。二是各种淋证之间的相互转化，也可二种淋证或虚实同时并见，认识他们之间的关系，对临床有重要指导意义。

另外，淋证患者应避免劳累，禁食肥甘辛辣，注意个人卫生。

复习思考题

1. 试述淋证的临床特征及分类？
2. 简述各种淋证的临床特点？
3. 淋证与癃闭、尿血、尿浊如何鉴别？
4. 简述淋证的病因病机。
5. 试述各种淋证彼此之间的关系？
6. 对淋证如何进行辨证论治？
7. 淋证病人怎样进行调护？

癃　闭

〔概述〕

癃闭是指小便量少，点滴而出，甚则小便闭塞不通为主症的疾患。其中以小便不利，点滴而短少，病势较缓者为“癃”；以小便闭塞，点滴不通，病势较急者为“闭”。癃和闭虽然有区别，但都是指排尿困难，只有程度上的不同而已，故多合称为癃闭。

癃闭之名，首见于《内经》，该书对癃闭的病因病机、病位皆作了较为详细的论述。阐明了本病的病位在膀胱，病机是膀胱和三焦气化不利。《诸病源候论·小便诸候》中提出小便不通和小便难的病因都是由于肾与膀胱有热，《千金要方·膀胱腑》最早提出用导尿术治疗尿潴留小便难，《备急千金要方·闭塞》认识到本病有致死的严重后果。

朱丹溪认为小便不通有“气虚”、“血虚”、“有痰”、“风闭”、“实热”等多种不同的病因，根据辨证施治的精神，运用择吐法来治疗小便不通，开其上窍则下窍必利。

张景岳把癃闭的病因归纳为四个方面，尤其对气虚而闭的病理机转论述透彻。

至清代李用粹在《证治汇补·癃闭》篇归纳前人论述，把本病的病因分为7种，并提出具体治法，为癃闭的研究和治疗奠定了基础。

西医学中各种原因引起的尿潴留及无尿症，皆可参考本篇进行辨证施治。

〔病因病机〕

正常人小便的畅通，有赖于三焦的气化正常，而三焦的气化，又主要依靠肺气的宣降，脾气的运化，肾脏的启闭开阖功能来完成。所以本病除与肾关系密切外，还常和肺、脾有关。另外，肝气郁滞，尿路阻塞亦可影响三焦的气化而导致癃闭。兹将本病的病因病机分述如下：

一、湿热蕴结：素体湿热内盛，或嗜食辛辣厚味、酒浆而酿湿生热，湿热阻滞，下注膀胱，或他脏移热于膀胱，以致湿热蕴结，膀胱气化不利，小便不通，逐成癃闭。

二、肺热气壅：肺为水之上源，肺热素盛，或邪热袭肺，而致肺热气壅，肺气清肃无权，津液输布失常，水道通调不利，不能下输膀胱；又因肺热下移膀胱，导致上、下焦均为热邪闭塞，气化不行，癃闭乃成。

三、脾气不升：脾主运化升清。思虑劳倦，饮食不节，或久病体弱，年老体虚，均可致脾虚而清气不升，浊阴不降，小便因之不利。

四、肾元亏虚：肾主水。先天不足，后天劳伤，或年老体弱，久病体虚，均可致肾阳不足，命门火衰，则膀胱气化无权，而溺不得出；或因下焦湿热，日久伤阴，而致肾阴不足，所谓“无阴则阳无以化”，也可病癃闭。

五、肝郁气滞：肝主疏泄，有调畅气机，通利三焦，疏通水道的作用。七情内伤，肝郁气结，疏泄不及，则三焦气化不利，水道通调受阻，形成癃闭。又肝经绕阴器，抵少腹，这也是肝经有病，导致癃闭的原因。

六、尿路阻塞：瘀血败精，或肿块结石，阻塞及压迫尿路，以致排尿受阻，而形成癃闭。

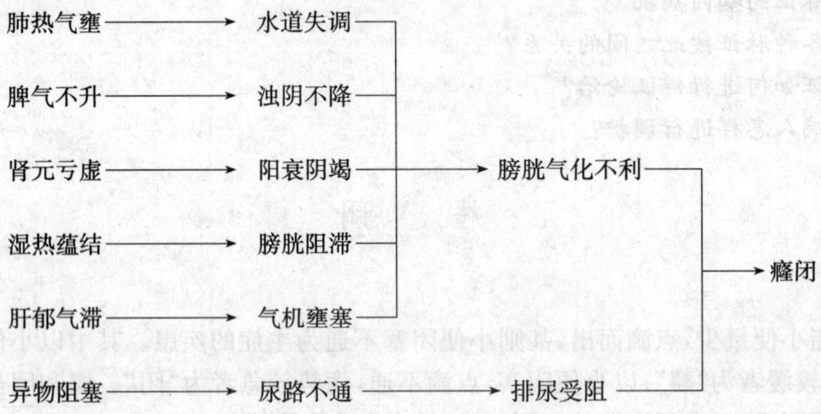

综上所述，癃闭的病位虽在膀胱，但与三焦、肺、脾、肾密切相关。上焦之气不化，当责之于肺，多因肺热气壅，水道通调受阻；中焦之气不化，当责之于脾，多因湿热蕴结，或脾土虚弱，而致清阳不升，浊阴不降；下焦之气不化，当责之于肾，多因湿热下注，或肾阳亏虚，气不化水，以上均可使膀胱气化失常，而形成癃闭。肝郁气滞，气机壅塞，或各种原因造成尿路阻塞，亦可发生癃闭。

〔辨证论治〕

一、辨证要点

癃闭的临床特点是小便点滴而下，或点滴全无，小腹胀或不胀，但尿道无疼痛感。起病可突然发作，或逐渐形成。病情严重时，可头晕、头痛、心悸、喘促、胸闷、恶心、呕吐、水肿，甚至神昏抽搐等症，因此对癃闭病人，必须及时给予有效的治疗，掌握辨治要点：

1. 辨有尿无尿：一般小腹胀痛，小便欲解不出，触叩小腹膀胱区胀满明显，为实音也，是尿潴留。如小便量少或不通，但无排尿感觉，或尿意不强，或小腹胀痛不著，触叩小腹部膀胱区亦无明显充盈征象，呈鼓音者，多是少尿或没尿。

2. 辨虚实：一般有尿者，多属实证；无尿或少尿者多属虚证。因湿热蕴结，肺热气壅，肝郁气滞，尿路阻塞所致者，多属实证；因脾气不升，肾元亏虚所致者，多属虚证。实证多发病急骤，小腹胀或疼痛，小便短赤灼热，舌苔黄腻或薄黄，脉弦涩或数；虚证多发病缓慢，神疲气短，语音低微，面色少华或晄白，排尿无力，点滴而下或全无，舌质淡，脉沉细弱。

3. 审轻重：通常癃者病势较缓，闭者病势较急。初起病“癃”，后转成“闭”者，为病势由轻转重；若初起病“闭”，后转成“癃”者，为病势由重转轻。癃闭如见小腹胀满疼痛，胸闷，气喘，呕吐等症，则病情较重；如见神昏，烦躁，抽搐等症，则病情危笃。

二、治疗原则

癃闭治则重在通利，并注意标本缓急。根据“腑以通为用”的原则，治疗本病着重于通，但通之法，有虚实之别。实证治宜清湿热，散瘀结，利气机而通水道；虚证治宜补脾肾，助气化，使气化得行，小便自通。此外，前人有“上窍开则下窍自通”理论，应开提肺气，即所谓“提壶揭盖”之法，疗治癃闭，每多获效。

同时，还要根据病因、病位进行辨证施治，切不可滥用通利小便之品。如由于饮水过少，汗出过多，或热病伤阴，而致小便不利，甚至癃闭者，宜用补阴之法，而毋妄投通利。

三、分型证治

(一)膀胱湿热

主症：小便点滴不通，或量极少而短赤灼热，小腹胀满。

兼证：口苦而黏，或口渴不欲饮，大便不畅。

舌脉：舌质红，苔黄腻，脉数。

分析：湿热蕴积于膀胱，气化不行，故小便不利而热赤，甚则闭而不通。湿热互结，气机不利，下焦气滞，故小腹胀满，大便不畅。湿热内盛，故口苦而黏。津液不布，故口渴而不欲饮。苔黄腻，舌红脉数，均因下焦湿热所致。

治法：清热利湿，通利小便。

方药：八正散加减。方中木通、车前子、萹蓄、瞿麦清热利湿，通闭利尿；山栀清化三焦湿热；滑石、甘草清利下焦湿热；大黄泻火通便。若舌苔黄腻而厚者，加苍术、黄柏以增强清热化湿有力。若因湿热煎熬尿液结成砂石，阻塞尿路者，可参考淋证之石淋治疗。若兼心烦，口舌生疮糜烂者，可合导赤散，以清心火，利湿热。若湿热久结下焦，灼伤肾阴，症见口干咽燥，潮热盗汗，手足心热，舌红少苔，或苔根黄腻者，可致用滋肾通关丸加生地、车前子、牛膝等以滋肾阴，清湿热而助气化。若湿热蕴结，三焦气化不利，尿量极少或无尿，面色晦滞，倦怠食少，胸闷烦躁，恶心呕吐，口有尿味，甚至神昏谵语，为尿毒内攻，宜用黄连温胆汤加车前子、白茅根、木通以和胃降浊，清热化湿；其病情严重者，可加用安宫牛黄丸以清热解毒，豁痰开窍；若大便秘结者，加生大黄以通便泄毒。

处方举例：

木通 6g、车前子(包煎)15g、萹蓄 12g、瞿麦 10g、生川军(后下)5g、滑石 10g、生甘草梢 6g、山栀 10g、黄柏 10g。

(二)肺热壅盛

主症：小便不畅，或点滴不通，或量少短赤，呼吸短促。

兼症：咳嗽咽干，烦渴欲饮。

舌脉：舌苔薄黄，脉数。

分析：肺热壅盛，失于肃降，不能通调水道，下输膀胱，则小便不畅，点滴不通，量少短赤。肺热气逆，则咳嗽，呼吸短促。肺热内郁，津失输布，则咽干，烦渴欲饮。苔薄黄，脉数，为热邪内盛之征。

治法：清肺热，利水道。

方药：清肺饮加减。本方用黄芩、桑白皮清泄肺热为主；辅以山栀清热，茯苓、木通、车前子清热利湿；佐以麦冬养阴清热，诸药配伍使上清下利，小便自通。若兼心烦，舌尖红，为心火旺盛，可加黄连、竹叶以清心火。若舌红少津，肺阴不足，加沙参、天花粉、玉竹以滋阴清热。若大便不通，加大黄、桔梗以宣肺通便。若兼头痛，鼻塞，脉浮，加薄荷、桔梗以宣肺解表。

处方举例：

桑白皮 15g、黄芩 10g、山栀 10g、木通 6g、车前子(包煎)12g、茯苓 12g、桔梗 6g、麦冬 10g、蝉蜕 6g、甘草梢 6g。

(三)肝郁气滞

主症：情志抑郁，或多烦善怒，小便不通，或通而不爽。

兼证：胸胁胀满或作痛。

舌脉：舌红，苔薄或薄黄，脉弦。

分析：七情内伤，肝失疏泄，气机郁滞，三焦气化不利，水液排出受阻，故情志抑郁，多烦善怒，小便不通，或通而不爽。肝脉抵少腹，贯膈布胁肋，肝郁气滞，则胁腹胀满作痛。脉弦为肝气盛，苔薄黄，舌红，为肝郁有化火之势。

治法：疏利气机，通利小便。

方药：沉香散加减。方用沉香、橘皮可疏达肝气；白芍、甘草柔肝缓急；当归、王不留行活血通气；配合石韦、滑石、冬葵子以通利水道。若胁腹胀满痛甚，加香附、郁金、乌药以增强疏肝理气之力。若烦躁易怒，舌红苔黄，为气郁化火，加丹皮、山栀、龙胆草以清肝火。若嗳气呕恶，为肝气犯胃，加苏梗、半夏以和胃降逆。

处方举例：

沉香粉 2g(冲服)、橘皮 10g、白芍 15g、香附 10g、石韦 10g、滑石 10g、冬葵子 10g、王不留行 10g、当归 10g、甘草 6g。

(四)尿路阻塞

主症：小便点滴而下，或尿如细线，甚则阻塞不通。

兼症：小腹胀满疼痛。

舌脉：舌质紫暗，或有瘀点，脉涩。

分析：因瘀血败精，或结石阻塞，致使尿路不畅或不通，故小便点滴而下，或尿如细线，甚则阻塞不通。浊瘀结石阻碍气机，则小腹胀满疼痛。舌质紫暗，或有瘀点，脉涩，为瘀阻气滞的征象。

治法：行瘀散结，通利水道。

方药：代抵当丸加减。本方用归尾、穿山甲、桃仁、大黄、芒硝重在通瘀化结。可加牛膝、红花、泽兰以增强活血化瘀作用。如尿路有结石，加金钱草、海金砂、滑石以排石利水。如久病气血两虚，面色不华者，宜加黄芪、归身、丹参以益气养血活血。如尿路阻塞，小便一时性不通，胀痛难忍者，加麝香末少许吞服，以行气活血止痛。如兼见血尿，可酌加琥珀粉、三七粉以活血止血。

处方举例：

当归尾 15g、桃仁 10g、炮山甲 6g、生大黄(后下)5g、牛膝 12g、金钱草 15g、石韦 12g、泽兰 10g、麝香 0.13g(冲)。

(五)中气下陷

主症：小腹坠胀，时欲小便而不得出，或量少而不畅。

兼症：神疲乏力，气短声低，纳少迟消，便意不尽，或久泄脱肛。

舌脉：舌淡，苔薄，脉弱。

分析：脾虚气陷，清气不升，浊阴不降，故小便不畅，欲出不得。脾气虚弱，气血乏源，故神疲乏力，气短声低。中气不足，运化无权，故纳少迟消。中气下陷，故便意频繁不尽，或久泄脱肛。舌淡，苔白，脉弱均为气虚之征。

治法：升清降浊，化气利水。

方药：补中益气汤合五苓散加减。补中益气汤能补中气，升清阳；五苓散能健脾祛湿，化气行水，两方合用，脾气升运，则浊阴易降，气化得行，则水道通利。纳少迟消者，加砂仁、神曲、麦芽以和中开胃；便意不尽，或久泄脱肛者，加枳壳15～30克，以助升举中气。

处方举例：

黄芪30g、白术10g、党参10g、茯苓15g、肉桂4g、陈皮10g、猪苓12g、泽泻12g、当归10g、升麻9g、柴胡3g、甘草6g。

（六）肾阳衰惫

主症：小便不通，或点滴不爽，排出无力。

兼症：腰膝酸软，形寒肢冷，面色㿠白，神气怯弱。

舌脉：舌质淡，苔白，脉沉细而尺弱。

分析：命门火衰，气化不及州都，故小便不通，或点滴不爽。肾元衰惫，则排尿无力，面色㿠白，神气怯弱。肾阳虚衰，不能温煦，故腰膝酸软，形寒肢冷。舌淡，苔白，脉沉细而尺弱，均为肾气不充之征。

治法：温阳益气，补肾利水。

方药：《济生》肾气丸加减。方中肉桂、附子温补肾阳，鼓舞肾气；六味地黄丸滋补肾阴；牛膝、车前子通利小便。若年高体弱，形神萎靡，腰脊酸痛，为元气大亏，病及督脉，加红参、鹿角胶、淫羊藿、仙茅以大补精血，助阳通窍。若肾阳衰惫，三焦气化无权，致小便量少，甚则无尿、呕恶、烦躁、神昏者，为尿毒内攻，可用《千金》温脾汤合吴茱萸汤以温补脾肾，和胃降逆。

处方举例：

熟地12g、山药15g、山萸肉10g、茯苓15g、泽泻12g、肉桂5g、制附片10g、牛膝10g、车前子（包煎）12g、巴戟天12g。

癃闭如能得到及时而有效的治疗，尿量逐渐增加，说明病情好转，甚至可以获得痊愈。如失治或治疗不当，症见头晕，心悸，胸闷，喘促，恶心，呕吐，水肿，乃至神昏，抽搐等，说明病情恶化，转为关格，若不及时进行抢救，可以导致死亡。

〔预防及护理措施〕

1. 锻炼身体，增强抵抗力。
2. 保持心情舒畅，切忌忧思恼怒。
3. 消除各种外邪入侵和湿热内生的有关因素，如忍尿、过食肥甘、纵欲过劳等。
4. 积极治疗淋证和水肿等疾患，对防止癃闭发生有重要意义。

〔典型病例分析〕

案一：张某某，男，70岁，工人。于秋分燥金当令之际来诊，主诉自去年患小便频数，时愈时犯，今夏某日突然小便不通，少腹憋胀疼痛难忍，口干不喜饮水，坐卧不宁，靠导管排尿至今已三日。诊得脉象沉细而数，舌苔白，大便干结。辨证：湿热蕴积，水热互结。立法：清利湿热，通利小便。

生地10g、黄柏6g、瞿麦12g、木通10g、竹叶9g、车前子12g、滑石12g、甘草梢6g。

二诊：服上方三剂，小便仍点滴全无，大便三日未行，舌苔转为黄燥，脉沉数，此湿热蕴结大肠，邪热上灼，肺津耗伤，大肠愈躁，须两顾之，急下存阴，佐以清热润肺。

熟军 9g、元明粉(另包)9g 分二次冲服、瞿麦 12g、萹蓄 12g、黄柏 6g、麦冬 15g、木通 10g、栀子 6g。

三诊：煎服一剂，大便通，小便剂，口干好转，少腹畅快，又进二剂，诸症若失。(《许玉山医案》)

按：素体湿热内居，稽留不去，故小便频数，时愈时犯；遇夏邪热内侵，湿热蕴积，水热互结，肠腑燥结。因肠燥而便不通，便不通则肺不降，肺不降则通调失职，故病癃闭。虽清利湿热，通利小便，但病本不在膀胱，治而不效，当泄下清肺，助肺肃降，佐以利水，大便通，则结滞之湿热得除，病豁然而愈。

癃闭是指小便量少，点滴而出，甚则小便闭塞不通为主症的疾患。临证时应与淋证进行鉴别，并注意辨清有尿与无尿。

癃闭乃由三焦气化功能失常所致。病位在膀胱，但和三焦、肝、脾、肺、肾均有密切关系。引起癃闭的病因病机有湿热蕴结、肺热气壅、肝郁气滞、尿路阻塞、中气下陷及肾阳衰惫。由前四种病因所致膀胱气化不利者，多属实证；由后两种病因所致膀胱气化无权者，多属虚证。

癃闭的辨证应根据证候首先分清虚实，然后权衡轻重缓急，进行有计划地治疗。治疗重在调节膀胱气化功能，实证宜清湿热，散瘀结，利气机而通水道；虚证宜补脾肾，助气化以利小便。在小便点滴不通的情况下，内服药缓不济急，可选用多种外治法来通利小便，一般先施针灸、按摩治疗；若尿闭已久，膀胱充盈，胀痛难忍，当用导尿法治疗。癃闭若因肿瘤或结石阻塞而致，针药不效者，应考虑外科手术治疗；若因肾功能衰竭而少尿或无尿者，病情复杂，治疗较难，预后不良。

复习思考题

1. 试述癃闭的含义。
2. 如何理解肺、脾、肾、肝在癃闭发病中的重要作用？
3. 以癃闭为例，阐述祖国医学“下病上治”和“欲降先升”的治疗原理？
4. 癃闭的辨证要点是什么？对癃闭怎样进行辨证论治？
5. 癃闭的预后如何？常用外治法有哪几种？

消　渴

〔概述〕

“消”有消谷、消水、消耗之意；“渴”指口渴能饮，饮不解渴而言。消渴是以多饮，多食，多尿，消瘦，或尿有甜味为特征的病证。古代医家根据本病的症状偏重不同，分为下、中、下三消。

西医学中的糖尿病，与本证的临床特点相合者，以及尿崩症具有多饮、多尿之症状者，均可参照本篇进行辨证论治。

〔病因病机〕

本病主要由于素体阴虚，复因饮食不节，情志失调，劳欲过度等所致。

一、饮食不节、积热伤津：长期过食肥甘，醇酒厚味，致脾胃运化失职，积热内蕴，化燥耗津，发为消渴。

二、情志失调、郁火伤阴：长期精神刺激，导致气机郁结，进而化火，火热炽盛，消烁肺胃阴津，发为消渴。

三、劳欲过度、肾虚精亏：房室不节，劳欲过度，损耗阴精，肾阴亏虚，虚火内生，则"火因水竭而益烈，水因火烈而益干"，终因阴虚火旺，上蒸肺胃，遂致肾虚与肺燥胃热俱现，发为消渴。

素体阴虚，是消渴发生的基本因素。既可因先天禀赋不足，也可以由于后天长期失于调养而渐成。

综上所述，消渴的病机，主要有以下几个特点：

阴虚为本，燥热为标：消渴的病机主要为阴津亏损，燥热偏旺，两者往往互为因果，燥热甚则阴愈虚，阴愈虚则燥热愈甚。病变的脏腑虽与五脏均有关，但主要在于肺、胃、肾，而以肾为关键。肺主治节，为水之上源，肺受燥热所伤，治节失职，水液直趋下行，故小便频数量多，肺不布津，故口渴喜饮。胃为水谷之海，胃为燥热所伤，胃火炽盛，故消谷善饥，大便干结。肾主水藏精寓元阴元阳，肾阴亏损，虚火内生，燥热伤肾，气化失常，开阖失司，封藏主权，故小便量多频数，精微下注而小便味甜。三脏之中，虽所伤有所偏重，但往往又互相影响。如肺燥阴虚，精液失于滋布，则胃失濡润，肾失滋源。胃热偏盛，则可灼伤肺津，耗伤肾阴。而肾阴不足，阴虚火旺，亦可上炎肺、胃。日久可见肺燥、胃热、肾虚常同时存在，多饮、多食、多尿亦常相互并见。

气阴两伤，阴阳俱虚：消渴一病，迁延日久，阴损及阳，津亏气弱，可见气阴两伤或阴阳俱虚，甚则表现为肾阳虚衰之候。亦有初起即兼有气虚或阳虚者，多与患者素体不足，后伤饮食或情志、劳倦，虽伤其阴，易及气及阳。但后者临床上较为少见。

阴虚燥热，致变证百出：消渴之病，由其阴虚燥热，可变生他证。如肺失滋润，日久可并发肺痨；肾阴亏损，肝火涵养，肝肾精血不能上承于目，则可并发白内障、雀目、耳聋；燥热内结，营阴被灼，络脉瘀阻，蕴毒成脓，发为疮疖、痈疽；阴虚燥热内炽，炼液成痰，痰阻经络，而见四肢麻木疼痛，或痰瘀互组而见心痛等。痰蒙清窍而为中风偏瘫。阴损及阳，脾肾衰败，水湿潴留，泛滥肌肤，则成水肿。若阴津极度耗损，痰火上蒙，虚阳浮越，可见面红，头痛，烦躁，恶心呕吐，目眶内陷，唇干舌红，息深而长，甚则昏迷，最后可因阴竭阳亡而见昏迷，四肢厥冷，肺微细欲绝等危象。

消渴病因病机示意图

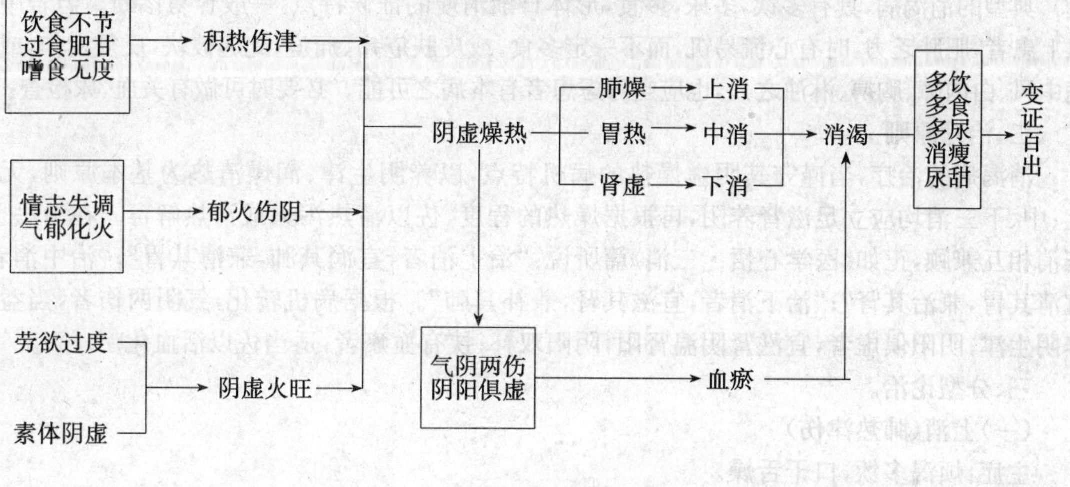

此外，消渴发病常与血瘀有关。血瘀的产生，主要因为阴虚内热，耗津灼液，而致血虚血瘀，或病损及阳，以致阴阳两虚，阳虚而寒凝，亦可导致血瘀。血瘀更使水津不布，而消渴愈甚。

〔**辨证论治**〕

一、辨证要点

对于消渴的辨证，首先当辨三消主次，以及区别阴虚与燥热的标本轻重。消渴虽有上、中、下三消之分，肺燥、胃热、肾虚之别，实际临床所见，常常是三多症状同时并存，只是有程度上的轻重不同。其以多饮为主，而多食、多尿为次者称为上消，以多食突出，而多饮、多尿不著者称为中消；以多尿为重，而多饮、多食较轻者称为下消。由于本病以阴虚为本，燥热为标，两者互为因果，常因病程长短和病情轻重的不同，而阴虚和燥热之表现则各有偏重，大体初病多以燥热为主，病程较长者则阴虚与燥热互见，日久则以阴虚为主，进而由阴损及阳，导致阴阳两虚之证。

其次当重视发病年龄，了解预后转归。本病一般多发于中年以后，但也有青少年罹患此病者。由于发病年龄不同，则病情的发生发展、轻重程度及预后转归有差异。年龄越小者，一般发病急，发展快，病情重，症状多具有典型性，预后较差，这与幼年儿童为“稚阴稚阳”之体，机体生理特点为易虚易实有关；中年之后发病者，一般起病较缓，病程较长，部分患者之临床表现不具有典型性，其临床表现有的类于虚劳，常有痈疽、肺痨、心、脑、肾、眼等并发症出现。因此必须重视此病的发病年龄，这对了解预后转归，确定治疗手段，有极其重要的意义。

再者当注意辨识消渴的危重证候。消渴日久，或因治疗不当，或因感受他病，或因妊娠、分娩等，均可使其消渴症状加重。若见面红，头痛，烦躁，恶心呕吐，厌食，唇舌樱红而干，呼吸加深加快，且有烂苹果的味道，甚或思睡，神昏，为阴津极度耗失，阴不敛阳，虚阳浮越，痰火欲蒙心窍的严重证候，最后可因阴竭阳亡而见昏迷、四肢厥冷、脉微细数欲绝等危象。消渴若见严重痈疽、肺痨、泄泻亦易出现危候。

还有消渴与瘿病之初容易混淆，临床上当注意区别。西医的甲亢，属中医瘿病范畴。其病以情绪极易急躁，多食善饥，形体日渐消瘦，心慌心悸，眼突，颈前一侧或两侧肿大为特征。其中多食善饥，消瘦为主症，而突眼、颈肿未显出时，极似消渴病的中消，但其病机略有不同。瘿病为痰气郁结，日久化火，心肝火旺，心胃阴虚，病变脏腑主要在肝、心，而连及胃。临床上若从症状、病史难以辨别时，可做必要的血、尿等化验检查。

典型的消渴病，具有多饮，多尿，多食，形体日渐消瘦的证候特点，一般容易诊断。但若中年以上患者，肥胖乏力，时有心慌易饥，而不一定多食，或皮肤疮疖、痈疽，此起彼伏，反复发作，或已病中风、白内障、胸痹、淋浊之人，也应当考虑患者有本病之可能。必要时可做有关血、尿检查。

二、治疗原则

消渴病的治疗，当谨守其阴虚燥热的病机特点，以养阴生津、润燥清热为基本原则，无论上、中、下三消均应立足滋肾养阴，再根据燥热的程度，佐以清热泻火或清热解毒。在治法上，三消相互兼顾，正如《医学心悟·三消》篇所说：“治上消者，宜润其肺，兼清其胃”；“治中消者，宜清其胃，兼治其肾”；“治下消者，宜滋其肾，兼补其肺”。根据病机转化，气阴两伤者，当益气养阴生津；阴阳俱虚者，宜滋肾阴温肾阳，阴阳双补；挟有血瘀者，适当佐以活血化瘀。

三、分型论治

(一)上消(肺热津伤)

主症：烦渴多饮，口干舌燥。

兼症：尿量频多，形体日渐消瘦。

舌脉：舌边尖红，苔薄黄，脉洪数。

分析：肺热炽盛，耗液伤阴，故口干舌燥，烦渴多饮。肺主治节，燥热伤肺，治节失职，水不化津，直趋于下，故尿频量多。津液流失，故形体日渐消瘦。舌边尖红，苔薄黄，脉洪数，是内热炽盛之象。

治法：清热润肺，生津止渴。

方药：消渴方加味。方中重用花粉以生津清热，佐黄连清热降火，生地黄、藕汁等养阴增液。

加减：应酌加葛根、麦冬、元参以加强生津止渴，养阴润躁之力。

若脉洪数无力，烦渴不止，小便频数，乃肺肾气阴两虚，可用二冬汤化裁。方中用人参（亦可用沙参代）益气生津，二冬、花粉、黄芩、知母清热解渴。

若苔黄燥，烦渴引饮，脉洪大，乃肺胃热炽，耗损气阴之候，可用白虎加人参汤以清泄肺胃，生津止渴。

处方举例：

天花粉 20g、葛根 10g、沙参 15g、元参 12g、天麦冬各 10g、知母 10g、生石膏（先下）30g。

（二）中消（胃热炽盛）

主症：多食善饥，大便干燥。

兼症：形体消瘦。

舌脉：苔黄燥，脉滑实有力。

证候分析：胃火炽盛，腐熟水谷力强，故多食易饥。阳明热盛，耗伤津血，无以充养肌肉，故形体消瘦。胃津不足，大肠失其濡润，故大便干燥，甚或秘结不行。苔黄燥，脉滑实有力，是胃热炽盛之象。

治法：清胃泻火，养阴增液。

方药：玉女煎加栀子、黄连治之。方中石膏、知母清肺胃之热；生地黄、麦冬益肺胃之阴；黄连、栀子清热泻火；牛膝引热下行。

加减：若大便秘结不行，可用增液承气汤以增水行舟，润燥通腑，待大便通下后，再转用上方治疗。

处方举例：

生地黄 15g、生石膏（先下）30g、知母 10g、牛膝 10g、麦冬 10g、元参 10g、焦山栀 10g、黄连 4g。

（三）下消

1. 肾阴亏虚

主症：尿频量多，手足心热。

兼症：尿混浊如脂膏，或尿甜，口干唇燥，甚或五心烦热。

舌脉：舌红，脉沉细数。

分析：肾虚无以约束小便，故尿频量多。肾失固摄，水谷精微下注，故小便混浊如脂膏，有甜味。手足心热，五心烦热，口干唇燥，舌红，脉沉细数，是肾阴亏虚，虚火妄动之象。

治法：滋阴固肾。

方药：六味地黄丸化裁。方中山药、山萸肉用量宜大，因山药能养脾阴而摄精微，山萸肉能固肾益精，不使水谷精微下注；熟地黄滋肾填精，三药合用，以达到三阴并补之功。又配茯苓淡渗脾湿，以助山药之益脾。泽泻清泄肾中相火，并防熟地之滋腻。丹皮清泄肝火，又制山萸肉之温，共为佐使。临床实践证明，本方对消渴确有治疗和巩固疗效的作用，适合消渴病人长期服用。

加减：若阴虚火旺，症见潮热烦躁，失眠，遗精，舌红，脉细数者，宜养阴清热，固精潜阳，可加知母、黄柏、五味子、龙骨、牡蛎、龟板等。

若尿量多而混浊如脂者，宜益肾缩泉，加益智仁、桑螵蛸、五味子、蚕茧、五倍子等。

若气阴两虚，伴困倦乏力，气短懒言，舌淡红者，宜酌加党参、黄芪等益气之品。

处方举例：

生熟地各 12g、山萸肉 12g、山药 12g、丹皮 10g、麦冬 10g、五味子 10g、泽泻 10g、元参 12g。

2. 阴阳两虚

主症：小便频数，饮一溲二，形寒畏冷。

兼症：小便混浊如膏，面色黧黑，耳轮焦干，腰膝酸软，阳痿不举。

舌脉：舌淡苔白，脉沉细无力。

分析：肾失封藏，固摄无权，故小便频数，混浊如膏。下元虚惫，约束无权，而致饮一溲二。水谷之精微随尿液下注，无以熏肤充身，故面色黧黑不荣。肾主骨，开窍于耳，腰为肾之府，肾虚故耳轮焦干，腰膝酸软，命门火衰，宗筋弛缓，故见形寒肢冷，阳痿不举，舌淡苔白，脉沉细无力，是阴阳俱虚之象。

治法：温阳滋肾固摄。

方药：《金匮》肾气丸化裁。方用附子、肉桂以温补肾阳，六味地黄丸药物以调补肾阴。

加减：若阴阳气血俱虚，可用鹿茸丸治之。方中用熟地、麦冬、元参、山萸肉、地骨皮、五味子滋补肾阴，益精生血；鹿茸、补骨脂、肉苁蓉以滋肾助阳；人参、黄芪益气；茯苓淡渗；鸡内金助运化；牛膝引药入肾。全方气血阴阳双补，滋而不滞。

若饮一溲二，可于上两方酌加覆盆子、桑螵蛸、金樱子等以补肾固摄。

处方举例：

熟地 15g、山萸肉 10g、元参 12g、补骨脂 10g、苍术 6g、黄芪 15g、山药 12g、五味子 10g、肉桂 3g、丹参 12g。

以上各种证型的消渴，如出现血瘀之证，可加用丹参、山楂、红花、桃仁等活血化瘀药，以提高治疗效果。

（四）兼症

白内障、雀目、耳聋，是肝肾精血不足，不能上承耳目所致，宜滋补肝肾，可用杞菊地黄丸或羊肝丸治之。

疮疡、痈疽：初起热毒伤营，治宜解毒凉血，用五味消毒饮加味。病久气营两虚，脉络瘀阻，蕴毒成脓，治宜益气解毒，用黄芪六一汤合犀角丸酌加金银藤、连翘等。

如并发肺痨、水肿、中风、淋证、厥证等，可参照有关各篇进行辨证论治。

（五）重危证

1. 虚阳浮越：症见烦渴加重，头痛，恶心呕吐，唇红舌干，呼吸深快，脉细数无力。治宜育阴潜阳，用生脉散加山萸肉、天冬、牡蛎、龟板等急煎服，或中西医结合治之。

2. 阴欲竭、阳欲亡：症见昏迷，四肢厥冷，脉微细欲绝。治当益气敛阴，回阳救脱。以生脉散合参附汤加减，并采用中西医结合，积极抢救。

消渴的治疗，也可在辨证论治基础上，酌情配合一些单方草药，以提高疗效。除药物治疗外，要避免精神紧张，节制性欲。饮食方面，以清淡为宜，不可过饱，一般以适量米类，配以蔬菜、豆类、瘦肉、鸡蛋等为宜。禁忌辛辣刺激之品。

〔预防及护理措施〕

1. 注意休息，不过劳，病重者应卧床休息。

2. 精神恬淡，节制性欲，戒烦躁，忌忧郁。

3. 饮食有节，每日主食少于5两，多食蔬菜，忌食辛辣厚味及含淀粉多的食物，禁烟戒酒。

4. 注意个人卫生，防止并发症的发生。

〔典型病例分析〕

案一：张某某，男，52岁，干部。

患者二个月来，自觉烦渴多饮（每日约1000毫升），多食尚饥（饭后2小时即有饥饿感），口唇干裂，大便秘结，舌质红，苔薄黄，脉数。

辅助检查：空腹血糖：220mg%，尿糖：（+++）。

中医诊断：消渴（胃火炽盛）。

西医诊断：糖尿病。

治则：清胃泻火，益气养阴。

方药：玉女煎化裁。

石膏20g、知母20g、黄芩10g、黄连10g、栀子5g、生地15g、花粉20g、玄参15g、党参20g、黄芪100g、麦冬20g、五味子10g。

上方随症加减，25剂后，空腹血糖：120mg%，尿糖：（—），症状消失。（庞妹弘，辨证治疗消渴病15例《黑龙江中医药》1988，(1)：21)。

按：本案经辨证属中消，胃火炽盛型，治疗当以清胃泻火，益气养阴为法，药用石膏、知母清肺胃之热，生地、麦冬、玄参、五味子、花粉益肺胃之阴，黄连、黄芩、栀子清热泻火，党参、黄芪益气，使胃火降，阴液存，诸症除。

消渴是以多饮、多食、多尿、消瘦为特征的病证。素体阴虚复加饮食不节，情志失调，劳欲过度为其病因，阴虚燥热为其主要病机，亦有气阴两伤，阴阳俱虚者。阴虚燥热又可引起多种病理变化，故消渴并发症很多。

消渴的病位在肺、胃、肾，而以肾为重。临床辨证时，首当区别上、中、下三消及阴虚与燥热的主次，其次重视发病年龄，以了解预后转归，再当注意辨识危重证候，及区别消渴与瘿病之初，并对中年以上人群，注意从易发兼症如疮疖此起彼伏、白内障等，发现消渴患者。

治疗上以养阴生津、润燥清热为基本原则，无论上、中、下、三消均应立足于滋肾养阴，佐以清热，其他情况均酌情兼顾。还当配合单方草药，结合生活调理，以提高疗效。另外，要注意对虚阳浮越，阴欲竭、阳欲亡等危重症的抢救。

复习思考题

1. 试从临床表现来阐述消渴病的病机重点是阴虚燥热,并说明阴虚与燥热的关系。

2. 为什么说消渴的病位在肺、胃、肾?

3. 试述上、中、下三消的辨证论治。

4. 消渴病的合并症有哪些?重危证有何表现?

痹　证

〔概述〕

痹证是指由于风、寒、湿、热等外邪侵袭人体,闭阻经络,气血运行不畅,引起肌肉、筋骨、关节的疼痛、麻木、重着、肿胀、活动不利,甚或灼热的疾患。仲景有风湿、湿痹、历节的论述;后世又有历节风、白虎风、白虎历节风、痛风、鹤膝风、鼓槌风等病名,均属痹证范围。

《黄帝内经》以感受风寒湿邪之偏盛,将痹证分为行痹、痛痹、着痹。后世又增加热痹一类。另外,以感邪季节和受邪病位之异,有骨、筋、脉、肌、皮痹等五体痹之称,而五体痹久不已,可以病及五脏,发展成五脏痹,如临床上常见的心痹,表现为"脉不通,烦则心下鼓,暴上气而喘,嗌干善噫,厥气上则恐";肾痹症见"尻以代踵,脊以代头"等。这对我们认识痹证的临床特征,演变过程极为有益。

西医学中风湿性关节炎、类风湿性关节炎、骨性关节炎、坐骨神经痛、肩关节周围炎、痛风等疾病,均可参考本证进行辨证论治。

〔病因病机〕

痹证的发生,主要是在正气不足之际,感受风、寒、湿、热之邪所致。现简述于下:

一、正气不足,卫外不固:腠理不密,从而使外邪得以乘虚而入,客于肌肉、筋骨、经络之间,阻遏气血的正常运行。正气不足与素体虚弱,劳逸不当,缺少锻炼,或妇女经期、产后有密切关系。

二、风寒湿邪,侵袭人体:若天暖汗出,当风而卧,易感风邪;若天寒地冻,寒邪直入,易受风寒;若久居湿地,冒雨涉水,则易致湿邪侵入。若感受风热之邪,与湿相合,而致风湿热合邪为患;也有风寒湿痹日久不愈,邪郁化热,也可成风湿热而伤人。

正气不足,外邪侵袭是痹证病因,其中外邪入侵是外因,是条件;正气不足是内因,是基础。内外合邪,方可致病。人体阳气偏盛,或阴虚火旺者,或感受风湿热之邪,易转化成风湿热痹;若人体阳气偏虚,或感受风寒湿之邪,易转化成风寒湿痹。风寒湿痹与风湿热痹,两者之间,在某些条件作用下可以互相转化。此外,无论风寒湿痹或风湿热痹,经久不愈,经络气血凝滞,易产生痰瘀互结之证,如皮肤瘀斑、皮下及关节周围结节,或关节畸形等。再者,由于邪气阻滞经络,瘀血不去,新血则不生,再加之关节不利,活动减少,亦易引起气血耗伤,甚或肝肾亏虚之证。终至痹证迁延不愈,复感于邪,病由体及脏,而成脏腑痹,其中以心痹、肾痹居多。

总之,痹证初起,以邪实为主,反复发作;而病久则病渐及脏,邪恋正虚,虚实挟杂,寒热错综。

痹证病因病机示意图

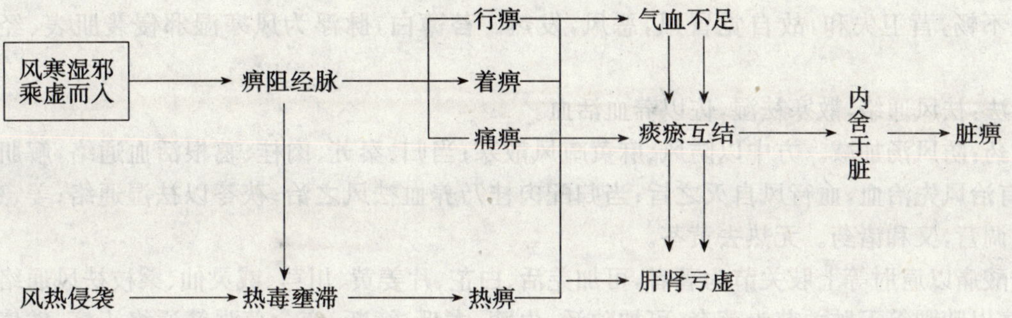

〔辨证论治〕

一、类证鉴别:本病与痿证的鉴别,缘于两者的症状都在肢体、关节,而且可以互相转化。但痹证是以筋骨、肌肉、关节的酸痛、重着、肿胀、屈伸不利为主要临床特点。虽有时亦兼见酸麻不仁,但无瘫痿的表现。而痿证则以肢体痿弱不用、肌肉瘦削为特点,肢体关节一般不痛。

痹证日久,肢体因疼痛而少动,肌肉可见枯瘦,关节多见变形、僵硬,然亦有间见痿软者,故痹而致痿者临床可见。痿证体虚,若复感于邪,客于经脉,气血痹阻不通,亦可引发痹证,故痿而兼痹者临床也有之。

二、辨证要点

(一)首辨风寒湿痹与风湿热痹:前者唯肢体、关节疼痛、肿胀、窜走不定,而无焮红灼热之症;后者以关节红肿灼热烦痛为特点。

(二)辨风、寒、湿之偏盛:风邪偏盛则肢体、关节酸痛游走不定;寒邪偏盛则肢体、关节疼痛剧烈、固定不移;湿邪偏盛则肢体、关节肿胀重着、酸痛不仁。

(三)辨痰瘀互阻经脉:多为痹证日久,关节肿大,甚至强直畸形,屈伸不利,舌紫苔腻,脉细涩等。

(四)辨虚实:痹证初起,肢体、关节疼痛持续不休,甚伴寒热者,多属实证:痹证久治不愈,反复发作,肢体、关节疼痛虽不著,但兼见气血不足或肝肾亏虚见症,如神疲乏力,腰膝酸软,五心烦热等,多属虚证或虚实挟杂。

三、论治要点:痹证之发,责之风、寒、湿、热邪侵袭所致,故治疗总以祛风、散寒、祛湿、清热以及舒经通络为基本原则。后期兼见虚损者当配合补益之剂。《医学心悟·痹》对治痹作了概括,指出:"治行痹者,散风为主,而以除寒祛湿佐之,大抵参以补血之剂,所谓治风先治血,血行风自灭也。治痛痹者,散寒为主,而以疏风燥湿佐之,大抵参以补火之剂,所调热则流通,寒则凝塞,通则不痛,痛则不通也。治着痹者,燥湿为主,而以祛风散寒佐之,大抵参以补脾之剂,盖土旺则能胜湿,而气足自无顽麻也。"可供临证时参考。

四、分型证治

(一)风寒湿痹

1. 行痹

主症:肢体关节酸痛,游走不定。

兼症:恶风发热,或自觉关节冒风,关节屈伸不利。

舌脉:舌淡红,苔薄白,脉浮。

分析：风寒之邪客于经脉，阻痹气血运行，而致肢体关节酸痛，关节屈伸不利。行痹以风邪偏盛，风性善行而数变，故关节疼痛游走不定，时左时右，忽而上肢，忽而下肢。肢体经脉气血不畅，营卫失和，故自觉冒风，恶风，发热。苔薄白，脉浮为风寒湿邪侵袭肌表、经脉之象。

治法：祛风通络，散寒祛湿，佐以养血活血。

方药：防风汤加减。方中以防风、麻黄疏风散寒；当归、秦艽、肉桂、葛根活血通络，解肌止痛，古有治风先治血，血行风自灭之旨；当归配肉桂乃养血祛风之治；茯苓以祛湿通络；姜、枣、草和中调营，又和诸药。无热去黄芩。

若酸痛以肩肘等上肢关节为著者，可加羌活、白芷、片姜黄、川芎、威灵仙、桑枝祛风通络止痛；酸痛以膝踝等下肢关节为著者，可加独活、牛膝、木瓜、续断、鹿含草强筋通络止痛；酸痛以腰脊关节为著者，可加杜仲、桑寄生、骨碎补、淫羊藿补肾通经止痛，也可以独活寄生汤化裁为治。

若风寒湿三邪杂至，关节肿胀，苔薄黄，为邪郁化热，可用桂枝芍药知母汤化裁，寒热并用，通痹止痛。

处方举例：

防风 10g、秦艽 10g、羌活 10g、独活 10g、赤芍 12g、当归 10g、威灵仙 15g、桂枝 6g、麻黄 5g、桑枝 30g、地龙 10g。

2. 痛痹

主症：肢体关节疼痛剧烈，痛有定处，得热则缓，遇寒痛甚。

兼症：关节僵硬，不可屈伸，皮色不红，触之不热。

舌脉：舌淡红，苔薄白或白润，脉浮紧。

分析：风寒湿邪痹阻经脉，而以寒邪偏盛者，缘于寒为阴邪，其性凝滞、主收引，故痛有定处，疼痛剧烈。经脉气血得热则流畅，通则不痛，故痛减；经脉气血遇寒则凝涩，不通则痛，故痛甚。寒凝阳痹，气血不畅，故局部不红不肿，触之不热，关节僵硬，不可屈伸。苔薄白或白润，脉弦紧，均为寒凝痛剧之象。

治法：温经散寒，祛风除湿。

方药：乌头汤加减。方中乌头、麻黄温经散寒，除湿止痛；黄芪宜生用，益气固表，兼能利血通痹；芍药、甘草化阴通络，缓急止痛。若寒重痛甚，可加桂枝或肉桂、细辛，草乌与川乌同用，以增强温经散寒之力；若痛痹经久不愈，可酌加骨碎补、补骨脂、巴戟天、鹿角霜等温肾助阳之品。

若平素阳虚，寒痹难愈者，也可以阳和汤化裁为治。

处方举例：

制川乌 5g、制草乌 5g、麻黄 5g、赤白芍各 10g、生甘草 10g、桂枝 10g、生黄芪 30g、生姜 3 片、大枣 7 枚。

3. 着痹

主症：肢体关节肿胀、重着、疼痛，肌肤麻木不仁。

兼症：周身酸困，倦怠，手足沉重，活动不利。

舌脉：舌淡红，苔白腻，脉濡缓。

分析：感受风寒湿邪而以湿邪偏盛，湿性重浊黏滞，留着化迟，故肢体关节肿胀、重着、疼痛。湿阻经络，气血行涩，故肌肤麻木不仁。湿属阴邪，阳气不展，故周身酸困、倦怠，手足沉重，活动不利。苔白腻，脉濡缓为湿浊不化之象。

治法：除湿通络，祛风散寒。

方药：薏苡仁汤加减。方中苡仁、苍术除湿通络；羌活、独活、防风虽为祛风之药，以风能胜湿，故祛风除湿。川乌、麻黄、桂枝温经散寒除湿通络。当归、川芎辛温通脉，养血活血；生姜、甘草和中化浊。若湿重肿甚者，可加萆薢、木通、木瓜、防己以利湿通络。若肌肤不仁，可加白术、防风、芍药或海桐皮、豨莶草以去肌表之风湿，使营卫调和，气血通畅。

若痹证初起，风寒湿邪在表，无汗表实，可用麻黄加术汤微发其汗，或用五积散加减调治。有汗表虚者，可用桂枝附子汤为治。

处方举例：

薏苡仁 30g、萆薢 10g、苍术 10g、羌活 10g、独活 10g、防风 10g、防己 10g、麻黄 5g、桂枝 10g、当归 10g、川芎 10g。

（二）风湿热痹

主症：关节红肿、灼热、疼痛，痛甚拒按，得冷稍舒，可见于一个或多个关节。

兼症：发热，恶风，汗出，口渴，烦闷不宁。

舌脉：舌红，苔黄燥，脉滑数。

分析：邪热壅遏经络、关节，气血瘀滞不通，故关节红肿、灼热，烦痛难忍，病可犯及一个或数个关节。关节热蕴不散，气血壅滞，故疼痛怕按、拒按，按之痛甚，得冷稍舒。邪热不净，营卫不和，故发热，恶寒。邪热内传，里热炽盛，故壮热不解，汗出，口渴喜饮，烦闷不宁。舌红，苔黄燥，脉滑数亦属热蕴湿遏之象。

由于风湿热痹患者，或由于邪气过胜，或人体阳气偏盛，全身及局部症状均较严重，发病较急，且极易内舍脏腑，以致病情多变。

治法：清热通络，祛风除湿。

方药：白虎桂枝汤加味。方中以白虎汤清热除烦，养胃和中；桂枝疏风通络。若咽喉肿痛，可加青果、元参、桔梗清利咽喉，或用六神丸含化服。若邪热偏盛，发热恶风，可加金银藤、连翘、虎杖、山栀清热解毒。若壮热、口渴，除重用生石膏外，可加鲜芦根、天花粉、元参、生地泄热生津。大便秘结者，可加山栀、大黄、元明粉泄热通腑。若关节烦痛明显者，可加桑枝、豨莶草、威灵仙、秦艽、乳香、没药，以及地龙、蜈蚣、祁蛇、乌梢蛇等通络止痛。若关节红肿灼热明显者，加丹皮、生地、赤芍、紫草等凉血解毒。

若关节红肿热痛、苔黄而腻者，也可用宣痹汤化裁为治。方中防己、晚蚕砂、苡仁、赤小豆祛风除湿，通利经络；连翘、山栀、滑石清热利湿。本方清轻宣泄，使经络中之湿热得除，气血畅行，痹痛得止。若病在下肢者，还可配用三妙丸以增强清化下焦湿热之力。

若关节红肿，疼痛剧烈，筋脉拘急，日轻夜重，壮热烦渴，舌红少津，脉弦数者，为热毒化火，深入筋骨，津伤阴耗，治宜清热解毒，凉血止痛，可用犀角散合白虎汤化裁治之，还可酌加生地、丹皮、玄参、麦冬滋阴凉血；加木通、苡仁、木瓜、蚕砂清热除湿，通络止痛。若犀角药源不足，也可用水牛角取代，但用量宜大。

处方举例：

生石膏（先下）30g、知母 10g、紫草 10g、连翘 10g、金银藤 30g、桂枝 10g、赤白芍各 12g、木通 6g、生甘草 10g、生苡仁 30g、粳米 10g。

(三)尪痹

尪痹，是指痹证迁延日久，肢体瘦削而关节肿大、畸形、强直为临床特点的病证，为近年来国内临床与学术研讨中被承认的病名。与《黄帝内经》所述“尻以代踵，脊以代头”的“肾痹”有相似之处。在此专论，以利于临床研治的发展。

主症：痹证久治不愈，关节肿大、畸形、僵直，屈伸不利，甚则全身关节畸形、强直。

兼症：肢体关节酸痛明显加重，多昼轻夜甚，阴雨天寒痛剧，自觉疼痛发自骨内，初起早晨关节发僵，逐渐终日关节不灵。常伴腰膝酸软，倦怠乏力，喜暖畏寒，或女子月经不调，男子遗精、阳痿。

舌脉：舌质或红、或淡、或黯、或有瘀斑，苔或白或黄，脉多沉细弦，且尺弱。

分析：肾内寄元阴元阳，藏精，生髓，主骨，是为先天之本。肝藏血、主筋。肝肾同源，精血互生。若先天不足，后天失养，肝肾亏虚，筋骨不健，而易感邪为病。故平素肝肾亏虚之人，感受风寒之邪，则邪易深入筋骨；亦有痹证日久，暗耗真阴，使邪气渐入者。精血不充，筋骨失荣，故骨松筋挛，久则骨节变形、僵硬而屈伸不利，终至肢体废用。寒邪深入，其性收引、凝滞，故疼痛剧烈，痛发于骨，喜暖畏寒，阴雨天寒之时尤甚。昼属阳主动，夜属阴主静。动则气血流通，静则气血行涩，故疼痛昼轻夜甚，晨起肢体僵硬，而活动后逐渐轻便。腰为肾府，肝主筋，肝肾不足故腰膝酸软，倦怠乏力。女子冲任失养，故月经不调；男子肾精失摄，故见遗精、阳痿。偏阴虚者舌红，偏阳虚者舌淡，精血不足而络脉瘀阻者舌黯，甚或有瘀斑、瘀点。寒湿胜则苔白或腻，邪郁化热则苔黄而腻。脉沉主里，细主不足，弦主疼痛，而尺脉弱者为肾虚之象。

治法：补肾散寒为主，佐以祛风除湿，养肝荣筋，通经活络。

方药：经验方治尪汤加减。本方由桂枝芍药知母汤合《简易方》虎骨散化裁而成。方中用补骨脂、川断、制附片、熟地黄补肾散寒，桂枝、赤白芍调和营卫；骨碎补、炙虎骨祛骨风壮筋骨；淫羊藿、独活、威灵仙温肾阳祛风湿；防风、麻黄疏散风寒；苍术燥湿理脾；炙山甲、伸筋草、松节通经活络，舒筋利节；知母清虚热，并能制桂附等辛热之偏；牛膝补肝肾通经络，引药入肾。若腰膝酸痛明显，则去苍术，加桑寄生、狗脊、鹿衔草，或重用川断、怀牛膝、补骨脂，杜仲。若肢体挛缩，拘急，加生苡仁、木瓜、炙甘草，重用白芍。若肌肉瘦削，肢体倦怠，加黄芪、党参、白术。若关节肿大，胀痛较甚，下肢浮肿，加萆薢、防 己、生苡仁、百蔻仁，重用威灵仙。若痹证日久，病入血络，或有瘀血征象，加红花、地龙、乳香、没药。若寒热错杂，治宜补肾散寒，佐以清热除湿通络，则于主方中减温热药量，加生地、黄柏、金银藤、络石藤以温清并用；若寒已化热，又当按热痹处理，重用补益肝肾药，如生地、鸡血藤、首乌藤、露蜂房。若病久不愈，也可加祁蛇、乌梢蛇、全蝎、蛴螬。

处方举例：

熟地 12g、补骨脂 10g、骨碎补 10g、川断 15g、桂枝 10g、制附片 6g、赤白芍各 5g、麻黄 5g、炙山甲 10g、威灵仙 12g、独活 10g、防风 10g、生苡仁 15g、牛膝 15g、炙甘草 6g。

各种痹证迁延日久，正虚邪恋，病入血络，血瘀行涩，津凝为痰，终致痰瘀痹阻，症见疼痛时轻时重，关节肿大，皮色不泽，甚至关节畸形、强直，屈伸不利，舌质紫黯，或有瘀点、瘀斑，脉细涩等，治宜化痰祛痰，搜风通络，用桃红饮加穿山甲、地龙、地鳖虫等养血活血，化瘀通络；加白芥子、竹沥汁、生姜汁、南星化痰通络散结；加全蝎、乌梢蛇等虫类药搜风通络止痛。

痹证久治不愈，除风寒湿邪闭阻经络关节的症状以外，由于正气暗伤，还会出现气血不足或肝肾亏虚的症状。治疗时，当宜标本兼顾，攻补兼施，即在祛风散寒除湿的同时，或佐以补益气血，或佐以滋养肝肾。补益气血，多用四君、四物、养荣、归脾化裁；滋养肝肾，多用左归、右归加减，独活寄生汤、健步虎潜丸也可选用。若痹久内舍于心，症见心悸气短，动则益甚，面色少华，舌淡，脉虚数或结代者，治宜益气养心，温阳复脉，用炙甘草汤加减。

本病除内服药物治疗外，针灸、推拿、熏洗等法配合使用，多有裨益。

〔预防及护理措施〕

1. 病之初起，肢体关节疼痛剧烈，关节肿胀、活动不利，发热较高时，应卧床休息，并注意患病病位的体位，使之舒适而减轻疼痛。

2. 病情稳定，肢体关节疼痛、肿胀减轻以后，可适当增加活动，循序渐进，以增强体力而不致过劳，特别注意恢复关节功能。

3. 住室宜温暖、空气新鲜，尤宜注意患肢保暖，减少疼痛，利于疾病恢复，防止反复。

4. 饮食应注意增加营养，以增强人体抵抗力。少食辛辣刺激性食物，痛痹者忌食生冷，宜多食牛羊肉等温性食物；热痹者宜多食蔬菜水果。

5. 可以药袋热熨、膏药外敷，或药浴、蒸汽浴，必要时配合针灸、推拿治疗。

6. 出现合并症时，及时诊治。

〔典型病例分析〕

案一：苏某某，女性，31岁。

产后3个月，上街逢大雨被淋，当夜无感觉，次日即不能起床，腰以下如瘫痪状，两腿疼痛不能转动，只能仰卧，不能翻身。经检查，腰骶关节处外部不红不肿，亦无压痛，脉象两关弦虚，两寸尺均无力。依据以上症状，显然是由于产后气血虚受风寒，与内湿结合而为痹。治拟温经散寒，调和营卫，以黄芪桂枝汤和术附汤加减，处方：

黄芪、桑寄生各15g，桂枝、白术、生姜各9g，川附片、炙甘草各6g，炒苡仁30g，红枣4枚。服后腹内觉热，次日即痛减，两日后月经来潮，小腹有轻微痛，此为产后第一次行经。三剂后能独自来门诊，切脉弦兼数，方予当归、川芎、秦艽、白术、川牛膝各6g，白芍、桂枝、生地、桑寄生各9g，黄芪15g，杜仲12g，防风5g，细辛、炙甘草各3g，调和气血，并祛风湿。连进三服，痛再减，脉象渐趋缓和，基本已告痊愈。后因素有头晕、耳鸣等肝肾不足症状，继续与天麻丸、虎骨木瓜丸及大活络丹等调理。

按：本例产后未满百日，受大雨，风寒湿三气同时侵袭，故以温经散寒，调和营卫法治之，三剂即见明显效果，经行痛轻，再三剂则痹痛告愈。

痹证是临床常见病证。正气不足为其发病内因，而感受风、寒、湿、热等外邪为致病外因。内外相合而为病。痹证以肌肉筋骨关节的疼痛、酸楚、重着、麻木及关节肿大、屈伸不利为特征。病情常与气候变化有明显关系。痹证病机主要为经络痹阻，气血运行不畅。临床一般分为风寒湿痹和风湿热痹两大类，近年来对尪痹的研治不断深入，丰富了痹证的内涵。风寒湿痹中，风偏胜者称行痹，以疼痛游走不定为特点；寒偏胜者称痛痹，疼痛剧烈，痛有定处为特点；湿偏胜者称着痹，疼痛重着不移，关节肿胀，肌肤麻木为特点。风湿热痹，常见关节红肿灼热疼痛。尪痹，多属久病，疼痛发自骨内，昼轻夜重，关节肿大、畸形，甚则人体变形。

治疗痹证，应辨清正邪盛衰，根据病程长短，病势缓急，病情轻重，以及证候特点，审明虚实寒热，标本缓急。一般初病多实，实者治以祛邪、通经活络；久病虚实挟杂，治以扶正祛邪、通经活络，或祛邪行瘀散结，兼顾扶正。正所谓急则治标，缓则标本兼顾。治疗痹证的基本治法是祛风、散寒、除湿、清热以及通经活络。结合病情辅以化痰散结、活血祛瘀、健脾益气、温阳补肾、补血养肝等。同时，对不同部位的疼痛，配伍适当的引经药，以提高疗效。如痛在上肢选用羌活、川芎、姜黄、桂枝；痛在下肢选用牛膝、独活、木瓜、木通；痛在颈项选用葛根；痛在腰脊选用桑寄生、杜仲、狗脊、鹿衔草等。治疗中还应时时注意调护脾胃，方能有利于痹证的治疗和恢复。

另外，在痹证的治疗中，由于风寒湿痹疼痛剧烈，常选用附子、乌头等以祛风除湿，温经止痛。但附子、乌头均系辛热有毒之品，一般不宜大量服用或长久服用，服用时剂量宜从少量开始，逐渐加量。凡入煎剂，药量在 10 克以上时，要久煎（先煎 30～60 分钟），或与甘草同煎，或用蜜煎，以缓和其毒性。服药后患者若有唇舌发麻，手足麻木，恶心，心慌，脉迟等中毒症状时，应酌情减轻剂量，或立即停药，必要时应及时采取解救措施。对于痹证之病程较久，常用药物治疗不效的抽掣疼痛，肢体拘挛者，常配伍虫类搜剔经络药物，如白花蛇、乌梢蛇、穿山甲、蜣螂、地龙、蜂房、全蝎、蜈蚣之类，以通络止痛。因为这类药物大多性偏辛温，作用较猛，有的也有不同程度的毒性，对胃肠还有刺激，故使用时也不宜用量过大或久服，宜于入丸剂为优，中病即止。

痹证治疗过程中，注意加强身体锻炼，避免感受风寒、潮湿，增减衣被适时令，对预防复发和调治极为重要。痹证治疗及时者一般预后良好，但本病易复发，多缠绵。久病不愈，痰瘀痹阻，出现关节畸形，以及内舍于脏，证属气血不足，肝肾亏虚者，病多深重，常不易恢复，预后亦差，当结合本书有关章节积极调治。

复习思考题

1. 试述痹证的病因病机。
2. 风寒湿痹如何辨证论治？
3. 风湿热痹如何辨证论治？
4. 痹证而兼痰瘀痹阻、气血不足、肝肾亏虚者如何诊治？
5. 痹证内舍于脏，多见哪些证候？
6. 治疗痹证，如何应用综合疗法？
7. 治疗痹证，选用附子、乌头及虫类药时，应注意什么？

痿证

〔概述〕

痿证是以肢体筋脉弛缓，软弱无力，或者肌肉萎缩的一种病证。临床上可表现为全身肌肉萎缩和无力，也可表现为局部的肌肉萎缩。以双下肢痿弱，行走乏力或者不能行走时多见，故有“痿躄”之称。“痿”指肢体痿弱不用，筋脉弛纵不收；“躄”是指下肢软弱无力，不能步履。

根据痿证的临床特征，现代医学的脊髓炎，急性感染性多发性神经根神经炎，进行性肌营养不良、重症肌无力，周期性麻痹，进行性脊髓性肌萎缩，肌萎缩侧囊硬化症，癔病性瘫痪等均可参考本证进行辨证治疗。多发性硬化、脊髓空洞症等多合并有感觉障碍，如以肢体无力、肌肉萎缩为主症时，则亦可参考本节内容进行辨证。

痿证病因病机示意图

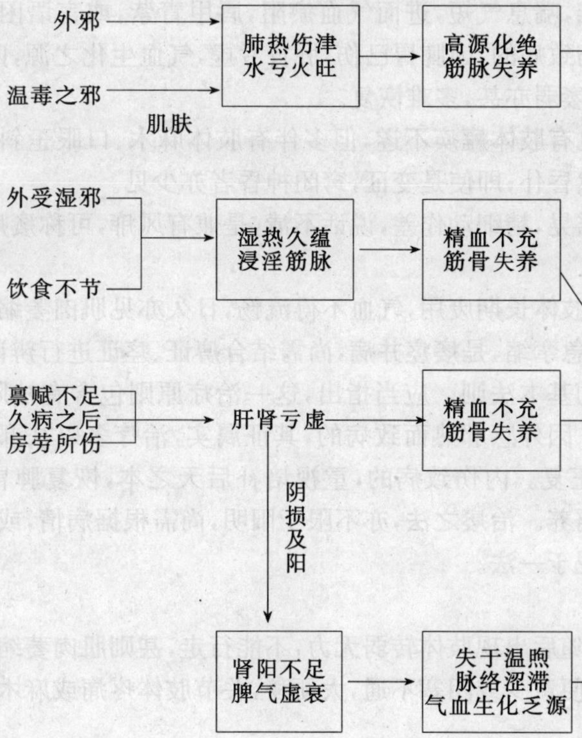

〔病因病机〕

一、肺热伤津:由于正气不足,卫外不固感受湿热毒邪,或风寒之邪,入里化热,高热不退,或病后低热不退,余邪未尽,或五脏之病,移热于肺,肺受热灼,津液耗伤,筋脉失于濡养,导致手足痿弱不用,而成痿证。肺为华盖,又为娇脏,位置最高,受脏腑上朝之清气,禀清肃之体,不耐邪侵,凡六淫邪气,一有所著,即能致病。肺朝百脉,具有输布水谷精微的作用,热邪伤肺,气耗阴伤,肺不能发挥其输布水谷精微的作用,因而四肢百脉皆失濡养,而致筋脉弛纵,发为肢体虚弱而成痿证。

二、湿热浸淫:久处湿地,或冒雨露,感受外来之湿邪,湿留不去,郁久化热;或湿热之邪内侵,困扰脾胃,流注下焦;或饮食不节,如过食肥甘,嗜烟酒,多饮辛辣,损伤脾胃,湿浊停聚,失于运化,湿蕴日久,气机郁滞,郁而化热,以致湿热浸淫筋脉,气血不得流通,筋脉肌肉失于营养,因而弛纵不收,成为痿证。

三、脾胃虚弱:脾胃为后天之本,气血津液生化之源,五脏六腑皆禀气于胃,四肢筋骨肌肉皆赖以荣养。如素体脾胃虚弱或因劳倦,或因病后,后天已伤,胃虚不能受纳;脾弱不能运化,为胃行其津液,则四肢不得禀水谷精微,久失所养,则宗筋弛纵,肉削筋枯,渐而成痿。

〔辨证论治〕

痿证为临床常见病症之一,主要表现为肢体酸软弱无力和肌肉萎缩。究其病因病机,有外感内伤之不同,证有虚实之不同。由于外受温热之邪而发病的,常发生于湿热病中或病后,迅速出现肢体的痿弱不用;湿热浸淫,亦属新病。外邪引发者,起病多急,其证属实,病情变化亦快。脾胃虚弱,肝肾亏虚者,病史较长,缓慢起病,渐进加重,以双下肌肉萎缩和力弱为多见。其证多虚,有时亦见虚中挟实。外感致病的,如治疗及时,热清湿去,气血流畅,筋脉通利,则肢体痿弱无力诸症逐渐恢复，病势为顺，预后多好。如因邪盛正衰，热伤气阴，湿热留滞，筋脉不利，亦可出现变证，表现为呼吸困难，喘息气短，进而气血瘀阻，唇甲青紫，或言语困难，大汗淋漓，肢冷脉微，转为亡阳之证。内伤致病的，因脾胃已伤，肝肾亏虚，气血生化之源，四肢筋脉不得濡养，如正气不复，则津血日枯，痿弱亦甚，多难恢复。

本证应与中风相鉴别。中风也有肢体瘫痪不遂，但多伴有肢体麻木、口眼歪斜，且起病时鲜有外感六经病证。痿证多无突然昏仆；即使是变证，窍闭神昏者亦少见。

如肢体无力，兼有震颤，走路摇晃，精细动作差，说话不清，是兼有风痱，可称痿痱并病。应结合风痱进行辨证治疗。

如因痹病而致肢体不能活动，肢体长期废用，气血不得流畅，日久亦见肌肉萎缩，是痿痹并病。如兼有肢体关节强痉不舒，拘急挛缩，是痿痉并病，尚需结合痹证、痉证进行辨证论治。

“治痿独取阳明”是治疗痿证的基本法则。应当指出，这一治疗原则包含有祛阳明之邪和补阳明之虚两种不同的治疗方法。因外感邪热而致病的，其证属实，治疗多以祛邪为主，或清阳明实热，或清热利湿，务使邪清正复。内伤致病的，重视培补后天之本，恢复脾胃的运化功能，务使气血得以生化，筋脉赖以濡养。治痿之法，亦不限于阳明，尚需根据病情，或滋补肝肾，或养血通经，当随证而立，不可拘泥于一法。

一、肺热伤津

主症：病起发热，或高热不退，随后出现肢体转弱无力，不能行走，甚则肌肉萎缩。

兼症：心烦口渴，咳呛咽干，小便黄少或闭塞不通，大便秘，关节肢体疼痛或麻木不仁。

舌脉：舌红苔黄，脉数或细数。

分析：肺主卫外，卫外不固，感受湿热毒邪，温热之邪犯肺，肺热伤津，津伤液少，不能正常地输送到周身以温润肌腠和皮毛，筋脉失养，故肢体痿弱不用，肌肉萎缩。心烦口渴咽干，均为热盛伤津的表现。热邪犯肺，气机不利，故而呛咳。肺与膀胱通气化，在水液代谢中发挥重要作用，为水之上源。肺热津伤，水精不布，水道不通，膀胱气化失常，因而小便黄少或闭塞不通。肺与大肠相表里，肺热移于大肠，又因津伤液枯，大肠传化失司，腑气不通，故大便秘结。舌红，苔黄，脉细数，均为阴伤津枯，邪热内炽的表现。

治法：清热润燥，养肺生津。

方药：清燥救肺汤加减。方中人参、麦冬养肺生津；生石膏、桑叶、麻仁清热润燥；杏仁宣肺。若高热，口渴，汗出，可加知母、银花、连翘清热祛邪。热甚，重用石膏、枇杷叶、阿胶清肺养阴，还可加桑白皮、玄参、生地等清肺养阴之品。若咳呛少痰，酌加贝母、全瓜蒌。若身热已减，口燥咽干，食欲不振，舌红少苔，证属肺胃阴伤，宜用益胃汤加薏仁、白术、山药、谷芽之类，益胃生津，补阳明之阴。

如经及时治疗，肺热解，毒邪祛，气阴渐复，则筋脉得以濡养，痿弱肢体逐渐恢复，二便亦可通利。若是毒热邪盛，难以速去，气阴大伤，形体败坏，则可出现变证，表现为喘息气短，进而唇甲青紫，吞咽困难，言语不利，大汗淋漓，四肢厥冷，进而阴竭阳亡。变证的出现，是由于毒热之邪耗伤正气，气阴俱衰，由肺及肾，肺肾俱病，肾主水，肺为水之上源，肺津伤，不能下荫于肾，火邪伤肾，肾为火炽，肾阴亦涸，不能上济于肺，则肺脏更燥，即是所谓高源化绝。肺重气，肾为气之根，肺主呼气，肾主纳气。肺气大伤，终必及肾，肾不纳气，有升无降，则喘促气急。肺朝百脉，肺佐心主治节，百脉亦有赖心肺推动而正常循行。肺气衰，血瘀脉阻，故唇甲青紫。吞咽困难，言语不利，是舌本不利，因手太阴肺经脉抵舌本主咽喉，是少阴肾脉挟舌本，手少阴心脉系舌本。津伤气弱，经脉不利，心肺肾俱损，故气虚汗多，又使阴津更伤，阴竭阳亡，阳气虚脱转为寒证。治疗上，宜急予回阳固脱之剂，参附汤、生脉散之剂皆可选用。

处方举例：

生石膏（先下）30g、麦冬 10g、桑叶 6g、桑皮 10g、阿胶 10g、苡仁 30g、连翘 10g、杏仁 10g、生甘草 10g。

二、湿热浸淫

主症：肢体困重，甚则肿胀，痿软无力，麻木不仁，尤以双下肢为常见。

兼症：或有发热，甚则喘息，呼吸困难，小便赤涩热痛，汗出，二便闭塞不通，吞咽困难。

舌脉：舌质红，苔黄腻，脉滑数。

分析：湿热浸淫，内蕴不清，肺受热乘则津伤，脾受湿淫而湿浊益甚。湿为阴邪，其性重浊，湿浊下沉，浸渍肌肤，故见肢体困重。湿热内停，阻碍气血津液流通，故肢体肿胀，麻木不仁。湿热郁蒸，浸淫筋脉，肢体筋脉弛纵不收，故软弱无力，久则可见肉痿筋消。湿热交阻于营卫可见身热，壅滞于胸膈而气机不利则胸脘痞闷。湿热下注膀胱，致使气化失常，小便赤涩不利。舌苔黄腻，脉滑而数均是湿热内蕴的表现。

治法：清热利湿。

方药：加味二妙散。方中黄柏清热，苍术燥湿，萆薢、防已清利湿热，当归、牛膝养血通络。如肢体困重、肿胀，舌苔厚腻，为湿重，可加茯苓、滑石等淡渗之剂，还可加木通、苡仁、木瓜等利湿通络。兼有胸脘痞闷，为湿阻气机不畅，可加厚朴、藿梗等理气化湿。夏秋之季，可加藿香、佩兰芳香化湿。形体消瘦，心烦，舌边尖红，或中剥无苔，脉细数，为热邪偏重，热甚阴伤，阴虚挟有湿热，徒清热，则阴更伤，惟养阴则湿热益甚，宜于上方中去苍术之温燥，酌加生地、麦冬等以养阴清热。如肢体麻木不仁，关节运动不利，舌质紫暗，脉涩，为内有瘀血阻滞，加红花、赤芍、丹参、木瓜、地龙等以活血通络。腰胁下肢发凉，为湿热之邪阻滞经脉，阳气不得温煦，宜去黄柏，加桂枝温经通脉，重者可用附子、肉桂。

如经积极治疗后，湿去热清，则气血流畅，筋脉得养，病情渐向愈。若是湿邪流注筋脉，重浊黏滞，不易速去，困扰脾土，中焦失于运化，则脾不举四肢，四肢虚弱困重；又因热灼阴伤，正气大衰，肺不主气，喘息气急，进而血脉瘀滞，阳气衰绝，为病热逆转，又宜益气回阳，参附汤主之。

处方举例：

黄柏 10g、牛膝 12g、苍术 9g、苡仁 30g、茯苓 20g、半夏 6g、木瓜 20g、地龙 9g、滑石（包煎）15g、生甘草 10g。

三、脾胃虚弱

主症：肢软无力，劳累及活动后加重，或肌肉萎缩，逐渐加重。

兼症：食少便溏，神疲乏力，面色不华，或痰涎壅盛，声音嘶哑。

舌脉：舌淡苔薄白，脉细或重按无力。

分析：脾胃为后天之本，如脾胃虚弱，则气血化源不足，脉不得养，筋不得荣。初则肢软力弱，不耐劳作，久则脉痿筋消，肌肉瘦削。脾不健运，湿浊内停，清阳之气不升，故而食少便溏。神疲乏力，脉细，均由脾胃虚弱，气血生化不足引起。脾为生痰之源，脾虚痰浊内生，痰阻舌本，故可出现声哑。

治法：健脾益气。

方药：参苓白术散加减。方中党参、白术山药、扁豆、莲子肉均为健脾益气之品；茯苓、苡仁健脾利温；砂仁、陈皮和胃理气；食少纳呆，加鸡内金；肢冷畏寒，加附子、干姜以温脾阳。若是病久体弱，气血两虚者，又宜加黄芪、当归、白芍等补养气血。

如经治疗，脾胃阳气渐复，气血得以生化，筋脉肌肉得以濡养，逐渐恢复正常功能，诸症悉除。如因饮食失节，寒温不适，喜怒忧思，劳役过度，则脾胃更虚，或因复感时邪，正气更伤，则痿弱益重，亦可累及肺肾，出现喘息气短，言语困难，此即李东垣所谓，胃病之后，"气短、气夺，而声哑喘急，此肺之胃败也"，终至五脏俱衰，多难救治。

处方举例：

党参 10g、白术 12g、茯苓 20g、山药 10g、陈皮 10g、苡仁 30g、砂仁 6g、当归 10g、黄芪 15g、制附片 6g、干姜 3g、炙甘草 10g。

四、肝肾亏虚

主症：起病缓慢，下肢痿软无力，腰背酸软。

兼症：头晕目眩，耳鸣，遗精或二便失禁，或筋惕肉瞤，或吞咽呛咳，言语不清，或月经不调，或见肢体肌肉萎缩，舌肌颤动。

舌脉：舌红少苔，或舌体瘦小，舌面少津，脉细数或沉细。

分析：先天不足，或后天失养，或房劳所伤，肝肾亏虚。肝血虚，血不养筋则萎；肾精亏，肾不主骨则骨弱。肝肾亏虚，筋骨经脉皆不充养，因此渐而成痿。腰为肾之府，精髓不足，腰脊失养，故见腰脊酸软。肾主骨生髓，通于脑，肝肾不足，髓海空虚，因而头晕目眩，耳鸣不止。肾虚精关不固，则遗精。肾虚二便失司，膀胱失约，二便失禁。如因肝肾不足，内风时起，则可见筋惕肉瞤。冲任失养则月经不调。吞咽咳嗽，言语不清，总因肝肾不足，舌本病变引起。舌红少苔，脉细数，均为肝肾不足，阴虚内热的表现。

治法：补益肝肾，滋阴清热。

方药：虎潜丸加减。方中虎骨、牛膝，强壮筋骨；锁阳温肾益精；当归、白芍养血柔肝；黄柏、知母、熟地、龟板滋阴清热。若面色萎黄，心悸气短，脉细弱者，酌加黄芪、党参、何首乌等以补气养血。如阴虚有热，宜去锁阳、干姜。若久病阴损及阳，肌肉萎缩，肢体发凉，时而冷汗出，小便清长，舌质淡暗，脉沉细或沉弦。此系命门火衰，失于温煦，血络瘀阻而成，治宜温肾阳，益筋骨，活血络，选用验方加味金刚丸为主方。方用巴戟天、杜仲、肉苁蓉、淫羊藿、菟丝子补肾阳强筋骨，制马钱子、木瓜、牛膝益肝肾舒筋脉，天麻，蜈蚣、僵蚕、乌蛇祛风活络，萆薢、乌贼骨和胃祛湿。还可酌加当归、白芍养血柔肝，地龙、红花活血通络。因病久，需常服，以丸药为宜。

处方举例：

黄芪 15g、锁阳 10g、补骨脂 12g、仙灵脾 10g、制附片 6g、巴戟天 10g、当归 12g、白芍 12g、熟地 9g、牛膝 12g、黄柏 3g、白术 10g。

痿证的治疗，除服药以外，配合针灸、推拿、按摩，适当进行功能练习，加强肢体的活动，对于促进功能恢复，防止因肢体的痿废不用引起的挛缩变形是有帮助的。

〔预防及护理措施〕

罹患本病之后，多渐进加重或稳定于一定程度，恢复起来较为困难，因此与其治疗于已病之后，莫如预防于未病之前，这也符合中医学不治已病治未病的思想，为了预防本病的发生，应保持生活节律，谨慎起居，勿长期坐卧湿地，饮食合理，富于营养，清洁卫生，勿伤脾胃，勿过劳作，清心节欲，免伤肝肾，及时治疗内伤及外感发热等疾患。注意身体锻炼，古语云："流水不腐，户枢不蠹。”经常活动有利于肢体肌肉的功能正常。

既病之后，首先应对疾病有正确的认识，保持乐观向上、与疾病作斗争的信心，并坚持长期治疗，长期锻炼。护理人员应帮助患者树立对待疾病的正确态度，对于痿缩的肢体及肌肉加强主动和被动活动。可配合按摩，每天上下午各一次，尽量使患病的肌肉充分活动，注意其饮食的营养，因患者一般身体较为虚弱，当注意勿外感风寒湿热之邪，否则会加重病情的进展，且难以治疗。卧床的患者，应防止褥疮的发生，应勤翻身拍背，按摩受压的骨突部，注意大小便，勿浸渍受压的肌肉，尿失禁或难以排出者可留置尿管。对能部分活动的患者，注意不要因为活动受限而悴伤、碰伤及出现其他意外事故。

〔**典型病例分析**〕

有一5岁小儿，感冒后发热4天，最高体温达40℃，经治疗后热退，10余天后出现左腿走路无力，呈跛行，渐渐走路困难，肌肉萎软无力，西医诊断为“脊髓灰质炎”，予加兰他敏1mg/次肌注，日两次，口服维生素B族，并嘱家长延中医治疗。患者来诊时，面色略显皖白，食欲差，口唇干，舌红苔少，脉细，左小腿肌肉松软，其时尚未见萎缩，走路跛行，诊为“痿证”，证属肺胃阴伤，治疗宜清肺余热，滋养肺胃，处方予桑皮、阿胶、麦冬、桑叶、生苡仁、白术、谷麦芽、鸡内金等。服药10余剂后食欲转佳，舌淡红，苔薄白，走路仍呈跛行，考虑此时肺胃阴伤已复，以脾胃虚弱为主，乃改以健脾养胃，兼及肝肾。处方予党参、白术、茯苓、苡仁、白扁豆、青陈皮、黄柏、川断、怀牛膝。连服20余剂，诸证平稳，走路较前有力，但左小腿肌肉明显松弛。略改前方后嘱家长配丸剂，继服数月，未再来诊。

按：此患者外感高热之后出现肢体软弱无力，乃外邪侵肺，肺热伤津，津液失于敷布，肌肤不得濡养，其时当清泻肺热，养阴生津。但患者来诊时高热已退，主见舌红苔少，食欲差，属肺之余热未尽，伤及肺胃之阴津，滋养肺胃之后，症已平稳，根据“治痿独取阳明”的法则，改以调理脾胃。下肢为肾所主，脉筋为肝所司，故又佐以益肾调肝之品，诸症平妥。后以丸剂久服以收功，并嘱家长加强患肢的活动。

痿证主要以肢体筋脉弛缓、软弱无力，或者肌肉萎缩为主要临床表现，以下肢痿弱无力或不能行走为多。致病或为肺热叶焦，失于濡润，或以湿热浸注，气血不通，或以脾胃虚弱，化源枯竭，或以肝肾亏虚，筋无所主，即总以肢体筋脉肌肉失于濡养为主。治疗的基本法则是“治痿独取阳明”，重视调理脾胃功能。因外感邪热致病者，其证属实，治以祛邪为主，或清阳明实热，或清热利湿；内伤致病者，重视培补后天，恢复脾胃的运化功能。治疗常选用清燥救肺汤、参苓白术散、加味二妙散、虎潜丸等。现代医学多种神经肌肉疾病，见有肌肉、肢体无力和萎缩者，均可参考本证辨治。

复习思考题

1. 痿证的病因有哪些？
2. 常见的痿证有几个主要证候？怎样进行治疗？
3. 如何正确理解和运用“治痿独取阳明”的原则？

内伤发热

〔概述〕

凡以内伤为病因，脏腑功能失调，气血阴阳亏损为病机的发热，称之为内伤发热。其临床主要特征为起病缓慢，病程较长，一般以低热为多，有时也见有高热，或自觉发热，或五心烦热而体温并不升高，并在发热同时多伴有内伤虚损或肝郁、血瘀、湿郁的见症。

内伤发热是具有独立性的证候，作为一个症状也可伴见于一些慢性疾病之中，本篇所讨论的是以内伤为病因，发热为主症的病证。

西医学中的功能性低热、肿瘤、血液病、结缔组织疾病、内分泌疾病、结核病、慢性感染性疾病所引起的发热，以及某些原因不明的发热，具有内伤发热的临床表现时，均可参照本篇进行辨证论治。

〔病因病机〕

内伤发热主要由情志、饮食、劳倦等内因所引起，也有少数始为外感，久则导致脏腑气血阴阳失调而产生。若由于脏腑气血阴阳亏虚而产生的发热，多称为虚热、虚火，为虚证；若由于气机郁结，瘀血停滞，饮食积滞，湿热阻滞等引起的发热则多为实证或虚实夹杂证。病及的脏腑随内伤发热的各种类型而异，现分述如下：

一、阴精亏虚：素体阴虚，或热病日久伤阴，或久泻，或误用、过用温燥辛散药物等，导致阴精亏虚，水不制火，阳气相对偏亢而引起发热，此称之为阴虚发热。

二、中气不足，过度疲劳：饮食失调，或病后失于调养，以致脾胃虚弱，中气不足，而引起发热，通常称之为气虚发热。其病机或为气虚而虚阳外越；或为气虚而阴火上冲；或为气虚而卫外不固，营卫不和。阴火是对阳火而言，阳火是元气的别名。阴火泛指虚火、邪火。中气不足，气虚下陷，虚火或邪火得以上乘。

三、营血亏虚：久病心肝血虚，或脾虚不能生血，或因出血、产后或手术后失血过多，造成营血亏虚。血本属阴，阴血不足，无以敛阳，而导致阳浮发热，此称之为血虚发热。血虚发热多以气血两虚或阴血两虚出现。

四、肾阳虚弱：平素阳气不足，或寒证日久伤阳，或误用过用寒凉药物，导致肾阳虚弱，寒气内盛。格阳于外，即虚阳浮于外而发热。脾胃气虚日久，亦可导致脾肾阳虚而发热。此皆称为阳虚发热。

五、肝经郁热：情志抑郁，肝气不能条达，气郁化火而致发热，或恼怒过度，肝火内盛以致发热，此皆称为肝郁发热。因这种发热和情志不遂有关，故又称“五志之火”。

六、瘀血阻滞：由于情志、劳倦、外伤、出血等原因导致瘀血产生，瘀血停积行体内，阻滞经络，气血运行不畅，壅遏不通因而引起发热，通常称瘀血发热。

七、湿浊郁蒸：湿邪内郁或化热熏蒸所造成的发热，可有外感与内伤之别。内伤者多由脾胃气虚，脾运不健，水湿停留，久则郁而化热，湿热蕴蒸而致，通常称湿郁发热。

综上所述，内伤发热的原因可分为虚实两大类，属虚者不外气、血、阴、阳不足，属实者以情志为病，瘀血停滞、湿浊郁蒸为多。而临床上虚实相兼，或由两种病机同时引起的发热也屡见不鲜，如气郁血瘀、气阴两虚、气血两虚、气虚湿阻等，都可同时引起发热。从病机的转化来看，久病往往由实转虚，由轻转重，其中以瘀血病久，损及气、血、阴、阳，分别兼见气虚、血虚、阴虚、阳虚者为多。气郁日久，正气亦虚，可成为气虚气郁的发热。若热伤阴津，又可转为气郁阴虚之发热。除此之外，湿浊久蕴、脾气虚弱，或湿浊内停、阴亦不足等发热，临证时也多见到。

内伤发热病因病机示意图

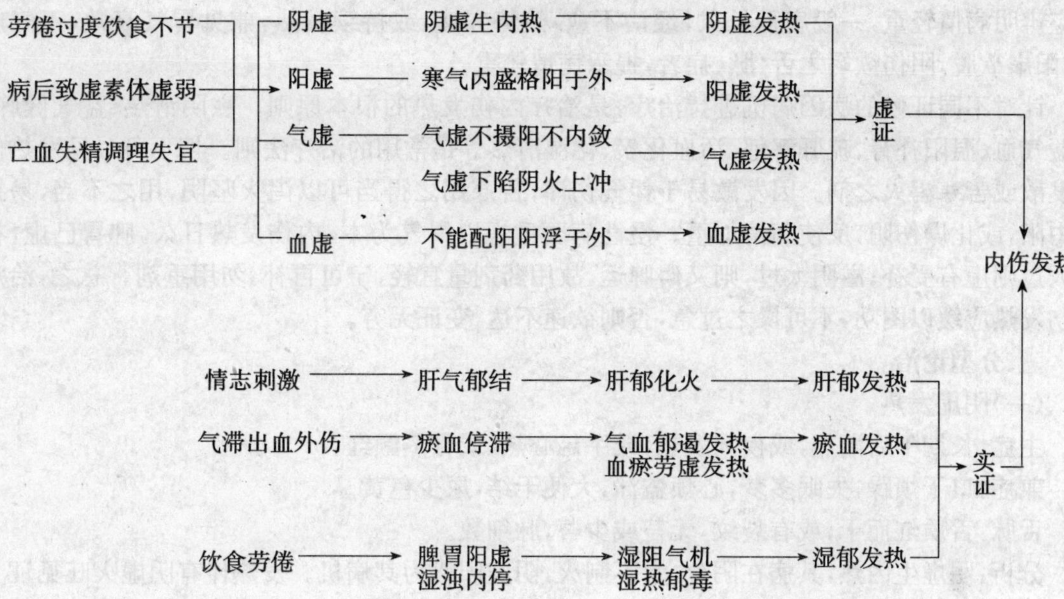

〔辨证论治〕

一、类证鉴别

内伤发热应与外感发热相鉴别，这主要通过四诊，注意起病、病因、病程、发热特点、伴随症、恶寒特点、舌脉等方面的不同，一般不难辨别。现将内伤发热与外感发热的主要区别列下表以示之：

类别 项目	内伤发热	外感发热
起病	多缓慢	多急骤
病因	内伤饮食情志劳倦	外感六淫邪气
病程	较长	较短
发热特点	①以低热为多，或自觉发热，或觉手足心热 ②热多有间歇，时作时止或无定时	①以高热为多见。 ②热多持续，外邪不解，发热不退。 ③温病发热，热势亢盛，易于传变汗出而热减
恶寒特点	发热时大多不恶寒，或感怯冷，得衣被则减	发热初期常伴恶寒，恶寒加衣被不缓解
伴随症	伴有内伤虚损症状，如头晕体倦，少气懒言，自汗盗汗等，汗出热不解	常伴有鼻塞流涕，头痛等表证
舌脉	苔少或无，或厚腻不退，舌质红或淡或有瘀象，脉虚弱或弦、涩。	苔薄白或薄黄，脉浮数滑紧等

二、辨治要点

对于内伤发热，首先应辨明病因病机及证候的虚实。虚证应注意区分气、血、阴、阳之虚孰轻孰重、五脏受损何脏为甚。实证应注意气郁、血瘀、湿郁孰最突出，是纯虚无实，纯实无虚，还是虚实夹杂。以及病机转化是因虚致实，或邪实伤正。这通过临床表现、病史，一般不难确定。再应辨明病情轻重，一般病程长久，经治不愈，热势亢盛，或持续发热，兼见胃气衰败，正气虚甚，阳虚欲脱，阴伤欲竭之舌、脉、症者，提示病情较重。

针对不同证候的病因病机进行治疗，是治疗内伤发热的根本原则。滋阴清热、益气健脾、补益气血、温阳补肾、疏肝解郁、活血化瘀、化湿清热等是常用的治疗法则。切不可一见发热便用发散或苦寒泻火之剂。因发散易于耗气伤津；苦寒用之得当可以泻火坚阴，用之不当，易损伤中阳，或化燥伤阴，反使病情加重。慢性病要重视以胃气为本，内伤发热日久，脾胃已虚，补益太过则虚有受补；滋阴太过，则又碍脾运，故用药剂量宜轻，宁可再补，勿用重剂。总之，治疗内伤发热应缓以图功，不可操之过急，否则欲速不达，变证无穷。

三、分型论治

(一)阴虚发热

主症：长期午后潮热，或夜间发热，或手足心热，或骨蒸颧红。

兼症：口干烦躁，失眠多梦，心烦盗汗，大便干结，尿少色黄。

舌脉：舌质红而干，或有裂纹，无苔或少苔，脉细数。

分析：阴虚生内热，其病在阴分，水不制火，阴虚阳盛为其病机。发热伴有阴虚火旺见证为特点。

阴精亏虚，虚火内炽，故见午后潮热或夜间发热，手足心热，骨蒸颧红。虚火上炎扰乱心神，则致心烦少寐多梦，内热逼迫津液外泄则盗汗。阴虚火旺，津亏失润，故口干咽燥，便干尿少。舌干红少苔甚至无苔，脉细数亦为阴虚火旺之象。

治法：益气健脾，甘温除热。

方药，补中益气汤加减。本方为益气升陷、甘温除热的代表方。方中以黄芪、党参、白术、甘草益气健脾；当归养血活血；陈皮理气和胃；升麻、柴胡既能升举清阳，又能透泄邪热。自汗多者，加煅牡蛎、煅龙骨，或浮小麦、糯稻根以固表收敛止汗。时冷时热、汗出恶风者，可加桂枝、芍药以调和营卫。胸腹痞满、舌苔白腻者，为挟有湿邪，可加苍术、厚朴以健脾燥湿，或加藿香、佩兰以芳香化湿；若湿浊有化热之势，口干苔稍薄黄，可加生炒苡仁、竹茹等化湿而不香燥之品。

处方举例：

党参10g、黄芪15g、白术10g、当归10g、茯苓10g、柴胡10g、升麻6g、陈皮10g、炙甘草5g。

(二)血虚发热

主症：发热多为低热，唇甲色淡，面色萎黄不华。

兼症：头晕眼花，身倦乏力，心悸不宁。

舌脉：舌质淡，脉细弱。

分析：血虚不能配阳为病机，发热伴有血虚见症为特点。

血本属阴，阴血不足，则无以敛阳，因而引起发热。血虚不能上滋头目、外濡肢体，故见头晕眼花，身倦乏力。血不养心，则心悸不宁。血虚不能上荣于面，血脉不充，故面色萎黄少华，唇甲舌淡，舌质淡，脉细弱。

治法：益气养血。

方药：归脾汤加减。本方补益心脾，益气生血，适用于心脾气血不足之证。方中黄芪、党参、白术、甘草益气健脾；当归、龙眼肉补血养血；酸枣仁、远志养心安神；木香健脾理气。因气血同源，血虚重症、急症，气随血脱伴见发热，因有形之血不能速生，无形之气所当急固，也可用当归补血汤为基础进行治疗。因精血互化，血虚阴 伤可同时兼见，可在益气养血的同时，加用滋阴养血之品，可用八珍汤化裁。

处方举例：

黄芪 20g、党参 10g、茯苓 10g、白术 10g、当归 10g、远志 10g、白芍 10g、夜交藤 20g、黄精 20g。

（三）阳虚发热

主症：发热而欲近衣被，形寒胀冷，四肢不温或下肢常冷。

兼证：头晕嗜卧，面色皖白，倦怠乏力，腰膝酸痛，五更泄泻，小便不利或小便频数。

舌脉：舌质淡胖，或有齿痕，苔白腻，脉沉细而弱，或浮大无力，或寸关浮大而尺弱。

分析：肾阳亏虚，虚阳外浮为病机，发热伴有肾阳虚衰见症为特点。

肾阳虚衰，失于温煦，故发热低欲近衣被，形寒怯冷，四肢不温。头为诸阳之会，腰为肾之府，肾阳亏虚，不能温养，故头晕嗜卧，面色皖白，腰膝酸痛。肾司二便，肾阳不足，黎明前阳气未振，阴寒较盛，则五更作泄。温化无能，开阖失司，故或为小便不利，或为小便频数。舌质淡胖，有齿痕，苔白腻，脉沉细弱，或浮大无力等皆为阳虚之象。

治法：温阳补肾。

方药：金匮肾气丸或右归饮加减。前方以六味地黄丸壮水之主，附片、肉桂补水中之火，温补肾阳，鼓舞肾气。古人称此方为“治肾命虚寒之正品，亦导龙归海之妙法”。后方右归饮，熟地、山药、山萸肉、枸杞子培补肾阴、肉桂、附子温养肾阳，炙甘草补中，杜仲强壮益精。若阳虚气弱，气短无力为著者，加人参、白术补益元气。火不生土，大便稀溏者，加干姜、白术温中健脾。五更泄泻者加五味子、肉豆蔻以补肾回涩。小便频数，或遗精滑精腰酸者，加补骨脂、芡实、金樱子等以涩精止泄。

处方举例：

制附片 10g、肉桂 6g、熟地 12g、山萸肉 10g、茯苓 10g、泽泻 10g、山药 10g、炒白术 10g、菟丝子 10g、杜仲 10g。

（四）肝郁发热

主症：时觉身热心烦，热势常随情志波动而起伏。

兼症：精神抑郁或烦躁易怒、胸胁胀闷喜叹息，口苦而干，妇女兼有月经不调，经来腹痛，或乳房发胀。

舌脉：苔薄黄，脉弦数。

分析：肝气郁结，气郁化火为病机，发热随情绪波动而起伏，多见于女性，伴有肝郁气滞见症为特点。

肝藏血，主疏泄，性喜条达，其经脉布胁肋，贯膈。肝气郁结，疏泄无权，气机不畅，故见精神抑郁或烦躁易怒，胸胁胀满，或月经不调，痛经，乳房发胀等症。叹息则气机可暂得舒展，故喜叹息。气郁化火而致发热，故身热心烦，且热与情绪相关，口苦口干。舌苔薄黄，脉弦数为郁火内蒸之象。

治法：疏肝解郁清热。

方药：丹栀逍遥散加减。本方具有疏肝解郁、养血清热之功，适用于肝郁血虚发热或月经不调之证。方中丹皮、山栀清肝泻热；柴胡、薄荷疏肝解热；当归、白芍养血柔肝；白术、茯苓、甘草培土健脾。若郁火内炽，面红目赤，心烦易急，尿赤便秘，舌红脉数者，可加龙胆草、黄芩、夏枯草、生地等以加强清热泻火作用，或用龙胆泻肝汤加减，以清郁火湿热。若气郁明显，胁痛乳胀尤甚，可加郁金、川楝子、香附、青皮、元胡等以理气止痛；妇女月经不调，可加泽兰、益母草调经活血。若气郁日久，热伤阴血，或素体阴虚而兼肝郁为患，宜用滋水清肝饮加减，以滋养肝肾，疏肝清热。此方以六味地黄丸壮水之主，丹栀逍遥散中生甘草、白术以减其温燥之性，妙在两者相合而用。若木郁克土，脾失健运，湿浊易停，症见舌苔厚腻，胸腹痞闷。气郁不振，为气郁挟有湿热痰浊，可改用越鞠丸或越鞠保和丸加柴胡、黄芩治之。

处方举例：

丹皮10g、栀子10g、当归10g、白芍10g、柴胡10g、茯苓12g、薄荷(后下)3g、郁金10g、黄芩10g。

(五)瘀血发热

主症：下午或夜晚发热，或自觉身体某些局部发热。

兼症：口干咽燥而不欲饮，肢体或躯干有固定痛处或肿块，或见皮肤粗糙，甚至肌肤甲错，面色萎黄或黯黑，或身有瘀斑、瘀点。

舌脉：舌质黯，或有瘀点、瘀斑，脉细涩。

分析：瘀血内停，气血郁遏为病机，发热伴见瘀血见症为特点。

瘀血内停，气血郁遏不通则发热；瘀血病在血分，属阴，故发热多在下午或夜间；瘀血停着之处，气血运行受阻，故痛处不移或有肿块瘀斑。因热郁营血，不在气分，故口干咽燥而不欲饮水。瘀血内阻，新血不生，气血不能荣于头面、肌肤，则见面色萎黄黯黑，肌肤粗糙，甚则甲错。唇舌紫黯，或有瘀点、瘀斑，脉细涩也为瘀血内阻之象。

治法：活血化瘀退热。

方药：血府逐瘀汤加减。方中桃红四物活血化瘀，四逆散疏利气机，桔梗、枳壳一升一降走气分，川芎、牛膝一升一降走血分，全方共奏理气活血之功。热甚者，加白薇、丹皮、大黄、地鳖虫以凉血活血清热。若畏寒肢冷，可加桂枝以温通血脉。气虚证亦见，可加黄芪以益气行血。胁下有瘀块者，可加鳖甲煎丸。

若有明确外伤史者，也可用复元活血汤加减治之。

处方举例：

桃仁10g、红花10g、当归10g、酒大黄6g、柴胡10g、枳壳10g、川芎10g、赤芍10g、白薇10g。

(六)湿郁发热

主症：低热，午后热甚，胸脘痞闷，发病缓慢。

兼症：口不渴，或饮入即吐，或呕吐，纳少，身重，大便稀溏或黏滞不爽。

舌脉：舌苔白腻或黄腻，脉濡数或沉滑。

分析：脾运不健，湿浊内生，郁而化热为病机，发热伴有湿浊或湿热内停见症为特点。湿为阴邪，自旺于阴时，故以午后发热明显。湿邪黏滞，故起病缓慢。湿阻气机，故见胸脘痞闷、身重。中焦停湿，故不思饮食，甚则呕恶，口不渴或饮入即吐。脾不健运，湿浊下渗则大便稀溏。

湿蕴化热，停滞肠中，亦可大便黏滞不爽。舌苔白腻，脉沉滑为湿郁之象。舌苔黄腻，脉濡数为湿郁化热之征。

治法：宣化畅中，利湿清热。

方药：三仁汤加减。方中杏仁宣降肺气，善开上焦；蔻仁芳化湿浊，和畅中焦；苡仁益脾渗湿，疏导下焦；配半夏、厚朴温燥湿浊；通草、滑石、竹叶清热利湿，共奏宣化畅中，利湿清热之功。湿郁化热，阻滞少阳枢机，症见寒热如疟，寒轻热重，口苦呕逆者，加青蒿、黄芩清解少阳，或用蒿芩清胆汤以清透肝胆湿热。湿热久郁，水谷精微不从正化，又每致湿热与阴虚并见，症见口干舌燥，苔黄厚，质红，可在化湿方中加麦冬、花粉等滋阴而不助湿之品，也可用青蒿、南沙参、丹皮加黄芩滑石汤化裁，以养阴化湿。

处方举例：

芦根 30g、滑石 12g、黄芩 10g、苡仁 20g、竹叶 10g、厚朴 6g、蔻仁 6g、青蒿 12g、通草 3g。

〔预防及护理措施〕

1. 针对可能导致内伤发热的病因，采取预防措施。如体质亏虚者，视其气、血、阴、阳之不足，及时调补。平素注意劳逸结合，避免过度疲劳。已有情志失调，或跌仆瘀阻，或湿浊内盛者，应及早审因治疗。

2. 坚定信心，减少思想负担，认真检查治疗。因内伤发热病情一般比较复杂，有时病程较长，甚至经年累日，缺乏战胜疾病的信心，或思想负担过重，更易使疾病加重。

3. 顾护脾胃。患 者饮食宜清淡而富有营养。治疗用药应保护脾胃健运。

4. 预防外感。注意保暖避风，尤其是有自汗、盗汗患者，外邪易乘袭卫表，故更应该注意。

5. 仔细观察，注意病机转化，更好辨证施治。

〔典型病例分析〕

案一：阴虚发热。卢某某，女，20 岁，知青，1976 年 8 月 31 日初诊。

一月来，午后低热，或隔日发，或数日不退。两颧潮红，手足心热，咽干口燥，经治未效。某结核病院诊断为肺结核。近日干咳无痰，胸痛，盗汗，骨节酸楚，周身乏力，失眠多梦，舌红少津，脉细数。肺热熏灼，清肃之令不行，肺阴亏耗，逐发本证，法当养阴清热。

银柴胡 15g、白芍 20g、白薇 15g、地骨皮 20g、青蒿 20g、知母 15g、元参 15g、鳖甲 25g、生牡蛎 50g。6 剂，水煎服。

9 月 9 日二诊：

上方服至 4 剂，低热即退，6 剂药后，余症大为减轻，再拟滋阴益气之方：

生地 15g、沙参 20g、麦冬 15g、党参 20g、五味子 10g、元参 20g、天冬 15g、山药 25g、生牡蛎 30g。6 剂，水煎服。

各症相继消失，又宗上方调治半月，身体康复，X 线透视示两肺清晰，无异常所见。

按：本例低热系《素问·调经论》所指之“阴虚则内热”之证，初以清骨散治其标，后以生脉散合增液汤固其本，层次分明。

内伤发热一病，由情志、饮食、劳倦、外伤等病因引起，临床表现以低热为多见。气血阴阳亏损，脏腑功能失调是其病机。临床辨证有虚实两类，虚者不外气血阴阳之不足，所致发热同时，必伴有气虚、血虚、阴虚、阳虚，或气血两虚、阴血两虚、气阴两虚、阴阳两虚的见证，实者主要有气郁发热、瘀血发热及湿郁发热发热同时必有肝气郁滞，瘀积内停，湿浊瘀阻的见证。针对病因病机确定相应治疗方法是治疗内伤发热的原则。但由于人体是一个统一整体，各种病机引起的发热常互相关联，或相互转化，彼此兼挟，因此必须用发展和相互联系的观点去看待和处理每个类型的内伤发热。不要一见发热日久就是内伤发热，也不要一见发热，不辨内伤、外感就用辛散或苦寒之剂，以酿成弊端无穷。

由于内伤发热病情比较复杂，病因常难一时明确，病程往往较长，有时可延续数年或反复发作，因此认真细致地观察，注意病机转化，及时调整治疗方案更为重要。在患者方面，若能注意劳逸结合，保持乐观情绪，饮食宜进清淡、富于营养，而又易于消化之品，防止外感，将有利于取得较好疗效。

复习思考题

1. 内伤发热的概念是什么？
2. 试述内伤发热的病因病机？
3. 如何鉴别内伤发热与外感发热？
4. 内伤发热常见有哪些证型？其辨证要点、治法及常用方剂是什么？
5. 内伤发热在辨证论治中应注意些什么？

方 剂 索 引

一 划

［1］ **一贯煎**（《柳州医话》）：沙参、麦冬、当归、生地黄、枸杞子、川楝子

二 划

［2］ **二冬汤**（《医学心悟》）：天冬、麦冬、天花粉、黄芩、知母、甘草、人参、荷叶

［3］ **二仙汤**（《中医方剂临床手册》）：仙茅、仙灵脾、巴戟天、黄柏、知母、当归

［4］ **二至丸**（《医方集解》）：女贞子、旱莲草

［5］ **二陈汤**（《太平惠民和剂局方》）：半夏、陈皮、茯苓、炙甘草

［6］ **二阴煎**（《景岳全书》）：生地黄、麦冬、枣仁、生甘草、玄参、茯苓、黄连、木通、灯心草、竹叶

［7］ **二妙丸**（《丹溪心法》）：黄柏、苍术

［8］ **二神散**（《杂病源流犀烛》）：海金砂、滑石

［9］ **十全大补汤**（《太平惠民和剂局方》）：熟地黄、白芍、当归、川芎、人参、白术、茯苓、炙甘草、黄芪、肉桂

［10］ **十灰散**（《十药神书》）：大蓟、小蓟、侧柏叶、荷叶、茜草根、山栀、茅根、大黄、丹皮、棕榈皮

［11］ **十枣汤**（《伤寒论》）：大戟、芫花、甘遂、大枣

［12］ **丁沉透膈散**（《太平惠民和剂局方》）：白术、香附、人参、砂仁、丁香、麦芽、木香、肉豆蔻、神曲、炙甘草、沉香、青皮、厚朴、藿香、陈皮、半夏、草果

［13］ **丁香散**（《古今医统》）：丁香、柿蒂、良姜、炙甘草

［14］ **七味都气丸**（《医宗已任篇》）：地黄、山茱萸、山药、茯苓、丹皮、泽泻、五味子

［15］ **人参养营汤**（《太平惠民和剂局方》）：人参、甘草、当归、白芍、熟地黄、肉桂、大枣、黄芪、白术、茯苓、五味子、远志、橘皮、生姜

［16］ **八正散**（《太平惠民和剂局方》）：木通、车前子、篇蓄、瞿麦、滑石、甘草梢、大黄、山栀、灯芯

［17］ **八珍汤**（《正体类要》）：人参、白术、茯苓、甘草、当归、白芍药、川芎、熟地黄、生姜、大枣

三 划

［18］ **三才封髓丹**（《卫生宝鉴》）：天冬、熟地黄、人参、黄柏、砂仁、甘草

［19］ **三子养亲汤**（《韩氏医通》）：苏子、白芥子、莱菔子

［20］ **三仁汤**（《温病条辨》）：杏仁、白蔻仁、薏苡仁、厚朴、半夏、通草、滑石、竹叶

［21］ **三圣散**（《儒门事亲》）：瓜蒂、防风、藜芦

［22］ **三拗汤**（《太平惠民和剂局方》）：麻黄、杏仁、生甘草

［23］ **大七气汤**（《医学入门》）：青皮、陈皮、桔梗、藿香、官桂、甘草、三棱、莪术、香附、益智仁、姜、枣

[24] **大半夏汤**(《金匮要略》):半夏、人参、白蜜

[25] **大补元煎**(《景岳全书》):人参、炒山药、熟地黄、杜仲、枸杞子、当归、山茱萸、炙甘草

[26] **大补阴丸**(《丹溪心法》):知母、黄柏、熟地黄、龟板、猪脊髓

[27] **大青龙汤**(《伤寒论》):麻黄、杏仁、桂枝、甘草、石膏、生姜、大枣

[28] **大定风珠**(《温病条辨》):白芍药、阿胶、生龟板、生地黄、火麻仁、五味子、生牡蛎、麦冬、炙甘草、鸡子黄、生鳖甲

[29] **大建中汤**(《金匮要略》):川椒、干姜、人参、饴糖

[30] **大承气汤**(《伤寒论》):大黄、厚朴、枳实、芒硝

[31] **大秦艽汤**(《素问病机气宜保命集》):秦艽、当归、甘草、羌活、防风、白芷、熟地黄、茯苓、石膏、川芎、白芍药、独活、黄芩、生地黄、白术、细辛

[32] **大柴胡汤**(《伤寒论》):柴胡、黄芩、半夏、枳实、白芍药、大黄、生姜、大枣

[33] **大黄甘草汤**(《金匮要略》):大黄、甘草

[34] **大黄附子汤**(《金匮要略》):大黄、附子、细辛

[35] **大黄硝石汤**(《金匮要略》):大黄、黄柏、硝石、栀子

[36] **大黄䗪虫汤**(《金匮要略》):地鳖虫、干漆、干地黄、甘草、水蛭、白芍、杏仁、黄芩、桃仁、虻虫、蛴螬虫、大黄

[37] **川芎茶调散**(《太平惠民和剂局方》):川芎、荆芥、薄荷、羌活、细辛(或香附)、白芷、甘草、防风

[38] **《千金》苇茎汤**(《备急千金要方》):鲜芦根、薏苡仁、冬瓜仁、桃仁

[39] **己椒苈黄丸**(《金匮要略》):防己、椒目、葶苈子、大黄

[40] **小半夏加茯苓汤**(《金匮要略》):半夏、生姜、茯苓

[41] **小半夏汤**(《金匮要略》):半夏、生姜

[42] **小青龙加石膏汤**(《金匮要略》):麻黄、桂枝、芍药、甘草、干姜、细辛、半夏、五味子、石膏

[43] **小青龙汤**(《伤寒论》):麻黄、桂枝、芍药、甘草、干姜、细辛、半夏、五味子

[44] **小建中汤**(《伤寒论》):桂枝、白芍、甘草、生姜、大枣、饴糖

[45] **小承气汤**(《伤寒论》):大黄、厚朴、枳实

[46] **小柴胡汤**(《伤寒论》):柴胡、黄芩、半夏、人参、甘草、生姜、大枣

[47] **小陷胸汤**(《伤寒论》):黄连、半夏、瓜蒌

[48] **小蓟饮子**(《济生方》):生地黄、小蓟、滑石、通草、炒蒲黄、淡竹叶、藕节、当归、山栀、甘草

四　划

[49] **天王补心丹**(《摄生秘剂》):人参、玄参、丹参、茯苓、五味子、远志、桔梗、当归身、天冬、麦冬、柏子仁、酸枣仁、生地黄、辰砂

[50] **天麻钩藤饮**(《杂病诊治新义》):天麻、钩藤、生石决明、川牛膝、桑寄生、杜仲、山栀、黄芩、益母草、朱茯神、夜交藤

[51] **无比山药丸**(《太平惠民和剂局方》):山药、肉苁蓉、熟地黄、山茱萸、茯神、菟丝子、五味子、赤石脂、巴戟天、泽泻、杜仲、牛膝

[52] **开噤散**(《医学心悟》):人参、黄连、石菖蒲、丹参、石莲子、茯苓、陈皮、冬瓜子、陈米、荷叶蒂

[53] **木防己汤**(《金匮要略》):木防己、石膏、桂枝、人参

[54] **木香顺气散**(《沈氏尊生书》):木香、青皮、橘皮、甘草、枳壳、川朴、乌药、香附、苍术、砂仁、桂心、川芎

[55] **止嗽散**(《医学心悟》):荆芥、桔梗、甘草、白前、陈皮、百部、紫菀

[56] **中满分消丸**(《兰室秘藏》):厚朴、枳实、黄连、黄芩、知母、半夏、陈皮、茯苓、猪苓、泽泻、砂仁、干姜、姜黄、人参、白术、炙甘草

[57] **五子衍宗丸**(《丹溪心法》):枸杞子、覆盆子、菟丝子、五味子、车前子

[58] **五生饮**(《世医得效方》):生南星、生半夏、生白附子、川乌、黑豆

[59] **五仁丸**(《世医得效方》):桃仁、杏仁、柏子仁、松子仁、郁李仁、橘皮

[60] **五汁安中饮**(验方):韭汁、牛乳、生姜汁、梨汁、藕汁

[61] **五皮散**(《中藏经》):桑白皮、橘皮、生姜皮、大腹皮、茯苓皮

[62] **五苓散**(《伤寒论》):桂枝、白术、茯苓、猪苓、泽泻

[63] **五味消毒饮**(《医宗金鉴》):金银花、野菊花、蒲公英、紫花地丁、紫背天葵

[64] **五积散**(《太平惠民和剂局方》):白芷、橘皮、厚朴、当归、川芎、白芍药、茯苓、桔梗、苍术、枳壳、半夏、麻黄、干姜、肉桂、甘草、姜

[65] **五磨饮子**(《医方集解》):乌药、沉香、槟榔、枳实、木香

[66] **六一散**(《伤寒标本心法类萃》):滑石、甘草

[67] **六君子汤**(《医学正传》):人参、炙甘草、茯苓、白术、陈皮、制半夏

[68] **六味地黄丸**(《小儿药证直决》):熟地黄、山药、茯苓、丹皮、泽泻、山茱萸

[69] **六磨汤**(《证治准绳》):沉香、木香、槟榔、乌药、枳实、大黄

[70] **升降散**(《寒温条辨》):炒僵蚕、蝉蜕、姜黄、大黄

[71] **化肝煎**(《景岳全书》):青皮、陈皮、芍药、丹皮、栀子、泽泻、贝母

[72] **化积丸**(《类证治裁》):三棱、莪术、阿魏、海浮石、香附、雄黄、槟榔、苏木、瓦楞子、五灵脂

[73] **牛黄清心丸**(《痘疹世医心法》):牛黄、朱砂、生黄连、黄芩、栀子、郁金

[74] **丹参饮**(《医宗金鉴》):丹参、檀香、砂仁

[75] **丹栀逍遥散**(《医统》):当归、白芍药、白术、柴胡、茯苓、甘草、煨姜、薄荷、丹皮、山栀

[76] **乌头汤**(《金匮要略》):川乌、麻黄、芍药、黄芪、甘草

[77] **乌头赤石脂丸**(《金匮要略》):蜀椒、乌头、炮附子、干姜、赤石脂

[78] **乌头桂枝汤**(《金匮要略》):桂枝、芍药、甘草、生姜、大枣、乌头

[79] **乌附麻辛桂姜汤**(《成都中医学院戴云波方》):川乌、附子、麻黄、细辛、桂枝、干姜、甘草、蜂蜜

[80] **乌梅丸**(《伤寒论》):乌梅、黄连、黄柏、人参、当归、附子、桂枝、蜀椒、干姜、细辛

[81] **少腹逐瘀汤**(《医林改错》):小茴香、干姜、延胡索、没药、当归、川芎、肉桂、赤芍药、蒲黄、五灵脂

[82] **水红花膏**(《景岳全书》):红蓼子、大黄、朴硝、山桃、石灰、酒酵

[83] **水陆二仙丹**(《证治准绳》):金樱子、芡实

五　划

[84] **玉女煎**(《景岳全书》):石膏、熟地黄、麦冬、知母、牛膝

[85] **玉枢丹**(《百一选方》):山慈姑、续随子、大戟、麝香、腰黄、朱砂、五倍子

[86] **玉屏风散**(《世医得效方》):黄芪、白术、防风

[87] **正气天香散**(《证治准绳》引刘河间方):乌药、香附、干姜、紫苏、陈皮

[88] **石韦散**(《证治汇补》):石韦、冬葵子、瞿麦、滑石、车前子

[89] **龙虎丸**(验方):牛黄、巴豆霜、辰砂、砒石

[90] **龙胆泻肝汤**(《兰室秘藏》):龙胆草、泽泻、木通、车前子、当归、柴胡、生地黄(近代方有黄芩、栀子)

[91] **左归丸**(《景岳全书》):熟地黄、山药、山茱萸、菟丝子、枸杞子、川牛膝、鹿角胶、龟板胶

[92] **左归饮**(《景岳全书》):熟地、山萸肉、杞子、山药、杜仲、甘草、附子、肉桂

[93] **左金丸**(《丹溪心法》):黄连、吴茱萸

[94] **右归丸**(《景岳全书》):熟地黄、山药、山茱萸、枸杞子、杜仲、菟丝子、附子、肉桂、当归、鹿角胶

[95] **右归饮**(《景岳全书》):熟地、山萸肉、杞子、山药、茯苓、甘草

[96] **平胃散**(《太平惠民和剂局方》):苍术、厚朴、橘皮、甘草、生姜、大枣

[97] **平喘固本汤**(《南京中医学院附院验方》):党参、五味子、冬虫夏草、胡桃肉、沉香、灵磁石、坎脐、苏子、款冬花、法半夏、橘红

[98] **甘麦大枣汤**(《金匮要略》):甘草、淮小麦、大枣

[99] **甘草干姜汤**(《金匾要略》):甘草、干姜

[100] **甘草泻心汤**(《伤寒论》):炙甘草、黄芩、大枣、干姜、半夏、黄连、人参

[101] **甘遂半夏汤**(《金匮要略》):甘遂、半夏、芍药、甘草

[102] **甘露消毒丹**(《温热经纬》):滑石、茵陈、黄芩、石菖蒲、川贝母、木通、藿香、射干、连翘、薄荷、白蔻仁

[103] **四七汤**(《太平惠民和剂局方》引《简易方》):苏叶、制半夏、厚朴、茯苓、生姜、大枣

[104] **四妙丸**(《成方便读》):苍术、黄柏、牛膝、苡仁

[105] **四君子汤**(《太平惠民和剂局方》):党参、白术、茯苓、甘草

[106] **四味回阳饮**(《景岳全书》):人参、制附子、炮姜、炙甘草

[107] **四物汤**(《太平惠民和剂局方》):当归、白芍药、川芎、熟地黄

[108] **四神丸**(《证治准绳》):补骨脂、肉豆蔻、吴茱萸、五味子、生姜、大枣

[109] **四逆散**(《伤寒论》):炙甘草、炒枳实、柴胡、芍药

[110] **四逆汤**(《伤寒论》):炙甘草、干姜、生附子

[111] **生脉散**(《备急千金要方》):人参、麦冬、五味子

[112] **生铁落饮**(《医学心悟》):天冬、麦冬、贝母、胆星、橘红、远志、石菖蒲、连翘、茯苓、茯神、玄参、钩藤、丹参、辰砂、生铁落

[113] **失笑散**(《太平惠民和剂局方》):五灵脂、蒲黄

[114] **代抵当丸**(《证治准绳》):大黄、归尾、生地、穿山甲、芒硝、桃仁、肉桂

[115] **白头翁汤**(《伤寒论》):白头翁、秦皮、黄连、黄柏

[116] **白金丸**(验方):白矾、郁金

[117] **白虎汤**(《白虎汤》):知母、生石膏、炙甘草、粳米

[118] **白虎加人参汤**(《伤寒论》):知母、石膏、甘草、粳米、人参

[119] **白虎加桂枝汤**(《金匮要略》):知母、石膏、甘草、粳米、桂枝

[120] **半夏白术天麻汤**(《医学心悟》):半夏、白术、天麻、陈皮、茯苓、甘草、生姜、大枣

[121] **半夏泻心汤**(《伤寒论》):半夏、黄芩、干姜、人参、炙甘草、黄连、大枣

[122] **半夏厚朴汤**(《金匮要略》):半夏、厚朴、紫苏、茯苓、生姜

[123] **半夏秫米汤**(《内经》):半夏、秫米

[124] **半硫丸**(《太平惠民和剂局方》):半夏、硫黄

[125] **归脾汤**(《济生方》):党参、黄芪、白术、茯神、酸枣仁、龙眼、木香、炙甘草、当归、远志、生姜、大枣

[126] **加味二妙散**(《丹溪心法》):黄柏、苍术、当归、牛膝、防已、萆薢、龟板

[127] **加味四斤丸**(《三因极一病证方论》):肉苁蓉、牛膝、菟丝子、木瓜、鹿茸、熟地、天麻、五味子

[128] **加味四君子汤**(《三因方》):人参、茯苓、白术、炙草、黄芪、白扁豆

[129] **加味四物汤**(《金匮翼》):白芍、当归、生地、川芎、蔓荆子、菊花、黄芩、甘草

[130] **加味甘麦大枣汤**(《妇科辑要》):甘草、小麦、大枣、芍药、紫石英

[131] **加味金刚丸**(《验方》):巴戟天、杜仲、肉苁蓉、淫羊藿、菟丝子、制乌前子、木瓜、牛膝、天麻、蜈蚣、僵蚕、乌蛇、萆薢、乌贼骨

[132] **加味泽泻汤**(《验方》):泽泻、生白术、钩藤、珍珠母、药花、川牛膝、灵磁石。

[133] **加味桔梗汤**(《医学心悟》):桔梗、甘草、贝母、橘红、银花、苡仁、葶苈子、白芨

[134] **加味清胃散**(《张氏医通》):生地、丹皮、当归、黄连、连翘、犀角、升麻、生甘草

[135] **加减承气汤**(验方):大黄、风化硝、枳实、礞石、皂角、猪胆汁、醋

[136] **加减泻白散**(《医学发明》):桑白皮、地骨皮、粳米、甘草、青皮、陈皮、五味子、人参、白茯苓

[137] **加减葳蕤汤**(《通俗伤寒论》):玉竹、葱白、桔梗、白薇、豆豉、薄荷、炙甘草、大枣

六 划

[138] **百合固金丸**(《医方集解》引赵蕺庵方):生地黄、熟地黄、麦冬、贝母、百合、当归、炒芍药、甘草、玄参、桔梗

[139] **百部煎剂**(验方):百部30g,切碎加水200ml,煎半小时左右,煎至30ml,于临睡前作保留灌肠,连续10~12天为一疗程(此为小儿童,成人量加倍)。

[140] **地黄饮子**(《宣明论》):生地黄、巴戟天、山萸肉、石斛、肉苁蓉、五味子、肉桂、茯苓、麦冬、炮附子、石菖蒲、远志、生姜、大枣、薄荷

[141] **地榆散**(验方):地榆、茜根、黄芩、黄连、山栀、茯苓

[142] **芎芷石膏汤**(《医宗金鉴》):川芎、白芷、石膏、菊花、藁本、羌活

[143] **芍药汤**(《素问病机气宜保命集》):黄芩、芍药、炙甘草、黄连、大黄、槟榔、当归、木香、肉桂

[144] **芍药甘草汤**(《伤寒论》):白芍药、炙甘草

[145] **过敏煎**(《验方》):柴胡、白芍、防风、五味子、乌梅

[146] **如金解毒散**(《景岳全书》):桔梗、甘草、黄芩、黄连、黄柏、山栀

[147] **至宝丹**(《太平惠民和剂局方》):朱砂、麝香、安息香、金银箔、犀角、牛黄、琥珀、雄黄、玳

瑁、龙脑

[148] **羊肝丸**(《类苑方》):夜明砂、蝉蜕、木贼草、当归、羊肝

[149] **交泰丸**(《韩氏医通》):黄连、肉桂

[150] **安宫牛黄丸**(《温病条辨》):牛黄、郁金、犀角、黄连、朱砂、冰片、珍珠、山栀、雄黄、黄芩、麝香、金箔衣

[151] **安神定志丸**(《医学心悟》):茯苓、茯神、远志、人参、石菖蒲、龙齿

[152] **当归芍药散**(《金匮要略》):当归、芍药、茯苓、白术、泽泻、川芎

[153] **当归六黄汤**(《兰室秘藏》):当归、生地黄、熟地黄、黄连、黄芩、黄柏、黄芪

[154] **当归龙荟丸**(《宣明论方》):当归、龙胆草、栀子、黄连、黄芩、黄柏、大黄、青黛、芦荟、木香、麝香

[155] **当归补血汤**(《内外伤辨惑论》):黄芪、当归

[156] **竹叶石膏汤**(《伤寒论》):竹叶、石膏、麦冬、人参、半夏、粳米、炙甘草

[157] **竹沥达痰丸**(《古今医鉴》):青礞石、沉香、大黄、黄芩、竹沥、半夏、橘红、甘草、姜汁、茯苓、人参

[158] **竹茹汤**(《本事方》):竹茹、半夏、干姜、甘草、生姜、大枣

[159] **朱砂安神丸**(《医学发明》):黄连、朱砂、生地黄、归身、炙甘草

[160] **血府逐瘀汤**(《医林改错》):当归、生地黄、桃仁、红花、枳壳、赤芍药、柴胡、甘草、桔梗、川芎、牛膝

[161] **舟车丸**(《景岳全书》引刘河间方):甘遂、芫花、大戟、大黄、黑丑、木香、青皮、陈皮、轻粉、槟榔

[162] **导赤散**(《小儿药证直诀》):生地黄、木通、竹叶、甘草

[163] **导痰汤**(《济生方》):半夏、陈皮、枳实、茯苓、甘草、制南星

[164] **防己黄芪汤**(《金匮要略》):防己、白术、黄芪、甘草、生姜、大枣

[165] **防风汤**(《宣明论方》):防风、当归、赤茯苓、杏仁、黄芩、秦艽、葛根、麻黄、肉桂、生姜、甘草、大枣

[166] **防风通圣散**(《宣明论方》):防风、川芎、当归、芍药、大黄、芒硝、连翘、薄荷、麻黄、石膏、桔梗、黄芩、白术、栀子、荆芥穗、滑石、甘草、生姜

[167] **阳和汤**(《外科全圣集》):熟地黄、白芥子、鹿角胶、姜炭、麻黄、肉桂、生甘草

七　划

[168] **六君子汤**(《医方集解》):人参、白术、茯苓、甘草、黄芪、山药

[169] **麦门冬汤**(《金匮要略》):麦冬、人参、半夏、甘草、粳米、大枣

[170] **麦味地黄丸**(《医级》):熟地黄、山萸肉、山药、丹皮、泽泻、茯苓、麦冬、五味子

[171] **苍术二陈汤**(《杂病源流犀烛》):苍术、白术、茯苓、陈皮、甘草、半夏

[172] **牡蛎泽泻散**(《伤寒论》):煅牡蛎、泽泻、蜀漆、炒葶苈子、炒商陆、海藻、栝蒌根

[173] **苏子降气汤**(《太平惠民和剂局方》):苏子、橘皮、半夏、当归、前胡、厚朴、肉桂、甘草、生姜

[174] **苏合香丸**(《太平惠民和剂局方》):白术、青木香、犀角、香附、朱砂、诃子、檀香、安息香、沉香、麝香、丁香、荜茇、苏合香油、熏陆香、冰片

[175] **杞菊地黄丸**(《医级》):枸杞子、菊花、熟地黄、山茱萸、山药、泽泻、丹皮、茯苓

[176] **杏苏二陈丸**(验方):杏仁、半夏、陈皮、茯苓、苏子、甘草

[177] **杏苏散**(《温病条辨》):杏仁、紫苏叶、橘皮、半夏、生姜、枳壳、桔梗、前胡、茯苓、甘草、大枣

[178] **更衣丸**(《先醒斋医学广笔记》):芦荟、朱砂

[179] **妙香散**(《沈氏尊生书》):山药、茯苓、茯神、远志、黄芪、人参、桔梗、甘草、木香、辰砂、麝香

[180] **连朴饮**(《随息居重订霍乱方》):制厚朴、黄连、石菖蒲、制半夏、炒豆豉、焦栀子、芦根

[181] **连理汤**(《张氏医通》):人参、白术、干姜、炙甘草、黄连、茯苓

[182] **吴茱萸汤**(《伤寒论》):吴茱萸、人参、生姜、大枣

[183] **沉香降气散**(《张氏医通》):沉香、砂仁、甘草、香附、川楝子、玄胡索

[184] **沉香散**(《金匮翼》):沉香、石韦、滑石、当归、橘皮、白芍、冬葵子、甘草、王不留行

[185] **沙参麦冬汤**(《温病条辨》):沙参、麦冬、玉竹、桑叶、甘草、天花粉、生扁豆

[186] **沙参清肺汤**(验方):北沙参、生黄芪、太子参、合欢皮、白芨、生甘草、桔梗、苡仁、冬瓜子

[187] **良附丸**(《良方集腋》):高良姜、香附

[188] **启膈散**(《医学心悟》):沙参、茯苓、丹参、川贝、郁金、砂仁壳、荷叶蒂、杵头糠

[189] **补天大造丸**(《医学心悟》):人参、白术、当归、枣仁、炙黄芪、远志、白芍、山药、茯苓、杞子、紫河车、龟板、鹿角、大熟地

[190] **补中益气汤**(《脾胃论》):人参、黄芪、白术、甘草、当归、陈皮、升麻、柴胡

[191] **补气运脾汤**(《统旨方》):人参、白术、茯苓、甘草、黄芪、陈皮、砂仁、半夏曲、生姜、大枣

[192] **补阳还五汤**(《医林改错》):当归尾、川芎、黄芪、桃仁、地龙、赤芍、红花

[193] **补肝汤**(《医宗金鉴》):当归、白芍、川芎、熟地、酸枣仁、木瓜、炙甘草

[194] **补肺汤**(《永类钤方》):人参、黄芪、熟地、五味子、紫菀、桑白皮

[195] **牡蛎散**(《太平惠民和剂局方》):煅牡蛎、黄芪、麻黄根、浮小麦

[196] **皂荚丸**(《金匮要略》):皂荚、大枣

[197] **身痛逐瘀汤**(《医林改错》):秦艽、川芎、桃仁、红花、甘草、羌活、没药、香附、五灵脂、牛膝、地龙、当归

[198] **附子理中丸**(《太平惠民和剂局方》):炮附子、人参、白术、炮姜、炙甘草

[199] **附子粳米汤**(《金匮要略》):炮附子、粳米、半夏、甘草、大枣

[200] **阿魏膏**(《景岳全书》):羌活、独活、玄参、官桂、赤芍、穿山甲、苏合油、生地、豭鼠矢、大黄、白芷、天麻、红花、麝香、土木鳖、黄丹、芒硝、阿魏、乳香、没药

[201] **附子泻心汤**(《伤寒论》):大黄、黄连、黄芩、炮附子

[202] **纯阳正气丸**(成药):陈皮、丁香、茯苓、茅术、白术、藿香、姜半夏、肉桂、青木香、花椒叶、红灵丹

八 划

[203] **青娥丸**(《太平惠民和剂局方》):补骨脂、杜仲、胡桃肉、大蒜头

[204] **周氏回生丹**(《全国中药成药处方集》)五倍子、檀香、木香、沉香、麝香、雄黄面、公丁香、甘草、续随子霜、大戟、山慈姑、冰片、朱砂面、神曲面

[205] **泽泻汤**(《金匮要略》):泽泻、白术

[206] **苓甘五味姜辛汤**(《金匮要略》):茯苓、甘草、五味子、干姜、细辛

[207] **苓桂术甘汤**(《金匮要略》):茯苓、桂枝、白术、甘草

[208] **枕中丹**(《备急千金要方》):龟板、龙骨、远志、菖蒲

[209] **虎潜丸**(《丹溪心法》):龟板、黄柏、知母、熟地黄、白芍药、锁阳、陈皮、虎骨、干姜

[210] **河车大造丸**(《扶寿精方》):紫河车、熟地黄、杜仲、天冬、麦冬、龟板、黄柏、牛膝

[211] **泻心汤**(《金匮要略》):大黄、黄芩、黄连

[212] **泻白散**(《小儿药证直诀》):桑白皮、地骨皮、生甘草、粳米

[213] **羌活胜湿汤**(《内外伤辨惑论》):羌活、独活、川芎、蔓荆子、甘草、防风、藁木

[214] **定志丸**(《备急千金要方》):党参、茯神、石菖蒲、远志、甘草汤泡,一方有茯苓、白术、麦冬

[215] **定痫丸**(《医学心悟》):天麻、川贝、胆南星、姜半夏

[216] **定喘汤**(《摄生众妙方》):白果、麻黄、桑白皮、款冬花、半夏、杏仁、苏子、黄芩、甘草

[217] **实脾饮**(《济生方》):附子、干姜、白术、甘草、厚朴、木香、草果、槟榔、木瓜、生姜、大枣、茯苓

[218] **知柏地黄丸**(《医宗金鉴》):知母、黄柏、熟地黄、山萸肉、山药、茯苓、丹皮、泽泻

[219] **金水六君煎**(《景岳全书》):当归、茯苓、半夏、熟地黄、陈皮、炙甘草、生姜

[220] **金佛草散**(《太平惠民和剂局方》):旋覆花、麻黄、前胡、荆芥穗、炙甘草、姜半夏、赤药、生姜、大枣

[221] **金箔镇心丸**(《太平惠民和剂局方》):紫河车、山药、牙硝、炙甘草、人参、茯苓、朱砂、冰片、麝香、金箔

[222] **金铃子散**(《素向病机气宜保命集》):金铃子、延胡索

[223] **《金匮》肾气丸**(《金匮要略》):桂枝、附子、熟地黄、山萸肉、山药、茯苓、丹皮、泽泻

[224] **金锁固精丸**(《医方集解》):沙苑蒺藜、芡实、莲须、龙骨、牡蛎、莲肉

[225] **炙甘草汤**(《伤寒论》):炙甘草、人参、桂枝、生姜、阿胶、生地黄、麦冬、火麻仁、大枣

[226] **驻车丸**(《备急千金要方》):黄连、阿胶、当归、干姜

[227] **参附汤**(《妇人良方》):人参、熟附子、姜、枣

[228] **参苏饮**(《太平惠民和剂局方》):人参、苏叶、葛根、前胡、法半夏、茯苓、橘红、甘草、桔梗、枳壳、木香、陈皮、姜、枣

[229] **参苓白术散**(《太平惠民和剂局方》):人参、茯苓、白术、桔梗、山药、甘草、白扁豆、莲子肉、砂仁、薏苡仁

[230] **参蚧散**(《济生方》):人参、蛤蚧

九　划

[231] **春泽汤**(《医方集解》):白术、桂枝、猪苓、泽泻、茯苓、人参

[232] **柏叶汤**(《金匮要略》):侧柏叶、干姜、艾叶、马通汁

[233] **枳术丸**(《内外伤辨惑论》):白术、炒枳实

[234] **枳实导滞丸**(《内外伤辨惑论》):大黄、枳实、黄芩、黄连、神曲、白术、茯苓、泽泻

[235] **荆防败毒散**(《外科理例》):荆芥、防风、羌活、独活、柴胡、前胡、川芎、枳壳、茯苓、桔梗、甘草

[236] **茵陈五苓散**(《金匮要略》):茵陈蒿、桂枝、茯苓、白术、泽泻、猪苓
[237] **茵陈术附汤**(《医学心悟》):茵陈蒿、白术、附子、干姜、炙甘草、肉桂
[238] **茵陈蒿汤**(《伤寒论》):茵陈蒿、山栀、大黄
[239] **茜根散**(《景岳全书》):茜草根、黄芩、阿胶、侧柏叶
[240] **牵正散**(《杨氏家藏方》):白附子、僵蚕、全蝎
[241] **胃苓汤**(《丹溪心法》):苍术、厚朴、陈皮、甘草、生姜、大枣、桂枝、白术、泽泻、茯苓、猪苓
[242] **济川煎**(《景岳全书》):当归、牛膝、肉苁蓉、泽泻、升麻、枳壳
[243] **《济生》肾气丸**(《济生方》):地黄、山药、山茱萸、丹皮、茯苓、泽泻、炮附子、桂枝、牛膝、车前子
[244] **《活人》败毒散**(《南阳活人书》):人参、羌活、独活、前胡、柴胡、川芎、枳壳、桔梗、茯苓、炙甘草、生姜
[245] **养心汤**(《证治准绳》):黄芪、茯苓、茯神、当归、川芎、炙甘草、半夏曲、柏子仁、酸枣仁、远志、五味子、人参、肉桂
[246] **养胃汤**(《证治准绳》):沙参、麦冬、玉竹、生扁豆、桑叶、甘草
[247] **举元煎**(《景岳全书》):人参、炙黄芪、炙甘草、炒升麻、炒白术
[248] **宣白承氣汤**(《温病条辨》):生石膏、生大黄、杏仁粉、括蒌皮
[249] **宣痹汤**(《温病条辨》):防己、杏仁、连翘、滑石、薏苡仁、半夏、蚕砂、赤小豆皮、栀子
[250] **神术散**(《医学心悟》):苍术、陈皮、厚朴、甘草、藿香、砂仁
[251] **神犀丹**(《温热经纬》):犀角、石菖蒲、黄芩、生地黄、银花、金汁、连翘、板蓝根、豆豉、玄参、天花粉、紫草
[252] **香连丸**(《太平惠民和剂局方》):黄连、木香
[253] **香苏散**(《太平惠民和剂局方》):香附、紫苏茎叶、陈皮、甘草
[254] **香附旋覆花汤**(《温病条辨》):生香附、旋覆花、苏子霜、苡仁、半夏、茯苓、橘皮
[255] **香薷饮**(《太平惠民和剂局方》):炒扁豆、厚朴、香薷
[256] **香砂六君子汤**(《时方歌括》):木香、砂仁、陈皮、半夏、党参、白术、茯苓、甘草
[257] **复元活血汤**(《医学发明》):柴胡、栝楼根、当归、红花、甘草、穿山甲、大黄、桃仁
[258] **顺气和中汤**(《证治准绳》):黄芪、人参、白术、陈皮、当归、芍药、炙甘草、升麻、柴胡、蔓荆子、川乌、细辛
[259] **保元汤**(《情爱心鉴》):人参、黄芪、肉桂、甘草、生姜
[260] **保和丸**(《月溪心法》):神曲、山楂、茯苓、半夏、陈皮、连翘、莱菔子
[261] **独参汤**(《景岳全书》):人参
[262] **独活寄生汤**(《备急千金要方》):独活、桑寄生、秦艽、防风、细辛、当归、芍药、川芎、干地黄、杜仲、牛膝、人参、茯苓、甘草、桂心

十　划

[263] **秦艽鳖甲散**(《卫生宝鉴》):地骨皮、柴胡、秦艽、知母、当归、鳖甲、青蒿、乌梅
[264] **真人养脏汤**(《证治准绳》):诃子、罂粟壳、肉豆蔻、白术、人参、木香、官桂、炙甘草、生姜、大枣
[265] **真武汤**(《伤寒论》):炮附子、白术、茯苓、芍药、生姜

[266] **桂枝汤**(《伤寒论》):桂枝、芍药、生姜、炙甘草、大枣

[267] **桂枝甘草龙骨牡蛎汤**(《伤寒论》):桂枝、炙甘草、龙骨、牡蛎

[268] **桂枝加厚朴杏仁汤**(《伤寒论》):桂枝、芍药、炙甘草、生姜、大枣、厚朴、杏仁

[269] **桂枝芍药知母汤**(《金匮要略》):桂枝、芍药、炙甘草、麻黄、白术、知母、防风、炮附子、生姜

[270] **桂枝茯苓丸**(《金匮要略》):桂枝、茯苓、牡丹皮、炒桃仁、芍药

[271] **桃花汤**(《伤寒论》):赤石脂、干姜、粳米

[272] **桃仁红花煎**(《素庵医案》):丹参、赤芍、桃仁、红花、制香附、延胡索、青皮、当归、川芎、生地

[273] **桔梗白散**(《外台秘要》):桔梗、贝母、巴豆

[274] **桔梗杏仁煎**(《景岳全书》):桔梗、杏仁、甘草、银花、贝母、枳壳、红藤、连翘、夏枯草、百合、麦冬、阿胶

[275] **栝蒌桂枝汤**(《金匮要略》):栝蒌根、桂枝、芍药、甘草、生姜、大枣

[276] **栝蒌薤白半夏汤**(《金匮要略》):栝蒌、薤白、白酒、半夏

[277] **栝蒌薤白白酒汤**(《金匮要略》):栝蒌、薤白、白酒

[278] **柴胡桂枝干姜汤**(《伤寒论》):柴胡、桂枝、干姜、黄芩、栝蒌根、牡蛎、炙甘草

[279] **柴胡疏肝散**(《景岳全书》):柴胡、枳壳、芍药、甘草、香附、川芎

[280] **柴胡清骨散**(《医宗金鉴》):秦艽、鳖甲、柴胡、地骨皮、青蒿、知母、胡黄连、薤白、甘草、童便、猪脊髓、猪胆汁

[281] **柴胡四物汤**(《素问病机气宜保命集》):川芎、熟地黄、当归、芍药、柴胡、人参、黄芩、甘草、半夏釉

[282] **柴胡白虎汤**(《重订通俗伤寒论》):柴胡、石膏、天花粉、粳米、黄芩、知母、甘草、鲜荷叶

[283] **柴枳半夏汤**(《医学入门》):柴胡、黄芩、半夏、栝蒌仁、枳壳、桔梗、杏仁、青皮、甘草

[284] **凉膈散**(《太平惠民和剂局方》):大黄、朴硝、甘草、栀子仁、薄荷叶、黄芩、连翘、竹叶、白蜜

[285] **润肠丸**(《沈氏尊生书》):当归、生地、麻仁、桃仁、枳壳

[286] **涤痰汤**(《济生方》):制半夏、制南星、陈皮、枳实、茯苓、人参、石菖蒲、竹茹、甘草、生姜

[287] **消渴方**(《丹溪心法》):黄连末、天花粉末、生地汁、藕汁、人乳汁、姜汁、蜂蜜

[288] **益气聪明汤**(《证治准绳》):黄芪、人参、升麻、葛根、蔓荆子、芍药、黄柏、炙甘草

[289] **益胃汤**(《温病条辨》):沙参、麦冬、生地黄、玉竹、冰糖

[290] **调胃承气汤**(《伤寒论》):大黄、炙甘草、芒硝

[291] **调营饮**(《证治准绳》):莪术、川芎、当归、延胡、赤芍药、瞿麦、大黄、槟榔、陈皮、大腹皮、葶苈、赤茯苓、桑白皮、细辛、官桂、炙甘草、姜、枣、白芷

[292] **调营敛肝饮**(《医醇賸义》):当归、白芍、蛤粉炒、阿胶、枸杞子、五味子、川芎、枣仁、茯苓、陈皮、木香、生姜、大枣

[293] **射干麻黄汤**(《金匮要略》):射干、麻黄、细辛、紫菀、款冬花、半夏、五味子、生姜、大枣

[294] **皱肺丸**(《百一选方》):五味子、人参、桂枝、款冬花、紫菀、白石英、羯羊肺、杏仁

[295] **逍遥散**(《太平惠民和剂局方》):柴胡、白术、白芍药、当归、茯苓、炙甘草、薄荷、煨姜

[296] **通幽汤**(《兰室秘藏》):生地黄、熟地黄、桃仁泥、红花、当归、炙甘草、升麻

[297] **通窍活血汤**(《医林改错》):赤芍药、川芎、桃仁、红花、麝香、老葱、鲜姜、大枣、酒
[298] **通瘀煎**(《景岳全书》):归尾、山楂、香附、红花、乌药、青皮、木香、泽泻
[299] **桑白皮汤**(《景岳全书》):桑白皮、半夏、苏子、杏仁、贝母、黄芩、黄连、山栀
[300] **桑杏汤**(《温病条辨》):桑叶、杏仁、沙参、浙贝母、豆豉、山栀、梨皮
[301] **桑菊饮**(《温病条辨》):桑叶、菊花、连翘、薄荷、桔梗、杏仁、芦根、甘草
[302] **桑螵蛸散**(《本草衍义》):桑螵蛸、远志、菖蒲、龙骨、人参、茯神、当归、龟板

十一划

[303] **理中丸**(《伤寒论》):人参、白术、干姜、炙甘草
[304] **黄土汤**(《金匮要略》):灶心黄土、甘草、干地黄、白术、炮附子、阿胶、黄芩
[305] **黄芩滑石汤**(《温病条辨》):黄芩、滑石、猪苓、茯苓皮、大腹皮、白豆蔻仁、通草
[306] **黄连解毒汤**(《中药制剂手册》):黄连、黄芩、黄柏、栀子、升麻、金银花、防风、炒牛蒡子、大黄、当归、赤芍药、甘草
[307] **黄连上清丸**(《古今医方集成》):黄芩、黄连、黄柏、栀子、菊花、桔梗、薄荷、川芎、大黄、连翘、当归、葛根、玄参、花粉、姜黄
[308] **黄连阿胶汤**(《伤寒论》):黄连、阿胶、黄芩、鸡子黄、芍药
[309] **黄连香薷饮**(《类证活人书》):黄连、香薷、厚朴
[310] **黄连清心饮**(《沈氏尊生书》):黄连、生地黄、当归、甘草、酸枣仁、茯神、远志、人参、莲子肉
[311] **黄连温胆汤**(《千金方》):半夏、陈皮、茯苓、甘草、枳实、竹茹、黄连、大枣
[312] **黄芪六一汤**(《太平惠民和剂局方》):黄芪、甘草
[313] **黄芪汤**(《金匮翼》):黄芪、陈皮、火麻仁、白蜜
[314] **黄芪建中汤**(《金匮要略》):黄芪、白芍、桂枝、炙甘草、生姜、大枣、饴糖
[315] **黄芪鳖甲散**(《卫生宝鉴》):黄芪、鳖甲、天冬、地骨皮、秦艽、柴胡、紫菀、半夏、茯苓、知母、生地、白芍、桑白皮、人参、肉桂、桔梗、甘草
[316] **黄病绛矾丸**(验方):厚朴、茅术、陈皮、甘草、绛矾、红枣
[317] **栀子柏皮汤**(《伤寒论》):栀子、甘草、黄柏
[318] **栀子清肝汤**(《类证治裁》):栀子、丹皮、柴胡、当归、芍药、茯苓、川芎、牛蒡子、甘草
[319] **控涎丹**(《三因极一病证方论》):甘遂、大戟、白芥子
[320] **鹿角胶丸**(《医学正传》):鹿角胶、鹿角霜、熟地黄、川牛膝、白茯苓、菟丝子、人参、当归、白术、杜仲、虎胫骨、龟板
[321] **鹿茸丸**(《沈氏尊生书》):鹿茸、麦冬、熟地黄、黄芪、五味子、肉苁蓉、鸡内金、山萸肉、补骨脂、人参、牛膝、玄参、茯苓、地骨皮
[322] **麻子仁丸**(《伤寒论》):麻子仁、芍药、炙枳实、大黄、炙厚朴、杏仁
[323] **麻杏石甘汤**(《伤寒论》):麻黄、杏仁、石膏、炙甘草
[324] **麻杏苡甘汤**(《金匮要略》):麻黄、炙甘草、薏苡仁、杏仁
[325] **麻黄加术汤**(《金匮要略》):麻黄、桂枝、炙甘草、杏仁、白术
[326] **麻黄汤**(《伤寒论》):麻黄、桂枝、杏仁、炙甘草
[327] **麻黄连轺赤小豆汤**(《伤寒论》):麻黄、杏仁、生梓白皮、连轺、赤小豆、甘草、生姜、大枣

[328] **麻黄附子细辛汤**(《伤寒论》):麻黄、附子、细辛

[329] **旋复代赭汤**(《伤寒论》):旋覆花、代赭石、人参、半夏、炙甘草、生姜、大枣

[330] **旋覆花汤**(《金匮要略》):旋覆花、新绛、葱

[331] **羚羊角汤**(《医醇賸义》):羚羊角、龟板、生地、丹皮、白芍、柴胡、薄荷、蝉衣、菊花、夏枯草、石决明

[332] **羚羊钩藤汤**(《通俗伤寒论》):羚羊角、桑叶、川贝、鲜生地、钩藤、菊花、白芍药、生甘草、鲜竹茹、茯神

[333] **清金化痰汤**(《统旨方》):黄芩、山栀、桔梗、麦冬、桑白皮、贝母、知母、栝楼仁、橘红、茯苓、甘草

[334] **清肺饮**(《证治汇补》):茯苓、黄芩、桑白皮、麦冬、车前子、山栀、木通

[335] **清胃散**(《兰室秘藏》):当归、生地黄、牡丹皮、升麻、黄连

[336] **清骨散**(《证治准绳》):银柴胡、胡黄连、秦艽、鳖甲、地骨皮、青蒿、知母、甘草

[337] **清震汤**(《素问病机气宜保命集》):升麻、苍术、荷叶

[338] **清暑益气汤**(《温热经纬》):西洋参、石斛、麦冬、黄连、竹叶、荷梗、知母、甘草、粳米、西瓜翠衣

[339] **清热镇惊汤**(《医宗金鉴》):石决明、紫石英、龙胆草、山栀、木通、生大黄、干姜、柴胡、硃麦冬、天竺黄、胆南星、远志、菖蒲、明天麻、勾藤

[340] **清燥救肺汤**(《医门法律》):桑叶、石膏、杏仁、甘草、麦冬、人参、阿胶、炒胡麻仁、炙枇杷叶

[341] **银翘散**(《温病条辨》):金银花、连翘、豆豉、牛蒡子、薄荷、荆芥穗、桔梗、甘草、竹叶、鲜芦根

[342] **猪苓汤**(《伤寒论》):猪苓、茯苓、泽泻、阿胶、滑石

十二划

[343] **葱豉汤**(《肘后备急方》):葱白、豆豉,或加葛根、升麻,或加麻黄

[344] **葱白七味饮**(《外台秘要》):葱白、葛根、麦门冬、干地黄、豆豉、生姜、甘澜水

[345] **葛根汤**(《伤寒论》):葛根、麻黄、桂枝、生姜、甘草、芍药、大枣

[346] **葛根芩连汤**(《伤寒论》):葛根、黄芩、黄连、炙甘草

[347] **葶苈大枣泻肺汤**(《金匮要略》):葶苈子、大枣

[348] **葱豉桔梗汤**(《通俗伤寒论》):葱白、豆豉、薄荷、连翘、栀子、竹叶、桔梗、甘草

[349] **越婢加术汤**(《金匮要略》):麻黄、石膏、甘草、大枣、白术、生姜

[350] **越婢加半夏汤**(《金匮要略》):麻黄、石膏、生姜、大枣、甘草、半夏

[351] **越鞠丸**(《丹溪心法》):川芎、苍术、香附、炒山栀、神曲

[352] **椒目瓜蒌汤**(《医醇賸义》):川椒目、瓜蒌仁、葶苈子、桑白皮、苏子、半夏、茯苓、橘红、蒺藜、生姜

[353] **硝石矾石散**(《金匮要略》):硝石、矾石

[354] **紫金丹**(《普济本事方》):砒、豆豉

[355] **紫雪丹**(《太平惠民和剂局方》):滑石、石膏、寒水石、磁石、羚羊角、青木香、犀角、沉香、丁香、升麻、玄参、甘草、朴硝、朱砂、麝香、黄金、硝石

[356] **黑锡丹**(《太平惠民和剂局方》):黑锡、硫黄、川楝子、胡芦巴、木香、炮附子、肉豆蔻、阳起石、沉香、茴香、肉桂、补骨脂

[357] **痛泻要方**(《景岳全书》引刘草窗方):白术、白芍、防风、炒陈皮

[358] **温胆汤**(《备急千金要方》):半夏、橘皮、甘草、枳实、竹茹、生姜、茯苓

[359] **温脾汤**(《备急千金要方》):附子、人参、大黄、甘草、干姜

[360] **滋水清肝饮**(《医宗已任篇》):生地黄、山茱萸、茯苓、归身、山药、丹皮、泽泻、白芍、柴胡、山栀、酸枣仁

[361] **滋肾通关丸**(《兰室秘藏》):知母、黄柏、肉桂

[362] **程氏萆薢分清饮**(《医学心悟》):萆薢、车前子、茯苓、莲子心、菖蒲、黄柏、丹参、白术

[363] **犀角地黄汤**(《备急千金要方》):犀角、生地黄、丹皮、芍药

[364] **犀角散**(《备急千金要方》):犀角、黄连、升麻、山栀、茵陈

[365] **犀黄丸**(《外科证治全生集》):犀黄、麝香、没药、乳香

[366] **疏凿饮子**(《世医得效方》):商陆、泽泻、赤小豆、椒目、木通、茯苓皮、大腹皮、槟榔、生姜、羌活、秦艽

[367] **普济消毒饮**(《东垣十书》):黄芩、黄连、连翘、玄参、板蓝根、马勃、牛蒡子、僵蚕、升麻、柴胡、陈皮、桔梗、甘草、薄荷

十三划

[368] **搐鼻散**(《医学心悟》):细辛、皂角、半夏

[369] **暖肝煎**(《景岳全书》):肉桂、小茴香、茯苓、乌药、枸杞子、当归、沉香、生姜

[370] **新加香薷饮**(《温病条辨》):香薷、鲜扁豆花、厚朴、金银花、连翘

[371] **辟瘟丹**(验方):羚羊角、朴硝、牙皂、广木香、黄柏、茅术、茜草、黄芩、姜半夏、文蛤、银花、川连、犀角、川朴、川乌、玳瑁、大黄、藿香、玄精石、郁金、茯苓、香附、桂心、赤小豆、降香、鬼箭羽、朱砂、毛茨姑、大枣、甘遂、大戟、桑皮、千金霜、桃仁霜、槟榔、蓬莪术、胡椒、葶苈子、牛黄、巴豆霜、细辛、白芍、公丁香、当归、禹余粮、滑石、山豆根、麻黄、麝香、菖蒲、水安息、干姜、蒲黄、丹参、天麻、升麻、柴胡、紫苏、川芎、草河车、檀香、桔梗、白芷、紫菀、芫花、雌黄、琥珀、冰片、陈皮、腰黄、斑蝥、蜈蚣、石龙子

[372] **解语丹**(《医学心语》):白附子、石菖蒲、远志、天麻、全蝎、羌活、南星、木香、甘草

十四划

[373] **槐角丸**(《丹溪心法》):槐角、地榆、黄芩、当归、炒枳壳、防风

[374] **酸枣仁汤**(《金匮要略》):酸枣仁、知母、川芎、茯苓、甘草

[375] **膏淋汤**(《医学衷中参西录》):山药、芡实、龙骨、牡蛎、生地黄、党参、白芍

[376] **膈下逐瘀汤**(《医林改错》):五灵脂、当归、川芎、桃仁、丹皮、赤芍药、乌药、延胡索、甘草、香附、红花、枳壳

十五划以上

[377] **增液汤**(《温病条辨》):玄参、麦冬、生地

[378] **增液承气汤**(《温病条辨》):大黄、芒硝、玄参、麦冬、生地黄

[379] **薏苡仁汤**（《类证治裁》）：薏苡仁、川芎、当归、麻黄、桂枝、羌活、独活、防风、川乌、苍术、甘草、生姜

[380] **橘皮竹茹汤**（《金匮要略》）：人参、橘皮、竹茹、甘草、生姜、大枣

[381] **黛哈散**（验方）：青黛、海蛤壳

[382] **藿香正气散**（《太平惠民和剂局方》）：藿香、紫苏、白芷、桔梗、白术、厚朴、半夏曲、大腹皮、茯苓、橘皮、甘草、大枣

[383] **礞石滚痰丸**（《养生主论》）：青礞石、沉香、大黄、黄芩、朴硝

[384] **鳖甲煎丸**（《金匮要略》）：鳖甲、乌扇、黄芩、柴胡、鼠妇、干姜、大黄、芍药、桂枝、葶苈子、石韦、厚朴、丹皮、瞿麦、紫葳、半夏、人参、䗪虫、阿胶、蜂房、赤硝、蜣螂、桃仁

[385] **癫狂梦醒汤**（《医林改错》）：桃仁、柴胡、香附、木通、赤芍药、半夏、大腹皮、青皮、陈皮、桑白皮、苏子、甘草

[386] **薯蓣丸**（《金匮要略》）：薯蓣、人参、白术、茯苓、甘草、当归、芍药、川芎、干地黄、阿胶、麦冬、杏仁、桔梗、豆黄卷、防风、柴胡、桂枝、神曲、干姜、白敛、大枣

[387] **镇肝熄风汤**（《医学衷中参西录》）：淮牛膝、龙骨、生白芍、天冬、麦芽、代赭石、牡蛎、玄参、川楝子、茵陈蒿、甘草、龟板

[388] **蠲痹汤**（《医学心语》）：羌活、独活、桂心、秦艽、当归、川芎、炙甘草、海风藤、桑枝、乳香、木香